Gender, Race, and Politics
in the Midwest

Blacks in the Diaspora

Darlene Clark Hine, John McCluskey, Jr., and David Barry Gaspar,
GENERAL EDITORS

Gender, Race, and Politics in the Midwest

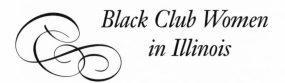 *Black Club Women in Illinois*

Wanda A. Hendricks

Indiana University Press

BLOOMINGTON & INDIANAPOLIS

The paper used in this publication meets the minimum requirements of American National Standard for Information Sciences—Permanence of Paper for Printed Library Materials, ANSI Z39.48-1984.

MANUFACTURED IN THE UNITED STATES OF AMERICA

Library of Congress Cataloging-in-Publication Data

Hendricks, Wanda A.
    Black club women in the Midwest : agents of social and political change / Wanda A. Hendricks.
        p.   cm. — (Blacks in the diaspora)
    Includes bibliographical references and index.
    ISBN 0-253-33447-0 (cl. : alk. paper). — ISBN 0-253-21233-2 (pa : alk. paper)
    1. Afro-American women—Illinois—Societies, clubs, etc.—History. 2. Afro-American women—Illinois—Political activity—History. 3. Afro-Americans—Illinois—Social conditions. 4. Afro-Americans—Illinois—Politics and government. 5. Illinois—Race relations. I. Title. II. Series.
F550.N4H46   1998
305.48'896'0730773—dc21   98–3091

1   2   3   4   5   03   02   01   00   99   98

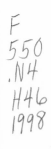

12260807

CONTENTS

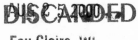

ACKNOWLEDGMENTS

During the years that I have worked on this book, I have incurred numerous debts to archivists, librarians, scholars, family, and friends. I received much support from several staff members at the Illinois State Historical Library in Springfield. Kathryn M. Harris shared her expertise on both local and state history, unearthed numerous buried documents, and became a cherished friend. Cheryl Pence was especially helpful in locating records in some of the most obscure places. Christine Henderson at the Illinois State Library in Springfield, and Louise Ogg, Marsha Davis, and Pat McAllister at the Cairo Public Library in Cairo assisted in uncovering the life stories of many of the African American women who appear in this book. I also owe a debt to the staff at the Carter G. Woodson Public Library, the Chicago Historical Society, and the Joseph Regenstein Library in Chicago.

I am grateful to Arizona State University for its assistance through a Faculty Grant-in-Aid and a Women's Studies Summer Research Award. I am also grateful for financial assistance from the American Association of University Women and Purdue University. The AAUW and the David Ross Dissertation Fellowships granted me the time to do the necessary research for this project.

Many wonderful colleagues deserve special thanks. I owe a special note of gratitude to my mentor and colleague Darlene Clark Hine at Michigan State University, who shared her insights, offered words of encouragement, and helped me realize the possibility of a life in the academy. Moreover, she always believed that this project was very important to the emerging scholarship about African American women. Nancy Gabin at

Purdue University shared her knowledge of women's history and stimulated my thought processes. I thank Wilma King at Michigan State University and Glenda Riley at Ball State University for reading the manuscript and for their insightful comments. Robert May, Raymond Dumett, Harold Woodman, and James Davidson at Purdue University provided much-needed support during my graduate student days. My colleagues in the Association of Black Women Historians, especially Sylvia Jacobs, Valinda Littlefield, Linda Reed, Jacqueline Rouse, Stephanie Shaw, Rosalyn Terborg-Penn, Lillian Williams, and Deborah Gray White, proved to be invaluable sources of professional and personal growth. Over the years I have also received assistance from Julia Kirk Blackwelder at Texas A & M, David Goldfield at the University of North Carolina at Charlotte, and Marjorie Spruill Wheeler at the University of Southern Mississippi.

My family and friends have always been my strongest support network. Like the women in this book, my mother, Velma G. Hendricks, and my grandmother, Lucinda Stewart, triumphed over seemingly insurmountable odds. My mother's resilience when my father, Joshua J. Hendricks, died ensured that the family of five children remained as healthy and happy as possible. When my mother died only four years later, my grandmother kept her promise to raise her five grandchildren and provide them with the necessary skills to survive and prosper.

From the moment I began this journey, the unconditional love of my niece April K. Hendricks and my nephew Joshua J. Hendricks III sustained me in immeasurable ways. My dearest friend, Beverly Glover Logan, shared her optimism when I had lost mine, and she housed, fed, and hugged me when necessary. Her husband and daughter, Larry Logan and Victoria Logan, also shared in this journey by being very patient and generous with their time. My cousin Sharon Adams McLean advised me and graciously shared her thoughts about the project. Without the support of a wonderful circle of friends—Felix Armfield, Brenda Brock, Mary Campbell, Vickie Crawford, Deborah Fortune, Grace Gouveia, Donna Hall, Laura Adair Johnson, Lois

Kennedy, Carolyn Powell, Pamela Smoot, and Nancy Spencer—my life both professionally and personally would have been sorely limited. Most of all, I am indebted to my staunchest supporter, Weston James, who died too soon to realize his own dream of seeing this work completed.

INTRODUCTION

This book explores the significance of the social and political grassroots movement led by African American club women in Illinois from 1890 to 1920. It looks at the unique structures, ideologies, strategies, and tactics that differentiated this movement from and linked it to the national black club women's movement during the period. By focusing on the ways in which efforts at the state level intersected with those on the national stage, this study demonstrates that the limitations imposed on these women by racism and sexism did not hinder them from effecting social and political change. In addition, it shows the crucial role that regional differences played in shaping the ideologies and institutions that sustained and nourished black communities throughout Illinois.

This study focuses on Illinois because there was an unprecedented proliferation of black female clubs there, and because the women who joined these associations faced numerous challenges that were unique to their region of the country. Illinois was one of several Midwestern states affected by a burgeoning industrial economy and by the massive movement of African Americans. Like other states in the area, it was mostly rural but was dominated by a large city. While the black population gradually increased during the twenty-six years from 1890 to 1916, it mushroomed between 1916 and 1920. By 1920, the number of black residents was triple that of 1890. And because the number of blacks living in rural areas was steadily declining, the state became one of the most urbanized black regions in the nation. Chicago's population, for example, more than doubled during those years.[1] With that urbanization came a variety of problems associated with growth. Poverty, overcrowding, and high mortality rates plagued the many blacks who sought shelter in the state.

Many of the blacks who migrated to Illinois prior to the turn of the century were attracted by the state's reputation for racial tolerance. Indeed, few legal, social, and political restrictions greeted migrants. Yet Illinois was the site of some of the worst race riots in the nation during the first two decades of the twentieth century.

For black female activists, the confluence of these circumstances presented some unique challenges and opportunities. By 1920 they had helped to establish the largest national network of black club women in the country, created scores of women's associations, developed a political network, and cast ballots for the first black elected to Chicago's city council. In Chicago alone, there were more than seventy social and political clubs.[2] Even in rural areas, where there were fewer clubs, women participated and demonstrated a commitment to the community, providing valuable service to those in need.

It was a genuine concern for the problems faced by blacks in both rural and urban areas that drew women to association building. When the call went out for a national network of black women to be formed, club women in Illinois eagerly joined. The creation of the National Association of Colored Women (NACW) in 1896 was both an affirmation of their efforts and a method of organizing women's clubs nationwide in the struggle for voting rights and health and educational programs for women and their communities. Three years later, one of the largest state organizations of black club women, the Illinois Federation of Colored Women's Clubs (IFCWC), was born.[3] Its primary goals were linking the state's women to the NACW, elevating the image of black womanhood, providing social and economic services to blacks throughout the state, and contributing to the welfare of African American women.

The IFCWC united the voices, resources, and skills of hundreds of women in the state. Its multiple layers of local and regional organizations united middle-class women from every area into the largest African American social welfare agency in the state. Like the NACW, the IFCWC adopted a constitution, bylaws, and a motto, opened its membership to any woman with the financial resources and the time to commit to uplift, provided for the cultural benefit of its members, and developed strategies to nourish the black community. Because the number of black women in rural and urban areas shifted over time, the club made no distinctions between those areas heavily or less populated by blacks when it planned its annual meetings. Conventions were held in northern, central, and southern cities and towns such as Peoria, Springfield, Evanston, Jacksonville, Quincy, Danville, Champaign, Bloomington, Monmouth, Rock Island, Moline, Galesburg, and Carbondale. But because nearly 80 percent of blacks resided in urbanized areas by the second decade of the twentieth century, members did adapt by reflecting the changes in the election of officers and in the types of programs they created.

A variety of women sought membership in the association. Almost all were middle-class and educated. Many were native to the state, while others were migrants. Most had some connection with the community in which they resided through both secular and religious work. They all pledged to be dedicated soldiers in the struggle against inequality. It was these members who enabled the IFCWC and regional and local affiliates to create, support, and manage an extensive list of social, cultural, and political agencies. The IFCWC had a large following, claiming nearly eighty groups by 1921, with at least ten members in each.

While the migration that brought so many black Southerners to the state came to represent both an escape from oppression and a promise of opportunity, it presented major challenges to the reform network of club women. The social programs organized by these women became vital to the survival of the black community. Largely through their own volunteerism and fundraising, they combated the problems of homelessness, unemployment, illiteracy, high mortality, and inadequate health care that plagued African Americans. They opened kindergartens, day nurseries, orphanages, settlement houses, homes for the elderly, recreation centers, and medical care facilities. Another consideration was providing decent housing for homeless women and girls. As the migration escalated, morality was increasingly an issue for black women. To halt the assault on their Victorian womanhood, these middle-class women vigorously led a campaign to rid the African American community of the image of female impropriety. They located housing for prostitutes, homeless women, and young female migrants. They also built and supported institutions specifically for them, or directed them to the appropriate authorities for help.

The simultaneous explosion of industrialization, urbanization, and immigration from eastern and southern Europe exacerbated tensions between blacks, immigrants, and whites. Competition for space and heightened racial animosity made Illinois almost as inhospitable to blacks as the South. Slums flourished in Chicago and East St. Louis. White ward bosses prevented African American men from achieving any tangible political gains. In Springfield and Cairo it was much the same. African Americans too often occupied substandard housing, paid higher rents, were forced to accept the lowest-paying jobs, and received little aid from social service agencies. Pervasive fear and resentment on the part of whites led to an alarming increase in violent crimes in the state. With little being done to relieve tensions, lynchings and race riots escalated.

The vigorous efforts to end violent attacks against blacks in the Midwest also led to an energetic campaign for the enfranchisement of women and the political empowerment of the African American populace. The race riot in Springfield in 1908, the impetus for the creation of the National Association for the Advancement of Colored People (NAACP), signaled that racial polarization had reached its highest level. The number of race riots in Illinois had increased dramatically since the turn of the century. It was the riot in Springfield, however, that elicited the loudest public outcry, because this disturbance symbolized the extent to which racial animosity and violence had grown, and illustrated the alarming rate at which lynchings and riots were spreading throughout the nation. In response, progressive whites, prominent black club women, and black men organized the NAACP. Its support of black rights, anti-lynching legislation, and woman suffrage impelled Illinois resident Ida B. Wells-Barnett to sign the initial call and participate in the association's first conference. The IFCWC endorsed the organization as well.

Through the pages of the journal *The Crisis*, the editor, William E. B. DuBois, nationalized the dual plight of African American women and averred that female enfranchisement could be a potentially powerful force for the African American population. DuBois theorized that the African American female vote was both an opportunity for the black populace to increase their political standing in a racist society and an opportunity for African American women to become equal partners with white suffragists in the fight for women's rights. Since leading white suffrage organizations in the North had increasingly begun to campaign for membership among Southern white women, who adhered to a policy of white supremacy, the NAACP's platform was significant: for the first time, a group integrated by race and gender was publicly endorsing the franchise both for black men and for women.

The ideology of expediency adopted by the National Woman Suffrage Association (NAWSA) had a profound effect on its state affiliates and on black women. The predominantly white suffrage organizations in Illinois embraced black women for the most part, but they were also bound by the dictates of their national affiliations. In other words, national policy often overshadowed state policy. In 1913, for example, there was a nationally sponsored suffrage parade in Washington, D.C., in which suffragists from every state were invited to participate. Before the procession began, Wells-Barnett and a few of her white colleagues questioned the validity of NAWSA's policy of allowing the individual state suffrage associations to make their own decisions concerning the admittance of black members. They felt that this policy essentially sanctioned the Jim Crow practices of the South, practices that had been enforced during the late nineteenth century and bolstered by the Supreme Court's *Plessy v. Ferguson* decision in 1896. By custom and law, Southern suffrage affiliates of NAWSA could maintain their practice of racial segregation even during the parade. As a matter of fact, political expediency necessitated that any racially integrated affiliated organizations conform to the Southern standard.

The majority of Wells-Barnett's white colleagues voted to acquiesce to the demand of NAWSA that the marchers be separated by state and race so that the Southern participants would not be offended. Wells-Barnett was to march at the back of the procession with all the other black women, not with her state contingent.[4] One of the most outspoken advocates of female suffrage now found herself being rejected by those who had enlisted and utilized her services as a lecturer for the cause. The action both illuminated the complicity of local suffrage chapters in the national organization's Jim Crow agenda and demonstrated the attempt to bifurcate gender and race. Despite the racist overtones of the larger suffrage movement, black women in Illinois continued to ally themselves with local white suffragists and build strong political networks.

In 1913, the Illinois legislature approved the Presidential and Municipal Suffrage Bill, which gave women in the state the right to vote in municipal elections. Its passage propelled Illinois into the national spotlight as the first state east of the Mississippi River to politically empower a substantial female voting constituency. This legislation opened the way for African American female voters in racially segregated urban wards to play a profound role in the electoral process. By the second decade of the century, they had created their own political culture, organizing associations and developing the skills to become actively involved in black political life.

So politicized, by 1915 club women were moving into important roles in the state's fifty-year celebration of black emancipation. During the planning stages of the festivities, African American club women secured administrative posts on committees of interest to them, and eventually, through successful lobbying, they gained a place on the planning board as well. When suffrage legislation made it possible for African American women to become equal partners with men in the public arena, they formed suffrage clubs, cast ballots, entered public debates on major issues, and voiced their opinions on the importance of holding politicians accountable for their actions. Because much of their rhetoric was shrouded in the Victorian ideology of the day, which demanded that women bear the moral responsibility for society, they successfully circumvented most major attacks from black males.

The successful alliance between black men and women forced the powerful Republican machine on Chicago's south side to re-evaluate its policies concerning African Americans. The Second Ward was home to the majority of African American men and women in the city by the second decade of the twentieth century, and racial segregation on the south side had created the largest concentration of African American women voters in the state. As the population continued to grow and women gained access to the ballot, prominent black men and white Republicans pursued a politically expedient policy that actively pursued the black female vote. In 1915 the policy paid major dividends, as Oscar Stanton DePriest was elected the first black alderman in the city. His victory was the result of the political empowerment of women, the migration of blacks before and during World War I, residential segregation, and a heightened sense of race consciousness.

The "race woman's vote" continued to play a significant political role, ensuring that African American men maintained a lock on at least one city council seat. With the passage of the Nineteenth Amendment, black women's expanded political power contributed to an increase in the number of black state legislators, and helped DePriest to become the first black United States representative elected from the North.

Through their club work and political involvement, African American women helped to advance the chances for eradication of social and political forces oppressive to the Illinois African American community. They shared equally with their men in defining the direction of black life during one of the bleakest eras. They instituted welfare programs and sought social justice to redress the inequities within American society. At the height of the migration, these race-conscious women embraced politics to further their cause. The marriage of the public domain of politics with the personal space of domesticity came to symbolize both a civic duty and an obligation to the race. Ultimately, they promoted an African American–based movement built around a racially conscious ideology, successfully blending their private world of club work with the public world of political activism.

Gender, Race, and Politics
in the Midwest

ONE

The Movement to Organize Race Women

Planning for the World's Columbian Exposition, to be held in Chicago in 1892, got under way in 1890. The fair, dedicated to commemorating the four hundredth anniversary of the founding of America by Europeans and celebrating the accomplishments of Americans, presented black women activists in the city with the opportunity to lay the foundation for a social and political movement that would last well into the twentieth century. To expose their exclusion and increase their visibility, African American club women pushed for greater involvement in fair activities by petitioning the governing body over women's exhibits. As a result of the criticisms leveled at the all-white governing body, Chicago resident Fannie Barrier Williams was appointed to an administrative post.

Black female activism at the exposition also inspired a campaign to organize a national movement of African American women. As a result of her polemical pamphlet documenting racism at the fair and her international campaign against lynching, Chicagoan Ida B. Wells's character was subsequently viciously attacked in the white press. Feeling the sting, black women across the nation called for their loosely tied web to form a powerful association of "race women" dedicated to combating racism and sexism, serving the needs of black women, and uplifting the race. This call eventually ignited an unprecedented growth in local and regional associations of club women in Illinois and across the nation.

From the beginning, the exposition was mired in controversy. For white Americans, the fair represented an outlet for showcasing the cultural and technological superiority of the United States. It reminded African Americans, however, of their second-class status. (The style of the buildings was the first indication that blacks would play a limited role in the activities: all of the buildings were to have white exteriors.)[1] Financed partly with funds appropriated by Congress, the fair was to be governed by at-large national committees representing each state and territory. Because of the inclusion of the historic Woman's Building, there were two committees, one all-male and the other all-female. At the outset, however, these committees reflected the racism that pervaded the country: the female committee had one black member, while the male committee had none. An editorial in the December 1890 *Indianapolis Freeman* chastised President William Harrison for the oversight. "The Negro is surely no useless part of the great American people," the editor lamented. "[But the fact that] no Negro is on the commission implies that no one Negro in any state of the Union had the required qualities to represent one-fourth of his state or one-eighth of the nation."[2] Eventually a token African American male was appointed as an alternate.[3]

As residents of the host city, African American women in Chicago felt that despite the one position accorded them on the national committee, they were being deliberately snubbed by those fair personnel who would be orchestrating local preparations. In addition to the at-large female committee, the fair commission appointed a nine-member Board of Lady Mangers to oversee the concerns of women, particularly the Woman's Building. Final approval for space in the building rested with this powerful group of women. Headed by wealthy socialite Bertha Honore Palmer, this nine-member board from Chicago had no African American women on it.

The women also objected to the fact that there had been no attempt to procure works by African American women for the Woman's Building. Angered by the insensitivity of the board, the Woman's Columbian Association, a black women's group in the city, delivered a resolution to Palmer in November 1890:

> Whereas no provisions have as yet, been made by the World's Columbian Exposition Commission for securing exhibits from the colored women of this country, or the giving of representation to them in such Fair, and WHEREAS under the present arrangement and classification of exhibits, it would be impossible for visitors to the Exposition to know and distinguish the exhibits and handwork of the colored women from those of the Anglo-Saxons, and because of this the honor, fame and credit for all meritorious exhibits, though made by some of our race, would not be duly given us, therefore be it RESOLVED, that for the purpose of demonstrating the progress of the colored women since emancipation and of showing to those who are yet doubters, and there are many, that the colored women have and are making rapid strides in art, science, and manufacturing, and of furnishing to all information as to the education and industrial advancement made by the race, and what the race has done, is doing, and might do, in every department of life, that we, the colored women of Chicago request the World's Columbian Commission to establish an office for a colored woman whose duty it shall be to collect exhibits from the colored women of America.[4]

While struggling to clear the racial obstacle in their path to participation in the exhibition, the members of the Columbian Association were also pressuring the board to recognize their contributions as women. The dual nature of their complaint frustrated the board, because to recognize black female womanhood meant to acknowledge black women's rightful place in the Woman's Building. Unprepared to deal with the issue, the board did not grant black women a seat; nor was a black woman appointed to collect the works of African American women.

But the resolution did prompt discussion among board members. As a result of their deliberations and, as scholar Anne Firor Scott suggests, their profound sense "that educated prosperous white women like themselves not only would but should set the agenda for the burgeoning woman's movement," they appointed Mary Cecil Cantrill, a Southern white woman, to represent the interests of African American women.[5] The appointment of Cantrill drew angry protests from African Americans. As the *New York Age* opined in October 1891,

> As to the merits of the controversy we are free to say that we are in sympathy with the "colored women" as against the "lady managers" on general principles. In the first place, a "colored lady" should have been placed on the Board just as a "colored man" should have been placed upon the Board of Commissioners. We don't know Mrs. CANTRILL. We are sure she is a splendid woman, as Mrs. LOGAN and Mrs. BRAYTON vouch for her. But why she should have been placed in charge of the interests of the colored women does not appear on the face of matters. She cannot know as much about our "women" as what they are capable of as Mrs. GEORGE L. RUFFIN of Massachusetts, Mrs. PHILIP A. WHITE of New York, Mrs. BLANCHE K. BRUCE of the District of Columbia and Indiana, Miss IDA B. WELLS of Tennessee, and a hundred other "women" of the race we could name.[6]

A similar criticism from the Woman's Columbian Auxiliary Association, another group of Chicago club women, forced the board to reconsider its earlier appointment. After much deliberation, members agreed to select a black woman for a post within the organization. They chose black socialite Fannie Barrier Williams of Chicago to assist in supervising installations in the Woman's Building.[7]

Williams was certainly qualified for the position, and she represented the best of African American womanhood. But her appointment served primarily to quiet the controversy for the Board of Lady Managers. Williams was chosen by the board primarily because she had not publicly vocalized her sentiments, and because she represented the black female aristocracy, who were thought to have more in common with the white socialites than with the majority of African American women. As a member of the exclusive "Elite 400," she belonged to a culturally distinct group of some of the wealthiest blacks in Chicago. This class distinction afforded her the necessary acceptance of the board because her background was similar to theirs. Moreover, she had grown up in a small, predominantly white New York town, where her father was a successful entrepreneur and her mother was a homemaker. From childhood to adulthood, she had had sociable relations with whites. Educated and refined, she was married to a prominent attorney in the city.[8] Thus Williams was chosen to help board members feel comfortable with their decision to appoint an African American woman to a position. Williams represented the best of the African American women for the members. They also hoped that her genteel demeanor would be less apt to produce hostile behavior. So to pacify black women and the black community, the board embraced Williams, later appointing her the secretary of the Art Department of the Woman's Branch of the Congress Auxiliaries.[9]

Williams's appointment and her friendship with a number of prominent white women secured her a spot at the Departmental Congress of the National Association of Loyal Women of American Liberty at the World's Congress of Representative Women on May 17, 1893. As one of the few black women present, she spoke before an audience of women from the United States, England, Germany, France, Finland, Denmark, Greece, Sweden, and Canada. In her presentation, titled "The Intellectual Progress and Present Status of the Colored Women of the United States since the Emancipation Proclamation," she challenged her predominantly white female audience to both acknowledge the existence of black women and understand that the commonality of gender played a much greater role in their lives than the divisive factor of race. "Less is known of our women than of any other class of Americans," she lamented. "No organization of far-reaching influence for their special advancement, no conventions of women to take note of their progress, and no special literature reciting the incidents, the events, and all things interesting and instructive concerning them are to be found among the agencies directing their career." She found it curious that "there has been no special interest in [African American women's] peculiar condition as native-born American women. Their power to affect the social life of America, either for good or for ill, has excited not even a speculative interest."[10] For that matter, resources "relative to colored women are not easily obtainable," while for white women "nearly every fact and item illustrative of their progress and status is classified and easily accessible."[11]

Her remarks were intended to raise the level of gender consciousness and place African American women at the heart of the contextual debate about the feminine role in American society. Because there had been little interest in their activities, she argued, African American women remained invisible. This produced a denial of black female citizenship and legitimized black women's omission from the general discourse on women and the larger women's movement. As women in Victorian America, African American females embodied all the qualities of respectable middle-class women. They were religiously astute, benevolent, educated, and moral. "Our women show a progressiveness parallel in every important particular to that of white women in all Christian churches," Williams noted. And in the twenty-five years since slavery, "conditions discouraging in the extreme, thousands of our women have been educated as teachers. They have adapted themselves to the work of mentally lifting a whole race of people so eagerly and readily that they afford an apt illustration of the power of self-help. Not only have these women become good teachers in less than twenty-five years, but many of them are the prize teachers in the mixed schools of nearly every Northern city."[12]

On the myths surrounding the morality of African American women, Williams said, "I regret the necessity of speaking to the question of the moral progress of our women, because the morality of our home life has been commented upon so disparagingly and meanly that we are placed in the unfortunate position of being defenders of our name." The malicious attacks on black womanhood, she continued, "are impertinent and unjustly suggestive when they relate to the thousands of colored women in the North who were free from the vicious influences of slavery. They are also meanly suggestive as regards thousands of our women in the South whose force of character enabled them to escape the slavery taints of immorality."[13] This public defense of black women's morality highlighted the concerns of the nation's black female middle class about stereotypical views of impropriety.

Williams's "progress" speech fit the themes of all the speeches made by African American women. Anna J. Cooper and Fannie Jackson Coppin followed Williams with more discussion of the progress of black women. Sarah J. Early delivered the address "The Organized Efforts of the Colored Women of the South to Improve Their Condition." Hallie Q. Brown supplemented Early's speech. Frances E. W. Harper spoke on "Woman's Political Future."[14]

Williams was chosen out of all the black female participants to speak to the World's Parliament of Religions a few months later. There she opined that "it is a monstrous thing that nearly one-half of the so-called Evangelical churches of this country, those situated in the South, repudiate fellowship to every Christian man and woman who happens to be of African descent." For African Americans, "the golden rule of fellowship taught in the Christian Bible becomes in practice the iron rule of race hatred." "Can religion help the American people to be consistent and to live up to all they profess and believe in their government and religion?" she asked. Yes, she concluded—if it was reinforced by "the gentle power of religion that all souls of whatever color shall be included within the blessed circle of its influence. It should be the province of religion to unite, and not to separate, men and women according to superficial differences of race lines."[15]

Williams's deliveries at both the National Congress and the World's Parliament of Religions catapulted her into national prominence. Over the next few decades, her services as a speaker, writer, and organizer were sought by both black and white audiences. As an African American woman, she used those forums to debunk myths, highlight the concerns of middle-class

African American women, and explain the issues facing the black populace.

Another African American woman who gained a reputation as a strong advocate for black rights and women's rights at the fair was Ida B. Wells. Though not a resident of the state at the time of the fair, she later became one of its most prominent citizens. An anti-lynching crusader, a club woman, and a political activist, she epitomized the defiant attitude that characterized only a small group of black activists in the late nineteenth century.

Wells's presence at the fair resulted from her passion for exposing racial injustice. Having had firsthand experience dealing with racism, she led a campaign against lynching. Some personal battles with racism and discrimination and the knowledge that the fair would attract both a national and an international audience encouraged her to take her crusade there. Her uncompromising and nonconformist style set her apart from club women such as Williams. Though she had published and lectured and was nationally recognized, Wells was not embraced by the Board of Lady Managers, or, for that matter, by any other fair administrative unit. Often on the receiving end of criticism from her black colleagues, she charted her own course.

Financed by several club women, Wells wrote, produced, and sold the pamphlet *The Reason Why the Colored American Is Not in the World's Columbian Exposition*. It was published on August 30, 1893, and twenty thousand copies surfaced during the exposition. Frederick Douglass, former minister to Haiti, provided Wells with a desk at the Haitian building on the fairgrounds, where American and foreign visitors could purchase the booklet. The inclusion of essays by Douglass, Ferdinand Barnett, a lawyer in the city, and I. Garland Penn, a journalist and editor, contributed to the pamphlet's popularity.[16]

In *The Reason Why*, Douglass discussed the shift from slavery to the entrenchment of discriminatory laws. Wells presented a statistical and descriptive account of lynchings. Penn acknowledged the impressive progress of emancipated blacks despite overwhelming odds. Barnett addressed the disappointment of blacks at being purposefully excluded from the fair.[17] He concluded that the failure of black representation was "not of our own working and we can only hope that the spirit of freedom and fair play of which some Americans so loudly boast, will so inspire the Nation that in another great National endeavor the Colored American shall not plead for a place in vain."[18]

The African American community was divided over the publication and distribution of the pamphlet. Some condemned it, attacking Wells's motives. Opponents also questioned the use of hard-earned money for such a venture. Philanthropic gestures toward building up the black community, they believed, would better serve African Americans. Supporters, on the other hand, championed Wells and Douglass's efforts and called for increased financial patronage. They believed that protest, not accommodation, would pave the way for equitable social, economic, and political resources. Further, they encouraged the distribution of the pamphlet in national and international markets.[19]

Wells's denouncement of the designation of August 25 as "Colored People's Day" at the fair also stirred debate. According to Wells, the true purpose of this "Negro Day" was to "appease the discontent of colored people over their government's attitude of segregation." For her, acceptance of the offer meant acquiescence to the system of Jim Crow. So she encouraged blacks to boycott the exposition on that particular day.[20]

Controversial actions had always limited Wells's ability to work closely with other blacks and whites who did not share her views. Her assertiveness, independence, and outspokenness ran counter to the female mores of the Victorian era and often left her isolated and marginalized. A product of Southern white racism and the ideology of white supremacy that governed the social, economic, and political lives of blacks and whites alike, Wells developed these characteristics early in life. Born July 16, 1862, in Holly Springs, Mississippi, she was the eldest of the eight children of Jim Wells, the son of his master and a slave woman, and Lizzie Warrenton, a former Virginia slave.[21]

Life in Mississippi was not easy. Post–Civil War era Mississippi accorded few opportunities to African Americans. Though black Mississippians were a majority during the late nineteenth century, they continued to be subjected to systematic disfranchisement, Jim Crow segregation, and racial discrimination. White supremacists thwarted most educational, political, and economic opportunities for them. By 1890, few African Americans voted; most were still tied to sharecropping and tenant farming, and separate, inferior facilities were very much a part of their lives.[22]

Despite the inhospitable surroundings, the Wellses were able to educate their children. In 1866, the Freedman's Aid Society established Shaw University in Holly Springs, later renamed Rust College, for freed people. As an interested father and community activist, Jim Wells became a trustee at Shaw. Lizzie Wells, who had had no formal education, often accompanied her children to classes so that she could learn to read and write.[23]

In 1878, yellow fever swept through the area and changed Ida Wells's life drastically. Her father, her mother, and a nine-month-old sibling died in the epidemic. The care of the other children then fell on sixteen-year-old Ida's shoulders.[24] Financially responsible for the family, she passed the teacher's exam for the county schools and gained employment at a school six miles from her home, with a monthly salary of twenty-five dollars. A year later, invited by her mother's sister in Memphis, Tennessee, Wells left Holly Springs. She took the two younger girls with her to Memphis, leaving a sister and two brothers with relatives. As a teacher in the Shelby County school district, she earned a higher salary than in Mississippi.[25]

In the post-Reconstruction era, Memphis, like much of the South, implemented a program built on the usurpation of African American rights, a pervasive system of Jim Crow rules. By 1883 the U.S. Supreme Court, in a series of cases, had upheld the right of Southern states to enforce laws that violated the civil rights gained by African Americans after the Civil War. Deeply disturbed over the events leading to the restoration of white supremacy, Wells challenged the legality of the system. In May 1884, she boarded a train owned by the Chesapeake and Ohio Railroad and chose a seat in the ladies' coach. Though informed by the conductor that as an African American woman she could not sit in the car reserved for white females, Wells stood her ground and refused to move to the all-black Jim Crow car. Rather than allow Wells to remain seated, the conductor attempted to forcefully remove her. In retaliation, she bit his hand. Refusing to be outdone, the conductor sought the aid of the baggage man. The two men then dragged Wells from the coach.

In retaliation, she hired a black lawyer and sued the railroad. Disappointed with his services, she turned to a white lawyer. The victory, with its settlement of $500, was bittersweet. The state supreme court reversed the ruling of the lower court. Though disappointed, Wells understood that hers was "the first case in which a colored plaintiff in the South had appealed to a state court since the repeal of the Civil Rights Bill by the United States Supreme Court," and if she had won, it "would have set a precedent which others would doubtless have followed."[26] The case and its outcome served as a springboard for her career fighting racism and discrimination. Over the years, she pushed the system to its limit by persistently defending her rights as an African American woman. She advocated protest, demanded equality, and sought redress for crimes committed against her race.

One of the mediums she used to publicize her message was the newspaper. Realization of the power of the printed word came when she joined a lyceum of public school teachers that met on Friday afternoons. After each program, the meeting was closed with a reading of a weekly, the *Evening Star.* The *Star* disseminated news about important events, included biographies of influential blacks in the area, and provided literary notes. Reaching hundreds, it was an important source of communication in the black community. So when the editor of the paper returned to his position in Washington, D.C., Wells assumed the post. She continued her membership in the lyceum and accepted responsibility as the weekly reader of the paper. Wells later proudly claimed that membership in the lyceum grew because "they came to hear the *Evening Star* read."

One of the people who heard Wells's readings was a local Baptist minister who published the weekly *Living Way*. Impressed by her oratorical style and her editorship, he invited her to write for his paper. She accepted the offer because she had "an instinctive feeling that the people who had little or no school training should have something coming into their homes weekly which dealt with their problems in a simple, helpful way." Her weekly column, written under the pen name "Iola," reached mostly rural, uneducated people, so she wrote "in a plain, common-sense way on the things which concerned our people." Her popularity grew, and over the years she contributed articles to local and national publications such as the Memphis *Watchman*, the *New York Age*, the *Indianapolis World*, and the Chicago *Conservator*.[27]

In 1889 she bought a one-third interest in the Memphis *Free Speech and Headlight*. F. Nightingale and J. L. Fleming attended to the public relations and financial end of the business, while Wells edited the paper. (Wells and Fleming later purchased Nightingale's share.) Early on, she spent much of her time writing about Jim Crow schools. She abhorred the poor conditions in local schools for black children. Inadequate buildings and improperly trained teachers exacerbated already deteriorating conditions. Reactions to her exposés were overwhelmingly negative. Conservative blacks distanced themselves from her, and the white school board refused to renew her contract for the following year. Despite the setback, she believed that her action was "a blow against glaring evil and I did not regret it."[28]

Without financial support, Wells searched for new endeavors. She spent much of the summer of 1890 seeking subscribers for the *Free Speech* throughout the Delta region in Mississippi, Arkansas, and Tennessee. Reacquainting herself with the people of Mississippi, she attended political meetings, church conventions, and Masonic meetings. While in Mississippi, she learned that three of her colleagues in Memphis had been lynched. This horrible episode led Wells into another realm of journalism, investigative reporting.[29]

The events surrounding the deaths of Thomas Moss, Calvin McDowell, and Henry Stewart on March 9, 1892, forced Wells to challenge her own perceptions about black-white relations. The three men had successfully managed a grocery business, the People's Grocery, in a heavily populated black section just outside Memphis. Their fates were sealed when a competing white grocery store owner, accompanied by a police deputy, visited the store and harassed two of the African American owners. An altercation ensued. McDowell knocked the white grocer down and confiscated his gun. Stewart and McDowell were charged with assault and battery and were arrested. McDowell later posted bond, and they were released. The following Saturday night, the white grocer and a mob of white men entered through the back door of the store. Fearful of retribution, the African American men inside fired several shots at the intruders. Three of the white men were wounded. Chaos erupted when news spread that several black men had been dragged from their homes and questioned or incarcerated. Eventually, Moss, McDowell, and Stewart were indicted and thrown in jail. During the night they were removed from the jail, shot, mutilated, and hanged.[30]

The African American community responded in several ways. The *Free Speech* ran an editorial that indicted the entire white community for the deaths of the three men and encouraged blacks to leave the city:

> The city of Memphis has demonstrated that neither character nor standing avails the Negro if he dares to protect himself against the white man or become his rival. There is nothing we can do about the lynching now, as we are out-numbered and without arms. The white mob could help itself to ammunition without pay, but the order was rigidly enforced against the selling of guns to Negroes. There is therefore only one thing left that we can do; save our money and leave a town which will neither protect our lives and property, nor give us a fair trial in the courts,

but takes us out and murders us in cold blood when accused by white persons.[31]

Pushed by fear, many black Memphis residents heeded the call of the *Free Speech* and migrated to Oklahoma. So many departed that there was a rapid drop in black ridership on the City Railway Company's trains. As a result, profits decreased for the owners of the Railway Company and other businesses heavily trafficked by African Americans. Concern over the massive out-migration forced mainstream white newspapers to discourage such moves and declare Oklahoma to be a major disappointment and plagued by hardships.

Wells refused to bow to pressure from white business owners to join them in their efforts to terminate the movement. Lost profits, she believed, were a small price to pay for the lives of three responsible citizens. She even visited several black churches, urging members "to keep on staying off the [railway] cars," and she "rejoiced" when many more blacks sought refuge in Oklahoma.[32]

Wells also decided to do her own investigation of the murders. The fates of Moss, McDowell, and Stewart forced her to question the rationale of lynchers and to reassess her own ideas about the reasons for lynchings. Like most Americans, black and white, she had been heavily influenced by myths that suggested that lynchings happened to accused rapists—that is, black men who raped white women. The men brutally murdered in Memphis, however, did not fall into that category. They were outstanding community citizens whose only crime was competing with a white grocer. This realization compelled Wells to examine previous lynching cases. After extensive research, she concluded that more often than not, the cry of rape served as a device for racist white men to legitimize the elimination of African American competitors.

She subsequently wrote a scathing editorial: "Eight Negroes lynched since last issue of the *FREE SPEECH*. Three were charged with killing white men and five with raping white women. Nobody in this section believes the old thread-bare lie that Negro men assault white women. If Southern men are not careful they will over-reach themselves and a conclusion will be reached which will be very damaging to the moral reputation of their women."[33] The editorial attacked Southern white male honor and suggested that white women could be attracted to black men. It infuriated the white community.

Fortunately, when the editorial appeared, Wells was en route to Philadelphia to attend the African Methodist Episcopal General Church Conference. Warnings from an enraged white mob persuaded the co-owner of the paper, J. L. Fleming, to flee. The mob destroyed the newspaper office and in their rage threatened Wells's life should she dare return to Memphis. Exiled from her home, she moved to New York, joined the staff of the *New York Age*, and continued her exposés on lynchings.[34]

Wells had met the editor of the *Age*, Timothy Thomas Fortune, in the summer of 1888 and maintained her contact with him. When Fortune called for the formation of the National Afro-American League, she supported him. Through the *Age*, Americans were alerted to the inherent problems of disfranchisement, lynching, inequitable distribution of educational funding, the convict lease system, and Jim Crow.[35]

Wells's research on lynching culminated in the pamphlet *Southern Horrors: Lynch Law in All Its Phases*, published in October 1892. She prefaced it with "Somebody must show that the Afro-American race is more sinned against than sinning, and it seems to have fallen upon me to do so." She was determined to prove that blacks were not a "bestial race" and to "arouse the conscience of the American people to a demand for justice to every citizen."[36]

In her crusade to alert the world to the plight of blacks in the United States, Wells became a lecturer. On October 5, 1892, Victoria Earle Matthews, a social worker who had established the White Rose Working Girls Home for young African American women, and Maritcha Lyons, a schoolteacher, invited Wells to Lyric Hall in New York City to speak to approximately 250 women. Her topic was lynching.[37] The speech in New York offered her the chance to expose this heinous practice to a national audience. But it was not easy. Upon approaching the lectern at Lyric Hall, Wells recounted later, "A panic seized me. I was afraid that I was going to make a scene and spoil all those dear good women had done for me. I kept saying to myself that whatever happened I must not break down, and so I kept on reading. I had left my handkerchief on the seat behind me and therefore could not wipe away the tears which were coursing down my cheeks." Bewildered, disconcerted, and annoyed by this emotional demonstration, "I was mortified that I had not been able to prevent such an exhibition of weakness."[38] Rather than being offended, the audience seemed captivated by her uncharacteristic public display of a "woman's weakness," and they listened intently. The emotional interlude successfully awakened the assembly to the serious state of the African American community, particularly the male population.[39]

In appreciation, Wells received five hundred dollars and a gold brooch in the shape of a pen, symbolic of her newspaper reporting skills.[40] The event also launched her public speaking career. Invitations poured in from around the country, and by the close of the year, it was evident that she had a secure position as a spokesperson for African American rights.[41]

Wells's speech challenged its listeners to become involved in issues of relevance to the black community. Soon afterward, several women formed clubs of their own. Victoria Earle Matthews organized the Women's Loyal Union of New York, and Josephine St. Pierre Ruffin went back to Boston and established the Women's Era Club.[42] Moreover, Ruffin, an active club woman and suffragist and her daughter, Florida Ruffin Ridley, began publication of a monthly newspaper, the *Woman's Era*, which disseminated news by and about black women throughout the country. As a vital component of the African American women's clubs, the *Era* circulated in Boston, New Bedford, Providence, New York, Chicago, Washington, and Kansas City.[43] Several women, including the co-chair of the New York rally, Victoria Earle Matthews, and Chicago resident and club woman Fannie Barrier Williams, reported news from cities around the country on a monthly basis. Articles focused on local club activities, child welfare issues, and woman suffrage.[44]

Williams regarded the journal as a "rallying" instrument for black women, because it provided them with the opportunity to voice "words of hope, courage and high resolves in a journal that seems to spring out of the very heart and peculiar needs of our women." Hundreds of black women viewed the journal, Williams insisted, "as the first intimation of the wideness of the world about them and the stretch of human interest and sympathy."[45]

Wells, meanwhile, made plans to take her crusade to an international audience and began looking for a new home. She chose Chicago, which offered a vibrant black population and a freedom of expression that she found exciting. Her first endeavor was the creation of the first black women's club in the city, the Ida B. Wells Club. Known as the mother of the women's clubs in Illinois, it placed African American women squarely in the reform movement in the Midwest and served as a model for many newly created associations.[46]

When she traveled to England and Scotland in 1893 and 1894, Wells helped launch several anti-lynching clubs. On the second tour of England, in hopes of persuading the English to exert international pressure on the American government to end lynchings and discrimination, she harshly criticized the activities of prominent white leaders considered to be favorable toward the causes of blacks, arguing that they did not take a strong enough stance on lynching, and that their silence on the issue sanctioned mob violence. In addition, she denounced those among them who spoke to racially segregated audiences, saying that their actions condoned racial segregation and strengthened arguments for intolerance.[47] Disguised as friends, she insisted, these white leaders were reaping the loyalty of African Americans and the praise of the white community.

The accusations reverberated throughout the black and white communities and elicited swift rebuttals. Several African American leaders chastised Wells and sent a letter to the *Era* in defense of one white spokesperson in particular, Francis Willard. As president of the Women's Christian Temperance Union (WCTU), an organization that attracted and included many black women, Willard had demonstrated an unquestioned commitment to the African American community. Nevertheless, the *Era* supported Wells and suggested that even Willard had not publicly condemned one of the most atrocious crimes against African Americans, lynching.[48]

Denunciation of Wells and her speeches was immediate. The president of the Missouri Press Association, John Jacks, published a letter that he had sent to Florence Belgarnie, an Englishwoman who had a keen interest in the causes of black Americans. Jacks's letter condemned the activities of Ida B. Wells and characterized black women as "having no sense of virtue and altogether without character."[49]

It was through the pages of the *Era* that many African American women learned of Jacks's comment. His venomous defamation of black womanhood angered African American women, and in defense they rallied once again. Exploiting the contents of the letter, the *Era*'s editor, Ruffin, issued an urgent call for a national congress of black women. She believed that Jacks's letter represented not just his own views, but those of much of white America. The legacy of slavery legitimized the idea that black women were "for the most part ignorant and immoral." She sent copies of the letter to black women nationwide, calling for a national conference:

> Although this matter of a convention has been talked over for some time, the subject has been precipitated by a letter to England, written by a Southern editor, and reflecting upon the moral character of all colored women; this letter is too indecent for publication, but a copy of it is sent with this call to all the women's bodies throughout the country. Read this document carefully and use discriminately and decide if it be not time for us to stand before the world and declare ourselves and our principles. The time is short, but everything is ripe and remember, earnest women can do anything.[50]

Women in Illinois eagerly responded to the call to action. Fannie Barrier Williams led the appeal for the formation of a national organization. According to Williams, Jacks's letter had "stirred the intelligent colored woman of America as nothing else had ever done."[51] "In spite of its wanton meanness," Williams continued, the letter "was not without some value in showing to what extent the sensitiveness of colored women had grown. Twenty years prior to this time a similar publication would scarcely have been noticed, beyond the small circles of the few who could read, and were public-spirited. In 1895 this open and vulgar attack on the character of a whole race of women was instantly and vehemently resented, in every possible way, by a whole race of women conscious of being slandered." Women were encouraged to hold mass meetings nationwide "to denounce the editor and refute the charges" of immorality.[52] Like Ruffin, Williams believed that an umbrella association would provide black women with the knowledge they needed for social welfare work and the power to defend black womanhood. "In order to equip ourselves with knowledge, sympathy, and earnestness for this work," she told a Memphis, Tennessee, audience, "we need the soul-strengthening influences of organization. Women unorganized in the presence of the heart-stirring opportunities are narrow, weak, suspicious, and sentimental. . . . Women organized for high purposes," by contrast, "discover their strength for large usefulness, and encircle all humanity with the blessedness of their sympathy."[53]

For Williams, women were the "spirit of reform incarnate," and it was only through them that African American women and their communities would be saved from the wretchedness of discrimination and poverty. Women's spirit of reform "impresses its reforming influence upon every existing evil, and its protecting power of love hovers over every cherished interest of human society. All combined institutions of Church, State, and civic societies do not touch humanity on so many sides as the organized efforts of women," she declared.[54]

On July 29, 30, and 31, 1895, the first national conference of African American women was held in Boston. The impressive array of speakers included Booker T. Washington, Margaret Murray Washington, Timothy Thomas Fortune, Henry B. Blackwell, William Lloyd Garrison, Jr., and Anna Julia

Cooper. Topics varied from "Women and the Higher Education," "Industrial Training," and "Individual Work for Moral Elevation," to "The Value of Race Literature" and "Political Equality and Temperance."[55] Ida B. Wells, however, was not there. Married only a month before, to Chicago lawyer and newspaper publisher Ferdinand Barnett, Wells was suffering from exhaustion, and did not attend the conference.[56]

Members at this meeting agreed to form a permanent organization, the National Federation of Afro-American Women (NFAAW), headed by the wife of Booker T. Washington, Margaret Murray Washington. The creation of the new national organization fostered a rift between the Boston group and a Washington-based black women's club. The Colored Women's League led by Mary Church Terrell, considered itself the first national black women's organization and protested the activity of the NFAAW. On July 19, 1896, the NFAAW convened for its first annual meeting in Washington, D.C., at the 19th Street Baptist Church, shortly after the league had held its annual meeting. The following day, seven members from the two organizations agreed to meet at the church; they resolved to drop the individual names of their organizations and unite under the name the National Association of Colored Women.[57]

Black women's clubs from every region quickly joined the NACW. From Illinois, the Ida B. Wells Club sent its president, Wells-Barnett, as a delegate to the first meeting. With a new baby in tow and accompanied by a nurse, she attended the historic event.[58] Other Illinois clubs present included the Phyllis [Phillis] Wheatley Club and the Y.P.S.C.E. of Quinn Chapel.[59] Each paid the two dollar membership fee and was listed in the first directory of delegates. The Woman's Civic League, Wayman Circle, Progressive Circle of King's Daughters, Hyde Park Woman's Club, North Side Woman's Club, and Peoria Woman's Club joined later.[60]

The National Association held its first biennial meeting in Nashville, Tennessee, in 1897 and elected Mary Church Terrell president. Illinois sent Connie Curl, president of the Civic League, and Elizabeth Lindsay Davis, president of the Phyllis

Wheatley Club, as delegates to the meeting. Part of their responsibility was to invite the NACW to hold its second biennial meeting in Chicago.[61]

Successful in the bid and cognizant of the need to unite factions on both the national and local levels, several Illinois club women organized under the name the Women's Conference. Attempting to connect the national movement with the local one, they sought to elect a recognizable, well-respected, supportive leader to represent them. They chose Fannie Barrier Williams as president. Over the ensuing months, the group mapped out their plans. Williams appointed a receiving committee composed of Agnes Moody, Rosa Moore, Albert Hall, Anna Douglas, Birdie Evans, Mary Davenport, and Elizabeth Lindsay Davis. They represented the Ida B. Wells Club, the Phyllis Wheatley Club, the Civic League, the Progressive Circle of King's Daughters, the Ideal Women's Club, and the G.O.P. Elephant Club of Chicago, and the Julia Gaston Club of Evanston. The four-day conference, August 14–17, 1899, was to be held in Chicago.[62] For the members of the Women's Conference, this was an exciting time. Publicity from the alliance with the still-novel NACW put them in the national spotlight and generated enormous interest statewide. Unquestionably, these Victorian African American women reflected "the Vision of the progressive Future."[63]

Wells-Barnett did not attend the Chicago rally. Instead, she joined forces with old colleague Timothy Thomas Fortune in preparing for the Afro-American Council Conference, to be held August 17–19 at Bethel AME Church in Chicago. Since the conference opened on the same day that the NACW gathering ended, a few NACW members attended the council meeting.[64]

The NACW's conference in Chicago gave black women in Illinois a place to network, creating opportunities for them in the process. Over the years, several women gained administrative positions within the organization. Connie Curl, former delegate to the Tennessee biennium, was elected recording secretary; Elizabeth Lindsay Davis became national organizer;

Eva Jenifer served as chair of Ways and Means and as parliamentarian; Agnes Moody was second vice president; Agnes E. Payton became corresponding secretary; and Theresa G. Macon served as recording secretary.[65]

The formation of the NACW was an aggressive response to the demands of African American women. Insisting on visibility, responding to the deteriorating conditions in the African American community, and defending black womanhood, these activists created the largest African American organization in the country. The association expanded the range of pursuits for African American women, yielded enormous profits, and played a major role in redefining the concept of a black female sphere by providing a basis of organized reform and widening the scope of black women's work. As a result, the numerous associations already in existence flourished, and new ones sprang up across the nation.

The formation of the NACW energized African American club women in Illinois. They began to focus on increasing the localized volunteerism of women and solidifying their forces. Clubs proliferated throughout the 1890s. They concentrated on self-development and literary and cultural activities, as well as benevolence. By the turn of the century, female activists had brought together a group of like-minded black Illinois women and joined the ranks of those creating state associations.

TWO

"Loyalty to Women and Justice to Children"

THE ILLINOIS FEDERATION OF
COLORED WOMEN'S CLUBS

The members of the Women's Conference Committee who gathered in October 1899 at Institutional Baptist Church in Chicago were meeting to explore the feasibility of becoming part of the national club women's movement.[1] They strategized about how to create a state federation that would consolidate the efforts of the state's black female activists as well as be a viable means of stimulating the growth of more clubs committed solely to racial uplift. United by racial pride and inspired by the success of the NACW, these women created a state superstructure consisting of an army of organized black women from a network of local and regional clubs. The members decided from the outset that the current name of their group, the Women's Conference Committee, while demonstrating their gender consciousness, reflected neither their race consciousness nor their regionalism. Perceiving themselves as representative of educated, moral African American women providing racial leadership in a Midwestern state, the committee adopted the name the Illinois Federation of Colored Women's Clubs (IFCWC).[2]

The actual creation of the IFCWC took more than a year to complete. On November 21, 1900, the members finally agreed on a mission statement, adopted a constitution, and elected officers.[3] Unfortunately, the sources needed to reconstruct the deliberations over that year and the day-to-day inner workings of the IFCWC over the next twenty years remain elusive, primarily because minutes, reports, and correspondence do not exist. But Elizabeth Lindsay Davis's *The Story of the Illinois Federation of Colored Women's Clubs* and a small cache of material (including a constitution, bylaws, and some records of regional organizational development) housed with the Illinois Association of Club Women and Girls Papers do provide important details on the significant role that the IFCWC played in Illinois history and in the national African American club women's movement of the period. Published in 1922, *The Story* documents the activities of more than fifty clubs, provides biographies of more than seventy members, and describes ten community-improvement projects undertaken by affiliates of the organization. Both the book and the papers list convention schedules and the names of elected officers and include the constitution and bylaws adopted by the federation. Further, Davis's impressive work illuminates how wide-ranging the membership and the activities of the IFCWC became over time. It also suggests that the members of the federation were a sophisticated group who shared a common vision of racial uplift and self-improvement.[4]

One of the first orders of business at the initial meeting was to develop a governing document. The constitution and bylaws set out the structure of the organization. Its twelve articles dealt with the election of officers and their terms, membership criteria and dues, and a list of permanent benevolence departments. After determining that officers would serve one-year terms, be eligible for two successive terms, preside over state conventions, and act as delegates to the NACW conventions, members voted on the first slate of administrators.[5] Precisely how they decided among women who had equally impressive skills as club women, and who in all probability had forged strong friendships, is difficult to determine from the limited records available. The women chose as president Mary

Jane Jackson of Jacksonville. A native Illinoisan, she had grown up in the northwestern town of Galesburg and later migrated to Jacksonville, a community in central Illinois, then to Chicago. The wife of a minister, she had much experience in aiding the black community. She was heavily involved in both church auxiliaries and secular club women's organizations. At one time, she had held membership in the West Side Woman's Club and was elected first vice president of the Phyllis Wheatley Club.[6]

In addition to the president, other first officers were elected, including five vice presidents: Cordelia West of Chicago, first vice president; Katherine Tillman of Chicago, second vice president; M. V. Baker of Evanston, third vice president; Julia Gibson of Peoria, fourth vice president; and Julia Duncan of Springfield, fifth vice president. Other officeholders included Margaret Anderson of Chicago, recording secretary; Jennie McClain of Springfield, assistant secretary; Sarah Floyd of Peoria, treasurer; and Elizabeth Lindsay Davis of Chicago, organizer.[7]

At the second three-day annual convention of the IFCWC, held October 9–11, 1901, in Peoria, Jennie McClain from Springfield was elected president, serving until 1903. Subsequent presiding officers reflected a cross-section of state affiliates: Fannie Hall Clint, Chicago, 1904–1905; L. L. Kinnebrew, Jacksonville, 1905–1906; Annie M. Peyton, Chicago, 1907–1908; C. B. Knight, Alton, 1908–1909; and Eva Monroe, Springfield, 1909–1910. By the second decade, however, when the black population in Chicago had swelled to historic proportions, women in the city gained a monopoly on the top post. Elizabeth Lindsay Davis, who became president in 1910, served two terms, as did Ida D. Lewis and Theresa G. Macon, locking the presidency up until the 1916 election.[8]

The Chicago hegemony in the presidential office, however, did not translate into dominance of the other posts. Although the first election favored Chicago women (first vice president, second vice president, recording secretary, and organizer), and for twenty years at least two or more members of the board were residents of the city, women from Alton, Aurora, Bloomington, Canton, Champaign, Danville, Du Quoin, Galesburg, Joliet, Lovejoy, Moline, Monmouth, Peoria, Rock Island, and Springfield gained other leadership positions.[9] The strategic inclusion of women from all geographical areas of the state reflected the quest to maximize resources and an attempt to minimize the impact of the largest and most organized group of club women on the less influential club women in other regions of the state.

Over the years, other executive board positions were added. By 1907, the heads of the Ways and Means Committee and the Social Improvement Committee began to take active roles in the decision-making process. Eventually, a chaplain, a parliamentarian, a statistician, and a historian were also included.[10]

Membership in the IFCWC was selective and was designed to attract middle-class race women with the economic means and the time to volunteer. In order to join, individuals had to pay a five dollar fee, and women's clubs had to have at least ten members, incorporate social and benevolent components, and pay a two dollar fee. Individuals maintained life member status as long as they remained financially stable in a local club. Privileges included all the rights of a regular elected delegate. In addition, city and district federations with a membership of ten or more clubs were granted admittance. The fee of two dollars entitled them to one delegate for every ten clubs.[11]

Another important order of business during early deliberations was choosing a motto that would symbolize their mission and uniquely characterize the middle-class women who sought membership in the federation. Self-help and racial uplift drove them to be community developers and reformers, but it was the importance of advancing and improving the lives of women that led them to adopt the slogan "Loyalty to Women and Justice to Children."[12] The motto reflected the group's concern about the negative impact of race and gender discrimination on black women's lives and their goal of defending black womanhood. It also expressed their interest in influencing the lives of the children of the black community.

Every aspect of the organization's outreach was governed

by its mission. Effecting social change and providing the opportunity for uplift were the motivating forces behind the establishment of twenty-four standing committees that tackled domestic, educational, and cultural issues unique to women. There were arts, crafts, and music departments, which encouraged the growth of clubs such as the Imperial Art Club of Chicago, the Art and Study Club of Moline, the Domestic Art Club of Bloomington, the Progressive Art Club of Rock Island, and the Social Art and Literary Club of Peoria, where members read the classics, did needlework, and listened to classical music.[13] Committees on hygiene, temperance, and civic responsibility were set up to teach women about the necessity of cleanliness, abstention from alcoholic beverages, and the importance of self-help. The mothers' department instructed black women about child rearing and other domestic duties associated with the family.[14] To be sure, the dissemination of these middle-class Victorian values reflected an attempt by the club women to direct, and to a degree control, people's lives, and suggests that they believed that it was their job to be the moral caretakers and uplifters of the masses.

As a philanthropic agency, the IFCWC also funded several projects. The primary criterion for beneficiaries was that the objective had to coincide with the mission of assisting women and children. For more than twenty years, the IFCWC provided financial resources to the YMCA, the YWCA, the Phyllis Wheatley Home, the Amanda Smith Orphanage, the Old Folk's Home, Provident Hospital, and various day nurseries in Chicago. Other contributions went to the Lincoln Colored Home in Springfield, Yates Memorial Hospital in Cairo, the Lillian Jameson Home in Decatur, the Home for Dependent Children in Bloomington, the Woman's Aid Community House in Peoria, and the Iroquois Home for girls in Evanston.[15]

In keeping with its mission, the IFCWC also funded educational programs. With the goal of establishing more kindergartens and making them an integral part of the public schools, the federation allocated 20 percent of its funds for providing financial assistance in the form of educational scholarships to ensure that several African American youth could attend college. In addition, a special-purpose fund went toward increasing the number of African American kindergarten teachers.[16]

The federation also set aside funds for members who were "financially unable to attend" the annual convention. The Pioneer Fund provided transportation costs and afforded those women who otherwise would not splurge on such a luxury the opportunity to travel to many parts of the state. This assistance proved fruitful. Black women in Chicago, Peoria, Springfield, Evanston, Jacksonville, Quincy, Danville, Champaign, Bloomington, Monmouth, Rock Island, Moline, Galesburg, and Carbondale increasingly organized local clubs to assist the masses. Moreover, the conventions provided an arena for dialogue between members on civic, social, and economic matters. State delegates described and discussed the programs in their local organizations, and NACW delegates reported on the activities of the national organization. Officers unveiled plans for future projects.[17]

The IFCWC adapted to the social and economic changes in black lives. The increased demands on the organization's resources by the large numbers of migrants attracted to Illinois by economic opportunity in several major industries challenged club women to develop more sophisticated ways to simultaneously recruit members, expand their resource base, and aid the masses, particularly those in urban areas. To that end, regional districts were created that divided the state into three sections. These sub-federated organizations were modeled after the IFCWC in that they were overlapping networks of localized clubs situated in the northern, central, and southern regions of the state. Each had its own governing body and bylaws, and each acted as a philanthropic, benevolent, and/or cultural agency. These sub-federations provided the opportunity to engage as many club women as possible in the reform efforts, to encourage the creation of clubs in rural and urban areas where women had not yet organized, and to acquaint women with the various strategies used by area clubs as well as those throughout the state and the nation.[18] An additional benefit was a reduction in travel expenses. The regional associations allowed those who could not afford to attend IFCWC conventions to stay abreast of important issues.

The oldest and largest district was organized in the spring of 1906. Thirteen clubs met in March at the Frederick Douglass Center in Chicago to unite club women in the city. Soon after, the following associations joined the new City Federation of Colored Women's Clubs (CFCWC): the Ida B. Wells Club, the Phyllis Wheatley Club, the Women's Civic League, the Frederick Douglass Center Women's Club, the Necessity Club, the Mother's Union Club, the Cornell Charity Club, the Julia Gaston Club, the Volunteer Workers' Club, the North Side Woman's Club, the Ladies' Labor of Love Club, the Imperial Art Club, and the Progressive Circle of King's Daughters Club. The group adopted the motto "From Possibilities to Realities" to reflect their mission statement: "To promote the education and welfare of women and children. To raise the standard of the home. To secure and enforce civil rights for minority groups and to foster interracial understanding, so that justice and goodwill might prevail among all people." A popular association among women in the city, the CFCWC included more than seventy women's clubs on its roster nearly ten years after its inception.[19]

Elected to serve as the first CFCWC president was Cordelia West, who had migrated to Chicago from Evanston, Indiana, sometime during the last half of the nineteenth century. Her three-year term lasted from 1906 to 1909. As an active club woman, West at one time presided over the Ida B. Wells Club and the Volunteer Workers Club. She also held the offices of first vice president (1900), chair of the Ways and Means Committee (1901), organizer (1902, 1914, and 1915), and parliamentarian (1918) of the IFCWC. Soon after the state legislature passed the suffrage amendment, enfranchising women, she became heavily involved in Chicago politics.[20]

In 1921, under the reign of Irene Goins, the CFCWC incorporated and became the Chicago and Northern District Association of Colored Women.[21] Subsequent presidents of the organization included Annie Peyton, Fannie Turner, Theresa G. Macon, Clara Johnson, Jessie Johnson, and Martha Walton.[22]

Throughout its existence, the CFCWC assisted more than three thousand individuals and contributed to numerous institutions and causes. Among them were the Amanda Smith Home, the Phyllis Wheatley Home, the Frederick Douglass Center, the Chicago Peace and Protective Association, the Equal Suffrage Association, the League of Women Voters, the Women's Legislative Congress, the NAACP, the Chicago Urban League, and Provident Hospital.[23]

More than a decade passed before the Central District was created. On March 22, 1918, several women met at Wards AME Chapel in Peoria to organize the Central District Federation. Membership areas included Peoria, Macomb, Galesburg, Bloomington, and Canton. Service activities increased thereafter among the local club women of central Illinois. Early presidents served one-year terms and included Julia Lindsay Gibson, treasurer of the IFCWC from 1914 to 1915, Mildred Farral, and Victoria Thomas, who served as statistician of the IFCWC from 1920 to 1921.[24]

The Southern District was organized at the AME Church in Du Quoin. This district focused much of its attention on the development of Yates Memorial Hospital at Cairo, which served African Americans on the Illinois-Missouri border. The five hundred women who belonged to the district held membership in the Carrie Lee Hamilton Club in Colps, Douglass Parent Teachers in Mounds, the Hallie Q. Brown Club in Du Quoin, the Community Club in Carbondale, the Community Club in Elkville, Garrison Parent Teachers in Cairo, the Yates Woman's Club in Cairo, the Silver Leaf in Mounds City, the Benevolent Workers in Marion, the Woman's Club in Lovejoy, the Sojourners Club in Carbondale, Woman's Opportunity in Mounds, the Woman's Club in Sparta, the Sunbeam Club in Marion, the Sunshine Club in Harrisburg, and the Mary Q. Waring Club in Murphysboro.[25]

The women drawn to the IFCWC shared a number of characteristics. Each had a profound belief that only through collective effort was it possible to uplift and improve the community. Almost all were well educated, with many holding academic and professional degrees. They were also quite religious. With few exceptions, they had ties with and maintained membership in various churches throughout the state. It was through their participation in church auxiliaries that most of them honed the administrative and social-service skills that they used in creating their clubs.[26] Lillian E. Jameson, for example, a former resident of Evansville, Indiana, acquired her initial experience through her church Sunday school. As a teacher, she gained public-speaking and organizational skills. She transferred those abilities to various secular club pursuits, such as campaigning and winning the presidency, chairing the Executive Board, and becoming the organizer for the IFCWC.[27] Jennie E. Lawrence's father was a Presbyterian minister. Accustomed to strict supervision and a rigid daily schedule, Jennie was well prepared for the superintendency of the Phyllis Wheatley Home.[28] Jennie Coleman McClain's volunteerism in both the Union and Zion Baptist churches provided her with the skills she needed to help found the Springfield Colored Woman's Club and govern the IFCWC for two terms in 1901 and 1902.[29]

The women's religious affiliations also influenced their fundraising pursuits, because religious institutions often were instrumental in the success of their operations. Some clubs sought much-needed monetary assistance from area congregations for homes for orphans and the elderly. For example, St. Paul, St. John, Union Baptist, and Pleasant Grove churches contributed to the annual year-end fundraising for Springfield's Lincoln Colored Home. Other churches were called upon to house kindergartens and provide shelter for African American children, such as that at Bethel AME Church in Chicago. The establishment of an IFCWC committee on religion attested to the desire on the part of the club women to nurture their religious beliefs and integrate them with their secular pursuits.[30]

Although most of the women attracted to the IFCWC and its affiliates shared some basic similarities, the group was not homogeneous. Some of the members were native Illinoisans, while others, though longtime residents, had migrated to the state. While some were considered to be in the middle class, a few belonged to an elite group of the wealthiest African Americans in the area. Most belonged to the professional class of teachers and small business owners, but some were essentially socialites who were not employed outside the home.

Fannie Barrier Williams best exemplifies the elite group. Born February 12, 1855, into a prominent free black family in Brockport, Fannie was perhaps one of the wealthiest and most "cultured" of the IFCWC members. She and her two siblings were educated in the small town, with seemingly few problems assimilating into the white community. The Barrier family appreciated "the refinements of life, were public spirited and regarded as good citizens."[31]

As the only black family in Brockport for many years, the Barriers enjoyed financial and social success. From all indications, Harriet Prince Barrier was not employed outside the home. Anthony Barrier made a successful living as a barber and coal merchant. As a man and a property owner, he shared in the leadership of the community. He held key positions as clerk, trustee, treasurer, and deacon. Both parents taught Bible classes at the predominantly white church the family attended.[32]

Though surrounded by whites, Fannie and her siblings faced no social or educational barriers. "During our school days," Fannie recalled, "our associates, schoolmates and companions were all white boys and girls. These relationships were natural, spontaneous and free from all restraint. We went freely to each other's houses, to parties, socials and joined on equal terms in all school entertainments with perfect comradeship." Carried into adulthood, these memories had a strong influence in shaping her views about race and class in American society.[33]

After graduating in 1870 from the State Normal School at Brockport, Barrier devoted her time to teaching. One of her first jobs was in the South. "Race instinct" inspired her to join the other black and white Northern women who were venturing south to educate the newly freed African Americans. The experience was anything but pleasant. Influenced by life in

Brockport, she strongly believed that class distinctions outweighed race in relationships. Outside the borders of her Northern haven, however, she came face to face with Jim Crow. In the South, she "began life as a colored person, in all that term implies."[34]

Caught in the racist and sexist web of post-Civil War Southern culture, Barrier found that her background and views were a liability. Her elite status meant little to Southern whites. Embittered by the experience, she angrily wrote, "No one but a colored woman, reared and educated as I was, can ever know what it means to be brought face to face with conditions that fairly overwhelm you with the ugly reminder that a certain penalty must be suffered by those who, not being able to select their own parentage, must be born of a dark complexion."[35] So traumatized by the mores of the South, Barrier realized that in order to survive, "everything that I learned and experienced in my innocent social relationships in New York State had to be unlearned and readjusted to these lowered standards and changed conditions. . . . [Even the] Bible that I had been taught, the preaching I had heard, the philosophy and ethics and the rules of conduct that I had been so sure of, were all to be discounted."[36] "Instead of there being a unity of life common to all intelligent, respectable and ambitious people," she lamented, "down South life was divided into white and black lines, and . . . in every direction my ambitions and aspirations were to have no beginnings and no chance for development."[37] Thus Barrier discovered that the idyllic childhood and the breeding, wealth, and education that had ensured her elite status in Brockport had also insulated her from the realities of American life. "I never quite recovered from the shock and pain of my first bitter realization that to be a colored woman is to be discredited, mistrusted and often meanly hated."[38]

Frustration coupled with indignation compelled her to move to more hospitable surroundings. Washington, D.C., offered a large African American elite community and respectable employment. She became a teacher in Washington, socialized with other "aristocrats of color," and met a promising young law student, S. Laing Williams. A native of Georgia and a former Alabama schoolteacher, he had graduated from the University of Michigan in 1881. When they met, he was employed at the Pension Office and was attending Columbian University Law School in Washington. Upon completion of his law degree in 1887, the couple married and moved to Chicago. The Williamses moved quickly up the social ladder. He became a prominent lawyer and was later appointed the first black assistant district attorney in Chicago by President Taft in 1909, primarily on the recommendation of Booker T. Washington, the director of the Tuskegee Institute in Alabama. She became an active reformer and club woman.[39]

She joined the elite literary Prudence Crandall Study Club and played a key role in establishing a nurses' training program at Provident Hospital. Little is known about the study club except that it was an exclusive upper-class literary society with twenty-five members. The hospital was established in 1891, and through the agitation of Williams, a training school for black nurses was added. As a result, Provident became one of only a few places in the United States where African American women could be trained as nurses.[40]

The national prominence that Williams achieved in 1893 as one of the few African American female participants in the Columbian Exposition in Chicago illuminated her early position as a race woman. When she told the audience that "except for teaching in colored schools and menial work, colored women can find no employment in this free America. They are the only women in the country for whom real ability, virtue, and special talents count for nothing when they become applicants for respectable employment," she was attempting to counteract the negative image of African American women generated by white society and challenging the racial status quo. It was, she insisted, "the blighting thrall of prejudice," not the lack of a work ethic, that hindered hundreds of African American females.[41]

Because of her performance, several of her white friends chose her to integrate the elite white Chicago Woman's Club in the fall of 1894. Carefully scrutinized and rigorously investigated, the women admitted to the club were white and usually wealthy. Celia P. Woolley, author, lecturer, and Unitarian minister; Ellen Henroten, former president of the Chicago Woman's Club and the Board of Lady Managers; Grace Bagley, a prominent club woman in Chicago; and two others must have known the enormous significance of introducing Williams's name to the membership committee. Her credentials were impeccable: she already belonged to the exclusive elite black female literary association, the Prudence Crandall Study Club; she was married to a prominent lawyer; and she had been nominated by leading white Chicago women. Nevertheless, she was African American.

When the club deliberated over the nomination for fourteen months, it must have seemed like déjà vu for Williams.[42] Culture, class, and intellect guaranteed nothing for an African American woman in Victorian, Jim Crow America. For despite their locale, Midwesterners largely shared the Southern perspective of an African American female's place. Some members of the club refused to address the issue because they felt that "the time had not come for that sort of equality." For Williams, the agony over the debate surrounding her confirmation resembled the "anti-slavery question" because it "was fought over again in the same spirit and with the same arguments." "This simple question," she concluded, "was the old bugbear of social equality." In contrast to her Southern experience, however, these Midwestern women did admit her, because, she asserted, "the common sense of the members triumphed over their prejudices."[43] It is unclear how effective she was within the confines of the club or in opening the door for other black women. Obviously, however, class and gender played as significant a role as race in her admittance. She was a middle-class woman of African American ancestry. Over the next two decades, Williams was involved in many activities. She assisted Woolley in the creation of the Frederick Douglass Center, contributed articles to several journals, and lectured extensively.[44]

Less well known but also a member of the "Elite 400,"

Fannie Emanuel was born in 1871. Like Williams, she migrated to Illinois and found Chicago a hospitable place. Marriage to businessman William Emanuel in 1888 provided her with a stable financial situation and enabled her to pursue several opportunities. She enrolled in the Graham Taylor School of Civics and received her M.D. in 1915 from the Chicago College of Medicine. While attending school, she operated a charity home for children, the Emanuel Settlement Home. Additionally, she was actively involved in the club movement. She was a member of the Board of Directors of the Phyllis Wheatley Club, served in 1901 as recording secretary for the IFCWC, and was elected president of the Alpha Suffrage Club and the Frederick Douglass Woman's Club.[45]

Elizabeth Lindsay Davis, on the other hand, was part of the growing professional middle class. The eldest daughter born to Thomas and Sophia Jane Lindsay in Peoria County, Illinois, in 1855, she enrolled at Bureau County High School in Princeton at the age of ten. One of three blacks to graduate from the institution, Davis became a teacher. Traveling extensively throughout the Upper South and the Midwest, she held positions in Kentucky, Iowa, Indiana, and Illinois. When she married William H. Davis of Frederick, Maryland, in 1885, she quit teaching and devoted her time to church service and club work. An ardent believer in reform and social uplift, Davis embraced the idea that the best women of the race should be at the forefront of reform.

Her interest in local issues was demonstrated with the establishment of the Chicago Phyllis Wheatley Women's Club in 1896, of which she served as president for twenty-eight years. In 1908 this organization opened the Phyllis Wheatley Home for young black females seeking refuge from a life on the city streets. Active in other clubs, Davis held memberships in the Woman's City Club, the Chicago Forum League of Women Voters, the Woman's Aid, the Giles Charity Club, the E. L. D. Study Club, and the Service Club.

As national organizer for nine years, state organizer for six years, state president from 1910 to 1912, and historian of the

NACW and IFCWC, Davis made immense contributions to both organizations. Her documentation of the movement in *The Story of the Illinois Federation of Colored Women's Clubs* constituted the first record of women's clubs in the state. *Lifting As They Climb*, published in 1933, was the first national history of the black female club movement.[46]

Another middle-class professional was Susan Allen. Born in Galesburg, Illinois, she was a member of one of the first families to settle in Knox County. Her parents played an instrumental role in organizing the first Methodist church in the county. Educated in the Monmouth public schools, Allen became a missionary. While rearing her children, she maintained an active schedule. She championed temperance and female suffrage and held membership in the Republican Club. She served as president of the Autumn Leaf Club and assisted in the creation of the Woman's Progressive Club. In 1910 and 1911, she held the post of third vice president of the IFCWC.[47]

Native Illinoisan Jennie Coleman McClain was born in Springfield on February 12, 1855, to Laundrum and Melissa Coleman. After completing high school, she moved to Missouri and taught school. She returned to Springfield sometime during the last decades of the nineteenth century and remained there for the rest of her life. Committed to religious endeavors, McClain assumed an active role in the church. She was treasurer of the Union Baptist Sunday School, secretary of the Zion Baptist Sunday School, and assistant secretary and vice president of the Wood River Baptist Sunday School Convention. Strongly committed to the welfare of children, McClain held a seat on the executive board of the Lincoln Colored Home in Springfield. At the age of fifty-four, she was elected the Grand Most Ancient Matron of the Heroines of Jericho Lodge, one of the most distinguished honors for a member. Other lodge work included serving as grand lecturer in the Grand Chapter Order of the Eastern Star. In the IFCWC, she was elected chair of the Committee on Constitution and By-Laws, assistant secretary, and president.[48]

Connie Curl-Maxwell, from Cincinnati, Ohio, came to Illinois via a long trail of job opportunities in the South and the Midwest. After graduation, she secured teaching positions in Cincinnati, Keokuk, Iowa, and Louisville, Kentucky. Upon her arrival in Chicago, she became an active club woman. She organized and became the first president of the Woman's Civic League and a member of the Phyllis Wheatley Home Association. In addition, she served as the recording secretary of the NACW from 1899 to 1900.[49]

The mobilization of these middle- and upper-class African American women was based on a shared belief that they had to collectively tackle the issues contributing to the destruction of the African American community. They saw their social welfare crusade as improving both their own lives and the lives of those around them. Equally devoted to uplifting the community and to aiding themselves, they found that participation in the club movement offered them a rare opportunity to associate with like-minded individuals who also were seeking collective advancement. Thus the IFCWC was organized to maintain a resource network of reliably skillful black females who could help lift the masses while elevating the image of middle-class black womanhood.

When the IFCWC incorporated in 1912, members were also turning their attention to discussions of female enfranchisement on the state level. At the Rock Island convention that year, the keynote address was "Why Women Should Vote."[50] The interest of the IFCWC was piqued for two reasons: the first was the growing national campaign by the National Association for the Advancement of Colored People, the NACW, and white female suffrage groups to enfranchise women in the eastern states; the second was their own local interest. The female suffrage legislation pending in the state assembly would have a major impact on organized club women, further enhancing their ability to serve the community. When the legislation passed in 1913, the newly enfranchised club women adapted. As the first and largest group of black women in the country to obtain suffrage, they joined forces with Western black club women, who had already enjoyed that privilege. By 1915 the Northwestern Federation of Colored Women's Clubs was born.[51]

Throughout its tenure, the IFCWC remained a grassroots organization. Committed to empowering affiliates, club women met the social, political, and economic challenges faced by blacks in both rural agricultural areas and urban industrialized areas. The unification of local and regional affiliates into a centralized association harnessed the inventiveness, the spirit, and the essence of black reform-minded progressive women while expanding interest, commitment, and funds. In turn, black women gained considerable administrative skills, friendship, and the satisfaction that they had indeed uplifted the race.

The organization had a strong foundation, enduring well into the second half of the twentieth century and remaining responsive to the needs of blacks. Club women continued to extend social services to the black community long after the reform years ended. In August 1931, the federation changed its name to the Illinois Association of Colored Women. In December 1954, it became the Illinois Association of Club Women. With the change, a junior association known as the Illinois Association of Club Girls was added. Girls ages nine to seventeen and a young adult group, ages eighteen to twenty-five, were trained to incorporate volunteerism into their daily lives and embrace racial uplift.[52]

The creation and development of the IFCWC was a response to the increasing demands on African American women in the state. The organization enlarged their sphere of influence, contributed to their sense of sisterhood, and provided them with the resources they needed to assist the African American populace. Including more than eighty clubs by 1922, the IFCWC was unquestionably a powerful force: it was the largest organization in the state championing the rights of blacks, and the most comprehensive welfare agency meeting their needs. Through more than two decades of extensive social service work, the organization successfully increased the level of racial consciousness, contributed to improving the lives of the poor, and provided black women with a sense of comradeship that enhanced their own lives. Moreover, the members of the IFCWC successfully addressed issues concerning poor black women and bridged the barriers between urban and rural women.

THREE

Agents of Social Welfare

Industrial growth exploded during the Progressive Era in Midwestern states such as Illinois, and with the rapid advances and changes in manufacturing came a need for additional labor. African Americans both from Southern states and from within Illinois sought economic opportunities in these industries. As a result, the state's black population increased, and there was a dramatically altered pattern of black settlement. In 1890, 57,028 blacks resided in Illinois. By 1920 that number had more than tripled, to 182,274. Moreover, the percentage of blacks residing in rural areas dropped steadily—from nearly 40 percent in the last decade of the nineteenth century, to 28 and then 22 percent during the first two decades of the twentieth century.[1] With approximately 80 percent of African Americans in 1920 situated in urban enclaves, where there were few social programs to aid them, the social welfare network of black club women became not only a means of improving the quality of life, but also a necessity for survival.

Many of the blacks who migrated to the state prior to 1916 did find gainful employment. Yet for most blacks there were few other long-term tangible benefits. Racism, segregation, and discrimination blocked any chance of significant advancement.

Because many of the black migrants who settled in urban centers came from rural Southern environments, they were, as Fannie Barrier Williams explained, "utterly incapable of adapting themselves to the complex conditions of city life. They come for more liberty, and alas, many of them find it all too soon and to their lasting sorrow. They come for better homes, only to find unsanitary tenements in the black belts of the city. Some of the more competent come with high hopes of easily securing employment in some of the higher class occupations, but they find themselves shut out by a relentless prejudice, drifting at last into the easy path of immoral living."[2] While Williams's remarks denote her own class bias, they nevertheless demonstrate that African Americans in Northern urban centers such as Chicago often found themselves at the bottom of the employment scale. While a few others found jobs in the factories, labor unions usually excluded them, a fact that further eroded their economic power.

Eventually, the only housing areas open to them were the urban ghettos. Segregated by race and economic status, the majority of these areas set aside for African Americans lacked adequate shelter, educational institutions, recreational programs, and decent health-care facilities. Black deaths in Northern and Midwestern cities increased because of the high incidence of tuberculosis, venereal diseases, infant cholera, and pneumonia. Although the rates of death for both blacks and whites declined steadily after the turn of the century, historian Florette Henri contends that "the black death rate was consistently higher and diminished less rapidly" than the death rate for whites. In 1910, nonwhites died at a higher rate: 21.7 per 1,000, as opposed to 14.5 per 1,000 for whites. Although the disparity was reduced in 1920, the death rate for nonwhites continued to be greater than that for whites, 17.7 to 12.6, respectively.[3]

Restrictions based on race were not limited to urban areas. Racially segregated neighborhoods, exclusion from better economic opportunities in the factories, and the denial of services by social welfare agencies in rural communities exacerbated the plight of blacks. Hoping to find better housing and employment, many rural blacks joined a large intra-state migration. Their move to more urbanized areas aggravated the difficulties for both the newcomers and the natives.

To answer the needs of the increasing number of poor blacks who descended on the state prior to the Great Migration of the second decade of the twentieth century, African American club women, on the city, regional, and state level, created a remarkable network of social agencies. They organized and maintained kindergartens, established a large number of homes for the aged, the infirm, and the orphaned, and opened, staffed, and operated medical facilities. They also "rescued" young women from a life of immorality, provided libraries and recreational facilities, and responded to the health concerns of black men and women.[4]

Because there were so many demands on the club women, fundraising was a full-time activity. Maintaining their allegiance to the self-help philosophy, the women looked primarily to the African American community for assistance. They generated funds from membership dues, bake sales, talent shows, and musical presentations. Church congregations contributed money for the upkeep of orphanages and homes for the elderly. The women also turned to the philanthropic arm of the NACW and wealthy African Americans in Illinois. The African American community provided other types of aid as well: Churches donated space to house kindergartens and recreation centers, and the services of church personnel to teach and maintain the programs. Doctors and nurses donated their time and energies to taking care of the sick. Others in the community presented women's clubs with much-needed furnishings, blankets, rugs, utensils, and clothing.

Because of the enormous burden placed on the limited resources of the African American community, black women also found it necessary and often prudent to seek the aid of white philanthropists. Influential whites provided the requisite funds for sustaining the services black women offered the masses. Too, they often became a political voice for these second-class citizens.

Two of the most important programs initiated by club women were in child and elderly care. The kindergarten at Bethel AME Church and the day nurseries maintained by the Phyllis Wheatley Club and the Necessity Club in Chicago demonstrate the commitment of black women to the young. The Amanda Smith Home in Harvey, the Lincoln Colored Home in Springfield, and the Home for the Aged and Infirm in Chicago exemplify their zealous mission to help the elderly, infirm, and orphaned.

The club women in Chicago took the lead in developing day care for black children. One of the first projects of the Ida B. Wells Club, founded in 1893, was the establishment of a kindergarten at Bethel AME Church. Only a few of the private kindergartens established in the "Black Belt," the Second Ward, admitted African American children. But increased demand, coupled with long waiting periods, such as at Armour Institute, remained a deterrent to black parents seeking early educational training for their children. Recognizing the void, the members of the Ida B. Wells Club sought aid from Reverdy C. Ranson, pastor of Bethel from 1895 to 1900. The group, the minister, and two African American women trained to teach kindergarten opened an alternative school for African American children in the mid-1890s. The lecture room at Bethel served as the classroom for half-day sessions.[5]

Other clubs followed a similar route. In 1904, the Phyllis Wheatley Club established a day nursery at Trinity AME Mission in the Second Ward. With $1,000, the Necessity Club purchased and remodeled a building in the ward, opening the Necessity Day Nursery in 1920.[6]

As the number of black migrants in Illinois rose, so did the number of orphaned children and elderly. Amanda Smith led the fight to obtain adequate facilities for orphaned children in Harvey. The eldest of thirteen children, Smith was born in slavery on January 23, 1837, in Long Green, Maryland. Her father, eager to free himself and his family, labored in the fields for his master by day, then hired himself out at night. With his income he first bought his own freedom, then purchased that of his wife and children. The family subsequently moved to Pennsylvania.

Commitments to education and religion shaped Smith's life. Though not formally educated, she did learn to read at an early age. As a young child, assisted by her mother, she practiced forming words from the one source of literature in her home, the newspaper.[7] Religion also played a major role in her life. In the mornings, the family would gather around the table after breakfast as her father read the Bible. Influenced by her early life, Smith married a deacon in the Methodist Episcopal Church in 1859. During their marriage, she worked as a washerwoman and became a devoted follower of Christianity. After the death of her husband in 1869, she pursued a career as an evangelist. For almost two decades, she dedicated her life to being a Protestant missionary and lecturer, proselytizing in New York, England, Africa, and India.[8]

In 1892, Smith settled in Chicago. When she arrived in the city, the number of homeless black children was still on the rise. Three years later, at the age of fifty-eight, she invested her life savings, $10,000, in some land in Harvey, a suburb of Chicago, as a site for the future Amanda Smith Orphan Home. Nearly four years later, the home opened to five orphaned children. As one of the few orphanages for black children in the state, with ties to the Cook County Juvenile Court, it continued to experience increased enrollment. Less than five years after it had opened, thirty children found refuge there. Support from Smith's savings, the sale of her autobiography, *Amanda Smith's Own Story*, and her newspaper, the *Helper*, evangelistic work, and donations from black and white friends kept the orphanage afloat in its first years. But the lack of consistent long-term financial support finally took its toll. Restricted growth and an inefficient staff limited the home's success. In 1905, ten years after it had opened, the constant shortage of funds and inadequate staff led state inspectors to suggest that the orphanage be closed. Practicality prevailed, however. It was the only facility in the area serving African American children, and the state could hardly do without it.

By 1913, the orphanage was granted a state charter. In honor of Smith's contributions and in recognition of its new mission as a home for orphaned and delinquent girls, it was renamed the Amanda Smith Industrial School for Girls. Nearly forty girls between the ages of four and seventeen attended the school by 1917. Smith, however, had relinquished the helm. Failing health forced her into retirement in Sebring, Florida. She died February 23, 1915. Three years later, the home was destroyed in a fire.[9]

Another champion for the orphaned was Eva Carroll Monroe, who was less than thirty years of age when she opened the Lincoln Colored Old Folks' and Orphans' Home. Born in Kewanne, Illinois, in 1868 (or 1869) to Richard and Mary Glenn Carroll, Monroe learned early about responsibility. After the death of her mother in 1880, she gained custody of six younger siblings. In the mid-1890s she settled in Springfield and worked for a while at a sanatorium.

Over the next three decades, Monroe became deeply involved in the black women's club movement. She joined the Illinois Federation of Colored Women's Clubs and served as president from 1909 to 1910. She represented the federation at the national conventions in Salt Lake City in 1909 and in Kansas City in 1916. She was the only black woman on the executive board of the State Department of the Illinois Woman's Relief Corps. In 1915, the Illinois Commission of the National Half-Century Anniversary of Negro Freedom made Monroe vice chairman of its Department of Sociology. In addition, she held memberships in the WCTU and the Phyllis Wheatley Home Association of Chicago.[10]

Springfield, located in Sangamon County, had a large number of dependent black children. Most were undernourished, inadequately clothed, and homeless. The only facility in the city for orphans, the Home for the Friendless, was restricted to whites. Distance and lack of space rendered the Amanda Smith

Home ineffectual. Recognizing the enormous need, Monroe and her sister, Ollie Price, solicited money from the black community for the down payment on an old, dilapidated brick house on South Twelfth Street in Springfield. On March 8, 1898, Monroe named the structure the Lincoln Colored Home, moved herself, Price, four children, and one elderly woman into the building, and thereby started the first orphanage and elderly home for African Americans in the county.

The Lincoln Colored Home experienced the same financial woes that had plagued the Amanda Smith Home. Depleted funds and the lack of consistent outside financial resources remained a problem. Monroe and Price solicited help from black and white friends and acquaintances. Donations of furniture, bedding, carpet, and coal made the home habitable and sufficiently comfortable for the residents. By the end of the year, however, the sisters were behind on their mortgage payments, and unsanitary conditions remained a problem. When foreclosure seemed imminent, the wife of a former mayor, Mary Lawrence, paid off the mortgage of $1,400 and had the building deeded to her. Lawrence's philanthropic role was strengthened by her friendship with city officials and acceptance in the white community. Until her death in 1904, she was an indispensable financial and political ally for Monroe, the home, and the African American community.[11]

In addition to Lawrence's support, Monroe and a small group of middle-class black women met in August 1899, at the home of Julia Duncan, to discuss organizing a black women's club that would be dedicated to keeping the home open, providing necessities to the residents, increasing awareness of the black orphan problem in Sangamon County, and seeing to the cultural welfare of African American women. The club adopted the name the Springfield Colored Woman's Club. Duncan, the granddaughter of Sangamon County's first black settler, William Florville, was elected president.[12]

The club immediately elected a board of officers and board of directors to set policies and act as liaison between the club, the home, and the black community. The first board of officers included Julia Duncan, president, Sadie Demeny, vice president, Mattie Johnson, secretary, Martha Hicklin, treasurer, Ollie Price, matron, and Eva Monroe, solicitor. The board of directors consisted of Jennie McLain, Lizzie Taylor, Hattie Manuel, Anna Donegan, Etta Taylor, and Sarah and Alice Wilson.[13]

To help the club reach its goals, each member selected a benevolent or social section. The Philanthropic Section developed methods of raising much-needed capital. The Home Culture and Social Purity Section educated members about domestic and moral issues. The Mother's Division and Juvenile Section provided lessons in parenting skills. Cultural activity was the province of the Musical and Education sections.[14]

Through annual dues, a ten cent tax on each member, and solicitations from the community, the club raised $360.50 for the home in its first year. Over the next decade, more than $3,000 was contributed. Members sold tickets to musical programs, held bake sales, and solicited financial support from individual blacks and whites, churches, businesses, and clubs in the city. In addition, members donated food, bed linen, crutches, medicine, and a washing machine.[15]

Members also sought assistance from African American churches. Their monthly visits increased awareness of the goals of the home and the club, as well as encouraged African Americans as a group to commit to their own community development. And in all probability, since many of the women were members of the churches, they found receptive audiences in the congregations. The "small sum" received from the worshipers "soon counted up," related club historian Jennie McClain. As a result of the success, club members tapped into this resource on an annual basis.[16]

In addition, they harnessed the support of other black women's clubs, individual black men, and black men's clubs in the city. For example, a women's club, the Don't Worry Club, assisted in the home's annual fundraising fair. Donations from individual black men helped to purchase shingles for the building. A men's club called the Douglass Club performed a drama, which generated $300.[17]

They also solicited the aid of one of the black newspapers, the *State Capitol*, which urged the black community to support the home because it was "a colored institution entirely managed by colored ladies." A year after Monroe opened the home, the paper published a patron donation list so that "the public can see who are and who are not doing anything for their race." Perhaps the editor imagined that interest in the project would increase if it was endorsed by the local media, or that public embarrassment would force non-contributors to donate.[18] Whatever the motive, this strategy suggests that black community values and mores rested on the philosophy of empowerment and self-help.

Though no records exist of white patrons, McClain notes that white Springfield residents, including Lawrence, came to the home's aid. During a matching campaign, nearly $500 was raised. Mary Lawrence later contributed an additional $800.[19]

The Springfield Colored Woman's Club also looked to the IFCWC as a source of funding. After the state convention in Springfield in August 1902, the IFCWC adopted the Lincoln Colored Home as a project and contributed to its fund on an annual basis.[20]

Ultimately, the stability and upkeep of the home remained in the hands of Monroe. As solicitor, she was responsible for administering and canvassing for funding. To that end, she traveled throughout the state, attending social events and making speeches. Northwest of Springfield, she visited the cities of Galesburg, Havana, Monmouth, Peoria, Quincy, and Rock Island. Beardstown, Decatur, and Jacksonville were the cities on her itinerary for the central areas. Southwest of Springfield, she spoke to audiences in Alton and Edwardsville. In addition, she traveled as far as Joliet, in the northeastern part of the state. Monroe also canvassed outside Illinois, in places such as Fort Madison and Davenport, Iowa.

Her productive campaigns heightened awareness of the home's existence, which led to a rise in applications. Soon a larger and more modern structure was needed. After enough money had been successfully secured, primarily from Lawrence, and the dilapidated old structure had been demolished, construction began on a new building in 1903. Residents lived in tents on the property during this time. A limited supply of water, carried in by the boarders, contributed to poor sanitary conditions. Alarmed by the situation, club members requested that Mary Lawrence intercede on their behalf. Lawrence spoke with the white district alderman, and within a few days a water system was installed.[21]

On New Year's Day 1904, residents celebrated the opening of a modern three-story brick building. There were almost eight times as many boarders as in earlier years. In addition to Monroe and her sister, the new Lincoln Colored Home housed eight elderly women and twenty-nine children. Growth, however, remained a problem for the home. Diminishing space and financial resources eventually forced the board to curtail Monroe's travels. Solicitations and applications were now limited to Springfield.[22]

Soon after the new building was dedicated, Lawrence died. With her death, Monroe, the Springfield Colored Woman's Club, and the African American community lost a valuable ally. For years, Lawrence had influenced white residents and government officials on behalf of African Americans. Funding from the white patrons had flowed in annually, and city officials had remained on friendly terms with Monroe at the insistence of Lawrence. She was a critical link between the black and white communities: when she donated money and furnishings to aid the home, her white colleagues did the same. As she had requested, and in her memory, Lawrence's daughter, Susan L. Dana, was deeded the property and donated $7,000 to the home. Dana continued to make contributions over the years, but her preoccupation with personal issues overshadowed her involvement with the home.

The Springfield Colored Woman's Club and the Lincoln Colored Home began a series of outreach programs for the community. The Mary A. Lawrence Club was formed to provide monthly literary and educational programs for boarders and patrons. The home also hosted the Crispus Attucks Camp for black youth. The 1913 dedicatory exercises of the camp included an address by the governor of Illinois, Edward F. Dunne. During the same year, Monroe secured a charter for the Mary A. Lawrence Industrial School for Colored Girls and the Lincoln Industrial School for Colored Boys.[23]

In the 1920s, the Lincoln Colored Home became part of the Springfield Council for Social Agencies. State guidelines then governed its administration. By the early 1930s, criticism of Monroe's administration surfaced. Depending on the generosity of the African American community and white philanthropists, the facility had operated on a shoestring throughout its history. Because of the Depression, even with financial help from the Service Bureau for Colored Children, in all probability the home continued to operate on limited funds. And in all probability, Monroe's inadequate training exacerbated the distress. As the push to professionalize social service work escalated, Monroe's obsolete late-nineteenth-century training rendered any credentials she may have acquired invalid. Because of her enormous commitments, she had little time and few financial resources to enroll in classes to improve her skills.

Charges of understaffing and operating an unsanitary facility continued to hound Monroe, but she managed to keep the home open. By the mid-thirties, however, she finally succumbed to the bureaucracy, and the home was closed by the bureau. The children and the elderly were moved to another site under the direction of Family Services of Sangamon County.

Eva Monroe remained in the home until she was hit by a car in the late 1940s. She spent months in the hospital and died January 31, 1950, while being taken to a home for the elderly at Quincy, Illinois. The Lincoln Colored Home was sold at public auction on April 17, 1944.[24]

During the same year that Monroe had begun her search for housing for orphans in Springfield, a fire destroyed the homes of seven elderly black citizens in Chicago. This prompted Grabrilla Knighten Smith and Fannie Mason, two Chicago club women, to seek funds from women's clubs and churches to open the Home for Aged and Infirm Colored People of Chicago in 1898. By 1899, thirteen men and women resided in the facility, and a permanent board of trustees was appointed.

As in Springfield, the Home for Aged and Infirm Colored People spawned the organization of a black women's club to act as custodian and fundraiser. In 1904, the Volunteer Workers for the Home for Aged and Infirm Colored People was organized to work exclusively for the home. Workers raised money, donated food and clothing, ran errands, and served dinners. They purchased a steam-heating plant at a cost of $342 and built a separate stairway leading to the men's quarters for better accessibility.

In order to broaden their philanthropic efforts to reach more underprivileged African Americans, the Volunteer Workers adopted new bylaws in 1911 and became the Volunteer Workers Charity Club. The new organization widened its sphere and donated time and money to several other services: the Amanda Smith Home, the Phyllis Wheatley Home, and Provident Hospital. Its financial support helped to purchase larger quarters for the Home for Aged and Infirm Colored People in 1921.[25]

Other projects were also initiated. For example, the Colored Old Folk's Home Association of East St. Louis expanded its services by opening an orphanage on May 5, 1920, in a rented building. The Labor of Love Club in Chicago installed a bathroom in the Home for Aged and Infirm Colored People. In addition, several clubs, including the Cornell Charity Club, the East Side Woman's Club, and the Union Charity Club, donated money for the maintenance of housing facilities.[26]

The Progressive Era, which ushered in one of the "most zealous and best recorded campaigns against prostitution," offered African American women another avenue for curtailing moral evil in their communities. A consequence of rapid growth, particularly in urban areas, prostitution represented for black middle-class women the corruptibility of young, poor black women and lent support to the demoralizing stereotype of black females. Thus, prostitution reform involved a campaign against the popular myths of promiscuity and immorality that had plagued black women throughout their lives. The ultimate goal, of course, was to uplift the race by elevating and bestowing dignity on black womanhood.[27]

For black women, the attack on prostitution was important for two reasons. First, as Victorian women and as moral caretakers, they felt that it was their duty to attack the underside of American life. Abolishing prostitution meant protecting the home from negative outside forces. Restraining the sexual appetites of men was viewed as a priority. Second, the legacy of slavery had generated stereotypes of black women which were directly opposed to the ideal moral Victorian woman. Because African American women were labeled as licentious, sensual, and promiscuous by mainstream society, they were "prey for the men of every race," suggested Nannie Burroughs, a national lecturer and active club woman. Consequently, most middle-class black women struggled throughout the late nineteenth and early twentieth centuries to dispel the myth.[28]

As the largest metropolis in the state, Chicago presented the biggest challenge to the eradication of prostitution. City authorities, including police, often cooperated with prostitutes and pushed the red-light districts into or near black neighborhoods to keep them away from commercial and white residential areas. Consequently, blacks received little support in their efforts to clean up their streets. The lack of aid prompted Fannie Barrier Williams to complain that she and other law-abiding black citizens were forced to "witness the brazen display of vice of all kinds in front of their homes and in the faces of their children." It was these "trying conditions" under which Victorian black women lived, Williams insisted, that motivated them to organize crusades against prostitution.[29]

Black girls who were "led unawares into disreputable homes, entertainment and employment because of lack of the protection that strange girls of the other Races enjoy" found a cadre of black club women committed to preventing them from falling victim to "the hand maid of shame."[30] Club women took young women into their homes, appointed task forces to study the problem, built recreational and housing facilities, instituted programs, and taught classes on the duties of women.

Members of a task force formed by several black women's clubs in Chicago concluded that a shelter was needed for homeless young girls. Lula Farmer, Anna Dunmore, Laura Manning, Naomi Fenwick, and the well-known black educator Dr. Anna Cooper found that because the YWCA and similar white organizations providing services for single women restricted those services to whites, many black girls were turning to a life on the streets. The task force recommended that accommodations be purchased in a "desirable neighborhood" to protect young girls from "human vultures ever ready to destroy young womanhood."[31]

The Phyllis Wheatley Home, which opened in 1908, was a direct result of the increasing number of African American female migrants who were seeking employment and housing. To deter them from the temptations of life in saloons and prostitution, the Phyllis Wheatley Club, established in 1896, raised funds to provide employment services, recreation, and lodging for as many as three hundred girls over an eight-year period. In an ongoing effort to maintain the home, a philanthropic arm, the Phyllis Wheatley Home Association, was created in 1909. It was successful in its mission, and the home grew rapidly. By 1915, a new facility was built to accommodate the swelling female population.[32]

Women in other parts of the state also joined in the pro-morality and anti-prostitution crusade. The Big Sister Club of Decatur, founded in 1913, initially dedicated resources to supplementing rental payments, working with the juvenile court system by vouching for young girls sentenced to jail, and placing dependent youth in homes. By 1918, however, the club was limiting its work to aiding dependent women and their children. It opened the Lillian Jameson Home, named in honor of a fellow colleague, which provided low-cost shelter for estranged girls and women who needed a safe environment.[33] In Evanston, Eva Rouse, president of the Iroquois Community League, initiated the construction of a recreation center for girls. The Iroquois Community League Home opened in 1923 and was promoted as a place where girls could find "healthful recreation, Christian guidance, and protection."[34]

In rural areas such as Rock Island and Mounds, women's clubs also provided a safe and secure environment. The Juvenile Department of the Progressive Art Club in Rock Island reported rescuing several girls from prostitution. The Silver Leaf Club pleaded for leniency in juvenile court for a few delinquent youth and placed girls in the homes of club members when necessary.[35] The Springfield Colored Woman's Club did the same; for example, Julia Duncan offered room and board to a young girl brought before the club at one of its Monday night meetings.[36]

Few concrete conclusions can be drawn about the success of the campaign against prostitution among black women, or about the success of the moral and Christian values that middle-class women sought to instill in their charges. Increasing migration and ongoing racial and gender discrimination continued to contribute to the high unemployment and poverty levels among black women. Other black women could not "rescue" all of them. As a result of limitations placed on them by outside forces, newly arrived young girls were often easy prey for aggressive recruiters. Many also found themselves at the mercy of the juvenile court system, with few alternatives available. Moreover, because of blacks' limited political clout, red-light districts in their neighborhoods withstood even the most zealous efforts. The secrecy surrounding the business of prostitution, scanty records, and the failure of the club women to list the numbers of girls they "saved" add to the difficulty of ascertaining whether the club women could claim any substantial victory.

The nationwide settlement house movement of the late nineteenth and early twentieth centuries attracted African American women as well. Their interest contributed to the nearly one hundred settlements operating in the United States by 1900. Distressed over the filth, squalor, and poverty in American cities, these women dedicated their lives to combating problems.

The settlements provided temporary and permanent shelter, employment, education, and recreation.[37]

The two most prominent and renowned settlements in Illinois were Hull House, founded by Jane Addams, and Graham Taylor's Chicago Commons. But because white settlement workers were not free of prejudices, few houses accepted African American residents. Even the YMCA, the YWCA, and the Salvation Army discriminated against blacks, despite the fact that African Americans accounted for a disproportionate percentage of the unemployed, underemployed, and impoverished. Women such as Williams demanded to know what migrating blacks were supposed to do when they could not find employment or adequate housing upon entering the city. "Go to the Young Men's Christian Association?" Williams quipped. "That exists only for the benefit of white young men."[38]

Wells-Barnett voiced a similar accusation: "While every other class is welcomed in the Y.M.C.A. dormitories, Y.W.C.A. homes, the Salvation Army and the Mills hotels, not one of these will give a negro a bed to sleep in or permit him to use their reading rooms and gymnasiums. Even the Women's Model Lodging House announces that it will give all women accommodations who need a place to sleep, except drunkards, immoral women and negro women. What then is the negro to do?"[39]

The Frederick Douglass Center, the Negro Fellowship League, and the Wendell Phillips Settlement filled the void, becoming the most prominent settlements in black Chicago. In 1904, Celia Parker Woolley, a white Unitarian minister who had moved to Chicago in 1876, called a meeting of several black leaders, including Ferdinand and Ida Wells-Barnett, George Cleveland Hall, a prominent physician, and S. Laing Williams, a lawyer and the husband of Fannie Barrier Williams, to discuss the feasibility of opening an interracial settlement in the Second Ward. The black leaders applauded the settlement idea, believing that it would be an important asset to the community. The Frederick Douglass Center, dedicated to promoting amicable relations between whites and blacks, opened in 1905. It incorporated and was governed by an interracial board.[40]

Woolley and her husband lived at the center and monitored daily operations. Blacks and whites worked together in recreational groups, religious services, boys' clubs, and athletic programs. The Douglass Women's Club was formed as a result of the center's activities to improve the lives of women. A white woman, Mrs. George Plummer, acted as president, and Ida B. Wells-Barnett was vice president.[41]

Wells-Barnett left the center a few years after its inception because of an ideological disagreement with Woolley and other whites associated with the project. She argued that the white administrators patronized blacks and "were not willing to treat us on a plane of equality with themselves." So she solicited money from Victor Lawson, the publisher of the *Chicago Daily News*, and organized the Negro Fellowship League in May 1910.

The league launched a newspaper, the *Fellowship Herald*, in 1911, and provided lodging, recreational facilities, a reading room, and an employment agency for primarily new migrant men from the South. Like the Phyllis Wheatley Home, the league acted as a referral service for men seeking jobs. By the end of the first year, Wells-Barnett claimed, it had helped 115 black men find employment. The league also acted as a political agency, fighting discrimination on several fronts. It sponsored lectures and conferences on racial discrimination in employment and on race riots, particularly the East St. Louis Riot of 1917.

As an advocate for temperance, Wells-Barnett argued that the league's purpose went beyond that of a social center. It was important because "all other races in the city are welcomed into the settlements, YMCA's, YWCA's, gymnasiums and every other movement for uplift [because] their skins are white. Only one social center welcomes the Negro, and that is the saloon." The league, then, was to play an important role in curtailing the vices of alcoholism and vagrancy among black men.

Dwindling funds, however, limited the success of the Negro Fellowship League. After 1912, Victor Lawson completely withdrew financial assistance. In addition to feeling that the league should be self-supporting, Lawson felt that other facilities established for blacks were sufficient to meet the social, economic, and cultural demands of the African American community. The YMCA for black men opened in 1913, and the Chicago Urban League was established in 1916. This lack of funds, coupled with waning public support, forced Wells-Barnett to move the league to smaller quarters. Determined to maintain the association, she financed it with money earned from her appointment as a probation officer. She subsequently used the league as a reporting station for her probationers. After she lost her job, the league disbanded.[42]

On the west side of Chicago, a group of blacks and whites established a settlement house in 1908 for the enrichment of black life. The Wendell Phillips Settlement was similar to the Douglass Center in that it had an interracial board of directors and relied on white financial support. Julius Rosenwald, a wealthy philanthropist, contributed 25 percent of the operating budget for the settlement from 1912 until its closing in the twenties. Under the administration of black social worker Birdye Henrietta Haynes, one of the first graduates of the Chicago School of Civics and Philanthropy, the settlement provided recreational activities for more than three hundred children.[43]

In rural communities, inadequate funding deterred African American women from building large facilities. But because they too had an interest in "rescuing" children from the juvenile court system and from the other corruptible vices, they rented or purchased houses for recreation. The Woman's Aid Club, a group with branches in several cities and towns, was in the forefront of the battle. For example, the Woman's Aid Club of Danville purchased the Woman's Aid Club House in 1907 to hold club meetings and to serve as a recreation center for youth, and the Woman's Aid Club branch of Peoria bought a nine-room house for similar purposes.[44]

One of the most important reform activities of African

American women was health care. Preventive medical care was virtually nonexistent for blacks. They were excluded from most hospitals, or assigned to small, inadequate facilities. Most white doctors were reluctant to treat black patients for fear of white retaliation or because of their own prejudices. Consequently, the black community was responsible for constructing facilities and for training its own people. Hospitals providing care for African Americans opened in Philadelphia, Chicago, Savannah, and many other cities across the country. Staffed by black doctors, nurses, and administrators, these institutions supplied both the black community and the national health care profession with trained personnel.[45]

The Nurses Training School at Provident Hospital in Chicago and Yates Memorial Hospital of Cairo exemplify the concerns of black women about the inadequacy of medical treatment facilities available for black Americans. Black women assisted in developing programs, opening hospitals, providing funding, and administering services.

In 1891, Dr. Daniel Hale Williams founded Provident Hospital and successfully made it a model of black and white cooperation. It had an interracial staff, admitted patients of all races, and was governed by an interracial board of trustees. In its first five years, Provident served more than six hundred patients. It also offered one of the few schools in the nation at which black women could train for a nursing career. Although trained nursing had become an acceptable profession for white women by 1870, racial discrimination severely limited the entry of black women into the field. They were refused admission to nursing schools and nurses' associations. Aware of these obstacles, Fannie Barrier Williams assisted Daniel Hale Williams with the planning of the nurses' training program at Provident. She served as a consultant and fundraiser.

Women from twenty-four states, Canada, and the West Indies enrolled in the new two-year nursing program. Students attended daily classes and performed regular hospital duties. In addition, they visited the poor and the infirm who were unable to enter the hospital, and they administered medicine and medical advice. By 1913, 118 nurses had graduated. Many went to work in the South. Others practiced in the North.

The success of the nursing program at Provident prompted Daniel Hale Williams to establish a similar school at Freedmen's Hospital in Washington, D.C. Opened in 1894, it provided health-care services to blacks and was another option for black women seeking a career in nursing.[46]

Blocked from joining the national organizations created by white women, nurses from Provident and Freedmen's were integral in the establishment of the National Association of Colored Graduate Nurses (NACGN). It was organized in 1908 with twenty-six charter members. The NACGN played a major role in establishing a professional identity for African American women in health care.[47]

Another health-care facility in Illinois was Yates Memorial Hospital in Cairo. Located in the southern part of the state, on the Kentucky-Missouri border, Yates Memorial was one of three hospitals in Cairo, and the only one that served the more than five thousand blacks in Cairo and the surrounding area. The hospital opened in December 1916 under the direction of the Yates Woman's Club, the oldest (est. 1905) black women's organization in the city. The president of the club for eleven years, Florence Sprague Fields, initiated the project. She served as superintendent of the hospital until the late teens or early twenties. Fields, her husband, Williams H. Fields, a surgeon, and the other black physician in Cairo, E. S. Dickerson, probably staffed the hospital.

Like most facilities in the black community, Yates was plagued by financial limitations. Fundraising drives were essential for its survival. The Yates Club held musicals and bazaars to encourage black support and ensure "efficient and fair treatment, highly skilled medical service and a congenial environment" regardless of economic status. Yates Memorial remained open until 1928.[48]

The social agency demonstrated by black club women between 1890 and 1915 made them the largest providers of social welfare services to African Americans in the state. They created, modified, and transformed their reform programs to fit the needs of most black Americans. In doing so, they laid the foundation for the delivery of basic social welfare services to blacks long before federal or statewide assistance was available. Black women decided what was most critical, and they raised the money, built the buildings, solicited white aid, and administered to the needy. They implemented these programs, as Fannie Barrier Williams asserted, "in the same independent spirit" as they had the black female club movement.[49] Clearly their "independent spirit" produced tangible benefits in education, orphanages, homes for the elderly, homes for girls, settlement houses, health care, and recreational centers. Moreover, these women played a major role in raising the level of race consciousness and instilling race pride. Self-determination motivated them to sponsor picnics and open playgrounds for children, and to take care of the elderly. It was their commitment to Victorian mores and the negative images of African American women that persuaded them to rescue young African American women from the streets.

To enhance their reform efforts, club women would embrace yet another aspect of progressivism—female suffrage. When the national drive for the franchise gained momentum during the second decade of the twentieth century, black Illinois club women joined in the push. Some joined forces with white state suffragists, while others continued to work in groups stratified by race and gender. Regardless, both groups recognized that enfranchisement offered organized black club women the chance to further entrench themselves in both the local and the state communities. For them, exercising the franchise would strengthen their expanding visibility, reinforce their ability to do social service work, and limit the escalating violence directed against blacks in the Midwest.

FOUR

Race Riots, the NAACP, and Female Suffrage

THE NATIONAL MOVEMENT

In 1909, Ida B. Wells-Barnett boarded a train in Chicago bound for Cairo, a small river town located at the southern tip of the state. She was going there to investigate the lynching of a black man.[1] As the most active anti-lynching crusader in the country, Wells-Barnett had learned through her investigations that racial hatred and mob violence had long been a painful part of Illinois history. The steady pace of African American out-migration from the South between 1890 and 1910, coupled with a pervasive fear of economic competition, succeeded in transferring problems once believed limited to Southern culture to Middle America. During the first decade of the twentieth century, the heightened racial tensions between African Americans and whites led to an alarming increase in violent attacks against blacks. Fearing the lynchings and beatings, and forced out of towns and cities throughout the region, many blacks fled.

The brutal crimes directed against blacks in Illinois proved to be a watershed in race relations. Between 1900 and 1915, the quality of life for African Americans in the state deteriorated. At least twelve lynchings took place, and the number of racially motivated incidents continued to climb. In each case the victim was an African American man. Yet the entire black community was affected, because the rioting occurred in their neighborhoods, bringing with it property damage and loss of life.

The first of these incidents occurred on June 6, 1903, in Belleville. David Wyatt, a black teacher, was hanged, doused with kerosene, and set on fire for shooting a white superintendent who refused to renew his teaching certificate. Later that summer, John Metcalf of Danville, accused of murdering a white man, was hanged from a telephone pole while a mob of citizens fired shots at his body. Unsatiated, the mob then dragged Metcalf's body to the county jail and burned it.

Before it became the site of yet another mob murder, Cairo, situated at the convergence of the Mississippi and Ohio rivers, had bustled with river and railway commercialism during the second half of the nineteenth century. By 1890 its population stood at more than ten thousand, of which African Americans accounted for more than one-third.[2] The majority of the black populace consisted of Southern migrants who had come seeking economic opportunity, social equality, and political freedom. Illinois offered them jobs, equal access to education and public accommodations, and voting privileges.[3] As a result, many African Americans found success in Cairo. John J. Bird won an appointment to the Trustee Board of the Illinois Industrial University at Champaign. William H. Fields opened a medical practice. Others gained employment as police officers, mail carriers, and state civil servants.[4] Yet Cairo, like other Midwestern towns, was not free of racial problems. In 1909 William James, a black coal driver, was arrested and charged with the rape and murder of Anna Pelley, a saleswoman in a local store. A white mob dragged James out of the jail, hanged him, and shot him several times. Mob participants also cut out his heart and chopped it into pieces, carrying them away as souvenirs, then torched his body. There were no arrests.[5]

The most famous and one of the most brutal racially motivated incidents occurred in the state capital, Springfield. In the summer of 1908, Joe James, a young African American drifter, allegedly stabbed to death Clergy A. Ballard, a white middle-aged miner. Reportedly caught in the bedroom of Ballard's sixteen-year-old daughter, James attempted to flee, struggling with Ballard in the process. He then stabbed the miner several times. A few hours later, Ballard died of his wounds. Before James was taken into custody, a group of Ballard's friends and relatives severely beat him. Admittedly too intoxicated at the time of his arrest to remember the crime or the beating, James steadfastly maintained his innocence. He remained in jail for the next few months.

The James-Ballard incident represented more than a simple case of assault, murder, and random violence. According to scholar Roberta Senechal, it indicated a pervasive attitude that "emphasized the issues of black crime and miscegenation, reflecting white concerns about the social control of blacks in the North." James's alleged rape of a white woman heightened white men's anxieties about maintaining the innocence and virtuousness of the mothers of their race, who symbolized piety. James had defiled this romanticized ideal. Moreover, James was not a model citizen. A vagrant who drank excessively and a man with questionable associates, he epitomized the stereotypical African American male criminal.[6] For Springfield residents, he was the convenient scapegoat for their mounting apprehension caused by the influx of African Americans into the Midwestern region. Fears of race mixing and competition for jobs played on xenophobic tendencies. Pent-up racial fears eventually spilled into the streets of the city in the form of a race riot.

Nearly five weeks after James's arrest, just before midnight on August 13, 1908, a white woman, Nellie Hallam, reportedly was assaulted and raped by a black man. She told police that when the man entered her bedroom, he grabbed and gagged her. He then dragged her into an outside building, where the alleged assault took place. When the ordeal ended, Hallam's screams alerted neighbors, who promptly summoned the police. On the basis of a positive identification by Hallam, the police arrested George Richardson. Interestingly, he became the jailmate of Joe James.

Within hours after the Hallam assault was reported, an angry crowd gathered outside the jail. To ensure the safety of the prisoners, the sheriff, aided by a local citizen, put James and Richardson on a train to the state prison in Bloomington, Illinois. The crowd grew and became violent after learning that the perpetrators of the crimes were no longer in the city jail. Incensed, they attacked the restaurant of the man who had helped the prisoners escape to Bloomington. Looting, shooting, burning, and destruction of property continued well into the night.

Still unsatiated, the mob turned their rage on the black citizens of Springfield, destroying black-owned businesses and homes, and killing several African Americans. Scott Burton was beaten unconscious, then lynched, and his body was mutilated. William Donegan, nearly eighty years old, was also beaten and lynched. Though still alive when he was rushed to the hospital, he died the next day. By the time that 3,700 militia had arrived to restore order, four whites were included among the dead, and more than a hundred were injured. The property loss totaled approximately $120,000. Scores of white citizens were arrested; only a few were ever taken to trial, however, and for the most part they pleaded guilty to a lesser charge and received fines. Nellie Hallam retracted her previous accusation against George Richardson but refused to identify the person who really had assaulted her. There were rumors that she had concocted the story to cover up an adulterous affair.[7]

Throughout the riot, Joe James, the young man arrested earlier in the summer for murder, remained incarcerated. The court convened in mid-September to determine his guilt or innocence. In light of the riot and James's dubious status as an alcoholic drifter, Senechal argues that because "the press and city authorities worried that his acquittal might spark yet another riot, his conviction appears to have been a foregone conclusion for many in Springfield." An all-white jury convicted him on mostly circumstantial evidence and sentenced him to death. The following month, James was executed.[8]

The black residents of Springfield remained ambivalent

about living there. Some left the city permanently, while others who had sought refuge with friends and relatives during the riots returned weeks later to reclaim their lives. Public denunciation from the local black community was sparse. Speaking for the larger community, the black weekly *The Forum* called the acquittals of the rioters a "farce" and a "travesty."[9] Nearly seven years later, the paper was still asserting that "there is entirely too much prejudice and hatred," and that "the future is ominous."[10]

For whites in the city, the riot served notice that racial segregation was necessary for calm. This practice legitimized discrimination against blacks and encouraged their exclusion from restaurants, theaters, and hotels. It continued throughout much of the first half of the twentieth century.[11]

The riot in the state capital, a historic Northern city that was preparing to celebrate the centennial of the birth of Abraham Lincoln, the president who issued the Emancipation Proclamation, did generate an enormous outcry from an outraged national black and white community. The riot seemed the epitome of race hatred and represented the culmination of years of white rage aimed at the African American population. African Americans constituted significantly less than a tenth of the population of Springfield, only 2,961 of the 51,678 residents; they resided primarily in the densely populated wards one and six, commanded little political and economic power, and in this case could not possibly have represented a threat to white supremacy.[12]

Noted crusader and reporter Ida B. Wells-Barnett, when asked for comments, was hard-pressed to deal adequately with the riot, especially since blacks "had not yet perfected an organization which was prepared to take hold of this situation, which seemed to be becoming as bad in Illinois as it had hitherto been in Georgia."[13] Her personal response to the ordeal was to create a local forum for young African American males, in which they could openly discuss the atrocities directed at them. The forum later became known as the Negro Fellowship League.[14]

Wells-Barnett was not alone in her assessment that the state had become a hostile environment for African Americans as a result of deteriorating race relations. The official journal of the Niagara Movement, *The Horizon*, concluded that Illinois had become "infected with the mob spirit" evident throughout the country.[15] William English Wallings, a wealthy former slave owner from Kentucky, a socialist, writer, and settlement-house worker, arrived in Springfield in the aftermath of the riot. He maintained that whites not only had abdicated their duty to protect citizens but also had closed their eyes to "the whole awful and menacing truth—that a large part of the white population of Lincoln's home . . . have initiated a permanent warfare with the negro race." White Illinoisans, he argued, justified their mob actions by fooling themselves into believing that the problem was not racially motivated but one that lay with the criminal elements. In reality, whites had adopted and embraced an approach "like that of the South, on which it is modeled." Lynchings, race riots, and acquittals of white murderers symbolized the white South's ideology of supremacy. The events in Springfield resembled white Southern attempts to control black Southerners. Wallings concluded, "Race hatred . . . is really the cause of it all."[16]

Wallings issued a nationwide call for concerned parties to address white rage and to unite blacks and whites in meaningful dialogue with hopes of curtailing these problems. Mary White Ovington, a Unitarian socialist and social worker in New York, and Henry Moskowitz, a New York social worker, accepted the challenge. By January 1909, Oswald Garrison Villard, grandson of abolitionist William Lloyd Garrison, had joined the group. The four adopted three primary goals: to increase white awareness of the race problem; to bring about effective political changes for the benefit of the black community, including woman suffrage; and to hold a national conference to address those concerns.

For the first National Negro Conference, Wallings and his colleagues called on several noted leaders, including Booker T. Washington, W. E. B. DuBois, Mary Church Terrell, and Ida B. Wells-Barnett. DuBois, Terrell, and Wells-Barnett accepted the invitations. Washington, the leading African American spokesperson, did not.[17]

Unimpressed with the group's leaders and their activities, Washington continued to advocate accommodation over protest, vocational training over intellectual development, and provisional franchise over full political rights for men and women.[18] Nevertheless, Oswald Villard, a friend of Washington, attempted to win the Tuskegee educator's support. Villard believed that in order for the organization to be successful, it was imperative for black leaders from all arenas to take part in it. Perhaps to appease Washington—especially since Washington's antitheses, W. E. B. DuBois and Ida Wells-Barnett, were participants—Villard steadfastly maintained that "there is not the slightest intention of tying this movement with either of the two factions in the negro race. It is not to be a Washington movement, or a DuBois movement."[19]

Despite Villard's claims, the presence of DuBois and Wells-Barnett, neither of whom espoused the ideology of accommodation to white interests, signaled to Washington the direction of the conference. He decided that the new organization would be a radical political movement and would dismantle the limited gains that Southern blacks had achieved under his accommodationist approach. Washington tactfully declined the invitation, stating that his participation "might restrict freedom of discussion, and might, also, tend to make the conference go in directions which it would not like to go."[20]

The majority of those invited to the conference, Washington charged, really did not understand Southern culture as he did, and could not truly aid black Southerners. "There is a work which those of us who live here in the South can do, which persons who do not live in the South cannot do. If we recognize fairly and squarely this, then it seems to me that we have gone a long ways." Washington criticized the group for its opposition to his strategies of accommodation and warned that the newly formed association might create more problems than solutions. He "recognized the value of some agitation and criticism, but not to the extent of having our race feel that we can depend upon this to cure all the evils surrounding us." In the long run, he believed, the group would not survive, and he would continue to reign in black circles.[21] Washington's refusal to join the association, coupled with the fact that accommodation subsequently produced few gains and in effect contributed to the violence against blacks, paved the way for a stronger protest group to take charge and lead blacks into the second decade of the twentieth century. Although Washington remained a powerful figure among white philanthropists, his prominence in the African American community had been severely challenged.

Those who spoke at the conference echoed the sentiments of Wells-Barnett. Calling lynching a national crime, she lambasted white Springfield residents and the legal system in the city. She argued that both had ceased to be a credible source of support for the African American citizens of Springfield. The need to subordinate blacks and preserve white supremacy had been the rationale for the lynching of two men, the forced out-migration of blacks from their homes, and the acquittal of murderers, "all because a white woman said a Negro had assaulted her." The riot and the increasing number of lynchings, she declared, showed the pervasiveness of white racism and underscored black Americans' subordinate place in the United States. Moreover, these acts demonstrated how negative racial attitudes had infiltrated a judicial system that was supposed to protect all its citizens. Murderers were not prosecuted because they were white, while black lives were at the mercy of perpetrators who trampled on their civil rights.[22]

Soon after the formation of the National Association for the Advancement of Colored People (NAACP), Wells-Barnett offered a solid approach to fighting racial violence. Enfranchisement, she believed, was the answer. The disfranchised were, quite simply, marginalized, and pawns in the hands of those with political power. Mobilization in an organization such as the NAACP, coupled with political empowerment, would generate social and economic opportunity as well as stop racially motivated violence. Pressure from interracial groups and the election of black officeholders who would push for the passage of anti-lynching legislation would bring an end to mob rule.[23]

Other women joined Wells-Barnett in her push for mobilization and political activism. Nearly one-third of the sixty people who signed Wallings's call to action were women. They held positions on the executive and general committees and on the board of directors.[24] Because of the roles occupied by women in the organization, the association was forced to address women's causes as humanitarian issues rather than as issues unique to women.[25] In addition to assisting in the creation of the NAACP, Illinois club women joined the ranks of blacks nationwide who endorsed or held membership in the association. As branches opened across the country, club women supported those as well. In 1911, the IFCWC endorsed the NAACP. Fannie Barrier Williams and Mary F. Waring joined the successful cooperative efforts of numerous African Americans in Chicago in opening a branch there.[26] Club women sought membership in the organization primarily because it championed racial cooperation and furthered the cause of blacks and women in the political arena.

W. E. B. DuBois launched a massive campaign for the enfranchisement of Southern blacks and of women in every region of the country. A longtime protest activist, DuBois had always propagated his views on the disfranchisement of black men in the South and on his belief in equal suffrage for women. He believed that when the Fifteenth Amendment was reinstated, black men's vote would deter white manipulation, open doors to educational opportunity, and renew self-respect among the black masses. Disfranchised blacks, DuBois asserted, were "a provocation, an invitation to oppression, a plaything for mobs and a bonanza for demagogues."[27]

Relentless in his crusade against political oppression, DuBois constantly and consistently agitated for change. The publication in 1910 of the first official journal for the NAACP, *The Crisis*, provided him with another vehicle to further his own method of protest.[28] Throughout much of the first two decades of the twentieth century, DuBois argued that the inequities that plagued African Americans were humanitarian problems that had evolved from racism. He warned that "the caste system which attempts to exclude Negroes from the benefit of the general social and political organization of a great modern state is strong and growing both north and south, and is not only a hindrance to Negro Americans but a serious menace to American democracy."[29] The "problem," he had long believed, was that the white community did not seem to understand that the obstacles for blacks were human problems bound by poverty and ignorance, and were not defined solely by race: "There is in America today, no human problem of advance and uplift which does not in a more or less subtle way involve the Negro American and his condition." And as long as black Americans were "systematically degraded," he declared, such degradation would also affect "large numbers of [their] fellow white citizens."[30]

DuBois was even more relentless in his devotion to a federal amendment to enfranchise women, especially African American women. Early on, he recognized the potential benefit of black women's attaining the vote, particularly in Southern states. "Votes for women, means votes for Black women," he stated in 1912. Total political empowerment for blacks required the cooperative effort of black men and women. "Nothing human must be foreign, uninteresting or unimportant," he told his male readers, because "whatever concerns half mankind concerns us."[31] Therefore he urged black men to modify their Victorian political ideas about a woman's place, because blacks could ill afford to adhere to a white male ideal of a woman's sphere in a racially segregated, politically disfranchised society.

Scholar Deborah Gray White suggests that many men, threatened by women's push into the male domain, were reluctant to ally themselves with women. She argues that whereas women's status in the black community derived primarily from their club network, the political arena afforded black men their only public means of exercising real power. Men's organizations seldom did public domestic housekeeping, except in connection with women's efforts, because that duty was thought to be among women's natural abilities. For men to move into that arena meant redefining gender roles. So men secured their position in the community in the only public venue left solely to them precisely because women lacked the ballot.[32]

DuBois was sympathetic to male fears, such as those expressed in an Illinois black weekly:

> After all, when you take a close analytical view of [the] situation, you will find that the addition of women to the suffrage arena has not improved the "reformation" very preceptably [sic].
>
> It is true, that in some inconsequential localities the results from the women's vote have been improved, that is the "drys" have gained, and certain issues, supposed to be "reformatory" have carried which would not have carried had women not been voting. But by their influence and logical reasoning, the government was intended to be run by the men, assisted by the "ladies." We challenge any one to prove that granting to women the franchise has made any permanent reforms. The tendency to the world is to reformation.[33]

He assured his male audience that politically active black women would not seriously encroach upon the separate sphere ideology; instead, their work would further the betterment of the entire race. "The enfranchisement of these women will not be a mere doubling of our vote and voice in the nation" but would represent "stronger and more normal political life, the rapid dethronement of the 'heeler' and 'grafter' and the making of politics a method of broadest philanthropic race betterment, rather than a disreputable means of private gain."[34]

In 1915, DuBois presented "A Symposium of Leading Thinkers of Colored America" to his readers, both to placate male egos and to substantiate his view that political activism and racial progress were linked. He introduced the ideas of some of the most distinguished women in the country. The guests included Mary B. Talbert, vice president-at-large of the NACW, Nannie H. Burroughs, secretary of the Woman's Auxiliary to the National Baptist Convention, Josephine St. Pierre Ruffin, Mary Church Terrell, and Illinoisan Dr. Mary F. Waring. Each

appealed to the common sense of enlightened, racially conscious African American men by suggesting that the notion of
separate spheres had no place in the African American community. The shared experience of racism proved that the concept was antithetical to race progress.

For Talbert, the issue was the dual discrimination of racism
and sexism. She wrote:

> It should not be necessary to struggle forever against popular
> prejudice, and with us as colored women, this struggle becomes
> two-fold, first, because we are women and second, because we
> are colored women. Although some resistance is experienced in
> portions of our country against the ballot for women, because
> colored women will be included, I firmly believe that enlight-
> ened men, are now numerous enough everywhere to encourage
> this just privilege of the ballot for women, ignoring prejudice of
> all kinds.[35]

Burroughs suggested that the ballot offered African American women a weapon against sexual assault. Stigmatized as immoral and promiscuous, black women often found little justice
against their attackers in the courts. For Burroughs, the franchise would "bring to her the respect and protection that she
needs," because it would be "her weapon of moral defense."[36]

Terrell also invited African American men to consider the
absurdity of opposing female suffrage. "Precisely the same arguments used to prove that the ballot be withheld from women
are advanced to prove that colored men should not be allowed
to vote. The reasons for repealing the Fifteenth Amendment
differ but little from the argument advanced by those who oppose the enfranchisement of women." She concluded, "Nothing could be more inconsistent than that colored people should
use their influence against granting the ballot to women, if they
believe that colored men should enjoy this right which citizenship confers."[37]

Waring argued that the ability to make sound decisions
should be the only requirements for enfranchisement. "The
ability to weigh the merits of the persons to fill office and the

value of ordinances which govern the people, requires a knowledge of men and affairs. A trained mind, no matter in what profession, is more capable of making logical deductions; therefore the people naturally turn for information to the enlightened. The question of sex is of no importance," she wrote.[38] "The work of the professional woman just as that of the professional man places her in a position to help the many with whom she necessarily comes in contact, and therefore her influence is a power to be reckoned with." "Trained judgement," she continued, "is needed every where and it should always be armed with the ballot."[39] For Waring, education, economic standing, and expertise in assisting others, not sex, were the factors that should determine voting competency.

By suggesting that the needs of black women were essential to the welfare of the race, the women assured black men that they were not seeking to usurp men's power in politics. None of the women proposed the formation of a party of black women for the purpose of developing African American female politicians. They made it clear that black women posed no threat to the inside players in the political realm—men. Instead, they proposed the promotion of female political activists, whose goal it would be to curb the negative effects of racism and sexism on the African American community as a whole.

But to gain suffrage, African American women had to cross race lines and join forces with white women, who also were fighting for enfranchisement. Well aware of this double-edged sword, DuBois highlighted the hazards of racial alliances for his national audience. On the basis of the history of the white female suffrage movement, he questioned the political motives of many white suffragists, because, he maintained, they espoused the same racist views as white men. In an effort to gain the approval of the white male electorate, white female suffragists not only challenged the validity of granting the ballot to blacks but also questioned the franchise for the poor. He warned that white female suffragists "have continually been in great danger of asking the ballot not because they are citizens, but because they occupy a certain social position, are of a certain grade of intelligence, or are 'white.'" These factors often resulted in discrimination and continued ostracism of African American women in their club activities and rhetoric.[40]

African American female suffrage advocates had long known what DuBois printed for his audience. The historical evidence showed clearly that the "race question" had created barriers between black and white suffragists and plagued the movement until the passage of the Nineteenth Amendment. Indeed, in her pioneering studies, historian Rosalyn Terborg-Penn asserts that for black women, "discrimination . . . was the rule rather than the exception within the women's rights movement."[41] The women who gathered at Seneca Falls in 1848 launched the national woman suffrage movement and adopted two primary goals: suffrage for all women and the abolition of slavery. These goals, however, changed soon after slavery ended. In 1869, with the passage of the Fifteenth Amendment, which granted suffrage to black men, white feminists became disillusioned. Black men won the right to vote, but white women did not. The black vote and women's suffrage became two separate issues.

Internal disagreement over the issue gave rise to two groups, the National Woman Suffrage Association (NWSA) and the American Woman Suffrage Association (AWSA). NWSA, led by Elizabeth Cady Stanton and Susan B. Anthony, believed that suffrage for women, specifically white women, took priority over the disfranchisement of black men. AWSA, led by Lucy Stone and her husband, Henry Blackwell, promoted universal suffrage.

In 1890 the two groups merged, becoming the National American Woman Suffrage Association (NAWSA), and new strategies were adopted. The new suffrage argument, which appeared at the beginning of the Progressive Era, ceased to advocate suffrage as a reform and a right for women, but instead advocated it as a means to reform and as an expression of the duty of women. Stressing the differences between men and women rather than the similarities, the rhetoric emphasized women's special skills as nurturers and caretakers. Moreover, white suffragists divorced themselves from issues concerning blacks, adopting racist and nationalist arguments in an effort to dissociate the suffrage movement from the mid-nineteenth-century abolitionist movement. The new policy actively courted white Southern women and embraced the states' rights stance taken by most Southerners. In effect, this action by NAWSA repudiated the political freedoms of minority males and advocated the withholding of suffrage from minority women.[42]

By 1893, NAWSA was openly and actively pursuing a policy of white supremacy by calling for the disfranchisement of black and immigrant male voters through an educational qualification. At the annual convention, the association passed a resolution:

> Resolved, that without expressing any opinion on the proper qualifications for voting, we call attention to the significant facts that in every State there are more women who can read and write than all negro voters; more white women who can read and write than all negro voters; more American women who can read and write than all foreign voters; so that the enfranchisement of such women would settle the vexed question of rule by illiteracy, whether of home-grown or foreign born production.[43]

The adoption of this resolution suggests that the common bond of being middle-class, native-born, white Anglo-Saxon Protestants superseded citizenship rights and shifted the argument from what the vote could do for women to what white women could do with the vote. This new argument became known as expediency.[44]

By the second decade of the twentieth century, it was becoming increasingly clear that NAWSA would not change its policy. As the opportunities for suffrage extended beyond the Western states, African American women remained vigilant in scrutinizing the activities of white women. White women continued to sidestep the race issue in order to placate their Southern white colleagues. During the presidential reign of Anna Shaw from 1910 to 1915, NAWSA consistently defended its policy and suggested that if African American women "do not belong to us," then "it is merely because they have not organized and have not made application for membership."

NAWSA's platform, Shaw argued, was to seek avenues for attaining "justice to women, white and colored." Despite the challenges of African American women, she refused to admit that the association's states' rights policy was an endorsement of Jim Crow, though she did concede that state branches retained the right to reject black membership. "I do not feel that we should go into a Southern state to hold our national convention and then introduce any subject which we know beforehand will do nothing but create discord and inharmony in the convention." These strong-arm tactics, she concluded, "would do more to harm the success of our convention . . . than all the other things that we do good."[45]

The centralized bureaucracy of the national organization also ensured a unity of purpose among the many local suffrage branches. State affiliates were often forced to adhere to the national association's racist policy. Although Midwestern and Northern suffragists often admitted black females into their clubs and did not publicly endorse a policy of white supremacy, they nevertheless, perhaps by default, embraced white Southern supporters and never publicly denounced white supremacy. In other words, state organizations sidestepped the issue primarily because they did not want to lose their ties with the national organization. Most white suffragists believed that ratification of a federal amendment was possible only through organized regional efforts. Alienating the large Southern constituency would surely doom the passage of a federal amendment that needed ratification by thirty-six states.

Because the major suffrage clubs in Illinois did include black women in their membership, there was little debate about the role of race in the state or the national movements. After the passage of the 1913 Illinois suffrage bill, the two most prominent white suffrage leaders and their organizations channeled most of their energies into getting legislators to endorse the Nineteenth Amendment while ignoring the brewing debate over the inclusion of African American women in the national suffrage association. The chair of the Suffrage Amendment Alliance, Catharine W. McCulloch, for example, indicated in a letter to Senator Lawrence Y. Sherman in 1916, "You may be interested to know that in Illinois we are pushing for the submission of an Illinois Suffrage Amendment so that we may no longer present to the world the absurd picture of being able to vote for May-or and Alderman but not for Constable."[46] Grace Wilbur Trout of the Illinois Equal Suffrage Association encouraged the senator to help make Illinois "the first state to ratify the Federal Suffrage Amendment."[47] Silence on the race question, however, did not eliminate the controversy. Tacit acceptance of the states' rights policy reinforced NAWSA's platform and increased the likelihood of racial conflict at nationally sponsored functions when black female suffragists demanded the same treatment as their white counterparts.

The ideological split between the roles of the state and national suffrage organizations highlighted both implied and overt attempts to bifurcate gender and race. The unwillingness of the state and national community of white suffragists to coordinate a comprehensive plan that would include black women's concerns reflected their belief that black women were no more than marginal to their cause. Caught between the bureaucracy of state and national white suffragists, African American female activists viewed the hypocrisy in NAWSA's fight for "woman" suffrage as DuBois did—as "not only a hindrance to Negro Americans but a serious menace to American democracy," because the expediency argument revealed that "the Negro problem is the door which bars progress in the United States and which makes us liars and hypocrites."[48] Like DuBois, race women believed that "every argument for Negro suffrage is an argument for woman's suffrage; every argument for woman suffrage is an argument for Negro suffrage."[49] For those reasons, race women became active political agents.

FIVE

"I Am Doing It for the Future Benefit of My Whole Race"
AGENTS OF POLITICAL INCLUSION

Social agency coupled with political astuteness brought Illinois club women their greatest successes. As black women became increasingly aware of political issues, they joined and created organizations devoted to enhancing their political power. Heartened by the passage of the Woman's Suffrage Act in 1891, various other legislation that expanded women's opportunities in electing members on school boards and university trustees, and the Presidential and Municipal Suffrage Bill in 1913, black women both joined their white female colleagues on the front lines of the suffrage battle and sought alternative ways to expand opportunities for their race.

Ida B. Wells-Barnett, for example, traveled the state delivering political speeches for the Women's State Central Committee.[1] Surprised at the fact that, during her many trips, "in only a few instances did I see any of my own people," she posited that "if the white women were backward in political matters, our own women were even more so." A lack of the skills needed to understand the political process, she reasoned, hindered African American women from full participation in civic affairs.[2] Wells-Barnett strongly supported the notion of a correlation between lynching and disfranchisement. In her essay

"How Enfranchisement Stops Lynching," she argued that because the majority of blacks were without the ballot, they could
do little to white supremacists who committed violent attacks.
Political empowerment would help lead to the election of representatives sensitive to African American issues and to the passage of anti-lynching legislation.[3]

Fannie Barrier Williams held membership in and served as
secretary and vice president of the Illinois Woman's Alliance,
an interracial state umbrella association consisting of suffrage,
social, temperance, and labor organizations.[4] Excited at the
prospect that women might be granted unrestricted suffrage,
she made this enthusiastic prediction in November 1894:

> American women are beginning to see the end of their years
> of struggle for equality of suffrage. The arguments are nearly all
> in and the signs of favorable verdict are everywhere apparent to
> those who understand the trend of things.
>
> Fragmentary suffrage, now possessed by women in nearly
> all the states of the union, carries with it the triumph of the prin-
> cip[le] contended for, and [whether] its extension to complete
> enfranchisement of women will be realized depends largely upon
> the use we make of our present gains. The false reasoning of the
> opposition having been overcome, we have now to fight only the
> prejudices in opposition. When the opposing man sees women
> actually voting, and looks in vain for the evils predicted, his preju-
> dices will yield and he will gladly join the forces that are fast
> making for their complete emancipation.[5]

Williams's projection was incorrect, of course. It would take
almost twenty-six years for women to obtain suffrage by federal mandate, so the "fragmentary suffrage" conceded by state
governments to appease female suffragists would continue to
be the only way for the majority of women to gain any measure
of political empowerment.

Williams believed that full suffrage would be the turning
point for African American female reformers in their quest for
racial uplift. Complete enfranchisement would further their
moral mission by providing them with the means to repair the

damage caused by black men who had failed in their duty to the race. "Must we begin our political duties with no better or higher conceptions of our citizenship than that shown by our men when they were first enfranchised? Are we to bring any refinement of individuality to the ballot box? Shall we learn our politics from spoilsmen and bigoted partisans, or shall we learn it from the school of patriotism and an enlightened self-interest?" she asked. Suggesting that black men were pledging their allegiance to parties over the race, she warned black women that "if our enfranchisement means only a few more votes added to the republican and democratic sides, respectively, of political issues, there certainly has been no gain for the cause of principle in American politics." Enfranchisement, she concluded, was the opportunity for black women to become "corrective forces" in the political arena. If they chose instead to follow the same path as men, "there will be much disappointment among those who believed that the cause of temperance, municipal reform and better education would be more surely advanced when the finer virtues of women became a part of the political forces of the country."[6]

Other women, under the auspices of the IFCWC, began to actively lobby the governor and members of the legislature. Concerned over the "alarming increase" in discrimination, the IFCWC voted at its 1913 convention to send letters to each member of the Illinois House and Senate demanding some redress. Two years later, the federation appointed a committee to appeal to the state legislature to appropriate monies "to build suitable housing" for the state's growing number of young female wards. By 1916, like many progressive women across the nation, the IFCWC members were pressing hard for the endorsement of Prohibition. In 1919, the club turned its attention to the economic plight of blacks by seeking to increase employment opportunities for African Americans. It created a committee "to urge the appointment of a Colored Home Visitor in the department of State Welfare." Delegates were exhorted to educate themselves and their club members on political issues and, of course, to register to vote.[7]

The IFCWC also enlarged both its political and its social sphere by establishing a coalition of women in the Midwest. At the state meeting held in Moline in 1914, the federation adopted the following resolution:

> Whereas, the women of the Western Country are becoming to be recognized as a power because of their political franchise, and the old adage "In Union There Is Strength" has been found to be true in what ever line it has been tried, and since that Constitutional privilege has been granted to the women of Illinois and other states hereinafter named, it is highly necessary that the women of the Northwest join themselves together in a compact body, the better to work, to promote religious, social and civic conditions and to make a stronger protest against unwise legislation.[8]

A committee composed of Joanna Snowden Porter, Melissa Elam, Jessie Johnson, Eva Monroe, Carrie Lee Hamilton, Elizabeth Lindsay Davis, and Infelice B. Thompson was appointed to determine the feasibility of such an alliance. The following year, at St. Marks ME Church, the Northwestern Federation held its first meeting. Women from Indiana, Illinois, Iowa, Kansas, Kentucky, Michigan, Minnesota, Missouri, Ohio, Wisconsin, and Wyoming convened. Some of the most notable attendants were Hallie Q. Brown from Ohio, former dean of women at Tuskegee Institute, president of the Ohio Federation of Colored Women's Clubs, and NACW president from 1920 to 1924, and Lucy Thurman, a Michigan resident and a former national superintendent of and spokesperson for the Women's Christian Temperance Union.[9]

This was not the first such regional federation—there already was a Northeastern Federation in existence. What was unique about the new Northwestern Federation was its geographical scope and the fact that the women openly acknowledged that the shared empowerment of the franchise distinguished them from any other group. The organization included eleven very large Midwestern states. Suffrage for women in Wyoming had come as early as 1890, while Kansas and Illinois women gained the right to vote in 1912 and 1913, respectively. Between 1918 and 1920, with the exception of Iowa, the remaining states followed suit. Each state, because of industrial growth, attracted large numbers of African American migrants, and along with them came the typical problems caused by overcrowding and poverty. The consolidation of Midwestern women's efforts enlarged their sphere of influence by combining their resources and enhancing their ability to ensure better social, economic, and political opportunities for the race.

One approach taken by the women to the problems plaguing the black community involved bringing politicians and corporate executives around to a position of sympathy to the needs of African Americans. Club women on the local level employed moral suasion and grassroots direct action to this end. The club women's primary duty, Elizabeth Lindsay Davis argued, was to focus the attention of corporate heads and philanthropists on "the serious consequences of present day industrial and social unrest, the crime, disease, and poverty emanating from bad housing and unwholesome environment," and to "train their hands to give systematically to the cause of human betterment."[10] The affiliates of the IFCWC joined the national club women's movement (NACW) and set up departments to monitor companies that discriminated against black men and women. As purchasers of many products and services, they found that a boycott was one of the most effective means of conveying their dissatisfaction with company policies.[11]

The IFCWC also became a formidable lobbying organization on behalf of African American women. Its effectiveness in this regard was most clearly evidenced during the planning stages of the historic Illinois National Half-Century Exposition commemorating fifty years of freedom for African Americans. In mid-summer 1913, Illinoisans began preparations for celebrating the progress of African Americans since the end of slavery. On July 1, Governor Edward F. Dunne appointed a nine-member commission to govern and organize the exposition. The state legislature appropriated twenty-five thousand dollars for the venture. The month-long event, to be held in

Chicago, was scheduled to begin on August 1, 1915. Its mission was "not to emphasize differences, and to formulate platforms," but "to come together in a spirit of human brotherhood and to work for those things about which there exists no difference of opinion."[12] The experiment in racial cooperation was endorsed by President Woodrow Wilson and two former presidents, Theodore Roosevelt and William Howard Taft. There were honorary vice presidents from all over the country. The governors of Arizona, Colorado, Iowa, Kansas, Kentucky, Louisiana, Michigan, Minnesota, Ohio, Oklahoma, Oregon, Pennsylvania, New Mexico, Texas, West Virginia, Wisconsin, and Wyoming appointed delegates to attend the exposition. The Advisory Council included representatives from as far away as Rhodesia and Liberia, Africa.[13]

Because the exposition was devoted to the progress of the race, African American women secured influential positions in the departments that addressed their concerns. Black women were appointed to administrative positions in four of the twelve units. Mary F. Waring served as vice chair of the Department of Education. Eva T. Jenifer was appointed vice chair of the Department of Industry, with Elizabeth Lindsay Davis serving as her first assistant. The Miscellaneous Department was headed by Sarah F. Sheppard. Theresa G. Macon took the helm of the Department of Social Progress, while Fannie Barrier Williams served in the Bureau of Literature under Macon's direction.[14] The movement of black women into positions of influence and power in the exposition shows quite clearly how they combined their efforts in the cause of mobilizing and gaining assignments for their allies. They thereby had major input into the implementation of policies, procedures, and programs and how those would be delivered to the masses.

But club women did not secure a position on the highest administrative board, the commission appointed by the governor. His recommendations included four white men—the Reverend Samuel Fallows as president, plus John Daley, W. Duff Piercy, and Medill McCormick; one white woman—Susan Lawrence Joergen-Dahl; and four African American men—A. J.

Carey, George W. Ford, R. R. Jackson, and Thomas Wallace Swann.[15] As with the board appointments at the World's Columbian Exposition twenty-three years earlier, African American women had been ignored. Joergen-Dahl, like Mary Cantrill on the earlier fair's Board of Lady Managers, was chosen to represent the interests of all women, including black women.

Joergen-Dahl's appointment caused some controversy, although she appeased some African American club women. Because of her family's long, cordial history with African Americans in the state's capital, Springfield, that city's club women warmly embraced her. Joergen-Dahl's relationship with blacks was primarily a legacy of her parents' political and philanthropic aid. Her father, Rheuna Lawrence, was a Republican who won the mayoral seat in 1891. He developed close political ties with blacks as they in turn supported his political aspirations.[16] Joergen-Dahl's mother, Mary Lawrence, held the deed to the Lincoln Colored Home. The creation of the Mary A. Lawrence Industrial School for Girls by Eva Monroe and of the Mary A. Lawrence Woman's Club in 1915 by a group of African American club women attested to the strong ties that the family continued to have with the home and with black women in the city.[17] As the only child, Susan inherited her parents' holdings and their ties to the African American community upon their deaths. She continued to contribute to the home throughout the next several decades, and in May 1913 she sang at the Lincoln Colored Home's own celebration of the fiftieth anniversary of black freedom.[18] When her husband died that year, she held a segregated service for African Americans at her home. Approximately three hundred blacks attended.[19]

Because of Joergen-Dahl's warm reception by the Springfield club women, her appointment was endorsed by the IFCWC.[20] But those who had no ties to the Springfield community found the recommendation disconcerting. Ida B. Wells-Barnett was so outraged that she altered an address that she was to give on the morning that the names appeared in the newspaper. "Instead of giving my scheduled address," she wrote, "I lectured about the appointment of that commission and how

Negro women, who were the only organized force in the state for civic work, had been ignored." Her impassioned speech, she claimed, aroused many of the women and compelled them to write to the governor demanding that a black woman be appointed to the committee.[21]

Whether or not Wells-Barnett overstated her role in the matter, black club women jumped at the opportunity to appoint one of their own when Joergen-Dahl resigned. Succumbing to an exhaustive schedule of traveling to Chicago, Peoria, and New York for the exposition, and fatigue caused by a relapse from a severe cold she had contracted earlier, she, upon the advice of her physician, removed herself from the commission. The IFCWC quickly mustered its forces and recommended that Dr. Mary F. Waring take Joergen-Dahl's place. The governor accepted the recommendation, and Waring took her seat in early 1915.[22]

Waring, a Chicago resident, was one of the IFCWC's best representatives. A longtime member of the IFCWC, she had been elected to serve as chair of the executive board, corresponding secretary, treasurer, and statistician. A graduate of Louisville National Medical College and Chicago Medical School, she held a teaching post at the Wendell Phillips School, chaired the Health and Hygiene Committee of the NACW, and served as the administrator of the Dunbar Sanatorium. An active club woman, she founded and presided over the Necessity Club, which operated a day nursery in Chicago, and was elected president of the Woman's Second Ward Suffrage League.[23]

Political activism among African American women intensified after a shift in the balance of political power to the Progressives in the state legislature resulted in a successful outcome for those in the state's Equal Suffrage Association. On May 7, 1913, the Illinois Senate passed the Presidential and Municipal Suffrage Bill by a vote of twenty-nine to fifteen. On June 11, the House, by a vote of eighty-three to fifty-eight, approved the measure. Before the month ended, the legislature had ratified the bill, which granted partial suffrage to female citizens twenty-one years of age or older. Illinois became the first state east of the Mississippi River to enfranchise its female populace.[24]

The suffrage bill was limited in scope and pushed women voters toward municipal affairs. Women could not vote for the highest elected state officials, such as governor and lieutenant governor, or for any members of the legislature; nor could they vote for those in top judicial positions, such as county or district judges. But what seemed restrictive on the surface ultimately became the catalyst in transforming the nature of city politics. Specifically, the bill allowed women to vote in all elections governed by the state constitution, including those for presidential electors, mayors, aldermen, municipal court judges, sanitary trustees, and most local officers.[25] Having a smaller pool of candidates from which to choose gave women the opportunity to pool their resources and become intimately familiar with individuals and their platforms. Locked out at the state level, they became actively involved in local elections, and with their knowledge and interest, they could be either powerful allies or formidable foes. The number of voters doubled in many areas, forcing politicians to alter their platforms and cater to the needs of their new electors. For the first time, women had a direct voice in the governance of their own wards and neighborhoods.

Club women seized the opportunity to promote their causes. In Peoria, the Woman's Aid Club, under the leadership of Elizabeth Lindsay Davis, investigated jails and juvenile courts and joined with other groups in demanding the establishment of the Peoria County Detention Home. The Frederick Douglass Center Woman's Club of Chicago held meetings twice a month to discuss political and social equality issues. The Elizabeth Lindsay Charity Club, also in Chicago, provided information on legal counsel.[26] Near the end of the decade, women in Springfield began strongly pushing for a gender-integrated law enforcement staff. In a letter sent to the sheriff, they requested that a woman fill the post of deputy.[27]

Black women in Springfield also allied themselves politically with men who were endorsing a second power generator for the city to lower the cost of electricity in black homes. The reserve generator, a *Forum* editorial suggested, would appeal to the industrialized woman because it would provide not only lighting but also electricity for irons, toasters, and washing machines.[28]

Individuals became much more politically sensitized, and increased their activities as well. Sadie Lewis Adams, for example, served on the election board, attended the National Equal Rights League and the Illinois Equal Suffrage League conferences, and held offices in the Alpha Suffrage Club.[29] Ella G. Berry became a state organizer of African American women for the National Republican Party.[30]

But it was in Chicago where women's grassroots political progress was most evident. In many ways the club women awakened the black community to its ability to determine how best to advance the race. Black women's entrance into municipal politics simultaneously boosted both gender and racial consciousness. The development of suffrage clubs heightened awareness and sensitized the community to race and gender issues, permanently changing the political climate. To a large degree, club women came to symbolize the black community's political liberation from white ward bosses.

The suffrage legislation resulted in a doubling of the African American vote. For the first time, black men and women shared the same space in municipal affairs, contributing to the creation of a political agenda that was racially based and gender-inclusive, and that encouraged racial responsibility. There were 17,845 African American males of voting age out of a citywide male constituency of 700,590 in 1910. Whereas only 2.5 percent of black males were eligible to vote in 1910, that number jumped to nearly 5 percent, or 42,837, by 1920. Black women twenty-one and older totaled 39,035 by 1920, or 4.7 percent of the female constituency.[31] The notion of a black political force became a real possibility, as these high numbers of African American women and men could wield considerable power if they voted as a bloc. Congregated in densely populated segregated wards, enfranchised black women would be able to dynamically converge with an astute and racially conscious black male voting populace to pursue a self-directed political agenda.

Club women in Chicago established the most and the largest gender-segregated suffrage clubs in the nation. The Alpha Suffrage Club, the Aloha Political Club, the Colored Woman's Party of Cook County, the Mary Walker Thompson Political Club, the 3rd Ward Political Club, and the Woman's 25th Precinct Political Club were a few of the organizations that resulted from women's interest in politics. Little is known about most of these clubs. Some acted primarily as the female counterparts to Republican male political associations.[32] Others, such as the Aloha Political Club, the Colored Woman's Party, and the Alpha Suffrage Club, were autonomous organizations concerned chiefly with educating black women in civic affairs and advancing women's opportunities in municipal reform.

Led by Josephine Crawford, the Aloha Political Club was organized sometime before the 1914 aldermanic primary. Members participated in suffrage parades and worked toward electing an African American to the city council.[33] The Colored Woman's Party in Chicago's Thirtieth Ward, also established in June 1914, was a non-partisan organization whose members pledged "to vote for the best men at all elections regardless of their politics." It boasted a membership of nearly one hundred politically active women. The first slate of officers included Blanch M. Gilmer, president; Katherine Johnson, first vice president; Carrie Warner, second vice president; Charlotte Ross, treasurer; Maud Johnson, recording secretary; Susan A. Woodland, corresponding secretary; Mary Perryman, financial secretary; and Laura Smith, chaplain.[34]

One of the most important African American suffrage clubs in the state was the first one, the Alpha Suffrage Club (ASC), which was established in January 1913 by Wells-Barnett and a white colleague, Belle Squire, a member of the No Vote No Tax League.[35] The alliance between the two women was symbolic of the cooperation between black and white state suffragists. At the organizational meeting, Squire encouraged this cooperation by declaring, "The time has come when we suffragists must broaden our views and enlist all women to our cause, re-gardless of race or color, if we are to be successful." For that reason, she added, "We want every colored woman in Chicago to become a suffragist. We need them and they need us."[36]

From the beginning, Wells-Barnett assumed leadership of the organization. She made sure that it remained controlled by blacks, and that they made all the decisions. All of the elected officers were black, and the meeting place was located in the heart of one of the largest black communities in the city, the Second Ward. The first officers included Ida B. Wells-Barnett, president; Mary Jackson, vice president; Viola Hill, second vice president; Vera Wesley Green, recording secretary; Sadie Lewis Adams, corresponding secretary; Laura Beasley, treasurer; and K. J. Bills, editor. Three years later, Wells-Barnett and Beasley remained in their posts as president and treasurer, while Adams had replaced Jackson as vice president. Other officers included F. D. Wyatt, secretary; J. E. Hughes, assistant secretary; and W. N. Mills, corresponding secretary.[37]

The forums at ASC meetings provided honored guests and political candidates with an engaging audience. Jane Addams of Hull House, a longtime advocate of female suffrage; Elizabeth Lindsay Davis, former president of the IFCWC; and George C. Hall, chief of staff at Provident Hospital, were among the many who interacted with individual members. The political candidates who visited the forums discussed their platforms and sought votes. The exchange proved beneficial to both groups.[38] The women learned canvassing techniques, met candidates seeking office, and developed analytical skills. In turn, the can-didates gained insight into the issues important to women. The popularity of the club was so great that less than three years after its establishment, it claimed a membership of nearly two hundred women.

One of the first official acts of the ASC was to send Wells-Barnett to the nationally sponsored suffrage parade in the nation's capital on March 3, 1913. Unfortunately, it proved to be one of the most divisive public occasions in the suffrage movement's history. As a black woman, Wells-Barnett was forced to challenge the Jim Crow policy of both the national and the state suffrage organizations, and her white colleagues learned the painful lesson that they had little control over the institutional policies of the national suffrage organization. In a show of solidarity, black and white women joined in the parade down Pennsylvania Avenue in Washington, D.C. Representing almost every state in the union, the marchers highlighted the demand for female enfranchisement. Interestingly, in this demonstration of gender unity, African American women were relegated to the back of the line, regardless of state residency. This instance of discrimination exemplified the contradiction between the ideal of gender equality and the reality of racism within the suffrage movement.

Like many African American women nationwide, Wells-Barnett had long been an advocate of female suffrage. And like so many others, she expressed an enthusiastic interest in the parade. As the founder of the first African American female suffrage organization in Illinois, she traveled to Washington to join with other women from her state. To her surprise, however, as the sixty-five delegates from Illinois prepared for the march along Pennsylvania Avenue, Grace Wilbur Trout, president of the Illinois Equal Suffrage Association and chairperson of the Illinois delegation, informed the group that "many of the eastern and southern women have greatly resented the fact that there are to be colored women in the delegations." Because of their concern, she stated, "Mrs. Stone of the National Suffrage Association and the woman in charge of the entire parade has advised us to keep our delegation entirely white. So far as Illinois is concerned, we should like to have Mrs. Barnett march in the delegation, but if the national association has decided it is unwise to include the colored women, I think we should abide by its decision."[39]

Dismayed by the stance Trout had taken, Virginia Brooks, a colleague from West Hammond and a friend of Wells-Barnett, pleaded for a reconsideration. "We have come down here to march for equal rights," she declared. "It would be autocratic to exclude men or women of any color." She continued, "I think that we should allow Mrs. Barnett to walk in our delegation. If the women of other states lack moral courage, we should show them that we are not afraid of public opinion. We should stand by our principles. If we do not the parade will be a farce."[40]

While the delegates pondered Brooks's recommendation, Wells-Barnett, her cheeks stained with tears and her voice quavering, told the group, "The southern women have tried to evade the question time and again by giving some excuse or other every time it has been brought up. If the Illinois women do not take a stand now in this great democratic parade then the colored women are lost."[41] After listening to Wells-Barnett and objections from Brooks, Trout reconsidered her position. "It is time for Illinois to recognize the colored woman as a political equal and you shall march with the delegation," she told Wells-Barnett.[42]

Trout's words were bittersweet. One of the delegates immediately pulled her aside and explained that she could not make such a promise without consulting with the NAWSA leadership first.[43] While Trout went to confer with the officials, the other delegates discussed the situation. Though some were sympathetic to Wells-Barnett, they were unwilling to challenge the national segregationist policy. One delegate told the group that although "it will be undemocratic if we do not let Mrs. Barnett march with us," obedience and expediency ranked higher than democratic principles. "We should not go against the law of the national association," she declared, because "we are only a small part in the great line of march, and we must not cause any confusion by disobeying orders."[44] When Trout returned, it was to renege on her earlier promise. "I am afraid," she told Wells-Barnett, "that we shall not be able to have you march with us." "Personally," she continued, "I should like nothing more than to have you represent our Illinois suffrage organization. But I feel that we are responsible to the national association and cannot do as we choose. After talking again with Mrs. Stone, I shall have to ask you to march with the colored delegation. I am sorry, but I feel that it is the right thing to do."[45]

Angry and deeply disappointed in her colleagues, with

whom she had worked so closely on the suffrage issue, Wells-Barnett told Trout and the other delegates, "I shall not march at all unless I can march under the Illinois banner. . . . When I was asked to come down here I was asked to march with the other women of our state, and I intend to do so or not take part in the parade at all." In response, one member of the group retorted, "If I were a colored woman, I should be willing to march with the other women of my race." Wells-Barnett replied, "There is a difference, . . . which you probably do not see. . . . I shall not march with the colored women. Either I go with you or not at all. I am not taking this stand because I personally wish for recognition. I am doing it for the future benefit of my whole race."[46]

When Wells-Barnett later disappeared from the parade site, her colleagues assumed that she had admitted defeat and decided not to march at all. But as the delegates began moving down Pennsylvania Avenue, she quietly stepped out from the crowd of spectators and joined them. So important was the event that a photograph of her, flanked by two white Illinois women, Belle Squire and Virginia Brooks, appeared in the *Chicago Daily Tribune*, giving the event and its participants local and national exposure.[47] As the marchers proceeded, none of the Southerners defected, perhaps in part because they were not aware of the event until after the paraded had ended. At any rate, the press coverage underscored the tenuous place that black women nationwide held in the suffrage movement, and it probably convinced many whites, despite NAWSA's insistence, that "the Negro question" and female suffrage were not separate issues.

Wells-Barnett's ordeal was a clear indication of discriminatory policy. It was the fear of antagonizing Southern white women, whose support was worth more to NAWSA's cause than the support of African American women, that prompted Wells-Barnett's Illinois colleagues to deny her participation. Viewing black women as a threat to white supremacy, white women in the South rejected the legitimacy of black female state delegates' marching with white state delegates. As historian Steven Buechler argues, Southern white women required absolute control of black women's visibility within the movement in exchange for their own participation. In an attempt to convince state legislatures that African American suffrage and women suffrage were unconnected, they devised a strategy to "maximize white women's votes, minimize black women's votes, and leave restrictions on black male voters intact."[48] Wells-Barnett's inclusion in the state delegation to the parade threatened to impede that tactic by lifting the veil of Jim Crow and opening the door to other African American women. NAWSA's acquiescence to Southern white women and the submission of the white Illinois delegates clearly proved that the racist agenda was expedient.

It also demonstrated the benefits that white state suffragists were reaping by following NAWSA's policy. They could discriminate against African American women on racial grounds while simultaneously embracing them along gender lines. They could enlist the aid of black women such as Wells-Barnett in their cause while denying them access to the national arena. Wells-Barnett had participated in the state movement for more than twenty years. In the late 1890s she had toured for the Women's State Central Committee, making political speeches. Although she was often the only African American present at these meetings, she enjoyed them. She received no salary for her commitment, and she had to nurse her six-month-old child during one of the trips.[49] For Wells-Barnett and the countless African American women like her, the complicity of state suffrage clubs in the racist policy adopted by NAWSA was a cruel blow.

Wells-Barnett was not afraid to confront the duplicity. In many ways, she defined the battle for African American women by raising questions concerning her right as a state citizen, an (African) American, and a woman to participate in the struggle for universal suffrage. As an Illinoisan, she held membership in integrated clubs and spoke on behalf of all women gaining the ballot. As an American, however, she failed to persuade suffragists on a national level to embrace her as an African American woman seeking the vote for all women. Despite the setback, Wells-Barnett did affirm black women's place in the fight for the ballot by marching despite her anger. She and her two white colleagues provided a better model of gender unity than NAWSA or the state delegates could offer.

Recognition of the valiant efforts of Wells-Barnett, Squire, and Brooks came from black club women. When the trio returned to Chicago, members of the ASC and the Progressive Club celebrated their triumphant return at Quinn Chapel on Monday evening, April 7, presenting the three to a crowd of spectators. For an admission fee of twenty-five cents, the audience heard speeches from the women, were entertained by a choir, received refreshments at a reception, and contributed to the reimbursement of expenses incurred by Wells-Barnett.[50]

The promotion of black female political activism in Chicago had other immediate effects as well. Like the Aloha Political Club, the ASC made no secret of the fact that its members, while non-partisan, supported the candidacy of an African American for the city council. Black male politicians who had long been disgruntled about their lack of power within the white-dominated Republican Party viewed the female vote as an opportunity to shed their confinement by both the party line and the party's patronizing posture. The first viable black candidate ran as an independent early in 1914, less than a year after the Presidential and Municipal Suffrage Bill was passed.

SIX

The Politics of Race

CHICAGO

In October 1914, Fannie Barrier Williams, a resident of Chicago's Second Ward, wrote in the *Southern Workman*,

> A new and important responsibility has come to Chicago women in the franchise. It is believed that this power granted to the women of the state of Illinois is going to lift colored women to new importance as citizens. They appreciate what it means and are eagerly preparing themselves to do their whole duty. They believe that they now have an effective weapon with which to combat prejudice and discrimination of all kinds.[1]

The franchise for African American women in the Second Ward indeed became "an effective weapon" in the divisive arena of patronage politics in Chicago, one that challenged the Republican Party's white leadership and enabled both women and black male Republicans to become aggressive participants in municipal politics.

They succeeded primarily because most of the African Americans in Illinois lived on the south side of Chicago, mainly in the Second Ward. In 1910, African Americans constituted 25 percent of the 42,801 residents of that ward, and by 1915 that proportion had risen to nearly 40 percent of the 63,342 residents.[2] This high concentration gave African American voters a large enough voting bloc that Republican Party leaders were forced to nominate blacks to key elective offices.

Several other factors contributed to their success. African American women who joined the racially based coalition canvassed the neighborhood seeking voters who would cast their ballots for "race man" candidates. The black press, particularly the *Chicago Defender*, aroused public interest in the possibility of black representation on the all-white city council and highlighted the participation of women in the election process. And the predominantly white Republican machine, adopting a pragmatic agenda, delivered on a promise to support an African American nominee for alderman.[3]

Despite the fact that African American male voters tended to be loyal Republicans, the Party of Lincoln had conceded few key political positions to them. Instead, white party bosses manipulated and monopolized the Second Ward, denying autonomy to the African Americans living there, downplaying concerns unique to the segregated black neighborhood and stifling the political voice of thousands.

As the black population in Chicago continued to increase, still concentrated in the Second Ward, black Republicans escalated their vocal protests about the party's failure to place African Americans in key areas that more directly affected the masses. They believed that accommodating to the interests of the Republican machine was depriving them of the opportunity to use politics as a vehicle for the public expression of grievances, particularly racial ones, and denying them any hope of representative government.

The discourse about black representation centered on the powerful post of alderman. Aldermen assisted in planning the city budget, granted franchises to businesses, appointed officials to municipal posts, and supervised administrative policies for the wards in the city. An African American alderman, then, could play an important role in achieving better social, political, and economic conditions for blacks in the city.[4] But white patriarchs had always held that position, governing the ward according to the dictates of the machine. Therefore, if blacks hoped to have any political clout, they had to enlarge their sphere of influence either within the party structure or outside to gain control of the aldermanic post.

A leading critic of the machine was Edward Wright. A lawyer, Wright was born in New York City in 1864 and settled in Chicago in the mid-1880s, at the age of twenty. Over the course of a decade, his loyalty earned him several positions. He was appointed to the State Central Committee, and by 1887 he held a post in the county clerk's office. The following year he became the first black bookkeeper and railroad incorporation clerk in the office of the secretary of state in Springfield, Illinois. He later moved back to Chicago, to the city clerk's Office. In 1894, Wright made an unsuccessful bid for the nomination of county commissioner. Two years later he ran again and was victorious, becoming only the third African American to fill the post.[5]

Wright and some other disgruntled colleagues spent much of the first decade of the twentieth century building a strong black coalition within the Republican ranks. Their primary goals were to force change from within and to develop their own monopoly over the predominantly black ward. In 1910, Wright stepped out of the shadows of the machine and declared himself a candidate for alderman. Securing the black vote and garnering support from sympathetic whites would be imperative to his success. Black males of voting age constituted only about 28 percent of the population of the ward, making it essential for him to receive some white votes or hope that the white vote would be split among the other candidates.[6] Although his chances for victory were slim, his supporters believed that he would be the first black alderman, and that his election to the city council was in the best interests of Chicago's black community within municipal government.[7]

Wright's detractors, however, worried that his bid would lead to the loss of the few favors granted to blacks by the Republican machine. Wedded to the party's patronage policy, they hesitated to ostracize themselves and refused to endorse

Wright's candidacy. Rather than expressing concern about blacks' dependence on the limited favors provided by the white ward boss, the opposition highlighted the long history of Republican assistance. For them, Wright's bid for this post would divide a fragile community already heavily stressed by poverty, crime, and overcrowding.

Wright's campaign had its early boosters as well. The black press chastised his detractors and non-voters alike, promoted the cause of male responsibility, and appealed to African American pride. A headline in one of the major black newspapers, the *Chicago Defender*, asked, "Do You Want a Colored Alderman?" To elect one, the paper contended, men who had never used their power at the ballot box would have to think about the consequences of their actions. The opportunity to elect a black alderman depended on their vote. Black men should go to the polls, not just to vote for Wright as an individual, but primarily "for the sake of the race of which you are a part, of which your fathers, mothers, sisters and children are members." The paper called upon black men to "arouse from your slumber and realize that on your shoulders rests a responsibility as a man . . . and help push the cause of the Negro forward by securing every position of advantage possible."[8]

The *Defender's* focus on advancing "the cause of the Negro" played to the race consciousness of African American men of voting age by linking the race man concept to civic duty. True citizens, the *Defender* made clear, must set aside all other considerations to "fight for the common cause, a Negro in the City Council." The paper instructed "good people of color, men of influence, apostles of civil rights and advocates of political liberty, [to] get together and get together quickly and nominate and elect a Negro alderman."[9] The message was clear: African Americans were not rejecting the party, but instead were opting for one of their own, a candidate who could voice their unique concerns.

But it was virtually impossible to win without the machine's support. Those who nominated and campaigned for Wright were well aware that unless he emerged as a dark horse candidate, he would not be able to beat the favored ward nominee, Wilson Shufelt. At best, they hoped for a respectable showing. Wright did not win. But neither did he finish in last place. The recorded vote was Wilson Shufelt, 3,619; John Montgomery, 2,376; Edward Wright, 1,583; and Edward Wentworth, 1,081. Wright's third-place showing was indeed a respectable achievement.[10] His candidacy attracted attention, was endorsed by the major black newspaper, and earned him a significant number of black votes despite his lack of recognition by the machine. He may not have won the election, but the votes he got revealed a discontent among the black masses. A vote for Wright was the clearest way they could voice their dissatisfaction.

An ambitious Wright ran again in the 1912 aldermanic primary. This time, however, some of the black politicians who had previously supported him backed away from his candidacy. Their marginal status within the party structure and their reluctance to alienate themselves from the machine, a powerful political ally, governed their decision. Without key black Republican support for Wright, his defeat was inevitable.[11]

Nevertheless, the 1910 and 1912 contests were successful in highlighting black dissatisfaction and making it an issue within the Republican ranks. The actions of black Republicans and the increased interest of black males in the electoral process emphasized the necessity for the machine to change its tactics if it was to maintain a monopoly over the predominantly African American ward.

The passage by the Illinois General Assembly of the state woman suffrage amendment in 1913 marked the entrance of black women onto the political battlefield.[12] Initial concerns among men about women's participation in civic affairs diminished as politicized women assured their male counterparts that their interests lay in bolstering, not usurping, men's role in the public domain of politics.

The struggle over the female vote began a year after the suffrage amendment was passed. When the Republican machine endorsed the candidacy of incumbent Hugh Norris in the February 1914 primary, it expected African American women as well as most men to cast their ballots for him.[13] Many black Republicans, however, saw the female vote as a means of electing a race man to the city council. They backed William Randolph Cowan, a prominent African American real estate businessman who was running as an independent, and pushed hard for women to join their crusade.

While many professional politicians hailed the new gender-integrated electorate, other ward men challenged women's incursion into their domain. As members of the Alpha Suffrage Club marshaled their forces and canvassed the black community to register women for the primary, some men "jeered at them and told them they ought to be at home taking care of the babies." Others accused them of "trying to take the place of men and wear the trousers."[14] The criticism had an impact on these Victorian club women. In public declarations, they reasserted their established roles and their view of the franchise as a way to extend their moral duty to the race. In an attempt to calm these men's fears about women's newly acquired role, Fannie Barrier Williams assured them that "there need be no anxiety as to the conduct of these newly made colored citizens. They have had a large and varied experience in organizations and we expect to see in them an exhibition of the best there is in the colored race."[15]

Ida B. Wells-Barnett made no such pronouncements. Instead, she insisted that those women who questioned the legitimacy of their place in the political arena must remain focused on the goal of electing a black man. Because of her loyalty to the "race man" concept, she refused to allow black women in the ASC to cave in to male pressure. She urged each of the workers to return to her neighborhood and continue registering women. Under Wells-Barnett's tutelage, most of the women stuck to their convictions, continued the registration efforts, and in the process realized the importance of their participation in politics. When forms were counted after the primary, some 7,290 female and 16,327 male voters had registered.[16] Wells-Barnett proudly proclaimed that as a result of the respectable showing by women, "our men politicians were surprised because not one of them, even our ministers, had said one word to influence women to take advantage of the suffrage opportunity Illinois had given to her daughters."[17]

Other African Americans, however, particularly women, fought gallantly for the election of the white candidate, Hugh Norris, arguing that remaining loyal to the white Republican machine was the most expedient means of achieving equality for the community.[18] Several days before the February primary, the Second Ward held a Republican rally for Norris. A prominent Chicago club woman, Marie Mitchell, presided. When Edward Wright disrupted the meeting and attempted to speak on behalf of William R. Cowan, Mitchell exercised her political clout, reportedly chastising Wright on the grounds that "if he could not be a gentleman in the presence of the ladies present; that they would vote against him if he ever ran for office; in this city or county."[19] The incident served to bolster Norris's campaign and established Mitchell as a major political leader in the black community. About two weeks after the meeting, Mitchell and several other club women created their own female Republican suffrage organization. As president, Mitchell led the women in resolving that

> WHEREAS In that through organization comes to all classes of Citizens that which they fail to secure through independence of action, and since the Second Ward organization has presented the name of Hon. Hugh Norris as being a fit person to succeed himself in the City Council,
> THEREFORE be it resolved that this Auxiliary club join hands with the main body, and cast our lot with theirs in the endorsement of Mr. Norris for the place he has so honestly . . . filled for the past two years, believing that he possess the sterling work, honesty of purpose, and all those qualities which warrant us in using all our influence in re-electing him to the City Council.[20]

Affirmation of the white Republican candidate did not suggest that Mitchell and her cohorts were any less "race women" than Wells-Barnett and her backers. On the contrary, they, like their counterparts, based their advocacy on what they believed was best for the race. The difference lay in the strategies of the two camps. Norris supporters feared that attempts to force the Republican Party to back a black candidate were tantamount to political suicide for the community. African Americans had attained a large measure of influence in the Republican Party because it was one of the few political parties that actively recruited black members, provided employment opportunities, solicited black women's input, and served the neighborhoods. Upsetting this powerful group might mean a reduction in or even the termination of the limited flow of resources. Ultimately, for this group, the concept of the "race man" went beyond traditional notions of color to include one who could clear a path for African Americans to derive benefits from an oppressive system. Pro-Norris constituents echoed the *Broad Ax*'s warning that Cowan backers did not "realize the fact that they are engaged in mighty bad and dangerous business in stirring up racial strife or ill feeling setting the Whites and the Blacks against each other in their effort to establish the 'color line' in the great city of Chicago."[21]

Invigorated by the events at the Republican rally, the *Broad Ax* editorials, and black women's efforts to re-elect Norris, the ASC and other proponents of a black alderman increased their efforts. Exhorting women to "put a colored man in the city council," ASC members stepped up their canvassing efforts and campaigned vigorously for Cowan. Other Cowan supporters mastered the election laws with literature provided by the Board of Election Commissioners, then formed committees to instruct other black women about race politics. They adopted the slogan "Race interest first, last and all the time." While polling potential black voters, many female solicitors discovered that many women knew about Cowan and were impressed that a race man was in the running. They concluded that "the candidate's name did not matter, so long as he was a Republican and an Afro-American."[22]

The *Chicago Defender* captured the sentiments of many women with its sensationalized headlines for February 21, 1914:

"Women to Show Loyalty by Casting First Ballot for Cowan for Alderman," "Second Ward Women Determine to Use Their Power to Better Themselves and Strengthen the Race," "Asserted Men Needed Their Assistance," and "Garbage Question, Children's Playgrounds, Ventilation in Public Places, Supervision of 'Movies' Important Matters to Them." The paper triumphantly predicted that black women would become "the balance of power" in the aldermanic campaign and would "see their first vote make race history in Chicago."[23]

On primary day, almost three thousand women cast ballots in the Second Ward. While William Cowan lost the election, to the disappointment of the Suffrage Club women, he amassed 45 percent of the votes—and many of those votes came from women. According to the *Defender*, this showed that black women understood better than their men the interconnection between duty and politics: "They were actuated by principle in politics just as they are in everything else. . . . The women's vote was a revelation to everyone, and after analysis shows them still actuated by the sense of duty to do more." Only through the women, the paper said, could the ward "be purified." Concluding that because of women, "traitorous leaders are to be relegated to the background and citizens of strength and character are to take their places," the *Defender* vigorously promoted both Victorian ideals and female participation in the electoral process.[24]

The female vote even compelled the *Broad Ax* to acknowledge that "Cowan and his followers woke things up . . . for he received 2700 votes[,] more than one thousand of that number being cast by the ladies." The vote "plainly brought to the front one thing and that is that within the next two or four years at the longest a high class popular solid Colored man of affairs can and will be elected to the city council from that ward." If only three hundred of the black votes for Norris had been transferred to Cowan, the paper concluded, "nothing could have prevented him from breaking into the city council."[25]

Impressed by women's strong crusade for Cowan, many black men began to adjust to the new sexual context of local politics. Black Republicans saw that female suffrage might provide them the leverage they needed to achieve the coveted prize of alderman. Loyalists to the race man concept adopted the women's strategies, welcomed women into their fold, and agitated the Republican ward machine. Second Ward political organizations began advertising their weekly meetings in local black newspapers, hoping to appeal to a larger audience. In all probability, these meetings were gender-integrated. The purposes of the gatherings were threefold: first, they provided an opportunity for black men and women to speak about issues of interest to blacks; second, "County Commissioners Night" and "Municipal Judges Night" allowed black women and men to listen to and question candidates; and finally, stronger appeals could be made to women to register and vote.[26]

The machine was troubled by the newly unified male-female political strength in the ward. At an ASC meeting a few days after Cowan's defeat, a black Republican, Oscar Stanton DePriest, joined the president of the ward organization, Samuel Ettelson, in an appeal for the women to campaign and vote for the machine candidate in the next election.[27] Women were urged not to support an independent candidate for alderman as they had in the Cowan primary, because doing so might split the black vote and lead to a win for the Democratic candidate. In turn, the party, "having realized that there was now a demand for a colored man, would itself nominate one at the next vacancy"—probably, they were told, in 1915. In November 1914, George Harding, a Second Ward alderman, was elected state senator. Keeping its promise, the organization pushed DePriest to the forefront by endorsing him as its candidate for alderman.[28]

Oscar Stanton DePriest was born in 1871 in Florence, Alabama. His father, Neander R. DePriest, a teamster and farmer, and his mother, Martha Karsner, a laundress, were former slaves who had joined the thousands of "exodusters" who left the South at the end of Reconstruction.[29] Because of a series of lynchings and economic hardships, they were forced to move the family from Florence to Salina, Kansas, in 1878. But racism and discrimination continued to haunt the family. As one of only two black families in Salina, they encountered open hostility from white schoolchildren and neighbors. Nevertheless, DePriest learned how to successfully maneuver his way in the predominantly white world. He attended Salina Normal School and studied business and bookkeeping. In 1889 he took those skills to Chicago, where he became a painter, decorator, and independent contractor. In 1903, he won $25,000 worth of contracts from the Chicago Board of Education. By the age of thirty-three, he was well entrenched in the Republican machine and had become the fourth African American to serve on the Cook County Board of Commissioners. As a two-term board member, DePriest attended to the needs of the poor by publicizing relief resources in the city and county.[30]

DePriest's success in the party was due primarily to patronage politics and his ability to build a viable black Republican faction. Between 1906 and 1910, he joined forces with Wright, and together they built a strong black group and successfully gained leverage with several factions within the party. But by 1912, personal jealousies had shattered the coalition. DePriest did not support Wright's second primary bid; instead, he shrewdly cultivated support for himself within the ranks of the party, becoming its choice for alderman in 1915.[31] He paid a price for his ambitions and maneuvering, however: his commitment to the race was often questioned by the masses, and other prominent black political figures publicly challenged him.

Despite the machine's endorsement of DePriest, his candidacy was contested. In fact, his nomination opened the door for other African American candidates seeking the coveted post. For the first time in Chicago's political history, three black candidates campaigned for alderman in the primary. Joining DePriest were Louis B. Anderson, a former journalist from Washington, D.C., and Charles Griffin, an insurance and real estate broker. Disgruntled with the expanded slate of black primary candidates and fearing a split black vote, DePriest attempted in January 1915 to limit the number of black candidates by arguing that he was the Republican organization's choice for alderman, so Anderson and Griffin should bow out of the race.[32] Neither Griffin nor Anderson withdrew.

Public denunciation of DePriest was swift. In a letter to the *Defender*, one reader cautioned that "the candidacy of Mr. Oscar DePriest, who is familiar with all the tricks of the game, and looked upon as one of the political leaders of the so-called black belt, should mark a new era in the political history of the intelligent self respecting Negroes of the Second ward. . . . Hypocritical boss-ridden demagogues have abandoned self-respect and race pride in order that their selfish aims may be obtained. Such men are unworthy of either confidence, or respect, and in my opinion can no longer control or influence the intelligent electorate of the Second ward."[33]

With the battle lines drawn, the candidates began seeking votes. One of the first forums for the three politicians was at the Alpha Suffrage Club's headquarters. The men presented their political platforms and entertained questions. Afterward, according to one historian, members passed a resolution to expel anyone who supported a white candidate.[34] The club also decided to "endorse" the Republican ticket and "our young giant Oscar DePriest for alderman of the Second Ward." They pledged "to leave no stone unturned" for his election, because "we realize that in no other way can we safeguard our own rights than by holding up the hands of those who fight our battles."[35] Other clubs in the ward were urged to "become a DePriest club," and the slogan "Elect Oscar DePriest to the City Council" was adopted.[36]

Some African American women opted to support the other candidates. With three blacks running in the primary, African American voters could focus on choosing the best "race" man as alderman. DePriest, some women felt, was not that person because he was an organization man first and a race man second, and would ultimately abandon his race if he was elected. As "one of the newly emancipated citizens of the Second Ward" explained, "The one thing above and beyond all, and to me of most concern, was to be sure that there would be one of our race nominated for this important office." But, she added, DePriest was not her favorite; rather, "Louis B. Anderson is the one candidate upon whom they can safely depend." Even though this woman endorsed Anderson, she still insisted that the way to achieve power in the black community was to get a black man in office. Consequently, she and other Second Ward women concluded that "there is too much at stake to vote for any other man but a race man."[37]

On February 27, 1915, Oscar DePriest was declared the winner of the Republican primary. He garnered 3,194 votes, to Anderson's 2,632 and Griffin's 1,432. Of the 7,258 votes cast, black females accounted for one-third: 1,093 of the votes for DePriest, 762 of those for Anderson, and 500 of those for Griffin. After the victory, DePriest called for unification among blacks in the ward: "To those who saw fit to support other candidates of them I have nothing to say save of the highest respect, but since they have acted in accordance with the spirit of the primary law and have failed of nomination of their choice, I now appeal to them, hoping that they will, as all good Republicans, give me in my coming fight for election their heartiest loyalty and support."[38]

Despite DePriest's appeal, dissent lingered. On February 28, Edward Wright, disgruntled over DePriest's victory and his own failed bids for the post of alderman, requested that the Political Equality League endorse William Cowan as an independent candidate against DePriest. As a member of the league and on behalf of the Alpha Suffrage Club, Ida B. Wells-Barnett repudiated the appeal. She argued that this scheme had been conjured up by "this nameless white man" who "had not been prompted by the desire to secure a better man for nomination. It simply was to get two colored men to fight against each other, and the result would be that neither one of them would secure the place." The league agreed, and the Wright-Cowan challenge ended.[39]

The contest between DePriest and three white candidates— Al Russell, Simon P. Gary, and Samuel Block—drew a large turnout. In April, thousands of African Americans in the Second Ward went to the polls to cast their ballots. When the votes were tabulated, Oscar DePriest was the clear winner, becoming the first black alderman of Chicago. He received 10,599 votes, to Russell's 6,893, Gary's 3,697, and Block's 433.[40]

DePriest's victory extended beyond the city. In the state capital, Springfield, the *Forum* complimented blacks in Chicago and proudly announced that "for the first time in her history, the second largest city in the Union has a Colored Council man, Oscar DePriest, from the 2nd Ward. This is quite an honor and adds much to the advancement, politically of the Colored people. . . . The Colored people of Chicago are to be congratulated for their pluck and aggressiveness. That Mr. DePriest will wear the honors worthily is beyond question."[41]

DePriest's victory also fostered public discussion of the significance of the female electorate. Women voters had been a decisive factor; without them, DePriest would not have won. Their ballots accounted for 3,899, or more than one-third, of the votes cast for him. Of the remaining votes, 2,313 went to Russell, 1,443 to Gary, and 187 to Block.[42] Again, more than a third of the votes for these candidates had come from women: 3,943 of 11,023. Aware of the debt owed to Second Ward women, DePriest asserted in the national black journal, *The Crisis*, "I favor extension of the right of suffrage to women" because the women in Chicago "cast as intelligent a vote as the men." Although there had been a certain degree of "timidity" during the first campaign in Chicago in which women were allowed to vote, women had educated themselves, and in the 1914 and 1915 campaigns, "the work of the women was as earnest and the interest as keen as that of the men and in some instances the partisanship was almost bitter." Moreover, in the campaign of 1915, "when colored men were primary candidates for alderman, the women of the race seemed to realize fully what was expected of them, and, with the men, rolled up a very large and significant vote for the colored candidates; and they were consistent at the election, contributing to a plurality of over 3,000 votes for the successful colored candidate in a field of five. Personally, I am more than thankful for their work and as electors believe they have every necessary qualification that the men possess."[43] DePriest's public advocacy of female suffrage signaled to other ambitious politicians that black women could be either their best ally or their most ardent foe. The ASC's earnest attempt to elect Cowan as an independent against the established party's candidate, and the fact that they had delivered on their promise to elect DePriest, showed these women to be as committed to the cause as male voters. A shrewd politician, DePriest appreciated their role in enabling him to make history; thus he had no objection to women's newly prominent place in the political landscape.

African American women won a considerable measure of acceptance in Chicago politics primarily because of their tenacity, the passage of a suffrage bill by the state legislature, the creation of organized suffrage clubs, and the development of a distinct politically conscious reform agenda. They appeased black men who felt threatened by their presence by highlighting woman's traditional role as municipal housekeeper, and they proved race loyalty by voting for the "race man." By blending what seemed to be the disparate concepts of race, gender, enfranchisement, and urbanization into a new paradigm for group politics, they were able to bridge gaps, merge voices, and consolidate energies into a powerful political bloc. As a result, gender conflict was suppressed, and a male-female alliance was created that kept in check the resistance of the Republican machine to the leadership of African Americans over their own people.

The racially charged events of 1914 and 1915 reflected the growing trend among African Americans toward self-determination and resistance. Determined that the kind of political exploitation that haunted thousands of blacks in the South would not be a part of the lives of urban Illinois blacks, those Second Ward residents of voting age pursued one objective—to make history by electing one of their own. This challenge to the Republican machine played a key role in the machine's re-engineering. Recognizing the shift in black ideology, the platform of white patriarchy gave way to one of pragmatic politics. The promise to back a black candidate in 1915 was a positive response to an increasingly concentrated black population, a rise in black assertiveness, and the extension of the vote to women. Moreover, by complying with the demands of the black press, black Republicans, and black women, the machine's endorsement of DePriest paved the way for the candidacy of other blacks in the Second Ward, as evidenced by the nominations of Anderson and Griffin. Had African Americans, particularly black women, failed to lead a vigorous grassroots campaign, cast ballots, influence black male voters, and cooperate with black Republicans in their efforts to elect a man of the race, it is unlikely that DePriest would have become the first African American alderman in Chicago.

As black women and men continued to migrate to the Chicago area, drawn by the promise of economic opportunity, African Americans remained a permanent fixture in municipal politics throughout the decade. The fact that they congregated primarily on the south side and harbored a "strong racial self-identification," scholar Dianne Pinderhughes argues, "minimized the extent to which intraracial conflicts invaded electoral politics. With increasingly large numbers of black Republican voters concentrated in the south side city council and state legislation districts, there were few head-to-head contests that divided the black vote and allowed the white candidate to win."[44]

SEVEN

"To Fill a Reported Industrial Need"
THE GREAT MIGRATION, RACE WOMEN, AND THE END OF AN ERA

The mass migration of African Americans out of the South, the riots that continued to plague the state, and the onset of World War I were sharp reminders to Illinois race women that their collective club activities had become indispensable to the sustenance and viability of black life. These events, more than anything else, boosted the resolve of club women and tested their endurance, as the migration simultaneously transformed and centered the state's black population, and the war accentuated both black patriotism and black anguish. The percentage of blacks in Illinois increased, from 2.5 percent to 3.7 percent, while that of whites decreased slightly, from 97.5 percent to 96.2 percent. And while nearly half of whites resided in rural areas, only 1 percent of the African American populace did so.[1]

Encumbered by their mostly rural and poor backgrounds, the migrants faced an uncertain future. As agents of uplift, race women were especially cognizant of the difficulties brought by the largest mass migration of African American people in history, and they were conscious of the dilemma that America's entrance into World War I posed for black citizens, who still had not attained equity. Race women met both challenges through collective action. They joined forces with newly created organizations, enhanced their own programs, and eagerly participated in the war effort.

Thousands of African Americans migrated to Illinois between 1915 and 1920, primarily, as Elizabeth Lindsay Davis says, "to fill a reported industrial need which was widely advertised in the south."[2] The Chicago *Defender*, one of the nation's major black newspapers, vigorously encouraged Southern blacks to head north. The advertisements generated interest in the Lower South states such as Alabama, Louisiana, Florida, and Mississippi, inspiring hope among people who continued to live under the oppressive system of Jim Crow. The possibility of an improvement in their economic standing and less discrimination induced many to make the trip to the Midwest.[3] Another reason was the railway lines that converged in Chicago, which provided easy access to the city for Southern black migrants seeking employment in the state's industries. By 1920, Illinois had a black population of 182,274, an increase of almost 74,000 over the black population in 1910.[4] In Aurora, the African American population more than doubled, from 293 to 627. In Danville, it jumped from 1,465 to 2,366; in East St. Louis, from 5,882 to 7,437; and in Peoria, from 1,569 to 2,130. The largest increase occurred in Chicago, from 44,103 to 109,458.[5]

Club women were especially interested in a unique aspect of this massive movement—the influx of black female migrants. Noted historian Darlene Clark Hine suggests that the significant rise in the number of female migrants—the "gender dimension"—marked this period of movement among African Americans as distinctive.[6] The black female population of Illinois alone jumped from 56,140 to 88,439 in a ten-year period. The number of black women twenty-one years of age and over was 60,604 by 1920. Most of these women were in the prime of their lives, ranging in age between eighteen and forty-four. As with the men, nearly 60 percent of them took up residence in Chicago, contributing to the city's entrenchment as the most metropolitan city in the state, as well as the city with the densest African American population.[7]

From the outset, women migrants faced greater challenges than their male counterparts. Desperate for employment opportunities and better wages, they willingly distanced themselves from both family and familiar surroundings.[8] "A woman traveling alone was surely at greater risk than a man," Hine argues. "After all, a man could and did, with less approbation and threat of bodily harm, spend nights outdoors. More importantly, men were better suited to defend themselves against attackers. However, given the low esteem in which the general society held black women, even the courts and law officials would have ridiculed and dismissed assault complaints from a black female traveling alone, regardless of her social status."[9]

Nevertheless, inquiries to the *Defender* suggest that the pull of the North was stronger than their fears. A fifteen-year-old in New Orleans with four younger siblings sought work to earn much-needed income for her family, requesting that "a pass" be sent ahead of time, and assuring prospective employers that "you will not be sorry I am not no lazy girl I am smart i have got very much learning but i can do any work that come to my hand to do."[10] A seventeen-year-old from Selma, Alabama, wrote, "I am a reader of the Chicago Defender I think it is one of the Most Wonderful Papers of our race printed. Sirs I am writeing to see if You will please get me a job. And Sir I can wash dishes, wash iron nursing work in groceries and dry good stores. Just any of these I can do. Sir, who so ever you get the job from please tell them to send me a ticket and I will pay them When I get their as I have not got enough money to pay my way."[11] A twenty-seven-year-old woman from Jacksonville, Florida, seeking "any kind of housework," dismissed any threat to her personal being because she believed that the North offered her better economic opportunity.[12]

Many of the women migrants would have brought children with them. An interested mother from Florida wrote, "I take grate pleazer in writing you as I found in your Chicago Defender this morning where you are secure job for men as I realey diden no if you can get a good job for me as am a woman and a widowe with two girls and would like to no if you can get one for me and the girls. We will do any kind of work and I would like to hear from you at once not any of us has any husbands."[13] And from Moss Point, Mississippi, a reader requested "in formation towards a first class cookeing job or washing job I wand a job as soon as you can find one for me also I wand a job for three young girls ages 13 to 16 years. Please oblidge."[14] It was a difficult situation for those who wanted to keep their families intact during the migration process. "I seen your name in the Chicago Defender," wrote one woman who was seeking refuge for her entire family. "I am real anxious to go north I and my family I am a married womon with family my husbon and 3 children my oders boy 15 younger 13 baby 4 my sister 20. I can wash chambe mad dishwasher nurse or wash and my boy can work my sister can cook or wash or nurse my husband is a good work and swift to lern we are collored pepel a good family wonts a job with good pepel pleasanser soon."[15]

But even for those who successfully made the journey, life was not easy. Alone in unfamiliar surroundings, many of these young women, often at the mercy of strangers, became easy prey for pimps and criminals. African American women often had difficulty obtaining adequate housing, and gainful employment, though somewhat diversified, continued to be concentrated in domestic service. Most became part of a larger group of what scholar Joanne J. Meyerowitz calls "women adrift." Separated from family, they joined the rapidly expanding female labor force. In Chicago alone, the number of single women, regardless of race, employed outside the home increased more than 1,000 percent between 1880 and 1930.[16] Limited access to child care, educational institutions, and social services restricted their children's opportunities for a better life.

To alleviate some of these problems, club women expanded their social services. The Lillian Jameson Home opened in Decatur in 1918 to help meet the needs of dependent black women and their children. The Community Club of Carbondale and the Benevolent Workers of Marion formed children's auxiliaries. The Sunshine Workers of Harrisburg, formed in 1919, maintained a bank fund specifically to aid children and the elderly at Christmas.[17] Because more than 60 percent of these women settled in Chicago, the club women there were the largest contributors to their welfare. They established charities such as the Diana Charity Club, the Gaudeamus Charity Club, and the Giles Charity Club to clothe and feed families. The Improvement Club provided counsel to mothers on the rearing of their children.[18] The Amanda Smith Industrial School for Girls continued its work in the suburbs of Chicago. The Alpha Home, the Old People's Home, the Old Soldiers' Widows Rest, and the Church of God and Saints of Christ Orphanage and Home also became part of the link between the community and the welfare work of club women.[19]

The club women did not limit their services to women. To meet the needs of the steady influx of African American men, the women augmented their social service network and forged alliances with agencies that dealt specifically with problems associated with minorities in urban areas. Club women looked favorably on the Urban League movement that had begun during the early part of the decade. By 1916, offices were established in East St. Louis and Chicago. Some women volunteered their services, while others contributed monetarily through clubs. For example, the Gaudeamus Charity Club made an annual contribution of five dollars to the Chicago branch.[20]

The Urban League was a refuge for those who were adrift, becoming one of the most important links in the migration process. Volunteers helped migrants obtain housing, offered work-related lectures, and investigated workers' complaints. The league also established day nurseries for children and contributed financially to settlement homes in the area.[21] Among the list of volunteers were club women Jennie Lawrence, Joanna Snowden-Porter, and Irene Goins.[22] They joined other workers in welcoming new migrants to the city. As the migrants disembarked from the trains, league members directed them to the homes of relatives or friends, or guided them to "proper homes for lodging." They also distributed business cards, offering the league as a troubleshooting, problem-solving agency for all new migrants.[23] Club women handed out their own business cards, referring the newcomers to similar city services and strongly encouraging a middle class code of conduct: "cleanliness, respect for public property, orderly conduct in the street and the best possible upkeep of the household."[24] Moreover, they urged young men and women to utilize the facilities of the YMCA for black men, which had opened in 1913, and the YWCA for black women, established in 1915.[25]

Lawrence, Snowden-Porter, and Goins had long been active in volunteerism and uplift work and were therefore proficient representatives of social activism. Involvement with the league was merely one aspect of their work. Lawrence was born in Salisbury, North Carolina, the daughter of a Presbyterian minister. After graduating from Scotia Seminary and Livingstone College, she migrated to Chicago, where she became a teacher, a social worker, and superintendent of the Phyllis Wheatley Home.[26] Snowden-Porter, a native of Chicago, was a member of the Juvenile Protection Association. An active club woman, she was elected treasurer of the Phyllis Wheatley Home and president of the Northwestern Federation, to which the IFCWC belonged. She also served as editor for the IFCWC from 1914 to 1916.[27] Goins was born in Quincy, Illinois, and attended schools there and in Springfield. She and her husband, Henry Sherman Goins, settled in Chicago in 1895. An entrepreneur, she had once owned a millinery business. Goins was active in club work, presiding over the City Federation of Colored Women's Clubs from 1919 to 1921, and serving as second vice president of the IFCWC from 1920 to 1922.[28]

Another important effort in aiding the migrants was the promotion of public health. The Department of Health and Hygiene of the IFCWC, at one time headed by Mary F. Waring, played a pivotal role in directing new migrants to health facilities. The federation contributed financially to Yates Memorial Hospital in Cairo, which cared for blacks living along the Illinois-Missouri border, and championed the health care provided by Provident Hospital in Chicago. By 1920, the IFCWC had become a bulwark in its emphasis on preventive medical practices. It strongly urged mothers to register the births of their babies so that the health records of all newborns would be available to parents and public health officials.[29] The goal was to reduce the number of major health problems associated with poverty and racism.

Related to their health concerns was the moral decline resulting from alcoholism and prostitution. Because of the devastating consequences of these vices for the black community, race women were urged to lead a vigorous campaign against them. In strong alliance with the Women's Christian Temperance Union's fight for Prohibition, the IFCWC recommended that "departments of Temperance and Child Welfare be particularly encouraged in every club in the State," and its members campaigned for the passage of the Eighteenth Amendment, ratified in 1919, which prohibited the sale or manufacture of alcoholic beverages.[30] The belief that only government legislation could bring tangible results led these women to conclude that closing down the saloons would move the red-light district out of their neighborhoods. Their hope was that a clean, wholesome environment would translate into an abatement in the vices that were destroying black families. Despite their best efforts, however, the red-light district remained centered in neighborhoods with limited economic and political clout.

The increase in and concentration of the black population did have a strong positive impact on both the local and the state levels. The vast majority of African Americans continued to flock to the racially segregated Second Ward in Chicago, which further strengthened the black electoral voice. Even when the district lines were redrawn during the 1920s, much of the black community remained concentrated in the Second and Third wards. Moreover, municipal suffrage for women, combined with the passage of the Nineteenth Amendment in 1920, helped blacks in Chicago to establish themselves within the city's political structure. The influx of female migrants increased the number of female voters, thus ensuring that black women would remain integral political players. And with the simultaneous rise in the number of black male voters, blacks were virtually ensured a prominent role in Republican circles. Dependent on black votes, the Republican Party could not retreat from continuing to support the candidacy of at least one African American in the Second Ward.

Even the problems stemming from DePriest's criminal indictments did not hamper support from black and white Republicans. Despite having been accused of gambling and bribery between 1915 and 1917, DePriest remained a favorite among many African Americans, primarily because racial polarization led to the belief that he had been deliberately persecuted by whites because he was the only black on the city council. Even though he was acquitted of the criminal charges, his solid base of support in the black community gradually began to erode, black Republicans began jockeying for his position within the party, and the machine's interest waned. Without the support of these two significant groups, DePriest's bid for an aldermanic post in 1918 and 1919 was doomed.[31] Nevertheless, the significance of his being the first race man to win a city post bore fruit in subsequent years.

By the end of the decade, African American politicians and their constituents had elected two more black aldermen. Louis B. Anderson was elected in 1917, and Robert R. Jackson in 1918.[32] Those successes, coupled with the continuous growth of the black population, spilled over into other areas. The election of white Republican Big Bill Thompson, dubbed "the Negro Mayor," increased the number of blacks in the city's legal department as well as the number of black police. With the support of Thompson, race women and men led a campaign to stop Chicago theaters from showing *Birth Of A Nation*, a racist film that glorified a united white South during Reconstruction.[33] Long after DePriest's victory, African American men and women continued to hold positions in city government, making it possible for blacks to reap some of the benefits of patronage politics.

African Americans sought political power on the state level as well. With the passage of the Nineteenth Amendment in 1920, black women were no longer limited in their political agency. Their entrance into the state electoral arena opened new doors for black politicians seeking to broaden their personal ambitions. The number of blacks in the legislature had increased to five by 1928, helping to shape the new political landscape of the state. Moreover, partly on the strength of black women's votes, Oscar DePriest, nearly thirteen years after his aldermanic success, was elected to the United States Congress. His victory represented a triumph both for black Illinoisans and for African Americans throughout the United States. A "race man" once again, DePriest was the first black elected outside the South, and the first in nearly three decades to be elected to the House. Continuing a tradition that had begun more than three decades before, race and club woman Sarah Gordon Walker created a social club in his honor, the Oscar DePriest Charity Club. Under the motto "We Help Ourselves Only As We Help Others," the club sought ways to improve educational opportunities and health-care facilities. It provided scholarships to public school students and contributed funds to Provident Hospital.[34]

While the rising black population and the movement of blacks into positions of influence on the local and state levels benefited many African Americans, it also generated enormous anxieties among white Illinoisans. Racial equality remained elusive, and race riots became common occurrences. Beyond their concern over the competition for employment and housing, whites in East St. Louis, for example, feared the political clout that blacks seemed to be gaining in the city. Newspapers incited whites by charging that Republicans in the city had imported Southern blacks to win elections in 1916. Indeed, by 1920, of the eight wards in East St. Louis, the majority of blacks resided in the Second Ward: 1,456 women and 1,545 men, for a total of 3,001. By comparison, there were only 3,773 native-born whites, plus 425 foreign-born whites.

Though outnumbered by native whites, the African American community held the edge in an important political category: Of the 1,837 women of voting age in the Second Ward, African American women accounted for 805, or 44 percent; native-born white women of native parentage accounted for

634, or 35 percent; and those of mixed parentage accounted for 242, or 13 percent. Foreign-born and naturalized women made up the remaining 156. Of 2,383 male voters, 951, or 40 percent, were black; 816, or 34 percent, were white men of native parentage; 256, or 11 percent, were whites of foreign or mixed parentage; and 241, or 10 percent, were foreign-born whites. The 119 naturalized men made up the remaining 5 percent.[35] Together, African American women and men totaled 43 percent of the voting-age residents of the ward. It would have been politically expedient for any party hoping to attract their vote to cater to their interests. Although blacks in the area did not wield the same kind of political clout as those in Chicago, they did constitute a political force.

Despite the fact that a one-year residency requirement kept many black migrants from the polls, a large number of whites chose to believe newspaper accounts of an alleged "colonization" attempt on the part of blacks who were wanting to take over the city. The real truth, Elliot Rudwick argues, is that employers, who often were Republicans, imported blacks as cheap labor.[36] The continued use of African Americans to replace striking white union workers further exacerbated racial tensions. By late May 1917, vocal protests against Southern black migration had escalated. One group filed a formal complaint with the city council, calling for a public meeting to voice their concerns. On the 28th of that month, frustrated with their lack of power over the situation and enraged by rumors that a mob of angry blacks had harmed whites in the area, some of the incensed workers retaliated. A mob of whites attacked and beat innocent blacks and demolished several African American businesses. The riots produced few substantial gains for white workers. Although those who participated received little punishment, and no effective measures were implemented by city officials to prevent future disorder, they nevertheless were not assured of job security, and employers continued to hire black migrants.[37]

The combination of angry white workers and heightened black fears increased the likelihood of more conflict. By mid-summer, those tensions boiled over into chaos. On July 2, city newspapers reported a shooting incident involving several police officers and black patrons in a black neighborhood. The following day, angry white mobs attacked and killed at least thirty-nine blacks, and did thousands of dollars' worth of damage to homes and businesses in black neighborhoods. Approximately nine whites were killed.[38]

In the aftermath, African American women in the city joined the Urban League in its efforts to tend to the needs of the black community. But the women and the league faced massive obstacles. The league was forced to close its doors because of waning white support, and black women were hampered by the chaos that had erupted in the city following the riot. Nevertheless, they continued their relief work. For example, the Colored Old Folk's Home Association dispensed clothing and household necessities to African Americans who had lost all their possessions in the riot. The IFCWC, on the other hand, denounced the mob actions of white East St. Louisans and sent a letter of protest to the governor and to President Wilson.[39] Other women voiced their protest and appeals in local newspapers. In the *Chicago Daily Tribune*, Ida B. Wells-Barnett editorialized that East St. Louis was simply a harbinger of the kind of violence that was likely to erupt in urbanized, racially polarized Chicago.

> With one Negro dead as the result of a race riot last week, another one very badly injured in the county hospital; with a half dozen attacks upon Negro children, and one on the Thirty-fifth street car Tuesday, in which four white men beat one colored man, it looks very much like Chicago is trying to rival the South in its race hatred against the Negro. Especially does this seem so when we consider the bombing of Negro homes and the indifference of the public to these outrages. It is just such a situation as this which led up to the East St. Louis riot two years ago. There had been a half dozen outbreaks against the colored people by whites. Two different committees waited upon Gov. Lowden and asked him to investigate the outrages against Negroes before the riot took place. Nobody paid any attention. Will the

legal, moral, and civic forces of this town stand idly by and take no notice here of these preliminary outbreaks? Will no action be taken to prevent these law breakers until further disaster has occurred? An ounce of prevention beats a pound of cure. And in all earnestness I implore Chicago to set the wheels of justice in motion before it is too late, and Chicago be disgraced by some of the bloody outrages that have disgraced East St. Louis.[40]

Wells-Barnett was clearly frustrated with the white administrators at the city and state levels. Her pronouncement that "an ounce of prevention beats a pound of cure" expressed her strong belief that redressing the crimes committed against African Americans would diminish the number of violent outbreaks in East St. Louis and other urban areas. But women such as she had little chance of forcing political leaders to heed their concerns, because they could not vote for state officials. At that time their political clout was still centralized in their own communities. As a result, administrators implemented no procedures for halting the attacks, and they worried little about the warnings of black women.

A race riot in Chicago—only one in a series of riots during the "Red Summer" of 1919—exemplified the heightened racial tensions throughout the nation.[41] Racial animosity boiled to the surface in Chicago late in July, when a young black boy was struck on the forehead by white onlookers while swimming in Lake Michigan. The young boy drowned, and the sensationalistic newspaper coverage further inflamed an already heated situation. Allegations that black men were retaliating by raping white women and murdering whites fueled the fire. For fourteen days in late July and early August, black and white Chicagoans battled. In the end, 38 were dead and 537 were injured. It was the African American community that suffered most: 23 of the dead and 342 of the injured were black.[42]

In the aftermath of the riot, club women stepped in to help. In Sparta, they distributed clothes, food, and money. Others denounced the riots and concluded that the cure for racial discord was the creation of "constructive program[s] to provide

proper housing, full recreational privileges and increased educational opportunities for all where they are now lacking." Had
programs geared to training the mind and the body been in
place before 1919, they believed, it would have been "impossible" for Chicago to have been one of the scenes of the rioting.[43] Some women, committed to racial cooperation and the
institution of change, joined forces with the Chicago Commission on Race Relations to study ways of reducing or halting
racial violence. Ella G. Berry, acting as one of the many investigators for the commission, found that many African Americans believed that race relations were deteriorating rapidly.[44]
One interviewee suggested that the race riot had resulted from
a heightened sense of black consciousness, increased migration, black participation in World War I, and white anxieties:

> The present relations between the races seem more tense than
> formerly. This is due to the fact that Negroes have developed
> within the past few years a greater race consciousness, a great
> race respect. The immigration from the South which permitted
> him to enter into the industrial life of the North with very few
> hindrances, to partake of its civic life without an ever-constant
> reminder of race, was one of the main factors in increasing race
> consciousness and race respect. Another factor was the treatment
> as equals and fellow human beings of the Negro soldiers by the
> French soldiery and people. These things have caused the Ne-
> gro to demand the respect which he is entitled to as a man and
> the privileges due him as a citizen. The whites at the present
> time still object to giving him these. This causes friction. I be-
> lieve, however, that it will be lessened as soon as the whites real-
> ize that these demands of the Negro will not be withdrawn but
> will continue to be made with greater insistence.[45]

Indeed, black participation in the war effort did have a major
impact. Black men joined and fought as part of the Illinois in-
fantries. For example, Ferdinand L. Barnett, Jr., the son of Ida
B. Wells-Barnett, entered the military in 1917.[46] The son of
Sadie Lewis and James P. Adams served in the 365th Infantry.[47]
For their sons, and because of their own patriotism, race women,

like most African Americans, championed the cause of democracy on the home front and "shared the glory won by our boys, who fought on the battle fields of France, first, to make the world a decent place for others to live in, second, to make it a safe place for themselves and theirs."[48]

On the state level, club women worked with the Woman's Committee of the Council of National Defense. In cooperation with the committee, the IFCWC registered women for war-relief work.[49] Federation members presented patriotic programs, made garments for soldiers, purchased and sent hundreds of cigarettes, and staffed the Red Cross and railroad canteens. They participated in the purchase of thrift stamps and liberty bonds, encouraged blacks to conserve the existing food supply, and continued social welfare reform work.[50]

The local efforts were equally impressive. The Gaudeamus Charity Club, the Young Matron's Culture Club, and the Union Charity Club of Chicago adopted the Eighth Illinois Infantry, which served with other African Americans on the French front.[51] The Duncan Auxiliary of Springfield and the Louise D. Marshall Auxiliary of Chicago were formed soon after the war ended, to continue assisting the African American men of the 8th Infantry.[52] In addition to providing care packages for healthy soldiers, black women saw to the needs of the disabled. Visits to hospitals and the provision of refreshments and cigarettes were daily activities. The dead were honored as well. The Louise D. Marshall Auxiliary raised one thousand dollars to improve the lighting in the armory and purchased flowers to be planted in memory of blacks who died in the war.[53]

The Peoria Woman's Aid Club invested money in war savings stamps and liberty bonds. The Springfield Colored Woman's Club, the Domestic Art Club of Bloomington, and the Violet Thimble Club of East St. Louis worked with the Red Cross to ease war-related problems. The Frederick Douglass Center Woman's Club in Chicago opened a war office for the Second Ward. The club registered women for service with the Woman's Committee, provided an exemption board for drafted men, managed a Red Cross auxiliary, distributed food, and operated a parcel post office for Christmas packages sent to soldiers.[54] Individuals such as Mary F. Waring also had a major impact. Professional expertise enabled Waring to supervise an auxiliary that knitted and sewed hundreds of garments for soldiers. She also served on the Illinois State Committee of the National Council of Defense, and she was appointed to the Mayor's Committee of Chicago to greet returning black soldiers.[55]

In spite of the hopes of African American men and women, the patriotism they showed during the war had little if any impact on race relations in the United States. Soldiers returned home in 1919 to find race hatred and intolerance. Nativism had gained a strong political voice, resulting in the passage of more restrictive immigration laws. The backlash against African Americans, Jews, and Catholics brought increasing demands for segregation and racial purity. The riots of 1919 and other violent attacks were manifestations of a larger climate of racial intolerance. Returning soldiers found few employment opportunities, and other blacks in Illinois and other Northern industrial areas, historian Florette Henri argues, "found themselves pushed out of jobs they had held during the war, especially the better jobs."[56] Along with the race riots, returning black soldiers were greeted with the rise of the new Ku Klux Klan, which was organized in 1915 and had dedicated itself to terrifying not only blacks but immigrants, Catholics, and Jews as well.[57] Even more disturbing to African American women was the subsequent creation of Women of the Ku Klux Klan. Like its male counterpart, the WKKK promoted racial purity, the superiority of Anglo-Saxon Americans, and segregation.[58]

To meet these new challenges, black women and men became more defiant and willing to challenge the social order. According to Allain Locke, it was a quest by African Americans to define themselves and control their own destiny. "This radicalism," Locke noted, meant "no limitation or reservation with respect to American life." He interpreted it as "a constructive effort to build the obstructions in the stream of his progress into an efficient dam of social energy and power."[59] That energy and power also contributed to the sudden rise of Jamaican-born Marcus Garvey. Garvey's flamboyant style and fiery speeches inspired blacks to rise up and determine their own path. He successfully coordinated the largest economic movement of blacks in history through the Universal Negro Improvement Association (UNIA), which enabled blacks to own and operate stores, laundries, and restaurants. In 1919 he opened the first of his Liberty Halls in New York, where nightly mass meetings were held to instill race pride and encourage black community identity, solidarity, and unity. Garvey denounced organizations such as the NAACP and the Urban League because he felt that they were white-run and offered little help to the black masses. As a Washingtonian, he believed in segregation and championed economic prosperity. Unlike his predecessor, however, who had been an outspoken critic of white supremacy, Garvey believed that most white Americans felt an affinity with Klan ideology.[60]

Garvey's huge following included nearly nine thousand women and men from Illinois.[61] Although few prominent blacks publicly embraced his movement, Ida B. Wells-Barnett did. It was his philosophy of self-determination rather than his segregationist rhetoric that attracted her. She shared his belief that blacks had to organize for themselves and had to take the lead in fighting for their own independence from white oppression. She did not hesitate to speak to UNIA audiences when requested to do so by Garvey. She hailed Garvey as the person who had "made an impression on this country as no Negro before him had ever done. He has been able to solidify the masses of our people and endow them with racial consciousness and racial solidarity."[62] By the mid-twenties, Garvey had been indicted, imprisoned, and deported for mail fraud. But Wells-Barnett continued to appreciate the fact that his strong will, much like her own, and his unprecedented ability to inspire blacks had provided the basis for African American advancement in a racist culture: Had he enjoyed "the support which his wonderful movement deserved, had he not become drunk with power too soon, there is no telling what the result would have been."[63]

Unlike Wells-Barnett, most club women distanced themselves from Garvey and his segregationist ideas. They believed that as race women they could encourage race consciousness and self-determination while also soliciting assistance from white-controlled groups. They were assimilationists, not segregationists. Thus they did not denounce the Urban League and the NAACP, because these organizations assisted them in their pursuit for racial equality. When the Woman's Opportunity Club of Mounds, for example, held a "colored doll contest" to generate funds for future projects, it saw itself as "instilling Race pride," not supporting racism.[64] When the IFCWC strongly recommended "that all clubs urge their members to read race literature," it was attempting to instill self-esteem and championing race pride for black achievements, not denigrating the literary talents of white authors. And to counteract the rhetoric and actions of Garvey and other segregationists, the IFCWC encouraged "the organization in every community of committees on inter-racial relations."[65] For women who viewed their club activities and their association with whites as a necessary part of their "race work," these assertions reflected both the twenty year continuity in their commitment to uplift and their recognition of their own vulnerability in a racist and sexist culture.

Conclusion

What began in 1890 as a protest against the underrepresentation of African American women on the planning committee for the nation's celebration of its founding grew into a grassroots movement to empower both African American women and all African Americans. The voluntary association movement that gained momentum in Illinois during the late nineteenth century became a link in a chain that had originated with the national black women's club movement. The creation of the IFCWC and its network of local and regional affiliates broadened the base and the vision of the middle-class women who cultivated, nurtured, and maintained the clubs and provided a viable means of sustaining, supporting, and improving the lives of the African American masses.

Dominated by a single huge metropolitan community that was surrounded by small rural communities, the state of Illinois presented unique challenges and offered numerous opportunities for club women. Chicago housed the majority of both the poorest and the wealthiest blacks in Illinois, segregated its communities by race, and offered the greatest number of employment opportunities in the state. Because it required the most in the way of charitable resources, the city was home to the largest regional black female association, the largest number of clubs, and the most politically powerful group of black women in Illinois. The lack of available resources makes it impossible to ascertain whether women debated among themselves about Chicago's influence. What is clear, however, is that women in the metropolis as well as in the rural areas understood that it was because of racism and sexism, not regional residence, that blacks were denied equal opportunity.

Through mutual association, club women inserted themselves into first the social and then the political infrastructure of black communities, making their activism vital to these communities' survival. Establishing a network of social agents in both rural and urban areas, they fed, clothed, housed, and provided medical services to thousands of poor blacks. These successes prompted Elizabeth Lindsay Davis to write, "Our women in this State are alive three hundred and sixty-five days in the year, their hearts filled with enthusiasm and inspiration, each doing her level best to make the world better because she has lived."[1]

Because they were oppressed and marginalized on the basis of both their race and their sex, club women decided that their movement, while primarily emphasizing black women's empowerment, would cut across the lines of gender, class, and race. Black men, though not members of their associations, were expected to contribute equally in their attempts to further racial progress. The women encouraged and accepted both financial contributions and public support. Although they acknowledged the inherent differences between men and women, they rejected any notion that race women could not be social and political partners with their men.

Though some men resisted women's entrance into the male domain of the voting constituency, most recognized what club women had before the dawn of the new century—that it was a prerequisite for any kind of political success. Although race women had become sociopolitical agents by 1913, they still yielded to Victorian mores that dictated that as women, they attempt to usurp neither the prominent political role that black males played nor their limited gains. To assuage male egos, Fannie Barrier Williams reassured the men of Chicago that they need have "no anxiety as to the conduct" of black female voters. The implication, of course, was that the women would not attempt to publicly challenge male leadership. Still, the members of the Alpha Suffrage Club were "jeered" by some men when they tried to register voters.[2]

This kind of discrimination from black men did receive attention from women. While they chastised their men and sometimes questioned their moral character, they continued to adhere to their philosophy about their place as women. Although they didn't seek political office, their supporting roles as club organizers and canvassers were equally important. As race women, they did not believe that it was necessary to dispossess black men of their valued position in order to be successful. But they did believe that it was essential to augment that role with female political and social activism in order to achieve racial progress. Instead of challenging black men for organizational leadership, they politicized by developing female-centered organizations that addressed their unique concerns, just as they had done in their social welfare work. They tended to vote along race lines, just as their men did. And like most women, they benefited from the political process by being able to highlight issues relevant to the lives of families and communities.

While these women were middle-class, they catered to the needs of the poor. Because residential segregation did not afford the middle class the opportunity to insulate themselves from the poor, club women could not have distanced themselves from those who needed to be helped even if they had wanted to. That is not to suggest that they did not favor imposing their mores on the masses; rather, the majority of their clubs were founded for the purpose of service rather than purely for cultural enrichment. Even the few cultural clubs that developed eventually added social service work to their missions.

Club women eschewed the black nationalist and separatist ideology in favor of interracial cooperation despite discrimination and their own reservations. They interacted with whites both out of necessity and out of a genuine belief that collaboration between the races was important. Lacking economic clout, they enlisted the financial aid of white philanthropists. Lacking political influence, they accepted assistance from white women. Out of political expediency, they supported the candidacy of white male Republicans for upper-level administrative positions. And they joined white female organizations. Yet they espoused a racially conscious agenda by maintaining their commitment to self-determination and by creating and joining racially segregated clubs.

Ultimately, these social and political agents believed that their efforts would further the cause of racial equality. Neither the rise in racial tensions nor their own dual oppression as black women could dampen their resolve. If anything, the heightened tensions, coupled with the increased demands of a migrating populace, reinforced the club women's resolve to continue their public protest and their mutually interdependent activities. These women succeeded in spite of the racism and sexism that shaped their life experiences. It was not the push of external constraints that motivated them in their reform work; rather, it was the pull of internal forces that encouraged them to develop and maintain clubs and institutions that could provide a service to the community and nourish their desire to be good race women.

NOTES

INTRODUCTION

1. *Thirteenth Census of the United States, 1910*, p. 477; *Fourteenth Census of the United States, 1920*, p. 244.
2. Anne Meis Knupfer, *Toward a Tenderer Humanity and a Nobler Womanhood: African-American Women's Clubs in Turn-of-the-Century Chicago* (New York and London: New York University Press, 1996), p. 36.
3. Ibid.
4. *Chicago Daily Tribune*, 4 March 1913.

ONE. THE MOVEMENT TO ORGANIZE RACE WOMEN

1. Arna Bontemps and Jack Conroy, *Anyplace but Here* (New York: Doubleday, Doran and Co., 1945; reprint ed., New York: Hill and Wang, 1966), pp. 88–93; John G. Cawelti, "America on Display: The World's Fairs of 1876, 1893, 1933," in *The Age of Industrialism in America*, ed. Frederic Cople Jaher (New York: Free Press, 1968), pp. 317–363; Elliot M. Rudwick and August Meier, "Black Man in the 'White City': Negroes and the Columbian Exposition, 1893," *Phylon* 26 (1965): 354; Anne Massa, "Black Women in the 'White City,'" *Journal of American Studies* 8 (December 1974): 319; Jeanne Madeline Weimann, *The Fair Women* (Chicago: Academy Chicago, 1981), pp. 103–124; Anna R. Paddon and Sally Turner, "African Americans and the World's Columbian Exposition," *Illinois Historical Journal* 88 (Spring 1995).
2. *Indianapolis Freeman*, 27 December 1890.
3. Rudwick and Meier, "Black Man in the 'White City,'" pp. 354–355.
4. Ibid.
5. Massa, "Black Women in the 'White City,'" p. 323; Anne Firor Scott, *Natural Allies: Women's Associations in American History* (Urbana and Chicago: University of Illinois Press, 1991), p. 130; Gayle Gullett, "'Our Great Opportunity': Organized Women Advance Women's Work at the World's Columbian Exposition of 1893," *Illinois Historical Journal* 87 (Winter 1994): 270–272.
6. *New York Age*, 24 October 1891.
7. Paddon and Turner, "African Americans and the World's Columbian Exposition," p. 24; a detailed description and analysis of Williams's life is in chapter 2.
8. Fannie Barrier Williams, "A Northern Negro's Autobiography," *The Independent* 14 (July 1904): 91; Anne Meis Knupfer, *Toward a Tenderer Hu-*

manity and a Nobler Womanhood: African American Women's Clubs in Turn-of-the-Century Chicago (New York and London: New York University Press, 1996), pp. 34–35.

9. Massa, "Black Women in the 'White City,'" p. 334; Weimann, *Fair Women*, pp. 117–119.

10. Fannie Barrier Williams, "The Intellectual Progress of the Colored Women of the United States since the Emancipation Proclamation," in *The World's Congress of Representative Women*, ed. Mary Wright Sewall (Chicago: Rand, McNally and Co., 1894), p. 696.

11. Ibid., p. 698.

12. Ibid., pp. 698, 699.

13. Ibid., pp. 702–703.

14. Sewall, *The World's Congress of Representative Women*, pp. 433, 696–729.

15. Fannie Barrier Williams, "What Can Religion Further Do to Advance the Condition of the American Negro?" in *The World's Parliament of Religions*, 2 vols., ed. John Henry Barrows (Chicago: Parliament Publishing Co., 1893), vol. 2, p. 1115.

16. Alfreda Duster, ed., *Crusade for Justice: The Autobiography of Ida B. Wells* (Chicago: University of Chicago Press, 1970), pp. 115–117; *The Baltimore Afro-American*, 29 April 1893.

17. Ida B. Wells, *The Reason Why the Colored American Is Not in the World's Columbian Exposition* (Chicago, 1893).

18. Ibid., p. 81.

19. Rudwick and Meier, "Black Man in the 'White City,'" p. 356.

20. Duster, *Crusade*, pp. 118–119. Wells later regretted her public denunciation, because her friend, statesman and orator Frederick Douglass, successfully highlighted the successes as well as the problems and concerns facing black people on that day.

21. Duster, *Crusade*, pp. 7–8.

22. See Neil R. McMillen, *Dark Journey: Black Mississippians in the Age of Jim Crow* (Urbana: University of Illinois Press, 1989).

23. Ibid., p. 9; N. F. Mossell, *The Work of Afro-American Women* (Philadelphia: George S. Ferguson Co., 1894), p. 32.

24. Duster, *Crusade*, pp. 9–16; Monroe A. Majors, *Noted Negro Women: Their Triumphs and Activities* (Chicago: Donohue and Henneberry, 1893; reprint ed., Nashville: Fisk University Library Negro Collection, 1971), pp. 187–188.

25. Duster, *Crusade*, pp. 16–18.

26. Ibid., pp. xvii, 18–20; Mildred Thompson, "Ida B. Wells-Barnett: An Exploratory Study of An American Black Woman, 1893–1930" (Ph.D. dissertation, George Washington University, 1979), pp. 26–28.

27. Duster, *Crusade*, pp. 22–24; Thompson, "Ida B. Wells-Barnett," pp. 29–31; Majors, *Noted Negro Women*, p. 189.

28. Duster, *Crusade*, pp. 35–37, 39.

29. Ibid., pp. 37–42.

30. Ibid., pp. 47–51; Ida B. Wells, "Southern Horrors: Lynch Law in

All Its Phases," in *On Lynchings* (New York: New York Age Printing, 1892; reprint ed., New York: Arno Press, 1969), pp. 18–19; David M. Tucker, "Miss Ida B. Wells and Memphis Lynching," *Phylon* 32 (1971): 115–116.

31. Duster, *Crusade*, p. 52.

32. Ibid., pp. 53–58.

33. Ibid., pp. 65–66.

34. Ibid., pp. 61–67.

35. Ibid., pp. 71, 77; Thompson, "Ida B. Wells-Barnett," pp. 36–37, 58; Emma Lou Thornbrough, "The National Afro-American League, 1887–1908," *Journal of Southern History* 27 (1961): 504.

36. Wells, "Southern Horrors," Preface.

37. Duster, *Crusade*, p. 78; Paula Giddings, *When and Where I Enter: The Impact of Black Women on Race and Sex in America* (New York: William Morrow and Co., 1984), p. 30.

38. Duster, *Crusade*, pp. 79–80.

39. Ibid., p. 80.

40. Ibid.

41. Ibid., pp. 80–82.

42. Ibid., p. 81; Tulia Kay Brown Hamilton, "The National Association of Colored Women, 1896–1926" (Ph.D. dissertation, Emory University, 1978), p. 13.

43. *Woman's Era*, May 1894; Hamilton, "The National Association," p. 13; Giddings *When and Where I Enter*, pp. 30, 83.

44. *Woman's Era*, November 1894. Reporters included Fannie Barrier Williams, Chicago; Josephine Silone Yates, Kansas City; Victoria Earle Matthews, New York; Mary Church Terrell, Washington; Elizabeth Ensley, Denver; and Alice Ruth Moore, New Orleans.

45. *Woman's Era*, 1 June 1894, p. 5.

46. Elizabeth Lindsay Davis, *The Story of the Illinois Federation of Colored Women's Clubs* (Chicago, 1922), pp. 26–28.

47. Duster, *Crusade*, pp. 112, 136, 151; Giddings, *When and Where I Enter*, pp. 89–92; *Woman's Era*, August 1894.

48. *Woman's Era*, July 1895.

49. Fannie Barrier Williams, "The Club Movement among Colored Women of America," in *A New Negro for a New Century: An Accurate and Up-to-Date Record of the Upward Struggle of the Negro Race*, ed. Booker T. Washington (Chicago: American Publishing House, 1900), pp. 396–397; Elizabeth Lindsay Davis, *Lifting as They Climb* (Washington, D.C.: The National Association of Colored Women, 1933), pp. 14–15; Hamilton, "The National Association," p. 14.

50. Davis, *Lifting*, pp. 14–15, 18.

51. Williams, "Club Movement among Colored Women," p. 397.

52. Ibid.; *Woman's Era*, May 1894.

53. Fannie Barrier Williams, "Opportunities and Responsibilities of Colored Women," in *Afro-American Encyclopedia; or, The Thoughts, Doings, and Sayings of the Race*, ed. James T. Haley (Nashville: Haley and Florida, 1895), p. 153.

54. Ibid.

55. *Woman's Era*, August 1895; Davis, *Lifting*, p. 16; Williams, "Club Movement among Colored Women," pp. 397, 400.

56. Duster, *Crusade*, pp. 239, 242.

57. Davis, *Lifting*, pp. 20–21; Thompson, "Ida B. Wells-Barnett," pp. 131–135; Hamilton, "The National Association," pp. 16–21; Beverly Jones, "Mary Church Terrell and the National Association of Colored Women, 1896–1901," *Journal of Negro History* 67 (1982): 21–22.

58. Duster, *Crusade*, p. 243.

59. Davis, *Illinois Federation*. Phillis Wheatley was a famous black female poet. The clubs often named in her honor used the spelling Phyllis instead of Phillis.

60. Davis, *Lifting*, p. 11; "The Negro in Illinois," Writers Project of the Works Progress Administration, George Cleveland Hall Library, Chicago, Illinois, n.d.

61. Davis, *Illinois Federation*, pp. 2, 51; "The Illinois Federated Club Movement," Illinois Association of Club Women and Girls, Inc., Papers, p. 1, Illinois State Historical Library, Springfield, Illinois.

62. Davis, *Lifting*, pp. 2, 33, 132; *The Broad Ax*, 15 July, 12 August 1899; "The Illinois Federated Club Movement," p. 1.

63. Williams, "Opportunities and Responsibilities," p. 161; Davis, *Lifting*, p. 33; Davis, *Illinois Federation*, p. 1.

64. *The Broad Ax*, 29 July 1899; Duster, *Crusade*, pp. 258–260; Thornbrough, "National Afro-American League," pp. 503–504.

65. Davis, *Lifting*, pp. 33–37; Giddings, *When and Where I Enter*, p. 106; Davis, *Illinois Federation*, p. 51.

TWO. THE ILLINOIS FEDERATION OF COLORED WOMEN'S CLUBS

1. This meeting set the stage for an unprecedented number of black club women in the Midwest to become actively involved in the national black club women's movement.

2. Elizabeth Lindsay Davis, *The Story of the Illinois Federation of Colored Women's Clubs* (Chicago, 1922), p. 2; "The Illinois Federated Club Movement," Illinois Association of Club Women and Girls, Inc., Papers, p. 1, Illinois State Historical Library, Springfield, Illinois. For a discussion of the Midwestern experience of black club women, see Darlene Clark Hine, "Black Women in the Middle West: The Michigan Experience," in *Black Women and the Re-Construction of American History* (Brooklyn, N.Y.: Carlson Publishing, 1994), pp. 59–85; Stephanie J. Shaw, in "Black Club Women and the Creation of the National Association of Colored Women," in *"We Specialize in the Wholly Impossible": A Reader in Black Women's History* (New York: Carlson Publishing, 1995), pp. 433–447, argues that the NACW was not the beginning of the black women's club movement. The NACW originated from the grassroots efforts of club women who had already created and developed clubs of their own. See also Anne Firor Scott, "Most Invisible of All: Black Women's Voluntary Associations," *Journal of Southern His-*

tory 56 (1990): 3–22, about the marginalization of black women's associations in the larger club women's movement.

Elizabeth Lindsay Davis refers to this organization as the Illinois Federation of Colored Women's Clubs, while the incorporation papers filed on September 5, 1912, refer to the organization as the Illinois State Federation of Colored Women's Clubs. I have chosen to use Davis's reference throughout the book.

3. Davis, *Illinois Federation*, p. 123.

4. See Davis, *Illinois Federation*, and Illinois Association of Club Women and Girls, Inc., Papers.

5. Davis, *Illinois Federation*, p. 121.

6. Ibid., p. 42; Anne Meis Knupfer, *Toward a Tenderer Humanity and a Nobler Womanhood: African American Women's Clubs in Turn-of-the-Century Chicago* (New York and London: New York University Press, 1996), p. 150.

7. Davis, *Illinois Federation*, p. 110.

8. *The Broad Ax*, 19 October 1901; Davis, *Illinois Federation*, pp. 113–114.

9. Davis, *Illinois Federation*, pp. 113–114.

10. Ibid., pp. 111–118.

11. Ibid., p. 120.

12. Ibid., p. 37.

13. Ibid.

14. Ibid., p. 122.

15. Ibid., p. 4.

16. Ibid., p. 3; "Constitution, Article III, Funds," Illinois Association of Club Women and Girls, Inc., Papers.

17. "Constitution, Article III, Funds;" Davis, *Illinois Federation*, pp. 110, 122.

18. Davis, *Illinois Federation*, pp. 119, 121; "Constitution, Article III, Membership," Illinois Association of Club Women and Girls, Inc., Papers.

19. "Fifty Year History of the Chicago and Northern District Association of Colored Women, Inc.," Illinois Association of Club Women and Girls, Inc., Papers, p. 7.

20. Ibid., p. 23; Davis, *Illinois Federation*, pp. 60, 110–118.

21. "Fifty Year History," p. 25; Davis, *Illinois Federation*, p. 67.

22. "Fifty Year History," pp. 24–25.

23. Davis, *Illinois Federation*, pp. 9–10.

24. Ibid., pp. 3, 9.

25. Ibid., pp. 3, 20.

26. See, for example, Evelyn Brooks Higginbotham, *Righteous Discontent: The Women's Movement in the Black Baptist Church, 1880–1920* (Cambridge, Mass.: Harvard University Press, 1993), for a discussion of the role that the religious movement among African American women, particularly in the Baptist church, played in the women's club movement during the Progressive years.

27. Davis, *Illinois Federation*, pp. 47–48, 116–117.

28. Ibid., p. 55.

29. Ibid., pp. 42, 110–111.

30. *The Forum*, 11 December 1909; Davis, *Illinois Federation*, p. 122.

31. Fannie Barrier Williams, "A Northern Negro's Autobiography," *The Independent* 14 (July 1904): 91. For a discussion of the black elite, see Willard B. Gatewood, *Aristocrats of Color: The Black Elite, 1880–1920* (Bloomington: Indiana University Press, 1990), and Darlene Clark Hine, ed., *Black Women in America: An Historical Encyclopedia* (New York: Carlson Publishing, 1993), s.v. "The Middle Class," by Sharon Harley.

32. Williams, "A Northern Negro's Autobiography," p. 91.

33. Ibid.; Bert James Loewenberg and Ruth Bogin, eds., *Black Women in Nineteenth-Century American Life: Their Words, Their Thoughts, Their Feelings* (University Park: Pennsylvania State University Press, 1976), p. 263; Edward T. James, Janet Wilson James, and Paul S. Boyer, eds., *Notable American Women, 1607–1950: A Biographical Dictionary*, 3 vols. (Cambridge, Mass.: Belknap Press of Harvard University Press, 1971), vol. 3, p. 620; Elizabeth Lindsay Davis, *Lifting As They Climb* (Washington, D.C.:The National Association of Colored Women, 1933), p. 266.

34. Williams, "A Northern Negro's Autobiography," p. 91. Williams reveals few other details about her Southern ordeal. She does not divulge where she went or when she visited the region.

35. Ibid., p. 91.

36. Ibid.

37. Ibid., pp. 91–92.

38. Ibid., p. 92.

39. Loewenberg and Bogin, *Black Women*, p. 263; James, James, and Boyer, *Notable American Women*, pp. 620–621; N. F. Mossell, *The Work of Afro-American Women* (Philadelphia: George S. Ferguson Co., 1894), pp. 111–112; Harold Gosnell, *Negro Politicians: The Rise of Negro Politics in Chicago* (Chicago: University of Chicago Press, 1935), p. 217; Allan H. Spear, *Black Chicago: The Making of a Negro Ghetto, 1890–1920* (Chicago: University of Chicago Press, 1967), pp. 69–70; Gatewood, *Aristocrats*, p. 267.

40. Adade Mitchell Wheeler and Marlene Stein Wortman, *The Roads They Made: Women in Illinois History* (Chicago: Charles H. Kerr Publishing Co., 1977), pp. 70–71; Hine, *Black Women in America*, s.v. "Fannie Barrier Williams," by Wanda Hendricks; Darlene Clark Hine, *Black Women in White: Racial Conflict and Cooperation in the Nursing Profession, 1890–1950* (Bloomington: Indiana University Press, 1989), p. 28; Jay David, ed., *Black Defiance: Black Profiles in Courage* (New York: William Morrow, 1972), pp. 64, 70.

41. Fannie Barrier Williams, "The Intellectual Progress of the Colored Women of the United States since the Emancipation Proclamation," in *The World's Congress of Representative Women*, ed. Mary Wright Sewall (Chicago: Rand, McNally and Co., 1894), pp. 700, 705–711; see also Anne Massa, "Black Women in the 'White City,'" *Journal of American Studies* 8 (December 1974): 319–337, and Jeanne Madeline Weimann, *The Fair Women* (Chicago: Academy Chicago, 1981).

42. Chicago Woman's Club Papers, Boxes 20, 45, 46, Chicago Historical Society, Chicago, Illinois; Fannnie Barrier Williams, "The Club Movement among Negro Women," in *The Colored American from Slavery to Hon-*

orable Citizenship, ed. J. W. Gibson and W. H. Crogman (Atlanta: J. L. Nichols and Co., 1903), p. 217.

43. Williams, "Club Movement among Negro Women," p. 218; Williams, "A Northern Negro's Autobiography," p. 94.

44. See, for example, "The Frederic Douglass Centre," *The Voice of the Negro* 1 (December 1904): 601–604; "The Need for Social Settlement Work for the City Negro," *Southern Workman* 33 (September 1904): 501–506; "The Negro and Public Opinion," *The Voice of the Negro* 1 (January 1904): 31–32; "A Woman's Part in a Man's Business," *The Voice of the Negro* 1 (November 1904): 543–547; "The Colored Girl," *The Voice of the Negro* 2 (June 1905): 401–403; "Social Bonds in the Black Belt of Chicago," *Charities* (7 October 1905): 40–44; "Colored Women in Chicago," *Southern Workman* 63 (October 1914): 564–566.

45. Davis, *Illinois Federation*, pp. 65, 110–111; Knupfer, *Toward a Tenderer Humanity*, p. 147.

46. Davis, *Lifting*, pp. 203–205; Sylvia G. L. Dannett, *Profile of Negro Womanhood* (Chicago: Educational Heritage, 1964), p. 249; *The Broad Ax*, 3 February 1900.

47. Davis, *Illinois Federation*, pp. 73, 113.

48. *The Forum*, 2 October 1909; Davis, *Illinois Federation*, p. 42.

49. Davis, *Illinois Federation*, p. 51.

50. "Incorporation State of Illinois Department of State," Illinois Association of Club Women and Girls, Inc., Papers; Davis, *Illinois Federation*, p. 125.

51. Davis, *Illinois Federation*, pp. 33–34.

52. "Incorporation State of Illinois Department of State."

THREE. AGENTS OF SOCIAL WELFARE

1. *Thirteenth Census of the United States, 1910*, p. 477; *Fourteenth Census of the United States, 1920*, p. 244.

2. Fannie B. Williams, "The Need for Social Settlement Work for the City Negro," *Southern Workman* 33 (September 1904): 502.

3. Florette Henri, *Black Migration: Movement North, 1900–1920* (New York: Anchor Press, 1976), pp. 108–113.

4. Elizabeth Lindsay Davis, *The Story of the Illinois Federation of Colored Women's Clubs* (Chicago, 1922); see also Elsa Barkley Brown, "Womanist Consciousness: Maggie Lena Walker and the Independent Order of Saint Luke," *Signs: Journal of Women in Culture and Society* 14 (1989): 610–633.

5. Alfreda Duster, ed., *Crusade for Justice: The Autobiography of Ida B. Wells* (Chicago: University of Chicago Press, 1970), pp. 249–250; Evelyn Brooks Higginbotham, *Righteous Discontent: The Women's Movement in the Black Baptist Church, 1880–1920* (Cambridge, Mass.: Harvard University Press, 1993), pp. 173–174.

6. Davis, *Illinois Federation*, pp. 16, 26–27, 197.

7. Bert James Loewenberg and Ruth Bogin, eds., *Black Women in Nineteenth-Century American Life: Their Words, Their Thoughts, Their Feelings* (University Park: Pennsylvania State University Press, 1976), pp. 30–31.

8. Ibid., p. 143.

9. Edward T. James, Janet Wilson James, and Paul S. Boyer, eds., *Notable American Women, 1607–1950: A Biographical Dictionary*, 3 vols. (Cambridge, Mass.: Belknap Press of Harvard University Press, 1971), vol. 3, pp. 304–305; Booker T. Washington, "Negro Women and Their Work," in *The Story of the Negro: The Rise of the Race from Slavery*, 2 vols. (New York: Outlook Co., 1909; reprint ed., New York: Peter Smith, 1941), vol. 2, pp. 321–322; Davis, *Illinois Federation*, pp. 70–71; H. F. Kletzing and W. H. Crogman, eds., *Progress of a Race; or, The Remarkable Advancement of the Afro-American* (Atlanta: J. L. Nichols, 1897; reprint ed., New York: Negro Universities Press, 1969), p. 446; Ann Meis Knupfer, *Toward a Tenderer Humanity and a Nobler Womanhood: African American Women's Clubs in Turn-of-the-Century Chicago* (New York and London: New York University Press, 1996), pp. 76–81; Elizabeth Lindsay, *Lifting As They Climb* (Washington, D.C.: The National Association of Colored Women, 1933), pp. 293–294.

10. Davis, *Illinois Federation*, pp. 44–45; Melinda Fish Kwedar, *Unsung Heroines: A Salute to Springfield Women* (Springfield: Sangamon County Historical Society, 1977), pp. 10–11.

11. *The Forum*, 21 November 1908; Esther M. Phillips, "The Lincoln Colored Home 'in Reality,'" Family Service Center of Sangamon County Papers, Illinois State Historical Library, Springfield, Illinois, pp. 4–6; Colored Children's Service Bureau Records, Family Service Center of Sangamon County Papers, Illinois State Historical Library, Box 60; Carmelita Banks, "The Lincoln Colored–Kren Home," Vertical File–Negroes–Springfield, Illinois, 1989, Sangamon Valley Collection, Lincoln Library, Springfield, Illinois, pp. 2–3; Benjamin Brawley, *Women of Achievement* (Chicago: Woman's American Baptist Home Mission Society, 1919), p. 11.

12. Jennie Coleman McClain, *The Springfield Colored Woman's Club* (Hamann Print, n.d.), n.p.; Banks, "The Lincoln Colored–Kren Home," p. 3; Davis, *Illinois Federation*, pp. 21, 53; *Directory of Sangamon County's Colored Citizens* (Springfield: Springfield Directory Co., n.d.); "Black and Beautiful: Springfield's Heritage," February 1984, Lincoln Library, Springfield, Illinois, Clippings File; Kwedar, *Unsung Heroines*, p. 10.

13. H. W. Washington, "Helping Each Other," *Springfield's Voice* (24 April 1975): 7; Phillips, "In Reality," pp. 3–4; McClain, *Springfield Colored Woman's Club*.

14. McClain, *Springfield Colored Woman's Club*.

15. *The Forum*, 31 July 1909; McClain, *Springfield Colored Woman's Club*.

16. McClain, *Springfield Colored Woman's Club*.

17. Ibid.

18. Ibid.; *State Capitol*, 13 January 1899.

19. Ibid.

20. Davis, *Illinois Federation*, pp. 4, 42, 102; McClain, *Springfield Colored Woman's Club*; Family Services Center of Sangamon County Papers.

21. Ibid.; Washington, "Helping Each Other," p. 7.

22. Phillips, "In Reality," p. 4.

23. McClain, *Springfield Colored Woman's Club*; Davis, *Illinois Federation*,

pp. 28- 29, 44–45; Kwedar, *Unsung Heroines,* p. 10; Phillips, "In Reality," pp. 4–6.

24. Kwedar, *Unsung Heroines,* p. 10; Banks, "The Lincoln Colored–Kren Home," p. 4; "Black and Beautiful," p. 1; Washington, "Helping Each Other," *Springfield's Voice,* p. 7.

25. Davis, *Illinois Federation,* pp. 32, 56, 99–101.

26. Davis, *Illinois Federation,* pp. 8, 10, 13, 24, 28.

27. See, for example, Ruth Rosen, *The Lost Sisterhood: Prostitution in America, 1900–1918* (Baltimore: Johns Hopkins University Press, 1982), pp. xi, 51–52; Mark Thomas Connelly, *The Response to Prostitution in the Progressive Era* (Chapel Hill: University of North Carolina Press, 1980), pp. 92, 100, 195–196.

28. See Deborah Gray White, *Ar'n't I a Woman? Female Slaves in the Plantation South* (New York: W. W. Norton and Co., 1985), pp. 27–61; N. H. Burroughs, "Black Women and Reform," *The Crisis* 10 (August 1915): 187.

29. Allan H. Spear, *Black Chicago: The Making of a Negro Ghetto, 1890–1920* (Chicago: University of Chicago Press, 1967), pp. 25–26; Fannie Barrier Williams, "Social Bonds in the Black Belt of Chicago," *Charities* 15 (7 October 1905): 40–41.

30. Fannie Barrier Williams, "The Need For Social Settlement Work for the City Negro," *Southern Workman* 33 (September 1904): 502; see also Joanne J. Meyerowitz, *Women Adrift: Independent Wage Earners in Chicago, 1880–1930* (Chicago: University of Chicago Press, 1988), chapters 2 and 3. For a discussion on black female migration to the Midwest, see, for example, Darlene Clark Hine, "Black Migration to the Urban Midwest: The Gender Dimension, 1915–1945," in *The Great Migration in Historical Perspective: New Dimensions of Race, Class, and Gender,* ed. Joe William Trotter, Jr. (Bloomington: Indiana University Press, 1991), pp. 127–146.

31. Davis, *Illinois Federation,* p. 17; W. E. B. DuBois, ed., *Efforts for Social Betterment* (Atlanta: Atlanta University Press, 1909), p. 100, quoted in Dorothy C. Salem, "To Better Our World: Black Women in Organized Reform, 1890–1920" (Ph.D. dissertation, Kent State University, 1986), p. 176.

32. Davis, *Illinois Federation,* pp. 16–17, 95–96; Knupfer, *Toward a Tenderer Humanity,* pp. 81–84; Spear, *Black Chicago,* p. 102.

33. Davis, *Illinois Federation,* pp. 7, 47–48, 97; see also Meyerowitz, *Women Adrift,* pp. 21–42.

34. Davis, *Illinois Federation,* pp. 61, 98.

35. Ibid., pp. 19, 21.

36. McClain, *Springfield Colored Woman's Club.*

37. See Elisabeth Lasch-Quinn, *Black Neighbors: Race and the Limits of Reform in the American Settlement House Movement, 1890–1945* (Chapel Hill: University of North Carolina Press, 1993); Sheila M. Rothman, *Woman's Proper Place: A History of Changing Ideals and Practices, 1870 to the Present* (New York: Basic Books, 1978), pp. 112, 117.

38. Williams, "The Need for Social Settlement Work," p. 504.

39. Quoted in Spear, *Black Chicago,* pp. 46–47.

40. Fannie Barrier Williams, "The Frederick Douglass Centre," *The Voice of the Negro* 1 (December 1904): 604; Williams, "The Need for Social Settlement Work," p. 504; Spear, *Black Chicago,* pp. 103–104; Davis, *Illinois Federation,* p. 66; Adade Mitchell Wheeler and Marlene Stein Wortman, *The Roads They Made: Women in Illinois History* (Chicago: Charles H. Kerr Publishing Co., 1977), pp. 70–71; Kathryn Kish Sklar, "Hull House in the 1890s: A Community of Women Reformers," *Signs* 10 (1985): 658–677; Louise C. Wade, *Graham Taylor: Pioneer for Social Justice* (Chicago: University of Chicago Press, 1964); Allen F. Davis, *Spearheads for Reform: The Social Settlements and the Progressive Movement, 1890–1914* (New York: Oxford University Press, 1967), pp. 12–13, 94–95.

41. Wheeler and Wortman, *The Roads They Made,* pp. 70–71; Mildred Thompson, "Ida B. Wells-Barnett: An Exploratory Study of an American Black Woman, 1893–1930" (Ph.D. dissertation, George Washington University, 1979), p. 182.

42. Wheeler and Wortman, *The Roads They Made,* p. 71; Thompson, "Ida B. Wells-Barnett," pp. 181–190; Spear, *Black Chicago,* p. 106; Duster, *Crusade for Justice,* pp. 279–309, 331–333; Knupfer, *Toward a Tenderer Humanity,* pp. 56–59; Thomas C. Holt, "The Lonely Warrior: Ida B. Wells-Barnett and the Struggle for Black Leadership," in *Black Leaders of the Twentieth Century,* ed. John Hope Franklin and August Meier (Urbana: University of Illinois Press, 1982), p. 55.

43. Spear, *Black Chicago,* p. 105; Iris Carlton-LaNey, "The Career of Birdye Henrietta Haynes, a Pioneer Settlement House Worker," *Social Service Review* 68 (June 1994): 254–263.

44. Davis, *Illinois Federation,* pp. 98–99.

45. Floris L. B. Cash, "Womanhood and Protest: The Club Movement among Black Women, 1892–1922" (Ph.D. dissertation, State University of New York, Stony Brook, 1986), pp. 33–34; Salem, "To Better Our World," p. 143; Bettina Aptheker, *Woman's Legacy: Essays on Race, Sex and Class in American History* (Amherst: University of Massachusetts Press, 1982), pp. 104–105; Darlene Clark Hine, *Black Women in White: Racial Conflict and Co-operation in the Nursing Profession, 1890–1950* (Bloomington: Indiana University Press, 1989), pp. 3–35.

46. Jay David, ed., *Black Defiance: Black Profiles in Courage* (New York: William Morrow, 1972), pp. 64, 70.

47. Ibid.; Spear, *Black Chicago,* pp. 56, 97–98; Robert McMurdy, "Negro Women as Trained Nurses: Experiment of a Chicago Hospital," *Survey* 31 (November 1913): 159–160; Kletzing and Crogman, *Progress of a Race,* pp. 440–441; Aptheker, *Woman's Legacy,* pp. 104–105; Hine, *Black Women in White,* pp. xix, 9, 26–28, 47.

48. Davis, *Illinois Federation,* pp. 26, 97, 112; John M. Lansden, *A History of the City of Cairo, Illinois* (Chicago: R. R. Donnelley and Sons, 1910; reprint ed., Carbondale: Southern Illinois University Press, 1976), p. 270; *Evening Citizen,* 26 February 1913; *Cairo Illinois City Directory,* 1909, 1917–1918, 1922, 1927, 1930; Brawley, *Women of Achievement,* p. 11; Shirley J. Carlson, "Black Migration to Pulaski County, Illinois, 1860–1900," *Illinois Historical Journal* 80 (1987): 44.

49. Fannie Barrier Williams, "The Club Movement among Negro Women," in *The Colored American From Slavery to Honorable Citizenship*, ed. J. W. Gibson and W. H. Crogman (Atlanta: J. L. Nichols and Co., 1903), pp. 204–205; see also Darlene Clark Hine, "Lifting the Veil, Shattering the Silence: Black Women's History in Slavery and Freedom," in *The State of Afro-American History Past, Present, and Future*, ed. Darlene Clark Hine (Baton Rouge: Louisiana State University Press, 1986), pp. 237–239.

FOUR. RACE RIOTS, THE NAACP, AND FEMALE SUFFRAGE

1. Alfreda Duster, ed., *Crusade for Justice: The Autobiography of Ida B. Wells* (Chicago: University of Chicago Press, 1970), pp. 309–320.

2. Hermann R. Lantz, *A Community in Search of Itself: A Case History of Cairo, Illinois* (Carbondale: Southern Illinois University Press, 1972), p. 49; *Gazetteer of the United States, Showing the Population of Every County, City, Town and Village According to the Census of 1890* (Chicago: George F. Cram, 1893), p. 60.

3. Shirley J. Carlson, "Black Migration to Pulaski County, Illinois, 1860–1900," *Illinois Historical Journal* 80 (1987): 40.

4. Ibid., p. 45; *Daily Telegram's Cairo City Directory for 1893* (Cairo, Ill.: Telegram Directory Publishers, 1893), p. 94.

5. Lantz, *A Community in Search of Itself*, p. 76; John M. Lansden, *A History of the City of Cairo, Illinois* (Chicago: R. R. Donnelley and Sons, 1910; reprint ed., Carbondale: Southern Illinois University Press, 1976), p. 277; Donald F. Tingley, *The Structuring of a State: The History of Illinois, 1899 to 1928* (Urbana: University of Illinois Press, 1980), pp. 290–292.

6. Roberta Senechal, *The Sociogenesis of a Race Riot: Springfield, Illinois in 1908* (Urbana: University of Illinois Press, 1990), p. 21.

7. James Crouthamel, "The Springfield Race Riot of 1908," *Journal of Negro History* 45 (July 1960): 165–178; Senechal, *Sociogenesis of a Race Riot*, chap. 1 and pp. 158–159, 168–173.

8. Senechal, *Sociogenesis of a Race Riot*, pp. 160–168.

9. *Springfield Forum*, 5 September 1908.

10. Ibid., 20 November 1915.

11. Ibid., pp. 182–183.

12. Senechal, *Sociogenesis of a Race Riot*, p. 60; Shelby M. Harrison, director, *The Springfield Survey of Social Conditions in an American City*, 3 vols. (New York: Russell Sage Foundation, 1920), vol. 3, pp. 23–25.

13. Duster, *Crusade for Justice*, p. 299.

14. Ibid., p. 300.

15. L. M. Hershaw, "Springfield," *The Horizon* 4 (August 1908): 9.

16. Charles Flint Kellogg, *NAACP: A History of the National Association for the Advancement of Colored People* (Baltimore: Johns Hopkins University Press, 1967), pp. 9–10; William English Wallings, "The Race War in the North," *Independent* 65 (3 September 1908): 529–530; "Black and Beautiful," Clippings File of Lincoln Library, Springfield, Illinois, February 1984.

17. Kellogg, *NAACP*, pp. 9–19, 45.

18. Louis R. Harlan and Raymond W. Smock, eds., *The Booker T. Wash-*

ington Papers, 13 vols. (Urbana: University of Illinois Press, 1981), vol. 9, pp. 700–701; vol. 10, pp. 7, 12, 25, 31–32; Louis R. Harlan, "Booker T. Washington," in *Black Leaders of the Twentieth Century*, ed. John Hope Franklin and August Meier (Urbana: University of Illinois Press, 1982), pp. 1–18.

19. Oswald Garrison Villard to Booker T. Washington, 26 May 1090, in *The Booker T. Washington Papers*, vol. 10, p. 116.

20. Booker T. Washington to Oswald Garrison Villard, 28 May 1909, ibid., p. 119.

21. Ibid.

22. Ida B. Wells-Barnett, "Lynching: Our National Crime," in *Proceedings of the National Negro Conference, 1909* (New York: Arno Press, 1969), pp. 174–176.

23. Ida Wells-Barnett, "How Enfranchisement Stops Lynching," *Original Rights Magazine*, June 1910, reprinted in Mildred I. Thompson, *Ida B. Wells-Barnett: An Exploratory Study of an American Black Woman, 1893–1930* (New York: Carlson Publishing, 1990), vol. 15 of *Black Women in United States History*, ed. Darlene Clark Hine, p. 269.

24. Kellogg, *NAACP*, pp. 16, 41, 43, 89.

25. Ibid., pp. 25–26, 298–308.

26. Davis, *Illinois Federation*, p. 125.

27. W. E. B. DuBois, "Politics and Industry," in *Proceedings of the National Negro Conference, 1909* (New York: Arno Press, 1969), p. 87; Kellogg, *NAACP*, pp. 48–49; W. E. B. DuBois, "Social Effects of Emancipation," *The Survey* 29 (1 February 1913): 571.

28. Wm. English Walling to W. E. B. DuBois, 8 June 1910, in *The Correspondence of W. E. B. DuBois*, ed. Herbert Aptheker (Amherst: University of Massachusetts Press, 1973), pp. 169–170.

29. DuBois, "Social Effects," p. 573.

30. DuBois, "National Negro Conference," *The Horizon* 5 (November 1909): 1.

31. W. E. B. DuBois, "Votes for Women," *The Crisis* 4 (September 1912): 234.

32. Deborah Gray White, "The Cost of Club Work, the Price of Black Feminism," in *Visible Women: New Essays on American Activism*, ed. Nancy A. Hewitt and Suzanne Lebsock (Urbana: University of Illinois Press, 1993), p. 253.

33. *The Forum*, 8 May 1915.

34. DuBois, "Votes for Women," p. 234.

35. Mary B. Talbert, "Women and Colored Women," *The Crisis* 10 (August 1915): 184.

36. N. H. Burroughs, "Black Women and Reform," *The Crisis* 10 (August 1915): 187.

37. Mary Church Terrell, "Woman Suffrage and the 15th Amendment," *The Crisis* 10 (August 1915): 191.

38. Mary Fitzbutler Waring, "Training and the Ballot," *The Crisis* 10 (August 1915): 186.

39. Ibid.

40. Philip Foner, ed., *The Voice of Black America: Major Speeches by Negroes in the United States, 1797–1971* (New York: Simon and Schuster, 1972), p. 237; Jean Fagan Yellin, "DuBois' Crisis and Women's Suffrage," *Massachusetts Review* 14 (1973): 368–369.

41. Rosalyn Terborg-Penn, "Discrimination against Afro-American Women in the Woman's Movement, 1830–1920," in *The Afro-American Woman: Struggles and Images,* ed. Rosalyn Terborg-Penn and Sharon Harley (New York: Kennikat Press, 1978), p. 17.

42. Aileen S. Kraditor, *The Ideas of the Woman Suffrage Movement, 1890–1920* (New York: Columbia University Press, 1965; reprint ed., New York: W. W. Norton, 1981), pp. 66, 163–218; Mari Jo and Paul Buhle, eds., *The Concise History of Woman Suffrage: Selections from the Classic Work of Stanton, Anthony, Gage and Harper* (Urbana: University of Illinois Press, 1978), p. 350; Marjorie Spruill Wheeler, *New Women of the New South: The Leaders of the Woman Suffrage Movement in the Southern States* (New York: Oxford University Press, 1993), esp. chap. 4. See also Barbara Hilkert Andolsen, *Daughters of Jefferson, Daughters of Bootblacks: Racism and American Feminism* (Macon, Ga.: Mercer University Press, 1986).

43. Kraditor, *Ideas of Woman Suffrage,* p. 328; Buhle, *The Concise History,* pp. 44–46.

44. For the history of the suffrage movement, see Eleanor Flexnor, *Century of Struggle: The Woman's Rights Movement in the United States* (Cambridge, Mass.: Belknap Press of Harvard University Press, 1959; revised ed., 1975; Kraditor, *Ideas of Woman Suffrage;* William O'Neil, *Everyone Was Brave: A History of Feminism in America* (Chicago: Quadrangle, 1971); Ellen Carol DuBois, *Feminism and Suffrage: The Emergence of an Independent Women's Movement in America, 1848–1869* (Ithaca: Cornell University Press, 1978).

45. "Suffering Suffragettes," *The Crisis* 4 (June 1912): 76–77; Terborg-Penn, "Discrimination against Afro-American Women," p. 25; W. E. B. DuBois, "Hail Columbia," *The Crisis* 5 (April 1913): 289–290; Yellin, "DuBois' Crisis," pp. 366–369.

46. Catharine W. McCulloch to Senator Lawrence Y. Sherman, 4 December 1916, The Lawrence Y. Sherman Papers, Box 116, Folder 8, Illinois State Historical Library, Springfield, Illinois.

47. Grace Wilbur Trout to Senator Lawrence Y. Sherman, 2 June 1919, The Lawrence Y. Sherman Papers, Box 116, Folder 9, Illinois State Historical Library.

48. Yellin, "DuBois' Crisis," pp. 366–369; W. E. B. DuBois, "Forward Backward," *The Crisis* 2 (October 1911): 243–244.

49. W. E. B. DuBois, "Woman Suffrage," *The Crisis* 9 (April 1915): 285.

FIVE. AGENTS OF POLITICAL INCLUSION

1. Adade Mitchell Wheeler and Marlene Stein Wortman, *The Roads They Made: Women in Illinois History* (Chicago: Charles H. Kerr Publishing Co., 1977), pp. 64, 106; Alfreda Duster, ed., *Crusade for Justice: The Autobiography of Ida B. Wells* (Chicago: University of Chicago Press, 1970), pp. 243–245.

2. Duster, *Crusade*, pp. 244–245, 345; Wanda A. Hendricks, "Ida B. Wells-Barnett and the Alpha Suffrage Club of Chicago," in *One Woman, One Vote: Rediscovering the Woman Suffrage Movement*, ed. Marjorie Spruill Wheeler (Troutdale, Ore.: NewSage Press, 1995), pp. 263–275.

3. Ida Wells-Barnett, "How Enfranchisement Stops Lynching," *Original Rights Magazine*, June 1910, reprinted in Mildred I. Thompson, *Ida B. Wells-Barnett: An Exploratory Study of an American Black Woman, 1893–1930* (New York: Carlson Publishing, 1990), vol. 15 of *Black Women in United States History*, ed. Darlene Clark Hine, pp. 269–274.

4. Ibid.

5. Fannie Barrier Williams, "Women in Politics," *The Woman's Era*, November 1894, p. 12.

6. Ibid.

7. Elizabeth Lindsay Davis, *The Story of the Illinois Federation of Colored Women's Clubs* (Chicago, 1922), pp. 126–127; *Chicago Record-Herald*, 20 August, 22 August 1913.

8. Davis, *Illinois Federation*, p. 33.

9. Ibid., p. 34; Darlene Clark Hine, ed., *Black Women in America: An Historical Encyclopedia* (New York: Carlson Publishing, 1993), s.v. "Hallie Quinn Brown," by Vivian Njeri Fisher; Cynthia Neverdon-Morton, *Afro-American Women of the South and the Advancement of the Race, 1895–1925* (Knoxville: University of Tennessee Press, 1989), p. 207.

10. Elizabeth Lindsay Davis, "Votes for Philanthropy," *The Crisis* 10 (August 1915): 191.

11. Emily H. Williams, "The National Association of Colored Women," *Southern Workman*, September 1914, p. 482; Davis, *Illinois Federation*, p. 126.

12. *First Annual Report, 1913–1914, the World's Most Unique Exposition*, Illinois State Historical Library, Springfield, Illinois, pp. 1, 17, 18.

13. Ibid., pp. 23–39.

14. Ibid., pp. 11–13, 21–22.

15. Ibid., p. 19.

16. Richard S. Taylor, *Susan Lawrence* (Springfield: Office of Research and Publications, Historic Sites Division, Illinois Department of Conservation, April 1982), pp. 11, 12, 15.

17. Ibid., p. 15.

18. Ibid., pp. 7, 14, 57–59.

19. Ibid., pp. 60–61.

20. Davis, *Illinois Federation*, p. 126.

21. Duster, *Crusade for Justice*, p. 362.

22. Ibid., p. 365; Taylor, *Susan Lawrence*, pp. 60–62; Davis, *Illinois Federation*, p. 126.

23. Davis, *Illinois Federation*, pp. 62, 114–117; Anne Meis Knupfer, *Toward a Tenderer Humanity and a Nobler Womanhood: African American Women's Clubs in Turn-of-the-Century Chicago* (New York and London: New York University Press, 1996), pp. 155–156.

24. Adade Mitchell Wheeler, "Conflict in the Illinois Woman Suffrage Movement of 1913," *Journal of the Illinois State Historical Society* 76 (Summer 1983): 106, 110; Anne Firor Scott and Andrew MacKay Scott, *One Half the*

People: The Fight for Woman Suffrage (Philadelphia: Lippincott, 1975; reprint ed., Urbana: University of Illinois Press, 1982), pp. 116–121; John D. Buenker, "Illinois and the Four Progressive-Era Amendments to the United States Constitution," *Illinois Historical Journal* 80 (Winter 1987): 222–225.

25. Carrie Chapman Catt and Nettie Rogers Shuler, *Woman Suffrage and Politics: The Inner Story of the Suffrage Movement* (Seattle: University of Washington Press, 1969), p. 193; "The Suffrage Conquest of Illinois," *Literary Digest* 46 (June 1913): 1409; Buenker, "Illinois and the Four Progressive-Era Amendments," pp. 210–211; Wheeler, "Conflict in the Illinois Woman Suffrage Movement of 1913," p. 97.

26. Davis, *Illinois Federation*, pp. 19, 29–30.

27. *The Forum*, 7 April 1917.

28. *The Forum*, 28 October 1916.

29. Davis, *Illinois Federation*, pp. 80–81.

30. Ibid., pp. 76–77.

31. *Thirteenth Census of the United States, 1910*, p. 505; *Fourteenth Census of the United States, 1920*, p. 274.

32. Ford S. Black, *Black's Blue Book: Directory of Chicago's Active Colored People and Guide to Their Activities, 1917* (Chicago: Ford S. Black, 1917), pp. 55–57; Ford S. Black, *Black's Blue Book: Business and Professional Directory* (Chicago: Ford S. Black, 1916), p. 55.

33. Black, *Black's Blue Book: Directory of Chicago's Active Colored People*, pp. 55–57; *Chicago Defender,* 21 February 1914; Black, *Black's Blue Book: Business and Professional Directory*, p. 55.

34. *The Broad Ax*, 20 June 1914.

35. Duster, *Crusade for Justice*, p. 345.

36. *The Afro-American Ledger* (Baltimore), 11 January 1913.

37. Katherine E. Williams, "The Alpha Suffrage Club," *Half Century Magazine*, September 1916, p. 12; *Alpha Suffrage Record*, 18 March 1914 [1915], Ida B. Wells-Barnett Papers, Joseph Regenstein Library, University of Chicago, Chicago, Illinois.

38. *The Broad Ax*, 10, 17 October 1914; 28 November 1914.

39. *Chicago Daily Tribune*, 4 March 1913.

40. Ibid.

41. Ibid.

42. Ibid.

43. Ibid.

44. Ibid.

45. Ibid.

46. Ibid.

47. Ibid.

48. Catt and Shuler, *Woman Suffrage and Politics*, pp. 241–242; Rosalyn Terborg-Penn, "Discrimination against Afro-American Women in the Women's Movement, 1830–1920," in *The Afro-American Woman: Struggles and Images*, ed. Rosalyn Terborg-Penn and Sharon Harley (New York: Kennikat Press, 1978), pp. 24–25; Aileen S. Kraditor, *The Ideas of the Woman Suffrage Movement, 1880–1920* (New York: Columbia University Press, 1965; reprint ed., New York: W. W. Norton, 1981), pp. 212–218; Steven Buechler, *The*

Transformation of the Woman Suffrage Movement: The Case of Illinois, 1850–1920 (New Brunswick, N.J.: Rutgers University Press, 1986), pp. 149–150, 226; Wheeler, "Conflict in the Illinois Woman Suffrage Movement of 1913," p. 106; Marjorie Spruill Wheeler, *New Women of the New South: The Leaders of the Woman Suffrage Movement in the Southern States* (New York: Oxford University Press, 1993); *Chicago Daily Tribune*, 3 March, 4 March, 1913.

49. Duster, *Crusade*, pp. 243–245.

50. *The Broad Ax*, 29 March 1913.

SIX. THE POLITICS OF RACE

1. Fannie Barrier Williams, "Colored Women of Chicago," *Southern Workman* 63 (October 1914): 566.

2. *Thirteenth Census of the United States, 1910:* The breakdown of the population was Native White–native parentage, 11,642; Native White–foreign or mixed, 11,225; Foreign-Born White, 9,118; Negro, 10,709; Indian, Chinese, Japanese, and all other, 107. Yearly census data for the area were kept by the *Chicago Daily News.* Corrections and updates can be found in James Langland, M. A. Compiler, *The Chicago Daily News Almanac and Year-Book for 1916* (Chicago: Chicago Daily News Co., 1915), pp. 585, 586. Also see Allan H. Spear, *Black Chicago: The Making of a Negro Ghetto, 1890–1920* (Chicago: University of Chicago Press, 1967), pp. 15 and 122, for population data from 1915.

3. See Wanda A. Hendricks, "'Vote for the Advantage of Ourselves and Our Race': The Election of the First Black Alderman in Chicago," *Illinois Historical Journal* 87 (Autumn 1994): 171–184.

4. Charles Branham, "Black Chicago: Accommodationist Politics before the Great Migration," in *The Ethnic Frontier: Essays in the History of Group Survival in Chicago and the Midwest*, ed. Melvin G. Holli and Peter d'A. Jones (Grand Rapids, Mich.: William B. Eerdmans Publishing Co., 1977), pp. 212–223, 241; Harold F. Gosnell, *Negro Politicians: The Rise of Negro Politics in Chicago* (Chicago: University of Chicago Press, 1935), p. 375; Spear, *Black Chicago*, pp. 125–126. Also see Dianne M. Pinderhughes, *Race and Ethnicity in Chicago Politics: A Reexamination of Pluralist Theory* (Urbana: University of Illinois Press, 1987), for an overview of Chicago politics.

5. Gosnell, *Negro Politicians*, pp. 82–83, 153–162; Spear, *Black Chicago*, p. 78. Also see D. A. Bethea, compiler, *Colored People's Blue Book and Business Directory of Chicago, Ill.* (Chicago: Celebrity Printing Co., 1905), pp. 127–129, Illinois State Historical Library, Springfield, Illinois, for a listing of Wright as a lawyer in Chicago.

6. *Thirteenth Census*, vol. II, p. 512.

7. St. Clair Drake and Horace R. Clayton, *Black Metropolis: A Study of Negro Life in a Northern City* (New York: Harcourt, Brace and Co., 1945; revised ed., New York: Harcourt, Brace and World, 1970), pp. 342–349; Gosnell, *Negro Politicians*, pp. 74–75; Spear, *Black Chicago*, pp. 122–123.

8. *Chicago Defender*, 29 January, 12 March, 2 April 1910; see also Mary E. Stovall, "The *Chicago Defender* in the Progressive Era," *Illinois Historical*

Journal 83 (1990): 159–172, for a discussion of editor Robert Abbott's contribution to black equality through his newspaper.

9. *Chicago Defender,* 29 January, 12 March, 2 April 1910.

10. *The Broad Ax,* 26 March, 9 April 1910; Gosnell, *Negro Politicians,* p. 156.

11. Gosnell, *Negro Politicians,* pp. 163–174; Spear, *Black Chicago,* pp. 122–123; Pinderhughes, *Race and Ethnicity,* p. 25; *Chicago Daily News Almanac and Year-Book for 1913* (Chicago: Chicago Daily News Co., 1912), p. 481. Wright's primary defeat opened the door to victory for the machine candidate. The final vote was Hugh Norris, Republican, 5,356; Raymond T. O'Keefe, Democrat, 1,603; George W. Doolittle, Progressive, 113; A. C. Harms, Socialist, 328; P. O. Jones, Independent, 476.

12. John D. Buenker, "Illinois and the Four Progressive-Era Amendments to the United States Constitution," *Illinois Historical Journal* 80 (Winter 1987): 210–227; Adade Mitchell Wheeler, "Conflict in the Illinois Woman Suffrage Movement of 1913," *Journal of the Illinois State Historical Society* 76 (Summer 1983): 65–114. See also *The Chicago Daily News Almanac and Year-Book for 1916,* pp. 585, 586; Spear, *Black Chicago,* pp. 15, 122.

13. *The Broad Ax,* 17 January 1914; Gosnell, *Negro Politicians,* p. 74.

14. Alfreda Duster, ed., *Crusade for Justice: The Autobiography of Ida B. Wells* (Chicago: University of Chicago Press, 1970), p. 346; Paula Giddings, *When and Where I Enter: The Impact of Black Women on Race and Sex in America* (New York: William Morrow and Co., 1984), pp. 119–121.

15. Williams, "Colored Women of Chicago," p. 566.

16. Duster, *Crusade,* p. 346; *The Chicago Daily News Almanac and Year-Book for 1915* (Chicago: Chicago Daily News Co., 1914), p. 632, Chicago Municipal Library, Chicago, Illinois.

17. Duster, *Crusade,* p. 346; *Chicago Defender,* 21 February 1914.

18. *The Broad Ax,* 21 February 1914; Elizabeth Lindsay Davis, *The Story of the Illinois Federation of Colored Women's Clubs* (Chicago, 1922), pp. 26, 60.

19. *The Broad Ax,* 21 February 1914.

20. *The Broad Ax,* 14 March 1914.

21. Spear, *Black Chicago,* pp. 43, 79, 82–83; *The Broad Ax,* 7 March 1914; Gosnell, *Negro Politicians,* pp. 67, 128.

22. Duster, *Crusade,* p. 346; *Chicago Defender,* 21 February 1914.

23. *Chicago Defender,* 21 February 1914.

24. Spear, *Black Chicago,* pp. 81–82; *Chicago Defender,* 7 March 1914.

25. *The Chicago Daily News Almanac and Year-Book for 1915,* p. 632; Spear, *Black Chicago,* p. 123; *Chicago Defender,* 21 February 1914; *The Broad Ax,* 28 February 1914.

26. *Chicago Defender,* 21 February and 7 March 1914; *The Broad Ax,* 17 October 1914.

27. Spear, *Black Chicago,* pp. 123–124; Duster, *Crusade,* p. 346.

28. Duster, *Crusade,* pp. 346–348; Gosnell, *Negro Politicians,* p. 170.

29. See Nell Irvin Painter, *Exodusters: Black Migration to Kansas after Reconstruction* (New York: Alfred A. Knopf, 1977; reprint ed., New York: W. W. Norton and Co., 1992), for a discussion of African American life in Kansas in the post-Reconstruction era. She suggests that geographical change

did not always alter the racial posture of whites. Nonetheless, African Americans, lured by the idea that life would be better, continued to leave the South.

30. Gosnell, *Negro Politicians*, pp. 163–195; Spear, *Black Chicago*, pp. 78–79; "Congressman DePriest Specialized in Being 1st," *Sun-Times*, 22 February 1990, African American Clippings File, Chicago Municipal Reference Library, Chicago, microfilm; Jim Bowman, "Oscar S. DePriest: Chicago's First Black Alderman Goes to Washington," *Chicago Tribune Magazine*, 15 January 1984, African American Clippings File, Chicago Municipal Reference Library, Chicago, microfilm.

31. Spear, *Black Chicago*, pp. 122–123.

32. Gosnell, *Negro Politicians*, pp. 30, 70, 104–105; Pinderhughes, *Race and Ethnicity*, pp. 77–78.

33. *Chicago Defender*, 16 January 1915.

34. Mildred Thompson, "Ida B. Wells-Barnett: An Exploratory Study of an American Black Woman, 1893–1930" (Ph.D. dissertation, George Washington University, 1979), pp. 199–200.

35. *Suffrage Record*, 18 March 1914 [1915].

36. Ibid.; *Chicago Defender*, 27 February 1915.

37. *Chicago Defender*, 16 January 1915.

38. Ibid., 27 February 1915; *The Chicago Daily News Almanac and Year-Book for 1916*, p. 567.

39. Duster, *Crusade*, p. 348.

40. *The Chicago Daily News Almanac and Year-Book for 1916*, pp. 567, 591; Gosnell, *Negro Politicians*, p. 171.

41. *The Forum*, 17 April 1915.

42. *The Chicago Daily News Almanac and Year-Book for 1916*, pp. 567, 591; Gosnell, *Negro Politicians*, p. 171.

43. Oscar DePriest, "Chicago and Woman's Suffrage," *The Crisis* 10 (August 1915): 179.

44. Pinderhughes, *Race and Ethnicity*, pp. 95–96.

SEVEN. THE GREAT MIGRATION,
RACE WOMEN, AND THE END OF AN ERA

1. *Fourteenth Census of the United States, 1920*, p. 244.

2. Elizabeth Lindsay Davis, *The Story of the Illinois Federation of Colored Women's Clubs* (Chicago, 1922), p. 38.

3. See, for example, James R. Grossman, *Land of Hope: Chicago, Black Southerners, and the Great Migration* (Chicago: University of Chicago Press, 1989). See also St. Clair Drake and Horace R. Clayton, *Black Metropolis: A Study of Negro Life in a Northern City* (New York: Harcourt, Brace and Co., 1945; revised ed., New York: Harcourt, Brace and World, 1970); "Documents: Letters of Negro Migrants of 1916–1918," *Journal of Negro History* 4 (July 1917): 290–340.

4. *Fourteenth Census*, p. 244; Donald F. Tingley, *The Structuring of a State: The History of Illinois, 1899 to 1928* (Urbana: University of Illinois Press, 1980), p. 281.

5. *Thirteenth Census of the United States, 1910*, p. 504; *Fourteenth Census*, pp. 244, 261, 262.

6. Darlene Clark Hine, "Black Migration to the Urban Midwest: The Gender Dimension, 1915–1945," in *The Great Migration in Historical Perspective: New Dimensions of Race, Class, and Gender,* ed. Joe William Trotter, Jr. (Bloomington: Indiana University Press, 1991), p. 132.

7. *Thirteenth Census,* p. 477; *Fourteenth Census,* pp. 244, 246, 261.

8. See, for example, Joanne J. Meyerowitz, *Women Adrift: Independent Wage Earners in Chicago, 1880–1930* (Chicago: University of Chicago Press, 1988), pp. 10–11; Florette Henri, *Black Migration: Movement North, 1900–1920* (New York: Anchor Press, 1976), pp. 95–96; Jacqueline Jones, *Labor of Love, Labor of Sorrow: Black Women, Work and the Family from Slavery to the Present* (New York: Vintage Books, 1986), pp. 152–195.

9. Hine, "Black Migration to the Urban Midwest," p. 132.

10. "Documents: Letters of Negro Migrants of 1916–1918," p. 316.

11. Ibid., p. 317.

12. Ibid., p. 315.

13. Ibid., p. 316.

14. Ibid.

15. Ibid., p. 318.

16. Meyerowitz, *Women Adrift,* p. 5.

17. Davis, *Illinois Federation,* pp. 7, 8, 21–22.

18. Ford S. Black, *Black's Blue Book: Directory of Chicago's Active Colored People and Guide to Their Activities* (Chicago: Ford S. Black, 1917), pp. 55–58.

19. Ibid., p. 68.

20. Davis, *Illinois Federation,* p. 14.

21. Arvah E. Strickland, *History of the Chicago Urban League* (Urbana: University of Illinois Press, 1966), pp. 44–55.

22. Ibid., pp. 29–30.

23. Ibid., p. 44.

24. Davis, *Illinois Federation,* p. 38.

25. Ibid., pp. 38–39; Allan H. Spear, *Black Chicago: The Making of a Negro Ghetto, 1890–1920* (Chicago: University of Chicago Press, 1967), pp. 100–101, 174.

26. Davis, *Illinois Federation,* p. 55.

27. Ibid., pp. 53, 115–116.

28. Ibid., pp. 67, 118.

29. Ibid., pp. 4, 37, 62, 97, 128; Spear, *Black Chicago,* p. 174. See, for example, Darlene Clark Hine, *Black Women in White: Racial Conflict and Cooperation in the Nursing Profession, 1890–1950* (Bloomington: Indiana University Press, 1989), for an overview of health care provided by black women.

30. Davis, *Illinois Federation,* p. 127; Adade Wheeler Mitchell and Marlene Stein Wortman, *The Roads They Made: Women in Illinois History* (Chicago: Charles H. Kerr Publishing Co., 1977), p. 109.

31. Harold F. Gosnell, *Negro Politicians: The Rise of Negro Politics in Chicago* (Chicago: University of Chicago Press, 1935), pp. 172–176; Dianne M. Pinderhughes, *Race and Ethnicity in Chicago Politics: A Reexamination of Pluralist Theory* (Urbana: University of Illinois Press, 1987), p. 149.

32. Gosnell, *Negro Politicians,* pp. 199–200.

33. Douglas Bukowski, "Big Bill Thompson: The 'Model' Politician,"

in *The Mayors: The Chicago Political Tradition,* ed. Paul M. Green and Melvin G. Holli (Carbondale: Southern Illinois University Press, 1987), p. 71; Gosnell, *Negro Politicians,* p. 39; Pinderhughes, *Race and Ethnicity,* pp. 95, 110–111.

34. Gosnell, *Negro Politicians,* pp. 180–187; "Fifty Year History of Chicago and Northern District Association," Illinois Association of Club Women and Girls, Inc., Papers, Illinois State Historical Library, Springfield, Illinois, pp. 75–76.

35. *Fourteenth Census,* p. 277.

36. Elliot Rudwick, *Race Riot at East St. Louis, July 2, 1917* (Carbondale: Southern Illinois University Press, 1964; reprint ed., New York: Atheneum, 1972), pp. 5–15; Tingley, *Structuring of a State,* pp. 287–290.

37. Rudwick, *Race Riot,* pp. 16–17, 27–35.

38. Ibid., pp. 38–57.

39. Ibid., pp. 154–156; Tingley, *Structuring of a State,* p. 308; Nancy J. Weiss, *The National Urban League, 1910–1940* (New York: Oxford University Press, 1974), pp. 141–144; Davis, *Illinois Federation,* pp. 24, 127.

40. *Chicago Daily Tribune,* 7 July 1919. See also Alfreda Duster, ed., *Crusade for Justice: The Autobiography of Ida B. Wells* (Chicago: University of Chicago Press, 1970), pp. 383–395.

41. John Hope Franklin and Alfred A. Moss, Jr., *From Slavery to Freedom: A History of African Americans,* 7th ed. (New York: McGraw-Hill, 1994), p. 349.

42. William M. Tuttle, Jr., *Race Riot: Chicago in the Red Summer of 1919* (New York: Atheneum, 1974), pp. 3–10, 32–66, 242. See also Carl Sandburg, *The Chicago Race Riots, July 1919* (New York: Harcourt, Brace and Howe, 1919; reprint ed., New York: Harcourt, Brace and World, 1969); The Chicago Commission on Race Relations, *The Negro in Chicago: A Study of Race Relations and a Race Riot* (Chicago: University of Chicago Press, 1922).

43. Davis, *Illinois Federation,* pp. 23, 40; Chicago Commission on Race Relations, *The Negro in Chicago,* pp. 494–495.

44. Chicago Commission on Race Relations, *The Negro in Chicago,* pp. 494–495.

45. Ibid.

46. Duster, *Crusade,* p. 366.

47. Davis, *Illinois Federation,* pp. 80–81.

48. Ibid., p. 35.

49. Ibid., pp. 35, 63, 81.

50. Ibid., pp. 35, 79, 89, 90. The work of Illinois women in World War I was paralleled in other areas. For Southern black women during the war, see William J. Breen, "Black Women and the Great War: Mobilization and Reform in the South," *Journal of Southern History* 44 (August 1978): 421–440.

51. Davis, *Illinois Federation,* pp. 8, 14, 28.

52. Ibid., pp. 53, 68.

53. Ibid., pp. 35, 68.

54. Ibid., pp. 12, 21–22, 29–30.

55. Ibid., pp. 62–63.

56. Henri, *Black Migration*, p. 313.

57. Ibid., pp. 316–317.

58. See Kathleen M. Blee, *Women of the Klan: Racism and Gender in the 1920s* (Berkeley: University of California Press, 1991).

59. Allain Locke, ed., *The New Negro* (New York: Albert and Charles Boni, 1925; reprint ed., New York: Atheneum, 1969), p. 12.

60. See Robert A. Hill, ed., *The Marcus Garvey and Universal Negro Improvement Association Papers*, 6 vols. (Berkeley: University of California Press, 1989); Lawrence W. Levine, "Marcus Garvey and the Politics of Revitalization," in *Black Leaders of the Twentieth Century*, ed. John Hope Franklin and August Meier (Chicago: University of Illinois Press, 1982), pp. 105–138.

61. Tingley, *Structuring of a State*, p. 309.

62. Duster, *Crusade*, pp. 380–381; Hill, *Marcus Garvey Papers*, vol. 1, pp. 328–331.

63. Duster, *Crusade*, p. 381.

64. Davis, *Illinois Federation*, p. 25.

65. Ibid., p. 128.

CONCLUSION

1. Elizabeth Lindsay Davis, *The Story of the Illinois Federation of Colored Women's Clubs* (Chicago, 1922), p. 106.

2. Fannie Barrier Williams, "Colored Women of Chicago," *The Southern Workman* 63 (October 1914): 566; Alfreda Duster, ed., *Crusade for Justice: The Autobiography of Ida B. Wells* (Chicago: University of Chicago Press, 1970), p. 346.

INDEX

Wanda A. Hendricks is Assistant Professor of History at Arizona State University, where she teaches courses on African American history. Her publications include articles and essays in *One Woman, One Vote: Rediscovering the Woman Suffrage Movement; African American Orators: A Bio-Critical Sourcebook;* and the *Illinois Historical Journal.*

The Sesquicentennial History of Illinois

Published for the

ILLINOIS SESQUICENTENNIAL COMMISSION

and the

ILLINOIS STATE HISTORICAL SOCIETY

by the

UNIVERSITY OF ILLINOIS PRESS

Urbana   Chicago   London

The Structuring of a State: The History of Illinois, 1899 to 1928

DONALD F. TINGLEY

LIBRARY OF CONGRESS CATALOGING IN PUBLICATION DATA

Tingley, Donald Fred, 1922–
The structuring of a State.

(The Sesquicentennial history of Illinois; v. 5)
Bibliography: p. 397
Includes index.
1. Illinois—History—1865–   I. Title.
II. Series.
F546.T56   977.3'04   79-14964
ISBN 0-252-00736-0

Contents

Preface

The history of Illinois is essentially the history of the United States. The politics, industrial growth, labor struggles, and cultural achievements of Illinois parallel those of the nation. Since state and local history can degenerate into antiquarianism unless care is taken to relate the specific to the general, I have attempted to show these relationships. Yet Illinois does have unique qualities. It is as different from California as Maine is from Mississippi, and it also differs from its Midwestern neighbors. Part of this difference comes from the great diversity of Illinois's resources and people.

Since 1900, historians and their readers have worried because history seemed inordinately concerned with politics. The need to put politics in perspective by showing greater concern for social and cultural history has been asserted in almost every journal and textbook on historical method. Historians have long noted the need for history from the ground up—for history of the real people of the world. I have tried to redress this imbalance by including material on what people were thinking and doing. The social and cultural sides of Illinois history must be examined to gain a true picture of the state. Many will relate to the statement of Finley Peter Dunne, Chicago writer, through his character Mr. Dooley: "I know histhry isn't true, Hinnissy, because it ain't like what I see ivry day in Halsted Sthreet. If any wan comes along with a histhry of Greece or Rome that'll show me th' people fightin', makin' love, gettin' marrid, owin' th' grocery man an' bein' without hard coal, I'll believe they was a Greece or Rome but not befure. Historyans is like doctors. They are always lookin' f'r symptoms. Those iv them that writes about their own times examines the toungue an' feels th' pulse an' makes the wrong diagnosis. Th' other kind of histhry is a post mortem examination. It tells ye what a country died iv. But I'd like to know what it lived iv."

As a lifelong resident of Illinois I am more inclined to be proud that Carl Sandburg, Benny Goodman, or John Walker came from my state than that Len Small, William Hale Thompson, or James Hamilton Lewis resided within its borders, but all six are important and each has his place in this book.

This project was financed by the Illinois Sesquicentennial Commission. The late Paul Angle, then director of historical publications for the commission, gave me remarkable aid and comfort, including some valuable short courses in historical writing. Eastern Illinois University provided a research grant and a reduced load for one year. The libraries of Eastern Illinois University (EIU) and the University of Illinois at Urbana were of great help, especially in dealing with some complex interlibrary loan problems. Much of the research for the volume was done at the Illinois State Historical Library and the photographs are credited to the Historical Library unless otherwise noted. William Keller, Sandra Stark, the late Paul Spence, Janice Petterchak, and Al von Behren of that library should be singled out for the special help they rendered. Graduate assistants in the EIU department of history, particularly Richard Morton, Mary Ellen Boyd, and Robert Gerling, aided with research. A legion of student typists have worked on the manuscript. Joyce Maurer deserves special thanks for typing the final drafts of the text, as does Mary Pearson for typing the bibliography. Catherine Cureton and Nancy Krueger of the University of Illinois Press were always helpful and saved me from many errors. Any errors of omission or judgment are my sole responsibility.

Donald F. Tingley

1

The State of the State: Illinois in 1900

As the nineteenth century closed, the citizens of Illinois could count great economic and population growth among their achievements. In the previous thirty-five years, Illinois, like the United States, had moved from a primarily rural, agricultural society to an urbanized, industrial one. Although the most casual observer could detect the crudities still apparent in politics, business, and society, change was in the air. New leaders appeared, and the new industrialists and politicians, although not always virtuous, exhibited a less selfish side than had their fathers. Poverty and social injustice contrasted with great wealth, but reformers with remedies appeared on the scene.

As January 1, 1900, approached, citizens argued about whether the new century started then or would actually begin on January 1, 1901. The *Chicago Tribune* took a middle-of-the-road stand with a cartoon showing Father Time looking at a sign, "Is '99 or 00 the end?" The caption read, "Father Time—'What Fools These Mortals Be.'"[1] The *Quincy Whig* believed that the new century would begin in 1901.[2] In any case, elaborate celebrations commemorated the beginning of the new year if not the new century. In Springfield the celebration reached a climax at the reception held at the executive mansion by Governor and Mrs. John R. Tanner. Holly and smilax, set off with scarlet flowers, decorated the mansion. In the state dining room, ropes of green dipped from each corner of the ceiling, meeting in the center over the mahogany table. Silver and cut glass covered the lace cloth. Mrs. Tanner wore a "white panne satin studded with French Crystals" as she and the governor received at the rear of the grand hall, while an orchestra played in the gallery at the second-floor landing.[3]

Earlier in the day, the governor greeted state employees and officers of the Illinois National Guard at the Leland Hotel. While there, he put in a surprise appearance at a dinner for employees of the *Illinois State Journal*. Asked to speak, he said that it was gratifying to see employer and employees "sitting at festal board" together because it was important for capital and labor to realize their mutual dependence. The governor added that if everyone was worth $100,000, no one would want to work for $1 or $2 per day, and everybody would have to do their own work. Labor was entitled to fair reward but capital deserved a reasonable return too. Having delivered this bit of orthodoxy, he wished the diners a happy new year and returned to the mansion.[4]

Elsewhere in the capital, Mrs. Logan Hay and her sister-in-law, Mrs. Stuart Brown, social arbiters of Springfield, received at their home. Others enjoyed parties, family reunions, balls, and dances. Several hundred young people of Springfield spent the afternoon and evening skating at Reservoir Park. Theatergoers viewed an operetta, "By the Sad Sea Waves," at Chatterton's Opera House. The *Journal* reported that the new year had "slipped in quietly" with few whistles blown.[5]

In Quincy, Mr. and Mrs. Frank H. Weems and their son, Milton, ushered in the new year with the greatest social event of the year. They held an afternoon reception and later a masked ball at the Baldwin Park Clubhouse. Three double arches of green decorated the clubhouse, and at the far end of the hall there was a large "W" woven in green with "1900" immediately below it. Holly, mistletoe, ilex, and rare vines were lit by arches of electric lights encased in Japanese globes and ornate lanterns. Dancers were dressed as Indians, dominoes, students in cap and gown, knights, school-girls, Chinese, one of Theodore Roosevelt's Rough Riders, and Santa Claus.[6]

Chicago greeted the new year with little noise, partly because of the cold weather. But a chorus of guns, revolvers, steam whistles, foghorns, fire tugs, locomotive whistles, and church bells sounded at midnight. The *Chicago Inter-Ocean* found it "rather half-hearted,"[7] but the *Tribune* thought there was too much "hideous din" and not enough of the genteel custom of calls of goodwill on New Year's Day.[8] The wealthier people of the Near South Side gave numerous parties. Harold Fowler McCormick and his wife, the former Edith Rockefeller, planned a large reception but recalled the invitations because of illness in the family and were able to receive only a few guests for a musical program. The cotillion of brother Cyrus Hall McCormick went off as scheduled.[9]

The Volunteers of America put on a meal of roast beef, turkey, and pork for a horde of "nervous, laughing, chafing arabs of the street" who ate as "if it were the first meal they had tasted for days." The band played to drown out the noise, and later in the day the Volunteers carried baskets of food to the poor. In the back room of his establishment, Chicago Avenue saloonkeeper Robert Briden fed turkey to fifty-seven prisoners just released from the Chicago Avenue Station. After the meal, the host made a speech in which he told his guests "of many ways by which they might better themselves."[10]

Looking back, the editor of the *Evening Citizen* (Cairo) found that the preceding twelve months had not been unusual but had been a year of "toil rather than achievement." There had been business prosperity with few calamities such as fires, failures, or disasters. The most exciting events of the year had been the visit of the gunboat *Nashville,* the assembly of the Illinois Medical Association in May, and the second annual street fair in October, all of which had "brought Cairo to prominence before the world."[11] Chicago reported prosperity for business, and the *Inter-Ocean* remarked, "Rarely have the most sanguine hopes and predictions found ampler realization." Most observers predicted continuation of the prosperity.[12]

The *Inter-Ocean* editorialized on the progress of the nineteenth century, noting that the United States had grown from sixteen states to forty-five and from a population of 5,000,000 to 75,000,000, "with the questions of a hundred years ago answered, and with the problems solved." The editor reported ethical and political progress as great as that in business and trade, and found the nation "as mighty in the arts of peace as in the achievements of war." He predicted that on January 1, 2000, the United States would be the most powerful nation in the world and the arbiter of the destinies of nations if it heeded the lessons of the previous century.[13]

Illinois, too, had grown. In fact it had undergone a drastic change in character by 1900. The twelfth census showed that for the first time more than half of the people of the state lived in towns of over 2,500 population. Illinois had become an urban state; the census showed that 54.3 percent of the 4,821,550 people lived in the cities, the largest of which was, of course, Chicago, with a population of 1,698,575. In any kind of statistical study, Chicago outdistanced its nearest competitor in the state. The next largest city, Peoria, was a poor second with a population of 56,000. The next ten cities were, in decreasing order of size, Quincy, Springfield, Rockford, East St. Louis, Joliet, Aurora, Bloomington, Elgin, Decatur, and Danville. All were in the northern half of the state except East St. Louis, which owed its growth, in part, to its neighbor across the Mississippi. Thus the major part of the population had also shifted to the north.[14]

The composition of the population at the turn of the century had changed. Most Illinoisians were now native-born Americans; less than 1,000,000, or about one-fifth of the total, were born abroad, although a sizable group had foreign-born parents. About three-quarters of the foreign-born lived in the cities. The Indian population hardly existed by this time, and there were only 1,503 Chinese and 80 Japanese. Perhaps the most striking fact, however, was that there were only 85,078 black persons in the state. Although some Blacks had resided in Illinois since slavery, and although contractors had brought in considerable numbers from the South to work on projects such as the drainage canal, the great migration of Blacks out of the South in search of better economic, social, political, and educational opportunities had not yet begun.[15]

Industry brought about the urbanization of Illinois. The total value of manufactured products produced in 1899 reached an astounding $1,250,000,000. Already Illinois could have boasted of being the "hog butcher of the world." Its packing plants produced 22.9 percent of the state's industrial total, with an annual product valued at $287,000,000. The packers employed 27,851 persons —7.1 percent of the work force of the state. The industry, proud of its efficiency, proclaimed accurately that it used all of the pig except the squeal. The census report for 1900 took note of this characteristic of the industry:

> Attention was early concentrated upon the by-products, and now the entire animal is utilized. The flesh is sold as meat, the blood is dried and sold for clarifying purposes, the entrails are cleaned and made into sausage casings, the hoofs are turned into neat's foot oil, the parings of the hoofs, hides, and bones are converted into glue, the finest of the fats are turned into butterine, lard, oils and the finest tallow, the cruder fats are made into soap grease, the hides are marketed for the manufacture of leather, the bones are used for the making of knife handles and for other purposes, the switches and tail ends are sold to hair mattress makers, and the short hair which cannot be dried and curled for sale to felt makers.

Chicago packed nearly 90 percent of the meat for Illinois and had no rival in the nation in this industry.[16] Five families, the Armours, the Swifts, the Cudahys, the Morrises, and the Wilsons, controlled most of the packing business. But statistics alone do not tell the story of an industry. Rudyard Kipling, in his unflattering description of Chicago, described the filth and gore of the killing floors.[17] As Upton Sinclair would soon show, the packers prepared meat for public consumption in unbelievably unsanitary conditions. The plants of "Packing Town" poured their refuse into the stagnant waters of Bubbly Creek, which ran alongside the yards and polluted the air with poisonous, gray smoke that darkened the city. The packers insisted on efficiency and thrift in the management of their plants. Gustavus Swift, in frock coat and cowhide boots, visited almost daily the point where the sewer from his plant dumped into Bubbly Creek, and woe to the superintendent who allowed even a trace of fat to go out through the sewer.[18] Packinghouse workers averaged a sixty-four-hour week in 1899 and were paid less than $500 per year.[19] These economies enabled a downtown store in Chicago to sell a Swift's Premium or Armour Star ham for 10.5 cents per pound, but few of the workers of the packinghouse could afford to buy it.[20]

Foundry and machine shop products constituted the second greatest industry. Small shops scattered throughout the state contributed an output of more than $63,000,000.[21] The closely related steel industry ranked third. Steel production grew in Illinois because of the ease with which Lake Superior ores could be brought by ship to the end of Lake Michigan to meet the trainloads of bituminous coal from the South. The first iron mill had been built on the north branch of the Chicago River in 1857. Later the industry expanded to the south side of the city.

Most of the steel production in Illinois in 1900 came from Judge Elbert H. Gary's Federal Steel, which he had put together through a succession of consolidations. Soon, with J. P. Morgan's help, Gary would add it to the Carnegie interests in the East to put together the gigantic United States Steel Corporation. Inland Steel was in production in South Chicago and across the state line in Indiana. Granite City Steel had already made a beginning across the river from St. Louis.

By 1900 the mills turned out steel products valued at more than $60,000,000. Chicago was the third city in the nation in the production of iron and steel, and Joliet was eighth.[22] Some have described the use of iron and steel as a barometer of civilization. If this is the case, civilization was indeed on the rise, but (as in so many other areas of production) the workers paid a high price. The standard work week at the blast furnaces was eighty-four hours.

The distilleries gave Peoria its most important industry. The whiskey distillers prospered because of the location of the city in the midst of the Illinois corn fields, adjacent to an abundant supply of cold water (for cooling the mash), and close to the coal fields. By 1900 Peoria ranked first in the nation in this industry. Illinois whiskey nearly equaled in value the steel production of the state.[23]

In 1900 the production of agricultural implements rose, particularly in Moline and Chicago, to more than $42,000,000. Among these manufacturers the McCormick and Deering interests in Chicago, the Deere Company, and the Moline Plow Company in Moline produced the most. Situated in the heartland of agricultural production, near the sources of iron and steel, Illinois had long been important in this industry.[24] Ranking in the top dozen Illinois industries were printing and publishing, men's clothing, flouring and grist mills, and the manufacture of railroad cars, glucose, furniture, and dairy products (cheese, butter, and condensed milk).[25]

Although the number of farms and farmers was declining in 1900, nearly half of the people lived in rural settings and more men made their living from farming than from any other industry. More than a quarter-million farms produced grain and livestock to the amount of $345,649,611, a sum greater than that originating in any other single industry.[26] Machinery revolutionized farming. Due to mass production the price of tools that the farmer used was quite cheap. In 1900 a twelve-inch walking plow sold in Springfield for $10, and such a plow, pulled by two horses, turned the soil of much of the ten million acres planted in corn the year before. Other tools sold for similarly low prices; the farmer could buy a gang plow for $47, a corn planter for $32, a disc for $20, or a ninety-tooth harrow or riding cultivator for $14.50.[27]

It is possible to describe the average farmer of 1900. His farm contained 124.2 acres, with a value per farm of $7,588. This sum represented $5,732 invested in land, $952 in buildings, $170 in implements, and $734 in livestock.[28] The statistical farmer produced grain and livestock worth $1,300, of which $300 represented grain fed to the livestock. This left him about $1,000 in cash. The farmer and his family supplied most of the labor for producing crops. Fertilizer was virtually unknown beyond the manures produced on the farm. The Illinois farmer in 1900 paid only $3 for fertilizer, a kind of tribute to the marvelous fertility of Illinois soil but a fact which explains why the farmer could boast of only forty bushels to the acre in his corn crop and about thirteen bushels to the acre in his wheat.[29]

The products of Illinois farms included a wide range, but more than 80 percent of the farmer's income came from livestock, hay, and grain. Illinois farmers planted about 10,000,000 acres in corn, nearly 2,000,000 acres in wheat, and about 4,500,000 acres in oats.[30] Illinois farmers sold some $69,000,000 worth of livestock and slaughtered another $10,000,000 worth on their farms. Thus they contributed largely to the Chicago meat-packing industry. There were more hogs and half as many cattle as people in Illinois in 1900.[31] Although the average farmer worked nearly 125 acres, many tilled less. Nearly 20,000 farmers worked farms of under twenty acres and another 40,000 ranged from twenty to fifty acres. More than 1,000 farms in Illinois in 1900 reported no cash income. On the other hand, only 6.8 percent reported a product valued at more than $2,500.[32]

Illinois did not rank high in the extractive industries. Bituminous coal, just then beginning to be used for coking and the most important of the mining industries, employed some 36,000 people and mined 32 million tons of coal. About half the counties reported some coal mining. Some cement, lead, zinc, and fluorspar were mined, but only in small quantities which, while important locally, did not contribute much to the general wealth of the state. The oil and gas industry had not yet been developed, although there were a few producing gas and oil wells in Montgomery County.[33]

As the citizens of Illinois from Chicago, Springfield, Quincy, or Centralia opened their newspapers on the first day of 1900, they found exciting political news. They had become accustomed to the idea that the United States was now an imperial power, but there was trouble in the Philippines and the English faced problems with the Boers in South Africa. The interests of the Illinois citizenry on the national and international scene were in the hands of the venerable Senator Shelby Cullom and his colleague, Senator William Mason. The good, gray, bearded Cullom, orthodox in his Republicanism, supported the policies of President William McKinley in extending the responsibilities of the United States over the world, but Mason, also a Republican, was an outspoken critic of McKinley's policies, as well as of the fight of the British against the Boers. While they expected that Democrats like William Jennings Bryan would criticize McKinley's policies, Republicans took it badly that one of their own would be so ill-advised. Mason's stand soon brought the wrath of Republican groups and newspapers down on his head. The Old Tippecanoe Republican Club of Chicago voted to demand his resignation from the Senate and expelled him from the club. Senator Mason, when informed of this development, remarked that if he had known he was a member of this organization, he would have resigned and saved them the trouble of expelling him.

Mason's nemesis in this incident was a Colonel McWhorter, who had introduced the expulsion motion. Mason said he knew McWhorter as "a professional deadbeat" and "political toucher" who had once sent a representative to ask Mason for $25. Mason had replied that he would "chip in a dollar if the colonel would take a bath," but McWhorter's representative, according to Mason, had replied that this was asking too much. Mason closed with the statement, "Meanwhile, I am for liberty and self-government in Cuba, the Philippine islands, South Africa, and Chicago, McWhorter or no McWhorter." The *Chicago Tribune* was nearly as bitter about Mason as McWhorter and the Old Tippecanoe Club but thought it was too much to hope that he would resign. The *Tribune* commented, "He will cling to his office like a child to the breast of his mother."[34]

"Uncle Joe" Cannon, not yet Speaker of the House but a veteran of more than twenty-five years of service, led the Illinois delegation in the House of Representatives. The delegation contained fourteen Republicans and eight Democrats and included William H. Lorimer, the "blond boss" of Chicago. Governor Tanner, finishing his term in the governor's mansion, had announced that he would not seek renomination. In Chicago, the office of mayor was held by a young, handsome, urbane, occasional reformer, Carter Harrison. Harrison, a Democrat, was serving his second two-year term, well on his way to matching the record of his father who had served five terms in office before being assassinated during the World's Columbian Exposition.[35]

Doubtless the best-known politician of Chicago or Illinois in 1900 was "Bathhouse" John Coughlin, who, with his diminutive colleague, Michael "Hinky Dink" Kenna, ruled Chicago's Loop and the wild area to the south which comprised the first ward. Bathhouse John, his sartorial splendor now nationally known, had recently returned from Saratoga and Gotham, where he had educated the effete East in matters of dress. He had also achieved a fraudulent fame as a writer of ballads. His first effort, "Dear Midnight of Love," came to public attention in 1900. Of his ballad he said, "It's a hummer. It's a sample of pure, high-class ballad, and is bound to be popular. There's nothing like it in print now." The editor of the *Tribune* commented wryly that this last statement was doubtless correct and suggested that the alderman should be the first to sing it in public with his "silvery tenor voice." The editor noted that although most of Bathhouse's midnight experiences had "savored of the hilarity of the saloon," the sentiment of the ballad would probably be acceptable. With tongue in cheek, the *Tribune* predicted a great literary career for Bathhouse: "It is late in his life for genius to manifest itself, but there have been such instances, and Bathhouse John may yet be known not only in modest ballads but in the higher flight of the cantata or in the imperial themes of the symphony."[36]

Bathhouse and Hinky Dink, well-known as grafters and collectors of tribute from saloonkeepers, madams, and flophouse keepers in the first ward, had helped Mayor Harrison thwart the stranglehold of Charles Tyson Yerkes on the street railways of Chicago. For this they became good friends of the mayor and could, when it was useful, pose, however unconvincingly, as reformers. The "Bath" and the "Hink" reflected much that was bad in municipal politics, but they also represented a kind of comic relief from it all, and they were no more corrupt than many of their aldermanic colleagues. For all their graft, they did feed the hungry and, for a price, looked out for the interests of their constituents. Compared with some of their successors, they were shining lights. Paul Douglas could say later that they compared pretty favorably with some of the respectable people who would not have shaken their hands.[37]

Perhaps the greatest local story at the opening of 1900 was the completion of the sanitary canal linking the South Fork of the Chicago River with the Illinois River. For decades the Chicago River, a stagnant, turgid, filthy piece of water, hardly moved. After several years of construction, the great engineer Isham Randolph completed the canal. The Illinois River towns and St. Louis howled with anguish, believing they would be inundated with Chicago garbage and sewage. To threats of legal suits Randolph asserted calmly that the moving water would soon clear itself.

As many as 15,000 men worked on the canal at the height of construction. Blacks and immigrants worked on the project at the wage of 15 cents an hour. The *Tribune* noted the wage with approval and said that the project had been possible because there had been no interference by labor unions, thus allowing "absolute free trade in labor." Citizens along the project complained of drunkenness and disorder, but this problem was alleviated by the contractors' construction of camps where the laborers lived. The contractors charged so much for room and board that the laborers had very little left to get drunk on.

Chicagoans hung over the bridges to watch the miraculous cleaning of the water. When someone caught a fish off the Wells Street bridge after a few days, it was a cause for excitement. Commented the *Tribune,* "If the water is not yet desirable as a beverage, it is at least up to the mild requirements of a Lake Michigan bullhead." Randolph, whose assurances proved to be accurate, was indeed a man to be respected.[38]

Culturally, Illinois left something to be desired, but in Chicago Theodore Thomas was conducting the symphony orchestra which he had brought to great heights; by 1900 it was possible for Chicagoans to hear first-rate classical music.[39] The opera fared less well in Chicago, and the town was defensive about this in the face of Eastern criticism. A New York company had lost money during the 1899–1900 season, and when an article appeared condemning the lack of musical taste of Chicago and its inadequate support of the company, the *Tribune* pointed with pride to the symphony and informed the East that, after all, opera had little significance in the long run.[40] The Art Institute was in its permanent home and showing many fine exhibits of painting.

Downstate, the musical fare was likely to be less stimulating. Perhaps the best program in Quincy in 1900 was by John Philip Sousa and his band in their last American performance before setting off to play in France.[41] The most popular musical entertainment seemed to be the minstrel shows, such as Harry Martell's production in Centralia, "The South Before the War." The show was said to have "Three Score Sweetest Voices in one grand swelling chorus, thirty champion buck and wing dancers" with "sensational situations, heartfelt-harmony, and realistic scenery."[42] In Quincy, John W. Sham was including Belle Davis, "The Star of Her Race," as well as "Rag time fancies, polite vaudeville, Grand opera and Coon songs as they never were sung before."[43]

The pattern for higher education in Illinois was set for the next four decades. At the University of Chicago William Rainey Harper was collecting his famous faculty, including such figures as Albert Michelson in physics, John Merle Coulter in botany, J. Lawrence Laughlin in economics, and Albion Small in sociology. President Harper announced at the beginning of 1900 that he was within

$300,000 of matching a $2,000,000 contribution by John D. Rockefeller, the most recent of several monumental gifts from that source. At the same time, Northwestern opened a drive to raise $1,650,000 for new buildings and endowment of chairs of instruction. Among the buildings listed on the program were a natural history museum, gymnasium, library, and chapel.[44] The University of Illinois, under the presidency of Andrew Sloan Draper, was shaking off the trade school image. Apparently this fact had not been communicated to Governor Tanner, because in the appropriations the previous year he had vetoed $99,000 of the building funds allocated by the legislature. Among those items vetoed was $20,000 for the library, but he allowed $75,000 for the agriculture school. The appropriation for the university's operating budget was $135,000 per year. Four normal schools were operating in 1900: Northern at DeKalb, Southern at Carbondale, Normal at Normal, and Eastern at Charleston. The legislature had appropriated funds for the Western Illinois Normal School, but a site for it had not yet been selected. The operating budgets for Northern, Normal, and Eastern were each $33,000, while Southern got $26,723.22.[45]

Athletics were beginning to intrigue the populace, and the sports page was an important part of the daily newspaper. George Huff, presiding over the program in Urbana, announced plans to build one of the largest stadiums in the country. Amos Alonzo Stagg, head football coach, was probably the most famous man at the University of Chicago. The great football teams were still in the Ivy League, but the Western Conference was organized, and Northwestern, Illinois, Chicago, Michigan, Wisconsin, and Iowa were fielding football teams. There was concern about professionalism, and the *Tribune* warned that it would ruin athletics if other branches were allowed to become professional as had baseball. Much of the athletics was in the hands of the private clubs such as the Chicago Athletic Club, where Mayor "Big Bill" Thompson got his first fame as an athlete. Otherwise, on the sports pages there were accounts of boxing, horse racing, track, poker, whist, and chess. The last three of these occupied about as much space as college athletics.[46]

These scattered observations suggest that by 1900 many of the patterns of the state were developing. As a leader in industrial and agricultural production, Illinois was producing great riches. To many in Illinois, as in the nation, this was an age of contentment and confidence and a time of well-being. In these euphoric days before world wars and the widespread use of the draft to support those wars, there was no need to be concerned about foreign affairs. Political campaigns brought controversy over the question of imperialism, which the Republicans said did not exist. On the other hand, the Democrats accused the Republicans of tyrannical imperialist policies. But by and large these problems did not affect the average person very much.

The rich had every reason for complacency with the great progress. For George M. Pullman, Gustavus Swift, Philip Danforth Armour, and others of the favored group, there was no reason to doubt that everything was bright and rosy or that the world should be grateful to them for the progress. It was easy to jump to the conclusion that wealth was the product of hard work, thrift, and loyalty to one's employer or class, and, conversely, that anyone who was poor deserved his lot because he was lazy, unthrifty, and lacking in loyalty. These ideas were common among those who had "arrived" as well as among those who hoped shortly to "arrive." To a generation that had grown up on a steady diet of Horatio Alger's books, many who had not and would never arrive at wealth and position were led to believe that they could do so by promoting these qualities.

Already in 1900, however, others were beginning to doubt the doctrines of orthodoxy as pronounced by the rich and their defenders. Labor leaders told their adherents that all was not well and that they ought to have a greater share of what they produced. Reformers of all kinds held that changes were needed. Settlement-house workers such as Jane Addams and Graham Taylor managed to make reform a respectable posture and were welcome not only among the poor people of the slums where both lived but also in the drawing rooms of millionaires. There were a few radicals (though not as many as the conservatives always feared) who proposed that there should be a complete overturn of the system. These radicals ranged from men who had become disillusioned with trade union methods and had turned socialist, like Eugene Debs, to rich men such as Joseph Medill Patterson, who turned socialist and announced that there was no hope of reform under the system as it existed. Writers such as Henry Demarest Lloyd, lawyers such as Clarence Darrow, and politicians such as John Peter Altgeld raised the question of reform in varying degrees.

The political leaders of Illinois failed to inspire much hope for a better day. Politicians fought out the issues on the basis of personalities and political self-seeking that promised little reform.

Some politicians lacked ability or honesty or both, but many decent political figures worked for the public interest. Even if honest, however, many adhered to the status quo and the shibboleths of conservative doctrine so that even where their intent was good, they had little vision to bring to the solution of the problems. Illinois was already taking on the image of political buffoonery and corruption that was to stain its reputation for many years. Senator Shelby Cullom, Congressman Medill McCormick, and some of the congressional delegation worked in the best interests of their constituents. Some governors could boast of honest and even progressive administrations. But in the thirty years following 1900 William H. Lorimer and Frank L. Smith were denied seats in the U.S. Senate, and a grand jury indicted Governor Len Small for fraud, giving the state a bad reputation.

Various institutions moved to reduce the cultural lag between the East and the Midwest. William Rainey Harper had already made progress in developing the University of Chicago, and the University of Illinois was beginning to cast off its agricultural school image. Northwestern already had something of a national reputation. Other educational institutions, such as McKendree, Shurtleff, Illinois College, and Knox, some of them nearly a hundred years old, were doing their best to raise the educational level. Better transportation helped reduce a similar lag between Chicago and downstate Illinois by bringing a wider audience to the glories of the Art Institute and the symphony.

At the turn of the century there was great change in the air, especially in material progress. It was a time of confidence and optimism. Although the distribution of the wealth produced by the material progress was not equitable, even the poor hoped for better days to come. Notably, there was little regimentation of workers and little governmental or private regulation of business. This would change in the next three decades.

1. *Chicago Tribune,* Jan. 1, 1900, p. 13.

2. *Quincy Daily Whig,* Jan. 4, 1900, p. 4.

3. *Chicago Daily Inter-Ocean,* Jan. 2, 1900, p. 4; *Illinois State Journal* (Springfield), Jan. 2, 1900, p. 5.

4. *Illinois State Journal,* Jan. 1, 1900, p. 2.

5. Ibid., Jan. 1, 1900, p. 6; Jan. 2, 1900, p. 5.

6. *Quincy Whig,* Jan. 2, 1900, p. 1.

7. *Inter-Ocean,* Jan. 1, 1900, p. 9.

8. *Chicago Tribune,* Jan. 2, 1900, p. 12.

9. Ibid., Jan. 1, 1900, p. 15; Jan. 7, 1900, p. 39.

10. *Inter-Ocean,* Jan. 1, 1900, p. 9; Jan. 2, 1900, p. 4.

11. *Evening Citizen* (Cairo), Jan. 1, 1900, p. 2.

12. *Chicago Tribune,* Jan. 1, 1900, p. 18; *Inter-Ocean,* Jan. 1, 1900, p. 8.

13. *Inter-Ocean,* Jan. 1, 1900, p. 8.

14. *Fourteenth Census of the United States,: 1920 State Compendium: Illinois* (Washington, D.C., 1924), p. 8.

15. *Twelfth Census of the United States: Population* (Washington, D.C., 1900), p. xx.

16. *Twelfth Census of the United States: Manufactures* (Washington, D.C., 1900), pp. 161, 163–64.

17. *From Sea to Sea* (New York, 1899) quoted in Charles N. Glaab, ed. *The American City* (Homewood, Ill., 1963), pp. 340–43.

18. Louis Franklin Swift, *The Yankee of the Yards: Biography of Gustavus Franklin Swift* (Chicago, 1927), pp. 3–4, 11–12.

19. Paul Brissenden, *Earnings of Factory Workers 1899–1927* (Washington, D.C., 1929), p. 386.

20. *Chicago Tribune,* Jan. 1, 1900, p. 14.

21. *Twelfth Census of the United States: Manufactures,* p. 164.

22. Ibid.; Victor S. Clark, *History of Manufactures in the United States,* 3 vols. (New York, 1929), II, 235–38, III, 45–47.

23. *Twelfth Census of the United States: Manufactures,* pp. 164, 1069; Clark, *History of Manufactures,* III, 275–78.

24. *Twelfth Census of the United States: Manufactures,* pp. 164–65.

25. Ibid.

26. *Abstract of the Twelfth Census of the United States,* (Washington, D.C., 1900), pp. 226, 236–37.

27. *Illinois State Journal,* Feb. 16, 1900, p. 3.

28. *Thirteenth Census of the United States: Agriculture* (Washington, D.C., 1912), p. 652; *Abstract of the Twelfth Census of the United States,* pp. 226–37.

29. *Illinois Agricultural Statistics, Circular 445* (Springfield, Ill., 1949), pp. 15, 19.

30. *Abstract of the Twelfth Census of the United States,* pp. 252–53, 258–59.

31. *Illinois Agricultural Statistics, Circular 445,* pp. 81, 86.

32. *Abstract of the Twelfth Census of the United States,* pp. 226, 232–33.

33. Ibid., p. 432.

34. *Inter-Ocean,* Jan. 28, 1900, p. 9; Jan. 29, 1900, p. 1. *Chicago Tribune,* Jan. 16, 1900, p. 6; Jan. 31, 1900, p. 6.

35. *Biographical Directory of the American Congress 1774–1961* (Washington, D.C., 1961), p. 263. Shelby M. Cullom, *Fifty Years of Public Service* (Chicago, 1911), p. 446. Carter H. Harrison, *Growing up with Chicago* (Chicago, 1944), pp. 141, 253.

36. *Chicago Tribune,* Jan. 5, 1900, p. 6.

37. Lloyd Wendt and Herman Kogan, *Bosses in Lusty Chicago: The Story of Bathhouse John and Hinky Dink* (Bloomington, Ind., 1967), pp. x.

38. *Chicago Tribune,* Jan. 7, 1900, p. 36. *Inter-Ocean,* Jan. 3, 1900, pp. 1, 6. *The Book of Chicagoans, 1917* (Chicago, 1917), p. 557.

39. John H. Mueller, *The American Symphony Orchestra: A Social History of Musical Taste* (Bloomington, Ind., 1951), pp. 101–6.

40. *Chicago Tribune,* Feb. 6, 1900, p. 6; Apr. 15, 1900, p. 40.

41. *Quincy Whig,* Feb. 27, 1900, p. 3.

42. *Centralia Sentinel,* Mar. 9, 1900, p. 1.

43. *Quincy Whig,* Feb. 3, 1900, p. 4.

44. *Chicago Tribune,* Jan. 5, 1900, p. 6; Apr. 1, 1900, p. 1.

45. *Laws of the State of Illinois, Passed by the Forty-first General Assembly* (Chicago, 1899), p. 55; *Illinois Blue Book, 1928–29* p. 358.

46. *Illinois State Journal,* Jan. 8, 1900, p. 6. *Chicago Tribune,* Jan. 7, 1900, pp. 17–20; Feb. 8, 1900, p. 6; Feb. 14, 1900, p. 6; Mar. 3, 1900, p. 6.

2

The Growth of Industry

Students of U.S. history have heard the years after 1900 described as the progressive era, a period in which "trustbusting" was a major feature. Actually, in Illinois, as in the nation as a whole, the trusts continued to grow, and there were more at the end of the progressive era than at the beginning. It is true that Theodore Roosevelt, the "Great Trust-buster," made some inroads into industrial concentration, but his efforts only slightly curtailed the growth and consolidation of industry into ever larger companies. Industrialists found that the concentration of industry under a single management effected economies of production, transportation, warehousing, and finance.

The industrial concerns that grew large during the nineteenth century were frequently the creation of a single man or family who treated them like a personal barony, to be manipulated to the satisfaction of its owner. In their drive for power and wealth, industrialists engaged in competitive activities ruinous to themselves as well as to the public. Long before the end of the nineteenth century, they had tired of this game and sought ways to eliminate competition. By doing so, they could raise prices and avoid disastrous price wars.

The private company no longer sufficed to carry on the business of these mammoth concerns. Soon after the end of the nineteenth century, most of the older men who created the industrial development of Illinois in its earliest years disappeared from the picture. By 1900 Cyrus McCormick, inventor of the reaper, and John Deere, who had perfected new methods of making plows, had been dead for years. George Pullman died in 1897, Philip Danforth Armour in 1901, and Gustavus Swift in 1903. Financial greats of

Illinois such as Potter Palmer, Marshall Field, and Levi Z. Leiter had little time left.

In many instances, these men left dynasties which carried on the family business. This was especially true in the farm implement and meat-packing businesses. There seemed to be no end to the young Swifts and Armours to carry on the packing business or to McCormicks in the farm machinery industry. In the case of George Pullman, his sons were a disappointment to him, but one of his daughters married Frank Lowden, who, until he went into politics, carried on in the tradition of his father-in-law. Although Pullman opposed the marriage of his daughter to the young corporation lawyer, he found that Lowden was a man after his own heart. Lowden had been the attorney for big corporations before his marriage to Florence Pullman, but, backed by Pullman's money, he became involved in larger and larger enterprises such as the incorporation of the National Biscuit Company, the Shelby Steel Tube Company, and the American Radiator Company.[1]

The men of the younger generation, J. Ogden Armour, Louis Swift, and Cyrus Hall McCormick II, were a different breed of men than their fathers and grandfathers. The older generation consisted of practical men who knew every detail of the business they created. Gustavus Swift started as a butcher and could slaughter and dress a beef as well as any of his employees. His sons would not have considered the possibility.[2]

Many of the newer industrialists were no less rapacious than their fathers, but their operations were not as rough. Financing of the old companies had been shaky, and control had often been concentrated in the hands of a single individual, but this began to change in the new generation. Companies were incorporated, which spread the ownership. Control was maintained within the family but usually a manager with a reputation as a financial wizard was employed. In some cases, control of the companies migrated to the money center in New York, concentrated in the hands of J. P. Morgan or others of his kind. Gustavus Swift's son reported that his father borrowed from nearly every bank north of the Ohio River. He said the elder Swift scattered his loans deliberately to ensure that his notes would never all be called at once.[3] As the money market changed in the twentieth century, it was possible to finance operations with corporate stock and bond issues. The census figures for 1900 show that corporations had almost complete control of the state's productive capacity. In that year the total value of the industrial production of Illinois reached

$1,250,000,000. Corporations produced 73 percent of the total, although they represented only 10 percent of the establishments in the state. By 1910, corporations produced 83 percent of the total. This development of corporate enterprise continued throughout the early years of the twentieth century, although it was more pronounced in some industries than in others. For example, by 1910 corporations provided more than 90 percent of all production in foundries, machine shops, meat-packing establishments and manufactories of paint and varnish.[4]

One of the remarkable industrial consolidations in Illinois took place in the steel business. Elbert H. Gary, a former judge of a county court from suburban Naperville, provided the leadership for this consolidation. Judge Gary, a puritanical, dapper man of whom J. P. Morgan's daugher said he was "too plausible," proved to be adept at financing and running great corporate enterprises.[5] The steel industry in Chicago began with the founding of the North Chicago Rolling Mill, which rolled the first steel rails in America in 1865. By 1882 the company had four blast furnaces in operation, another under construction, and had started a new plant at South Chicago. Steel men had built the first Bessemer converters at Joliet around 1873. There were several other iron and steel mills in the area, and by 1879 the annual production of these mills was about 22,000,000 tons. They combined Lake Superior ore, Connellsville coke, and nearby limestone to produce the steel. In 1889 much of this productive capacity was formed into the Illinois Steel Company, which joined the old North Chicago Rolling Mills (including a plant at Milwaukee), the South Chicago Works, the Union Iron and Steel Company, and the Joliet Works. This company brought together capital of $25,000,000 and increased the amount in 1891 to $50,000,000. Altogether Illinois Steel had fourteen furnaces on blast, producing some 650,000 tons of pig iron. It operated four Bessemer converters capable of turning out 750,000 tons of ingot a year. It also owned extensive coal lands, coke ovens, miles of railroad, and mills for rolling rails, rods, plates, and structural shapes. The combined organization created the biggest steel capacity in the world. From time to time new mills and furnaces were added, and eventually the rail mill at North Chicago was abandoned entirely as the area became more congested.[6]

In 1898 Judge Gary entered the steel picture in Illinois, putting together the Federal Steel Company, which included Illinois Steel Company, Minnesota Iron Company, Lorain Steel Company of

Lorain, Ohio, and Johnstown, Pennsylvania, and the Chicago Outer Belt Railroad. Gary combined a capital of $200,000,000 in Federal. The company controlled some of the richest ore lands in the Lake Superior region, as well as transportation facilities from mines and coke ovens to the mills. The charter of Federal Steel gave it the privilege of mining, manufacturing, transporting goods and passengers on land or water, building any houses, structures, vessels, ships, boats, railroads, cars or other equipment that might be needed and maintaining and operating railroads and steamship lines. Thus, at the turn of the century Judge Gary and his Federal Steel Company (with Morgan backing) controlled much of the productive capacity in the West.[7]

The only rival to Judge Gary's company was the immense holding of Andrew Carnegie in the East. Carnegie had confined his operation to the Pennsylvania area where he provided raw material for rolling mills all over the country. In line with the attempt to achieve monopolies in all aspects of industry, men began to envision combining the Carnegie interests and the Federal Steel Company to avoid a competitive struggle and price war, which would be disastrous to the industry. An example of the threat of competition in the steel industry was the problem of manufacturing and selling steel rails. Since 1885 there had been a pooling arrangement where, by common agreement, the producers of rails set the price of the product and the output allotment of each company in advance. The leaders in this pool were Carnegie and Illinois Steel. The rail mills dissolved the pool around 1900, thus creating the threat of a price war. Some of Gary's associates began to cancel orders with the Carnegie company for steel for rolling wire, rails, and steel hoops.[8]

Carnegie prepared to retaliate by building his own rolling mills to produce these items and sell them competitively with the companies which were attempting to cut him out of ingot production. Gary and others convinced Morgan that there needed to be further consolidation to prevent problems in the steel industry. Morgan, remembering the price wars among the railroads, gave his blessing to this project. Gary's representatives approached Carnegie, who, after some hesitation, agreed to sell his holdings for an astounding $492,000,000. The result was the organization of the United States Steel Corporation, which included Carnegie's holdings, the Federal Steel Company, the National Steel Company, American Steel and Wire, and the Rockefeller ore holdings in Minnesota. Capitalized at

$1,400,000,000, the United States Steel Corporation had in its empire blast furnaces, Bessemer converters, open-hearth furnaces, rolling mills, ore, coal and limestone lands, 112 steamships, and 1,000 miles of railroad. It boasted a capacity of over 7,000,000 tons of pig iron, more than 9,000,000 tons of raw steel, and more than 7,000,000 tons of finished steel. Even so, the United States Steel Corporation could never achieve a monopoly. The company produced 68 percent of the rails rolled in the United States, 60 percent of the structural steel, 60 percent of the wire, 95 percent of the nails, nearly all barbed and woven wire, 95 percent of the bridges, and half of the coke. Later it constructed a huge steel plant at Gary, Indiana, just over the state line from Chicago. Then, as a result of Theodore Roosevelt's "rule of reason," it was allowed to add the Tennessee Coal, Iron and Rail Company in the South. In the first decade of its existence, United States Steel mined 181,000,000 tons of ore, produced 95,000,000 tons of pig iron, and some 86,000,000 tons of rolled and finished steel.[9]

This gigantic corporation brought much of Illinois steel production under one management, but control and ownership migrated to the East Coast, the money center of J. P. Morgan and his associates. Gary continued as an important factor in the company, but Carnegie's base of operation was now New York, although he still held many directorships in Illinois banks and industrial companies as one of J. P. Morgan's minions.[10] In 1900 Chicago was the third city in the nation in steel and iron production with $31,000,000 of such products; Joliet was eighth with a production of $13,000,000. Chicago held this position through 1910, but by 1914 had slipped to fourth place as Cleveland increased its production.[11] Many other cities had steel and iron production. East St. Louis was important, as was Granite City, and Waukegan had steel and rolling mills.[12] The Inland Steel Company operated rolling mills at Chicago Heights. The Keystone Steel and Wire Company grew up at Peoria from a consolidation of the Keystone Fence Company and the Atlas Company.[13] By 1910 iron and steel production in Illinois was in excess of $86,000,000. In 1914, just prior to World War I, Illinois ranked third in the nation in blast furnace production with some $25,000,000 in value. The state was third that year in iron and steel rolling mills, which turned out a product of $64,995,121.[14]

Steel is basic to many industries, and a number of factories came to Illinois because of its availability. This development of corporate enterprise continued throughout the early years of the twentieth century. The picture of the great corporations that controlled the steel production of Illinois presents a dilemma, however. On the one hand, this tremendous production brought progress and added to the material wealth of the state. On the other hand, a tremendous price was paid in human sacrifice for this progress. Laborers in the blast furnaces worked an eighty-four-hour week, twelve hours a day every day of the week. The lot of the laborer in the rolling mills was somewhat better, but workers in both the blast furnaces and the rolling mills made only $500 a year for their share of the riches produced.[15] Without question the consolidation of the steel mills brought wealth to men like Morgan and Gary, but the workers in the steel mills profited little by what they produced.

Another Illinois industry that went through the process of consolidation was the farm implement business. Prior to the beginning of the twentieth century, Illinois ranked first in the nation as a producer of agricultural implements. There were several reasons for this. First, the location of the state in the center of a great farming area of the United States provided a market. Second, proximity to the steel mills meant easy access to the necessary raw materials. And finally, the state's central location put the industry within reach of other major farming areas. In 1900 Illinois produced 41 percent of the agricultural implements made in the United States. This represented $42,000,000 worth of implements produced in 94 establishments around the state. The implement business was constantly growing, and by 1910 the industry was producing more than $57,000,000 worth of farm implements. By 1914 the value of the production had reached more than $65,000,000, and throughout the whole period Illinois ranked as the top producer in the country. Several cities ranked high in the production of agricultural machinery. Chicago achieved first place in the state, dealing primarily in harvesting machines such as reapers, mowers, and binders. Moline was second, manufacturing plows, cultivators, and other tillage implements. Springfield, Freeport, Rock Island, Canton, and Rockford were also important in this production.[16]

The best-known figures in the farm machinery business were Cyrus McCormick, who developed the reaper, and John Deere, who improved the plow. Both men had been mechanics, adept at developing new products in the farm machinery business. Both had died by 1900 and their businesses were operated by their children. The greatest of all the consolidations, the International Harvester Company, grew out of McCormick's reaper business, which since 1844 had been directed by his son Cyrus.[17] Also important in Chicago in the manufacture of reapers, mowers, and similar machines was Charles Deering, who organized the Deering Company and brought it to great heights. Deering and McCormick were the chief competitors in harvesting machines, and prior to the turn of the century had engaged in some major price wars.[18]

In June, 1902, fearing further disastrous competition, McCormick went to New York to seek the aid of Morgan in avoiding further difficulties. He talked there with the youngest of the Morgan partners, George Perkins, who suggested merging the McCormick company into a larger concern. This came as a blow to McCormick because his was a family business which stood as a monument to his father. Several conferences followed and Perkins called in other implement manufacturers to point out how they could effect economies. Perkins believed the industry could improve sales efficiency by eliminating many of the 40,000 implement dealers in the United States. Morgan, in Europe at the time, kept in touch, encouraging consolidation; eventually he supplied the International Harvester name. Subsequently the Morgan Interests paid $60,000,000 for the assets of the companies making up International Harvester, including the Milwaukee Harvester Company, the Plano Company, the Champion Company of Springfield, and the Deering and McCormick interests.[19]

The new company produced less than the component parts because they had been overproducing for the market. For five years before consolidation the average number of binders produced had been 152,000, while for the first ten years after the consolidation of International Harvester, the average was 91,000. Where before, the average had been some 217,000 mowers a year, now it was only 170,000.[20] In addition to the original companies that made up International Harvester, in 1903 the D. M. Osborne Company of Auburn, New York, which made tilling and harvester machines, was added. In 1904 the Keystone Company of Rock Falls, Illinois, with a line of tilling and hay tools, was incorporated. And in that same year International Harvester brought the Webber Wagon Company of Chicago, the Camp Manure Spreader Company, and a nearly defunct company called Aultman-Miller of Akron, Ohio, into the company. Also incorporated into International Harvester was the Warder, Bushnell and Glesner Company, which had originated in Springfield, Ohio, but whose headquarters were in Chicago. At the outset International Harvester was a holding company whose entire stock was voted by a trust made up of McCormick (president), Deering (chairman of the board), and Perkins (representing the Morgan interests).[21] Although Gary was Deering's lawyer, he seems to have taken no part in the amalgamation of the farm implement business.[22] The annual output after consolidation was about 8,700,000 machines. Since the parent plant and the home office of the company were maintained in Chicago, control of International Harvester did not migrate out of the state as was the case with United States Steel. McCormick continued as president of the company until 1918, when his brother Harold Fowler McCormick succeeded him. International Harvester also expanded into new products and areas. In 1908 it began tractor production and eventually made the transition from steam to gasoline-powered tractors. The result was its Farmall tractor, the second most popular in the country for many years and a common sight on Illinois farms. International Harvester also made one abortive attempt to build pleasure cars, and moved into truck production, which proved to be highly successful.[23]

With so much suspicion of big business during the progressive era, it was inevitable that such a large company would come under the scrutiny of federal officials. After a few years, International Harvester found itself in the courts for violation of the Sherman Anti-Trust Act. The U.S. District Court of Minnesota handed down an opinion in 1914 that the company had violated that act in the consolidation of 1902. International Harvester appealed to the U.S. Supreme Court, first arguing the case in April, 1915. The court could not agree and it was necessary to reargue in 1917. There was still no agreement. The court postponed the case in 1918 and after this the company agreed to a consent decree whereby it divested itself of some of its holdings. The divestment applied to the Osborne, Champion, and Milwaukee reaper companies. International Harvester also had to abide by a limit of not more than one dealer per town. The court did, however, allow the company to make and sell plows, which it had not done before.[24]

Also involved in the consolidation of the farm implement business was the company of John Deere, developer and inventor of better methods of making plows. The original company had been incorporated in 1868, and in 1918 owned controlling interest in various branch distributing houses located in Minneapolis, San Francisco, Kansas City, Portland, and Dallas. These branch companies sold machinery manufactured not only by Deere but by allied and noncompeting companies like Deere and Manser of

Moline, which made corn planters and disk harrows, the Moline Wagon Company, which made farm wagons, the Union Malleable Iron Company of Moline, which made castings, the Dean Manufacturing Company of Otumwa, Iowa, which made hay tools, the Syracuse Chill Plow Company, which manufactured plows, the Kemp and Burpee Company of Syracuse, which produced manure spreaders, and the Van Brundt Manufacturing Company of Horicon, Wisconsin, which made grain drills. This loosely organized alliance failed to achieve the desired results. After the turn of the century, Charles Deere, son of the founder, assumed the leadership of the company. He became ill, however, and did not have the strength and energy to carry through plans for consolidation. After his death in 1907, his son-in-law William Butterworth established a committee to direct its reorganization. Appointed to the committee was George Peek, a collateral relative of the Deere family who had been in their employ for a number of years and who was later to be quite prominent in the politics of farm legislation. Eventually the committee effected a unification of the companies that had cooperated with Deere, believing that under this reorganization Deere would be able to compete better against rivals like International Harvester. By 1911 it had completed the reorganization, and Deere and Company, a holding and operating firm, was able to produce and distribute a more complete line of farm machinery and to compete in an advantageous way.[25]

The Moline Plow Company, incorporated in Illinois and wholly owned by John N. Willys of Moline, produced a significant amount of farm implements. This independent company competed with Deere and International Harvester for a share of the market. It manufactured plows, planters, and cultivators in Moline, and passenger vehicles at Freeport in a subsidiary called the Henny Buggy and Freeport Carriage Company. It also made wagons, manure spreaders, hay loaders, side delivery rakes, and scales at Stoughton, Wisconsin, drills and seeders in Minneapolis, plows at the Acme Steel Company in Chicago, and operated a harvesting machine plant in Poughkeepsie, New York. After World War I, with the Moline Plow Company in serious financial trouble, Willys prevailed upon George Peek to take over as president of the company. Unfortunately the company was on the verge of financial ruin. It was virtually bankrupt when Peek took it over, and in the depression years immediately after the war, 1920 and 1921, the business of selling farm machinery fell off drastically. For the next three or four years Peek struggled valiantly to put the company back on its feet but was unsuccessful.[26]

The slaughtering industry was for many years by far largest in Illinois. In 1900 the production of the Illinois slaughterhouses reached $250,000,000, or 20 percent of the total industrial production of the state. By 1910 the product value of the slaughtering industry had increased to $389,000,000. Almost all of this was produced by four or five great companies, the Swifts and the Armours being the largest, but with the Morrises, Cudahys, and Wilsons also accounting for a substantial amount. There were several smaller organizations around the state, but they accounted for only a tiny portion of the total production.[27] In spite of the corporate nature of this industry, however, it was never able to consolidate its operation as the steel or farm implement businesses did. This was partly because the slaughtering business created a very bad image for itself. The pioneers of the meat-packing industry, Gustavus Swift and Philip Danforth Armour, had built the industry by developing new techniques and methods. Gustavus Swift, hardly more than a village butcher in Massachusetts, emigrated to the Midwest shortly after the Civil War, developed the refrigerator car, and, after a struggle, convinced Easterners that they could buy and eat midwestern beef cheaper than their own locally killed beef.[28] Rudyard Kipling made a devastating attack on the packinghouses of Chicago in 1899, and Chicago reacted with its usual feeling of pride against Kipling's denunciation of the packing industry. A year later, a public relations statement by the meat-packing industry pointed out that it was sending 40,000 dressed beef quarters to England each week using the cold storage methods developed by Swift. The *Tribune,* delighted with this information, said there had never been a better example of poetic justice. The Englishmen who had pointed the finger of scorn at the stockyards were now dependent upon them for roast beef.[29]

In 1900 the head of Armour and Company was Philip Danforth Armour, a profane, expansive man fond of telling questionable stories. Armour was filled with the clichés of orthodoxy. He encouraged loyalty, promptness, thrift, and hard work on the part of his employees, and was fond of passing out money to surprised employees who had been seen doing something worthwhile. It was not unusual for him to hand a surprised employee 50 cents, $1, or occasionally even $5 for having been at work early or having performed some other item of service beyond the call of duty. He often paid a nickel for a newspaper when it only cost a penny, and he gave money to apple women and other unfortunates whom he saw on the streets. Like many other industrialists of the time,

Armour enjoyed putting money into philanthropic enterprises. The Reverend Frank Gunsaulus, of Plymouth Church, one Sunday preached a sermon on the subject "What I Would do with a Million Dollars" in which he outlined a plan for technical education for boys who were too poor to go to college. Armour, who was in the congregation, offered Gunsaulus $1,000,000 provided he would run the school. The result was the Armour Institute of Technology, which provided technical education for a great many poor boys of Chicago.[30]

The years around 1900 were tragic ones for the Armour family. The bad image that plagued the slaughtering industry was beginning to catch up with Philip Armour. During the Spanish-American War, Armour had sold beef to the Army, and many soldiers had become ill from it, bringing about the "embalmed beef" scandal. While some of the bad beef came from Libbey, McNeill and Libbey (which was allied with the Swift interests), it was palatable compared with that which came from Armour. Apologists for Armour have said that the scandal contributed to his death. In 1899 a former Armour employee named Dolan had made an affidavit that conditions at the Armour slaughterhouses were bad and that diseased animals were used. It was found that Armour later tried to bribe Dolan with $5,000 to get him to retract his statement, which left doubt in the minds of many about Armour and Company.[31] There were frequent charges of selling spoiled meat—in Minnesota in September, 1900, for example.[32]

In January, 1900, while Philip Danforth Armour was spending the winter in Pasadena, his son, also in California, died very suddenly at the age of thirty-one. Young Philip Armour had been made a partner in the Armour Company at the age of twenty-five, and at the time of his death was engaged in merger discussions with the other packers, hoping to put together a great meat trust. The senior Armour himself had only a short time longer to live: he died almost exactly a year after the death of his son, at his home on Prairie Avenue in Chicago. This brought the eldest son, J. Ogden Armour, to the presidency of the company.[33]

The second well-known company in the meat-packing business was Swift, which had been founded by Gustavus Swift at about the same time and in about the same way that Armour had founded his firm. And though Armour was an expansive man, and the elder Swift a kind of Puritan, they shared many of the same values. P. D. Armour believed in the virtues of thrift, hard work, promptness, and loyalty; if one wanted rapid promotion with Gustavus Swift's company he had to possess these virtues. In the year 1902 there was a continued effort at consolidation, but Gustavus Swift died the next year and his place was taken by his eldest son, Louis.[34]

The third of the three great companies was the Morris Company, which was in the hands of Edward and Nelson Morris.

In 1902 packers established the National Packing Company, which initiated consolidation of some thirty of the smaller packers, hoping that once this combination had been made, National could acquire Armour, Swift, and Morris. As Louis Franklin Swift said in his biography of his father, "Consolidation was in the air and it seemed to be the thing to do." But public opinion was so strong against consolidation of the meat-packing industry that the company had trouble surviving. And as time went on, the reputation of the industry worsened.

J. Ogden Armour, in a book defending the packing industry, quoted a letter that he had received from a Presbyterian minister in Michigan:

> When Marshall Field died the other day, the entire country mourned. No one denied his right to the millions he amassed honorably, but were you to pass away tomorrow, the news would be received with general satisfaction from one end of the country to the other. No business besides your own would suspend operations for an hour. It should be a bitter thing for you to realize the loathing and destestation in which you are held in every place where your unfair, small souled, cruel methods are becoming known.[35]

Another letter which Armour received referred to "your continuous gorging upon the sweat and blood of the people in the nation."[36]

One of the greatest blows to the power of the packing industry came with the publication of Upton Sinclair's novel *The Jungle* in 1906. In this novel, Sinclair recounted the horrible working conditions of the immigrant workers who slaved in the packinghouses. He told of the hazards and drudgery of the work, of how the workers, through countless days, months, and years of toil in steamy, disease-ridden places, became victims of tuberculosis, of how they had their fingers or hands cut off in machinery. He described the hands of some, crisscrossed with knife cuts from which they contracted blood poisoning. He wrote of others falling into the vats, from which they went out to the public in lard pails with no trace of them ever found. In addition to the miseries of the packing-town workers, Sinclair also told the story of the diseased meat industry: meat from diseased cattle and hogs being sold to the public and spoiled meat being ground up into sausages and offered as desirable items. He told of dead rats, rat poison, and rat dung being ground up into the sausage in the same way. Sinclair, a socialist, had intended to bring the bad working conditions of the people employed by the packers to the attention of the public. But what caught the public imagination and sparked further distaste for the packers was the description of the filthy meat sent out to the public table. Sinclair's book had a great impact, bringing about a Federal Meat Inspection Act which after a time improved the quality of the meat the public bought.[39]

J. Ogden Armour made an effort to reply to Sinclair in a series of articles in the *Saturday Evening Post,* which was under the editorship of George Horace Lorimer, a former Armour employee. Unfortunately for Armour, not many people believed what he said.[38] Armour also tried to still the criticism of Sinclair and others by flooding the country with advertising which lauded the cleanliness and soundness of the Armour operation.[39]

In the meantime, the federal government made a number of efforts to limit the so-called beef trust. Eventually the packers were brought to heel by the federal courts. In 1905, in a famous case involving Swift and Company, Justice Oliver Wendell Holmes, although he was generally not a proponent of the Sherman Anti-Trust Act, issued an injunction restraining the activities of the company. This was a landmark case because, for the first time, the court ruled that the purchase, processing, and sale of meat came within the "current of commerce." Therefore the federal government could regulate the industry. There was also some effort to secure criminal convictions of individual offenders, but here the government made a number of errors which hindered the prosecution of the beef trust. Theodore Roosevelt's administration had established the Bureau of Corporations to investigate the trusts. In the ensuing scrutiny the testimony of a number of important witnesses was required. The law gave these witnesses immunity from further prosecution for offenses disclosed in their testimony. The Federal District Court in Chicago ruled that by giving testimony on their own bad habits, the meat-packers had immunity from any punishment under the anti-trust laws. Thus the government could do little to curb the packers.[40]

The Jungle came out while the Department of Justice was prosecuting these anti-trust cases and this brought action on other fronts. The disclosures horrified Theodore Roosevelt and the result was the Meat Inspection Bill, which ended some abuses. Thus in the face of possible government action and public opposition, the meat packers were forced to cease consolidation attempts.[41]

As time went on, the two newer companies, Wilson and Cudahy, grew almost as large as the older firms of Armour, Swift, and Morris. These five companies controlled the production and distribution of about 75 percent of the fresh meat entering the general trade of the United States. They also controlled meat imported from Latin American countries. In addition, they were among the largest distributors of butter, eggs, and canned goods as well as products such as breakfast food and staple groceries. Thus, although the meat-packers were never able to consolidate in the same manner as the steel or farm machinery business, they controlled the bulk of the production in the United States.[42]

Other areas of Illinois industry were involved in the process of consolidation into virtual monopolies. The Pullman Company, for example, had a monopoly of the sleeping-car industy long before 1900, but Pullman died that year, leaving a somewhat chaotic situation in the company.[43] Robert Todd Lincoln and Norman B. Rheam settled his estate, receiving a fee of $425,000 for their work,[44] and, in spite of the opinion of Carter Harrison the younger about Lincoln ("A man of mediocre attainments puffed up with pride almost to the exploding point by the brilliance of his parents, who left to his own devices, would never have arisen above the common place"),[45] the two men subsequently played a major part in managing the company, as did Frank Lowden, who kept a hand in because of his wife's inheritance of company stock. Like so many other companies, the Pullman enterprise had started out as the personal empire of a single man who had devised the product involved. Now, although much of the stock of the company was in the hands of Pullman's heirs, ownership was scattered and control of the company passed to other men—a pattern common in the annals of industry of this era.[46]

Also involved in the consolidation of industry was the distilling business, which, organized into the Distilling Company of America, brought together a capital of $125,000,000. Important independent distillers in Kentucky, Pennsylvania, and Maryland provided competition for the new company. Rum, made principally in New England (as it had been since colonial times), also represented competition. The industry was an increasingly important one in the country: in the twenty-five years before prohibition, the per capita consumption of alcoholic beverages increased 55 percent, from fifteen gallons per person to twenty-six.[47] Peoria had long been important in the distilling of alcoholic beverages because of its location in the middle of the corn belt, with an adequate supply of the coal and cold water essential for processing. Most of the spirits were distilled from local corn, but some rye whiskey was also produced. In 1900 Peoria was the first distilling city in the nation by a wide margin, and in malt liquors it was fourth.[48] The Illinois production of distilled liquors in that year represented nearly 40 percent of the nation's total. In 1910 Illinois produced 27 percent of the total, three-fourths of the value of which represented a federal excise tax of more than $42 million. The distilling industry was, therefore, a considerable contributor to the revenue of the United States.[49]

In addition to the large industries in steel, harvesting, slaughtering, distilled liquors, and Pullman cars, there were many other industries of significance in Illinois, and Chicago in almost all of these was the first city in the state in terms of total manufacturing production. In 1910 Chicago produced more than two-thirds of the total industrial output of Illinois. Besides steel, slaughtering, and farm implements, it produced more than three-fourths of the men's clothing, printing and publishing, lumber, and electrical products of the state.[50] In 1910 the second city in manufacturing was Peoria, which in addition to distilling, was important in slaughtering, cooperage, printing and publishing, agricultural implements, breweries, and flour mills, producing a total of $63,000,000 worth of goods. The third city for manufacturing in Illinois was Joliet, about half of whose total produce was steel.

The fourth largest manufacturing city in Illinois in 1910 was Rockford, which was important for furniture, the knitting of various products for clothing, the production of agricultural implements, and the products of foundries and machine shops. Moline was fifth in manufacturing in Illinois and in addition to the farm implements for which it was so well known, it contributed carriages and wagons and foundry and machine-shop products. It had its own steel and rolling mills and by 1910 was producing automobiles. The sixth city in manufacturing was Waukegan, where the steel business was also important. There were several rolling mills, and the manufacture of various glucose products was also important. The seventh city was East St. Louis, which turned out flour and grist mill products and operated foundries, machine shops, and steel and rolling mills. There were firms that produced chemicals, meat, paint, paper, and wood pulp products.

The eighth manufacturing city in Illinois was Quincy, where there were foundries and machine shops, factories making stoves and furnaces, meat-packing and food-preparation establishments, and breweries. The ninth manufacturing city was Elgin, already well known for the manufacture of clocks and watches. This city also operated foundries and machine shops, condensed milk factories and printing and publishing businesses. The tenth city was Aurora. Repair shops for the steam railroads, foundry and machine shops, and manufacturers of bicycles and motorcycles operated there.[51]

Some smaller cities were also industrially significant. In 1910 Decatur manufactured the products of flour and grist mills and machine and foundry shops. Springfield produced agricultural implements, boots, shoes, and watches. Freeport turned out carriages and wagons, windmills, and patent medicines. Rock Island had its share of the agricultural implement business and also produced lumber, oilcloth, and linoleum. La Salle was active in the smelting and refining of zinc (in which Illinois ranked high), and in cement. Building and repairing railroad cars was important in Bloomington, Danville, Mattoon, and Galesburg. Jacksonville produced men's clothing; Lincoln, coffins, burial cases, undertakers' goods, and mattresses and springs for beds.[52] The list could go on almost indefinitely. Not all of these were large consolidations of industry, it should be noted. Often an industry that contributed substantially to the total production of Illinois (e.g., the machine shops and foundries) consisted of hundreds of establishments under separate ownership which felt no need to consolidate as steel and harvester companies had done.

An interesting aspect of the consolidation of industry in Illinois is where the capital came from. The Chicago Clearing House Association included sixteen banks, a decline from twenty-four a few years before. This reduction had come about due to mergers. In 1911 the country had become concerned about the money trust, and there was a major congressional investivation by the Pujo Committee, which was particularly interested in the involvement of J. P. Morgan in so many big industries. Upon investigating the question of interlocking directorates, it found that the Chicago banks had close connections with industry and with the Morgan interests.[53]

One of the banks that fell under the scrutiny of the Pujo Committee was the First National Bank of Chicago, which had a capital stock of $20,000,000 and deposits of $117,000,000. The Pujo Committee found that First National held twenty-nine directorships in six banks and trust companies including not only other Chicago banks but also the Chase National of New York, the First National of New York, and the New York Trust Company. It held two directorships in a life insurance company, fifteen directorships in fourteen railroads, including a number of those that served the Chicago area such as the New York Central, the Erie, the Baltimore and Ohio, the Chicago, Burlington and Quincy, the Great Northern, and the Wabash. First National also held nine directorships in seven producing and trading companies, including such important Chicago companies as the International Harvester Company, the Pullman Company, United States Steel Corporation, and the National Biscuit Company. The combined capital of these companies in which the bank directorships was more than $2,000,000,000.[54]

Also important among Chicago banks was the Continental Commercial Bank of Chicago, with a capital of $21,000,000 and deposits of $182,000,000. This bank held twenty-four directorships in six banks, including the New York Trust Company, the National City Bank of New York, and the Astor Trust Company. These six banks had resources of $506,000,000, giving the Continental Commercial access to tremendous resources. In addition, Continental Commercial held two directorships in two insurance companies, including the Equitable Company, one of Morgan's, and eleven directorships in nine railroads and nine directorships in seven producing companies. These last included three directorships on the board of Armour and Company and directorships in International Harvester, Pullman, and United States Steel. In addition it held posts in various public utilities, including the Chicago Elevated Railway Company and Commonwealth Edison.[55]

The Illinois Trust and Savings Bank of Chicago had twelve directorships in nine banks and trust companies, including the First National of Chicago, the Chase National of New York, and the First National of New York. It held one directorship in a life insurance company, five directorships in five railroads, and four directorships in three producing and trading companies, including two seats on the board of directors of the Pullman Company. It also held six directorships in four public utilities, including Commonwealth Edison and the Chicago Elevated Railway Company.[56]

A list of the various industrialists who served on the board of directors of these banks looks like a Who's Who of industrial development in Chicago. On the board of directors of the First National Bank of Chicago were Harold Fowler McCormick, brother of Cyrus Hall McCormick, and Charles Deering. In addition there were James J. Hill, who ran the Great Northern Railroad, Edward Morris of the meat-packing industry, and Norman B. Rheam, who was a part of the Pullman organization.[57] Louis Franklin Swift, who by the time of the Pujo investigation had succeeded his father as head of Swift and Company, was on the board at the National Bank of the Republic.[58] At the Merchants Loan and Trust Company, the names of Cyrus Hall McCormick, E. H. Gary, and E. L. Ryerson, who was also in steel, appeared on the list of the board of directors.[59] Robert Todd Lincoln, Gary, F. E. Weyerhauser of the lumber family, E. A. Cudahy, and J. Ogden Armour of packing were on the Continental Commercial Bank of Chicago board.[60]

It is interesting to compare the experiences of some of the older industrialists in financing their companies with those of their sons and grandsons. According to the younger Swift, Gustavus Swift was constantly warding off bankers to keep his company from being thrown into bankruptcy. By comparison, the younger meat-packers had excellent financial connections. J. Ogden Armour, for example, had directorships in many banks, most of them in the Midwest, including the National Bank of the Republic in Chicago and the Stockyards Saving Bank in Omaha. He also held a directorship in the National City Bank in New York. Edward Foster Swift was a director of the Illinois Trust and Savings Bank, the Ft. Dearborn National Bank, and the Livestock Exchange National Bank. Edward Morris, Jr., held directorships in five banks, and his brother Nelson had directorships in three banks, including the First National of Chicago. Edward Cudahy, Sr., had directorships in four banks, mostly in Omaha and Wichita, but he was also a director of the Continental Commercial Bank of Chicago. Edward Cudahy, Jr., had directorships in two banks in Omaha, and Joseph Cudahy had a directorship in the National Bank of the Republic. The Wilson family had directorships in five banks, including the First National Bank of Chicago and the Guaranty Trust of New York.[61]

These connections created a change in the industrial pciture of Illinois and Chicago. The same process developed over all the nation, making the operation of industrial concerns more secure, and enhancing the personal security of the people involved. At the same time the industry/bank connection tended to take control of industry out of the hands of the founding families. The control of many areas of industrial production had been taken from the so-called practical men by lawyers and bankers. Where Andrew Carnegie or his counterparts in Illinois Steel or Federal Steel had been competent to go into a mill, look at a process, and judge whether it was running efficiently, it is doubtful whether Elbert H. Gary knew much about the technical side of the industry, but he was adept at finance and squeezing profits from the business. Men who knew the business only as paid employees ran the mills and factories. Operation from the top was largely financial, and the technological side of the business was left to engineers and superintendents.

This dispersal of company control caused considerable changes in the attitudes of management. Where Carnegie or others of his generation had been quite willing to fight if threatened by competition, new directors and industrial managers tended to find ways to avoid fighting. In the steel business the annual dinners which Judge Gary held to announce the prices of steel for the coming year were well known. Gary would announce the price that United States Steel would charge for a particular steel product and the rest of the industry would go along—only the public suffered. The consumer paid for these arbitrary decisions while the companies protected themselves from competition.

As the old industrial families got wealthier, they sent their sons to eastern prep schools like Phillips Andover, and then to the Ivy League universities of Harvard, Yale, and Princeton. The young Armours each spent some time at Yale;[62] the Cyrus Hall McCormick branch of the reaper family were graduates of Princeton and remained loyal alumni. Cyrus Hall McCormick II was later a trustee of the institution.[63] The sons of William Sanderson McCormick, Cyrus Hall McCormick's brother, graduated from Yale. In this branch of the McCormicks were such figures as Joseph Medill McCormick and Robert Rutherford McCormick, who, through the combination of a small portion of the reaper fortune and the *Chicago Tribune* money inherited from their maternal grandfather, Joseph Medill, became important in their own right.[64] This new generation of industrialists and financiers tended to have an outlook different from that of their fathers. Through the influence of education, they were smoother and less inclined to engage in the rougher side of business. Many had the privilege of the "grand tour" of Europe. Young Philip Danforth Armour owned a great art collection acquired in Europe after his short stay at Yale. Armour came back to Chicago in 1895, married, and together with his brother, J. Ogden Armour, bought entire block on Michigan Avenue so the two could build their houses side by side. Young Philip Armour reportedly spent $600,000 building his home. In 1895 this was a tremendous sum of money, perhaps as good an example as any of the conspicuous consumption that Thorstein Veblen was writing about in those years at the University of Chicago.[65]

In addition to whatever educational and cultural advantages these young men had, their fortunes now represented "old money." They had never know what it was like to be poor in the way their fathers could keenly remember. The result was that they squeezed their businesses, their labor, and their consumers less overtly than their fathers had. At the same time, the younger industrial leaders better understood finance and maintained financial connections superior to those available to their fathers. They often consummated fortunate marriages which combined large fortunes. Harold Fowler McCormick married Edith Rockefeller, coupling the sizeable McCormick family fortune with that of John D. Rockefeller.[66] In another branch of the family, Joseph Medill McCormick married Ruth Hanna, daughter of Marcus Alonzo Hanna.

In addition to the interlocking directorate that existed among the corporation executives, there was an interlocking social directorate as well. Beyond the social circuit presided over by such eminent women as Mrs. Potter Palmer and Mrs. Edith Rockefeller McCormick, there was another aspect to the social situation. An examination of biographical material relating to the various industrialists in Chicago shows that most of the men who ran the business of Chicago and Illinois were members of certain exclusive clubs. Almost all were members of the Union League Club. Most were members of the Hamilton Club, the leading social group of the Republican Party, and many were members of clubs dedicated more or less to athletic activities, such as the Onwentsia Golf Club. Many had summer places near this club at Lake Forest. A few belonged to the Chicago Athletic Club or the Illinois Athletic Club. Through the Hamilton Club, they made contributions to the dominant Republican party and their voices were heard within it. There were almost no Democrats among them; only Cyrus Hall McCormick belonged to both the Union League Club and the Iroquois Club, the Democratic organization. The McCormicks had long been Democrats, having come from Virginia, and Joseph

Medill always referred to the elder Cyrus Hall McCormick as a copperhead during the Civil War era.[68] Many others were members of various clubs of some special interest, such as the Commercial Club, the Chicago Club, or the (Jewish) Standard Club.[69]

These gentlemen saw each other regularly not only at meetings of the board of directors of their now interlocked companies and banks but also at lunch at the Union League or one of the other clubs. They tended, as befitting the nobility of the economic world, to rally around when festive occasions occurred in any of the families. When Frank Lowden, the still impecunious young lawyer, married the daughter of George M. Pullman, the wedding was a grand affair. Besides many of the local celebrities such as the Marshall Fields, the Robert Todd Lincolns, the Philip Armours, and the Shelby Culloms, from out of town came the Andrew Carnegies, the John D. Rockefellers, the Henry Flaglers, and the Steven B. Elkinses, not to mention three Supreme Court justices, Brown, Field, and Harlan, former President and Mrs. Benjamin Harrison, the widow of another president, Mrs. Ulysses S. Grant, and the widows of the Republican candidates of 1884, Mrs. James G. Blaine and Mrs. John A. Logan. Thus, socially, the rich had established their political connections well.[70]

These millionaires also all tended to live in the same areas of the city. The six or seven blocks along Prairie Avenue, known as Millionaires' Row were indeed remarkable.[71] The Lowdens bought a residence at 1912 Prairie Avenue, only a block from Mrs. Lowden's father, George M. Pullman.[72] Many other wealthy people lived along the same street or a block west on Michigan Avenue. There was an area called McCormickville on Rush Street.[73] Thus, these millionaires lived together in almost complete segregation from the world in their town houses or on the fine estates near Lake Forest, isolated from the unpleasantness of the world. It did not concern them that the squalor and vice of the red light district was a scant four blocks away from Prairie Avenue.

So these millionaires saw each other regularly in their business enterprises or at lunch at the various elegant clubs to which they belonged, and congregated together on social occasions. Many of them went to church and listened to the same kinds of noncontroversial sermons that the Armours heard from Reverend Frank Gunsaulus, and in the end most of them were buried near each other in Graceland Cemetery under similarly elaborate tombs and mausoleums.

Any effort to evaluate the effects of the ever-increasing con-

solidation of business in the twentieth century brings the historian into a position of ambivalence. Professor Robert Wiebe notes that in spite of all the connections, financial and social, of the business interests, many divisions still existed. Businessmen were divided along sectional lines and between the small towns and the cities. But the business community was united by one goal: the desire for profits. Anything or anyone who threatened this was the enemy and was dealt with as ruthlessly as necessary. The big companies and their managers called the tune in labor costs, pricing of goods, and consolidation.[74]

Gabriel Kolko points out that most businessmen after the beginning of the twentieth century believed that consolidation and bigness were necessary, inevitable, rational, and desirable. Kolko believes that much consolidation came about because of the increasing market for industrial stocks and that the consolidation grew not so much out of a desire to control but from an effort to stabilize and bring an end to the chaotic situation in business.[75]

It is true that consolidation brought efficiency, but only up to a certain point. General Motors found by 1923 that centralization brought problems and reversed the process by bringing about decentralization of management of its component companies. Kolko also points out that total control was impossible because of the fluidity of the economic situation and the rapidly shifting markets. The growth of industry brought benefits in jobs created, in new products, and in a higher standard of living. These benefits were achieved at a heavy cost in human resources—the broken lives of workers through low pay, long hours, and disgraceful living conditions. It is not the business of the historian to describe what might have been, but there remains the question of whether or not too high a price was paid for progress.[76]

1. William T. Hutchison, *Lowden of Illinois: The Life of Frank O. Lowden*, 2 vols. (Chicago, 1957), I, 48, 50-64.

2. Louis Franklin Swift, *The Yankee of the Yards: Biography of Gustavus Franklin Swift* (Chicago, 1927), pp. 7–9.

3. Ibid., pp. 27–32.

4. *Abstract of the Twelfth Census of the United States* (Washington, D.C., 1900), pp. 334–35; *Thirteenth Census of the United States: Manufactures* (Washington, D.C., 1912), p. 267.

5. Ida M. Tarbell, *The Life of Elbert H. Gary: The Story of Steel* (New York, 1925), pp. 18–19; David Brody, *Labor in Crisis: The Steel Strike of 1919* (New York, 1965), p. 19.

6. Victor S. Clark, *History of Manufactures in the United States*, 3 vols. (New York, 1929), II, 235–38; *Twelfth Census of the United States: Manfactures* (Washington, D.C., 1902), p. 164.

7. Clark, *History of Manufactures*, III, 45–47.

8. Ibid., pp. 96, 118, 122–23.

9. Ibid., pp. 54–64.

10. Tarbell, *Life of Elbert H. Gary,* pp. 95–96.

11. Ibid.

12. *Twelfth Census of the United States: Manufactures,* pp. 190–91, 1067; *Thirteenth Census of the United States: Manufactures,* pp. 265, 266; *Abstract of the Census of Manufacturing, 1914* (Washington, D.C., 1917), p. 267.

13. *Poor's Manual of Industrials, 1914* (New York, 1914), pp. 531–32, 2212.

14. *Abstract of the Census of Manufacturing, 1914,* p. 267.

15. Paul H. Douglas, *Real Wages in the United States 1890–1926* (New York, 1966), p. 623; Paul F. Brissenden, *Earnings of Factory Workers 1899–1927* (Washington, D.C., 1929), p. 386; *Thirteenth Census of the United States: Manufactures,* p. 262.

16. *Twelfth Census of the United States: Manfactures,* pp. 184–85, 190–91; *Thirteenth Census of the United States: Manfactures,* pp. 254–56, 265–66.

17. Cyrus McCormick, *The Century of the Reaper* (New York, 1931), p. 90.

18. Ibid., pp. 94–106.

19. Ibid., pp. 111–17; Clark, *History of Manufactures,* III, 146–47.

20. McCormick, *Century of the Reaper,* p. 121.

21. Ibid., pp. 118, 122–23.

22. Tarbell, *Life of Elbert H. Gary,* p. 95.

23. McCormick, *Century of the Reaper,* pp. 130, 132–33, 145, 157.

24. Ibid., pp. 164–72; United States *vs.* International Harvester Company, 24 U.S. 693 (1927).

25. Gilbert C. Fite, *George N. Peek and the Fight for Farm Parity* (Norman, Okla., 1954), pp. 26–27.

26. *Poor's Manual of Industrials, 1914,* pp. 677–78; Fite, *George N. Peek,* pp. 36–37.

27. *Twelfth Census of the United States: Manufactures,* pp. 163–64; *Thirteenth Census of the United States: Manufactures,* pp. 265–70.

28. Swift, *Yankee of the Yards,* pp. 65–81.

29. Kipling is quoted in Charles N. Glaab, *The American City* (Homewood, Ill., 1963), p. 339; *Chicago Tribune,* Mar. 9, 1900, p. 12; Mar. 10, 1900, p. 12.

30. Cora Lillian Davenport, "The Rise of Armours, an American Industrial Family" (M.A. thesis, University of Chicago, 1930) pp. 27–28, 32–33.

31. Ibid., pp. 25–36, 74–75.

32. *Chicago Tribune,* Sept. 15, 1900, p. 3.

33. *Chicago Daily Inter-Ocean,* Jan. 28, 1900, p. 28; Davenport, "Rise of the Armours," p. 31; J. Ogden Armour, *The Packers, the Private Car Lines and the People* (Philadelphia, 1906), p. v.

34. Swift, *Yankee of the Yards,* pp. 82–101, 209.

35. Armour, *The Packers,* pp. 167–68.

36. Ibid., p. 171.

37. Upton Sinclair, *The Jungle* (New York, 1965), pp. 91–96, 130–32.

38. Stewart Holbrook, *The Age of Moguls* (Garden City, N.Y., 1953), pp. 110–11.

39. Davenport, "Rise of the Armours," p. 77.

40. Carl Brent Swisher, *American Constitutional Development* (New York, 1943), pp. 509–10; Swift and Company *vs.* United States, 196 U.S. 375 (1905).

41. Swisher, *American Constitutional Development,* p. 511.

42. Clark, *History of Manufactures,* III, 265.

43. Stanley Buder, *Pullman: An Experiment in Industrial Order and Community Planning* (New York, 1967), pp. 210–11; Almont Lindsey, *The Pullman Strike* (Chicago, 1942), pp. 341–43.

44. *Inter-Ocean,* Jan. 6, 1900, p. 1

45. Carter H. Harrison, *Stormy Years* (Indianapolis, 1938), p. 276.

46. Hutchison, *Lowden of Illinois,* I, 64–66.

47. Clark, *History of Manufactures,* III, 275–78.

48. *Twelfth Census of the United States: Manfactures,* p. 1069.

49. *Thirteenth Census of the United States: Manfactures,* p. 256.

50. Ibid., p. 265.

51. Ibid., pp. 264–66.

52. Ibid.

53. *Chicago Banker,* 6 (Sept., 1900), p. 27.

54. *Money Trust Investigations before a Subcommittee of the Committee on Banking and Currency: Interlocking Directorates,* 3 vols. (Washington, D.C., 1913), III, 19–20.

55. Ibid., III, 18–19.

56. Ibid., p. 20.

57. Ibid., p. 66.

58. Ibid., p. 77.

59. Ibid., p. 62.

60. Ibid., p. 77.

61. *The Book of Chicagoans, 1917* (Chicago, 1917), pp. 19, 164, 488–89, 663–64, 736.

62. Ibid., p. 19; *Chicago Tribune* Jan. 28, 1900, p. 8.

63. See Irving Dilliard, "When Woodrow Wilson Was Invited to Head the University of Illinois," *Journal of the Illinois State Historical Society,* 60 (Winter, 1967), pp. 370–76; *The Book of Chicagoans, 1917,* p. 454.

64. Frank C. Waldrop, *McCormick of Chicago: An Unconventional Portrait of a Controversial Figure* (Englewood Cliffs, N.J., 1966), pp. 18–19, 41–50, 51, 52–53.

65. *Chicago Tribune,* Jan. 28, 1900, p. 8; Feb. 27, 1900, p. 7; *Inter-Ocean,* Jan. 28, 1900, p. 13.

66. *The Book of Chicagoans, 1917,* p. 454.

67. Waldrop, *McCormick of Chicago,* p. 47.

68. *The Book of Chicagoans, 1917,* p. 454; Waldrop, *McCormick of Chicago,* p. 18.

69. *Chicago Tribune,* May 10, 1908, p. 7, p. 2.

70. Hutchison, *Lowden of Illinois,* I, 48–49.

71. A map and description are given in *Chicago Tribune,* Apr. 29, 1900, p. 5.

72. Hutchison, *Lowden of Illinois,* I, 63–64. Lowden sold the house in 1908 for $69,187. *Chicago Tribune,* July 24, 1908, p. 12.

73. Waldrop, *McCormick of Chicago,* p. 19.

74. Robert H. Wiebe, *Business Men and Reform: A Study of the Progressive Movement* (Chicago, 1962), pp. 10–15.

75. Gabriel Kolko, *The Truimph of Conservatism: A Reinterpretation of American History, 1900–1916* (Chicago, 1963), pp. 12–13, 19, 32–33.

76. Ibid., pp. 45, 54.

3

The Bountiful Land: Agriculture, Mining, and Oil

Illinois achieved greatness, in large part, because of the resources with which it was endowed by nature. Clarence W. Alvord referred to Illinois as "God's Meadow."[1] Its people, land, minerals, and petroleum contributed to its greatness. Without these benefits, the industrial, cultural, and political development would have been impossible.

Of these resources, the land and the farms on it were the most valuable. By 1900, less than half the people lived in rural areas and the percentage continued to decline during the first thirty years of the twentieth century. Yet throughout this period agriculture held its position as one of the most productive aspects of the state's economy. More people were engaged in farming than in any other single industry, although manufacturing as a whole outdistanced agriculture in the number of persons employed before the turn of the century. Through improved technology the Illinois farmer became more productive. Although the number of farmers declined in absolute numbers, farm production flourished, contributing food to the nation, as well as raw materials to industry.

It had long been thought that the ideal size for a family farm was 160 acres. This can be explained in part because the Homestead Act had set the allotment per settler at 160 acres. More important, however, a farm this size was regarded as about right for efficient family operation. Smaller farms could not be economically operated because the overhead did not decline in proportion to the smaller production of fewer acres.[2] The size of farms in Illinois averaged slightly under this ideal. Although there were many farms of 80 acres or less in the state, in 1900 the average was slightly over 124 acres. By 1910 it was 129, and in 1920 had grown to 135.[3] The 1930 census showed that the average farm in Illinois was slightly more than 143 acres.[4]

As the size of farms increased, the total number of farms decreased. In 1900 there were 264,151 farms. By 1910, this figure had dropped to 251,872. In the 1920 census there were 237,181,[5] and by 1930 this figure had fallen to 214,497.[6]

The value of farm property increased dramatically in the first two decades of the twentieth century but declined by the end of the 1920s. In 1900 the value of all farm property was over $2,000,000,000; by 1910 this had nearly doubled to $3,900,000,000. By 1920, because of the inflation caused by World War I, this figure reached $6,600,000,000. In 1925 the value of farm property declined to $4,600,000,000 and dropped to $3,700,000,000 by 1930.[7] The average value per acre of land was $46.17 in 1900. By 1910 this had risen $95.02 per acre and in 1920 the figure stood at $164.20.[8]

Land value per acre varied widely according to the location of the farm. In 1930, when the state average was $115.40 per acre, there were twenty-four counties in which the average was more than $150 per acre. The most valuable land lay in the northern part of the state. In Lake County, for example, land sold for $329 an acre. In DuPage County, it was $292 per acre, while in Macon County it was $205.60 per acre. The highly developed dairy industry was responsible for these prices. In the leading corn-belt counties, the price of land was somewhat lower than in the north. In McLean County, land was listed at $184.46 an acre. In Champaign County, it was $192.30 an acre. From the middle of the state to the southern tip of the state, however, the price of land declined drastically. In Hardin and Pope Counties, the average prices were $21.29 and $21.54 an acre respectively.[9]

A problem related to the declining number and the increased size of farms was farm tenancy. From 1900 to 1930 the number of farms operated by the owner steadily dropped, and the number of farm tenants correspondingly increased. In 1900 slightly over 39 percent of Illinois farms were farmed by tenant farmers; in 1930 more than 43 percent were operated by tenants.[10]

The increase of tenancy was viewed with concern. Some of the concern arose from those who held the Jeffersonian view that all virtue came from agrarian life. Others feared that tenant farming was bad for the land. Governor Frank Lowden referred to the system of giving tenant farmers one-year leases as "a conspiracy to ruin land." Lowden believed that such leases gave tenant farmers so little security, they had to work the land intensively to make a living. Lowden worked to compel landlords to give more favorable and longer-term leases and asked for legislation to compel owners and operators to improve the land.[11]

Landlords, like tenants, varied widely in their interest in the land. The retired farmer moved into town and rented his farm, often to a relative. Such landlords were often superior because they knew farming and had enough interest to oversee the land they rented. On the other hand, the investor or speculator, an absentee landlord, had little interest in the land other than the profit he could wring from it. Such a landlord, coupled with a bad tenant, was likely to reduce the value of land. Some landlords argued for a short-term lease as a necessity on the grounds that tenants were a sorry lot of people who could not be trusted. Therefore, it was best to have a short lease so that it could be broken at the end of any given year.

Tenants, plagued by the problem of moving every year or every few years, often did nothing to keep buildings in repair or to build up the land. Erosion and infertility resulted. Landlords frequently were shortsighted. Refusal to make improvements prevented tenants from operating the land at a profit.[12]

Some tenants operated on a sharecrop basis; others paid rent for their acreage. In 1900, 39 out of every 100 farms were tenant-operated. Of these, 14 were cash tenants and 25 were sharecrop tenants. Customarily sharecrop tenants got one-half of the corn and three-fifths of the oats produced, paying approximately $5 an acre for meadow or pasture. The landlord required the tenant to furnish horses, implements, seed, and labor. He might also be expected to pay the cost of threshing and harvesting and to deliver the landlord's share of the grain to the elevator. If the owner furnished the seed or the teams or tools to run the farm, he got a correspondingly higher proportion of the crop. Cash rentals ranged from $2 to $6 an acre, depending on the productiveness of the land.

Cash tenants complained that rents were raised more rapidly than the price of farm products or productivity of the land justified, and that the owner of the land was usually unwilling to do much to improve it. It was true, as the owners said, that some tenants were not competent. Others, however, were good farmers. Some had been farm laborers who saved money to buy equipment and take on a farm as a tenant farmer. Others were former landowners who had fallen on bad times and been reduced to tenant farmers. The climb from tenant to owner was difficult, but many tenants dreamed of becoming owners.[13]

Farm tenancy was higher on farms where the land was most valuable and productive. In 1920 there were twenty-seven counties in which more than 50 percent of the farms were operated by tenants. The highest percentage of tenant farming in Illinois in 1920 was in Ford County, where it exceeded 70 percent of the farms. In Livingston County, tenants operated more than 65 percent of the farms, and in Logan County the percentage was much the same. Of the counties in which 50 percent of the farms were tenant farms, only four were south of Decatur, and only two were south of U.S. highway 40.

On the other hand, twenty-one counties in Illinois had less than 30 percent farm tenancy. Of these, only Jo Daviess County, in the unglaciated area of the northwest corner of the state, was north of U.S. highway 40. The lowest rates of farm tenancy were in Pope and Johnson counties in the extreme southern portion of the state. In other words, in the most productive parts of the state there was a growing tendency toward farm tenancy.[14]

Among the reasons for the exodus from the farms was the increase in labor-saving farm implements. During the first thirty years of the twentieth century, Illinois farmers progressed from hand and horse-drawn implements to tractor-powered tools. The high cost of farm machinery was a factor in eliminating the smaller and less productive farmers from the land. In 1900, for example, the farmers of Illinois owned nearly $45,000,000 worth of implements, but in 1920 they owned more than $222,000,000 worth—a fivefold increase in two decades. During the '20s the figure declined, but in 1930 there were still more than $160,000,000 worth of implements on Illinois farms.[15]

The farmer was at the mercy of the weather and the costs of production. Young people left the farms because of the increased expense in getting started in farming and because the city seemed to offer higher wages. Also important in the decline of the number of farmers was the decline of rural towns. As the automobile made it possible to go to larger towns in the area, rural towns lost facilities and much of their charm.[16]

In the antebellum South, observers commented that cotton was king. It would be equally true to say that in the early years of the twentieth century, corn was king in Illinois. It was a rare farm that did not grow some corn each year. Farmers planted corn as a cash crop and as feed for their livestock. In 1900 farmers of Illinois planted 10,460,000 acres of corn. The corn acreage remained about the same each year until 1912, when it declined, and in 1927 the acreage was less than 8,500,000.

Average yields of corn fluctuated widely. In 1900 the yield was forty bushels per acre; in 1913, it was twenty-eight. The figure was somewhat above this in the 1920s, although in 1930 it was again down to twenty-six-and-a-half bushels per acre. The season average price per bushel ranged from 32 cents in 1900 to $1.47 in 1919 (at the height of wartime inflation). Throughout the 1920s the price was considerably below $1 per bushel, except for the year 1924, when production was off substantially.[17]

In 1909, livestock consumed more than two-thirds of the corn production, while in 1919 farmers fed less than 60 percent of their corn.[18] The most important crop grown in Illinois, both in acreage and value, corn produced more income and feed per acre for the farmer than any other crop. The importance of corn varied from area to area, but it occupied between 25 and 50 percent of the cropland used. Farmers planted corn as extensively as possible, depending on the fertility of the soil, the labor available, and the need for a feed crop. In 1929 in Champaign and Piatt counties, for example, 57.7 percent of the labor was used in growing corn.

Illinois was a leading state in the acreage, production, and value of corn. Although there were problems such as the corn borer, corn grew well in the Illinois soil and hot summer sun. Whether it was possible, as some farmers maintained, to hear corn growing on a hot July night, its growth was astounding.[19]

Corn was equal to about 50 percent of the value of all crops produced in Illinois, but only about 19 percent of it went into cash income from 1924–28. The sale of livestock and livestock products amounted to nearly 60 percent of the total cash income of farmers for the same period. In the east-central part of the state, farmers shipped nearly two-thirds of the corn grown out of the county where it was produced. In the western areas of Illinois, which produced a lot of livestock, only about 20 percent of the corn was shipped out of the county.[20]

The uses of corn depended on the local area, but in Illinois in 1929 more than 90 percent of the crop was harvested for grain, most of it husked from standing stalks. A small percentage was cut for silage or fodder while another small portion was "hogged down" or harvested by turning livestock into the fields. In the

Chicago dairy area, 17 percent of the corn grown was cut for silage and about 9 percent cut for fodder, but in the grain region of east-central Illinois, some 97 percent was husked from standing stalks. In west-central Illinois more than 7 percent of the crop was harvested by livestock.[21]

The corn shock was a common sight on Illinois farms in spite of the relatively small amount of corn harvested for fodder. Most farmers cut a little corn to feed to livestock. The common practice was to shock the corn by taking in fourteen hills of corn each way. A hardworking farm laborer could make twenty to thirty shocks per day.[22]

Through World War I corn was husked from the stalk by hand labor. One of the pleasant sounds of farm life was that of ears of corn hitting the bangboard of the wagon. Most of the corn was husked by the farmer and his family, although in the areas where corn was an important commercial crop, labor was hired for the harvest. The owner provided each workman with a wagon and a team, and the workman was expected to husk two loads per day, one in the morning and one in the afternoon. This not only involved taking the corn from the stalk but also hauling it and scooping it by hand into the crib. A good cornhusker could husk eighty bushels a day, although this amount varied according to the yield of the crop.

During the period under discussion, the rate paid for hand husking varied from 3 to 6 cents per bushel in east-central Illinois. (A cornhusker was almost always paid by the bushel.) Much of the labor was transient, and frequently the laborer got his room and board in addition to pay. Thus, taking into consideration the cost of boarding the laborer and keeping the horses and wagon to haul the corn, the cost of picking corn was approximately double the amount paid to the laborer. During the period 1920–28, taking into account both labor and overhead, the farmer of east-central Illinois paid 10.4 cents a bushel for his corn harvest.[23]

In 1900 the acres of wheat harvested amounted to 2,125,000 a figure close to the average for the period 1900–28. The wheat yield in 1900 was thirteen bushels per acre. From 1900–1928, the peak was twenty bushels per acre in 1918.

The price of wheat fluctuated considerably. In 1900 the season average price per bushel was 64 cents. Like all farm products, wheat reached its highest price in 1919, at $2.15 per bushel. The price declined during the 1920s, and by 1929 the season average price was $1.12.[24]

The oats production in acres harvested was more than double that of wheat. In 1900 there were 4,750,000 acres harvested, and the average harvest throughout the thirty-year period was a figure comparable to this.[25]

The soybean, ultimately an important crop in Illinois, was of no significance at this time. Virtually no soybeans were harvested in Illinois until 1916, when 1,000 acres were harvested. By 1930 this figure increased to 410,000 acres. The soybean gained in popularity and grew well in the Illinois climate. It was grown primarily for seed production but was also used as a hay crop for livestock. In addition, it was used for green manure when clover failed.[26]

Among other local crops of importance in Illinois, broom corn was grown in a few east-central counties. Eighty-three percent of the total in 1920 was grown in Coles, Cumberland, Douglas, Jasper, and Shelby counties. This crop amounted to 14,000 acres (compared with some 16,000 acres grown throughout the state), and represented a large portion of the world crop.[27] Apples were important in some of the western and southern counties. In 1920 seven counties grew more than 100,000 bushels. These were Adams, Calhoun, Jackson, Johnson, Marion, Pike, and Union counties. Some of the apples were used for local consumption and some were made into cider, but in 1920 about 70 percent were sold as a cash crop.[28]

In 1900 the dairy products sold amounted to some $29,638,619, a figure which had increased to $63,614,986 in 1919. In 1929 milk production totaled 506,374,072 gallons. The counties with the largest milk production were concentrated in the northern part of the state, serving the Chicago market. Counties that produced more than 8,000,000 gallons of milk in 1929 were Boone, Cook, De Kalb, Du Page, Henry, Iroquois, Jo Daviess, Kane, Lake, La Salle, McHenry, McLean, Madison, Ogle, Stephenson, Whiteside, Will, and Winnebago. Of these, only Madison County was outside the Chicago area, and it sent most of its production into St. Louis.[29]

A notable feature of Illinois farms in the first decades of the twentieth century was the single-family farm. There were exceptions throughout the state, but the general practice was for a farm to be family-sized and family-operated. The man and his wife carried on the work of the farm, their labor supplemented by the children. Small boys of the family started their day along with the adults at daybreak, slopping the hogs, feeding them corn, currying and harnessing the horses, taking care of the cows, and helping with the milking. All participated in patching fences, cutting brush, chopping weeds out of the corn, and hoeing the family garden.[30] Occasionally the farmer hired a young man or a young woman to help in the fields or the house. Employees of this kind were never thought to be inferior, and in many instances became sons-in-law or daughters-in-law. Working as a hired man was the accepted method by which a young man got started as a farmer.[31]

Transients added to the labor force during the busy season. Harvest crews were a necessary evil which caused anxiety. They were likely to be a motley group ranging from hobos to college boys, often a noisy, hard-drinking lot. The women of the family were faced with feeding the thresher crew or the cornshuckers. Harvesting was a dawn-to-dark task, and all were relieved when it was over. Transients were supplemented with neighbors who traded labor for the season. In the broom-corn area each fall the "Broom-corn Johnnies" appeared, a nomadic, often drunken lot, regarded with contempt by the more stable farmers.[32]

The farm family, a nearly self-sufficient entity, paid little for food. To obtain the food or clothing that they could not produce on the farm, they sold or traded chickens, eggs, vegetables, butter, cream, or cowhides. Nearly all of these were produced as incidental to the chief cash crop. If the family lived near a village store or town, they took these items to the storekeeper and got due bills which could be used to buy things they needed.

In many communities the huckster wagon came to the farm. The huckster was an itinerant merchant, often a man who ran a store in one of the villages or small towns. He would load a wagon, especially fitted for the purpose, with all kinds of merchandise that the farm wife might need. This would include staples like salt and sugar, as well as needles and thimbles, blankets, pots, pans, and trinkets. In return, he took in trade surplus farm products as he went around the country. Some hucksters were unscrupulous businessmen who took advantage of the farm wife, but most were from nearby villages and were well known to the farmer and his wife. It was a banner day for children when the huckster wagon appeared. Besides relieving the routine of the day, the huckster often gave them candy or other treats.

Depending on location, the Illinois farmer spent his time providing his own fuel from the produce of the farm. One of the festive occasions was butchering day, usually carried out with the help of neighbors exchanging labor. The hogs were killed, scalded in a barrel, scraped, and hung. Eventually the pig would be cut up with little wasted—lard rendered, sausage ground and stuffed, and the children eating the cracklings. Also involved in farm life was the production of fruits and vegetables, much of which would be buried under a great mound of dirt and straw to prevent freezing in the winter. The farmer might also have special treats, including persimmon pudding, sassafras tea, or sorghum molasses depending on the season.[34]

There was livestock on almost every farm. Farm animals were treated well, often almost better than the family. The farmer depended on his animals for his living. It was common on the Illinois prairies to see farms where the barn appeared to be in better condition than the farmhouse.[35]

Horses were the most important livestock on Illinois farms in the first three decades of the century. After 1910, the number of horses declined due to the increasing use of the tractor, the automobile, and the truck. In 1900, there were 1,350,000 horses; by 1910, this number had increased to 1,450,000. In 1920, the number had decreased to 1,297,000, and by 1930, there were only 820,850 horses.[36] Horses served as draft animals for all purposes on the farm; mules were of relatively little importance. Very few of the horses were purebreds, but the most popular breed in Illinois was the Percheron, often crossbred with Shire or Belgian. The average weight of the horse was around 1,400 pounds. Horses were powered by produce, eating the corn and hay raised on the farm, and their manure was an important contribution to the fertilization of the farm.

The horse produced more efficiently on larger farms. On farms under 160 acres one study showed that the horse was able to produce 14.69 crop acres, but on farms over 240 acres the average rose to 21.38, nearly a 50 percent increase. Raising colts was a secondary source of income, but rarely did a farmer keep mares solely for breeding purposes. The farmer planned the breeding of his mares so that they would be able to put in full-time field duty during the busy season. The farmer sought to reduce the cost of supporting the horses and to get the largest amount of productive work from them. One study showed that on the average a horse put in 928 hours per year in the field, slightly less than three hours per day per horse, and it cost about 14½ cents an hour for horse labor. Again using averages, a study made of the efficiency of horse labor found that it took forty-six hours of horse labor to grow an acre of corn, eighteen hours to grow an acre of oats, thirty-eight hours to grow an acre of wheat, and twelve hours to grow an acre of clover. During the years 1913–18, a study was made of the cost of keeping horses, and it was found to range from $87 per year per horse in 1913 to $156.58 in 1918. From two-thirds to three-fourths of this cost represented feed. The rest of the cost involved labor, interest, shelter, harness, and other miscellaneous charges.[37]

In the early years of the twentieth century, horse labor made up a large part of the cost of the farmer's operation. Farmers still often used the single-bottom walking plow, but gradually the shift was made to the riding plow which turned two or three furrows. Plowing was one of the most important parts of the horse's activity. A man with three horses pulling a sixteen-inch sulky plow could turn a little over three acres of soil a day in the spring. On the other hand, a man with five horses pulling a gang plow with two fourteen-inch bottoms could turn a little more than five acres per day. With four horses pulling a twenty-foot harrow, a man could work forty acres per day. A man with an eight-foot binder pulled by four horses could cut almost eighteen acres of wheat per day.[38]

During the 1920s, the Illinois farmer used tractors more and more. The amount the tractor was used depended on the part of the state in which the farmer lived. In the cash-grain area of the prairie of east-central Illinois, tractors came into increasing use. In southern Illinois, where the productivity of the land was less and the farms were smaller, horses continued in use to 1930.

In a comparative survey done by the University of Illinois it was found that in 1920 the tractor was more profitable than the horse only in certain cases. The study divided all farm labor into nontractor work or that which could be done only by horses, doubtful tractor work where it seemed better to do it with horses, and tractor work where the tractor could unquestionably do the job better. Under purely tractor operations were included things like plowing, disking, harrowing, all operations which involved the preparation of the soil. In 1920 the tractor was regarded only as a traction device, a powerful and economical mechanical horse. The doubtful tractor operations involved such things as rolling, drilling small grains, harvesting corn with a corn binder, and harvesting the small grains, sorghum, and timothy. It was possible for the farmer to pull a binder with a tractor, but since the binder had to be operated by traction, it was a doubtful operation. To make it practical to haul grain on wagons with a tractor, a train of two or more wagons was needed. A number of things in 1920 could be done only by horse power. Among these were planting, cultivating, and husking corn, mowing hay, and hauling manure. It was believed that these things might be varied somewhat; the tractor could profitably pull the grain binder on a hot day when horses could not produce a good day's work. Otherwise it was not feasible to run a binder pulled by a tractor because this required a man on the binder as well as one on the tractor—by reducing horse labor, human labor was doubled.[39]

In the survey of 1918–19, the University of Illinois College of Agriculture studied 100 farmers in several east-central counties who owned tractors. It was found that of the 100 farmers, 30 had some previous tractor experience, 88 had some automobile experience, and 92 had some experience with other kinds of gas engines. The cost of operating the tractor was estimated at between $300 and $600 a year. The principal savings of the tractor came in the displacement of horses. It was estimated that a farm which produced 320 acres of crops needed sixteen horses. If the farmer added a tractor which could do the work of eight horses in plowing and disking, he could dispose of perhaps four horses and still have more traction force than before.[40]

The tractor saved little human labor, although in some tasks it could be run for longer hours, creating a savings over farming with horses. Most farmers believed that tractors did not increase yields but that they could plow deeper and faster. Other farmers used the tractor to do belt work in running grain dumps and cutting wood, not only on their own farms but on neighboring farms for hire as well. A few used their tractors for road grading, belt work on a thresher, cutting silage, and shelling corn. On the farms studied in 1918–19, farmers had used their tractors for only a little over two years in most cases, and their farms averaged 294 acres. The average cost of the tractor was $1,134.49 and there was an additional cost of $151.85 for plows. The estimated life of tractors was 5.8 years. Of the 100 tractors studied, 85 were three-plow, 10 were two-plow, and 5 were big enough to pull more than three-bottom plows.[41]

In 1920 the tractor was still a novelty, although a few manufacturers built tractors soon after the turn of the century. Hart and Parr, an Iowa firm, pioneered by building 16 tractors in 1901–02. Hart and Parr created heavy, durable tractors, half of which were still in operation in 1920.[42] Some companies produced steam tractors largely for threshing. One writer estimates that there were no more than 500 tractors in use in North America in 1906, but in that year eleven companies began manufacturing them.[43] To publicize the usefulness of tractors, manufacturers sponsored a series of plowing contests. The first was held in 1908 in Winnepeg, Canada, with 10 tractors competing, 5 gasoline and 5 steam. This contest proved that gasoline power was superior to steam power and spelled the doom of the steam tractor.[44]

International Harvester moved rapidly into the production of tractors. In 1909 Harvester entered two models in the plowing contest, a twenty- and twenty-five-horsepower, and won in both categories. In 1910, the company entered a tractor with a forty-five-horsepower engine. International Harvester built the Tractor Works at Chicago in 1910 to produce a mammoth sixty-horsepower tractor that weighed eleven tons. This powerful machine could pull an immense load. To demonstrate this, Harvester hitched three of their tractors to a fifty-five-bottom plow turning out a sixty-four-foot-wide strip of plowed ground.[45]

The tractor increased in importance as manufacturers reduced its weight while maintaining its power. The Bull Tractor Company produced the first small tractor in 1913. Called the Little Bull, the new machine weighed only 300 pounds and sold for $395. International Harvester followed with the production of a small tractor and Henry Ford brought out his low-priced Fordson tractor in 1915. The tractor industry began to learn the procedures of mass production from the automobile industry, making cheaper production possible.

The most important improvement in tractor production was the development of the power take-off. This device made it possible to use the tractor for more than just traction. Until this time, machines that were pulled had to be powered by friction through contact with the ground. On a binder, for example, in addition to the wheels that carried the weight of the machine there was a large wheel, called the bull wheel, which touched the ground. As the machine moved, contact with the ground caused the bull wheel to turn, providing power for the reel and cutting bar of the binder. With the power take-off, however, power could be transmitted directly from the tractor to the machine, resulting in greater efficiency of any implement. Until the development of the power take-off, the tractor had been limited to plowing, cultivating, and tillage. Now it could be used for all farm functions. By the end of the 1920s, the tractor industry had developed the small, all-purpose tractor which could do almost anything a horse could do. The International Harvester Farmall, the John Deere, and the Fordson provided the best examples of this development.[46]

Several organizations aimed at improving the efficiency of the farmer appeared during the first decades of the twentieth century. The University of Illinois Department of Agriculture increased its effectiveness through the use of demonstrations such as the Morrow Plots. These continuous cropping plots, in operation since 1876, afforded proof of the benefits of rotation and fertilization.[47] In 1902, the 4-H movement began in Winnebago County, where the County Superintendent of Schools, O. J. Kern, held meetings of boys for the purpose of improving their knowledge of scientific agriculture. The clubs sponsored speakers from the University of Illinois College of Agriculture; Dean Davenport of that college was one of the prime movers of 4-H. By 1904 there were a dozen clubs in that many counties and the state membership stood at 2,000.[48]

Will B. Otwell, a Carlinville nurseryman and secretary of the Macoupin County Farmer's Institute, provided impetus for the 4-H movement. He held a contest for the best corn yield on a controlled plot. This activity brought sufficient fame to Otwell so that Governor Richard Yates appointed him superintendent of the Illinois agriculture exhibit at the St. Louis World's Fair in 1904, where he created an exhibit out of the corn that boys raised over the state. Otwell coupled his program with the Winnebago County activities, and in 1915, when the Smith-Lever Act provided federal aid for these programs, 4-H began to flourish.[49]

The state government also made a number of efforts in the direction of better production for the farmer. The legislature passed a law in 1919 providing for tuberculin tests for cattle. This law was protested by many larger dairy farmers. Governor Frank Lowden lost a number of cattle from his farm, Sinnessippi. The first year he lost three carloads of milk cows that failed the test. By 1924, however, all his cows passed the test.[50] County fairs, subsidized by the state, also brought better farming methods to the attention of farmers; in 1900 fifty-five county fairs were operating in the state.[51]

In 1906 a group of Jackson County farmers formed the first unit of the Farmers Union at a meeting at the Grange Hall north of Murphysboro. Later that year two other groups met at Pincneyville and merged to form what was called the Illinois Farmers Union.[52] The Farmers Union, more radical than other such organizations, proposed to establish justice for the farmer by applying the golden rule. The union wanted to liberate farmers from the tyranny of mortgages, to assist members in buying and selling through cooperatives, and to provide scientific education and systematize production and distribution. They also wanted to eliminate

"gambling" on farm products through boards of trade. They hoped to bring farming up to the economic standard of other industries and to secure a better standard of living for farmers.[53]

President Charles S. Barrett summed up the philosophy of the Farmers Union in 1913. To the farmers he said, "You ought to sit at the first table, but you don't. Your clothes should be as good as any man wears, but they are not. Your home should be as well and comfortably furnished as other men's homes, but it is not. You should have the comforts and pleasures that others enjoy, but you don't. You and your family should go to resorts and rest as others do, but you don't."[54]

The membership of the Farmers Union in Illinois was never large, but they did sponsor a number of cooperatives. They hated the Farm Bureau and resisted the county agent system. One Farmers Union leader declared that the Farm Bureau was "ruled by Chicago grain merchants and Washington politicians."[55]

The Farm Bureau grew out of the county agent system, which developed early in the twentieth century. As early as 1901 the Illinois School of Agriculture organized an extension staff. In 1912 W. G. Eckhardt accepted a post as a full-time county farm adviser in De Kalb County and John Collier took a similar job in Kankakee County. These men were employed by county soil-improvement associations, which had worked for better fertility in their counties. Gradually other counties developed programs of this sort. In 1916 representatives of twenty of the twenty-two organized counties in Illinois held an organizational meeting for the Illinois Agricultural Association. They developed a constitution and set fees of $50 per county, soon raised to $100. Three years later a national meeting organized the American Farm Bureau Federation. Much of the membership at this meeting at the La Salle Hotel in Chicago represented Illinois (220 of the 500 delegates).[56]

The American Farm Bureau Federation was born out of the intolerance of the "Great Red Scare" as well as out of the needs of the farmers. At the opening meeting in Chicago, Henry J. Sconce, president of the Illinois Agricultural Association, said the meeting was timely because of the need for action against the industrial unrest that had been plaguing the nation since the armistice. "Is it any wonder that production has dwindled and the cost of living has so greatly increased?" he asked. "It is our duty in creating this organization to avoid any policy that will align organized farmers with the radicals of other organizations. The policy should be thoroughly American in every respect, a constructive organization

instead of a destructive organization."[57] Sconce was exceedingly conservative, and the *Prairie Farmer* of Chicago editorialized on that occasion as follows: "The American Farm Bureau Federation was launched at Chicago November 12–14, but it took to the water with its hull stove in and its engines hitting on two cylinders. Instead of being born of enthusiastic vision of big service to the business of American agriculture with which many of the delegates were inspired, it was born of the suspicion and conservatism which others brought to the meeting."[58]

Nonetheless, the Farm Bureau prospered. It started building a membership and set up cooperatives for buying fertilizer, twine, feeds, paints, tires, coal, and other products that farmers needed. It engaged in cooperative selling for the farmers and maintained a lobby in Washington. It supported the McNary-Haugen Bill of the '20s. In its organizational meeting, the Farm Bureau sang the praises of the American Legion and asked for the government to prevent outrages "against the flag and citizen." The Farm Bureau prospered because of its identification of farmers with the capitalist classes and against the laboring man. It also prospered because farmers had become accustomed to helpful county agents and cooperatives. For these reasons, the Farm Bureau grew more rapidly than the Farmer's Union. By 1925, ninety-five counties in Illinois had Farm Bureaus and employed farm advisers. The emergency of World War I gave additional funds for farm advisory work through the Smith-Lever Act. Farm advisers worked to persuade farmers to increase their use of fertilizer and to set up farm accounting programs, farm mechanics programs, and dairy and herd improvement associations.[59]

The farmer fared badly during the first thirty years of the twentieth century when his costs for implements and seeds increased more rapidly than the amounts he received for his produce. And when events caused farm prices to become inflated, his costs became even more so.

The most stable period for farm prices is generally considered to have been 1910–1914. The average prices of these years are used as a base for determining the relative wellbeing of the farmer at other times. In terms of this base price, the farmer was better off in 1914 than in any other year except the two war years of 1917 and 1919. In 1921–22 he was only about half as well off as in 1914. From 1910 to 1914 the price per bushel for corn averaged 58 cents. During the inflation of the war years, 1917–20, the price averaged $1.38 per bushel. By 1921, this price had dropped to 49 cents on the average.[60]

On the basis of averages corrected for the price level of produce, the farmer was less well off during the '20s, although the price received per bushel for corn averaged about the same as in 1910–14. To describe the situation another way, in the period 1921–28 it required 115 bushels of corn to purchase as many farm commodities as 100 bushels of corn paid for during the period 1900 to 1914. At the same time, it took 131 bushels of corn to buy as many commodities for family use or to pay a hired man's wages as 100 bushels bought in 1900–14. Taxes on farm property required 198 bushels to pay for as much as 100 bushels in 1900–19.[61]

In the 1920s some farm products sold remarkably well, but the more common crops did not measure up to the increase in the cost of supplies. Lambs, with the average of 1900–1914 equaling 100, brought 186, but corn and hogs were each 124 on that scale of 100 while beef cattle equaled 126. Horses were only 57 on that scale for 1921–28. Most of the things the farmer had to buy however cost considerably more than the average of the common crops would have brought. On the same scale, the same machinery would have cost 158, fertilizer 132, building materials 161, equipment and supplies 138, and seed 160. So even though the farmer's prices were higher, he could buy less. This was due to over-production. As the war ended, demand for many farm products declined, and the farmer found himself overproducing on the basis of the demands that had been made during the war.[62]

Other problems entered into reduction of the farm market in the '20s. The prohibition amendment brought decreased use of corn and other grains by the distillers. Distillers had found that for the small amount of legally manufactured industrial alcohol they could use cheaper raw materials such as blackstrap molasses. Before the war, distillers had used some 15 million bushels of corn and brewers another 15 million bushels.

The beginning of the use of corn for other products such as starch, corn sugar, and glucose offset these losses to a small degree, but these new industrial uses had not expanded enough to offset the decline in older uses.[63] The farmer had difficulty in reducing the acreage planted to corn since it was an essential part of the crop rotation. Farmers fed corn to meat animals and there were problems in estimating the necessary amount for feed, because the weather, always unpredictable, was the major factor in the yield of corn. The decline of horses on farms and in the cities also reduced the amount of corn and oats needed for feed, and although corn was widely used as feed for hogs, pork had fallen in popularity.

Similar problems with wheat and barley were encountered. The growth of commercial baking also had an adverse effect on the grain market because bakers made more economical use of flour than was common in home baking.[64]

The coal deposits of Illinois constituted another of its great natural resources. The deposits, estimated to have been as much as 200,000,000 tons, underlay more than two-thirds of the state. More than half of the counties mined coal. As early as the French period of Illinois, notice was taken of the coal deposits, and some coal was mined in Illinois as early as 1810, although commercial production had to wait until later in the nineteenth century. Geologists have numbered the veins of coal in Illinois from one through seven. These are in the order in which the coal was formed so that the number one seam is the deepest while the number seven seam is the most recent and the most shallow. The largest seams are those numbered five and six. By 1930 the number six seam accounted for nearly 67 percent of the total coal mined.[65]

In 1900 Illinois miners dug more than 32 million tons of coal. This figure represented the output of 875 mines employing more than 36,000 miners. Until 1916 Illinois ranked second in the nation in coal production with only Pennsylvania producing more. By that time Illinois produced 12.8 percent of the total tonnage mined in the United States. During the period 1916–1920 Illinois slipped to third place behind West Virginia but produced more than 14 percent of the total coal mined. In the period 1921–1925 Illinois still ranked third but was now producing 16 percent of the total tonnage. Between 1926–29 Illinois slipped to fourth place while Kentucky had moved into third place. In that period Illinois produced 11 percent of the U.S. total. During the years 1900–1911, 111 new mines opened in Illinois. During the period 1912–1930, there were 98 new mines.[66]

Coal mining in Illinois gradually moved from north to south. In 1881 La Salle County was the heaviest producer in the state. During the period 1893–1902 the first five counties in production, were, respectively, Sangamon, St. Clair, Macoupin, Vermilion, and La Salle. From 1903 to 1912 La Salle County slipped to tenth place while the first county in the state was Williamson followed by Sangamon, St. Clair, Macoupin, and Madison. In the period 1913–1922 Franklin County ranked first in production followed by Williamson, Sangamon, Macoupin, and St. Clair. By this time La Salle had slipped to seventeenth place. From 1923 to 1930 Franklin

County was first, Williamson was second, Macoupin third, Sangamon fourth, and Saline County had moved into fifth place. This phenomenon was brought about by a number of conditions. The coal in the northern fields, ranging from Will County to La Salle County, was a thin vein, while in the south the number six coal ranged from six to ten feet in thickness. The development of north-south railroads which handled the coal mined in the southern fields brought cheap haulage into the Chicago industrial market. And the better quality of coal in the southern counties promoted quicker development there.[67]

At the beginning of the twentieth century most of the mining was done with little mechanical labor. Haulage was carried on by mine mules, although a few mines used ponies. At least one mine used dogs for powering the cars and other mines used ropes for hand-pulling cars.[68] Most mules were stabled underground and never emerged from the damp darkness at the bottom of the shaft. In only a few mines were the mules brought up at the end of each working day, although studies showed that it added very little to the cost of coal per ton to stable them on top. Mules were a major item of expense in the mines. It was estimated in 1914 that a mine mule cost $175. The working life of the mule in the mine averaged three years. If he lived after this period, he could be sold for about $40. It cost about $11.50 a month to feed a mule corn and hay. Stabling mules in the mine presented a serious hazard because the practice of bringing hay into the mine created a danger of fire. Indeed, the Cherry Mine disaster, the worst of the period, was caused by such a fire.[69]

Even before 1900, some experiments used mechanical equipment in the mine. As early as 1877 an electric mine locomotive, called the Pioneer, was used. In 1891 another called the Terrapin Back was developed. In 1895 the predecessor of the modern mine locomotive was developed. But mechanized haulage in the mine developed slowly. In 1900 only seven mines used motor haulage. Twenty-seven mines used cable haulage, 374 used hand haulage, and 512 used horses or mules. By 1910, 106 mines, approximately 27 percent of the total, used motor haulage. By 1920 this had increased to the point where 276 mines, or 74 percent of the total, used some kind of locomotives in the mines. By 1930, 133 mines, representing 90 percent of the total, used motor haulage.[70]

The process of mechanization increased with the use of machines for undercutting the coal. Coal-cutting machines had been introduced as early as 1882. They required a skilled operator and an assistant. These men were paid by the cubic yard of coal cut from the face of the mine. Other miners were employed to fire the shots and load the coal; these men were paid by the ton. By 1900 about one-fifth of the mines used cutting machines, but by 1910 approximately 37 percent used this equipment. By 1920, 61 percent used undercutting machines, and by 1930 more than 75 percent used such machines. The same process occurred with the development of mechanical loaders for use in the mine, as well as on top, and by 1930 several mines had such equipment.[71]

There was also development of rapid hoisting processes. For example, the Old Ben No. 8 mine was able to hoist 4,428 tons in eight hours in 1914. In the same year the Superior Coal Company No. 2, at Gillespie, hoisted 5,133 tons in eight hours.[72] Where mine locomotives were used to haul from remote places of the mine to the hoisting shaft, mules sometimes pulled gathering cars from the side rooms. A number of hazards attended mechanized haulage. Electric locomotives required the running of electrical lines which could cause the electrocution of miners. Electric sparks sometimes set off explosions of gas in the mine. Gasoline locomotives emitted an exhaust which was sometimes explosive and created a need for extra ventilation. Cars sometimes ran over miners who could not hear them coming or who were unable to get out of the way.

The storage of powder and oil in the mines also caused hazards. In some places the coal dust was explosive and flammable and needed to be sprinkled down at regular intervals. Working with blasting powder was dangerous, and miners frequently opened metal kegs of powder with their pickaxes, causing sparks which exploded the powder. The miners were paid by the ton, so to make a modest subsistence, they had to work as fast as they could, often causing them to be careless.[73]

Many problems arose from bad mining practices; operators often used inadequate props and there were many falls, particularly if the blasting of the coal from the face was done carelessly. In many instances, miners failed to tamp the shots properly. A careful miner tamped the charge as firmly as possible with clay rather than coal dust and slack, called bug dust by the miners. A poorly tamped shot could result in a serious fire or explosion, and many a miner was killed because of these "windy shots." Miners also sometimes used too large a charge in order to get more coal down with each shot. Not only dangerous to the miner, this practice produced a poor quality of coal with too much slack. Excessive powder also had a tendency to crack the roof, which made for falls of the roof and often started fires on the face.[74]

From 1900 to 1920 the number of men employed in the mines increased. In 1900, including miners and workers on the surface, more than 39,000 men worked in the industry. By 1910 this figure had increased to 74,000. By 1920 more than 88,000 men were employed by the mines, but by 1930 the figure had declined to 56,000. As mechanized procedures were increasingly used in the mines, each man mined more coal. At the beginning of the century, the average tonnage per man per day in the mines was 3.5. By 1910 the average miner produced 3.9 tons per day. Ten years later this figure had risen to 5.3 tons per day. In the 1930s the average miner produced 8 tons per day. This meant that in thirty years the production per man more than doubled.[75]

Coal mining was the most dangerous occupation in Illinois. In the first three decades of the twentieth century, 5,337 men lost their lives in the mines. Defined as an accident in which more than two men lost their lives, mine disasters occurred fifty-seven times in Illinois between 1900 and 1930. Seven hundred and thirty men lost their lives in these tragic occurrences. Over ten were killed in each of eleven accidents, including the worst of all, the Cherry Mine fire in Bureau County.[76] This tragedy took place in 1910 at the St. Paul Coal Company No. 2 at Cherry. Two hundred and fifty-six miners lost their lives in a fire caused by taking hay into the mine. The car containing the hay was parked near an open flame which ignited the hay. In the panic someone pushed the car of burning hay into the draft of the ventilation system, in which the air was moving at 700 feet per minute. The flames caught the mine props in the roof on fire and shortly the whole mine was ablaze.[77]

Of the total number of fatalities in the thirty-year period, more than half were caused by roof falls brought about by improper use of mine props or excessively heavy blasting charges. The second highest number of fatalities came in haulage; over 18 percent of the fatalities were caused by men being hit by mine cars or caught in the locomotives. The third highest number, more than 10 percent, came from explosives. Other causes involved gas explosions, electrocution, and drowning.[78]

Although the miners were organized by the United Mine Workers, they were the most unfortunate group of workers in the state. Mine owners paid them by the ton and were often irresponsible and greedy. For example, Samuel T. Brush of Carbondale organized a company called St. Louis and Big Muddy Coal Company, financed mostly by out-of-state money. He started his operations in 1891 and made every effort to avoid unionization. After going through a large and expensive strike in 1899, he sold out to the Madison Coal Company, which allowed unionization of their plant, a typical company history of the times.[79]

Another of the famous operators was Joseph Leiter, who opened a mine at Zeigler in Franklin County. Leiter is of interest not only because of the Zeigler Coal Company but also because of his connections in Chicago. His father was Levi Z. Leiter, an associate of Marshall Field, one of the early developers of Chicago, and a financier of no mean talent. Joseph Leiter, an aggressive individual, once tried to corner the wheat market in Chicago, an episode which cost his father some 10 million dollars. The Leiters, father and son, became interested in coal mining through a new process of making coke utilizing Illinois coal. They bought 7,500 acres in Franklin County, where, at the time, there were no mines. They sank a shaft at Zeigler and brought in the best cutting and loading machines available, starting operation in 1904.[80] Although Leiter profited from the venture, there were many unfortunate aspects of the operation. The United Mine Workers waited until the day the mine was to open and then began a strike attended by bloodshed. Leiter incorporated the town and the coal mine in Delaware under the name of the Zeigler Coal Company, an enterprise in which the Leiters owned nearly all the stock.

After the conclusion of the strike, Leiter's trouble with the mine was not over. There were several disasters in the Zeigler mine and the blame for some of these, at least, was squarely on Leiter. The first of these problems arose on April 3, 1905, when a gas explosion killed fifty men in Leiter's mine. Subsequently a state mine inspector was killed in the investigation. On November 8, 1908, the mine caught on fire, but there were no immediate fatalities in this incident. State fire inspectors got agreement from the company to seal the mine for ninety days. It was hoped that lack of oxygen would put out the fire, and the mine could be reentered. But on January 10, 1909, the inspectors were called back to the mine; there had been an explosion which had killed twenty-six men— Leiter had failed to keep the mine sealed. Then the inspectors decided to seal the mine permanently or until they were sure the fire was out; but on February 9, less than a month later, they were called back. Another explosion had killed three more men. The owners had kept the mine sealed only twenty-one days and then had opened it again.[81]

A year later Leiter sold his interest in the mine to the Bell and Zoller Mining Company, which operated it for many years. In 1917, after Bell and Zoller had the mine, another explosion caused the death of three individuals. In spite of these disasters, however, this mine turned out to be profitable for its owners. By 1930 it had produced some 19 million tons of coal. The only mine that did better in total production was the Superior Coal Company No. 3 in Gillespie. It opened the same year as the Zeigler mine and by 1930 produced over 21 million tons of coal.[82]

As time went on corporate enterprise mined more and more of the coal and eliminated the individual owners such as Leiter. By 1930 the Peabody Coal Company owned twenty-three mines in Illinois: eight in Sangamon, five in Christian, four in Saline, two in Franklin, one in Vermilion, two in Williamson, and one in Madison County. A similar operation was carried on by the Old Ben Coal Company, which in 1930 owned twelve mines, nine in Franklin County and three in Williamson.[83] Old Ben owned some of the most productive mines of this period, acquiring some from other companies and in other cases starting new mines. Their Old Ben No. 8 at West Frankfort opened in 1910 and produced nearly 15 million tons of coal by 1930. Their second heaviest producer, Old Ben No. 11, produced more than 13 million tons by 1930.[84]

From time to time the state legislature tried to make the mines safer by legislation. The Constitution of 1870 provided power for the legislature to pass mine safety laws, and legislation in the nineteenth century provided for county mine inspectors, ventilation in the mines, escape shafts, and signals between the top and bottom of the shaft. In 1899 the legislature created a state mining board and provided that a certified mine manager had to be in charge of each mine.[85]

Responding to the hazards of handling explosives, in 1905 the legislature, during the Deneen administration, passed the "Shot-firers' Law." This act required that all mines in which more than two pounds of powder per shot was used must employ a shot-firer whose special job was to do all the blasting in the mine. Also in that session additional legislation tightened the requirements for signals in the shaft of the mine. There were provisions for a device to call for a stretcher or to reverse the ventilating fans. Women and children under sixteen were prohibited from working at manual labor in the mines. There was provision for ten inspection districts. Mine examiners were instructed to inspect each mine for air currents, recent falls, accumulation of gas, and other unsafe conditions.[86]

In 1907 the law provided for a state mining board appointed by the governor and consisting of five men—two practical miners, two coal operators (one an expert mining engineer), and a hoisting engineer. This board was given the power to administer examinations to mine inspectors, mine managers, and hoisting engineers; it became unlawful to employ any person in these jobs who was not certified by the board.[87]

Legislation further provided for the maintenance of fresh air in the mines and stables, for the mapping of mines, and for places of refuge in mine tunnels so that the miners could step off the tracks to avoid being hit by cars. The law in 1907 prohibited the storage of powder in mines and required miners to keep their lamps five feet away while opening a keg. Miners were forbidden to open kegs with their pickaxes, and it was required that the blast hole be tamped with copper tools rather than iron. There were requirements for the sprinkling of coal dust with water, and the law limited the amount of powder that could be used for a shot. In 1907 a mining commission of three miners and three owners was provided to investigate the methods and conditions of mining coal "with special reference to safety of human lives and property and the conservation of coal deposits."[88]

In 1909 a law requiring the University of Illinois to establish a Department of Mining Engineering was passed. In that year the law required that miners' compentency must be certified before their employment. The law provided that the county judge should appoint three miners as a committee to examine prospective miners. The examination cost one dollar, and only if the committee was satisfied as to the competency of the miner could he be employed. The mining board had the power to investigate reports of noncompliance with the law.[89]

In 1910 the Cherry Mine episode brought a renewed demand for safety legislation. Governor Charles Deneen called a special session of the legislature, which made provision for additional fire-fighting equipment in the mines and codified the mine laws. The law set detailed specifications for blasting powder and reaffirmed the powers of the state mining board to certify the competency of mine inspectors, managers, examiners, and hoisting engineers. The law provided for testing scales and regulating hoisting and required maps of the mines. It provided for signals in the shaft and control of the storage of oil and explosives. It also required safety lamps, regulated electricity in the mines, and provided for first aid and fire-fighting equipment as well as rescue stations. In 1913 legislation required owners of coal mines, steel mills, foundries, and machine shops to provide a heated washroom with lockers and hot and cold water for the benefit of employees.[91]

With the development of the Civil Administrative Code in 1917, there was provision for a Department of Mines and Minerals. The law provided for a director and assistant director, a mining board which included four members and the director, and a miners' examining board which included four members. In spite of all of this legislation, much of it reaffirmed session after session, there continued to be accidents and disasters.[92]

The chief development of mining in the 1920s came with the expansion of strip mining. In 1920 six-tenths of one percent (less than a half million tons) of the coal was mined by this process. By 1930 the strip mines produced more than 6 million tons of coal, which represented nearly 12 percent of the total production. Strip mining, a less complicated and much less dangerous operation, brought a wider use of machinery and a lower labor cost to the mine owners. The owner of a strip mine could count on a shorter interval between initial investment and full production. The strip mines recovered between 75 and 100 percent of all the coal in the seam, compared with 50 percent in shaft mines. And strip-mining equipment could be used for other purposes when the mine had been exhausted.[93]

Like the early shaft miners, an uninhibited, enterprising group, strip miners brought about new methods.[94] Strip mining required the seam of coal to be relatively shallow. To strip coal the ratio of the overburden to the thickness of the seam had to be 20 to 1 or less. In other words, operators could strip a three-foot seam of coal profitably if it lay no more than sixty feet below the surface. By the 1920s the operators had perfected equipment which made it possible to mine coal that far below the surface.[95]

The process of strip mining consists of cutting a trench along the edge of the coal bed and stripping away the overburden with a bulldozer, shovel, dragline, or other earthmoving equipment. Following this, a small power shovel is used to scoop the coal directly from the coal seam and load it into trucks which haul it to the washing or other preparation plants. The equipment used here was often equipment that had been used elsewhere; many of the shovels that were used to dig the Panama Canal ended up in Illinois strip mines. The stripping shovel was mammoth, often using a dipper which held thirty to thirty-five cubic yards of earth.[96]

Probably the greatest advantage in strip mining involved the safety factor. Very few lives were lost in strip mining: the mines required no timbering; there was very little blasting; and there was no accumulation of gas or other explosive materials.

There are some disadvantages in mining coal by this process, however. The chief drawback involves the destruction of the land, making it worthless for farming or most other uses, except perhaps recreation. Most of the cuts ultimately fill with water and can be used for fishing or boating, but the appearance of a stripped area can be one of great desolation.[97]

Petroleum constituted another of the natural resources of Illinois. Some oil was produced before 1900 but in such small quantities as to be of little concern. Significant production of oil started after drilling operations began in 1905. In 1906 the state produced 4.4 million barrels of crude oil. This expanded over the next few years until 1908, when 33.1 million barrels were pumped. Production then began to decline and went down slightly each year, until in 1929 producers pumped only 7.2 million barrels of crude oil. From 1907 to 1913 Illinois ranked third in the nation in oil production, behind California and Oklahoma respectively. After that time, as the oil production in Illinois declined, new fields were discovered in other states, and Illinois merited a lower rank each year.[98]

From the 1880s there were some producing oil wells, mostly around Litchfield in Montgomery County. In 1902 only 200 barrels were produced and used as an unrefined lubricant. No production at all was recorded in 1903 or 1904. In 1904, however interest in east-central Illinois revived. The first start in this field came at Oil Field, in Clark County, between Westfield and Casey, where a Pennsylvania group drilled a well that produced 35 barrels a day. During 1905 some 300 wells were drilled, extending the fields past Casey to Robinson in Crawford County. By the end of 1906 drillers had brought in a continuous field of oil wells some fifty miles long extending from western Clark County to northwestern Lawrence County.[99]

Standard Oil Company carried out much of the early exploration in Illinois. In 1906 it controlled 100 percent of the crude oil supply in the state. In the succeeding years, however, other companies—such as the Pure Oil Company and the Indian Refining Company of Lawrenceville—started drilling wells. By 1911 when the Standard Oil Company was broken up, it controlled 83 percent of the crude in Illinois. A number of independent operators also had some interest in this production.[100]

The shallow fields of southeastern Illinois produced only small amounts of oil compared with later discoveries. Lawrence County turned out to be the richest of the oil-producing areas of southeastern Illinois in this period. There the oil-bearing sands ranged from 450 to 1,985 feet deep and produced a quantity of high-grade oil. In 1913 prospectors found oil near Carlyle in southwestern Illinois. The Carlyle pool, in Clinton County, produced for several years, as did the Sandoval pool, in Marion County, which had 112 producing wells in 1913. A small amount of oil was found near Carlinville, in Macoupin County, which produced about 200 barrels per day during 1913.[101]

The thick oil in the northern part of the field contained asphalt and sulphur, while in the southern end of the eastern field, near Lawrence County, drillers found oil at a greater depth which was thinner and contained little sulphur. Most of the Illinois oils were easily refined.[102]

The early promoters of oil, a colorful lot, carried on a haphazard enterprise. The people who worked in the oil fields looked with doubt on the geologists. Most oil operators were practical men who had started as drill hands and possessed only limited education. Most of them could not understand a geological report, and most believed that geologists were fraudulent and of little help in prospecting. Men like Michael L. Benedum and Joseph C. Trees illustrate the nature of these plungers. Benedum was an operator and trader, while his partner, Trees, was an engineer. Trees had the ability to find oil and develop property, Benedum sold and traded, and through these combined skills they made money. Another colorful figure was Richmond Levering, who operated in the Bridgeport-Lawrenceville area. Levering was a personable plunger who paid little attention to details but could develop oil-producing property. He was for a number of years chief owner and president of the Indian Refining Company.[103] The oil-producing area in Clark County, around Casey, was brought in first by wildcatters, but soon men like James Donnell of the Ohio Oil Company, a subsidiary of Standard Oil, moved in.

The oil field business was a dangerous occupation. Illinois oil had a high paraffin content, and it was necessary to periodically shoot the wells with nitroglycerin. The technique, developed a number of years earlier, was a method of lowering a quantity of nitroglycerin into the well and setting it off. The resulting explosion would break open the pores of the sand and let the oil flow again. Some of the wells were shot with the astounding quantity of 200 quarts of nitroglycerin. The chief method of transportation in these early days was by wagon, and nitroglycerin was exceedingly sensitive. Any sudden jerk of the horses or the bump of an iron wheel into a hole or on a rock could set off the whole cargo. One historian of the oil fields says it was not uncommon to see a nitroglycerin wagon on the road one minute and a great explosion the next, after which wagon, horses, cargo, and driver would have disappeared. It took a special breed of man to put up with this life, and none of the oil field workers qualified as gentle types.[104] As the oil boom hit, rough characters, gamblers, sharpers, and speculators of almost every kind poured into Casey, Robinson, Bridgeport, and Lawrenceville.[105]

In the early part of this oil strike in east-central Illinois, the most important company was the Ohio Oil Company, at first a part of Standard Oil. Operators faced chaos in the oil fields in these early days because they could get oil out of the ground but had no way to get it to the refineries and markets. Standard owned refineries but the nearest was some 200 miles away, and it seemed an insurmountable problem to get the oil to them. They had built no pipeline except for a small number of gathering lines, and the railroad bed was unballasted so that roadbed often gave way under the weight of oil cars.

James Donnell of Ohio Oil went to the region and decided he could take advantage of this disparity of oil production and marketing. He did so by building tank farms at Martinsville-Casey and at Stoy, west of Robinson. Ultimately, the Ohio Oil tank farms contained nearly 1,000 tanks, each of which had a capacity of some 35,000 barrels. Donnell was able to buy a quantity of oil at the going price of 65 cents a barrel. When he finished a pipeline, he was able to sell the oil at $1.50 a barrel at its eastern terminus. He built the Illinois Pipeline Company, which went from Martinsville, Illinois, to Preble, Indiana, a distance of 191 miles. Here it joined the Indiana Pipeline Company, another subsidiary of Standard, to carry the oil to the refineries. This line was of eight-inch pipe, laid twenty inches underground, with pumping stations constructed along the way to push the oil through the pipe. No time or expense was spared in speeding this work to completion. Gangs of workers dug the trench for the pipe, often pulling it across streams, working up to their shoulders in water. When they came to railroad tracks or roadbeds, they burrowed beneath them. These pipeline workers were a hard lot of drifters, and they earned their money (25 cents an hour). The Ohio Oil Company's paymaster traveled around the country with his payroll in cash in a satchel. The pipeline, completed on Thanksgiving Day, 1906, went on-stream carrying the oil that Donnell had stored in his tanks. With transportation thus secured, the Ohio Oil Company branched out quickly in Illinois, purchasing oil from independent producers as well as drilling some 800 wells of its own.[106]

Standard Oil Company divested itself of the Ohio Company in 1911. Congress later passed the Hepburn Act, which put pipelines under the jurisdiction of the Interstate Commerce Commission. In 1914, the Supreme Court upheld the right of the government to regulate pipelines under the Hepburn Act, at which point the Ohio Company had to divorce itself from the Illinois Pipeline Company. Shareholders of the Ohio Company got shares of the Illinois Pipeline Company in proportion to the shares of the Ohio Company they held. Later the Ohio Company was able to buy back Illinois Pipeline Company when the government was less strict in the matters.[107]

There was relatively less interest of other major oil companies in the Illinois production. Shell Oil had an interest but its holdings were small because the Illinois wells produced only an average of ten barrels a day (compared with wells in Oklahoma which put out more than twenty barrels a day). The Shell Company investigated the holding of Richmond Levering around Lawrenceville but came to the conclusion that it would be better to buy Oklahoma oil and transport it to their Wood River refinery. Because of declining production in the first three decades, few major producers moved into drilling operations in Illinois. Ultimately, Richmond Levering lost his Indian Refining Company. It was nearly bankrupt from the early '20s on, and finally in 1931 Texaco bought this refinery.[108] Oil was an important part of Illinois' natural resources, but its production declined from 1910 to 1930. Later, new oil fields would be discovered to lift the production of oil in Illinois.

1. Clarence Walworth Alvord, *The Illinois Country 1673–1818* (Springfield, Ill., 1920), p. 1.

2. Theodore Saloutos and John D. Hicks, *Twentieth Century Populism: Agricultural Discontent in the Middle West 1900–1913* (Lincoln, Neb., n.d.), p. 13.

3. *Fourteenth Census of the United States, 1920: State Compendium: Illinois* (Washington, D.C., 1924), pp. 89–90.

4. *Fifteenth Census of the United States, 1930: Agriculture*, vol. II, part I, The Northern States (Washington, D.C., 1932), p. 568.

5. *Fourteenth Census, 1920: Illinois*, pp. 84–90.

6. *Fifteenth Census, 1930: Agriculture*, vol. I, Farm Acreage and Farm Volumes (Washington, D.C., 1931), p. 144.

7. Ibid., vol. ii, part I, The Northern States, p. 567.

8. *Fourteenth Census, 1920: Illinois,* pp. 89–90.

9. *Fifteenth Census, 1930: Agriculture,*   vol. II. part I, The Northern States, pp. 643–47.

10. Ibid., p. 567.

11. William T. Hutchison, *Lowden of Illinois: The Life of Frank O. Lowden,* (2 vols. (Chicago, 1957), I, 353.

12. Saloutos and Hicks, *Twentieth Century Populism,* pp. 14, 17.

13. Ibid., pp. 16–18.

14. *Fourteenth Census, 1920: Illinois,* pp. 100–109.

15. *Fifteenth Census, 1930: Agriculture,* vol. II, part I, The Northern States, p. 567.

16. Saloutos and Hicks, *Twentieth Century Populism,* pp. 24–27.

17. J. A. Ewing, comp, *Illinois Agricultural Statistics* (Illinois Department of Agriculture, Springifield, 1948), pp. 56, 16.

18. *Fourteenth Census, 1920: Illinois,* pp. 99; P. E. Johnston and K. H. Myers, "Harvesting the Corn Crop in Illinois: An Economic Study of Methods and Relative Costs," *University of Illinois Agricultural Experiment Station Bulletin 373* (Urbana, 1931), pp. 356–67.

19. Johnston and Myers, "Harvesting the Corn Crop," p. 355.

20. Ibid., pp. 356–57.

21. Ibid., p. 357.

22. H. R. Tolley and L. M. Church, "The Standard Day's Work in Central Illinois. Performance of Implements and Crews as Indicated by Reports from 600 Farmers in a Typical Corn-Belt Area," *U.S. Department of Agriculture Bulletin 814* (Washington, D.C., 1920), pp. 14–15.

23. Tolley and Church, "The Standard Day's Work," pp. 17–18; Johnston and Myers,"Harvesting the Corn Crop," pp. 359, 360, 362.

24. Ewing, *Illinois Agricultural Statistics,* pp. 19, 20; L. J. Norton and B. B. Wilson, "Prices of Illinois Farm Products from 1886 to 1929," *University of Illinois Agricultural Experiment Station Bulletin 351* (Urbana, 1930), pp. 504, 550.

25. Ewing, *Illinois Agricultural Statistics,* p. 25.

26. Ibid., p. 36; W. L. Burlinson and O. M. Allyn, "Soybeans and Cowpeas in Illinois," *University of Illinois Agricultural Experiment Station Bulletin 198* (Urbana, 1917), pp. 2–20.

27. *Fourteenth Census, 1920: Illinois,* pp. 120–129; *Illinois State Journal,* Jan. 8, 1900, p. 2.

28. *Fourteenth Census, 1920: Illinois,* pp. 120–129; *Fifteenth Census, 1930: Agriculture,* vol. II, part I, The Northern States, pp. 624–31.

29. *Abstract of the Twelfth Census of the United States, 1900* (Washington, D.C., 1900), pp. 252–53; *Fourteenth Census, 1920: Illinois,* p. 94; *Fifteenth Census, 1930: Agriculture,* vol. II, part I, The Northern States, pp. 632–36.

30. Soloutos and Hicks, *Twentieth Century Populism,* pp. 12–13.

31. Cyrus McCormick, *The Century of the Reaper* (New York, 1931), pp. 214–15; R. B. Best, *We Are What We Have To Be* (New York, 1965), pp. 123–25.

32. Best, *We Are What We Have To Be,* pp. 164–65, 286.

33. Ibid., p. 188.

34. John W. Allen, *Legends and Lore of Southern Illinois* (Carbondale, Ill., 1963), pp. 160–62, 164–65, 170–71.

35. Best, *We Are What We Have To Be,* p. 303.

36. *Fifteenth Census of the United States, 1930, Abstract* (Washington, D.C., 1933), p. 663.

37. W. F. Handschin, J. B. Andrews, and E. Rauchenstein, "The Horse and the Tractor: An Economic Study of Their Use on Farms in Central Illinois," *University of Illinois Agricultural Experiment Station Bulletin 231* (Urbana, 1921), pp. 176, 179, 882, 185, 188–94.

38. Tolley and Church, "The Standard Day's Work," pp. 2–3.

39. Handschin and Andrews, "The Horse and the Tractor," pp. 175, 203–25.

40. Ibid., pp. 210–11, 212.

41. Ibid., pp. 211, 212.

42. McCormick, *Century of the Reaper*, p. 155.

43. Ibid., pp. 153–54, 155–56.

44. Ibid., pp. 156–57.

45. Ibid., p. 158.

46. Ibid., pp. 159–60, 209–12.

47. E. E. DeTurk, F. C. Bauer, and L. H. Smith, "Lessons from the Morrow Plots," *University of Illinois Agricultural Experiment Station Bulletin 300* (Urbana, 1927), pp. 107–40.

48. Franklin M. Reck, *The 4-H Club Work* (Ames, Iowa, 1951), pp. 16–19.

49. Ibid., pp. 20–22, 109.

50. *Laws of the State of Illinois, Enacted by the Fifty-first General Assembly* (Springfield, 1919), pp. 211–12; Hutchison, *Lowden of Illinois* II, 498.

51. *Illinois State Journal*, Feb. 27, 1900, p. 5.

52. Roy V. Scott, "John Patterson Stelle: Agrarian Crusader from Southern Illinois," *Journal of the Illinois State Historical Society* 55 (Autumn, 1962), pp. 246–47; Allen, *Legends and Lore*, pp. 183–84; Saloutos and Hicks, *Twentieth Century Populism* p. 223.

53. Saloutos and Hicks, *Twentieth Century Populism*, pp. 230–31.

54. John A. Crampton, *The National Farmers Union: Ideology of a Pressure Group* (Lincoln, Nebr., 1965), p. 3.

55. Saloutos and Hicks, *Twentieth Century Populism*, pp. 230–31.

56. Orville Merton Kile, *The Farm Bureau through Three Decades* (Baltimore, 1948), pp. 25, 33, 45–46, 47–55.

57. Saloutos and Hicks, *Twentieth Century Populism*, pp. 255, 269.

58. Kile, *Farm Bureau*, pp. 54–55.

59. Saloutos and Hicks, *Twentieth Century Populism*, pp. 260, 261; Kile, *Farm Bureau*, pp. 67, 70; *Illinois Blue Book, 1925–26*, p. 357.

60. Norton and Wilson, "Prices of Illinois Farm Products," p. 495.

61. Ibid., p. 573.

62. Ibid., pp. 572–73.

63. Ibid., pp. 532, 536.

64. Ibid., pp. 527, 533, 534–35, 536.

65. "A Compilation of the Reports of the Mining Industry of Illinois from the Earliest Records to 1954," *Report of Illinois Department of Mines and Minerals 1955* (Springfield, 1955), pp. 13, 14, 19. Hereinafter referred to as "Compilation." Herman D. Graham, "The Economics of Strip Coal Mining with Special Reference to Knox and Fulton Counties, Illinois," *Bureau of Economic and Business Research Bulletin 66* (Urbana, 1948), p. 13n.

66. *Twelfth Census, 1900: Abstract*, p. 432; "Compilation," pp. 23, 54–57.

67. "Compilation," p. 16; Gilbert H. Cady, "Coal Resources of District I (Longwall)," *Illinois State Geological Survey Bulletin 10* (Urbana, 1915), pp. 15–16; John A Garcia, "A Mining Engineer's View of the Future of the Illinois Coal

Industry from the Standpoint of Recovery," *Illinois State Geological Survey Bulletin 60* (Urbana, 1931), p. 72.

68. "Compilation," p. 33; S. O. Andros, "Coal Mining Practice in District III," *Illinois State Geological Survey Bulletin 9* (Urbana, 1915), p. 23.

69. S. O. Andros, "Coal Mining Practice in District V," *Illinois State Geological Survey Bulletin 6* (Urbana, 1914), pp. 21, 30; S. O. Andros, "Coal Mining Practice in District II," *Illinois State Geological Survey Bulletin 7* (Urbana, 1914), p. 14, S. O. Andros, "Coal Mining Practice in District VI," *Illinois State Geological Survey Bulletin* (Urbana, 1914), p. 31. "Compilation," pp. 33, 86.

70. "Compilation," pp. 32, 33.

71. Ibid., pp. 31, 32, 34.

72. Andros, "District VI," p. 44; S. O. Andros, "Coal Mining Practice in District VII," *Illinois State Geological Survey Bulletin 4* (Urbana, 1914), p. 48.

73. Andros, " District VII," pp. 29, 35, 43; S. O. Andros, "Coal Mining Practice in District IV," *Illinois State Geological Survey Bulletin 12* (Urbana, 1915), pp. 48, 49.

74. Andros, "District V," pp. 17, 21, 23, 25.

75. "Compilation," pp. 18, 30.

76. Ibid., pp. 44, 113.

77. Ibid., pp. 86, 113.

78. Ibid., p. 145.

79. Paul Angle, *Bloody Williamson: A Chapter in American Lawlessness* (New York, 1952), pp. 90, 96–97, 116.

80. Ibid., pp. 118, 119.

81. *Chicago Tribune*, Aug. 5, 1904, p. 3; Aug. 8, 1904, p. 5; "Compilation," pp. 84, 113.

82. "Compilation," pp. 59, 84 113; Angle, *Bloody Williamson*, pp. 132, 133n.

83. "Compilation," pp. 54–57.

84. Ibid., pp. 45–57, 59.

85. Ibid., pp. 63–65.

86. Ibid., p. 65; *Laws of the State of Illinois Enacted in the Forty-fourth General Assembly* (Springfield, 1905), pp. 324–25, 326, 328–30.

87. *Laws of the State of Illinois Enacted in the Forty-fifth General Assembly* (Springfield, 1907), pp. 387–93.

88. Ibid., pp. 55–57, 349–400, 401–3.

89. *Laws of the State of Illinois Enacted in the Forty-sixth General Assembly* (Springfield, 1909), pp. 43, 284–86.

90. *Laws of the State of Illinois Enacted by the Forty-seventh General Assembly* (Springfield, 1911), pp. 385–427.

91. *Laws of the State of Illinois Enacted by the Forty-eighth General Assembly* (Springfield, 1913), p. 354.

92. *Laws of the State of Illinois Enacted by the Fiftieth General Assembly* (Springfield, 1917), pp. 22–24.

93. "Compilation," p. 20; Graham, "The Economics of Strip Mining," p. 25.

94. For example, see Paul Angle's description of William J. Lester, whose operation started the Herrin massacre. *Bloody Williamson*, pp. 11–12.

95. Graham, "The Economics of Strip Mining, pp. 11, 13.

96. Ibid., pp. 17–19, 27.

97. Ibid., pp. 7, 19–20.

98. Harold F. Williamson, Ralph L. Andreane, Arnold R. Daum, and Gilbert C. Klose, *The American Petroleum Industry: The Age of Energy, 1899–1959* (Evanston, Ill.,

1963), pp. 16, 302; Raymond S. Blatchley, "Petroleum in Illinois in 1912 and 1913," *Illinois State Geological Survey Circular 8* (Urbana, n.d.), pp. 3–4.

99. Raymond Foss Bacon and William Allen Hamor, *The American Petroleum Industry*, 2 vols. (New York, 1916), I, 236–37n.

100. Williamson et al., *American Petroleum Industry*, p. 7. Hartzell Spence, *Portrait in Oil: How the Ohio Oil Company Grew to Become Marathon* (New York, 1962), pp. 37–46, 60–62.

101. Bacon and Hamor, *American Petroleum Industry*, I, 77–78.

102. Ibid., I, 70.

103. Williamson et al., *American Petroleum Industry*, p. 45; Spence, *Portrait in Oil*, p. 109; Kendall Beaton, *Enterprise in Oil* (New York, 1957), p. 117.

104. Spence, *Portrait in Oil*, pp. 62–63; Bacon and Hamor, *American Petroleum Industry*, I, 330, 336.

105. Spence, *Portrait in Oil*, p. 61.

106. Ibid., pp. 61–62, 211–13.

107. Ibid., pp. 37–46, 213–15.

108. Beaton, *Enterprise in Oil*, pp. 117, 119.

4

The Position of Labor in Illinois

People in Illinois who worked with their hands for wages did not occupy an enviable position at the beginning of the twentieth century. Large corporations held much of the industry and the retail businesses in larger cities. Hired managers, who had no interest except increasing profits, ran these corporations. Employers paid low wages, and even when the laborer was able to improve his income, the cost of living generally rose faster than his income. He worked long hours that made recreation or rest impossible and often had inadequate food, housing, and clothing. The man who supported a family by working in a factory had to compete with women and children, often as young as ten years of age, who worked longer hours for lower wages. Industry imported immigrant laborers, who took submarginal wages. Long periods of unemployment, particularly in depression years, deprived laborers of even minimum decencies for their families.

Although working men had organized unions long before 1900, organized labor could muster little strength. Many citizens looked upon labor unions as radical organizations that sought to take away the freedom of both employers and employees. Writing in 1903, John Mitchell, one of the great labor leaders of Illinois, summed up the position of the working man:

Formerly and, in fact, until quite recently, all discussions upon the subject of labor, its rights, and duties assumed the working man to be a mere animate machine. The comparison was frequently made between the sale of labor and that of any other commodity, without reflection that the seller of a bushel of wheat cares not how, when, where or by whom it is consumed, whereas the seller of a day's labor may be affected throughout his life time by the manner, place, and circumstances of the use of that day's labor. The working man was considered a machine which cost so many dollars per day, which was to be used so many hours, which was to be given the smallest amount of care, attention, and fuel necessary to keep it in fair working order. He was an organism without a soul, composed, in fact, wholly of hands and stomach. Even now an employer speaks of so many hundred "hands" meaning thereby that number of individual workmen.[1]

In the years after 1900, retail store employees suffered the most. Observers agreed that a single woman could live in a city on no less than $8 per week. Yet thousands made less than that. John Glenn, secretary of the Illinois Manufacturers' Association, testified in 1913 that 57,000 women in Chicago were getting less than $5 per week.[2] Testimony of various owners of State Street stores confirmed Glenn's testimony. Barrett O'Hara, lieutenant governor of Illinois in the Dunne administration, conducted a vice investigation in the state in 1913. Many reformers believed that low wages frequently drove women into prostitution. O'Hara's committee conducted a thorough investigation of wages paid, and the report of the commission gives an excellent picture of wages for that era.

Officials of the State Street stores were called before the O'Hara Commission to testify on wages paid to their employees. Edwin F. Mandel, president of Mandel Brothers, who employed 1,866 women, told the committee that his company paid some employees as little as $3 per week. All those receiving this sum were under fourteen years of age. Mandel testified that the average wage paid to women in his store was $9.86 per week, but a substantial number got less than $7. The company paid a minimum of $5 per week for full-time work, and the average pay for all females in the store was $10.76 (this included buyers, managers, and others who were paid higher wages).[3]

James Simpson, vice-president of Marshall Field & Company, told the committee that competition kept wages down. He stated that doubling the wages of the 213 women who got $5 per week would only increase operating costs by $1,065 per week—an outlay which would not materially affect profits. But Simpson maintained that Field's could not pay more because of the competition. He insisted that his female employees were not badly treated, saying some worked only an eight-hour day. Field's gave employees two weeks paid vacation if they had been employed more than a year. Field's also kept a trained nurse in the store and had an arrangement with St. Luke's Hospital for taking care of employees who became ill. A lunchroom was maintained where food could be had for 10 or 11 cents a day.[4]

Edward J. Lehman, vice-president of the Fair Store, described a similar situation in his store. Lehman employed 1,705 women, a few of whom made as little as $3 per week. Those making $5 a week or less, called juveniles, were under eighteen years of age. Fifty-five percent of those making less than $5 were under sixteen. Approximately the same situation existed in most of the other stores along State Street including Carson, Pirie, Scott and Company, the Hub, and Siegel, Cooper, and Company.[5]

Testifying before O'Hara's committee probably pained Julius Rosenwald, the president of Sears, Roebuck and Company, more than the other store operators. Rosenwald, who had taken over the direction of Sears and developed it into a gigantic company, was gaining the reputation of a philanthropist but had to testify that even though his company made more than 7 million dollars profit in 1911, he paid wages as low as $5 per week. He also said that 1,465 of the 4,732 women employed by Sears got less than the $8 per week minimum (called "the bread line" by O'Hara). One woman said that those who were slow or careless were scolded to the point of tears. Another testified that in order to have water to drink during working hours, women had to pay 10 cents to the Sears company every two weeks.[6]

Montgomery Ward, chief competitor of Sears for mail-order business, could not boast of better conditions. Montgomery Ward paid women a minimum of $5 per week. Experienced women averaged $9.25 per week, but those who had been there a shorter period of time received only $8.80. Of the 1,973 inexperienced women, 233 got the minimum $5 per week, 572 received $6, 373 were paid $7, and 316 got $8 per week.[7]

In Peoria, the lowest paid women took home from $3.50 to $4 per week. Most of these women, sixteen years of age or below, worked as bundle wrappers, cash girls, or apprentices. It was estimated that the cost of living for a female in Peoria was a little less than in Chicago but, generally speaking, would still require $7 to $8 per week. In Springfield things were even worse. May Barnes, age sixteen, testified that she worked at the Boston Store as a cash girl for $2.75 for a week of fifty-seven hours.[8]

Male employees got more pay but still made little more than enough to survive on. Julius Rosenwald testified that he employed 4,171 men, of whom 1,289 were under age 21. The average wage for this younger group was $7.81 per week. The lowest figure he paid in this group was $5 per week for boys under sixteen. Boys over sixteen got $6 per week. The average salary for men over twenty-one was $18.82 per week. Sears made a distinction between married men and single men, giving married men a minimum of $12 per week.[9]

Marshall Field employed 3,510 men, paying them an average of $19 a week, not including section heads. This group included about 3,000 men over the age of twenty-one. These men worked as porters, elevator operators, salesmen, packers, and drivers. The lowest weekly wage paid to a married man was $12. Unmarried men between sixteen and twenty-one got $8 to $12 a week, while a few boys under sixteen got between $5 and $8 per week. Vice-president Lehman of the Fair Store testified that they paid their 417 salesmen an average wage of $14.48 per week. Some boys in the store got as little as $5 per week. John D. Pirie, Jr., vice-president of Carson, Pirie, Scott and Company, testified that among the 1,207 men they employed, the average weekly wage was $18.38. The lowest wage paid for adult males was $10 per week. He employed a few errand boys for as little as $4 per week.[10]

In other kinds of employment the wages varied a good deal for women. For example, George E. Munger, manager of a Chicago laundry which employed 186 women, testified that 93 got under $8 per week. Some earned $4 per week, although the average was $8.15. On the other hand, the female bookkeeper that had been with the laundry ten years made $21 per week. Two women who had been with him twenty and twenty-five years got $15 and $16 for a fifty-four-hour week. For the most part the women had to stand during the entire day. Munger testified that they were mostly Polish immigrants. Women working in laundries in Springfield took home an average of $6 per week.[11]

There were other kinds of employment where women made more. Jeanette Fullerton, a dramatic actress in a stock company in Peoria, testified that she was paid $40 per week. Fullerton, a leading lady, said that acting was the highest paid profession in the world for women. She testified that actresses were usually paid $35 to $75 per week.[12]

In Peoria, domestics and nurses in the Peoria State Hospital got from $20 to $75 a month. In addition to this, they got room, board, laundry, and free medical care. Ella Flagg Young, Chicago superintendent of schools, testified that elementary school teachers in her system got from $650 to $1,200 a year, averaging about $925. Manual-training teachers got a little more. Their pay ranged from $850 to $1,500 per year, with seven years experience necessary to make the top salary.[13]

Banks did not pay employees well. George Reynolds, president of the Continental Commercial Bank, testified that he employed 837 men, of whom 25 were getting $5 a week. He asserted that the average wage for men was $900 a year. John J. Mitchell, president of the Illinois Trust and Savings Bank, employed 217 people. He had 15 messengers who got as little as $42 per month. Clerks in the bank got as much as $120 a month. Bookkeepers averaged $90 per month. Women employees got only $80 per month; policemen employed by the bank got $81. Mitchell said the bank was careful about the amount paid to employees and believed an employee should not get married unless he was making an adequate salary. Mitchell recounted a story of a messenger, making only $50 a month, who married and was fired because the bank knew he could not support a wife on that salary. Bank officials were afraid he might steal to supplement his income.[14]

Theodore Robinson, vice-president of the Illinois Steel Company, a subsidiary of the United States Steel Corporation, testified that his company employed 22,000 people. The lowest wage paid for a ten hour day was $1.95 and the average was $2.74. This included some people such as highly skilled heaters in the rolling mills, who got $300 to $400 a month. He testified that the mill employed 150 women, including stenographers, typists, and telephone operators. For these, the average wage was $60.77 per month.[15] In a study of wages, Paul Douglas found that the average annual wage in the blast furnaces and rolling mills of the steel industry in 1900 was $561. This figure gradually rose. In 1905, the average annual wage in steel was $622. In 1910, it was $675. By 1915, with World War I imminent, the figure had risen to $766. This rise in wages took place in spite of the fact that the steel unions had been virtually destroyed by the steel magnates.[16]

A similar Douglas study of the packing industry showed that the average annual wage was $473 in 1904, $517 in 1908, $559 in 1912, and $727 in 1915.[17] Before the O'Hara Commission, C. L. Charles, an assistant superintendent of the Morris Packing Company, stated that in 1913 they paid the common laborer a minimum of 17½ cents per hour but paid women less. Louis Swift, president of Swift and Company, testified that they employed 399 female plant workers and paid an average wage of $7.59 per fifty-hour week. The lowest weekly wage paid was $6. M. D. Harding, a superintendent for Armour and Company, reported that they paid 840 women as little as 8⅓ cents per hour, or $5 per week, although the average weekly wage for all women employed at the plant was $7.19. He said 65 percent of these could sit during their work. Most of the women were Lithuanian, Slav, Bohemian, Serbian, and Polish immigrants. Harding said English-speaking women were given better jobs as the opportunity arose.[18]

Garment industries in Chicago treated their employees, for the most part women recently arrived in the United States, the worst both in terms of pay and working conditions. One of the worst of these was Rosenwald and Weil. Esther Berenson, Russian-born, age thirty-six had to be examined by the O'Hara Comission through an interpreter. She did not know the name of the firm she worked for but identified the location of Rosenwald and Weil. Married and the mother of three, she cleaned coats five days a week, 7:30 A.M.to 6:00 P.M., for $3.40 per week. Her husband earned $9 a week and she had one child, age sixteen, who also worked. Rebecca Shultz, age seventeen, Russian-born, who had been in this country nine months and spoke only Yiddish, also worked at Rosenwald and Weil. The company paid her $4 a week for basting coats ten hours a day. She lived with her brother in a rooming house where she paid $3.50 per week for room and board. Company officials of Rosenwald and Weil testified before the commission that the lowest wage in their factory was $2.60 per week. They commented that Esther Berenson would have made more except that she had not worked a whole week; she had worked only forty-seven hours. These men said that women earning $3.50 a week could save perhaps 25 to 30 cents a week after paying for their board, room, and clothes. This company employed 350 to 400 persons who were required to perform well and turn out a given amount of work to earn $3.50 per week.[19] Walter J. Rubens, of Rubens and Marble, manufacturer of underwear, testified that his company employed 186 women and paid a minimum of $5 per week for a fifty-four-hour week, yet 75 percent of the employees of Rubens and Marble got below the $8 minimum regarded as the level of decency.

In some cases, companies paid workers on a piecework system. Sarah Schwartz, age seventeen, testified that, in working for Nathan and Company as a machine operator making dresses, she was on piecework and sometimes made $10 a week. But she also said that at times the piecework rate was cut to the point where she could make only $2.50 to $3 per week. She had gone to work for Nathan and Company at age fourteen. She also testified that the foreman kept the record of earnings and she suspected that sometimes she had been cheated. She got 80 cents for making a dozen shirtwaists. She testified that the foreman was often overbearing toward the women and referred to them as "lousy Jews." Mrs. Siegel, another machine operator for Nathan and Company, testified she made $4 to $5.50 a week. She had a daughter who earned from $6 to $6.50 a week. The two of them were supporting an aged mother and five children.[20]

In Peoria the O'Hara Commission talked to industrialists and found that they paid about the same wages. Edward C. Heidrick, president of Peoria Cordage Company, testified that he employed 80 women and paid a minimum wage of $6 per week. He believed that a woman could live respectably on that wage. W. E. Persons, manager of the Larkin Company, which manufactured soap, toilet articles, and sundries, testified that they employed 316 women and paid a minimum of $5 per week. He reported that the highest paid wage in the factory was $17 a week. Of the females employed, 40 earned more than $8 per week. These women worked approximately a forty-seven hour week and were for the most part on piecework. Henry J. Kuch, a partner in Steuben and Kuch, manufacturers of tin cans and tinware, testified that they employed 56 women and paid them an average of $5.64 per week for an eight-hour day or $8.72 per week for a ten-hour day. This Peoria factory paid a minimum wage of $4 per week.[21]

The International Shoe Company in Springfield employed 258 women, most of them doing piecework fifty-nine hours a week. Women who worked for the company testified that they made wages of $4 per week and that working conditions were exceedingly bad. Pearl Briggs, age twenty-one, had been working since she was sixteen. She testified that the factory had a system of fines whereby workers were docked 10 cents from their wages if they were five minutes late to work. She worked at sewing shoe tips and had to sew seventy-two tips for five cents. If she ruined one, the company fined her 5 cents, which meant that she had to do seventy-two more shoe tips to break even. Miss Briggs earned from $2.75 to $5 a week. She and other women who worked for this company testified that the foreman shook them, threw shoes and boxes at them, and otherwise treated them in a brutal and inhuman fashion if they slowed down. Another woman testified that she had been poisoned from licking labels in the company's box factory.

A member of the O'Hara Commission expressed outrage at a system which charged women such excessive fines for mistakes. The superintendent replied, "What are you going to do when girls persist in doing things wrong?" One of the foremen in the factory said that the low wages were necessary, and if he could get labor even cheaper, he would do so immediately. When the commission questioned him on this point he said, "Yes, Sir; isn't it business to do it?" This foreman, William Alexander, Scottish-born, had been with International Shoe Company for a year and a half and was getting $20 a week at age twenty-seven.[22]

Paul Douglas examined the farm implement business and found that the wages there rose at about the same rate as in steel and meat-packing. The average annual wage in the manufacture of farm implements in 1900 was $531. In 1905, it had gone up to $574. In 1910 the wage was $572 per year on the average. By 1915 it had reached $745 per year.[23] The unionized industries paid better wages. In coal mining, where the union was well established, wage rates were determined biannually by agreements between miners and coal operators. The majority of the workers were paid by the ton of coal mined. Many miners were able to make as much as $5 a day when they were working. Unfortunately the mines operated irregularly, and in the year ending in June, 1913, the mines in Sangamon County operated for only 181 days. Mine owners paid others who worked around the mines—drivers, timbermen, and helpers—even less.[24]

In some other areas unions forced employers to pay better wages. Henry Blair, chairman of the board of Chicago Railways Company, testified that his company paid their 8,769 employers an average wage of $69.20 a month. They paid trainmen an average of $75.63 per month and track department workers, who handled construction and repairs, $42.63 per month. The highest paid people were the office workers, who got $91 per month.[25]

Paul Brissenden found that from 1899 to 1914 wages rose from an estimated full-time per capita earnings for male workers of $609 to $700 in 1904. In 1909, the figure climbed to $749, and by 1914 this figure had reached $854. Brissenden found that wages in Chicago were slightly higher than they were in Illinois as a whole. He also found that wages were higher in Illinois in the period from 1900 to 1925 than in any state east of the Mississippi. In the West, a few states paid higher wages, presumably because of the scarcity of labor.[26]

Paul Douglas found that between 1900 and 1915 the cost of living steadily rose. Taking the years 1890 to 1899 as the norm, he found the cost of living index had risen 58 percent by 1913. In this way, he found that although the weekly wage average of the worker had gone up, his real wages (in terms of buying power) were 5 percent lower in 1914 than for the decade of 1890 to 1899.[27]

The laboring man faced the problem of a long workweek. To a generation used to a standard forty-hour week, the hours worked in the years following 1900 seem impossible. In the sweated industries, employees worked a sixty-hour week, a ten-hour day, six days a week. Retail stores also required that their employees put in a sixty-hour week. In the steel industry many employees worked more than seventy-two hours a week. Three-fifths of those in the rolling mills worked at least that much, as did employees in the cement and gas industries. In a few industries, such as breweries, publishing and printing, and tobacco, employees worked forty-eight hours a week or less.[28]

Most workers could anticipate frequent periods of unemployment. The census of 1900 showed that of more than 400,000 engaged in manufacturing and mechanical pursuits, 64,000 were unemployed for periods ranging from one to three months during the previous year. More than 53,000 were unemployed for a period of four to six months the previous year, and 16,000 were unemployed for periods ranging upward from seven months.[29]

Paul Douglas and an associate also studied unemployment throughout the period. Their figures indicate that unemployment was common but varied from industry to industry. In manufacturing and transportation 6.3 percent of the workers were unemployed during 1900. In 1905, 4 percent were unemployed, while in 1910 only 3.7 percent were unemployed. But in the depression year of 1908, as many as 12 percent had been unemployed. In the building trades unemployment reached 26.7 percent in 1900. In 1905, it was 12 percent, in 1910, 20.2 percent, and in 1915, 31.5 percent. In coal mining the average of unemployment was high for the whole period. In 1900 it was 31 percent. In 1905, 30.8 percent were unemployed, while in 1910 it was 28 percent and in 1915, 31.7 percent.[30]

Child labor was a problem. Children working in the plants took jobs that men could otherwise have had. But far more important, hard work and long hours blighted the lives of children, making them liable to disease and crippling accidents. Children had no time to be children and had to forego education.[31] Hull House workers were perplexed when neighborhood children refused candy. They found that many of these children worked six days a week in a candy factory and could not stand the sight of candy.[32]

In 1899, the chief factory inspector of Illinois reported that 3.3 percent of the labor force in Illinois were children. In spite of laws prohibiting certain types of child labor, many children worked in such industries. An article in 1900 in the *Inter-Ocean* reported glaring abuses in the sweatshops. An article in the *Chicago Tribune* in 1908 pointed out that one manufacturer of mill machinery advertised his product as particularly well adapted for use by children.[33]

John Mitchell wrote bitterly in 1903 of the problem of child labor: "The utter ruinessness of this parasitic exploitation of children before they can arrive at strength or maturity should animate statesmen to legislate against this abomination and to destroy it root and branch. We are daily seeing the spectacle of children taken out of school and thrust into factories, with the result that a few years of ineffectual work are added and a great many years of productive and effective labor are lost."[34]

Most working people lived in inadequate housing. In spite of well-intended ordinances, landlords continued to rent decrepit and overcrowded housing. The Hull House district in 1910 contained ninety-one persons per acre while the average for the city of Chicago was only eighteen people per acre. As land became more expensive, real estate owners divided much of Chicago into standard lots of 25 by 100 feet and built shoestring buildings which covered most of the lot, eliminating light and ventilation and leaving little room for recreation. Children had to play in the streets. In the Hull House district more than 20 percent of the tenements covered 90 percent of the lot on which they stood. Another 25 percent covered 80 percent of the lot on which they stood, and 23 percent covered more than 70 percent of the lot. Often the owner constructed an additional tenement on the alley, sometimes converting an old stable. Among several bad areas in Chicago, the Hull House district, running east to the river and including the old ghetto, was particularly bad.

The Hull House district illustrates the changing character of the population of an area. After the Chicago fire, native Americans who lived there gave way to Irish and Germans, who in turn were replaced by Russians and Italians, and they by Greeks and Bulgarians. By World War I, Blacks and Mexicans had superseded these. The crowding in such an area was unbelievable. Investigators found four children sleeping in a room that had no windows and only 722 cubic feet of space. In another room five lodgers and a child crowded into a space which legally could be occupied by only three adults. One of the worst examples that investigators turned up in this crowded district was one in which the landlord had built a wide shelf over a basement stairway and closed it in to create a tiny, light-proof, air-proof room of only 125 cubic feet in which three men slept.

Refuse littered tenement areas, particularly in the early years when piles of horse manure were everywhere. Peddlers scattered refuse left from their operations. One description of the Hull House district went as follows: "Everywhere are rickety porches, stairs, and sheds, rotting clapboards and shingles, grimy, smoke covered and dingy from lack of paint." With all of the refuse and other problems that existed in these areas, rats were common. In the Hull House neighborhood some families slept with guns under their beds to shoot rats at night.[35]

Landlords overcharged for these substandard apartments, but they were cheaper than many other places, and the workers could afford them only by crowding. In the Hull House district in a survey of 1,768 apartments, investigators found a few apartments that rented for less than $5 a month; three-fourths of them rented for between $5 and $15 per month. Many tenements had toilet facilities in the yards or under porches or sidewalks. Often in bad repair, these community facilities froze during the winter. Many apartments had no sinks or running water. This primitive plumbing in an area so congested menaced the health of the community. Chicago outlawed outdoor privys but many still existed. Grace Abbott described a small tenement in which a Hungarian saloonkeeper, his wife, and three children lived on the first floor. The house had neither cellar nor basement, but in a low space under the house the family kept thirty chickens and twenty ducks. The family on the floor above had two children and eight lodgers. The only sanitary accommodation, except for four outdoor privies, was a hall closet which served not only the family and the lodgers but the patrons of the saloon as well.[36]

Many other areas, including Whiskey Row (in the stockyards area), Pilsen on the West side (which included a large Bohemian population), and the Polish neighborhood centering around St. Stanislaus Church, presented as dismal a picture. Conditions were also bad in South Chicago around the steel mills. Abbott described one situation in South Chicago where a man, his wife, their child, and three lodgers occupied a room at night containing 841 cubic feet, while four lodgers occupied the room during the day. It was common, especially among newly arrived immigrants, to rent out rooms in this way. The only group in worse condition than the newly arrived immigrants were the Blacks. Blacks, who began to come in large numbers only during and after World War I, lived in more decrepit houses than the poorest whites and paid higher rents. These conditions were true in Peoria and Springfield, as well as in Chicago. Any improvement over these conditions in smaller cities was only a question of degree.[37]

John Mitchell advocated that wages should be raised to the point where the average working man could own a comfortable, six-room house with a bathroom. Mitchell held that the American standard of living should mean, even to the unskilled workman, things like carpets, pictures, books, and furniture in a bright, attractive home. Mitchell believed every child should be kept in school until age sixteen. He estimated in 1903 that the least on which an unskilled workman could maintain such a standard of living was $600 a year. Others set the figure higher than this. Few unskilled workmen were able to achieve such a standard.[38]

The working man paid more for rent and food than others did and often got cheated even at the price he paid. A *Chicago Tribune* reporter checked 1,500 places in 1900 that sold coal by the basket. The poorest people could afford to buy only in small quantities. The reporter found that the purchaser usually got a short weight bushel of coal, often no more than ⅝ of a bushel. The *Tribune* took note of this editorially because the winter of 1899–1900 was especially cold. The *Tribune* said, "On the one side stand the short measure coal dealers, who sell baskets of coal containing only a little more than half a bushel at a price that would give them a large profit if the measure were an honest one. On the other side are the poor, who are forced to buy coal by the basket because they have not the means to buy it in larger quantities."[39]

Several organizations, including settlement houses, dedicated themselves to helping people in these ghettos. The idea of the settlement house originated in London with the founding of Toynbee Hall in 1884. By the end of the nineteenth century, settlements had been founded in various cities of the United States, including Boston, New York, and Chicago. Jane Addams founded Hull House, the best known, if not the most important, of the Chicago settlement houses. Graham Taylor founded Chicago Commons, and others created important settlement houses such as Northwestern University Settlement, the University of Chicago Settlement, Neighborhood House, Wendell Phillips Center, Frederick Douglass Center, and the Abraham Lincoln Center. The settlement houses carried on programs for aiding people in the neighborhood in which they worked. Hull House workers arranged a kindergarten to take care of children of working mothers. They also held classes in child care, teaching immigrant mothers the rudiments of nutrition, cleanliness, and cooking. They carried on classes in crafts to preserve the immigrants' native talents and taught vocational subjects to train people as a means to prepare them for a better way of life. They produced plays and musical performances, drawing on neighborhood talent.[40]

The settlement houses cooperated with the labor unions to get better wages and working conditions. Among the Hull House residents, Alzina Stevens supported labor unions and meetings. The settlement-house workers did everything they could to get legislation for protection of the workers. Florence Kelley, for example, was involved in getting the bill for the Children's Bureau passed through Congress.[41]

The Hull House group also organized the Immigrant Protective League in Chicago in 1908. The league met immigrants at the railway stations to see that they were not victimized. The league also aided in finding employment and housing for immigrants as they arrived in Chicago.

The Establishment usually regarded settlement-house workers as do-gooders who were undermining the fabric of society. However, settlement-house people were often able to show that it was to everybody's advantage to clean up bad neighborhoods. Florence Kelley pointed out that when a typhoid epidemic spread out of one of the foreign colonies into other sections, it was not the fault of the immigrants but the fault of impure water. She asserted that it was more reasonable to demand pure water than it was to demand the exclusion of the immigrants.[42] The typical settlement-house operation worked to improve the immediate neighborhood rather than attacking broader problems. By badgering local and state authorities to enforce the laws, they were often able to improve some things. The residents of Hull House established the first public playground in Chicago in 1893.[43]

By 1900 labor unions were demanding the improvement of working conditions and the increase of wages. In 1910, 5.5 percent of all persons gainfully employed in the United States were members of trade unions. The percentage for Illinois was about the same.[44] After the decline of the Knights of Labor in the latter part of the nineteenth century, the American Federation of Labor assumed leadership as the chief national labor organization. Under the leadership of Samuel Gompers, president for two generations, the union claimed most of the trade union members in the country. The AFL brought together a loose combination of national and international unions usually based on a particular craft, with various city centrals and state federations of labor. Power in the AFL lay with the national and international unions. After 1901, the federation, essentially conservative, maintained a definite bias against industrial unionism, although some industrial unions, such as the miners, affiliated from time to time. The AFL avoided politics and radicalism. Their insistence on organization by crafts left the unskilled workers of the country unorganized. Although there was no official national policy, many individual unions in the AFL refused to admit black members. This caused the Blacks either to form their own unions or remain unorganized.[45]

Within Illinois the AFL contained two major components, the Chicago Federation of Labor and the Illinois Federation of Labor. The Chicago Federation of Labor was an association of trade union groups operating in the city. Until 1906, the Chicago federation was in the hands of the so-called labor skates, dishonest labor leaders intent on feathering their own nests. Among these was Martin "Skinny" Madden, who had used the Chicago federation for his own benefit. In 1905 the members of the Chicago Federation of Labor, under police protection, elected John Fitzpatrick president of the federation.[46]

Fitzpatrick, one of several brilliant labor leaders in Illinois, was born in Ireland in 1871. Following the deaths of his parents, in 1882 he came to Chicago to live with an uncle. He worked in the stockyards, where he became a horseshoer and blacksmith and joined the International Union of Journeymen Horseshoers and later the Blacksmiths, Drop Forgers, and Helpers Union. He was identified with the horseshoers throughout his life. He served this union as business agent, treasurer, and president. Fitzpatrick, a physically powerful man, sober and industrious, championed the interests of the working man. He supported the union label movement and throughout his life was an Irish nationalist. Fitzpatrick, president of the Chicago Federation of Labor from 1906 to 1946, was interested in progressive unionism ahich, contrary to the national AFL policy, involved the union in politics. Edward Nockels, secretary of the Chicago Federation of Labor from 1903 to 1937, served with Fitzpatrick. Nockels was a gas fitter and electrical worker who, unlike Fitzpatrick, was a flashy individual, profane, eloquent, and radical.[47]

Broader based was the Illinois Federation of Labor, which had been founded in Chicago in 1884. All of the trades and the Knights of Labor were invited to the organizational meeting and 104 accredited delegates, about half from Chicago, met. The organizational meeting discussed a broad range of problems including child labor, female labor, convict labor, hours, wages, steam power and machinery, standard of living of working people, legislation (state, national, and municipal), political action, education, and land reform. They struggled over socialist and other radical ideas and rejected most. By 1890, the federation had almost expired because of internal struggles between the Knights of Labor, organized on an industrial basis, and the trade unions. The Haymarket Riot of 1886 caused dissension. There was a revival of the Illinois Federation of Labor in the 1890s under a movement sponsored by the printers, however.

Besides the problem of the mercenary leadership of the labor skates, Thomas J. Morgan injected another kind of dissension in the union with socialist proposals. Although Morgan was honest and devoted to the principles for which he stood, he caused trouble. There were other promoters of particular ideas, such as George Schilling, labor advisor to Governor Altgeld and head of the Bureau of Labor Statistics. Schilling believed in Henry George's theory of the single tax and injected this doctrine into labor councils.

For the first dozen years of the twentieth century, the Illinois Federation of Labor experienced solid growth. In the convention of 1900, held at Kewanee, 90 delegates elected T. J. O'Brien president. In 1913, 592 delegates, representing 37 central city groups and 350 locals, attended the convention held in Decatur and elected John Walker.[48] This growth was due to a number of things. Reform groups tried to keep the organization out of politics and to restrict the organization to workers only. As one delegate said in 1909, "I want to sit with printers that print, with cigar makers that make cigars, and with carpenters that use their saws and hammers."[49]

John Walker had been important in this growth because in 1908 he had brought the mine workers into the Illinois federation, substantially increasing the membership. Walker was born in Scotland in 1872. When he was nine, his father brought the family of eight children to the United States, where they settled near Braceville, Illinois. At age ten Walker began work in the mines at Coal City. He had little formal education, but his initiation into the problems of the working man began early. His father was blacklisted because of his union activities, so he went to Oklahoma territory to work in the mines. Walker was a robust, gregarious type and an admirer of John Mitchell, president of the United Mine Workers, himself an Illinois figure. Walker, long-time friend of Mary "Mother" Jones, organized a local of the UMW at Central City in 1896 and represented this local at the District 12 convention in Springfield in 1898. Walker became an international organizer and was president of the Danville subdistrict of the United Mine Workers. In 1904, District 12 elected him vice-president, and at various periods he held the post of president of District 12 (which consisted of the whole state). After the Cherry Mine disaster he was influential in getting mine legislation passed. Walker was president of the Illinois Federation of Labor from 1913 to 1930, except for one year. At first he supported political action by the unions but withdrew his support under pressure from the American Federation of Labor. Associated with Walker in the Illinois Federation of Labor was Victor Olander of the Lake Seamen's Union. As vice-president of the Illinois Federation, Olander rejected the progressive unionism of Fitzpatrick. More conservative than either Walker or Fitzpatrick, Olander rejected industrial unionism and stood firmly against the Russian Revolution.[50]

Several important Illinois unions never became a part of the various federations. This group included the Brotherhood of Locomotive Engineers, the Brotherhood of Locomotive Firemen and Enginemen, the Brotherhood of Railway Trainmen, which included conductors, baggagemen, brakemen, flagmen, and switchmen, and the Order of Railway Conductors. These unions, organized as mutual benefit societies, had become full-scale unions. John Mitchell regarded the failure of the railway brotherhoods to unite with other unions as "one of the most deplorable facts in the present status of labor organization in the United States." The railway brotherhoods included almost every worker in the railroad business. These unions took a conservative view toward strikes and generally required an apprenticeship for employment in the field. They advocated the open shop and emphasized the benevolent side of unionism.[51]

The unionization of the teamsters by the American Federation of Labor was made difficult by dissension and dual unionism in the early years. At first called the Team Drivers International Union, in its convention of 1901 the union raised dues. Immediately there was a split, with some locals leaving the group. The dissidents formed a new organization—the Team Drivers National Union—

which was important in Chicago, where most of the locals of the new group were located. From time to time, efforts were made to unite the Team Drivers International and the Team Drivers National unions. Problems arose from a bitter strike against Montgomery Ward in Chicago. As a result of this strike, Cornelius Shea, president of the Team Drivers National Union, was indicted for extortion. He was ousted from the presidency, and Daniel J. Tobin was elected in his place. Tobin served as president for more than forty years until he too was sent to jail. At this point, the union came to be known as the International Brotherhood of Teamsters and was a part of the American Federation of Labor.[52]

The Industrial Workers of the World was founded at a convention in Chicago in 1905. This union was organized by a group of radical labor leaders including Eugene V. Debs, by this time a leader of the socialists. Mary "Mother" Jones of the miners was the only woman invited. About 200 attended the conference, representing a variety of trades. Daniel DeLeon, William D. Haywood, and others noted for radicalism came to the organizational meeting as delegates. This union took on a radical cast, being willing at times to carry out sabotage as a means to achieve their end. The AFL opposed the IWW because the latter was organized on an industrial union basis.[53]

The Building Trades Council, an organization of all those involved in the construction business, was also important in Chicago. Council, organized in 1887, for a time dominated the construction business. A disastrous strike, called in 1900, caused its decline.[54]

Perhaps the best-organized group of working men in Illinois were the miners. The miners produced a number of noted labor leaders, including John Mitchell, who was born in 1870 in Braidwood. Mitchell, orphaned at the age of six, went to school irregularly and at age twelve entered the mines. He joined the Knights of Labor and went west, returning to Illinois three years later. He became adept in organizational activities, and in 1898 the United Mine Workers elected him vice-president; the following year they elected him president. Mitchell served in this capacity until 1908. In the anthracite strike of 1902 he established himself as a great labor leader and the United Mine Workers as a powerful union.[55]

By World War I, John L. Lewis was rising to prominence in mining circles. Born in Iowa in 1880, Lewis worked in mines all over the Midwest and West. These included coal mines in Iowa and Illinois, copper mines in Colorado, and coal mines in Montana. In

1909 he settled in Panama, Illinois, and his local elected him president. From this point he rose rapidly, holding a national position in the AFL after 1911. In 1916 he was president pro-tem of the United Mine Workers convention. In 1920 he was elected the ninth president of the UMW. He was not without opposition from his Illinois colleagues. Both John Walker and Frank Farrington carried on long feuds with Lewis, particularly over the question of autonomy of the districts.

The United Mine Workers provided a tremendous benefit for miners, who were engaged in the most hazardous industrial activities in the state. After the United Mine Workers had established themselves as a force in Illinois, mine workers were paid better. Mine operators were also forced to pay attention to safety devices.[56]

Needless to say, however, the unions met opposition. Industrialists and employers fought vigorously to keep their businesses free from union interference. Beyond this, many organizations of employers aimed at crippling the unions. Chief among these was the National Association of Manufacturers, which was organized in 1895. After 1902 the NAM took an aggressively anti-labor stance. By 1926, 229 member companies in Illinois had joined the NAM. The association created a department called the Industrial Relations Department to combat the closed shop and endorsed and worked with employer associations of particular industries. In 1907 the NAM organized the National Council for Industrial Defense, bringing together various employer associations to combat legislation favorable to the unions. This group took the view that labor unions were radical. In 1904 David M. Parry, NAM president, referred to the paramount question as being that of "lawless and socialistic unionism." In 1920 John Kirby, Jr., then president of NAM, said that all union leaders were reds.[57]

The NAM worked against strikes, boycotts, picketing, the closed shop, shorter working days, restriction of output, limiting of apprentices, and unified action of the unions. It opposed immigration restriction not as a liberal policy but to insure cheap, union-breaking labor. The NAM set itself up as a propaganda agency to educate the public against unions, developing what it called the American Plan, a device to fight the open shop. It entered politics wherever possible to get anti-union officials elected and to influence party platforms, pressure legislation, carry on lobbying, and get legislation favorable to the unions thrown out by the courts.[58]

The National Association of Manufacturers also developed the

Illinois Manufacturers' Association, a statewide counterpart to the national organization. In addition, the Chicago Employers' Association carried on similar programs. The Newspaper Publishers' Association, the Illinois Coal Operators, and the Interstate Coal Operators served the same purposes. The Metal Trades Association was another such group which became a national organization. Businessmen formed the Anti-Boycott League for the purpose of getting unions declared liable for damages under the Sherman Anti-Trust Act. Working uncompromisingly against the closed shop, the employer's associations expelled members who signed closed-shop agreements with their employees. These groups gave financial aid to employers who had trouble with unions and agreed to mutual aid in times of strikes. They advertised widely in newspapers to create a bad image for labor unions and to discredit union leaders by exploiting their mistakes in strikes or mismanagement of funds.[59]

Employers' groups kept blacklists of union organizers and worked to detach workers from their unions. Employers conducted trade schools to encourage people to take up a trade without going through a union apprenticeship. They employed strikebreakers and sluggers and established company unions. Employer's groups exerted pressure by using police and militia in strikebreaking and brought systematic appeals to the courts to hamper strikes by injunction. Employer's associations lobbied with legislatures to get laws unfavorable to the unions and entered politics to elect anti-union officials. They appealed to the press with attacks on unions, exploiting the violence of strikes. The employer's associations operated under the assumption that an employer has an absolute right to manage his business for his own benefit, as opposed to the welfare of his workers or the public. This involved the right to hire and fire at will, to pay as small a salary as possible, and to work employees as many hours as possible.[60]

Labor unions occasionally resorted to strikes to improve their wages and working conditions and started several spectacular strikes in Illinois in the years before World War I. Often the unions failed to win the strike, leaving workers in no better position than they were before. In 1901 the Amalgamated Association of Iron, Steel, and Tin Workers struck the United States Steel Corporation. The union believed it should challenge this newly organized giant before it got established. Although the strike was nationwide, the union's effort was not uniform. In Illinois they struck the Joliet plant but were unable to pull out the workers at South Chicago.

Weak in organization, the Amalgamated failed to gain full support from Samuel Gompers and the American Federation of Labor. J. P. Morgan and Judge Gary, leaders of the steel industry, showed their lack of sympathy with labor unions. The strike was broken and the Amalgamated was almost destroyed in the process. It would be another thirty-five years before there was real unionization in the steel industry.[61]

Shortly after winning the victory over the Amalgamated, the United States Steel Corporation in December, 1902, announced a profit-sharing plan whereby an employee could buy 7 percent preferred stock in the company in a quantity based on his income. The employees got the stock for a little less than market value. In May of 1906 United States Steel announced a safety program for employees and for many years led the country in industrial safety. In 1910 U. S. Steel introduced a pension system, a home-building program, vocational training, and medical facilities. All of this was a paternalistic effort to soothe the feelings of the workers so they would not join another union. Disheartened, labor leaders made little attempt to organize the steelworkers again until 1919. No successful attempt was made until the 1930s.[62]

Another spectacular strike came early in the twentieth century when the Butcher Workmen struck the meat-packers, principally in Chicago and East St. Louis. The packinghouses paid low wages; most of the workers in 1904 were receiving 18½ cents an hour. This wage was less than it seemed because of the irregularity of hours of employment. Employees might work fourteen hours a day in a busy season but at other times almost none. Even a full work week produced a wage of $7.40, which for a man with a family was almost intolerable. In 1904, the packers cut wages to 16½ cents an hour.[63]

Ernest Poole visited the stockyards area during the strike and described the living conditions. He said,

> To find what kind of living such a wage would give, I came a week ago to live in "Packing Town." I came in across Bubbling Creek, a waterway thickly coated with grease and filth and garbage, with carbonic acid gas boiling up from the impure masses below. From the bridge here the main street stretches away into "Packing Town." On the street, from the bridge I counted 27 saloons in one solid row. A few blocks to the left 20 tall slaughter house chimneys poured black smoke over the sky. To the right, one half mile are the great tracks of the Pennsylvania Railroad. The tracks of the Grand Trunk cross one half mile ahead. At midnight now I can hear the endless freight trains

go rumbling shrieking by. No wonder the three babies across the yard
waked up and are screaming. From this district the skilled workers
having won higher wages have moved out into better air. In here live
the unskilled men on $7.40 a week. Many by strict frugality have kept
their cottages comfortable and wholesome. Others live in wretched
basement rooms. A family of five in one room is not uncommon. The
more recent Polish and Slavonian and immigrant men live often in
boarding houses where one small bedroom does for four boarders.
On a night like this, such rooms are stifling and noisome from the
twenty chimneys and from Bubbling Creek. . . .Such living is what
comes from $7.40 a week. The demand that it may not be made worse
is not exorbitant.[64]

The packers took the view that the wage cut was necessary, a
matter of supply and demand. More workers were looking for jobs
than there were jobs and therefore the price of labor was going
down. As one official of the packers said, "It is hard that this wage
be reduced. But it can't be helped. It's simply the law of supply and
demand. The supply of labor is steadily growing larger. Had you
come here last week at 6 A.M. you would have seen over 5,000 men
looking for jobs. As the depression grows worse there will be
100,000 out of work in Chicago. They will crowd out here. They
won't demand 18½ cents they will be glad to get even 15 cents.
Why should we pay more than we have to? We certainly have a
right to hire cheap labor as cheap as we can."[65]

Poole put the point of view of the packers to one of the workman, who replied in this fashion: "It ain't right, I have worked six
years for the packers. If they got half shut down by the depression then I would have to suffer too. But they ain't shut down.
They are doing a big business. They are putting up prices higher
every year. Now, what I want to know is, ain't I a part of the show?
If I am, why shouldn't I get my share of their prosperity? At any
rate, why should I go down in wages just because the packers see a
chance to still make more money by squeezing me?"[66]

Poole found the men were victims of the wide variation in
working hours, never knowing from day to day whether they were
to work or not. The foremen treated the men with brutality, and
workers found themselves in competition with immigrants,
women, and boys. He thought it was up to the union to try to solve
the problem without violence, if possible.[67]

The packinghouse workers, mostly unskilled, had not organized
prior to 1900, except for some Knights of Labor assemblies and a
few independent unions. In 1897, they organized the Amalga-

mated Meat Cutters and Butcher Workmen of North America. Chicago figured prominently in the continuing organization of the Butcher Workmen. The stockyards in Chicago employed more than one-third of the total labor force in the packing industry. The packers, Armour, Swift, Morris, and Cudahy, all maintained headquarters in Chicago.[68]

Michael Connelly, president of the Butcher Workmen, organized the Chicago stockyards, slowly building support. By 1901 he had established several Chicago locals of the Butcher Workmen—among them locals of the hog butchers, sheep butchers, beef carriers, beef casing workers, and sausagemakers. Connelly promoted the idea that the union would bring better labor relations, and at first the packers seemed friendly. They took interest in the unskilled laborer, and it is to the credit of the Butcher Workmen that everybody, black or white, was welcome in the union. Settlement-house people helped in the organization. Mary McDowell, head resident of the University of Chicago Settlement, was active, particularly in organizing a women's local in 1902.[69]

During the second week of June, 1904, Connelly opened negotiations with the packinghouses. He asked for a 20-cents-per-hour minimum wage for the packinghouse workers. The going price for common labor in Chicago at that time was about 17 cents. Eventually Connelly cut his demand to 18½ cents for the industry, and for a time it seemed that they might get together as the packers came up a little and Connelly came down a little in his demands. But there was no bridging the gap between the union and the packers. On July 12, 1904, the workers struck. The *Chicago Tribune* reported that 20,000 men were on strike in Chicago and 5,000 in East St. Louis. The public expressed concern about the strike because of talk of meat shortages and threats of violence. Police arrested several people on the second day of the strike and the newspapers reported that black strikebreakers had been brought into the Morris plant. The packers began to increase prices on meat as shortages developed. On July 15, the police fired on strikers. Three patrolmen and one union man suffered injuries in quelling the riot near the stockyards. Again on July 18, riots broke out and seven were hurt.[70]

The teamsters refused to haul meat and the mechanical trades struck in sympathy with the packinghouse workers. During July the situation grew tense as the newspapers published daily stories that trainloads of black strikebreakers were being brought in. There were frequent clashes with police.[71] By August 2, it was reported that in Chicago 27,680 men were on strike, while 227 union men were still working as were 8,750 scabs. By August 5, the strikers faced a desperate situation. The *Tribune* reported that the saloons in the area were practically closed and the groceries were doing "penny trade." The *Tribune* went on to comment that foreign strikers were faring well, noting complacently, "When rent is only $1.50 a week and the necessaries of life are supplied by the relief bureau, few wants remain to drain the pocketbook. There is the daily can of beer to be purchased for the evening meal; a little tobacco—with the union label on it—for the men, and an occasional can of condensed milk for a sick child."[72]

During August the strikers and packers carried on a paper warfare, the strikers reporting progress while the packers stated that they had 29,660 scabs working for them on August 5. On August 20 the first death in the packinghouse strike occurred as strikebreakers fired on pickets. As the *Tribune* described it, the police were forced to "disarm many Negroes and foreigners." They went on to say that the police believed that "Lorney Everett, colored," was guilty of the murder.[73] Gradually the position of the Butcher Workmen worsened until finally on September 9, 1904, the union capitulated to the packers. Although Connelly tried to make the best of things, it was a disastrous defeat for the union. As the *Tribune* put it, "The striking butchers are willing to admit that they didn't make a killing this time."[74]

By the settlement the packers agreed to hire as many of the strikers as needed, giving preference on the basis of seniority, but also to keep on the strikebreakers if they wished to remain. The wages of skilled workers remained the same as before the strike. The packers agreed to try to keep the work week consistent so workers could depend on a certain amount of income. The packers established a ten-hour day and agreed not to employ women in the slaughtering department. The *Tribune* editorialized that the country was better off now that the strike was over. It believed the union had made a gross error in calling a strike at a time when there was a surplus of labor. The *Tribune* piously advised the strikers that they should try to get better wages or hours through negotiation, arbitration, and compromise rather than through a strike. On the other hand, they said employers who refused to treat workers reasonably brought about strikes, and they too lost. After 1904 there was a decline in union membership. In no case did the packers ever recognize the union.[75]

The Chicago teamsters carried out a strike in 1905 which grew out of a sympathy strike against Montgomery Ward. The Garment Workers struck Montgomery Ward and the strike dragged on for some time. The Chicago Federation of Labor asked the teamsters to help. They obliged and both sides dug in with organization and strike funds. Violence occurred as pickets attacked nonunion drivers, occasionally even where police were riding with the drivers. Federal Judge Charles Kohlsaat issued an injunction against the teamsters and a grand jury indicted several people, including Cornelius Shea, the president of the teamsters. Mayor Edward F. Dunne appointed a committee of five to settle the strike and added 1,000 policemen to handle the situation. Here, as was often the case, employers brought in black strikebreakers, which increased the bitterness in the strike. Governor Deneen refused to send troops to put down the strike so the sheriff of Cook County appointed 3,000 deputies for strike duty. More than 4,000 strikers left their jobs. It was estimated that employers lost 10 to 12 million dollars in business, 20 people died, 400 were injured, and police arrested 19 on charges of rioting. The teamsters strike ended on July 20, 1905, with little gain for either the garment workers or the teamsters.[76]

Workers in the men's clothing industry in Chicago walked off their jobs in 1910 to begin what turned out to be an important strike. In Chicago the men's clothing industry operated in two ways, by inside manufacture and by contract. The former, exemplified by Hart, Schaffner, and Marx, consisted of a factory system where the company made the entire garment in their shops. The second kind of production came through a system which farmed out various parts of the garment by contract. This was exemplified by an organization called the Chicago Wholesale Clothers Association. The workers were represented by an AFL union called the United Garment Workers, which was cautious and unaggressive. In September of 1910, Hart, Schaffner, and Marx cut wages and 1,200 workers went on strike. The United Garment Workers asked for recognition, higher wages, and abolition of payment by the workers for oil cans, bobbins, and spools. They also asked for time-and-a-half for overtime and better treatment by foremen. The president of the United Garment Workers, T. A. Rickert, arranged for arbitration. The workers felt little confidence in this procedure. John Fitzpatrick of the Chicago Federation of Labor organized commissaries to feed the striking workers. City Hall attempted mediation but was refused. In December police killed a picket; eventually 7 died and 874 persons were arrested.

The strike lasted 133 days and 40,000 workers were involved. Out of this strike emerged one of the great labor leaders of the nation, Sidney Hillman. Also active with Hillman in this strike were Frank Rosenbloom and Sam Levin, both of Chicago. Hillman and Levin, disgusted with the United Garment Workers, began setting up a new union. In 1911 the strike was settled satisfactorily to Hart, Schaffner, and Marx. The company agreed to improved sanitary conditions, a lunch period of forty-five minutes, equal division of work between the slack and busy seasons, arrangements for a grievance system, and a permanent board of arbitration. The workers got a 10 percent wage increase and a fifty-four-hour week with time-and-a-half for overtime.[77]

By 1914 Hillman and his followers were ready to separate from the United Garment Workers. On December 26, 1914, the garment workers formed the Amalgamated Garment Workers of America and elected Hillman president. This disturbed the American Federation of Labor, which regarded the Amalgamated as a prime example of dual unionism. John Fitzpatrick admired Amalgamated and supported it overtly when he could. In September, 1915, Amalgamated made an effort to control the entire men's clothing industry. They demanded a 48-hour week, no work on legal holidays with pay, time-and-a-half for overtime, a 25 percent increase in wages, closed shop, and abolition of fines and arbitrary discharge by the company. The employers rejected the demands, so on September 27, 25,000 garment workers struck. The union charged police brutality and nearly 900 people were arrested the first week. Fitzpatrick and Nockels were sympathetic to the strike and Mayor Thompson refused to intervene. The strike ended on December 12, 1915. The union did not get recognition from the companies but did get some concessions.[78]

Sidney Hillman emerged from the strike and organizational efforts as one of the ablest labor leaders in the country for several decades. Born in Lithuania, Hillman had studied to be a rabbi and managed to get a good education. Dissatisfied with the prospects in his country he migrated to England, and in 1907 e arrived in Chicago. He worked as a stock clerk for Sears, Roebuck and then apprenticed himself as a cutter in one of the factories of Hart, Schaffner, and Marx. He joined the strike of 1910 amost as a matter of course, being dissatisfied with working conditions. Later Hillman was involved with various employers of garment workers to increase the efficiency of the workers for the benefit of both workers and employers. The net result of this was the elimination of many jobs in the garment industries. Without question efficiency was increased, and those who retained their jobs were better paid. A fund was set up whereby people who lost their jobs through this new efficiency were paid $500 to tide them over.[79]

In addition to strikes, labor resorted to legislation and the courts as a means of solving their problems. In 1879, Illinois established a Bureau of Labor Statistics to gather information about labor problems. Laboring people regarded the right to organize a union as paramount. In 1893, the legislature passed a law making it legal to belong to a union, but the Illinois Supreme Court declared this law unconstitutional on the grounds that it invaded rights to life, liberty, and property, and constituted special legislation against employers. In 1897 the general assembly exempted labor unions from the state anti-trust law. The court declared this law unconstitutional on the grounds that it discriminated unfairly in favor of those who were exempted from the law. A number of laws prior to 1900 were aimed at harassment of unions. The Merritt Conspiracy Act and the Cole Anti-Boycott Act passed in 1887 were hindrances to labor. These laws, passed soon after the Haymarket Riot, declared most union acts conspiracies and all boycotts illegal. The courts upheld these laws. In 1912 for example, the state supreme court said, "The Court believes that what one individual may do a combination of individuals has a same right to do, provided they have no unlawful purpose in mind." Later the court limited the effect of this ruling by insisting that while a union member has the right to promote his ends by pursuing his calling as he thinks best, so also do nonunion workers or employers. The court held that lawful means to promote the common welfare is right but if the intent is to harm another, any action is unlawful. This made almost all union activities illegal. Strikes were held to be legal if the strike was carried out to further the interests of the workers in terms of wages and hours but workers could not strike to injure someone else. Since the court ruled that intent was all-important, it was never clear what union activities could be carried on. They held, for example, that an attempt to achieve a closed shop by a strike was illegal because of violation of the rights of an employer or of nonunion employees. In 1912 the court mandated that a strike to obtain a discharge of nonunion men did not constitute malice since no threat of violence was made.[80]

In 1902, the appellate court of Illinois ruled that picketing was legal if it was not accompanied by threat of intimidation or abusive language. It held that a large crowd could be interpreted as a threat to a prudent man even though the threat was not verbalized. The same court in 1905 reversed itself, holding that there could be no such thing as peaceful picketing. The Illinois courts insisted that an injunction could be issued to prevent any act that was punishable as a crime. They ruled that a conspiracy to ruin the business of an employer by picketing or boycott could be enjoined, and the injunction was used freely to prevent strikes. Laboring people protested the injunction on the grounds that it was punished by contempt proceedings, which did not require trail by jury. Thus, they said there were no safeguards in the case of injunctions. Labor unions regarded injunctions as disastrous because fighting them in the courts was expensive. Yet the courts, for all the restrictions they placed on them, never declared unions to be entirely illegal.[81]

In 1893 the legislature passed the Sweatshop Act, which prohibited the manufacture of clothing and cigars in apartments, tenement houses, or rooms used for eating and sleeping. The legislature intended this law to insure cleanliness for the benefit of the consumer as well as the worker. The law was not well enforced, however. Also in 1893, the general assembly passed the Factory Inspection Act, calling for a factory inspector, an assistant, and ten deputy inspectors. This slim force was expected to enforce the law throughout Illinois. In 1903 the law increased the number of deputy inspectors to eighteen, including seven women. The law divided the state into fifteen districts with at least one deputy in each district. In 1907, the Deneen administration established the Illinois Department of Factory Inspection, with a chief factory inspector and twenty-five deputy inspectors with salaries of $1,200 a year. The department had the power to appoint an attorney and enforce all laws applying to shops, factories, and mercantile places. The legislation also provided for an Occupational Disease Commission, which had to do with lead poisoning in the mining and smelting of lead and other occupational hazards such as carbon monoxide, poisons, and turpentine. The commission made various recommendations, and in 1911 the legislature passed the Occupational Disease Act, which ordered employers to protect employees, particularly those who worked with lead products, by providing the workers with protective clothing and respirators. The law also required that workers be examined by a physician once a month and that employers provide washrooms. Provision was made for ventilation and cleaning. The law made employers liable to fires and damages for death or injury to the health of an employee and required safety devices such as the boxing in of drive shafts to prevent workers from being injured. There were also provisions before 1900 for fire escapes and blowers to take away dust from grinders.[82]

In 1909 the legislature provided for an Industrial Commission. Governor Deneen appointed a responsible commission for this purpose with Edwin Wright, president of the Illinois Federation of Labor, as chairman. Upon their recommendation the legislature passed, effective January 1, 1910, the Health, Safety and Comfort Act. This provided for guards on belts and other moving equipment, adequate ventilation, toilet facilities for workers, washrooms, lunchrooms distant from poisonous substances, and better fire escapes. The act also required employers to provide seats for female employees. In 1903 a law required that vestibules of streetcars be closed in to protect conductors and motormen. In 1913 a similar law applied to autos and trucks to protect chauffeurs. In 1905, to protect railroaders, a law was passed requiring power brakes on trains, automatic couplers, secure grab irons on cars, regular inspection of equipment and regulation of the size and construction of cabooses. In 1915 a law required first aid kits and the instruction of engineers and trainmen in their use.

In 1907 a Building Construction Act provided for better scaffolds and safe hoists, cranes, and ladders. Enforcement of this law in Chicago brought a 60 percent drop in fatal accidents between 1906 and 1908. A 1915 law prohibited the use of basements for grinding, polishing, plating, or dipping materials in acids.

In 1903 the legislature passed a Miner's Wash House Act which provided for washrooms for miners to clean up in when they left the mines, but the Illinois Supreme Court declared this act unconstitutional in 1906 as constituting special legislation. In 1913 the legislature passed a general washhouse act which applied to all mines, mills, factories, foundries, or shops. There were to be hot and cold water and lockers for the men to use. This law was upheld by the Illinois Supreme Court in 1914.[83]

For a long time laboring men had faced the problem of competition from prison industries in Illinois. It was considered necessary to the well being and rehabilitation of prisoners that they do some kind of work. Often the materials that they made were sold in competition with private industry and free labor. In 1903, under Governor Yates, the Convict Labor Bill was passed which created a Board of Prison Industries whereby the produce of prisons was to be used only by state institutions or political subdivisions. In 1905 the legislature amended the act to restrict the use of tile or culvert pipe in road building. Organized labor, still not satisfied, wanted further extension and labeling of products as prison-made. In 1913 and 1915 laws permitted convicts to work on the roads.[84]

Workers also objected to the widespread use of child labor. Attempts to legislate child labor in Illinois prior to 1900 were ineffective. In the autumn of 1902, investigators found that 15,000 children under the age of sixteen were working in Chicago and that 20 percent of these were employed under false affidavits, signed by their parents, certifying that they were older than they really were. A child labor bill, introduced into the legislature by Representative Frederick L. Davies of Chicago, passed in 1903. Credit for passage of the bill is given to Jane Addams and other settlement-house workers such as Florence Kelley. The State Federation of Women's Clubs supported the bill, as did some 300 labor unions and the Chicago Federation of Labor. The Child Labor Law prohibited employment of children in virtually any kind of mercantile or manufacturing establishment, as well as in most service institutions, particularly theaters or places where intoxicating liquors were sold. No one could employ a child at a time when the public schools were in session nor before 7 A.M.or after 6 P.M. No child was permitted to work more than eight hours in one day or more than forty-eight hours in one week. The law specifically forbade children to operate dangerous machinery or handle poisonous substances or to do anything dangerous to life, limb, health, or morals. Employers could not employ females under sixteen in any capacity which required them to remain standing. The law was one of the most progressive in the United States and was soon extended to the mines (boys under sixteen could not be employed underground). The state appellate court upheld the act in 1904. As a result mine operators discharged 2,200 children from the mines.[85]

Many expressed concern over the inhuman conditions and hours under which women were forced to work. In 1903 the U.S. Supreme Court upheld an Oregon law regulating the working hours of women. This opened the way for legislation in other states. In 1909, during the Deneen administration, the general assembly passed a law providing for no more than a ten-hour day in factories and laundries where women worked. This legislation was supported by Jane Addams and the settlement-house people, the Women's Trade Union League, and labor leaders such as

Agnes Nestor. The Illinois Manufacturers' Association opposed the bill, as it did almost all legislation for the benefit of workers. In 1910 the Illinois Supreme Court upheld the law. The Women's Trade Union League worked unsuccessfully from 1912 to 1919 to get a minimum wage for women.

In 1910 the legislature created an Employer's Liability Commission. This commission reported 617 industrial fatalities in the state in 1910. A number of these cases went to court and some recovery was made for the workman's family, although in one case the amount recovered was only $120. In 1911 the general assembly passed the Workmen's Compensation Act, which provided for compensation for accidental death or injury suffered by an employee. The law required the employer to furnish first aid and pay medical bills. In case of death, the employer had to pay a widow or heirs four times the annual wage of the deceased but not less than $1,500 nor more than $3,500. In case of nonfatal accidents, the law required an employer to pay from $5 to $12 a week beginning on the eighth day after the accident for a period of up to eight years. For total disability the worker might receive a lesser sum after eight years but not less than $10 per month.[86]

Illinois established free state employment offices for workers beginning in 1899. The law required one agency in each city of over 50,000 population and three in a city of 100,000 or more. This office charged no fees, and employment officers were permitted to hire an interpreter for the benefit of immigrant laborers. Unions looked favorably on this law because it provided that the employment officers could not furnish laborers to employers who were under strike or locked out. The law regulated private employment agencies. Because of the provision which prohibited furnishing strikebreakers, the state supreme court declared the law unconstitutional. In 1903 the offices were reestablished without that provision and the act was effective. Illinois established three offices in Chicago and one each in Peoria, East St. Louis, Springfield, Rock Island–Moline, and Rockford. Between 1899 and 1928 the free employment offices placed more than 2 million people in jobs.[87]

In 1917 the general assembly tightened labor legislation by establishing the Illinois Department of Labor as a part of the Civil Administrative Code. Under this the Department of Factory Inspection enforced the Sweatshop Act, the Child Labor Law, the Women's Ten-Hour Law, the Health, Safety and Comfort Act, the Occupational Disease Act, the Wash House Act, and the Basement

Law. The director of labor headed the Department of Labor and supervised the secretary of the Bureau of Labor Statistics, superintendents of the free employment offices, and inspectors of private employment agencies. The law provided for a Factory Inspection Department, a State Board of Arbitration and Conciliation, and an industrial board. The law enjoined the Department of Labor to look after the welfare of wage earners, to improve living conditions, and to collect statistics. The Department of Mines and Minerals, established under the Civil Administrative Code, oversaw the mining board and mine inspectors. The law required this department to concern itself with mine safety and rescue and the welfare of miners. The Department of Trade and Commerce held power to look after safety features on railroads such as the automatic couplers, brakes, and hand grips. In the period after 1917 authority was centralized.[88]

World War I represents a watershed in the middle of the first thirty years of the twentieth century. The war disrupted life in Illinois, and laboring people were profoundly affected. Although the actual participation of the United States in this war amounted to only slightly more than a year and a half, pressure was brought to bear on the population by way of taxation and production of war materials and food supplies. Governor Lowden appointed a council of defense, which eventually had subdivisions affecting almost all Illinois citizens. The council was chaired by Samuel Insull and included labor leaders John Walker and Victor Olander. Of great importance on the national scene was the president's Mediation Commission appointed by Woodrow Wilson. John Walker of Illinois was one of the five members of this committee, which was chaired by Secretary of Labor William B. Wilson.[89]

Wages for labor improved during the war, and labor enjoyed nearly full employment. It is difficult to estimate whether the worker had more purchasing power, since the cost of living also rose. One student of the wages of this period, Paul Brissenden, estimated that in agricultural implement manufacturing the actual full-time annual wages for men were $992 in 1914 and $1,556 in 1919. In the needle trades it is estimated that the full-time estimated per capita annual wage for men making women's clothing went up from $1,167 to $2,334 between 1914 and 1919. At the same time, women in the same industry were getting only $499 in 1914 as compared with $998 in 1919. In the men's clothing industry, partly as a result of the organization of the Amalgamated Garment Workers, the average annual wage in 1914 was $936 versus $2,180 in 1919. In the same industry in 1914 women were paid $457 per year, while five years later they were getting $1,065. Brisenden estimates that during the period 1914 to 1919 the percentage of change in real earnings per capita in Illinois went up 19.5 percent.[90]

Most workers had not joined unions at the beginning of World War I, but in industries where organization existed, unions took advantage of war problems to improve their situation. Unions struck more often during the war than before or after. In 1914 there were 95 strikes in Illinois. In 1917 there were 282 strikes, in 1918, 284 strikes, in 1919, 267, and in 1920, 254. After the war the number decreased until in 1924 there were 80 strikes, in 1925, 84, and in 1926, only 72.[91] Conservatives used the wartime hysteria to do their best to break labor unions. Any radical view became unpopular, and it was alleged that ordinary labor leaders were radical, pro-German, or in any case un-American. Hysteria reached fever pitch during the war, and radical groups were persecuted for their beliefs. In the backlash of this hysteria, many moderate labor organizations were also suspect.

The packinghouse workers participated in one of the more spectacular strikes in 1917. The process of unionization in the packinghouses had declined during the period after the strike of 1904. By 1917 the Butcher Workmen could boast of only a small percentage of union workers in the stockyards. On June 15, 1917, William Z. Foster and John Fitzpatrick initiated organization of the yards; they formed the Stockyards Labor Council to coordinate the effort. Fitzpatrick served as president of the council and Foster the secretary-treasurer. By the end of October, 1917, they had organized 40,000 workers, about 50 percent of the labor force in the stockyards. The U.S. government regarded the packing industry as critical to the war effort. On Thanksgiving evening, 1917, union leaders called for a strike vote when the packers refused to negotiate. The union demanded union recognition, preferential shop, time-and-a-half for overtime, wage increases equaling $1 per day for time workers, 10 percent increase for piece workers, and equal pay for men and women.[92]

To avoid prolonged disruption of the industry, the president's Mediation Commission came to Chicago and held a meeting. The packers were on one side of the room and the union on the other, with Secretary of Labor William B. Wilson presiding in the middle. As the meeting started, one of J. Ogden Armour's lawyers began to speak out against any discussion with the union representatives.

John Fitzpatrick decided that this could not go on. He described the situation as he handled it:

> So I just stood up and said, "Gentlemen, it all seems to turn on whether or not Mr. Armour is going to meet anybody, and I want to say right here that I am now going to shake hands with Mr. Armour." So I just walked across that circle, had to walk about 20 feet over to where Armour was sitting, and I stuck out my hand. He got very red and looked up at me very funny and then he stood up very courteously and shook hands and said, "Of course I'll shake hands with Mr. Fitzpatrick." And then I went right on down that line of packers and shook hands with every one of them, and the lawyers argument in the whole conference went bust for 20 minutes. If the argument had gone on, we would have just got no where. But, after that 20 minutes of mix-up, we sat down and quickly arranged a conference with packers and union labor.[93]

After Fitzpatrick had broken the ice, the comission was able to settle some issues and got agreement that others were to be submitted to the arbitration of Federal Judge Samuel Alschuler in January, 1918. Judge Alschuler, a highly respected figure, had been the Democratic candidate for governor in 1900. His decision, announced on March 30, 1918, provided for an eight-hour day with ten-hours' pay, a forty-hour week with overtime pay, twenty-minute lunch periods, general wage increases, and the same rates for women as for men. The packing industry treated blacks and women equally with white males and the Butcher Workmen welcomed them in the union. As the packinghouse workers ratified the agreement, Fitzpatrick told them: "It's a new day and out in God's sunshine you men and you women black and white have not only an eight-hour day but you are on equality." Union membership surged after this victory. By November, 1918, the Butcher Workmen were paying per capita for more than 62,000 members to the American Federation of Labor.[94]

The packers did not recognize the union, which eventually caused trouble. A new agreement on February 15, 1919, gave 42½ cents an hour for minimum pay with time-and-a-half after eight hours. In the postwar period the Butcher Workmen faced the vital problems involved in the further organization of black workers. Substantial numbers of Blacks labored in the packinghouses prior to World War I. Many Blacks advanced into semi-skilled and skilled positions. In the prewar period, Blacks received higher wages than the immigrant workers, although lower wages than those paid to native-born whites. During the war, many Blacks migrated from the South to the urban areas of the North. The Chicago packing yards employed about 10,000 black workers by the end of 1918. This represented 20 percent of the work force. Unions found the newly arrived Blacks harder to organize than their urban counterparts. They came from rural backgrounds and had little knowledge of unions. Since they took home higher wages than formerly, they were likely to accept the status quo. The packinghouse operators played on the fears and prejudices of this group to prevent them from joining the union. The union made every effort to organize the newly arrived Blacks, but hope of doing so evaporated with the Chicago Race Riot which began on July 17, 1919. The Alschuler award continued until 1921, when the packers, feeling the pinch of the postwar depression, violated their agreement and cut wages. The workers struck the packers, and by January 31, 1922, the strike quickly collapsed. This left the packinghouse workers disorganized, and they were not brought under the umbrella of a union again until organization by the Congress of Industrial Organizations (CIO) in the 1930s.[95]

Labor made a massive attempt to organize the steel industry in 1919. After the collapse of the Amalgamated years before, steel workers had been virtually unorganized. Riding the crest of their success in the packing industry, Foster and Fitzpatrick made the first move to organize the steelworkers. As with the Butcher Workmen, they set up an organizing group called the National Committee for Organizing Iron and Steel Workers. The American Federation of Labor joined the effort for organization of the whole industry, and eventually the effort involved twenty-four craft unions. The steel operatives refused to negotiate and on September 22, 1919, some 279,000 men went on strike. Ultimately, as many as 360,000 were on strike. The union leaders established a commissary to feed workers. The operators still refused to negotiate, and gradually the strike began to disintegrate. By December 13, 1919, only 110,000 were still on strike, and on January 8, 1920, the leaders announced that the strike was at an end. The steel operators used the press, the courts, federal troops, state police, and public officers to break the strike. As was the case with the Butcher Workmen, the steelworkers remained virtually unorganized until the coming of the CIO in the late 1930s. The steel operators were utterly unsympathetic to the workers. John Fitzpatrick said, "When I think of those steel trust magnates and the conditions their workers live and work in and die in—why their hearts must be as black as the ace of spades."[96]

The miners ran into problems during the postwar period. The United Mine Workers had virtually 100 percent membership of all miners through World War I. After the war the miners were operating under a contract, the Washington Agreement, which was to last until April, 1920. The miners were faced with rising costs of living, and they began to demand revision of the Washington Agreement. The UMW elected John L. Lewis as their president. Lewis tried to initiate negotiations with the mine operators for a new contract before the expiration of the old one. The operators refused to negotiate, and a strike was called in the soft coal areas. President Wilson's attorney general, A. Mitchell Palmer, secured an injunction which ordered the union's officers to cease strike activities. This is the occasion when John L. Lewis issued his famous statement, "We can not fight the government." But in spite of his seeming capitulation, the miners refused to work. President Wilson entered the case and the workers were persuaded to accept a 14 percent increase in wages with arbitration of the other issues. Eventually the Bituminous Coal Commission gave the miners a 20 percent increase for monthly and day-rate men, while miners who were working on tonnage got a 30 percent increase to take effect in 1920. This was a major victory for the miners, but it was many years before they had another success. In the summer of 1920 the miners struck again, but upon appeal of President Wilson, John L. Lewis sent the miners back to work. This caused controversy within the UMW; the rank and file thought Lewis had sold out to the establishment. This marked the beginning of a long controversy which involved Frank Farrington, president of District 12, and John Walker, president of the Illinois Federation of Labor. Farrington demanded district autonomy in negotiation with operators, and Lewis consented temporarily.[97]

The public was usually against the UMW, but the Herrin Massacre brought so much adverse publicity to the union that it took many years to recover. The Herrin incident involved a strip-mining operation located halfway between Herrin and Marion (in Williamson County). The Southern Illinois Coal Company, owned by William J. Lester of Cleveland, Ohio, operated the mine. Lester employed fifty men, all United Mine Workers. On April 1, 1922, the soft-coal miners went on strike again, a few months after Lester had begun shipping coal from his mine. Lester was anxious to continue shipping in order to regain his investment as quickly as possible. The union gave him permission to repair the shovels used to dig the coal. Once this was done they gave him permission to uncover coal provided he did not ship. But Lester became greedy: on June 13 he fired the union miners and brought in fifty scabs and armed guards, and on June 16 he shipped sixteen cars of coal. Angry miners besieged the mine, and on June 22 the scabs surrendered to the union miners. The miners agreed to give them safe conduct out of the county, but as they made their way into Herrin, nineteen of the strikebreakers were killed. Several of the striking miners were brought to trial on charges of murder; all were found not guilty of the charges. The conservative *St. Louis Globe Democrat* called the incident "the most brutal and horrifying crime that has ever stained the garments of organized labor."[98]

From this point, the questions of better wages and working conditions, as well as the question of district autonomy, split the United Mine Workers. Lewis constantly made enemies within his union. By 1924, recognizing the serious position of the union, Lewis pulled it together and made a firm stand in negotiation. His efforts brought a three-year agreement, called the Jacksonville Agreement, which many miners regarded as unsatisfactory. By its terms the miners received a high wage when they worked but the mine owners were able to introduce labor-saving machinery with the result that many of the miners were either unemployed or underemployed. After the Jacksonville Agreement, miners worked an average of only 171 days a year.[99]

This situation caused further revolt against Lewis. The progressive miners opposed him within the union, and a communist group organized a rival union called the National Miners' Union. By 1929 the situation had grown intolerable in Illinois. Widespread rumors of corruption in District 12 spread through the coal fields. Lewis dismissed a number of the district officials on charges of corruption and replaced them with his own men. District 12 officials, led by Farrington, barred their offices to Lewis's men. At this point, Lewis revoked the charter of District 12, and Farrington, with rebel leaders from other states, made an effort to reorganize the UMW. The progressives' meeting at Springfield elected Alex Howatt of Kansas president of the reorganized union set up to rival Lewis's. Shortly after this the Progressive Miners Union was formed in the Belleville region, and this was to cause Lewis trouble for a number of years in the early 1930s.[100]

The problems of laboring people changed during the 1920s. Formerly European immigration created difficulties for the workers, but from 1910 to 1930 the number of foreign whites in Illinois increased by only about 16,000. Thus the competition afforded by cheap labor from abroad tended to slacken. Likewise labor suffered less from the competition of child labor in the 1920s because of the pressure of public opinion, child labor laws, and compulsory education laws. These gains were outweighed by the increased migration of Blacks from the South into urban areas of the North. The black population in Illinois in 1900 was 85,000. By 1930 the black population of Illinois had increased to more than 328,000. Of the Blacks living in Illinois in 1930, more than 75 percent were born in other states. This influx of Blacks started in World War I as new sources of labor were needed, and was in part responsible for the East St. Louis Race Riot in 1919.[101] It had been customary in industry to hire the most recent immigrants for the heaviest and dirtiest kinds of work. As a result there had been among the immigrants, as one writer describes it, "upward occupational mobility." Blacks were not subject to this upward mobility, and they tended to be kept in these poorer jobs on a more or less permanent basis.[102]

Women employed in industry in the northern areas provided further competition. During World War I the U.S. Employment Service placed 91,000 women in jobs in the twelve months preceding June 30, 1919.[103] This was done initially as a part of the war effort, but gradually the demand for jobs came to be a part of the new freedom for women. After the war, many women kept their jobs. Employers were willing to retain them because in most instances women worked more cheaply than their male counterparts and were less likely to join labor unions.

As the war closed, the shortage of labor ended. More than 200,000 men that had been drafted or had enlisted in the Navy came back into the labor market in Illinois as the demands on industry lessened. This left the labor market with a surplus caused by women who wanted to work, the returned servicemen, and the Blacks who had emigrated from the South.[104] Desiring to continue their wartime profits, employers capitalized on these changes and pushed for the open shop.

During the 1920s it was relatively easy to get capital for expansion of business. Industry used this new capital in many instances for labor-saving devices. From cigar-making machines to continuous strip-sheet rolling in the steel mills, mechanization was the order of the day. Capital for mechanization was cheaper than labor. The horsepower per worker increased 50 percent between 1919 and 1929. Productivity and efficiency became the rallying cry of industry during this time. With an engineer named Herbert Hoover in the Department of Commerce, the federal government was at the disposal of industry to make their operation efficient. This was the day of the efficiency expert and the industrial engineer; an engineer who could show an industrialist how to cut costs was the hero of the era.[105]

Labor unions experienced dissension as to the direction that labor ought to go. The American Federation of Labor held that unions should stick to craft union organization and pur ue a conservative policy of staying out of politics, but there were dissenters from the official policy. Fitzpatrick believed that the unions should organize a labor party to pursue some of their ends politically. On October 6, 1918, the Chicago Federation of Labor asked the president of the Illinois Federation of Labor, John Walker, to push for a labor party. In December the convention of the Illinois Federation of Labor endorsed a party organization and a platform which asked for a bigger voice in government, collective bargaining, an eight-hour day, minimum wages, equal treatment for men and women, a bigger voice in public education, the control of profit by the government, accident and health insurance, payment of war debts by inheritance and income taxes, and restoration of freedom of speech, assembly, and press. The Cook County Labor party was organized in December, 1918. This was followed by the Illinois State Labor party in April, 1919, and a National Labor party on November 22, 1918.[106] In 1919 Fitzpatrick was nominated for mayor of Chicago by the Cook County Labor Party. He received some 55,000 votes, about 8 percent of the total, and his party made the postelection claim that they had lost because of bad treatment by the press. They replaced the Socialists as the number three party in Chicago, however.[107]

The National Labor party attempted to broaden its base in 1920 when its national convention met in Chicago. The name was changed to Farmer-Labor party, and Parley P. Christensen was nominated for president and Fitzpatrick for senator. Walker was the party's candidate for governor. William Z. Foster, a Communist, tried to take the party in the direction of Marxism. Because of pressure by Samuel Gompers in the AFL organization, the Farmer-Labor party was virtually dead by 1924. The remnants endorsed Robert La Follette in his Progressive party bid in 1924.[108]

Labor unions in Illinois maintained a number of publications that were of importance during the 1920s. One of the earliest papers was the *New Majority*, first published on January 4, 1919.

This paper continued until 1924. Robert Buck, the editor, published book reviews, editorials, movie reviews, serialized novels, and labor news. In August, 1924, the name was changed to *Federation News*. In addition the *Federated Press* was established in 1915; it served as a news service for labor papers. This organization published a number of papers at one time or another in Illinois, among them the *Centralia Labor World* and the *Tri-City Labor News* in Christopher. These papers usually carried one page of local news and picked up the rest from the *Federated Press*. Another highly successful venture of labor in Illinois, the brainchild of Edward Nockels, secretary of the Chicago Federation of Labor, was the radio station WCFL, the first labor-owned radio station in the world, which began broadcasting on June 26, 1926.[109]

In the years during and immediately after World War I, the AFL continued its position of leadership among the national unions in the United States. Its peak membership came in 1920, when it had more than 4 million members. By 1924 it had declined to 2,865,000, and in the remaining years of the decade its membership never reached 3 million. During World War I the American Federation of Labor continued its conservative policies; at the outbreak of the war the federation had supported it, although many people within the union for one reason or another had not.[110]

Another crisis for unionism came with the Russian Revolution of 1917. At first Samuel Gompers, like most people, rejoiced at what seemed to be a moderate revolution overthrowing the czar to gain the rights of the people of Russia. As it became evident that the current of events in Russia had produced a communist revolution, the AFL began to shy away from this position and opposed the regime.[111]

Gompers suffered a challenge to his leadership in 1921 from John L. Lewis. Lewis, newly elected head of the United Mine Workers, was recognized as a forceful leader, but Gompers fended off his candidacy. Another source of agitation within the AFL came with the movement of progressive unionists for amalgamation—a demand for an industrial union. Leaders of the Chicago Federation of Labor, such as Nockels and Fitzpatrick, strongly favored this demand. The Chicago Federation of Labor tended to move a little leftward during World War I.[112]

In March, 1922, Foster called upon the executive council of the American Federation of Labor to merge the craft and amalgamated unions into industrial organizations. This was refused, and for a time the American Federation of Labor cut off its support of the Chicago Federation. In 1924 the American Federation came to the end of an era with the death of Gompers. Gompers's death came at a time when there was crisis within the labor movement because of the move for open shop by employers. Gompers became ill while attending a Pan-American Labor Federation Meeting in Mexico and was rushed back across the border so he could die on American soil. Upon Gompers's death, the American Federation of Labor elected William Green president, marking the beginning of a new era in the history of the AFL. Green was to head the union for nearly a generation.[113]

1. John Mitchell, *Organized Labor, Its Problems, Purposes and Ideals and the Present Future of American Wage Earners* (Philadelphia, 1903), pp. 154–55.

2. Barratt O'Hara, *Report of the Senate Vice Committee Created under the Authority of the Senate of the Forty-ninth General Assembly as a Continuation of the Committee Created under the Authority of the Senate of the Forty-eighth General Assembly, State of Illinois* (Chicago, 1916), p. 225. Hereafter referred to as O'Hara, *Report.*

3. Ibid., pp. 195–202.

4. Ibid., pp. 202–09.

5. Ibid., pp. 217–23, 236–37, 240, 260–65, 265–71.

6. Ibid., pp. 177–89.

7. Ibid., pp. 249–59.

8. Ibid., pp. 283–86, 295–98, 311–13, 322–27, 607–09.

9. Ibid., pp. 724–32.

10. Ibid., pp. 713–19, 719–32, 732–34.

11. Ibid., p. 681; Shelby Harrison, ed., *The Springfield Survey*, 3 vols. (Springfield, Ill., 1918), III, 179–80.

12. O'Hara, *Report,* pp. 309–10.

13. Ibid., p. 754.

14. Ibid., pp. 711–13, 734.

15. Ibid., pp. 739–47.

16. Paul H. Douglas, *Real Wages in the United States 1890–1926* (New York, 1966), p. 623.

17. Ibid., p. 623.

18. O'Hara, *Report,* pp. 698–710.

19. Ibid., pp. 386–87, 392–94, 411–13.

20. O'Hara, *Report,* pp. 375–86, 394, 400–401.

21. Ibid., pp. 281–82, 286–91, 343–44.

22. Ibid., pp. 618–54.

23. Douglas, *Real Wages*, p. 625.

24. Harrison, *Springfield Survey*, III, 178.

25. O'Hara, *Report*, p. 747.

26. Paul F. Brissenden, *Earnings of Factory Workers 1899–1927* (Washington, D.C., 1929), p. 386.

27. Douglas, *Real Wages*, pp. 130–31.

28. *Thirteenth Census of the United States Taken in the year 1910:* Manufacturers, Reports by States (Washington, D.C., 1912), p. 262.

29. *Twelfth Census of the United States: Occupations* (Washington, D.C., 1900), p. 262.

30. Paul H. Douglas and Aaron Director, *T e Problem of Unemployment* (New York, 1934), pp. 26–28.

31. Mitchell, *Organized Labor,* p. 139; *Chicago Tribune,* June 7, 1908, part 5, p. 1.

32. Allen F. Davis, *Spearheads for Reform: The Social Settlements and the Progressive Movement 1890–1914* (New York, 1967), p. 123.

33. *C icago Daily Inter-Ocean,* Jan. 1, 1900, p. 14; *Chicago Tribune,* June 7, 1908, part 5, p. 1.

34. Mitchell, *Organized Labor,* p. 139.

35. Edith Abbott, *The Tenements of Chicago, 1908–1935* (Chicago, 1936), pp. 63, 77, 93, 171, 175, 189, 191, 238, 262.

36. Ibid., pp. 210, 205–23, 277.

37. Ibid., pp. 58–59, 74–75, 99, 261–62, 293, 295, 305–40; Harrison, *Springfield Survey,* III, 117–18.

38. Mitchell, *Organized Labor,* pp. 116–18.

39. *Chicago Tribune,* Mar. 12, 1900, p. 1; Mar. 18, 1900, p. 40.

40. Davis, *Spearheads for Reform,* pp. 3–14, 40–42.

41. Ibid., pp. 103, 132–33.

42. Ibid., pp. 92–94.

43. Ibid., pp. 26, 27, 61, 75.

44. Paul H. Douglas, Curtice N. Hitchcock, and Wilfred E. Adkins, *The Worker in Modern Society* (Chicago, 1923), p. 562.

45. Ibid., pp. 549–51, gives an excellent sketch of the organization and method of the AFL. See also Sterling D. Spero and Abram L. Harris, *The Black Worker, the Negro and the Labor Movement* (Port Washington, N.Y., 1931), pp. 120–22; Paul Brissenden, *The I.W.W.: A Study of American Syndicalism* (New York, 1957), p. 83; John H. Keiser "John Fitzpatrick and Progressive Unionism 1915–25" (Ph.D. dissertation, Northwestern University, 1965), p. 29. The struggle between industrial and craft unions is treated in Robert Franklin Hoxie, *Trade Unionism in the United States* (New York, 1921). The standard history of the AFL in the period is Philip Taft, *The A.F.L. in the Time of Gompers* (New York, 1957).

46. Keiser, "John Fitzpatrick," p. 74; Eugene Staley, *History of the Illinois State Federation of Labor* (Chicago, 1930), pp. 195–96.

47. Keiser, "John Fitzpatrick," pp. 2–7, 11–12.

48. Staley, *History of the Illinois State Federation of Labor,* pp. 17–37, 59–83, 84, 99, 105–39, 178–80.

49. Ibid., p. 194.

50. John H. Keiser, "John H. Walker: Labor Leader from Illinois," in Donald F. Tingley, ed., *Essays in Illinois History* (Carbondale, Ill., 1968), pp. 24, 76–79.

51. Douglas, Hitchcock, and Adkins, *The Worker,* pp. 552–54; Hoxie, *Trade Unionism,* pp. 106–12; Mitchell, *Organized Labor,* p. 406; Taft, *The A.F.L. in the Time of Gompers,* pp. 462–63.

52. Taft, *The A.F.L. in the Time of Gompers,* pp. 109–13.

53. Brissenden, *The I.W.W.,* pp. 57–67, 83.

54. Selig Perlman and Phillip Taft, *Labor Movements,* Vol. 4 of *History of Labor in the United States, 1896–1932* (New York, 1935), pp. 83–96.

55. Charles A. Madison, *American Labor Leaders* (New York, 1950), pp. 165–66; Damon D. Watkins, *Keep the Home Fires Burning, a Book about the Coal Miner* (Columbus, Ohio, 1937), pp. 67–68. For an unfavorable view of Mitchell, see Mary

H. Jones, *Autobiography of Mother Jones* (Chicago, 1925), p. 242. Mother Jones said of Mitchell: "John Mitchell left to his heirs a fortune, and his political friends are using the labor movement to erect a monument to his memory, to a name that should be forgotten."

56. Watkins, *Keep the Home Fires Burning*, pp. 55, 74–77; Keiser, "John Walker," pp. 84–87, 90. See also Saul Alinsky, *John L. Lewis: An Unauthorized Biography* (New York, 1949).

57. Albion G. Taylor, *Labor Policies of the National Association of Manufacturers* (Urbana, Ill., 1928), pp. 12–16, 20, 23–24, 35–36, 42; Taft, *The A.F.L. in the Time of Gompers*, p. 262.

58. Taylor, *Labor Policies*, pp. 36–37, 57, 63–81, 82–94, 95–146.

59. Taft, *The A.F.L. in the Time of Gompers*, pp. 263–64; Hoxie, *Trade Unionism*, pp. 189–90.

60. Hoxie, *Trade Unionism*, pp. 190–203.

61. Perlman and Taft, *Labor Movements*, pp. 97–109; Harold U. Faulkner, *The Decline of Laissez Faire 1897–1917* (New York, 1951), p. 301; Ida M. Tarbell, *The Life of Elbert H. Gary: The Story of Steel* (New York, 1925), p. 159.

62. Taft, *The A.F.L. in the Time of Gompers*, pp. 272, 274–75; Perlman and Taft, *Labor Movements*, pp. 138–39; Tarbell, *Life of Elbert H. Gary,* pp. 165–66.

63. Ernest Poole, "The Meat Strike," *The Independent*, 57 (July 28, 1904), pp. 179, 181; David Brody, *The Butcher Workmen, a Study of Unionization* (Cambridge, Mass., 1964), pp. 50–58.

64. Poole, "Meat Strike," pp. 179–80.

65. Ibid., p. 180.

66. Ibid.

67. Ibid., p. 181.

68. Brody, *Butcher Workmen*, p. 34.

69. Ibid., pp. 34–35.

70. Ibid., pp. 50–58; *Chicago Tribune*, July 12, 1904, p. 1; July 13, 1904, pp. 1, 2; July 14, 1904, p. 3; July 15, 1904, p. 1; July 18, 1904, i. 1.

71. *Chicago Tribune*, July 19, 1904, p. 2; July 22, 1904, p. 1; July 24, 1904, p. 1; July 26, 1904, p. 1; July 27, 1904, p. 1; July 28, 1904, pp. 1, 4; July 29, 1904, p. 1; July 31, 1904, pp. 1, 2.

72. Ibid., Aug. 2, 1904, p. 1; Aug. 5, 1904, pp. 1, 3.

73. Ibid., Aug. 5, 1904, p. 1; Aug. 2, 1904, p. 1.

74. Ibid., Sept. 9, 1904, p. 1; Sept. 10, 1904, pp. 1, 6.

75. Brody, *Butcher Workmen*, pp. 59–61; *Chicago Tribune*, Sept. 10, 1904, p. 6.

76. Taft, *The A.F.L. in the Time of Gompers*, pp. 112–13; Perlman and Taft, *Labor Movements*, pp. 61–69; Faulkner, *Decline of Laissez Faire*, p. 300.

77. Madison, *American Labor Leaders*, pp. 337–42; Douglas, Hitchcock, and Adkins, *The Worker*, pp. 554–55; Perlman and Taft, *Labor Movements*, pp. 304–8; Keiser, "John Fitzpatrick," p. 30.

78. Perlman and Taft, *Labor Movements*, p. 313; Keiser, "John Fitzpatrick," p. 30.

79. Madison, *American Labor Leaders*, p. 338.

80. Earl R. Beckner, *A History of Labor Legislation in Illinois* (Chicago, 1929), pp. 16–17, 18, 23–24, 34–38, 488.

81. Ibid., pp. 40–42, 47–50, 50–54.

82. Ibid., pp. 223–28, 254–68.

83. Ibid., pp. 240, 244–47, 250–54.

84. Ibid., pp. 144–49.

85. Ibid., pp. 150–59; Davis, *Spearheads for Reform,* pp. 123–27.

86. Beckner, *A History of Labor Legislation,* pp. 188–209; Davis, *Spearheads for Reform,* pp. 138–47.

87. Beckner, *A History of Labor Legislation,* pp. 385–89, 423.

88. Ibid., pp. 501–2.

89. Arthur C. Cole, "Illinois and the Great War," in Ernest Ludlow Bogant and John Mabry Matthews, *The Modern Commonwealth 1893–1918* (Springfield, Ill., 1920), pp. 463–64; Marguerite Jenison, *The War-time Organization of Illinois* (Springfield, 1923), pp. 29–34, 38–281.

90. Brissenden, *Earnings of Factory Workers,* pp. 226, 394, 396.

91. Florence Peterson, *Strikes in the United States, 1880–1936* (Washington, D.C., 1938), p. 37.

92. Keiser, "John Fitzpatrick," pp. 34–38; Brody, *Butcher Workmen,* pp. 75–78.

93. Keiser, "John Fitzpatrick," p. 40.

94. Ibid., pp. 41–42; Brody, *Butcher Workmen,* pp. 78–82; Jennison, *War-Time Organization,* pp. 280–81.

95. Keiser, "John Fitzpatrick," p. 50; Brody, *Butcher Workmen,* pp. 85–87.

96. Keiser, "John Fitzpatrick," pp. 34, 36, 42–43, 47, 50; David Brody, *Labor in Crisis: The Steel Strike of 1919* (New York, 1965), pp. 62–86, 174. The quotation from Fitzpatrick is on p. 62.

97. Joseph G. Rayback, *A History of American Labor* (New York, 1959), pp. 307–8.

98. Ibid., pp. 308–9; Paul Angle, *Bloody Williamson: A Chapter in American Lawlessness* (New York, 1952), pp. 3–10, 11–12, 44–75.

99. Rayback, *A History of American Labor,* pp. 309–10.

100. Ibid., pp. 310–11.

101. Irving Bernstein, *The Lean Years: A History of the American Worker 1920–1933* (Baltimore, 1966), pp. 51–58, 55–56; Charles E. Hall, *Negroes in the Unived States 1920–1932* (Washington, D.C., 1935), pp. 9, 24.

102. Bernstein, *The Lean Years,* p. 51.

103. Jenison, *War-Time Organization,* p. 274.

104. Ibid., pp. 273–74, 374, 377.

105. Bernstein, *The Lean Years,* pp. 53–54.

106. Keiser, "John Fitzpatrick," pp. 118–27.

107. Ibid., pp. 127–28.

108. Ibid., pp. 130–40; Taft, *The A.F.L. in the Time of Gompers,* pp. 454–55.

109. Keiser, "John Fitzpatrick," pp. 159–63, 165.

110. Taft, *The A.F.L. in the Time of Gompers,* p. 362.

111. Ibid., pp. 444, 446, 448–49.

112. Ibid., p. 367.

113. Ibid., pp. 454–55, 486, 487.

5

The Robin's Egg Renaissance: Cultural Development

Illinois in 1900, still a raw, culturally underdeveloped area, was accumulating great wealth from industrial development, and some of its citizens acquired the leisure and money to turn their attention to cultural development. The fortunes amassed by the industrial giants paid for development in art, music, literature, and scholarship. In some instances this patronage of the wealthy excluded the lower classes from enjoying music and art. Even with massive support of music by the rich, the cost of tickets excluded the poorer people of Chicago and Illinois from concerts. However, libraries brought literature to them after a time, and the Art Institute of Chicago was open to the public at no charge.

A relatively small number of wealthy people contributed to the cultural advances. Examination of lists of the patrons of music, art, and literature reveals the same names again and again. In many instances it was the wives of the industrialists who poured money into cultural avenues; Mrs. Potter Palmer, for example, contributed heavily to art and music. Many of the social elite promoted culture as a matter of local pride, feeling their city should be as great as Boston or New York. Since art and music were highly regarded elsewhere, they reasoned, Chicago had to have as great a symphony or opera as other cities.

One of the earliest cultural developments in Illinois was the Art Institute of Chicago. The Institute, incorporated only a few years after the great fire of 1871, acquired some great works of art in its early years. In 1890, it purchased fifteen old Dutch masters including Rembrandt, Rubens, and Frans Hals. A great step in the development of the Art Institute came as a side effect of the Chicago World's Fair of 1893. Chicago's leaders believed something of permanent value should come out of the Columbian Exposition and decided on a permanent and elegant building to house the Institute. The city, the directors of the fair, and the trustees of the Institute, working cooperatively, made plans to build a permanent home for the Art Institute at the foot of Adams Street on Michigan Boulevard. The city granted 400 feet of frontage with the provision that the museum should be free to the public on Wednesdays, Saturdays, Sundays, and holidays. These agencies began construction with the understanding that the Columbian Exposition would use it during the fair, and then the Institute would take over the building permanently.[1]

By 1900 the Art Instutute was thriving. It elected Charles L. Hutchinson as president and he continued in this post until his death in the early 1920s. Among the other officers, trustees, and governing members were familiar names of Chicago finance and industry. Lyman Gage was the treasurer, and among the trustees were Martin Ryerson, Albert A. Sprague, Chauncy J. Blair, Stanley McCormick, Marshall Field, Robert Hall McCormick, and Carter Harrison, *ex officio*. Frank Lowden, Robert Todd Lincoln, Victor Lawson, P. A. Valentine, P. D. Armour, Hobart C. Chatfield-Taylor, Harold Fowler McCormick, Cyrus Hall McCormick, and Potter Palmer and his son Honore were among the governing members. In 1900 the Art Institute received the Nickerson Collection, which included several items of eastern art as well as modern paintings including Inness and Rousseau. They also received, as a part of a bequest of Mrs. E. S. Stickney, a painting by Whistler.[2]

The Institute had established the practice of having special exhibits throughout the year, and during the year ending June 30, 1900, it sponsored twenty-four special exhibits of paintings, sculpture, and prints. The trustees established lecture courses to instruct the public and maintained an art school. During 1900, 740 day students, 500 evening students, and 794 Saturday students attended classes.[3]

In July 1906, for 200,000 francs, the Art Institute purchased El Greco's great altarpiece called "The Assumption of the Virgin," a magnificent piece more than thirteen feet high and seven feet wide, painted in 1577. This painting may still rank as one of the most valuable items among the magnificent collections.[4]

The Art Institute promoted the work of American artists,

awarding endowed prizes each year. In 1909, Mrs. Potter Palmer established a gold medal with a prize of $1,000 in memory of her husband. This medal and cash prize were to go to the best work of art by a living American artist. It was also the Institute's practice to purchase paintings by Americans, and a number of Chicago artists profited as a result. The Institute acquired, for example, a collection of paintings and miniatures by Martha Baker, whose work was highly thought of at the time. While the Art Institute awarded generous prizes to American artists, Harriet Monroe said that the reason she established *Poetry Magazine* to aid poets was because they were less well rewarded than painters.[5]

In 1909 Institute patrons and members formed a group called the "Friends of American Art." Each of the 150 members agreed to give $200 annually to purchase works of art. The Friends elected William O. Goodman, an Institute trustee, first president. As the name implies, they purchased only American paintings, including those of James McNeill Whistler, Winslow Homer, and John Singer Sargent. Because of the generosity of this group, the Art Institute holds paintings by Gilbert Stuart, John Singleton Copley, Benjamin West, and later painters such as Mary Cassatt. During their first eight years the Friends gave the Institute eighty-six paintings, six pieces of sculpture, and thirty-six prints.[6]

Harriet Monroe, sponsor of *Poetry Magazine,* crusaded for recognition of modern art during the years she was art critic for the *Chicago Tribune.* She loved modern painting and held that just as experimentation was necessary in poetry, so also should there be experimentation in art. She was partial to modern artists such as George Bellows, George Inness, Albert Pinkham Ryder, Winslow Homer, and Childe Hassam. The first major exhibition of Bellows's paintings in Chicago was in 1911. Harriet Monroe said in the *Tribune* that Bellows was "a man who had something to say and a vigorous way of saying it."[7]

The *Chicago Tribune* sent Monroe to New York to review the Armory Show, and she had some part in bringing it to the Art Institute. The Armory Show, which came to Chicago in March and April, 1913, featured many daring innovations in cubism and other approaches. Duchamp's "Nude Descending a Staircase" shocked many, but Monroe defended it vigorously. She said that American art was much too conservative, "too pallid, moveless, photographic," and "anemic."[8]

The Armory Show, officially known as "The International Exhibition of Modern Art," aroused furor when it came to

Chicago. A group called the Association of American Painters and Sculptors, Inc., sponsored the exhibit of cubists, impressionists, and postimpressionists. Unable to get a showing for it in any New York gallery, it had been necessary to hold it in the Sixty-ninth Regiment Armory in New York, hence its name.[9] Chicago newspaper columists had a field day with the exhibit. "Nude Descending a Staircase" was variously described as a "blast in a shingle factory" and a "tornado in a lumberyard."[10] The exhibit was described as "weird school," "freak paintings," a "joke," and one writer asked did the exhibit "originate in an insane asylum?" Another said that van Gogh's "Bal Arles" was "van Gogh's recollection as he stumbled home through a fog about four in the morning. It is an indescribable medley of shapes and lights." Another warned, "Have your address about your person when you go to see the pictures, because your mind and memory may be gone when you come out of the exhibits."[11] Barrett O'Hara took his vice commission to see the exhibit to determine whether it was detrimental to public morality. Most viewers were baffled.[12]

Monroe, who was among the few defenders of the exhibit, wrote:

> For in a profound sense these radical artists are right. They represent the revolt of the imagination against nineteenth century realism: they represent disgust with the camera, outrage over superficial smoothness which covers up weakness of structure. They represent a search for new beauty, impatience with formulae, a reaching out toward the inexpressible, a longing for new versions of truth.
>
> Revolt is rarely sweetly reasonable: it goes usually to extremes, even absurdities. But when revolutionary feeling pervades a whole society or its expression in the arts, when the world seems moved by strange motives and disturbing ideals, then the wise statesman, the true philosopher is in no haste to condemn his age. On the contrary, he watches in all humility the most extreme manifestations of the new spirit eager to discover the deeper meaning in them.[13]

The director of the Art Institute received criticism for allowing the exhibit. In his report for the year, he commented:

> The International Exhitition of Modern Art, commonly called the "Cubist Show," held in March and April arrested a great deal of attention and attracted a great number of visitors. Question has been raised whether the Art Institute ought to exhibit the work of so extreme and radical a character; whether an established art museum ought not to adhere to recognized standards and refuse to exhibit works which at best represent but a small and eccentric group.
>
> The policy of the Art Institute, however, has always been liberal,

and it has been willing to give a hearing to strange and even heretical doctrines, relying upon the inherent ability of the truth to prevail. The curiosity of art circles here was much excited by the attention paid in Paris and New York to the various developments of modernist art, and there was no prospect of the works being seen here unless the Art Institute exhibited them.[14]

The list of artists represented includes Renoir, Manet, Gauguin, van Gogh, Matisse, Picasso, and Braque among the foreigners, and American artists Hassam, Ryder, Bellows, Henri, and Glackens, as well as many of lesser importance. Time justified the judgment of the promoters of the show. During the exhibit there were 188,650 visitors to the Art Institute, breaking all attendance records.[15]

Some remarkable bequests and gifts came to the Institute from individuals such as Edward V. Butler, a business executive of Chicago who was fond of collecting and donating paintings by George Inness. During the year 1910–11, he gave the Art Institute eighteen paintings. In 1911 and 1912, he added other paintings to the collection, which ultimately occupied a whole gallery.[16]

Perhaps the most valuable collection of paintings came from the estate of Mrs. Potter Palmer, who died in 1918. According to her will, the Art Institute was to receive paintings from her collection to the value of $100,000 to be selected by her sons, provided a special gallery was set aside for them. Ultimately, the two sons, Potter Palmer, Jr., and Honore Palmer, supplemented this generosity, and the institute received fifty-two paintings from the collection of Mrs. Palmer. The most valuable of these were forty-seven French paintings which included four Renoirs, three Corots, five Millets, two Manets, and six Monets. Also included were four American paintings and a portrait of Mrs. Palmer by Anders Zorn.[17]

Another important collection which went to the Art Institute was that of Mrs. W. W. Kimball, who died in June of 1921. In her will she bequeathed to the Institute twenty paintings valued at $1,000,000. Among these were paintings of the Barbizon school and a Rembrandt portrait of his father. Also included were works by English artists Sir Joshua Reynolds, J. M. W. Turner, John Constable, Gainsborough, Sir Thomas Lawrence, and George Romney, and some works of French painters including Corot, Monet, and Pissarro.[18]

The generosity of Chicagoans to the Art Institute did not stop with gifts of paintings. Friends of the Institute often bequeathed large sums of money for specific purposes or for the general use of the organization. One of the most generous of these gifts came from the will of George B. Harris, who died in 1918 and left a sum in excess of $1,000,000 for general purposes of the Institute.[19] As time passed, the original building underwent major additions. The Ryerson Library, Fullerton Hall, and the Goodman Theater were added and the Institute expanded across the Illinois Central tracks into the east part of Grant Park.

The Institute served Chicago and all of Illinois well, and now contains one of the great art collections in the United States. The Columbian Exposition provided a stimulus to the Art Institute, and in 1928 was already making preparations to aid in the World's Fair of 1933.

With the death of Charles L. Hutchinson in 1924, the Art Institute came to the end of an era. Hutchinson, president of the Institute since 1882, provided much of the leadership in building the collection. After his death, there was a shake-up in the officers of the Institute. Martin Ryerson, who had long been vice-president, became honorary president, and Frank G. Lowden and William O. Goodman became honorary vice-presidents. The active president was Potter Palmer, Jr. Robert Allerton and Cyrus McCormick, Jr. were vice-presidents, so the older men had given up active leadership. The general direction of the Art Institute did not change very much, however. The leadership emphasized collecting the best in the art world and raising money to finance the activities of the school and public lectures.[20]

Illinois produced a number of painters and sculptors, some of merit. The Art Institute held an annual exhibit of Chicago painters and various groups worked to encourage local talent. In addition to the Friends of American Art, another organization called the Municipal Art League purchased one canvas each year.[21] One Chicago painter, Grace Gassette, was included in the Armory Show.[22] Among the locally famous artists in the years before World War I, B. J. Nordfeldt, a friend and neighbor of Floyd Dell, painted in the Postimpressionist style. Martha Baker was called "the greatest living miniaturist."[23] William Claussen painted scenes of the Chicago River, and Pauline Fulmer was represented in a painting show at the Art Institute in 1913.[24] Among the sculptors was Stanislaus Szukalski, who claimed to have learned anatomy by dissecting the body of his father after he was killed in an accident. Szukalski maintained a studio in a loft over Wabash Avenue and was regarded as something of an oddity even among the avant-garde of the time. Harry Hansen described him thus: "Sculptor and philosopher, in velveteens; a big white collar,

Christopher Columbus haircut."[25] The most prestigious of all the artists was Lorado Taft, Chicago sculptor who had studied in Paris. His work is well known to most Illinoisians—the great statue of Black Hawk overlooking the Rock River, the *Alma Mater* in Urbana, and the *Fountain of Time* on the Midway in Chicago.[26]

An important school of architecture appeared in Chicago in the years after 1900. An important precursor of this group, John Wellborn Root, created the Columbian Exposition of 1893. Among the practicing architects in the years after 1900, Daniel Burnham (once Root's partner in an architectural firm) was, in the eyes of his fellow architects, the least creative. Nonetheless, he designed important buildings in Chicago and surrounding areas before his death in 1912 and deserves credit for the "Chicago Plan," which created the parks along the lake shore. Most regarded Louis Sullivan as more creative and original. Sullivan dismissed Burnham with the remark that he was "a colossal merchandiser." Sullivan, on the other hand, had a rather high opinion of Root, who died shortly after getting the Columbian Exposition under way.[27]

Harriet Monroe remarked that these architects made Chicago "the center of the rebellion against the historic styles in architecture." Sullivan was coming to the end of his career by the turn of the century. Only one great Sullivan project still remained to be done—the Carson, Pirie, Scott store, finished in 1904. Sullivan died in 1924, a victim of alcoholism.[28]

Sullivan was the teacher of Frank Lloyd Wright, the most important figure in Chicago architecture. Sullivan assigned Wright the task of designing family dwellings for the firm. This experience led Wright to design the "prairie house," his distinctive trademark after 1900. Wright referred to Sullivan as "the master" and gave him credit for his education.[29]

Much of the earlier building designs of homes, particularly the kind he called "General Grant Gothic" (such as the Potter Palmer mansion on North Lake Shore Drive), repelled Wright. He said the buildings of Sullivan, by comparison, stood clean and sharp. Wright, describing his efforts, told what needed to be done in order to build a distinctive house. He said:

> The first thing in building the new house, get rid of the attic, therefore the dormer; get rid of the useless false heights below it; next, get rid of the unwholesome basement, yes absolutely—in any house built on the prairie. Instead of the lean, brick chimneys bristling up everywhere to hint at judgment, I could see the necessity for one chimney alone, a broad generous one, or at the most two,

these kept low down on gentling sloping roofs or perhaps flat roofs. The big fireplace in the house below became now a place for a real fire. A real fireplace at that time was extraordinary. There were mantles instead. A mantle was a marble frame for a few coals and a grate or it was a piece of wooden furniture with tile stuck in around the grate. The whole set slam up against the plastered-paper wall, an insult to comfort. So the integral fireplace became an important part of the building itself in the houses I was allowed to build out there on the prairie.[30]

Examples of the "prairie house" were the Robie House in Chicago and the Dana House in Springfield. A historian of the Chicago School of Architecture said that the new school used

a simple cube, with a hip roof, the eves of which project boldly on all sides, its rectangular character is maintained consistently both in the banks of windows and the organization of the walls. Designed for a small family, the plan is simple: the living area is grouped around a central fireplace, the kitchen area is screened off in one corner of the square, while the dining and living rooms flow into each other; thus the cramped feeling that might result from such a small house thirty feet square is avoided.[31]

In 1900, Wright established his Oak Park studio, which became a center of training for a number of important architects in Chicago. Among those who followed Wright's lead were Myron Hunt, Robert Closson Spencer, Jr., Dwight Perkins, Arthur Heun, George Dean, Hugh Garden, George W. Maher, Birch Long, Max Dunning, and William Drummond.[32]

Also important in training architects was the Department of Architecture at the University of Illinois, the second such program developed in the country (the first being at the Massachusetts Institute of Technology). The development of the department at Illinois was largely due to the ability of its dean, Nathan C. Ricker. Ricker was as much a pioneer as Sullivan and Wright in the development of architecture in the Midwest, particularly in Illinois. Among the important architects produced by the department was Walter Burley Griffin, who graduated in 1898.[33]

Another of the great cultural events of Chicago, the state of Illinois, and the Midwest stemmed from the time of the Columbian Exposition of 1893. This was the formation of what was to become the Chicago Symphony Orchestra. There had been music of this kind in Chicago prior to the 1890s as traveling companies came to the city to perform, and from time to time local orchestras were formed by Germanic groups. These efforts were transitory, however, and the idea of a permanent Chicago orchestra had to wait until the end of the nineteenth century. The first conductor, Theodore Thomas, was among the traveling conductors who came to Chicago, so his musical abilities were known. Wherever he had gone with traveling orchestras, he thrilled audiences with the precision of his conducting. When Charles Norman Fay, a Chicago business executive and friend of Thomas, approached him in 1889 to come to Chicago to start an orchestra, Thomas quickly seized the opportunity. Then fifty-one years old, he was weary of traveling. He said he would have gone to hell if he had been offered a permanent orchestra there. The plan for founding an orchestra typified such things in Chicago. Fifty persons pledged $1,000 each to run the orchestra for three years. This small amount was calculated to do no more than absolutely necessary for the establishment of such an undertaking. The backers gambled that they would be able to find more backers when needed. In the original group were the familiar names of George Pullman, P. D. Armour, Marshall Field, Martin Ryerson, Cyrus Hall McCormick, and A. A. Sprague.[34]

Foreseeing a lack of talent in the city, Thomas brought along sixty musicians from New York to form a nucleus for the local group. Recognizing the resentment among local musicians, Thomas assured them that if they were adequate performers, they would be used. The orchestra staged its first concert in the Auditorium Theater. Designed by Louis Sullivan, the Auditorium was thought to have near-perfect acoustics. It seated 4,800 persons. Many times during the first years of the orchestra Thomas doubted its ability to survive, but because the deficits were small, it managed to hang on.[35]

Theodore Thomas was difficult to get along with; he was unwilling to bend to the press or to local personalities if doing so in any way interfered with his music. As it turned out, the Auditorium Theater was found to be a handicap. Although the acoustics were excellent, it was too large for a symphony. It was never possible to get 4,800 people in the same room at the same time to hear symphonic music, and the empty seats were depressing to the musicians. A lot of music was required to fill this great hall, and the orchestra never had money to hire enough musicians. In addition, the Auditorium was costly to rent and rehearsals often had to be held elsewhere.[36]

In 1899, Theodore Thomas announced that he intended to

resign. The trustees, fatigued with the situation, particularly with their obligation to cover the deficits, recognized that they must either abandon the orchestra or establish it on a firmer financial foundation. They decided to take the latter course by endowing the orchestra with a permanent building which would be a source of both income and security. The result was a campaign for donations to build Orchestra Hall. Completed by December, 1904, the building, designed by Daniel Burnham, was located at 220 South Michigan Avenue on land that once contained the stable for the Palmer House. The capacity of the hall was 2,500 persons, more appropriate to a symphony orchestra than the Auditorium Theater. Thomas, looking over the new home of his orchestra, said, "We are now in the same room as the audience."[37]

Orchestra Hall was completed about a year after the Iroquois Theater fire in which more than 600 Chicagoans died. This tragic event so shocked the world that many cities passed fire laws to protect against this kind of disaster. Orchestra Hall found itself a victim of these precautions, as fire laws took precedence over acoustical considerations. Concern for safety brought modifications, including reduction of the size of the stage. Because of these changes many complained that Orchestra Hall was acoustically inferior, and found the new facility disappointing. The building, ten stories high, contained office space for rental purposes as a means of support for the orchestra. In spite of the complaints, Orchestra Hall was a triumph for Thomas, although he did not live to enjoy it very long, dying only a few weeks after its dedication.[38]

Thomas, a skilled conductor, largely self-taught, maintained high standards and showed an iron will, never compromising with what he thought was the way music should be conducted. He made the claim that he was the only conductor who carried out the wishes of the composers in every detail. In recognition of his achievement, the trustees renamed the orchestra the Theodore Thomas Orchestra. This name continued until 1913, when the orchestra was renamed the Chicago Symphony Orchestra with the subtitle "Founded by Theodore Thomas."[39]

Since Thomas died in the midst of the 1904–5 season, it was necessary to replace him immediately. The trustees chose a young man named Frederick Stock. Stock, only thirty-two, was a violin player who had been assistant conductor for some years. Like Thomas of German birth, he studied with great teachers in Europe and was academically better prepared than Thomas. However, he had little experience as a conductor and put more of his personality into the music than Thomas would have thought of doing. Thomas played the music literally, while Stock was willing to embellish or edit the music as he felt necessary. Stock was usually on better terms with the public than Thomas, possessing ability to placate difficult patrons of the arts.[40]

Stock ran into trouble during World War I when prejudice ran high against Germans. Stock had applied for citizenship in 1895, but he had not carried through and his application had lapsed. When the outcry against everything German began, he removed himself from the orchestra until he achieved his citizenship. In a few months he had his papers and had composed a patriotic number entitled "March and Hymn to Democracy," which he played upon resuming the podium in August, 1918. While Stock was away from the orchestra, the group was conducted by Eric DeLamarter, a Chicago composer and organist. Stock returned amid the cheers of symphony patrons not only for his musicianship but also for his patriotism. Chicago had long been dependent on German musicians, and World War I emphasized the problems that this might create. In order to insure a supply of adequate musicians, the orchestra organized an apprentice ensemble called the Chicago Civic Orchestra. These apprentice musicians were sometimes conducted by Stock, DeLamarter, or George Tash, all members of the parent orchestra.[41]

The Chicago Symphony has always presented a broad repertoire. The reason for this varied fare goes back to Theodore Thomas. Thomas conducted many summer concerts which called for a broad range of music. While Thomas was unwilling to compromise with the music, he did, sometimes with condescension, play music of lesser stature in a frank compromise with the level of his audiences. The Chicago orchestra, always cosmopolitan, played the work of Americans, including local composers.[42]

Opera in Chicago followed a more hectic course. During the later years of the nineteenth century, traveling opera companies, some from New York, some from New Orleans, gave occasional performances. The dedication of the Auditorium Theater provided the occasion for one of the big operatic events in Chicago. Louis Sullivan and his partner, Dankmar Adler, designed the theater, and the engineering skill of Adler is said to have produced the near-perfect acoustics. A concert by Adelina Patti highlighted the opening of the theater, further glorified by the presence of President Benjamin Harrison and Vice-President Levi Morton. Harriet Monroe, already known as a poet, wrote an ode for the occasion. The company gave twenty-two performances during a four-week opera season.[43] The traveling opera companies did not always do well in Chicago, however, and in some instances, the season was a financial failure. In 1900, for example, impresario Maurice Grau, from New York, announced that he would never bring an opera company to Chicago again: "I have cut out Chicago; understand, cut out Chicago. Chicago does not want grand opera, repeat, and so I have done the only thing left to do. I have cut out the town absolutely! I have spoken."[44]

The *Chicago Tribune* reacted defensively to the announcement that there would be no more opera in Chicago:

> Would it not be more honest to admit that grand opera itself is in part a fad and a fashion instead of being one of the eternal verities upon which one may predicate culture and refinement. Why not confess frankly that the music drama is an artificial thing, that its charm is largely that of novelty, that the lasting element in it is solely in the music, that one may prefer to hear the music apart from the so-called dramatic part without being a barbarian, and that finally all refinement and culture are not confined to the few complacent persons who happen to enjoy nothing in music but the operas of Richard Wagner.[35]

Pointing with pride to the great successes of the Chicago Symphony, the *Tribune* thought the orchestra was proof enough of the cultural stature of Chicago.

Not until 1910 did Chicago begin to hear opera on a regular basis with its own company. Some years before, Oscar Hammerstein established the Manhattan Opera Company in New York to compete with the Metropolitan Opera Company, hoping to run the latter out of business. Hammerstein and his company performed French opera while the Metropolitan presented primarily Italian and German operas. After a struggle of several years, it became evident that the Manhattan Opera Company could not compete with the Metropolitan and Hammerstein sold out for $1,200,000 to the Metropolitan.[46]

Shortly afterward, Hammerstein appeared in Chicago and seemed to be thinking of establishing an opera company there. A group of Chicagoans decided to establish one on their own terms and bought what remained of Hammerstein's assets, including costumes, scenery, and scores. Many of the singers, managerial people, and conductors came to Chicago from the Manhattan Opera Company. The Chicago Grand Opera Company gave their first performance on November 3, 1910, with the production of

Verdi's *Aida*. The president of the company was Harold Fowler McCormick and the vice-president was Charles G. Dawes. The musical director was Cleofonte Campanini.[47]

A number of figures, musical and nonmusical, dominated the Chicago opera scene. Just as Harold Fowler McCormick dominated the financial side of Chicago opera for a dozen years, Mary Garden, a soprano who had grown up in Chicago, dominated it musically for twenty years. On the third evening of the new company's first season, Garden sang Debussy's *Pelléas and Mélisande* before a sold-out house. This opera became one of the most important in Garden's repertoire. Debussy himself had coached the soprano in this role and is said to have fallen madly in love with her. Some have said that Garden was not the greatest soprano of all time, but few doubt her ability as an actress both on and off the stage. Garden was born in Scotland but grew up in Chicago and studied music in Paris. She made her American debut with the Manhattan Opera Company in 1907 and from this time was a controversial figure. Some people thought as a musician she could do no wrong, while others thought she could do nothing right.

She created many tempestuous moments in Chicago circles.[48] During the first season she sang the title role in Strauss's *Salome*. In this performance, as in all her performances, she insisted on as much realism as possible. The opera was performed in French and what broke up Chicago was her rendition of the "Dance of the Seven Veils." Garden herself describes it in this way: "I had on enormous veils which I took off one by one and threw in Herod's face. With the very last veil, I enveloped myself entirely. Under that last veil was just the thinnest, thinnest muslin. As I ran from the cistern over to Herod, I thrust the last veil at him and knelt and said, 'I want the head of Jokanaan.'" The next morning Chicago found itself drawing up sides as to what had happened on the stage the night before. On the one hand the Puritans of the city thought it was a sinful spectacle. Chief of Police, Leroy T. Steward said: "It was disgusting. Miss Garden wallowed around like a cat in a bed of catnip. There was no art in her dance that I could see. If the same show were produced on Halsted Street the people would call it cheap, but at the Auditorium they say it's art." Garden, however, believed this was a narrow view. For the second performance, the house was packed and tickets sold at a premium. Arthur Farwell, president of Chicago's Law and Order League, protested, describing the performance as vicious and sinful. The third performance of *Salome* was canceled, and this opera was not heard again in

Chicago until Garden became the musical director of the opera in the early 1920's.[49]

There were many great figures in Chicago opera. Besides Garden, there was Maggie Teyte, a tiny woman with a big voice. Luisa Tetrazzini, the sister-in-law of the musical director Campanini, was also a woman with a big voice, but she had an enormous body to go with it. During the second season, Garden sang several roles, including the title role of Victor Herbert's *Natoma,* an opera set in California during the days of the Spanish occupancy.

The Chicago Opera supported American composers as well as classical ones. During its second season the most scandalous episode was the production of the opera *The Secret of Suzanne,* in which the singer in the title role was called upon to smoke a number of cigarettes on stage, bringing criticism from Chicago's Anti-Cigarette League, one of the reform movements of the time.[50]

In 1913, the opera promoted Campanini to general director as well as musical director. By this time Chicagoans owned all the stock of the Chicago Grand Opera Company and there was no longer influence from the outside. World War I brought problems, and in 1914 there was no opera season. This brought a reorganization of the company, then called the Chicago Opera Association, with Harold McCormick continuing as president and Charles Dawes as vice-president. Maestro Campanini continued as the general director. During the season of 1916–17 a young, unknown singer named Amelita Galli-Curci appeared in the Chicago Opera. Galli-Curci sang Verdi's *Rigoletto* and became an immediate sensation. She must be counted as one of the great opera singers of all time. In the meantime another singer, Rosa Raisa, appeared, and Garden, Galli-Curci, and Raisa divided most of the top roles among themselves. Garden sang mostly French operas, Galli-Curci was a coloratura, and Rosa Raisa was more important in dramatic works. Although each was a prima donna, they did not interfere with each other.[51]

The 1919–20 season featured the death and funeral of Campanini, events almost as spectacular as any of the operas he produced. He died of pneumonia during the middle of that season, and his funeral was held on the stage of the Auditorium Theater. His coffin was at center stage, brilliantly lighted with stands containing candles, his baton and scores resting nearby, and flowers everywhere. The opera company provided a musical funeral service. After this, the public filed by the coffin for three hours. Garden recalled, "After that, the curtain came down slowly, and that was the last we saw of Cleofonte Campanini,"[52]

The spring following Campanini's death, Harold McCormick told the company he would back the orchestra for only two more years. McCormick and his wife, Edith Rockefeller, had been paying the deficits of the opera company and announced that somebody else would have to take over. The last season the McCormicks backed was the season of 1921–22. They chose Mary Garden as general director. The McCormicks told Garden, who liked to be called Madame Directa, that they wanted to go out in a blaze of glory and expense was not to be considered. They wanted this to be the greatest opera season that Chicago, and perhaps the world, had ever known. "Madame Directa" traveled through Europe hiring talent, often paying above the going rates. By the time the opera season was ready to start, Garden had lined up talent far in excess of what was needed. The final roster indicated that she had hired seventeen sopranos, nine contraltos and mezzo-sopranos, thirteen tenors, eight baritones, nine basses, and five conductors—at least twice as many of each as needed. Edith Mason sang *Madame Butterfly*. "Madame Directa" herself sang *Carmen, Pelléas and Mélisande, Louise,* and *Le Jongleur de Notre Dame*. She also did *Salome* which had been banned for eleven years. Apparently the critical taste of Chicago had changed in the intervening years because there was no outcry against the performance this time.

Without question, Mary Garden had created a great season. In the spring of 1922, the management tabulated the final figures and gave McCormick the bill for the deficit for that season, a sum of $1,000,000. According to one historian of the Chicago Opera, "The tycoon's gentlemanly moan could be heard in every speakeasy in Chicago." Garden, on the other hand, commented, "If it cost a million dollars, I'm sure it was worth it."[53]

As the McCormicks gave up control of the opera, supporters devised a new plan for financing it. Typical of Chicago efforts, the plan brought together 500 guarantors who agreed to contribute a sum not to exceed $1,000 a year for the next five years. The Chicago Civic Opera went into operation in 1922. The new president was Samuel Insull, utilities magnate. Dawes again served as vice-president, and Harold and Edith McCormick chose to be relegated to the board of trustees. As might have been expected Insull made it clear that Chicago opera was to be run on a businesslike basis with a strict accounting system; he would not tolerate losses for which no one could account.[54]

The Chicago Civic Opera changed little from the Chicago Grand Opera in the performances that it gave, although it did offer more Italian operas. Almost immediately Insull devised a way to put opera on a paying basis in Chicago. In December of 1925 he revealed his plan. He proposed to build a great new opera house within a gigantic skyscraper. The opera house would occupy the ground floor, while the top floors would be leased as office space. The rent would cover the inevitable deficit of the opera. By the fall of 1927, Insull had completed plans for the building at 20 North Wacker Drive and construction began.[55]

On January 26, 1929, the Chicago Civic Opera Company gave its last performance in the Auditorium Theater with Gounod's *Romeo and Juliet,* sung by Edith Mason. After the performance the orchestra played "Home Sweet Home," the song Adelina Patti had sung at the dedication of the theater some forty years before. By the fall of 1929, the new structure was complete. In the forty-two-story building, the Chicago Civic Opera House and the smaller Civic Theater occupied the ground floor. The tower housed 729,000 square feet of office space. The building cost $20,000,000, half of which had been raised by subscription, the other half borrowed from the Metropolitan Life Insurance Company. The theater seated 3,471 people, with a main floor, two balconies, and thirty-one boxes. The house had a progressive lighting system so that lights could be directed to any part of the stage at any angle. The old scenery took on new life and dimension. The performers were intrigued with their new quarters, including the finest of dressing rooms and private bathrooms.[56] It is ironic that the company's fortunes fell on the same evil days as Insull's utilities empire. The new opera's first performance was in November, 1919, in the midst of the stock market crash.

The opera provided a number of amorous adventures for Chicago tycoons. Harold McCormick divorced Edith Rockefeller to enjoy a brief marriage with Ganna Walska, a Polish singer, whom he had employed to sing in the 1920 season. Charles Swift married Claire Dux, one of the sopranos of the opera company. J. Ogden Armour was much enamored with Mary Garden, and although he never quite got to the point of marriage with "Madame Directa," he did show up unexpectedly wherever she might be singing.[57]

No account of the musical activities of Illinois would be complete without some mention of the ten-week summer opera season offered at Ravinia on Chicago's North Shore. Usually the Chicago Symphony accompanied first-rate performances by famous artists.

These seasons began in 1911 under the sponsorship of Louis Eckstein.[58]

Several Illinois composers wrote serious music. One of these, John Alden Carpenter, a Chicago businessman, contributed several pieces of music based on impressionism as applied to American themes. Among the most commonly performed of his works are "Adventures in a Perambulator," "Concertina," and "Krazy Kat." "Adventures in a Perambulator," an attempt to capture some purely American impressions, was first performed by the Chicago Symphony in 1915. Percy Grainger first performed "Concertina" in Chicago, also in 1915. One historian described this work as consisting of "'Made in America' melodies and syncopated rhythms." Carpenter described the piece as "light-hearted conversation between piano and orchestra." His "Krazy Kat," a jazz pantomime based on the comic strip by the same name, was first performed in 1921. Walter Damrosch called Carpenter "the most American of composers." Influenced by Debussy, Carpenter applied great technical skill to American themes to produce a number of important works.[59]

Felix Borowski, an English-born Pole who taught at the Chicago Musical College and was a music critic for newspapers, contributed a number of compositions, including his "Adoration," most often heard as a violin solo. Gena Branscombe, a Canadian-born composer, studied with Borowski, and her symphonic suite, *Quebec*, was first performed in Chicago. Also associated with the Chicago Musical College were German composers Adolf Brune and Louis Falk. Composer Louis Campbell-Tilton, who was born in Chicago, also taught at the Chicago Musical College for a time. Harry Newton Redman, born in Illinois in 1869, composed several works, as did an ex-office boy from Chicago named Hamilton Forest, whose opera *Camille* was performed by Mary Garden in 1930–31, her last season. Cecil Burleigh, who grew up in Bloomington and also studied with Borowski, contributed several instrumental works.[60]

During the years before World War I, many young literary and artistic people flocked into Chicago. Because of their propensity for autobiography, we have a record of their lives while they were in Chicago. Most of these young people came from small towns, in Illinois, Ohio, Indiana, or Iowa. They were eager to seek their fortune and make their views known. Many were escaping overprotective mothers or ineffectual fathers; all hoped to escape the narrowness and dreariness they perceived in their small towns, and they came to Chicago because it was nearby and big enough so they could live anonymous lives. They joined bohemian groups which seemed to be the epitome of freedom. Young people in bohemias lived in a manner shocking to their conservative, middle-class neighbors and expressed themselves in ways that were often radical and, to parents, irresponsible. The literature they produced grated on ears used to a more genteel tradition, and their art and music was often incomprehensible to those who were accustomed to older, academic traditions.

Chicago provided a variety of cultural experiences about which small-town America could only dream. Almost all those who left reminiscences spoke of their rapture at seeing Isadora Duncan dance, listening to Theodore Thomas direct the symphony, or looking for hours at the Postimpressionist art in the Armory Show. The artists represented in this show seemed to these young people to express the same emotion in paint that they were expressing in poetry and prose. People like William Butler Yeats and Amy Lowell came to Chicago to see for themselves the literary revolution on Lake Michigan.

Many remembered Chicago for its dirtiness and brutality, but most remembered the city with love. Emanuel Carnevali remembered its softness, but he also remembered the dirt: "Chicago washes her dirty feet in the Michigan sea, and her feet are forever dirty."[61] Margaret Anderson spoke of Chicago in her memoirs: "Back in Chicago I began a marvelous life as literary editor. And I came to love Chicago as one only loves chosen—or lost—cities. I knew it in every aspect—dirt, smoke, noise, heat, cold, wind, mist, rain, sleet, snow."[62] Floyd Dell overlooked the ugliness in his autobiography: "I had been happy in Chicago; never would it seem to me a grey and ugly city. I loved the Lake, Michigan Boulevard with its open vista and its gleaming lights, the parks, even the preposterous loop district with its sudden architectural leap into the sky; I had seen beauty there, enough to fill my heart; there had been days and nights of talk and laughter; the years had passed in a golden glow of friendship; and it was a city haunted everywhere by memories of love, its pain and its glory. It had been a generous city to a young man. I would always be grateful for what it had given me."[63]

Even before 1900, Chicago had earned a considerable literary reputation. This reputation continued into the twentieth century and eventually flowered in what Sherwood Anderson called "the Robin's Egg Renaissance."[64] This fragile literary movement lasted little more than a decade, from about 1910 to about 1920. Among the earlier publishers, Stone and Kimball produced literary works, including a magazine of criticism called *The Chap Book,* published from 1894 to 1898. *The Chap Book* carried on laudable, critical fights, including a defense of Oscar Wilde in 1895. Stone and Kimball published books by such well-known figures as Eugene Field, Robert Louis Stevenson, William Butler Yeats, Maurice Maeterlinck, and Henrik Ibsen, as well as the complete works of Edgar Allan Poe. Stone and Kimball also published local writers such as Hobart Chatfield-Taylor, Robert Herrick, and George Barr McCutcheon.[65]

Francis Fisher Browne published *The Dial* in Chicago from 1880 until 1919. The magazine, under a new ownership, moved to New York in 1919. *The Dial* was not just representative of Chicago culture, although it published some local writers such as Hamlin Garland. Its attitudes were conservative, and when more radical magazines were founded in Chicago, *The Dial* carried on lengthy fights with them.[66]

The *Friday Literary Review,* a supplement of the *Chicago Evening Post,* reviewed books and provided a livelihood for many of the aspiring writers who came to Chicago. The usual practice was for the book reviewer to sell the book he reviewed and thereby earn enough to keep him alive.[67] Newspapers also carried book review sections. In 1912 Harriet Monroe founded *Poetry* magazine, which published otherwise unknown poets and, more important, paid them for their efforts. Monroe published her first issue of *Poetry* backed by the money of some of the old families of Chicago such as the Deerings, the Lowdens, the Palmers, and the McCormicks.[68]

Margaret Anderson founded another important magazine, the *Little Review,* during this period. Anderson came to Chicago to write and for a time was book review editor of a religious magazine; she also reviewed books for the *Friday Literary Review.* She wanted to found a magazine of her own which would not cater to the tastes of the masses. Anderson published new writers and counted among her triumphs the first United States presentation of James Joyce's *Ulysses.* [69]

The editors of *Poetry, The Dial,* and the *Little Review* carried on a running critical battle. Each criticized the other for the things they published. Each charged that credit was taken where credit was not due. These magazines and publishing houses created a literary tradition in Chicago that attracted the young writers. Here they could find a market for their writings, get encouragement, or perhaps review a few books for money.

A bohemia grew up in Chicago in much the same way that

Greenwich Village developed in New York, and much of the bohemian life around 1912 centered about the studios of Floyd Dell and his wife, Margery Curry. Dell was born in Barry, Illinois, and later lived in Quincy and Davenport, Iowa; like many others, he came to Chicago to engage in a literary career. Dell began his career on the *Friday Review of Literature* and eventually became editor. As editor, he brought his friend George Cram Cook, also from Davenport and a playwright and novelist, to Chicago to be his associate. Later Cook was succeeded by Lucien Cary, a critic of considerable reputation. After a time in Chicago, Dell married Curry, who also had literary ambitions. For a time they maintained an apartment which became a gathering place for the young literary crowd. They then moved to the corner of Fifty-seventh Street and Stony Island on Chicago's South Side. This corner was across from Jackson Park, near what had been the entrance to the Columbian Exposition of 1893. Here, one-story, basementless buildings had been constructed for small businesses serving the crowds who came to the exposition. These buildings featured wide front windows, made excellent studios, and, most important, could be rented for very little. Floyd Dell moved into a building on Fifty-seventh Street and his wife into another on Stony Island, separated from each other by the corner building but with connecting back entrances. (It was characteristic of the casual living of the time that husband and wife did not actually live together.) Here they created a kind of gathering place for other aspiring writers, many of whom are no longer known.

Nearly every writer of that era who lived in Chicago mentioned the pleasant times and great conversation that went on in these studios. They all came to visit Dell and Curry. Theodore Dreiser, Sherwood Anderson, Carl Sandburg, and most of the others eventually appeared there.[70] Anderson, who came to Chicago as a copy writer for an advertising agency, had already finished his first novel, *Windy McPherson's Son*. His brother, Karl, showed a copy of it to Curry, who in turn passed it on to Dell. They both liked the work, and Anderson was invited to the Fifty-seventh Street studio. Anderson describes how he stood outside listening to the party going on inside and was afraid to go in, feeling as he did that he was something of a fake and, as he put it, "a pimp for businessmen." He was plagued with doubts about his honesty, but the group accepted him.[71]

Writers also gathered at Schlogl's Restaurant on the north end of the Loop, where the newspaper writers congregated—men such as

Harry Hansen, Burton Rascoe, Ben Hecht, Justin Smith, and Sandburg. Sherwood Anderson liked this group, and Edgar Lee Masters found it congenial.[72]

At one time the fortunes of Margaret Anderson declined so drastically that she moved her living quarters and, to some degree, the editorial function of the *Little Review* to a tent on the shore of Lake Michigan near Ravinia. The tent became famous. Maxwell Bodenheim and Ben Hecht would walk out from Chicago and, if they found no one at home, pin poems to the tent for Anderson's consideration. At this point, Anderson had only one blouse and each morning she washed it in the lake before she went into the city for whatever business had to be done for the day.[73]

Writers also frequented the Dill Pickle Club, a place run by an ex-safecracker named Jack Jones who provided a place for writers to recite their poetry. Sometimes, when he was prospering, he would pay several dollars for a poem reading. As Jones told Sherwood Anderson, "I give them the high-brow stuff until the crowd grows thin, and then I turn on the sex faucet."[74]

One of the bohemians who remembered the Dill Pickle Club with fondness was Emanuel Carnevali. Carnevali, like many of his contemporaries, was always hungry. He recalled, "How many days of hunger in Chicago did I kill with sleep! . . . Sleep was then my greatest friend. I used to drown myself in sleep, terrible sleepless sleep, a sleep that was close to madness."[75] Since he was always hungry, Carnevali was appreciative of the help that he got from Jack Jones. He wrote years later of the club:

> This little club was the fair of freaks, the union of eccentrics, the forum of those who arrived at the wrong moment, were wrongly welcomed and came to the wrong place. The president of it was Jack Jones, the King of the Discontented and the Disconnected, and there he throned with his way of talking as funny as he was himself. He once gave me as much as seven dollars for reciting the part of Anatole in Schnitzler's *Wedding of Anatole* . . . . But I hope you are not dead, Jack Jones, because Chicago needs you. Chicago needs those two small rooms, one over the other, which were called the "Dill Pickle Club."[76]

The Dill Pickle Club was not the most attractive place, but it served a purpose. Carnevali described it thus:

> Tucker Alley was the apotheosis of all the strange alleys of Chicago. In their gutters cats come to die and there is always a stray dog nosing in the refuse, but Jack Jones brought his love into the

depths of this mysterious, cramped street. These stricken alleyways had lost even the sense of sight in the filthy dark; dirty children played in the rubbish; nothing beautiful ever passed that way except this fact which may be beautiful or not but which at any rate is true—one's back had to be bowed under a burden before one could pass through that little door that led to Tucker Alley. A burden of protest against man's foulness, or a burden of anguish or despair; but anyway a burden before one could enter the ranks of that high, pure army that waged its battle in Jack Jones' two rooms. In his little domain grew only stunted trees, but the strong manure of his remedies was good. He clothed those who had nothing, fed those who were in want, gave to those who begged the few dollars he could give in payment of the little speeches they made. What sort of business he actually did in his "Dill Pickle" I do not know. He was neither very rich nor very poor; this president of the disbanded whom he divided into groups, ate them, digested them, evacuated them, so that there was always room for more.[77]

A number of young poets gathered around Harriet Monroe and *Poetry* magazine. Unlike many of those she helped, Monroe came from an upper-class Chicago family, but her proteges were usually respectful of her. Lew Sarett, for example, said that he owed everything to Monroe, and Carnevali called her the "mother of poets."[78] Carnevali, a half-demented Italian, worked in some editorial capacity on *Poetry* magazine. He showed promise as a poet, spent a good portion of his life in mental institutions, and was always disreputable in appearance.[79] Maxwell Bodenheim was of a similar character. Bodenheim, who appeared in Chicago during the cultural renaissance, was a talented poet and anything but conventional. Ben Hecht described him in this way: "Maxwell Bodenheim in manner and appearance is the ideal lunatic. He is bowlegged and has pale green eyes. While uttering the most brilliant lines to be heard in American conversation, he bares his teeth, clucks wierdly with his tongue, and beats a tattoo with his right foot. He greets an adversary's replies with horrible parrot screams. Having finished an epigram of his own, he is overcome with ear-splitting guffaws.[80] Known as Bogie to his friends, he smoked an ill-smelling pipe with a long stem on which he tied a blue ribbon. He often wore one arm in a sling, although it was not broken. Bodenheim always had trouble surviving and occasionally read his poetry for money at the Dill Pickle Club. He sometimes published in the *Little Review*.[81] On one occasion Harriet Monroe appeared with some of her editorial staff, including Carnevali, at a party given by some of the literary people. Bodenheim was present at the party. Carnevali had just achieved a measure of local fame by being arrested for exposing himself to a policewoman in Lincoln Park. Bodenheim, apparently hoping to sell a poem, had been trying to be nice to Monroe, but he was incensed because he thought Carnevali's tactics were unfair. He said that anybody could be famous if he stooped to cheap publicity and went on to make lewd remarks which embarrassed Monroe and negated any good will that his transitory amiability might have achieved.[82]

Carl Sandburg, from Galesburg, a reporter for a socialist paper, had begun to write poetry immortalizing Chicago as the "city of big shoulders" and the "hog butcher of the world." Monroe referred to Sandburg as the "great slow-stepping Swede."[83] Edgar Lee Masters described him as he first met him when Sandburg came into his office: "He was taller than ordinary and with a martial bearing. His voice was deep and drowsy; and the smile on his large, loose mouth with its fleshy lips, broad and ingratiating. He wore steel-rimmed spectacles through which his gray-yellow eyes stared or grew luminous with sudden interest.[84]

Ben Hecht described Carl Sandburg as he remembered him from those days in Chicago:

> Carl Sandburg's manner is as distinct as a caricature. He draws his breath in between his teeth before speaking, inflates his chest, lifts up his shoulders, wags the upper part of his body from side to side, and talks with the brevity and importance of the Ten Commandments.
>
> Outwardly his senses are as blind as a bat. He sees black hair as green, looks at a young woman and says her age is fifty, reads preposterous meanings into handbills and colorless phenomena, and emerges from situations with humorously inaccurate memories of them.
>
> But Carl's inner response to life is a beautiful emotion—a fellowship set to music.[85]

Vachel Lindsay, the gentle boy from Springfield, whose domineering mother wanted him to be an artist and forced him into six years of art study, came to Chicago. Springfield neglected Lindsay, as did all of society, so that at first he had to trade his poems for bread. Later he made a bare living by reciting them around the country.[86] Monroe published "General William Booth Enters Heaven," and invited Lindsay to Chicago to recite "Congo" for William Butler Yeats. Yeats spoke glowingly of the works of the young poet. Monroe was pleased for she believed Lindsay was the best poet she published.[87] Lindsay loved Springfield and Illinois and all of America. He said that he would make Springfield a beautiful city, but he died in despair, drinking Lysol in his old family home near the governor's mansion.[88]

These young writers followed a pattern. The poets practiced imagism through the mechanism of free verse. The writers of prose, all naturalists, described society as it was, reducing their writing to the bare essentials, devoid of ornament. They wrote about the things that they saw and knew. They wrote about life as they believed it was. They used everyday language to describe the commonplace people and scenes with which they were familiar. The importance of the Chicago writers was noted by H. L. Mencken, who was likely to look upon most of his fellow writers with a jaundiced eye. Mencken wrote, "Find me a writer who is indubitably an American and who has something new and interesting to say, and who says it with an air, and nine times out of ten, I will show you that he has some sort of connection with the Abattoir by the Lake."[89]

Among the literary figures of Chicago, Henry Blake Fuller published several novels, but his best work was done by 1900. He realized the naturalism of the newer writers was more appropriate than the romantic stories that he had been writing. His pathetic swan song, as remembered by Sherwood Anderson, sums up all he found wrong with his own writing and all he saw in the younger writers:

> I am at bottom a Victorian. It got into me when I was a child. I can't escape it. I have a mind and an imagination. I have eyes to see, ears to hear. The wall we are building about ourselves must be broken down. We have come out of an age when we have presumed, for example, that all women, that is to say good women, never have any impure thoughts, never have any impure desires. I know it is all wrong, tht it would be sweeter and better, healthier for us all, to have more of the reality of life come into our writing, but I cannot do it.
> Nor can I go on writing the everlasting cheerful meaningless stuff we are expected to write.
> Therefore I quit.[90]

These new writers brought sex into their writing. Sherwood Anderson describes his reaction to the criticism of the sexuality in literature: "Criticism had been poured all over all my Chicago contemporaries from the start. We had the notion that sex had something to do with people's lives, and it had been barely mentioned in American writing before our time. No one had seemed to ever use a profane word and bring sex back to what seemed to us its normal place in the picture of life. We were called sex obsessed."[91]

These young writers revelled in the sexual freedom they assumed. Sherwood Anderson hints of nude bathing parties,[92] and Edgar Lee Masters boasts of amorous adventures in his memoirs.[93] Anderson also saw homosexuals for the first time and was intrigued. In his first major book,*Winesburg, Ohio,* he treated the subject of homosexuality and shocked many.[94] Anderson liked to go out in the evening with a large brass ring in his ear and was delighted with the stares that it brought.[95] Divorce figured large in the life of the bohemians. Dell divorced Margery Curry. Anderson divorced his first wife, Cornelia Lane, and married Tennessee Mitchell (though the newlyweds spent their honeymoon at Cornelia's house, and it was not uncommon for the three of them, with the children of both marriages, to go on vacations together).[96] The concept of marriage was changing.

Theodore Dreiser was a notorious libertine.[97] In his first book of importance, *Sister Carrie,* published in 1900 and suppressed, Dreiser dealt with illicit sex and illegitimacy.[98] He followed this with *Jennie Gerhardt,* a similarly descriptive book.[99]

Another characteristic of these writers was their portrayal of the big city, and their realistic or naturalistic descriptions of life. Masters's *Spoon River Anthology* shocked many, particularly the people of Lewistown, but he was making an effort to portray life as it was in a small town.

All of these writers had come from the small town environment; and they all were escaping it; they all were insisting on their freedom. Perhaps the greatest rebel of all was Margaret Anderson, who modestly described herself as "extravagantly and disgustingly pretty."[100] She made every effort to escape the conventional world. She came from a middle-class family in Columbus, Indiana. Her father was a successful businessman and her mother a clubwoman who wanted nothing more than for her to come back to Columbus and play bridge at the country club. By the time she graduated from Western College at Oxford, Ohio, she had decided that she wanted no part of that.[101]

Anderson entitled her autobiography *My Thirty Years' War,* and her description of her rebellion reads much like that of young people in any generation. She found herself boxed in by the attitudes of her Victorian family but refused to be cornered and live the life her family dictated. She rejected her family, much as they rejected her and her life-style. She refused to accept the conventional identity of wife, daughter, or sister. She lived the bohemian life and did what she could to further the arts, and although her own literary production was minor, she helped others.[102]

Edgar Lee Masters, writing of Vachel Lindsay, described the rebellion of youth in Illinois towns:

> There had been rebellion in Illinois on the part of the youth long before Lindsay's day. When I was a youth there, all of us who did not get jobs in the abstract office there to record real estate transfers, who did not become the manufacturers of cigars, or begin as clerks in the stores with the hope of one day owing the store, or take with alacrity to the practice of medicine or law, or raise chickens, or vegetables, or in short do something else which made us permanent denizens of our villages, were in rebellion. The church choked us to death, the constant ringing of prayer-meeting bells filled us first with melancholy, then with resentment; the moral intermeddlers which broke up every dance and frowned upon every amateur dramatic venture set our nerves to bristling with pugnacity. We had nothing but each other, and we were few. Except for the sustaining voices of Whitman and Emerson, we should have sunk to the dregs, worn out with the struggle against the prohibitionists and the Sunday school workers. A few of us survived and fought our way out. I am giving reminiscent pictures of my own town, where one aspiring girl wrote every week for one of the town's papers a column called "Culture's Garland," where another taught school and used her money to travel and read, and where another as a city editor castigated the forces of tyranny every week, and making himself bitter and doing no harm to those obtuse and stubborn souls.[103]

Many of these writers took up liberal causes and sometimes associated with various kinds of radicals. When Dell first came to Chicago from Davenport, he lived for a time at the Chicago Commons and there met many anarchists.[104] He later associated with these people and in time was a part of what H. L. Mencken liked to refer to as the "red ink fraternity."[105] When he left Chicago, he went to New York to live in Greenwich Village and to edit the *Masses*. During World War I he was arrested, tried, and acquitted for sedition because of the paper's antiwar editorial policy.[106] That Dell was a radical no one could deny, but he was what might be called an intellectual radical. Sinclair Lewis once referred to him as a "faun on the barricades."[107]

Sandburg was associated from the beginning with socialists. His poetry reflects his sympathy for the working man and the downtrodden. Sherwood Anderson was sometimes associated with radicals. He was friend of John Reed, who eventually became a Communist. Anderson reported that he himself was almost arrested during World War I.[108] Margaret Anderson was a close friend of Emma Goldman, an anarchist. Goldman visited at the famous tent on the North Shore and sometimes helped with the cooking.[109] Lucien Cary, of the *Friday Literary Review,* once said that Goldman was "a nice woman with ideas less radical than Emerson's and certainly less interesting."[110] William D. Haywood was also an Anderson guest on occasion.[111]

Joseph Medill Patterson, of the *Chicago Tribune* family, grandson of Joseph Medill and cousin of Robert R. McCormick, became disillusioned with the capitalist system as early as 1904 and announced that since reform was impossible, he was becoming a socialist. He wrote a novel, *A Little Brother of the Rich,* in which he promoted socialist doctrines and embarrassed his family.[112] He also embarrassed the socialists because they did not quite know what to do with a socialist who was so rich.

Many of the people in this group held pacifist views and opposed World War I. Never pro-German or un-American, they regarded war as immoral and opposed the destructiveness of it. Harriet Monroe was depressed when some of her young poets were killed in the war, men such as Joyce Kilmer, Alan Seeger, and Rupert Brooke.[113] Jane Addams of Hull House believed war was a terribly debilitating thing for a nation. She opposed it at every opportunity and starting in 1914 took the platform for pacifist causes. Congressman and one-time senator Billy Mason stood against the war in the most direct of terms. Most of the socialists took an antiwar position.[114]

This generation of young, talented people were rebels. They lived unconventional lives and proclaimed radical ideas. Although hardly revolutionaries, they often associated with those who were. That they came from small towns may explain their appreciation of the city. Often ill-educated, sometimes anti-intellectual, they were often provincial and frequently suspicious of the East. Yet many of them finally settled in New York, and a few became expatriates in the '20s.

Colleges and universities provided much of the cultural stimulus in downstate Illinois. The colleges brought an appreciation for things of the mind and spirit, providing contact with art, music, and literature, usually emphasizing scholarship rather than creative work. By 1900 the University of Illinois at Urbana was making every effort to upgrade its status in literature and the arts and shake off its cow-college image. Under the deanship of Professor Evarts B. Greene, himself a distinguished historian, the university elected William Abbott Oldfather, classicist, Stuart Pratt Sherman, professor of literature and literary critic, William Spence Robert-son, historian of Latin America, and Theodore Calvin Pease, Solon J. Buck, and Clarence W. Alvord, historians, to the faculty.[115]

Alvord took on the editorship of the *Collections of the Illinois State Historical Library* after 1909, as well as the editorship of the *Mississippi Valley Historical Review* and the *Centennial History of Illinois*. The Illinois Historical Survey opened under the adminis-tration of the graduate school in 1909. The university established a museum of European culture and a museum of classical culture in 1913. By 1915 the library, housed in Lincoln Hall, had a collection numbering 400,000 volumes. In 1909, the university began publication of a list of the printed works of its faculty; in 1914–15 this list had grown to thirty pages. In 1915 the University of Illinois began publication of *Studies in Language and Literature* under the editorship of Professors Flom, Oldfather, and Sherman, and in 1918 the University of Illinois Press was established. James Garfield Randall, historian of the Civil War and Lincoln biographer, came to Illinois in the same year.[116]

In the 1920s the university kept up its efforts to maintain its scholarship, bringing to Urbana distinguished men such as Frederick Charles Dietz, Thomas W. Baldwin, and Harris Fletcher. Dietz established himself as a scholar of the Tudor period of English history, Baldwin was the most distinguished Shakespeare scholar of his generation, and Fletcher gained a similar eminence in Milton studies.[117]

The other public institutions of higher education consisted of five normal schools, all of which became degree-granting institu-tions in the 1920s. These institutions, established largely for the training of teachers, initially for elementary schools, took little interest in scholarly activities and emphasized teaching skills. Scholarship and creative activity generally went unrecognized and unrewarded. Still, all offered courses in the classics, literature, history, art, and music. Because of low standards of admission, all maintained preparatory branches to prepare their students for college level courses. In the process, they brought a higher cultural appreciation to isolated parts of the state. The general assembly created the Illinois State Normal University in 1857. The legisla-ture provided for Southern Illinois Normal School at Carbondale in 1869, and it opened for classes in 1874. Eastern Illinois Normal School opened at Charleston in 1899 as did Northern Illinois Normal School at DeKalb. Western Illinois Normal School began classes in 1902.[118]

Various private colleges performed a similar service. By 1906, fifty-five private post-secondary educational institutions functioned in Illinois. Some of these, hardly more than vocational schools, trained young persons in the rudiments of business procedures; others, such as Knox College, founded in 1837, provided a higher level of scholarship and promoted cultural learning. Illinois College, Shurtleff College, and McKendree College celebrated their centennials in 1929.[119]

Illinois sponsored several cultural institutions, mostly in and around Springfield. The Illinois State Library grew from 70,000 volumes in 1919 to 106,000 volumes in 1929. Its extension service held 45,000 volumes for loan through local public libraries, of which there were 292 in 1919, at least 19 of which were built with funds furnished by Andrew Carnegie. The Illinois State Museum in Springfield displayed exhibits of natural science, crafts, and art. In 1919, it held an exhibition of Illinois artists. The Illinois State Historical Library, founded by the legislature in 1889, collected books and manuscripts relating to state history, and the Illinois State Historical Society functioned as a branch of the library to promote interest in the history of the state. The Illinois State Library, the Illinois State Museum, the Illinois State Historical Library, and the Illinois State Historical Society were housed in the Centennial Building, designated as the home of cultural affairs of the state after the centennial celebration in 1918. The Lincoln home became the property of Illinois in 1887 and New Salem was acquired in 1917.[120]

The concept of mutual self-help to enhance the cultural standing of a communnity has enjoyed a long and honorable history in the United States, and societies sprang up throughout Illinois for this purpose. Some promoted group study for members, amateur performances, or the pooling of resources to bring a professional artist or scholar to enhance the culture of a small town. In 1893 a Bloomington group founded the Amateur Musical Club, which brought professional musicians to the Coliseum, said to have near-perfect acoustics. They brought the Chicago Symphony to Bloomington, as well as opera stars such as Amelita Galli-Curci. Also in Bloomington the Philharmonic Society, founded in the 1920s, performed the *Messiah* annually. The music department of the Peoria Women's Club sponsored a chorus and an annual series of concerts with professional artists such as Josef Hoffman and Fritz Kreisler. Rockford had a seventy-piece symphony orchestra and a supporting choral group, and the Mendelssohn Club sponsored a concert series with national figures. Belvidere supported the Amateur Musical Club, and Havana had its Beethoven Club. By 1905, 97 percent of the public schools of Illinois taught music; by 1908, twenty-six conservatories, colleges, and universities offered music courses. Glee clubs and orchestras were common. Wherever German communities existed, there were singing societies such as the Liederkrantz at Belleville or the Highland Maennerchor Harmonie made up largely of German Swiss. The Highland Harmonie participated in singing festivals; one in Highland in 1905 featured a chorus of 800 voices.[121]

Similar societies devoted themselves to the appreciation of art. The Jacksonville Art Association was founded in 1873, the Lincoln Art Club in 1876, the Palladen of Bloomington in 1879, and the Art Club of Champaign in 1876. The Springfield Art Association, founded in 1877, is housed in the former home of Benjamin S. Edwards. The associations maintained permanent exhibits, hosted traveling shows, and held classes. The Harry and Della Burpee Art Gallery in Rockford provided a meeting place for literary and little theater groups as well as exhibiting a small permanent collection and traveling exhibits. In 1920, the All-Illinois Society of Fine Arts was founded to provide paintings for shows in the smaller towns of the Midwest, including Jacksonville, Aurora, and Rockford.[122]

Little theater groups modeled after that of Maurice Browne sprang up in the period after World War I. The art and literature department of the Peoria Women's Club performed a Shakespeare play annually, "with much spirit and intelligence." In Bloomington the Community Players, founded in 1923, performed current plays, and the Scottish Rite Players presented the American Passion Play every year. The Peoria Players Theatre was founded in 1919, using a converted firehouse as their theater.[123]

Many towns had literary societies devoting themselves to the study of literature or to readings by members. In Quincy, the Friends in Council, founded in 1866, boasted that it was the oldest women's literary club. In Jacksonville, the Literary Union, founded in 1864, promoted "knowledge and correct taste" for its members. Among the others were the Ladies Reading Circle of Mattoon, the Tuesday Club of Pana, and the Clionian of Pontiac.[124]

These efforts served to bring cultural matters to smaller towns and in some instances to bring professional musicians or paintings. Much of the reputation of Illinois rested on its material achievements in agriculture, industry, and transportation, but increasingly its accomplishments in performance, creativity, and scholarship brought fame, and for a brief time Illinois led the nation in cultural advances.

1. Clarence A. Hough, "The Art Institute of Chicago," *Art and Archaeology*, 12 (Sept.-Oct., 1921), pp. 145, 149; *Chicago Tribune*, July 22, 1900, p. 43

2. Art Institute of Chicago, *Twenty-first Annual Report of the Trustees for the Year Ending June 1, 1900* pp. 7, 17–18, hereafter referred to as *Annual Report*.

3. Ibid., pp. 27–30, 32–33, 38.

4. *Annual Report, for the Year ending June 1, 1907*, pp. 20–21, 59.

5. *Annual Report, for the Year Ending June 1, 1909*, p. 25; Harriet Monroe, *A Poet's Life: Seventy Years in a Changing World* (New York, 1938), pp. 240–41.

6. Lena M. McCauley, "Friends of American Art," *Art and Archaeology*, 12 (Sept.–1921), pp. 175–78.

7. Monroe, *A Poet's Life*, pp. 193–94, 204–5, 207; W. G. Rogers, *Ladies Bountiful* (New York, 1968), pp. 24, 33–34.

8. Monroe, *A Poet's Life*, p. 215.

9. *Chicago Evening Post*, Mar. 26, 1913, p. 7; *Chicago Daily Inter-Ocean*, Mar. 25, 1913, p. 5.

10. *Chicago Daily News*, Mar. 22, 1913, p. 2.

11. *Chicago Evening Post*, Mar. 22, 1913, p. 8; Mar. 26, 1913, p. 7; *Chicago Daily News*, Mar. 24, 1913, p. 4; *Inter-Ocean*, Mar. 30, 1913, p. M-5.

12. *Inter-Ocean*, Mar. 25, 1913, p. 5; Apr. 2, 1913, p. 10.

13. Monroe, *A Poet's Life*, p. 215.

14. *Annual Report, for the Year Ending 1912–1913*, pp. 36–37.

15. Ibid., p. 37.

16. *Annual Report, for the Year Ending 1910–11; 1911–12, pp. 59–62; 1912–13*, p. 61. Lena M. McCauley, "Some Collectors of Paintings," *Art and Archaeology*, 12 (Sept.-Oct., 1921), p. 169.

17. *Annual Report, for the Year Ending 1918*, p. 18; *for 1922*, p. 11; McCauley, "Some Collectors of Paintings," pp. 163–65.

18. *Annual Report, for the Year Ending 1922*, p. 11; McCauley, "Some Collectors of Paintings," pp. 162–63.

19. *Annual Report, for the Year Ending 1918*, p. 17.

20. *Annual Report, for the Year Ending 1924*, pp. 6, 21–23.

21. McCauley, "Friends of American Art," p. 178; *Annual Report, for the Year Ending 1913–14*, pp. 59–60; McCauley, "Some Collectors of Paintings," p. 172; Monroe, *A Poet's Life*, pp. 240–41.

22. *Chicago Evening Post*, Mar. 22, 1913, p. 8.

23. Floyd Dell, *Homecoming* (New York, 1933), pp. 211, 232–33.

24. *Chicago Tribune*, May 17, 1908, part 7, p. 8; Mar. 25, 1913, p. 7.

25. Ben Hecht, *A Child of the Century* (New York, 1954), pp. 238–40; Harry Hansen, *Midwest Portraits: A Book of Memories and Friendships* (New York, 1923), p. 101.

26. *Chicago Tribune*, Sept. 2, 1920, p. 2; David M. Mendalowitz, *A History of American Art* (New York, 1964), p. 486.

27. Louis H. Sullivan, *The Autobiography of an Idea* (New York, 1924), p. 293.

28. Monroe, *A Poet's Life*, p. 210; Mark L. Peisch, *The Chicago School of Architecture: Early Followers of Sullivan and Wright* (New York, 1964), pp. 25 -26, 27, 125.

29. Ibid., pp. 53–54.

30. Frank Lloyd Wright, *An Autobiography* (New York, 1943), pp. 108, 126.

31. Peisch, *The Chicago School*, p. 53.

32. Ibid., pp. 39–52; Thomas E. Tallmadge, *The Story of Architecture in America* (New York, 1927), p. 230.

33. Peisch, *The Chicago School*, pp. 7, 15.

34. John H. Mueller, *The American Symphony Orchestra: A Social History of Musical Taste* (Bloomington, Ind., 1951), pp. 101–3.

35. Ibid., pp. 103–4.

36. Ibid., p. 104.

37. Frank A. Randall, *History of the Development of Building Construction in Chicago* (Urbana, Ill., 1949), p. 225; Mueller, *American Symphony*, pp. 104–5.

38. Mueller, *American Symphony*, pp. 105–6. For the life of Theodore Thomas, see *A Musical Autobiography* 2 vols. (Chicago, 1905), and Rose Fay Thomas, *Memoirs of Theodore Thomas* (New York, 1911).

39. Mueller, *American Symphony*, p. 106.

40. Ibid., pp. 107–8.

41. Ibid., p. 108.

42. Ibid., pp. 110–11.

43. Ronald L. Davis, *A History of Opera in the American West* (Englewood Cliffs, N. J. 1965), pp. 30–36, 36–41. See also Ronald L. Davis, *Opera in Chicago* (New York, 1966).

44. *Chicago Tribune*, Apr. 15, 1900, p. 40.

45. Ibid., Feb. 6, 1900, p. 6.

46. Davis, *Opera in the American West*, p. 42; Vincent Shean, *Oscar Hammerstein I: The Life and Exploits of an Impresario* (New York, 1956), pp. 168–81.

47. Davis, *Opera in the American West*, pp. 42–43.

48. Mary Garden and Louis Biancoli, *Mary Garden's Story* (New York, 1951), pp. 1–7, 66–88, 107–57; Victor I. Serof, *Debussy, Musician of France* (New York, 1956), pp. 189–210.

49. Davis, *Opera in the American West*, pp. 44–45; Garden and Biancoli, *Mary Garden's Story*, p. 204.

50. Davis, *Opera in the American West*, pp. 46–47.

51. Ibid., pp. 48–49, 52; C. G. Le Massena, *Galli-Curci's Life of Song* (New York, 1945), pp. 9–10, 56–106.

52. Davis, *Opera in the American West*, pp. 52–53.

53. Ibid., pp. 55–59.

54. Ibid., pp. 61–62; John E. Hodge, "The Chicago Civic Opera Company, Its Rise and Fall, "' *Journal of the Illinois State Historical Society*, 55 (Spring, 1962), pp. 5–7.

55. Davis, *Opera in the American West*, pp. 62, 64.

56. Ibid., pp. 65–66.

57. Garden and Biancoli, *Mary Garden's Story*, pp. 194–208; Davis, *Opera in the American West*, p. 54; Arthur Meeker, *Chicago with Love: A Polite and Personal History* (New York, 1955), pp. 258–59.

58. John Tasker Howard, *Our American Music: Three Hundred Years of It* (New York, 1939), p. 463; John Tasker Howard and George Kent Bellows, *A Short History of Music in America* (New York, 1957), pp. 238–39.

59. Marion Bauer, *Twentieth Century Music, How It Developed, How to Listen to It* (New York, 1933), pp. 167–68; Howard, *Our American Music,* pp. 479–80; Howard and Bellows, *A Short History of Music in America,* pp. 228–29.

60. Howard, *Our American Music,* pp. 511, 512, 521–22, 541, 548, 551; Davis, *An Opera in the American West,* p. 66.

61. Emanuel Carnevali, *The Autobiography of Emanuel Carnevali,* comp. with Preface by Kay Boyle, (New York, 1968), pp. 158, 162.

62. Margaret Anderson, *My Thirty Years War* (New York, 1930), p. 32.

63. Floyd Dell, *Homecoming,* p. 244.

64. Sherwood Anderson, *Sherwood Anderson's Memoirs* (New York, 1942), p. 198.

65. Irving Howe, *Sherwood Anderson* (n.p., 1951), p. 57.

66. Margaret Anderson, *Thirty Years,* p. 28; W. G. Rogers, *Ladies Bountiful,* p. 28; Harriet Monroe, *A Poet's Life,* pp. 312, 314, 370.

67. Dell, *Homecoming,* pp. 189–90; M. Anderson, *Thirty Years,* pp. 36–38.

68. Monroe, *A Poet's Life,* pp. 242, 251–52.

69. M. Anderson, *Thirty Years,* pp. 12–25, 31; S. Anderson, *Memoirs,* p. 197.

70. Dell, *Homecoming,* pp. 189, 190, 207, 219–20, 232–33, 236–37; Howe, *Sherwood Anderson,* pp. 56–59; M. Anderson, *Thirty Years,* pp. 36–39; Hansen, *Midwest Portraits,* pp. 96–97.

71. S. Anderson, *Memoirs,* pp. 11–83, 234–35, 283; Howe, *Sherwood Anderson,* pp. 55–59, 64.

72. S. Anderson, *Memoirs,* p. 251; Bernard Duffey, *The Chicago Renaissance in American Letters: A Critical History* (Lansing, Mich. 1954), p. 138.

73. M. Anderson, *Thirty Years,* pp. 91–92; Howe, *Sherwood Anderson,* pp. 69–70.

74. Duffey, *The Chicago Renaissance,* p. 256.

75. Carnevali, *Autobiography,* p. 165.

76. Ibid., p. 168.

77. Ibid., p. 169.

78. Hansen, *Midwest Portraits,* p. 284; Carnevali, *Autobiography,* p. 156.

79. Ibid.

80. Ben Hecht, *Child of the Century* p. 331.

81. M. Anderson, *Thirty Years,* p. 59; Hansen, *Midwest Portraits,* pp. 97, 101.

82. Hecht, *Child of the Century,* pp. 222–23.

83. Monroe, *A Poet's Life,* p. 322.

84. Edgar Lee Masters, *Across Spoon River* (New York, 1936), p. 335.

85. Hecht, *Child of the Century,* pp. 331–32.

86. Edgar Lee Masters, *Vachel Lindsay, Poet in America* (New York, 1935), pp. 25–54, 229–49.

87. An account of the visit of Yeats is in Monroe, *A Poet's Life,* pp. 332–39.

88. Masters, *Vachel Lindsay,* pp. 335, 361–62.

89. Duffey, *The Chicago Renaissance,* p. 257.

90. S. Anderson, *Memoirs,* p. 459.

91. Ibid., p. 294.

92. Ibid., pp. 244–49.

93. Masters, *Across Spoon River,* pp. 224–44.

94. Sherwood Anderson, *Winesburg, Ohio,* ed. John H. Ferres (New York, 1966). See the story "Hands," pp. 27–34.

95. Howe, *Sherwood Anderson,* pp. 66–68.

96. Ibid., p. 83.

97. W. A. Swanberg, *Dreiser* (New York, 1965), *passim.*

98. Theodore Dreiser, *Sister Carrie* (New York, 1965), p. x.

99. Theodore Dreiser, *Jennie Gerhart* (New York, 1911).

100. M. Anderson, *Thirty Years*, p. 15.

101. Ibid., pp. 7–12

102. Ibid., pp. 3, 4.

103. Masters, *Vachel Lindsay*, pp. 99–200.

104. Dell, *Homecoming*, p. 181.

105. Swanberg, *Dreiser*, p. 189.

106. Dell, *Homecoming*, pp. 246, 310–28.

107. Howe, *Sherwood Anderson*, p. 68.

108. S. Anderson, *Memoirs*, p. 51,

109. Hansen, *Midwest Portraits*, p. 52.

110. M. Anderson, *Thirty Years*, pp. 83–84.

111. Ibid., pp. 72–75.

112. Joseph Medill Patterson, *A Little Brother of the Rich* (New York, 1908).

113. Monroe, *A Poet's Life*, pp. 340–61.

114. An account of the pacifism of Jane Addams, Congressman Mason, and various socialist groups is found in Arthur C. Cole, "Illinois and the Great War," in Ernest Ludlow Bogart and John Mabry Matthews, *The Modern Commonwealth 1893–1918* (Springfield, Ill., 1920), pp. 483–86.

115. Albert Nelson Marquis, ed. *Who's Who in America, 1940–1941* (Chicago, 1940), pp. 1972, 1032, 2197; Allan Nevins, *Illinois* (New York, 1917), 231.

116. Nevins, *Illinois*, pp. 231, 189, 290–91; *University of Illinois Studies in Language and Literature*, I (Urbana, 1915).

117. Marquis, *Who's Who in America, 1940–1941*, pp. 240, 773, 940.

118. For the development of the normal schools see: Helen E. Marshall *Grandest of Enterprises: Illinois State Normal University, 1857–1874* (Normal, 1956); Eli G. Lentz, *Seventy-five Years in Retrospect: Southern Illinois University, 1874–1949* (Carbondale, 1955); George Plochman, *The Ordeal of Southern Illinois University* (Carbondale, 1957) gives some of the earlier history but mostly deals with later developments; Earl W. Hayter, *Education in Transition: The History of Northern Illinois University* (DeKalb, 1974); Charles H. Coleman, *Eastern Illinois State College: Fifty Years of Public Service* (Charleston, 1950). For further insights into Eastern, see Henry Johnson, *The Other Side of Main Street* (New York, 1943) and Isabel McKinney, *Mr. Lord: The Life and Words of Livingston C. Lord* (Urbana, Ill. 1937). Victor Hicken, *The Purple and the Gold: The Story of Western Illinois University* (Macomb, 1970).

119. *Illinois Blue Book, 1907* (Springfield, 1908), pp. 372–73; Martha F. Webster, *The Story of Knox College, 1837–1912* (Galesburg, Ill., 1912); Arthur F. Ewert, "Early History of Education in Illinois—the Three Oldest Colleges, *"Illinois Blue Book 1929–30* (Springfield, 1929), pp. 301–34; Charles H. Rammelkamp, *Illinois College: A Centennial History, 1829–1929* (New Haven, 1929).

120. *Illinois Blue Book, 1905* p. 537; ibid., *1929–30*, pp. 421, 431, 435–41, 446–449; Roger D. Bridges, "The Origins and Early Years of the Illinois State Historical Society," *Journal of the Illinois State Historical Society*, 68 (Apr., 1975), pp. 98–120; *New Salem: A Memorial to Abraham Lincoln* (Springfield, 1934), p. 2.

121. H. Clay Tate, *The Way It Was in McLean County, 1972–1822* (Bloomington, Ill., 1972), pp. 261–62; Federal Writers Project, *Illinois: A Descriptive and Historical Guide* (Chicago, 1939), pp. 141, 367, 373, 619–20; Belle Short Lambert, "The Womens Club Movement in Illinois," *Transactions of the Illinois State Historical Society*, 9 (1904), pp. 331–32; James M. Rice, *Peoria: City and County, Illinois* (Chicago, 1912), pp. 427–28; A. P. Spencer, *Centennial History of Highland, Illinois, 1837–1937* (Highland, 1937), pp. 122–25.

122. Federal Writers Project, *Illinois*, pp. 115,373, 394; Lambert, "Women's Club Movement," p. 317.

123. Federal Writers Project, *Illinois*, p. 362; Tate, *The Way It Was*, p. 262; Rice, *Peoria* p. 427.

124. Lambert, "Women's Club Movement," pp. 317–18; Charles H. Rammelkamp, "Four Historic Societies of Jacksonville, Illinois," *Journal of the Illinois State Historical Society*, 18 (Apr., 1925), pp. 205–8.

6

Progressivism, Bosses, and Factions: Politics

The political history of Illinois from 1900 to 1916 is a bewildering confusion of factions and bosses combined with occasional excursions into reform. Historians refer to the period as the progressive era. The term implies political reform, regulation of business, and legislation on behalf of working people, but historians disagree as to the nature of progressivism. George Mowry and Richard Hofstadter have pictured the progressive era as the product of urban, white, middle-class Protestant, Anglo-Saxon leaders.[1] More recently challenges have been made to this interpretation. John Buenker has demonstrated convincingly that progressivism would have been impossible in Illinois without the help of immigrant politicians (whom he calls the "new stock politicians").[2] Unquestionably, immigrant peoples provided legislators who contributed mightily to passage of progressive legislation in Illinois, and in many instances, progressive leadership came from the "new stock politicians."

Illinois, like most states, had a progressive period, and it is necessary to list the administrations of Governors Deneen, Dunne, and Lowden as reform periods. During the sixteen years from 1905 to 1921 when these men occupied the governor's mansion, the state saw reform measures in politics, industry, and labor. However, progressivism in Illinois never reached the heights that it achieved in Wisconsin or Oregon, for too often Illinois progressives were handicapped by bossism, corruption, and apathy. The political bosses of both parties supported progressive measures only when it suited their purposes or when it did not affect their political base.

Both the Democrats and Republicans were beset by factionalism, generally patched up at election time but often hindering party effectiveness. By 1900 Chicago and downstate factions split each of the parties. The factionalism did not stop with this division. The Republican party was split between downstate, Chicago, and what was called the federal crowd. The congressmen and senators who represented the state in Washington, particularly Joseph Cannon of Danville, for a period speaker of the House of Representatives, and Senator Shelby Cullom, who served the state for decades, led the federal crowd. Charles Gates Dawes, comptroller of the currency in the McKinley administration, who was often regarded as speaking for President McKinley, and Franklin MacVeagh, a Chicago financier and secretary of the treasury in the Taft administration, maintained a voice in that faction. The federal crowd carried more weight in national politics than in the state, but they exerted local influence in the interest of extending their political base. Dawes had political ambitions and made every effort to bend the party to his ends, but his political ambitions were often thwarted by other factions. Born in Ohio, the son of a Civil War general, Dawes graduated from Marietta College and entered the practice of law. He came to Evanston, where he engaged in business and became chairman of the Central Trust Company in 1902. After serving as a brigadier general in World War I, he held several minor offices. He reached the peak of his political career in 1924 when he was elected vice-president under Calvin Coolidge. He later served as ambassador to Great Britain.[4]

The Chicago branch of the Republican party was dominated for years by a political boss, William Lorimer. Lorimer, born in England in 1861, came to the United States while a small child. He had no regular education and worked his way up through business and the political jungle of Chicago. By 1895 Lorimer's political activities had gained him a seat in Congress, and he served from 1895 to 1901. He was defeated in that year but returned to Congress in 1903 and served until 1909. Lorimer had the reputation of being able to control Chicago, and many respectable political figures owed their start in politics to him. Governor Charles Deneen started as Lorimer's protégé, but as he gained his political feet he shook off Lorimer's control. The same was true of Frank Lowden. Later Lorimer promoted the career of William Hale "Big Bill" Thompson.[5]

The Democratic party in Chicago had a number of colorful figures. Among these was Roger Sullivan, whom many regarded as the worst kind of boss. Born of Irish immigrant parents at

Belvidere, Illinois, Sullivan was orphaned while quite young. Young Sullivan had difficulty getting along, and worked at a variety of things. He quickly took to politics, as did many of his Irish contemporaries. He held one minor office in Cook County but usually was behind the scenes. In the 1890s Sullivan organized the Ogden Gas Company and by manipulating the city council of Chicago became a rich man. He sold his interest in that company for $666,666. Later he organized other companies, including the Sawyer Biscuit Company and the Great Lakes Dredge and Dock Company, and was interested in banking. He was noted as a politician rather than as an industrialist, however, and had great influence with various factions in Illinois.[6]

Sullivan's greatest enemy in Illinois was Carter Harrison the younger. Harrison detested Sullivan and spent most of his life fighting him. Harrison, mayor of Chicago for five terms, had higher ambitions and from time to time had local support for the Democratic nomination for president. Harrison regarded Sullivan as a roughneck. Harrison was a powerful man in his own right and his faction fought for fifteen years with Sullivan's.[7]

Allied at first with Harrison was Edward F. Dunne. Like Sullivan, Dunne was the son of Irish immigrant parents but there the similarity ended. An attorney, Dunne had been educated at Trinity College in Dublin and had the distinction of having thirteen children. Although he was Harrison's associate early in the century, Dunne later became friendlier with Roger Sullivan, much to Harrison's disgust.[8] Among other figures of importance, Millard Dunlap of Jacksonville acted as the Illinois spokesman for William Jennings Bryan and was therefore important in the Democratic party.[9] Charles Boeschenstein, for many years a state central committeeman for the Democratic party in Illinois, served as its chairman for eight years.[10]

Particularly in Chicago, political clubs played an important role. The Union League Club, always important in Republican politics, was primarily a social club. The Standard Club, the Jewish club in Chicago, bore political influence from time to time. The Commercial Club was formed to promote the interest of the Republican party with the mercantile classes.[11] The chief Republican club was the Hamilton Club. It contained most of the leaders of the Republican party and served to bring businessmen and professional men into the political stream. The club raised money and otherwise promoted the party but its value was open to question.[12] Harold Ickes, always a rebel, described it this way: "The Hamilton

Club was always a hide-bound Republican organization, consisting in large part, of political mediocrities. All that was necessary to find favor in the eyes of its membership committee was to be a Republican. It was never interested in keeping its party clean."[13]

The chief Democratic club was the Iroquois Club. Founded in the 1880s, it included the leadership of the Illinois Democratic party. Like the Hamilton Club, it served to bring together business and professional men with political leaders and was influential in fund raising and promoting party views.[14]

The Sumner Club, a Republican organization for Blacks, aimed at keeping the black leadership of Chicago close to the Republican party.[15] Ethnic groups were important in the parties all over the state but particularly in Chicago. The Blacks of Illinois almost always voted Republican from 1900 until the depression and the New Deal because Blacks believed that the Republican party had been responsible for achieving their freedom from slavery. As far as the Blacks were concerned, the Republican party was still the party of Lincoln, and Republicans did give lip service to black causes. Thompson was regarded by many Blacks as important to their well-being and Lorimer courted the black vote, but on occasion it was possible for him to make a racist statement.[16]

Immigrant groups constituted an important voting element in Chicago, and politicians courted the ethnic groups. As the ethnic compositon of a neighborhood changed, each new group demanded to be cut into the political scene. The story is told of a Chicago ward that had been dominated by the Irish but through population shifts had become half Italian. The Italians demanded that they get at least one of the aldermen. An Irishman rose to the occasion with: "Well, ye got the Pope, ain't ye? Wot'n'll more d' ye want?"[17] Prior to the Civil War, Swedes, Germans, Irish, and Jews came to Chicago. These groups exerted influence in the policics of Illinois even before 1900. In the twentieth century, Italians, Poles, Czechs, Lithuanians, Yugoslavs, and East European Jews arrived in Illinois. The Swedes voted Republican from the beginning. They had opposed slavery, and Republicans welcomed them. The early Germans usually voted Republican, although because of their experiences in their homeland they tended to be more radical than Swedes. The early Jewish people of Chicago also tended to align themselves with the Republican party.[18]

Of the early immigrants only the Irish voted Democratic, but they did so devotedly and played a leadership role in the Democratic party from the beginning. A list of Illinois Democratic leaders after 1900 gives the impression that the party was an Irish party. Among the later immigrants party loyalty is less clear. the Czechs and Bohemians almost always voted Democratic from the time they arrived. The same can be said of the Poles, although they were less addicted to politics than the Czechs. The Italians fluctuated but basically tended to vote Republican. The Lithuanians were likely to cast a Democratic vote, while the Yugoslavs fluctuated in their political alliances.[19]

Even within these groups there was dissension. Both the Czechs and the Irish held ardent Democratic views, but they disliked each other and competed for leadership within the party. From 1900 to 1930 the Irish dominated the party leadership. This leadership ranged from well-educated progressives such as Governor Dunne to figures such as Roger Sullivan, Michael "Hinky Dink" Kenna, and his friend "Bathhouse" John Coughlin. Kenna and Coughlin got considerable publicity, but their power was limited to Chicago's first ward, where they were interested in milking as much graft as they could from the houses of prostitution, saloons, dance halls, restaurants, and even respectable businesses. They supported whatever and whoever seemed to promote their interests. During the early years of the century they supported Mayor Carter Harrison and his faction of the Democratic party. When pressures caused Mayor Harrison to close down the vice of the first ward, however, they hastily switched their allegiance to Roger Sullivan and his faction.[20]

As the election year of 1900 approached, Illinois (as well as the United States) was comfortably in the hands of Republicans. In Washington, William McKinley promoted the interests of conservatism while Illinois was represented in the national capitol by the venerable Shelby Cullom, a Republican from Springfield, and the colorful William E. Mason from Chicago. In the House of Representatives the Republicans outnumbered the Democrats two to one. There were several important Illinois figures among the congressional delegation, the most impressive being Joseph Cannon of Danville. Almost equally important was James R. Mann of Chicago. Mann had the reputation of being an astute debater and parliamentarian. One historian described him thus: "He spoke there so often that he seemed to dwell on the floor, where his fierce scowl and sharp sarcasm made him a really fearsome creature to many of his colleagues." Mann was a contradictory figure. It was said he was a man of conscience who sometimes worked for decent reforms. On the other hand, he could seem to accept proposals of his opponents and then manipulate them through Congress in such a way that they lacked substance once passed.[21]

In Springfield, Governor John R. Tanner had, after a lackluster administration, announced that he would not run for reelection. He was ill during the early months of 1900, but he coveted a senate seat.[22] Newspaper columnists and other interested parties, speculating on who the candidates would be, watched for signs from the Iroquois Club as to the direction the Democrats might take. The Democrats were trying to shake off the free silver image of 1896 and move in the direction of respectability. The Iroquois Club split on the question of free silver and was reluctant to mention the issue but felt free to denounce the McKinley administration for its imperialism. Judge Edward F. Dunne, speaking to the Iroquois Club, declared that "Filipinos are being shot down for no greater crime than George Washington fought for in the Revolution— freedom." The Iroquois Club commemorated Jefferson's birthday in April of 1900 with Judge Dunne as the toastmaster. They honored Judge Murray Tuley, and the newspapers took note of the fact that several possibilities for governor attended the meeting. Among these, they spoke of Mayor Harrison and Adlai Stevenson, vice-president under Cleveland, Representative Samuel Alschuler of Aurora, Charles K. Ladd of Kewanee, and General Alfred Orendorf of Springfield. Alschuler spoke on Jefferson's ideas, Stevenson on party issues, General Orendorf on democracy, and Judge Worthington of Peoria on "A Democrat's Idea of Duty." Those at the speaker's table included Mayor Stevens of East St. Louis, Clarence Darrow, Millard Dunlap, and Chicago City Treasurer Adam Ortseifin.[23]

The Illinois Democratic convention met at the state house in Springfield on June 26, 1900. From the contenders for the gubernatorial nomination, the convention chose Judge Alschuler. Most of the ticket came from downstate, and it included Millard Dunlap. The *Tribune* thought that Alschuler would make a respectable candidate who would conduct a dignified campaign. Remembering Governor Altgeld with indignation, the *Tribune* said of Alschuler, "He will not froth and foam from Chicago to Cairo, as Mr. Altgeld four years ago."[24] The Democratic state platform denounced the administration of McKinley, imperialism, the gold standard, foreign alliances, the trusts, militarism, and government by injunction. On the other hand, they stood for equal rights for all, an interocean canal, and trial by jury in contempt cases, and demanded municipal ownership of public utilities and higher taxes

on corporation.[25] They denounced the administration of Governor
Tanner as "the most corrupt in the history of the state of Illinois."
They accused Tanner of extravagances and of favoring monopo-
lies and corporate enterprises. They favored the direct election of
U.S. senators and pledged their support to William Jennings Bryan
for president:

> We express our unqualified admiration for, and our devotion to,
> the man who for years has battled against the trusts, monopolies, and
> other public influences which are eating like a cancer into the heart of
> the Republic; a man who has succeeded in riveting the public gaze on
> their evil designs; a man who, by his patriotism and great ability has
> won the respect of even his enemies; who received six and one half
> millions unbought votes for the highest office in the gift of the
> American people, and who will in November next be placed in the
> office of which he was robbed in 1896 by a shameful system of
> corruption and debauchery; the foremost and beloved American of
> today William J. Bryan, and we pledge to him our loyal and
> unswerving support, and the delegates from the State of Illinois to
> the Democratic Convention are hereby instructed to vote as a unit for
> his renomination.[26]

Four years earlier the Democrats had been beset by serious splits,
so the attempt was made to recognize all factions in the delegation
elected by the state convention. Two delegates elected to the
national convention at Kansas City four years earlier had bolted
the party to support the Gold-Democratic candidate, John M.
Palmer of Illinois. Adlai Stevenson, a free-silverite, was similarly
recognized in this convention.[27]

The Democratic candidate for governor in 1900, Alschuler, a
lawyer from Aurora, was born in Chicago in 1859 of German-
Jewish parents. Later to be better known for his role as a labor
arbitrator and judge on the federal bench, at the time of his
nomination for governor he was serving in the general assembly.
Alschuler was a bachelor in 1900, a status he retained until 1923,
when he married at the age of sixty-two.[28]

Early in the year the Republican Cook County Central Committee announced that they would support Judge Elbridge Hanecy for
governor. This, in the eyes of the *Tribune*, meant Hanecy was the
candidate of Lorimer and linked him with Governor Tanner for
whom they had little use. Among others mentioned as possible
candidates for governor was Judge Orrin Carter. It turned out,
however, that Judge Hanecy was not acceptable to some, particularly the federal crowd. Dawes, said to be acting for President

McKinley, brought forth a dark horse candidate in the person of Richard Yates of Jacksonville. Frank Lowden, who opposed Tanner, turned to Yates when it seemed that he could not be stopped.[29]

The Republican convention, held in Peoria on May 8, nominated Yates on the fourth ballot as Lorimer switched to Yates when he found that Hanecy had no chance. Judge Carter tried to switch his vote to Owen Reeves, a Bloomington banker, but it was too late. Apparently some arrangement was made between the factions because a number of Tanner supporters were nominated for statewide office. Comptroller Dawes was the temporary chairman and former governor Joseph W. Fifer was permanent chairman. Fifer was a special friend of Shelby Cullom, who was endorsed by the Republican convention for reelection for senator. William Lorimer, angry at the interference of Dawes in the state convention, threatened to denounce the administration of McKinley.[30] The *Tribune* charged that state employees had been assessed 10 percent of their pay for the good of the party but that the money had been diverted into the Tanner-Hanecy campaign. It was charged that employees of the Kankakee State Hospital, already under the thumb of Len Small, were heavy contributors to this effort.[31]

The Republican state convention endorsed the gold standard policies of William McKinley as well as the protective tariff and imperialism:

> We heartily endorse the conservative and businesslike administration of Governor John R. Tanner. The state institutions under his administration have been managed in a manner that calls for the praise from all good citizens irrespective of political affiliation, and we commend him for his faithful adherence to the duties and obligations of his high office.
>
> We express our most hearty approval of the public career of our distinguished senior senator, Shelby M. Cullom, and declare it our desire that he shall be returned to the Senate of the United States.[32]

The Republican candidate for governor, Richard Yates, Jr., capitalized at every opportunity on the fact that he was the son of the Civil War governor of the same name. Over the years he had talked to Grand Army of the Republic posts and encampments at every opportunity. Yates was an attractive young man whose public service until 1900 was sparse, although he served with distinction later. At the time of his nomination for governor he was thirty-nine. One historian of the political scene of the time says of Yates: "In a candidate's role he had every qualification; but even some of his friends wondered if he had enough force and originality to be a statesman-like governor."[33]

The Republican national convention assembled in Philadelphia on June 19, 1900. The Illinois Republicans took a special train to the convention—a train which carried Lowden's private car. Graham Stewart became the national committeeman of the Republican party. Cannon and a few of the Illinois delegation supported Theodore Roosevelt for the vice-presidency, while others chose Senator Jonathan Prentiss Dolliver of Iowa. The campaign hinged on the prosperity issue. Lowden, as he left Chicago, told the Hamilton Club that Mary Elizabeth Lease, a former Populist orator, now imported her gowns from Paris and Jerry Simpson now wore socks, and there was much talk of the "full dinner pail" as the Illinois delegation went to Philadelphia. The convention nominated William McKinley for a second term and picked Theodore Roosevelt to run with him.[35]

The Democratic national convention met in Kansas City in July and the Illinois delegation was colorful as usual. Bathhouse John Coughlin and the Chicago delegation went to Kansas City to support Carter Harrison for president. Bathhouse wore one of his colorful outfits, including a ventilated straw hat with a purple band, checked trousers, and a blue-and-white-striped flannel coat. Carter Harrison might have gotten the position as vice-president but refused. He also protested the silver plank, which was put in the platform again. The convention nominated Bryan for a second try and Adlai Stevenson for vice-president. The *Tribune* said that Bryan was not pleased with Stevenson's nomination but that the candidacy of Stevenson had been necessary in order to head off the Harrison boom.[35]

Yates opened his campaign in Jacksonville, promising good legislation, good appointments, better parks, and public services. Billy Mason campaigned with Yates in September, confusing the issue by saying the Republican party intended no imperialist course. Lowden warned against free silver, while Yates said prosperity was the best argument for voting Republican. Yates closed out his campaign in November in Cook County, kissing babies and denying the charges of Alschuler that he was a tool of machine politicians. Everywhere Yates went in Cook County he was met by brass bands and occasionally by small boys shouting for Bryan.[36]

Yates, in an effort to meet all kinds of people, spoke at a black church at Dearborn and Thirtieth Street. On the last night of the campaign Yates spoke to South Side working people and endorsed the national Philippine policy and the prosperity brought by sound money. At the Illinois Central car shops a machinist shouted, "We voted for your dad, Dick, and we don't need speeches to make us vote for you." In South Chicago another enthusiast gave Yates a bouquet of yellow chrysanthemums and said to him, "Your father kept Illinois in the Union in '60, Judge, and you will take it back into the Union tomorrow."[37]

At the labor day parade in Chicago, 16,000 men marched before a reviewing platform containing Bryan, Alschuler, and Theodore Roosevelt. The *Tribune* complained that the program was in the hands of the Democrats, although Theodore Roosevelt spoke of the dignity of labor and "the right of the country to expect that every man do his share of work." Alschuler, as the campaign progressed, denounced the trusts and the militarism of the national administration and charged that, if elected, Yates would be controlled by Lorimer. Alschuler could speak German fluently and sometimes quoted Shakespeare in the campaign. Alschuler and Bryan had the support of the major Democratic factions. Carter Harrison denounced the trusts and imperialism as he spoke in their behalf, while John Peter Altgeld denounced the imperialism of the McKinley administration. At least one major newspaper in Chicago, *the Chicago Record,* edited by Victor Lawson, endorsed Alschuler over Yates.[38]

In the national campaign both parties campaigned heavily in Illinois, which was regarded as a key state. The chairman of the Republican National Committee, Marcus Alonzo Hanna, set up his headquarters in Chicago.

Late in the summer of 1900 there was a flurry of concern about anarchist threats. Fears were aroused by the assassination of King Humbert of Italy, an attempt to kill the Shah of Persia, and rumors of plots to assassinate President McKinley. There was a threat of violent action in Chicago. Lucy Parsons, wife of Albert Parsons, who had been hanged for complicity in the Haymarket affair, announced the renaissance of Chicago anarchy and a meeting to voice approval of the assassination of King Humbert. Chicago police moved quickly to abort this meeting, and Lucy Parsons and her friends were carted off in a patrol wagon and charged with disorderly conduct, obstructing the street, and resisting arrest.[39]

The Democrats proclaimed that a "full dinner pail" was insulting to the working man—that he wanted more and was deserving of more. On the other hand, the *Tribune* said:

This is a fair statement of the ambition of every American working man who is worthy to bear the name. It was endorsed by the Republican party the more sincerely because it has made it possible for him to realize them. Before any man can hope to enjoy the luxuries of life, he must first secure the necessaries. Before he can give his children the benefit of education he must first be able to feed them; the first ambition of every man who has settled the question of food, lodging, and clothing. Take away the full dinner pail and the working man finds himself fully employed in securing for his family the bare necessaries of life.[40]

The Republicans charged that Bryan was an exponent of populism and socialism which would destroy the Republican prosperity.[41]

Mary Elizabeth Lease, a former Populist rabble-rouser, was now speaking for the Republicans. She said the antiimperialist policy of Bryan was the same as copperheadism during the Civil War. She said Adlai Stevenson had been a copperhead in 1861 and was indeed still such.[42] The Tribune denounced Bryan's antiimperialist stand, saying, with pious racism, "When clothes are put on a monkey he does not become a human being. When a constitution similar to that of the United States is given some semi-civilized Malays a democratic form of government no more exists than it had existed before."[43]

The campaign was rough in 1900. Theodore Roosevelt came to Illinois for a tour. He attended church on a Sunday morning in October, and after services "a band of half-dozen or more dirty faced, tattered newsboys began to jeer him. The Governor said nothing although he looked volumes, and some men in the crowd drove the boys away. They retreated to the other side of the street where they stood cursing and shouting vulgar insults at Roosevelt." Roosevelt also did not escape the attention of Altgeld, who called him a "tinplate hero."[44]

Bryan came to Illinois, closing his campaign in Chicago. According to the Tribune, men threw eggs on him during his tour of the city. The Chicago Record endorsed Bryan but opposed his stand on free silver. The Tribune, on the other hand, thought free silver and Bryan were the "dead issue and the dead candidate."[45]

When the votes were counted on November 6, 1900, William McKinley had won the state as well as the nation. McKinley beat Bryan in Illinois by a little more than 94,000 votes. Woolley, the Prohibition candidate, got 17,000 cotes. Debs, the Socialist candidate, got 10,000 votes. In the gubernatorial race, Yates won over Alschuler by 62,000 votes. Alschuler carried the city of Chicago by 14,000 but lost in the county towns outside Chicago and lost badly in the downstate area. The Republicans controlled the state legislature by a substantial majority.[46]

The Yates administration was not especially distinguished. There were a few pieces of legislation that were of some importance. The Mueller Act authorizing municipal ownership of street railways was passed. There was also a constitutional amendment permitting some consolidation of offices in Chicago, which brought about increased efficiency. It was in the Yates administration that the first convict labor bill was passed.[47]

In the congressional races the parties split evenly, each holding eleven seats in the House of Representatives in the Fifty-seventh Congress. The Democrats elected congressmen from four of the Chicago districts and seven from the western and southern districts. Among the prominent Republicans elected were Joseph Cannon, James R. Mann of Chicago, Albert J. Hopkins of Aurora, Walter Reeves of Streator, and Vespasian Warner of Clinton. William Lorimer lost his seat to a Democrat.[48]

A major political struggle took place in 1901—the contest for senator. Cullom sought reelection, but for the first time he had a serious contest. Tanner had his heart set on succeeding Cullom. Cullom believed Tanner induced a number of others, including Congressmen Robert R. Hitt, Joseph Cannon, and George Prince, to enter the race. The Republican state convention in Peoria endorsed Cullom for reelection, but as it came time for the legislature to pick the senator, Cullom's opponents continued to line up members of the general assembly in their behalf. Cullom had taken the precaution of getting written pledges from various members of the legislature, however, and when the caucus of the Republicans took place, the senator was able to demonstrate his strength, and in the end his was the only Republican name presented to the committee.[49] In the meantime, however, Tanner had done his best to destroy the good name of Cullom. The *Daily Inter-Ocean* described a speech that Tanner had made in January of 1900 as consisting of "rasping criticism" which was "unmixed with qualifying phrases." Tanner charged that many young people, particularly in Sangamon County, had been voting for Cullom so long that they had grown old working in his behalf and had gotten nothing in return. Tanner said of Cullom: "In his career of 40 years of office holding he has cheated and deceived somewhere along the line, almost every Republican who has befriended him. He is known from one end of the state to the other as a wire puller, a foxy trader, always standing ready to trade off his friends for personal success. He has never been true to any principle. I have never known him to keep faith when it was to his personal and political interest to violate it."[50] Cullom answered this blast with moderation saying only that he regretted that Tanner had made such a speech.[51] As it worked out, Tanner was defeated and Cullom maintained his seat.

Two years later another struggle for the second Illinois senate seat took place. Senator Mason wanted to be reelected in January of 1903, and he opened headquarters at the state fair in 1902, passing out lapel buttons. But his candidacy was doomed because he had been critical of the McKinley administration for its imperialism. It is said that Comptroller Dawes really wanted the post and had McKinley's support, along with that of Senator Cullom and Republican National Committeemen Stewart, Lawrence Y. Sherman, Charles Deneen, and Roy O. West. Before Dawes could be elected, however, McKinley was shot and Theodore Roosevelt came to the presidency. Roosevelt did not like Dawes but was fond of Congressman Albert J. Hopkins. The Dawes support began to crumble as Lorimer and Governor Yates supported Hopkins. The Republican state convention endorsed Hopkins by a two-to-one vote as the general assembly elected him. Born in DeKalb County in 1846, Hopkins began the practice of law after graduating from Hillsdale College in 1870. From 1872 to 1876 Hopkins served as state's attorney of Kane County and in 1885 was elected to the House of Representatives to fill the unexpired term of Reuben Ellwood, serving eighteen years before capping off his career with a term in the Senate.[52]

In the off-year elections in 1902, the Democrats lost ground in the congressional delegation, electing only eight men to twenty-five seats. Lorimer regained a seat, and Cannon won handily in the eighteenth district. Among the notable figures elected to this delegation, Henry T. Rainey, Democrat from Carrollton, appeared for the first time. Rainey served continuously, except for one term, until his death in 1933; he was Speaker when he died.[53]

The Democratic state convention of 1904 met in Springfield on June 14. According to the *Tribune*, seven carloads of Sullivan Democrats and fourteen carloads of followers of William Randolph Hearst came to Springfield. The assembled Democrats paraded on the streets of Springfield under police protection. The Harrison group, which always tried to maintain an air of respectability, paraded in tall hats and long black coats with roses in their lapels. The *Tribune* said sourly, "Springfield feels somewhat like Cheyenne, Wyoming, used to when cowboys came to shoot up the town."

The convention spent much of its time on the question of whom the Illinois delegation should support for the presidency. The

Bryan faction of 1900, led by Millard Dunlap, supported William Randolph Hearst. The Hopkins-Sullivan-Brennan faction of Chicago joined in support of Hearst. Carter Harrison wanted the delegation to support Congressman James R. Williams as a favorite son. The convention was presided over by Frank J. Quinn of Peoria, who used a bung starter as a gavel. The convention approved a resolution offered by Clarence Darrow which committed the Illinois delegation to the Democratic national convention to vote for Hearst. The state convention nominated state Senator Lawrence Beaumont Stringer for governor and reappointed Roger Sullivan as their national committeeman. Senator Stringer, prominent citizen of Logan County, had served on the local bench and was in the state legislature for many years. The son of a minister, Stringer was born in 1866 in New Jersey. He graduated from Lincoln University with a bachelor's degree and after taking a law degree from Lake Forest University was admitted to the bar.[54]

The Democratic state convention in 1904 endorsed a primary election law, better auditing of public accounts, laws curbing corporations, regulation of utilities, a civil service law, suffrage for women, direct election of senators, and home rule for Chicago. They also took a shot at the Republican national administration by demanding rights for Puerto Ricans and Filipinos, saying that the Constitution must follow the flag, and by opposing the trusts and protective tariff.[55]

The Republican state convention of 1904 turned into an exciting endurance contest. Long before the convention met on May 12 in Springfield, men speculated on the name of the candidate for governor. The *Tribune* thought they could see Lorimer's fine hand promoting the interests of Congressman Lowden, the son-in-law of George Pullman. Linking Lowden with Lorimer and Doc Jamieson, the bosses of Cook County, the *Tribune* editorialized on the method of the bosses:

> These county job holders are the rank and file of the machine forces. They hustle on primary days, whether in rain or in shine; they never fail to make their adult male relatives vote; they never fail to persuade many of their intimate friends to vote, truly representing that the control of the primary district is essential to the retention of the job which is bread and butter. They are drilled and organized like an army of mercenaries; they leave nothing undone; they are the judges, clerks, and challengers at the polls; they have the saloon element with them. They are "good fellows" and "mixers." It is their business to make personal friendships, and they have, each of them, many friends.[56]

The *Tribune* published comments by Lincoln Steffens, who

proposed that the election of Charles Deneen would bring Illinois into line with other progressive states: "It is the great fight that is going on in all the cities and in all the states. In the whole country—namely the fight to determine what our parties are going to represent, the selfish brutal interests or just the common interests of us all. The Democrats of Missouri have answered. I am here . . . to tell the other states how the Republicans of Illinois handled it."[57]

The *Tribune*, noting that Deneen was a former Lorimerite while Lowden was still in Lorimer's camp, editorialized: "Lowden's victory will mean more power for Lorimer and Jamieson, more power for Lorimer and Jamieson means more exploitation of this community—more gas frontage and gas consolidation bills, more Allen bills, no civil service, no primary reform, more fat plastering contracts from state institutions, more fat coal contracts from county institutions, more fat dredging contracts from the drainage board, more Hanecys, more Bradens, more Nohes, Glades. . . . In short, even more flagrant corruption than heretofore." The *Tribune* was hard on Lowden in cartoons. For example, one McCutcheon cartoon portrayed "Bill Sikes" Lorimer boosting "Oliver Twist" Lowden into the window of the governor's office with the caption, "You slip in and open the back door for us." There was always a weeping Pullman porter in the back of cartoons depicting Lowden, pointing up his connection with the Pullman family.[58]

The convention elected as chairman Congressman Joe Cannon, whose gavel arm was badly swollen as the convention became deadlocked. Governor Yates had the most votes but far from a majority. He was trailed by Lowden, Deneen, Howland J. Hamlin, Sherman, and Vespasian Warner. After twelve hours the Republicans had cast fifteen ballots and there was no appreciable change in the lineup, although a new candidate, John Pierce, entered the picture. The Republicans continued wearily on, ballot after ballot, still desperately deadlocked, until on May 20 they recessed for ten days. By this time they had taken fifty-eight ballots and still no one had moved toward a majority. The *Tribune* editorialized that the deadlock in the state convention meant that the voters were taking over the process of nomination and proved that the bosses and the Washington crowd could no longer have their way with the nominating process. The *Tribune* believed the deadlock indicated clearly the need for a primary law.[59]

The convention reconvened on May 30 and took several more

ballots. It was not until June 3, on the seventy-ninth ballot, that Charles Deneen drew 957½ of the 1,205 votes present as Governor Yates withdrew from the race, throwing his support to Deneen. Lawrence Y. Sherman was nominated for lieutenant governor, and the 1904 convention marked the debut of Len Small of Kankakee in statewide politics. Small was a nurseryman and farmer in Kankakee County. Governor Tanner had appointed him a member of the board of trustees of the Kankakee State Hospital.[60]

Deneen was born in Edwardsville on May 4, 1863, the son of a professor of Latin and history at McKendree College. Deneen's father had served in the Civil War and the foreign service. Deneen grew up in an intellectual atmosphere and received a bachelor's degree from McKendree College in 1882. He attended the Union College of Law in Chicago after teaching in Newton and Godfrey. As a young lawyer in Chicago he taught evening classes to make ends meet. He entered the practice of law in Chicago in 1887. Making his way through ward politics, he was elected to the general assembly in 1892. In 1896 the voters elected him state's attorney for Cook County. Like many progressive leaders, he made his name in politics with that office. He was reelected state's attorney in 1900, and he remained active in Illinois politics for many years. By the time he was nominated for the governorship, Deneen had broken his relationship with Lorimer.[61]

Deneen, however, drew other supporters including his close friend and political manager, Roy O. West. West, born in Georgetown in 1868, graduated from DePauw University. West managed Deneen's campaign in 1904 and was elected chairman of the Republican State Committee at that time. Harold Ickes, who supported Deneen in 1904, said that Roy West "played a clever hand. He was noted for his 'affidavit face,' and he knew not only most of the devious tricks of the game but also the language of the political reformer. He could himself pose as a reformer when the state setting called for it."[62] Ickes also gave a good picture of Deneen: "Deneen gave a satisfactory account of himself during his years in office, even from the point of view of an impatient progressive like myself. I never was an enthusiastic Deneen man. I regarded him as too cold and cautious. He was altogether too conservative to suit me. He rarely took a step forward unless someone pushed him and then he took a quarter step. Not withstanding, he was a creditable public official and, according to his lights and within his limitations, rendered public service of a high order excepting only as to his grabbing fees during his eight years as states attorney—in total a tidy sum that had put him on his feet financially.""[63]

The Republican platform of 1904 asked for a compulsory primary election law and a new charter for Chicago. In praise of the Yates administration, the party commended the enactment of a convict labor law passed during his administration. They instructed their delegates to the Republican national convention to vote for Congressman Robert Hitt for vice-president.[64]

The Democratic national convention of 1904 convened in St. Louis, and Illinois sent its usual colorful delegates. Among them were Clarence Darrow and Samuel Alschuler on the one hand and Roger Sullivan and John Hopkins on the other. The Illinois delegates were instructed to vote for Hearst, although the Harrison faction joined with Millard Dunlap in an abortive attempt to block the seating of the Sullivan-Hopkins delegates. Bathhouse John Coughlin and Hinky Dink Kenna were among the delegates plugging for Carter Harrison, their hero and holder of Chicago patronage, as candidate for president. The Illinois delegation, under the unit rule, voted their 54 votes for Hearst. It was in vain, however, because Alton B. Parker of New York was nominated on the first ballot with some 655 votes to Hearst's 200.[65]

Elihu Root of New York presided as temporary chairman over the Republican convention of 1904 in Chicago, and Congressman Joseph Cannon took the gavel as permanent chairman. Most leading Republicans of the state were in the delegation, among them Lowden, Lorimer, Graham Stewart, Walter Reeves, Vespasian Warner, William E. Mason, Howland J. Hamlin, and Yates. Among the delegates were assorted industrialists such as Isaac Elwood of barbwire fame and Charles H. Deere of the farm machinery family, as well as professional men such as Fenton W. Booth of Marshall, attorney and judge. Cannon removed himself from the vice-presidency race early, so some of the Illinois factions supported Robert Hitt for the vice-presidency as instructed by the state convention. The race for the presidency was cut-and-dried, with the nomination of Theodore Roosevelt a certainty. The Illinois efforts to get one of their men into the vice-presidency failed as Roosevelt chose Fairbanks for the second place on the ballot.[66]

The Cook County Democratic Committee held a harmony meeting early in August to pull together its factions. There were pleas for unity by Roger Sullivan and State Chairman Charles Boeschenstein. Stringer started his campaign on September 1, setting out on the trail of his opponent, promising a lively campaign. Stringer based his campaign on charges of corruption leveled against the Republicans. He spoke about the spoils system and said that conditions in the state institutions were "unspeakably bad." He pledged himself to a "business administration" if elected. The Democrats opened their Chicago and Cook County campaign with a picnic on September 25. They planned a barbecue and beauty contest with athletic events, coupled with the political speeches. Elizabeth Stretch won the beauty contest over some fifty contestants, receiving a diamond-studded watch. Otherwise the rally failed to come off well. There was no food for the barbecue and there was a downpour. Stringer attacked the management of state charitable institutions, as well as the protective tariff.[67]

Throughout the campaign Stringer attacked the Yates administration, particularly corruption in the charitable institutions. He pledged himself to a merit system not only for the prisons but for every board and commission under the governor. Speaking in Oak Park, Stringer described his position as follows: "Whether I am elected or not, I will have the satisfaction of knowing that I have gone up and down the state telling the people of the wretched conditions which exist in the state service. Fifteen years ago Kankakee was the greatest insane asylum in the world. Now it is headquarters for political clubs. Governor Yates' methods of securing volunteer contributions to his campaign fund from state employees is highway robbery."[69] Stringer also devoted himself to the need for a new charter for Chicago. He charged that Deneen avoided the state issues and talked only about the national ones. Stringer also said that Deneen would have to follow the pattern of Yates because he would be a prisoner of his party, therefore he would lack the capability of passing a civil service law. The Stringer campaign did not catch on. There was noticeable scarcity of news about him in the metropolitan papers, and the *Tribune* said that in a poll they took on October 21, only 6 of 174 voters could identify Lawrence B. Stringer.[69]

Charles Deneen campaigned vigorously, speaking in each of the 102 counties in Illinois. He opened his campaign in the far south at Metropolis and Golconda, speaking to people who came to his meetings by rowboat and wagon. Meeting enthusiastic local politicians, he spoke of the need for a primary law in the state and against the imperialism of the Republican party, saying that the United States had conferred freedoms of speech, press, and religion on the lesser people and that these had been taken away.

In the meantime, Chairman Roy O. West charged that the Democrats were hoping to steal the state as Deneen, Sherman, and Yates met in Jacksonville and issued mutual compliments in a show of unity for the campaign. As he shifted his campaign to the north, Deneen made a plea for home rule for Cook County. The *Tribune* editorialized that Deneen was the equivalent of reformers Joseph W. Folk of Missouri or Robert La Follette of Wisconsin. The *Record Herald* editorially endorsed Deneen, saying his record as state's attorney had been a good one. The *Record Herald* took the position that leniency for criminals increased crime and that Deneen's good record was pointed up by the increased number of hangings at the Cook County Jail that year.[70]

In October the Hamilton Club chartered a special train to go to the World's Fair in St. Louis. From the train Sherman and Lowden addressed crowds along the way. In opening his Chicago campaign, Deneen spoke in favor of a new charter for Chicago, a civil service law, and a primary law. At the same time, he asked the voters to support Lorimer. By the end of the campaign Deneen's voice was worn out. He delivered seventy-six speeches in sixteen days at the end of his campaign.[71]

The national campaign in Illinois was of less interest in 1904. It was taken for granted that Roosevelt would carry Illinois, and Alton B. Parker did not come to the state to campaign. The most spectacular speaker for the Democratic national ticket was South Carolina Senator Benjamin F. Tillman, who came to speak in the stockyards area, expounding various Populist doctrines, including racist attacks on Blacks. Tillman said equality was for Whites, not Blacks. Democratic National Chairman Thomas Taggart also visited Chicago. The party held a reception for him in the Sherman House and a luncheon at the Iroquois Club. He was greeted by Sullivan, Boeschenstein, and Mayor Harrison. Many downstate Democrats, including Millard Dunlap and Frank Quinn, attended the rally. On two occasions during the campaign Parker summoned Mayor Harrison to New York for a conference. Apparently there were some efforts to get Parker to come to the state but he did not see fit to do so.[72]

The Socialists held a rally at the auditorium, where candidate Eugene Debs spoke to a crowd of some 4,000. Debs told the audience, "When Grover Cleveland sent troops to Illinois to violate the constitution and handcuffed John P. Altgeld, he had no more enthusiastic admirer than Theodore Roosevelt." There were hisses for Cleveland and cheers for Altgeld as Debs spoke.[73]

When the votes were tallied in the election of 1904, Theodore Roosevelt carried the state by nearly a two-to-one margin over Parker. Deneen carried the state by nearly the same margin over Stringer. The Cook County results were similar to the statewide election results. Debs got 70,000 votes, and Silas Swallow, the Prohibition candidate, got 35,000 votes.[74]

In the congressional election of 1904, the Republicans almost made a clean sweep of the delegation. Henry T. Rainey was the only Democrat elected. Lorimer and Cannon were returned to their seats, and Lowden was later elected to fill the seat of Robert R. Hitt of Mt. Morris, who died in office.[75]

In the off-year congressional elections of 1906, the Democrats regained some of their lost seats. They took two seats in Chicago, electing Adolph Sabath, from the Bohemian faction, for the first time. Downstate they got three seats, including the reelection of Rainey. Still, it was a poor showing since Republicans held twenty of the twenty-five seats.[76]

In 1907 the general assembly elected Senator Cullom for a fifth term. By this time the general assembly had enacted a preferential primary law to guide them on the election of U. S. senators. Former Governor Yates contended in the primary against Cullom, but the latter won by a considerable margin. When the legislature met in January of 1907, Cullom was the unanimous choice of the Republicans in the legislature.[77]

In 1908 Illinois held its first primary election for a full state ticket. In the Republican primary Deneen contested with Yates for the Republican nomination. It was thought by some that the Yates candidacy had the blessing of Lorimer and Doc Jamieson and note was taken that in a Yates rally in the Coliseum in June, Lorimer chaired the meeting. Yates denied the charge that the Illinois Central Railroad was financing his campaign. The *Tribune* saw the race as a choice between bossism, represented by Yates, Lorimer, and Jamieson, and clean government, represented by Deneen.[78]

Seven candidates sought the Democratic nomination for governor, possibly because many believed the split in the Republican party would make a Democratic victory in November possible. When the votes were counted after the primary, Governor Deneen had beaten Yates by only about 12,000 votes out of more than 400,000 cast. In the Democratic primary, Adlai Stevenson of Bloomington had a plurality of the Democratic vote; J. Hamilton Lewis ran a poor second. Stevenson had 80,000 votes while Lewis had slightly more than 30,000. Other candidates had a scattering of votes. The Republican primary endorsed Albert J. Hopkins for reelection as U. S. senator.[79]

The Democratic nominee for governor, Adlai Ewing Stevenson, was a familiar figure in Illinois politics. Now near the end of a long political life, Stevenson was seeking his first state office. He had held a number of national political offices—congressman, first assistant postmaster general during the first Cleveland administration, and vice-president during the second Cleveland administration. Regarded as an advocate of free silver, Stevenson won the vice-presidential nomination with Bryan in 1900. At the time of his nomination for governor, Adlai Stevenson was seventy-two years of age. It is said that his family tried to dissuade him from accepting the nomination on the grounds of his age. Stevenson's family was influential in Illinois affairs; his wife, Letitia Green, had helped found and served as first president-general of the Daughters of the American Revolution.[80]

Because of the use of the primary for nominating candidates, the state party conventions were reduced to drawing up a platform. The Democratic state convention came out against imperialism and Republicanism, denouncing the mismanagement of state and national affairs by the Republicans. They proclaimed that Adlai E. Stevenson was "a platform in himself." They portrayed Stevenson as a great patriot, a man of character, ability, and executive leadership. The Republican state convention commended the administration of Governor Deneen and pointed with pride to the record of progressive legislation and good administration. They endorsed Speaker Cannon for the presidency and spoke approvingly of the protective tariff, sound money, and the greatness of Theodore Roosevelt.[81]

The Democratic national convention in 1908 excited Illinois Democrats, particularly those from Chicago. The convention was held in Denver in July. The Chicago Democrats went to Denver by special train which had in the baggage car 800 quarts of champagne, 50 quarts of whiskey, 20 quarts of gin, and 8 crates of lemons. The Democrats, led by Hinky Dink Kenna and Johnny Powers, marched to the train with a forty piece band, all in top hats and swallowtail coats. Roger Sullivan chose to go by automobile caravan to Denver, taking along four Studebakers and a truck. Each of the cars seated seven. They planned to make between 125 and 150 miles per day. This move, according to the *Tribune*, was "establishing a new precedent in convention travel." Because of storms and muddy roads it took twelve days to make the trip. Upon checking in at Denver, most of the Chicago delegation went out to Colorado Springs, where Bathhouse John Coughlin had a summer home which he had purchased in 1902. The "Bath" had his place stocked with flowers and animals, including a slightly damaged elephant named Princess Alice, which the Bath had filched from the Lincoln Park Zoo. They were treated to a barbecue on the Bath's estate, complete with a carnival, and with champagne and beer to drink.[82] Bathhouse was very pleased to have his friends at Colorado Springs. According to the *Tribune*, Coughlin proclaimed, "Colorado is the most important geographical division of the known world outside of the first ward of Chicago. It is a section of great diversities like the first ward and a great range of climate and temperatures, also like the first ward. While there is nothing to compare with the variety of climate experience between the torrid regions of the 22nd Street and the rarified heights that occupy the Municipal Voters League, still Colorado has some high altitudes that are picturesque in their own crude way."[83]

After a fight in the delegation, Sullivan was reelected national committeeman over the protests of Millard Dunlap. Mayor Edward F. Dunne of Chicago was proposed for the post but beaten. Early at the convention several Illinoisians were mentioned as vice-presidential possibilities, among them Dunne, Judge E. R. Kimbrow, J. Hamilton Lewis, John Mitchell, Henry T. Rainey, Sullivan, and Stevenson. The convention nominated Bryan again. To run with him they chose John Kern of Indiana.[84]

The Republican national convention was held in Chicago in 1908. William Howard Taft was nominated on the first ballot by an overwhelming majority. The Illinois Republican delegation gave three votes to Taft and fifty-one to Congressman Joseph Cannon. Only a favorite son candidate, Cannon pledged his support to Taft and the *Tribune* editorialized in this way: "The Republican National Convention responsive to the will of the Republican party and to the best opinion of the country has selected as its candidate for the presidency the man best qualified, best equipped for the office. It has selected a man of action whose previous official experience and tried character qualify to enter upon the duties of the presidency as few if any of his predecessors are qualified." The *Tribune* predicted a large majority in Illinois for Taft.[85]

Illinois had a special interest in some of the minor parties in 1908. The Prohibition convention, for example, was held in Springfield. In their platform the Prohibitionists appealed for a Sunday closing law, economy in government, and the establishment of a postal savings bank. On the state level, they favored the initiative and referendum, abolition of the fee system for local officials, prevention of child labor, public ownership of public utilities, and woman suffrage. They nominated Eugene W. Chafin for president and Daniel R. Sheen for governor of Illinois.[86]

The Socialist convention of 1908 was held in Chicago in Brand's Hall, which was decorated with red flags although police prohibited the comrades from carrying red flags in a parade. G. T. Fraenckel of Chicago welcomed the delegates to the convention, saying "While the Socialists could not officially offer their freedom of the city, they already had the freedom of the jail." Millionaire Socialist J. Phelps Stokes and his wife, Rose Pastor Stokes, entertained on the eve of the convention. The *Tribune* sarcastically described the party:

> The feast was spread on long tables and crudely decorated but home-like room, wainscoted in red and with red and white decorations and pictures of Tolstoy, Karl Marx, and a few socialists of the common ordinary brand on the walls.
>
> There was plenty of plain food such as cream of tomatoes, roast veal with Spanish sauce, roast lamb, potato salad on lettuce, and comrade Stokes who would not attract any attention in a crowd, got away with it as if he relished everything. Nearly one half of those present were girl socialists—pretty girls at that, who look mighty scrumptious in their white shirtwaists and M. W. hats with big bunches of flowers on them. The comradesses who belong to the league make it popular with the comrades.

At the convention the Socialists nominated Eugene Debs for his fourth try at the presidency.[87]

In the state campaign of 1908 Republicans charged Adlai Stevenson with being a copperhead during the Civil War. They turned up a preacher from Metamora who said that Stevenson had been a leader of the Knights of the Golden Circle and that he spent only thirteen days in the Union Army between the time he was drafted and the time it took to hire a substitute. Republicans charged that if Stevenson were elected, Roger Sullivan would be the governor. The Republicans exploited antilabor stories about Stevenson. It was charged that he owned a coal mine near Bloomington in which he exploited his workers. They also brought up his reputation as a spoilsman while assistant postmaster general. There were charges that he exploited a building and loan association of which he had been a director, taking more from the company than his services were worth.[88]

The antilabor charges against Stevenson hurt him with working people. William Scaife, editor of the *United Mine Workers Journal,* reported that Stevenson had resisted unionization and that miners were threatened with arrest for even speaking of a union. The Illinois Federation of Labor endorsed Deneen. The Republicans carried the attack further by saying that Stevenson was sponsored by Francis Peabody, coal operator. In contrast they listed the impressive labor legislation under Deneen on the subjects of convict labor, mine safety, and protection of workers. The Republicans also used Roger Sullivan against Stevenson and Bryan. They argued that a vote for Stevenson was really a vote for Sullivan and that Stevenson favored big business interests, was against the primary law, and would put the institutions back in politics.[89]

On the other hand, the Democrats charged that Deneen had taken illegal or excessive fees while state's attorney by increasing certain kinds of indictment fees. They also charged that Deneen had abused the civil service law and permitted corruption in state institutions. The Democrats turned up a man named Ben Giroux who said that his son had died as a result of bad conditions at the Lincoln asylum. Stevenson pointed out that even though Deneen had made political hay of the primary laws, the Supreme Court declared unconstitutional both of the primary laws which he had signed. The Democrats charged that Deneen had not acted promptly and decisively in the race riot in Springfield during the summer of 1908.[90] However, black voters in the area of Thirty-eight and Dearborn endorsed Deneen's action in that riot. The Republicans came up with rumors that Lorimer and Sullivan were working on a deal to trade Bryan votes for Stevenson votes to defeat Deneen. Rabbi Emil Hirsch endorsed Deneen, telling his congregation that it was their "God-given duty" to vote for him. John Walker of the United Mine Workers also endorsed Deneen, saying Stevenson was a coal operator and no friend to labor. The Chicago Federation of Labor endorsed Stevenson.[91]

In the national campaign, Taft did not come to Illinois to campaign. Governor Charles Evans Hughes of New York spoke at the Coliseum under the auspices of the Hamilton Club in October. The Republicans staged an old-fashioned rally with red fire, marching clubs, torches, and bands. Taft received financial support from the wealthy of Chicago; Samuel Insull, John Shedd, and Norman B. Ream contributed heavily to the campaign. The Fat-Man's Taft Club was organized at the stockyards. Taft was said to weigh 297½ pounds but the average weight of the Fat-Man's

Taft Club was only 250 pounds. Blacks organized the Frederick Douglass Republican League to aid the Taft candidacy. W. N. Farmer of Chicago served as president of the organization and John G. Jones as secretary. Chairman of the executive committee was H. R. Parker. The black community of Chicago was not especially impressed with Taft and had become disenchanted with Theodore Roosevelt because of his dishonorable discharge of a black regiment in the Brownsville incident, so there was a threat that the Blacks would bolt the Taft ticket in 1908.[92]

Bryan came to Chicago and motored about the city, as the *Record Herald* put it, with Roger Sullivan, his "old time enemy and new time friend." Bryan spoke in Evanston and several places in Chicago, including the Pilsen Gardens in the midst of the Bohemian section, with Sullivan, Cermak, Sabath, and Dunne on the platform. Taft carried the state, although by a much smaller margin than Roosevelt had four years earlier. Taft had 630,000 votes while Bryan had 450,000.[93]

In a close state race, Governor Deneen won by a margin of 25,000 votes. Deneen had slightly more than 550,000 votes, while Stevenson had 527,000. Hinky Dink and Bathhouse John carried the first ward of Chicago for the Democrats. In their ward Bryan got 285 votes to 39 for Taft. The *Tribune* reported that Kenna and Coughlin were "up in the air" over one distressing aspect of the election. There had been eight Prohibitionist votes cast in the ninth precinct of the first ward, and Kenna and Coughlin, both saloonkeepers, were disturbed over how the enemy had infiltrated even to this small extent. The *Tribune* theorized that Deneen's poor showing in 1908 was due to the enmity of Lorimer, Yates, and Len Small but said that the enmity of such men was an honor to Deneen.[94]

In the congressional election of 1908, Republicans carried all but six of the twenty-five seats. The Democrats elected three in Chicago and three downstate, including Sabath and Rainey. Among the prominent Republicans elected were Speaker Cannon, Lowden, Fred Lundin, and utilities magnate William B. McKinley of Champaign.[95]

Shortly after Deneen's second inauguration, the time had come for the legislature to elect a U. S. senator. The Republicans had a majority in the general assembly. The Republican state convention endorsed Senator Albert J. Hopkins for reelection, and he had won the preferential primary. Starting on January 19, 1909, the legislature, in one of the most scandalous episodes in Illinois politics, balloted for 126 days and took ninty-five votes before they were able to elect a candidate. Several Republican candidates, including Senator Hopkins, former senator Mason, Congressman George Faust, and William G. Webster, sought the post. The Democrats also had candidates—Lawrence Stringer and Adison Blakely. Mason had been trying to reclaim his seat for some time but it was believed that Hopkins had the organization and would be the winner. As the deadlock continued, a new figure entered the scene in the person of Congressman Lorimer. On the ninety-fifth ballot, Lorimer was elected, receiving 108 votes, 55 from the Republicans and 53 from the Democrats.[96]

The outcome was a matter of public surprise. Governor Dunne explained it by the fact that, to the Democrats, Lorimer was "less offensively Republican" than the other candidates.[97] From the beginning there was talk of bribery, and on April 30, 1910, the *Chicago Tribune* published what was reported to be a confession of Charles A. White, a Democrat from the Forty-ninth district, that he had received $1,000 from Lee O'Neil Browne to vote for Lorimer. Subsequently several legislators made similar confessions. Lee O'Neil Browne was indicted by a Cook County grand jury but was acquitted. The charges and countercharges that arose caused shakeup in the Republican ranks in Illinois. In 1910 Theodore Roosevelt, already running for president in 1912, was speaking in Freeport and had been invited to have dinner at the Hamilton Club. He sent word that he would not come if William Lorimer was to be present. The Hamilton Club retracted Lorimer's invitation and Theodore Roosevelt ate with them.[98]

Subsequently a U. S. Senate investigating committee heard evidence in Chicago in October, 1910. The committee, chaired by Senator Julius C. Burrows, acquitted Lorimer on the grounds that he had a fourteen-vote majority and they could not prove that as many as fourteen people had been bribed. Senator Albert J. Beveridge of Indiana submitted a minority report that Lorimer had not been elected legally. Senator Lorimer made a moving speech in the Senate which brought several of his colleagues to tears. The Senate voted by forty-six to forty to let Lorimer keep his seat. His fellow Illinoisian, Shelby Cullon, voted with Lorimer.[99]

The issue did not die. Early in 1911 an Illinois Senate investigating committee found new evidence. Later the same year C. S. Funk testified that the International Harvester Company had been asked to contribute $10,000 toward a fund of $100,000 to elect Lorimer. The Illinois Senate committee, chaired by Senator

Douglas W. Helm, reported that Lorimer had been elected by corrupt methods. The Illinois Senate concurred by a vote of thirty to ten. Shortly after this, Senator Robert La Follette entered a motion in the U. S. Senate to reopen the Lorimer case. The Senate appointed a new committee, under the chairmanship of Senator William P. Dillingham, which recommended by a vote of five to three that Lorimer was entitled to his seat. At this point Senator John W. Kern of Indiana opened a floor fight to expel Lorimer. On July 13, 1911 the Senate voted by fifty-five to twenty-eight the following resolution: "Resolved, that corrupt methods and practices were employed in the election of William Lorimer to the Senate of the United States from the State of Illinois, and that his election, therefore, was invalid." This time Senator Cullom voted to expel Lorimer. Thus, Illinois was left with only one U.S. senator and a tarnished reputation in the political world. The Lorimer scandal added impetus to the movement for direct election of senators and caused Illinois to ratify the Seventeenth Amendment to the Constitution.[100]

In spite of charges made against it, the Deneen administration built an impressive record for itself in legislation, including many laws aimed at greater safety and protection for the laboring man. The first sentence in Deneen's first inaugural address reads, "Our state needs a compulsary primary election law." Almost immediately thereafter, a primary law passed the general assembly. The following year the law was declared unconstitutional by the Illinois Supreme Court on the grounds of illegal delegation of legislative authority. The court also argued that the law required a fee for filing in the primary which was a discrimination against the poor and that it also revised illegally the qualifications for state legislators.[101]

Five days later, on April 10, 1906, Governor Deneen called a special session of the general assembly for the purpose of passing another primary law. A new law was approved on May 23. The following year the law was declared unconstitutional by the Illinois Supreme Court by a seven-to-one vote on the grounds that it vested too much power in the hands of the county central committees to create delegate districts and was an illegal delegation of legislative power. On October 8, 1907, Deneen called another special session to study the primary law issue. On February 21, 1908, a third primary law was passed, and on June 16, 1909, the Supreme Court again declared it unconstitutional. Not until December 11, 1901, in still another special session of the general assembly, was a primary law passed which stood the test of the courts and continued in operation.[102] Primary election laws constituted one of the prime issues of the progressive era. Supporters hoped that taking the nominating process out of the state conventions would give the people a larger voice in the choice of candidates and thereby in their government. Although the primary democratized the nomination process, the bosses found ways to control the primaries.

The progressives also demanded a civil service law. The general assembly passed such a law in Illinois during the Deneen administration, placing some 4,700 out of 5,500 state employees under the protection of civil service. The law, passed in 1905, provided for a civil service commission of three members. The employees of state charitable institutions fell under its rules, and the law also mandated examinations as evidence of fitness for holding office. The statute made employees immune from political assessments and provided penalties for violation of their rights. In 1911 the act was extended to certain county positions and to the state parks and park districts.[103]

In the off-year elections of 1910, the Democrats improved their situation in the Congress, electing eleven of the twenty-five members of the House of Representatives. Among the familiar Republican names in the Sixty-second Congress were Mann, Cannon, and McKinley. Cannon lost his Speakership through the efforts of a coalition of Democrats and reform Republicans.[104]

The administration of state charitable institutions generated one of the greatest controversies in the early years of the twentieth century. In 1912, in a special session, the general assembly created a board of administration for these institutions. This board, appointed by the governor, held broad powers to inspect and administer the institutions. Supporters hoped this would keep them out of politics, providing better service for those committed to these institutions.[105]

By 1912 the primary election was well established in Illinois. Governor Deneen, announcing his candidacy for a third term, faced six opponents, including State Treasurer Small and former Governor Yates. After a bitter primary fight, Deneen won the nomination with a plurality of nearly 65,000 votes. In the presidential preferential primary, former President Roosevelt outpointed Taft and Senator La Follette by a clear majority.[106]

Edward F. Dunne announced early that he would be a candidate for the Democratic nomination for governor. Dunne was candid about his decision to make the race, believing several things boded well for the Democrats in 1912, although they had not elected a governor since Altgeld. Dunne thought the bad reputation the Republican legislature had gained for itself in the Lorimer affair would help the Democratic chances. In addition he counted on a split in the Republican party at the national level because of the deep-seated feud between Taft and Roosevelt. He also took into account the fact that Adlai Stevenson had given Governor Deneen a close race in 1908 and therefore chose as his slogan "jack-pottism," which had become the synonym for the sale of public office. As his opponent Dunne had Samuel Alschuler, the candidate in 1900 and a man of impeccable reputation. Ben F. Caldwell, the Democratic congressman from Sangamon County, was also a candidate. When the Democratic primary was over, Dunne had received 131,212 votes, Alschuler had 87,127, and Caldwell 71,972. In the Democratic presidential preferential primary, Champ Clark of Missouri carried the state over Governor Woodrow Wilson of New Jersey by a three-to-one majority.[107]

In their platform the Democrats condemned the extravagance of the Deneen administration and denounced jack-pottism, which they described as "a unique and newly coined disgrace of the splendid commonwealth of Illinois." They protested excessive taxation and demanded popular election of senators and a shorter ballot. They pledged the Democratic party to the enactment of legislation for building good roads. Republicans in their platform endorsed the administration of President William Howard Taft but spoke with affection of Theodore Roosevelt and expressed the preference of the convention for Roosevelt as the party's nominee for president. They pointed with pride to achievements of the previous four years, particularly passage of the civil service law and the primary law. They lauded the competent and honest administration of the charitable institutions and generally praised Deneen.[108]

The Republican national convention met in Chicago on June 18, 1912, and fifty-six on the fifty-eight Illinois delegates were instructed for Roosevelt on the basis of the preferential primary. Roosevelt did everything he could to hold the delegation and invited them to be his guests at Oyster Bay. When the convention met in the Coliseum, his difficulties began. President Taft controlled the machinery of the convention and most of the pro-Taft delegation were seated. The convention renominated Taft and Sherman, to the chagrin of Roosevelt and his followers.[109]

Delegates from twenty-two states held a meeting in Orchestra

Hall and decided to form a new party with Roosevelt as its leader. Roosevelt was present at this meeting and accepted the leadership in the new party. A call was put forth for a Progressive party convention to be held in Chicago on August 5, 1912. A number of prominent figures from Illinois were in this movement. Among these were Chauncey Dewey, Laverne W. Noyes, Harold Ickes, and Medill McCormick. The colorful Ickes, a lawyer, had entered municipal politics in Chicago and managed the unsuccessful mayoral campaigns of John M. Harlan in 1905 and Charles E. Merriam in 1911. He was an enthusiastic supporter of Theodore Roosevelt. The acid-tongued Ickes looked with contempt on Robert R. McCormick ("billious Bertie, the bingy bully") and his brother Medill. Both were actively connected with the *Tribune* and Ickes said they used to alternate month by month as editor so that "as to policy the paper was consistently inconsistent. One could always tell by reading it which genius was steering." The McCormicks split on the issue of Republican politics at this time. Robert R. McCormick stayed with the regular Republican nominee, Taft, while Medill joined the Progressive party and Roosevelt.[110]

Theodore Roosevelt proclaimed, "We are at our Armageddon and the battle is the lord's." The convention of the Progressive party, otherwise known as the Bull Moose party, nominated Theodore Roosevelt for president and Senator Hiram W. Johnson of California for vice-president. In the Progressive state convention, held in Champaign, Robert Merriam and Harold Ickes succeeded in getting the convention to nominate Frank Funk for governor. This was done over Medill McCormick's objection because he hoped to see Deneen reelected for a third term. Ickes and Merriam wanted to do as much damage as possible to Deneen because they blamed him for Merriam's loss in Chicago in 1911. It was with pleasure that Ickes watched Dunne beat Deneen. Ickes said it was "a victory that did my curmudgeonly soul no end of good."[111]

In the Democratic national convention of 1912 there was the usual fight within the Illinois delegation. Harrison, who had returned to Illinois after several years in California, was still opposed to anything Sullivan did. He therefore supported Champ Clark, Speaker of the House of Representatives, for president. Harrison did not like Woodrow Wilson, holding that his experience as a professor hardly qualified him for the presidency. Sullivan was more flexible, however, and just as it appeared that the convention was deadlocked, he shifted most of the Illinois delegation to Wilson, which gave Wilson the nomination over Clark. Sullivan's action represented something of a surprise to Illinois politicians because Bryan had earlier switched from Clark to Wilson, and Sullivan and Bryan had never been friendly. Harrison said bitterly that Sullivan worked in this campaign with his "inevitable working partners, the combination of Tammany, Norman Mack, the Pennsylvania grafters, the Western crew of big shot mercenaries, with the rag tag and bob tail, completely unsavory cabal hailing from Kentucky, Iowa, Minnesota, and all down the line." Harrison's influence had declined in his absence from the state. His candidate for governor, Alschuler, had been beaten by Dunne in the primary, and he was unable to hold the Illinois delegation for Clark.[112]

In the state campaign in 1912 most of the struggle came between Deneen and Funk. Dunne carried on a vigorous campaign but to be elected had to count on Funk taking votes from the normal Republican majority. Bryan came to Illinois and campaigned with Dunne, starting at his birthplace in Salem and visiting Mr. Vernon, McLeansboro, Carmi, Benton, and East St. Louis. The Democrats hit hard at the Republicans for Lorimerism and jack-pottism. They mailed out copies of Lorimer's speech in the Senate in which he implied that Governor Deneen had been involved in his corrupt election. Governor Dunne, making his campaign by automobile, visited most of the principal cities, remarking later that the campaign pointed up the abominable conditions of the roads and convinced him of the necessity for improved highway legislation. The Democratic party was free of partisan strife, and Dunne had the support of his primary opponents.[113]

Funk toured the state, also accusing Deneen of complicity in the Lorimer scandal, of an alliance with Roger Sullivan, and of making bad appointments and continuing some of Yates's worst appointments in office. Funk also charged Deneen with an alliance with Samuel Insull. Roosevelt came out strongly for Funk, sending a telegram to Medill McCormick saying, "Beat Deneen." As is often the case with reform movements, many celebrities were attracted to the Bull Moose campaign. Lillian Russell was in Chicago to sell "moose certificates" to raise money. There was a gala of artists and authors at the Lyric Theater with Edna Ferber selling tickets at the La Salle Hotel. A delegation of twenty-five original Rough Riders came to Chicago to support the campaign. An innovation of the 1912 campaign was the use of extensive newspaper advertising. The Progressives took full-page advertisements in metropolitan papers. A statement by Roosevelt declared, "There is no state in the union where it is more important than in Illinois that the progressive candidates for governor and state officers and for the legislature should be elected. The election of Frank Funk as governor will put an end to Lorimerism and 'jack-pottism' in Illinois." Roosevelt said Deneen's association with Lorimer made him "unfit to occupy a position of trust in the government." He reported that he felt "a very hearty contempt" for Deneen. On the eve of the election, to underscore their charges of corruption against the Republican party, the progressives hired a detective agency to watch for vote frauds. The action was taken by Medill McCormick at Roosevelt's suggestion.[114]

Governor Deneen lamented that men who claimed to be progressive ignored the progressive legislation of his administration. He said his administration had been on a business basis with not a single dollar misspent. The *Record Herald*, supporting Deneen, commented that a vote for Funk was a vote for Dunne. In another editorial they said that Deneen had had a clean administration and that his performance was "better than a team load of promises." The *Tribune* endorsed Deneen. Robert R. McCormick was chairman of a committee of 100 who called upon the voters to elect Deneen. Deneen closed his campaign pointing with pride to his record on labor, health, and safety. One of the issues of the campaign was the question of suffrage for women and this became closely identified with the social life of Chicago. Madame Schumann-Heink gave a concert at Orchestra Hall for the Illinois Equal Suffrage Society. Involved in this organization were socialites like Mrs. Edward Morris, Mrs. Julius Rosenwald, Mrs. Emmons Blaine, Mrs. Medill McCormick, Mrs. Cyrus McCormick, and Mrs. H. C. Chatfield-Taylor.[115]

In the presidential campaign of 1912, observers regarded Illinois as a critical state. The election turned on the questions of whether Wilson could hold Bryan's support of four years earlier and whether Roosevelt would take enough votes from Taft to elect Wilson. William E. Mason spoke on the prosperity theme, saying the election of Taft meant a continuation of Republican prosperity. He attacked the progressive platform, especially for recall of judges. As the polls began to show that Wilson would win and might even carry Illinois, the *Tribune* endorsed Roosevelt; the *Record Herald* made no endorsement but spoke approvingly of Wilson. The *Record Herald* said, "We can not have too many scholars and intellectuals in politics, provided they are hard headed, able and fit for political life."[116] As the campaign drew to a close, the leaders of the three parties predicted victory for their side. Mr. Dooley, the Irish saloonkeeper created by Finley Peter Dunne, commented on the predictions of the campaign managers:

> At th' Pri-grissive headquarters me frind George W. Perkins will overcome an impedymint in his speech an' tell ye that afther combin' over th' figures, he is lavin' headquarthers fr good, as he is afraid he will hurt himself laughin'. . . . Young Misther MacComb, th' sprite iv Dimmycratic headquarthers, gladdens the heart iv his followers with this inspirin' ballad: "Th' nation has spoken. All that now remains to be done is th' useless formality of addin' up th' figures. The Counthry has nobly responded to the appeals iv that jovyal prince iv good fellows an' divvle-may-care wag, Woodrow Wilson.
>
> Over at th' Raypublican headquarters Cheerful Charlie Hilles. . . . "It goes without sayin' that th' fewer th' number iv people you hear boastin' they'll vot fr William Haitch Taft th' larger his majority will be."
>
> Think iv bein' a Prohybition Candydate with no campaign manager an' nawthin' at all to cheer ye. I bet ye at this minyit while I'm talkin' th' campaign manager iv th' Prohybition party has got th' Prohybition candidate in a back-room an' is tellin' that th' Milwaukee brewers' union is secretly fr him because iv the horror they feel fr th' suds they make.[117]

The election of 1912 was an exciting one. As the polls closed, crowds gathered in the Loop for the returns. Bands played and peddlers did a rushing trade in banners. Throngs of people gathered at Hull House. For the society crowd of Chicago, the Saddle and Cycle Club brought in a special telegraph wire for the returns and served dinner to the accompaniment of an orchestra. The Onwentsia County Club served a game dinner while the returns came in. When the votes were counted, Dunne had won the race for governor. Deneen and Funk split the normal Republican vote between them, allowing Dunne to win both the state and Cook County by a plurality. Dunne had 443,000 votes, Deneen 318,000, and Funk 303,000. The Democrats, for the first time in many years, controlled the congressional delegation, winning twenty seats as compared with five for the Republicans and two for the Progressives. Cannon and McKinley, both prominent Republicans, were defeated. Cannon was defeated by Democrat Frank O'Hair of Paris. In the election for Congressmen-at-large, Democrats Lawrence Stringer and William Elza Williams won. In the presidential election Wilson carried Illinois by a plurality. Roosevelt carried Cook County but lost downstate.[118]

In the state legislature no party had a majority. The Democrats had more votes than either the Republicans or the Progressives but could not control the House. There was a struggle for control. Because of the deadlock in the legislature, Governor Dunne could not take his oath of office until February 3, 1913. The balloting had gone on since January, but it was not until early in February that the House was able to elect Representative William McKinley, Chicago Democrat, to the post of Speaker. The inauguration of Governor Dunne was held at noon before a joint session of the Senate and House. The oath of office was administered by Chief Justice Frank K. Dunn of the Illinois Supreme Court. Dunne was presented as the new governor of the state by Governor Deneen. That evening a public reception was held at the executive mansion and the Illinois Democrats attended to honor their first governor in the mansion since Altgeld. Dunne said they shook so many hands during the evening that both he and Mrs. Dunne had to have their right hands bandaged to relieve the pain.[119]

Because of the deadlock in the general assembly it was equally difficult to elect a senator. Illinois had to elect two senators, one to fill out the final year of Lorimer's term and the other as successor to Cullom, who had retired. In April of 1912, J. Hamilton Lewis of Chicago won the preferential primary for the Democrats and Lawrence Y. Sherman won the Republican nomination. The balloting in the legislature went on from February 11 to May 26, and it became necessary to arrange a compromise. With Governor Dunne taking a hand in the proceedings, it was arranged to elect Lewis to Cullom's seat and to elect Sherman for the short term.[120]

Lewis was prominent in Illinois politics for many years. A native of Virginia, he had grown up in Georgia and was admitted to the bar. He was elected congressman-at-large from the state of Washington and in 1903 moved to Chicago, where he set up a lucrative law practice. Sherman was born in Ohio, graduated from McKendree College, and practiced law in Macomb. He had held a number of state positions and served in the general assembly for four terms, including two as Speaker of the House of Representatives. A historian of the Republican party in Illinois describes Sherman in this way: "Mr. Sherman is one of the keenest intellects in the public service of Illinois today. He is a commoner of the old school; he has kept in touch with the people and believes in them, in their sense of justice and the accuracy of their judgment."[121]

Lewis, a tiny man, dressed in striking fashion. A *Chicago Daily News* reporter described his attire as he took the oath as senator: "Mr. Lewis was clad in a tight fitting dark grey cut-away suit, dark puffed tie, white vest, grey gloves, and a silk hat, and carried a silver-tipped cane, with a light lavender handkerchief peeping from the pocket of his coat." Senator Sherman was sworn in at the same time. The reporter commented, "The contrast between the two senators was most striking, Senator Sherman not only was devoid of whiskers of any sort, but his raiment consisted of a dark sack business suit, with a black string tie, and showed no form of outward adornment." For the first time since the ouster of Lorimer, Illinois had two senators.[122]

In the off-year election of 1914, the Republicans, no longer faced with challenge from the Progressives, regained most of the seats in the House of Representatives lost two years earlier. In the Sixty-fourth Congress, Illinois was represented by sixteen Republicans, including Mann, Cannon, and McKinley. The Democrats elected ten members, including Sabath and Rainey. The Progressives elected Ira C. Copley of Aurora.[123]

By the time Sherman's short senatorial term was completed, the states had ratified the seventeenth Amendment of the Constitution of the United States, requiring the direct election of senators. In the struggle within the Democratic party for the nomination, Carter Harrison, again mayor of Chicago, supported Lawrence Stringer. Harrison's former supporters Kenna and Coughlin deserted him because he had temporarily closed the houses of prostitution in the first ward. They supported Sullivan for the Democratic nomination. Lewis and Dunne joined Harrison in supporting Stringer because they thought one senator should be from downstate. Dunne later claimed that he supported Sullivan in the general election. The Republicans renominated Sherman as their candidate. The Progressives nominated Raymond Robbins, a settlement-house worker in Chicago. Sherman won the off-year election by about 25,000 votes, giving him a full term in the Senate.[124]

The Dunne administration was an illustrious one in the progressive tradition. He managed to get through the legislature the establishment of a state public utilities commission and the first law for building concrete highways in the state. Dunne brought a reorganization of the free state employment offices and, for the benefit of labor, secured legislative approval for a washhouse law and better legislation for protection of workers through safety appliances. The general assembly passed a law permitting woman suffrage in all elections for statutory offices and referendums. Dunne supported the establishment of the legislative reference bureau and provision for registration of lobbyists. Although Dunne tried desperately for the establishment of the initiative and referendum, it never passed the legislature.[125]

The Dunne administration created the Efficiency and Economy Commission to study reorganization of the state government. Governor Dunne was proud of institutional reform, which he believed eliminated cruelty and brought about honest administration. Dunne was particularly pleased that his administration was free of the kind of scandals that had in the past attended Illinois state government. He said, "And the proudest thing of all to me is that my administration as governor was free from graft, scandal and corruption of any kind or character." Although Dunne lacked a majority in the general assembly during his administration, he enjoyed a good relationship with the legislature. This is illustrated by a resolution in the Illinois Senate, dominated by Republicans, suggesting to President Wilson that he appoint Dunne to the Supreme Court of the United States.[126]

In the primary elections of 1916, Governor Dunne had token opposition from William F. Brinton and James Traynor. The Republican primary was more complicated. Nearly a year in advance, Frank L. Smith, a Dwight banker who had managed Taft's 1912 campaign, announced his candidacy. Frank Lowden's supporters began a campaign to get the nomination for him. In the preprimary struggles, the forces led by former Governor Deneen were important. A new figure had also entered the picture in Illinois Republicanism in the person of William H. "Big Bill" Thompson, who was elected mayor of Chicago in 1915. A windy buffoon, Thompson constituted a politically potent force in Illinois for two decades. Thompson had been born in Boston in 1867 and moved to Chicago as a small child. The son of a wealthy family, Thompson spent time in the West as a rancher and made a reputation in Chicago as an athlete. He founded the Chicago Athletic Club and was noted for his waterpolo, football, and sailing. He served briefly in local politics in Chicago around the turn of the century, but as mayor he was a political force, adding as well to the state's bad political reputation. Harold Ickes called him "William Hale Thompson the Gross" and "the Huey Long of his time and locale—without Huey's brains, however."[127]

In the primary election of 1916 an alliance was worked up between Lowden, Thompson, and Sherman, whereby Thompson got the satisfaction of playing kingmaker. Sherman was put on the Illinois primary ballot as the presidential candidate, and Lowden became the candidate for governor. The Deneen forces were unwilling to give up, and although they lost the organizational battle, Deneen persuaded Senator Morton D. Hull, a wealthy Chicagoan and former Progressive, to compete for the nomination against Lowden. Both Smith and Hull turned their oratorical guns against Lowden but to little avail. When the votes were counted, Lowden had a plurality. In the Democratic primary Dunne had more than a majority of the votes cast. In the presidential preferential primary Sherman got the nod from the Republican party, while Woodrow Wilson was on the ballot for the Democrats without opposition.[128]

At the Republican national convention, held in Chicago, all but two of the fifty-eight Illinois delegates supported Sherman on the first and second ballots, but he got only ten votes from seven other states. Theodore Roosevelt, who was coming back into the Republican party after the Progressive fiasco of 1912, would have liked the Republican nomination, but it was not to be. On the third ballot Charles Evans Hughes, a justice of the U. S. Supreme Court, was nominated for president, and Charles W. Fairbanks of Indiana was nominated to run with him. Hughes resigned from the Supreme Court to make the race. The Democratic national convention was held in St. Louis. There was no real contest in the convention and Woodrow Wilson was renominated. The Progressive party was dead by 1916, much to he despair of men like Harold Ickes. Medill McCormick returned to his old Republican alliance. Ickes, never fond of any of the McCormicks, said, "He was Medill-on-the-make. What he had done was to climb up over our shoulders and kick us in the face as he dived head long into the 'party of his fathers.'"[129]

Lowden based his campaign on the claim that he could run a more businesslike government than Dunne. One of the chief criticisms of Lowden was his close connection with big business through the Pullman Company, into which he had married, and the companies that he had helped to organize as a younger man. Lowden, who always went by the title of colonel because of his brief connection with the Illinois National Guard, hit at the increased expenditures of the Dunne administration. His supporters, who by now included Deneen, hit at the increased costs and mentioned that Dunne's administration was spending the frightening figure of $1,000 per hour. Medill McCormick charged that the cost of state government had risen 50 percent during the last four years.[130]

Accused of being dominated by big business, Lowden angrily

said that perhaps it was time that somebody with some business methods took part in state government. William E. Mason, a candidate for congressman-at-large, spoke for Lowden: "The Democratic party has the brain of a canary. The peacock is a lovely bird but it takes a stork to deliver." Lowden also sailed into Dunne for the patronage system, and spoke at length about a constitutional convention and the need for greater efficiency in government by consolidation of the agencies of government and reorganization of the government's finances. Both the *Tribune* and the *Herald* endorsed Lowden over Dunne. The *Tribune* said that although Dunne had a good and liberal administration, Lowden deserved support because of his call for a constitutional convention. They noted that Lowden had the support of the city hall crowd and Thompson, while Dunne had the support of some of the Sullivan crowd. They believed Lowden could shake off the influence of Thompson and Lundin easier than Dunne could shake some of his supporters. Much was made of the fact that although Lowden was rich, he was a self-made man, and his marriage to the wealthy Florence Pullman was ignored.[131]

The *Herald* played up this point and also said that the extravagance of the Dunne administration and weak appointments were enough to demand support for Lowden. Bryan spoke in the state for Dunne and Wilson, and as in earlier campaigns, worked in the area where he was born, starting out at Salem and speaking through southern and central Illinois. Roger Sullivan urged harmony in the party and supported Dunne, who also had the support of John Walker. Dunne tried to answer the charges of fiscal irresponsibility, saying that there was no deficit and the state was in good financial shape. As President Wilson passed through the state, Dunne boarded the train to identify himself with the president. Dunne, noting that Medill McCormick was on the campaign trail speaking for Lowden, quoted an editorial that McCormick had written in 1904 in which he denounced Lowden as the tool of the corporations and the political bosses. Dunne said Lowden had not changed—only McCormick had changed. Arthur Charles, chairman of the state Democratic Committee, tried to make a campaign issue of Lowden's connection with the Pullman Company. He noted that a Pullman porter got only $27.50 a month and depended on tips. This, Charles said, was Lowden's idea of a wage standard.[132]

In the presidential campaign of 1916 Republican speakers used two major issues. One was the high cost of living. A Hughes advertisement in the *Chicago Daily Tribune* said that a barrel of flour had gone up 110 percent during the Wilson administration. Ads urged a vote for Hughes and the protective tariff on the grounds that "Mr. Hughes never broke a promise." On the international scene, Republicans accused Wilson of cowardice and ineptness in handling foreign affairs. Roosevelt came to Chicago to speak for Hughes and talked to some 18,000 people. According to the account in the *Herald,* there was a thirty-four minute ovation for Roosevelt and only thirty seconds for Hughes. In the course of his speech Roosevelt said contemptuously of Wilson, "He speaks softly and carries a powder puff." Wilson was taken to task for what the *Tribune* regarded as weakness in Mexico, saying, "President Wilson has suggested only one distinct thought to the American people. That thought is he kept us out of war. That thought is yellow." On another occasion the *Tribune* said, "'Too proud to fight' and 'thank God for Wilson' are slipper phrases, soft cushioned phrases, pork chop phrases. They are phrases of a degenerating, demoralizing materialism, They are yellow phrases. They are dangerous, trouble involving phrases."[133]

William Jennings Bryan, campaigning for Wilson, said the campaign was essentially "a fight against privilege," remarking "Can money buy the governorship of Illinois? On the one hand you have Governor Dunne, a tried, honest efficient administrator, whose watch word is duty. For more than 20 years I have known him to be a fearless, independent friend of the people, and at all times when courage was needed to make a stand for popular rights. On the other hand there is an opposing candidate who is supported by the reactionary elements, the great corporate interests which are always seeking to control legislation and administration."[134] It has been said that Wilson tried to avoid using the slogan that he had kept us out of war. But the issue was used. One advertisement read: "You are working;—not fighting! Alive and happy;—not cannon fodder! Wilson in peace with honor? Or Hughes with Roosevelt and war?"

Wilson came to Illinois to speak during the campaign. He spoke to a crowd of some 15,000 at the Stockyards Pavilion. He addressed 4,000 Democratic women at the Auditorium. It was estimated that as many as 200,000 people saw him in a parade. When the votes were counted it was found that Lowden had defeated Dunne by nearly 150,000 votes, and Hughes carried the state by more than 200,000 votes over Wilson. As it turned out, the western states stayed with Wilson, who won the close election of 1916, although he lost badly in Illinois. Medill McCormick and William E. Mason were elected congressmen-at-large. The Democrats elected only six members to the Sixty-fifth Congress.[135]

Almost immediately after Lowden's inauguration as governor of Illinois, the nation and consequently the state were involved in the problems of World War I. Doubtless the Lowden administration was less effective in domestic problems within the state than it might have been otherwise. But Lowden, true to his promise, did bring about reorganization of State government. In the Dunne administration the legislature had appointed the Efficiency and Economy Commission, made up of four senators and four representatives with investigative powers to make recommendations for reorganization of state agencies. The committee had the assistance of Dr. John A. Fairlie, secretary of the Legislative Reference Bureau and political science professor at the University of Illinois. Lowden pledged himself to efficiency and economy and did his best to start this reorganization and support it.[136]

By overwhelming majority the general assembly passed the Civil Administrative Code in February, 1917, providing for nine departments of government, divided into ninety-six divisions, offices, and commissions. A number of boards and commissions were abolished or consolidated with others. The nine departments of government were the Departments of Finance, Agriculture, Labor, Mines and Minerals, Public Works and Building, Public Welfare, Public Health, Trade and Commerce, and Education. Each of these was to have a director and whatever assistants were necessary. This ended much duplication and inefficiency.[137]

Lowden had spoken of the need for a constitutional convention to reform the government of Illinois. The 1870 constitution was nearly fifty years old and seemed out of date for the needs of a highly industrialized state. Early in 1917, on the governor's recommendation, the general assembly passed a joint resolution calling for a referendum on the question of a constitutional convention. Shortly after this, the United States entered World War I, and the vote therefore did not take place until the general election of 1918, when the voters authorized the calling of a constitutional convention. The convention deliberated nearly two years before coming up with a document, which was submitted to the voters in December, 1922. The voters overwhelmingly rejected it for a variety of reasons, thus destroying one of Frank Lowden's dreams.[138]

In the off-year elections of 1918, the Republicans elected all but five of the twenty-five congressmen in the Sixty-sixth Congress. The Democrats held on to four seats in Chicago and that of Rainey downstate.[139]

From the beginning of the century through World War I, the Republicans dominated Illinois politics, except during the administration of Governor Dunne. Aside from the problem of Senator Lorimer, the period was one of better than average officeholders on both the state and national levels. It is true that some of the ward politics of Chicago left something to be desired and Len Small made his first appearance in politics, but Deneen, Dunne, and Lowden presented administrations which could be viewed with pride.

1. George Mowry, *The Era of Theodore Roosevelt* (New York, 1958), pp. 86–87; Richard Hofstadter, *The Age of Reform* (New York, 1955), pp. 182–87.

2. "The New-Stock Politicians of 1912," *Journal of the Illinois State Historical Society* (Spring, 1969), pp. 35–52; John Buenker, "Edward F. Dunne: The Urban New Stock Democrat as Progressive," *Mid-America* 50 (Jan., 1968), pp. 3–21; "Urban Immigrant Lawmakers," in Donald F. Tingley, ed., *Essays in Illinois History* (Carbondale, Ill., 1968), pp. 52–74.

3. William T. Hutchison, *Lowden of Illinois:The Life of Frank O. Lowden*, 2 vols. (Chicago, 1957), I, 93–95, contains an excellent analysis of the Republican factions.

4. For McVeigh see Edward F. Dunne, *Illinois: Heart of the Nation*, 5 vols. (Chicago, 1933), III, 16. For a sketch of Dawes see ibid., III, 11–12. Dawes wrote several autobiographical books: *A Journal of the McKinley Years* (Chicago, 1959); *A Journal of the Great War* (New York, 1923); *The First Year of the Budget of the United States* (New York, 1923); *Notes as Vice President* (Boston, 1935); *Journal as Ambassador to Great Britain* (New York, 1939); *A Journal of Reparations* (New York, 1939).

5. Carroll H. Wooddy, *The Case of Frank L. Smith, Study in Representative Government* (Chicago, 1931), pp. 147–55, is a good short account of Lorimer's career. The definitive biography of Lorimer is Joel A. Tarr, *A Study in Boss Politics: William Lorimer of Chicago* (Urbana, Ill., 1971).

6. Samuel Alvin Lilly, "The Political Career of Roger C. Sullivan" (M.A. thesis, Eastern Illinois University, Charleston, 1964); Dunne, *Illinois*, III, 274–75.

7. Carter H. Harrison, *Growing Up with Chicago* (Chicago, 1944), pp. 280–81.

8. Buenker, "Edward F. Dunne," pp. 3–4.

9. *Chicago Tribune*, June 28, 1900, p. 9; July 3, 1904, p. 2; July 7, 1908, p. 3; *Chicago Record-Herald*, Sept. 19, 1904, p. 7.

10. Dunne, *Illinois*, V, 420.

11. Charles E. Merriam, *Chicago, More Intimate View of Urban Politics* (New York, 1929), pp. 103, 111; *Chicago Tribune*, May 10, 1908, part 7, p. 2.

12. See the account of the "Appomattox Day" banquet of the Hamilton Club, *Chicago Tribune*, Apr. 8, 1900, p. 8; *Sunday Chicago Inter-Ocean*, Jan. 24, 1900, p. 6.

13. Harold Ickes, *Autobiography of a Curmudgeon* (Chicago, 1969), p. 147.

14. *Sunday Inter-Ocean*, Jan. 21, 1900, p. 5; *Chicago Tribune*, Jan. 24, 1900, p. 1; Apr. 10, 1900, p.1; Apr. 15, 1900, p. 4; July 1, 1900, p. 6.

15. *Sunday Inter-Ocean*, Jan. 14, 1900, p. 28.

16. John Myers Allswang, "The Political Behavior of Chicago's Ethnic Group, 1918–1932" (dissertation, University of Pittsburgh, 1957), p. 19.

17. Merriam, *Chicago,* p. 138; Lloyd Wendt and Herman Kogan, *Big Bill of Chicago* (Indianapolis, 1953), pp. 253–56; Harold F. Gosnell, *Negro Politicians, The Rise of Negro Politics in Chicago* (Chicago, 1935), pp. 38–39.

18. Alswang, "Political Behavior of Chicago's Ethnic Groups," pp. 7–8, 9, 17.

19. Ibid., 18–19.

20. Lloyd Wendt and Herman Kogan, *Bosses in Lusty Chicago: The Story of Bathhouse John and Hinky Dink* (Bloomington, Ind. 1967), pp. 192, 324.

21. *Biographical Directory of the American Congress 1774–1961* (Washington, D. C., 1961) p. 268; Blair Bolles, *Tyrant from Illinois* (New York, 1951) is the best biography of Cannon. For Mann see ibid., pp. 57–58. See also Charles A. Church, *History of the Republican Party in Illinois 1854–1912* (Rockford, Ill., 1912), pp. 197–98. For Cullom see Shelby M. Cullom, *Fifty Years of Public Service* (Chicago, 1911).

22. *Illinois State Journal* (Springfield), Jan. 3, 1900, p. 4; Mar. 12, 1900, p. 5; Mar. 14, 1900, p. 4; Cullom, *Fifty Years of Public Service*, p. 445; Dunne, *Illinois*, V, 48.

23. The *Sunday Inter-Ocean*, Jan. 21, 1900, p. 5; *Chicago Tribune*, Jan. 24, 1900, p. 4; Apr. 10, 1900, p. 1; Apr. 15, 1900, p. 4; July 1, 1900, p. 6.

24. *Illinois State Journal*, Mar. 8, 1900, p. 5; *Chicago Tribune*, June 27, 1900, pp. 1, 12; June 28, 1900, p. 9.

25. *Chicago Tribune*, June 28, 1900, p. 9; James D. Nowlan, comp., *Illinois Major Party Platforms 1900–1964* (Urbana, Ill., 1966), p. 9.

26. Nowlan, *Illinois Major Party Platforms*, p. 8.

27. *Chicago Tribune*, June 27, 1900, p. 1.

28. Ibid., June 27, 1900, p. 5; Dunne, *Illinois*, IV, 9; W. A. Townsend and C. Boeschenstein, *Illinois Democracy, History of the Party and Its Representative Members' Past and Present*, 4 vols. (Springfield, Ill., 1935), II, 59.

29. *Chicago Tribune*, Apr. 8, 1900, p. 4; Apr. 13, 1900, p. 6; Apr. 14, 1900, p. 1; Apr. 21, 1900, p. 1; Hutchison, *Lowden of Illinois*, I, 97.

30. *Chicago Tribune*, May 9, 1900, p. 1; May 10, 1900, p. 1.

31. Ibid., Apr. 15, 1900, i. 6.

32. Nowlan, *Illinois Major Party Platforms*, pp. 2–3.

33. Dunne, *Illinois*, III, 37; Hutchison, *Lowden of Illinois*, I, 97–98; *Chicago Tribune*, May 10, 1900, p. 3; May 12, 1900, p. 6; May 13, 1900, p. 8; Church, *Republican Party in Illinois*, p. 194.

34. *Chicago Tribune*, May 20, 1900, p. 47; Hutchison, *Lowden of Illinois* I, 98.

35. Wendt and Kogan, *Bosses in Lusty Chicago*, pp. 216–17; *Chicago Tribune*, July 5, 1900, p. 1; July 7, 1900, pp. 1, 12.

36. *Chicago Tribune*, Sept. 2, 1900, p. 1; Sept. 20, 1900, p. 4; Sept. 25, 1900, p. 4; Nov. 2, 1900, p. 4; *Chicago Record*, Nov. 3, 1900, p. 12.

37. *Chicago Record*, Nov. 5, 1900, p. 2; Nov. 6, 1900, p. 1.

38. *Chicago Tribune*, Sept. 4, 1900, p. 3; Sept. 12, 1900, p. 4; Nov. 1, 1900, p. 1; *Chicago Record*, Nov. 3, 1900, p. 12; Nov. 5, 1900, pp. 10, 14.

39. *Chicago Tribune*, Aug. 2, 1900, p. 3; Aug, 3, 1900, pp. 1, 3; Aug. 6, 1900, p. 1; Aug. 18, 1900, p. 1; Nov. 6, 1900, p. 2.

40. Ibid., Sept. 5, 1900, p. 6; Sept. 9, 1900, p. 2.

41. Ibid., Sept. 12, 1900, p. 12.

42. Ibid., Sept 21, 1900, p. 4.

43. Ibid., Sept. 11, 1900, p. 6.

44. Ibid., Sept. 1, 1900, p. 4; Oct. 8, 1900, p. 1.

45. Ibid., Nov. 2, 1900, p. 1; Nov. 4, 1900, p. 36; *Chicago Record*, Nov. 3, 1900, pp. 1–3.

46. *Chicago Record*, Nov. 7, 1900, p. 6; *Illinois Blue Book, 1903*, pp. 569–72.

47. Dunne, *Illinois*, II, 173, Church, *Republican Party in Illinois.*

48. *Illinois Blue Book 1927–28*p. 788.

49. Cullom, *Fifty Years of Public Service*, pp. 445–49; Hutchison, *Lowden of Illinois* I, 103; *Chicago Tribune*, Jan. 1, 1900, p. 6; Sept. 22, 1900, p. 4; *Chicago Record*, Nov. 8, 1900, p. 1.

50. *Inter-Ocean*, Jan. 12, 1900, pp. 1–2.

51. *Illinois State Journal*, Jan. 14, 1900, p. 3.

52. Church, *Republican Party in Illinois*, pp. 184–85, 196–97; Hutchison, *Lowden of Illinois*, I, 104–10; Nowlan, *Illinois Major Party Platforms*, p. 10.

53. *Illinois Blue Book 1927–28* p. 788. See also Robert A. Waller, *Rainey of Illinois, Political Biography, 1903–34* (Urbana Ill., 1977).

54. Carter H. Harrison, *Stormy Years* (Indianapolis, 1938), p. 233; *Chicago Tribune*, June 14, 1904, p. 2; June 15, 1904, p. 1; Dunne, *Illinois*, III, 250–51; Townsend and Boeschenstein, *Illinois Democracy, 4 vols.* (Springfield, Ill., 1935) IV, 8–10.

55. Nowlan, *Illinois Major Party Platforms*, pp. 23–26.

56. *Chicago Tribune*, May 1, 1904, p. 6.

57. Ibid., May 2, 1904, p. 6

58. Ibid., May 2, 1904, p. 6; May 6, 1904, pp. 1, 6; May 18, 1904, p. 1.

59. Ibid., May 7, 1904, p. 4; May 10, 1904, p. 1; May 11, 1904, p. 1; May 14, 1904, pp. 1, 2; May 15, 1904, p. 1; May 16, 1904, p. 6; May 18, 1904, p. 4; May 21, 1904, p. 1.

60. Ibid., June 1, 1904, p. 1; June 4, 1904, pp. 1, 2; Church, *Republican Party in Illinois*, pp. 199–200. For a complete account of the convention see J. McCan Davis, *The Breaking of the Deadlock* (Springfield, Ill., 1904).

61. For a sketch of Deneen see Dunne, *Illinois*, V, 456, or Church, *Republican Party in Illinois*, p. 203; *Chicago Record*, Nov. 8, 1900, p. 1.

62. *Republicans of Illinois, a Portrait and Chronological Record of Members of the Republican Party* (Chicago, 1905), p. 13; Ickes, *Autobiography of a Curmudgeon*, pp. 115–16, 118.

63. Ickes, *Autobiography of a Curmudgeon*, pp. 116–18.

64. Nowlan, *Illinois Major Party Platforms*, pp. 18, 21, 31.

65. *Chicago Tribune*, June 30, 1904, p. 5; July 3, 1904, p. 2; July 7, 1904, p. 2; July 8, 1904, p. 3; July 9, 1904, pp. 1, 4; Wendt and Kogan, *Bosses in Lusty Chicago*, pp. 242–43.

66. *Chicago Tribune*, May 12, 1904, p. 3; June 20, 1904, p. 1; June 21, 1904, pp. 1, 2; June 24, 1904, p. 1; Church, *Republican Party in Illinois*, p. 201.

67. *Chicago Tribune*, Aug. 3, 1904, p. 2; Sept. 4, 1904, part 1, p. 6; Sept. 27, 1904, p. 5; *Record-Herald*, Sept. 17, 1904, p. 2; Sept. 25, 1904, p. 2.

68. *Record-Herald*, Oct. 12, 1904, p. 2.

69. Ibid., Oct. 13, 1904, p. 3; Oct. 14, 1904, p. 2; Oct. 18, 1904, p. 4; Oct. 21, 1904, p. 2; Oct. 22, 1904, p. 4; Oct. 25, 1904, p. 4; *Chicago Tribune*, Oct. 21, 1904, p. 1; Oct. 29, 1904, p. 7; Nov. 1, 1904, p. 6.

70. *Record-Herald*, Sept. 3, 1904, p. 3; Sept. 12, 1904, p. 4; Sept. 24, 1904, p. 3; Oct. 5, 1904, p. 2; Oct. 6, 1904, p. 2; Oct. 7, 1904, p. 6; Oct. 12, 1904, p. 2; *Chicago Tribune*, Sept. 3, 1904, p. 1; Sept. 6, 1904, p. 3; Sept. 8, 1904, p. 5; Sept. 10, 1904, pp. 1, 5; Sept. 16, 1904, p. 6; Sept. 18, 1904, p. 1; Sept. 21, 1904, p. 5; Sept. 27, 1904, p. 3; Oct. 7, 1904, p. 6.

71. *Chicago Tribune*, Oct. 18, 1904, p. 5; Nov. 5, 1904, p. 4; Nov. 6, 1904, part 1, p. 4; *Record-Herald*, Oct. 13, 1904, p. 3; Oct. 18, 1904, p. 3.

72. *Chicago Tribune*, Sept. 30, 1904, p. 1; Oct. 7, 1904, p. 1; Oct. 13, 1904, p. 1; *Record-Herald*, Sept. 17, 1904, p. 2; Sept. 19, 1904, p. 7; Oct. 4, 1904, p. 2; Oct. 7, 1904, p. 1; Oct. 26, 1904, p. 3.

73. *Chicago Tribune*, Oct. 18, 1904, p. 4; *Record-Herald*, Oct. 18, 1904, p. 3.

74. *Illinois Blue Book, 1909*, pp. 449–52; *Record-Herald*, November 9, 1904, p. 1; Nov. 10, 1904, p. 3.

75. *Illinois Blue Book 1927–28* p. 788.

76. Ibid.

77. Cullom, *Fifty Years of Public Service,*pp. 450–52.

78. *Chicago Tribune*, May 10, 1908, p. 7; June 7, 1908, p. 6; June 23, 1908, pp. 1, 4, 5, 10; Aug. 2, 1908, Part 2, p. 1; Aug. 6, 1908, p. 8; Aug. 7, 1908, pp. 1, 8.

79. *Chicago Tribune*, Aug. 2, 1908, Part 1, p. 2; Aug. 10, 1908, p. 1; Aug. 11, 1908, p. 8; Church, *Republican Party in Illinois*, pp. 211–12; *Illinois Blue Book, 1909*, pp. 345–47, 355–57.

80. Dunne, *Illinois*, III, 59–61.

81. Nowlan, *Illinois Major Party Platforms*, pp. 40–44, 49–52, 53–55.

82. *Chicago Tribune*, May 3, 1908, p. 2; June 21, 1908, p. 1; June 29, 1908, p. 2; July 4, 1908, p. 5; Liffy, *Roger Sullivan*, p. 27; Wendt and Kogan, *Bosses in Lusty Chicago*, pp. 262–63.

83. Wendt and Kogan, *Bosses in Lusty Chicago*, pp. 255; *Chicago Tribune*, July 3, 1908, p. 2.

84. *Chicago Tribune*, July 7, 1908, p. 3; July 8, 1908, p. 3; July 10, 1908, p. 1.

85. Ibid., June 19, 1908, p. 1; Church, *Republican Party in Illinois*, p. 211.

86. *Chicago Tribune*, May 8, 1908, p. 4.

87. Ibid., May 8, 1908, p. 4: May 10, 1908, p. 4; May 11, 1908, p. 4; May 15, 1908, p. 2.

88. Ibid., Oct. 6, 1908, p. 8; Oct. 11, 1908, p. 4; Oct. 12, 1908, p. 5.

89. Ibid., Oct. 14, 1908, p. 2: *Record-Herald*, Oct. 19, 1908, p. 2; Oct. 20, 1908, p. 2.

90. *Chicago Tribune*, Oct. 27, 1908, p. 4; *Record-Herald*, Oct. 18, 1908, p. 7; Oct. 27, 1908, p. 2.

91. *Chicago Tribune*, Nov. 1, 1908, p. 4; Nov. 2, 1904, p. 1; *Record-Herald*, Oct. 27, 1908, p. 2; Oct. 29, 1908, p. 5; Oct. 31, 1908, p. 2.

92. *Chicago Tribune*, June 14, 1908, Section II, p. 4; June 16, 1908, p. 12; June 17, 1908, p. 7; June 20, 1908, p. 3; Aug. 2, 1908, p. 5; Nov. 21, 1908, p. 2; Nov. 24, 1908, p. 6; *Record-Herald*, Oct. 9, 1908, p. 5.

93. *Record-Herald*, Oct. 9, 1908, p. 5; Oct. 20, 1908, p. 5; Nov. 2, 1908, p. 5.

94. *Chicago Tribune*, Nov. 6, 1908, pp. 5, 8; *Record-Herald*, Nov. 5, 1908, p. 1; *Illinois Blue Book, 1909*, pp. 369–73.

95. *Illinois Blue Book, 1927–1928*, p. 788.

96. Dunne, *Illinois*, III, 36–37; *Chicago Tribune*, Aug. 2, 1908, Part 1, p. 2; Church, *Republican Party in Illinois*, p. 214; Alex Gottfried, *Boss Cermak of Chicago: A Study in Political Leadership* (Seattle, 1962), pp. 56–57.

97. Dunne, *Illinois*, II 181.

98. Church, *Republican Party in Illinois* pp. 214–15; Gottfried, *Boss Cermak*, p. 57; Tarr, *Boss Politics*, pp. 244–45.

99. Church, *Republican Party in Illinois* p. 215; Tarr, *Boss Politics*, pp. 233–67.

100. Church, *Republican Party in Illinois*, pp. 216–17; Tarr, *Boss Politics*, pp. 268–307.

101. Ibid., p. 206.

102. Ibid., pp. 207–8.

103. Dunne, *Illinois*, II, 179; *Laws of the State of Illinois Enacted by the Forty-fourth General Assembly at the Regular Biennial Session* (Springfield, 1905), pp. 113–22; *Laws of the State of Illinois Enacted by the Forty-seventh General Assembly* (Springfield, 1911), pp. 199–27.

104. *Illinois Blue Book 1927–28*, p. 788.

105. *Laws of the State of Illinois Enacted by the Forty-seventh General Assembly at the Third Special Session* (Springfield, 1912), pp. 66–86. 6,105:.

106. Dunne, *Illinois*, II, 312, 314–15; *Illinois Blue Book*, 1'13–14, p. 460.

107. Dunne, *Illinois*, II, 187, 308–14; *Illinois Blue Book*, 1913–14, p. 460.

108. Nowlan, *Illinois Major Party Platforms*, pp. 72–80, 81–84.

109. Church, *Republican Party in Illinois*, pp. 231–34; Dunne, *Illinois*, II, 315–16.

110. Dunne, *Illinois*, II, 316, V, 35; Ickes, *Autobiography of a Curmudgeon*, pp. 149, 167; Church, *Republican Party in Illinois*, pp 234–35.

111. Church, *Republican Party in Illinois*, p. 235; Ickes, *Autobiography of a Curmudgeon*, p. 162.

112. Harrison, *Stormy Years*, pp. 315–21.

113. Dunne, *Illinois*, II, 316; *Record-Herald*, Oct. 28, 1912, p. 2; Nov. 2, 1912, p. 2; *Chicago Tribune*, Nov. 4, 1912, p. 7.

114. *Chicago Tribune*, Nov. 2, 1912, pp. 5, 7; Nov. 3, 1912, p. 5; Nov. 4, 1912, p. 5; Nov. 5, 1912, p. 4; *Record-Herald*, Oct. 28, 1912, p. 2; Oct. 29, 1912, p. 4; Oct. 30, 1912, p. 5; Oct. 31, 1912, p. 5; Nov. 2, 1912, p. 2.

115. *Chicago Tribune*, Nov. 2, 1912, p. 5; Nov. 3, 1912, p. 1; Nov. 5, 1912, p. 4; *Record-Herald*, Oct. 29, 1'12, p. 5; Oct. 31, 1912, pp. 4, 5; Nov. 1, 1912, p. 6; Nov. 3, 1912, part VI, p. 2; Church, *Republican Party in Illinois*, pp. 222–24.

116. *Chicago Tribune*, Nov. 3, 1912, pp. 2, 3; *Record-Herald*, Oct. 30, 1912, p. 5; Nov. 3, 1912, p. 1; Nov. 11, 1912, p. 8.

117. *Chicago Tribune*, Nov. 3, 1912, part VIII, p. 1.

118. Ibid., Nov. 7, 1912, p. 6; *Record-Herald*, Nov. 5, 1912, p. 8; Nov. 6, 1912, p. 5; Nov. 17, 1912, part V, p. 6; *Illinois Blue Book, 1913–14*, pp. 565–66.

119. Dunne, *Illinois*, II, 317–18.

120. Dunne, *Illinois*, II, 366–67; *Illinois Blue Book, 1913–14*, p. 460; *Illinois Blue Book, 1925–26*, pp. 277–78; *Record-Herald*, Nov. 8, 1912, p. 4; Nov. 11, 1912, p. 4; N v. 12, 1912, p. 4; Nov. 18, 1912, p. 5.

121. Dunne, *Illinois*, III, pp. 3–4; Church, *Republican Party in Illinois*, pp. 203–4.

122. *Chicago Daily News*, Apr. 17, 1913, p. 1.

123. *Illinois Blue Book, 1927–28*, p. 788.

124. Dunne, *Illinois*, II, 367–68; Wendt and Kagan, *Bosses in Lusty Chicago*, pp. 324–25.

125. Dunne, *Illinois*, II, 318–30, 331, 333–34, 335–36, 337–38, 340–41, 342–46.

126. Ibid., II, 337–38, 349–58, 371, 372–75.

127. Hutchison, *Lowden of Illinois* I, 266–86; Ickes, *Autobiography of a Curmudgeon*, pp. 146, 172–73. For Thompson's career see Wendt and Kogan, *Big Bill of Chicago*, or John Bright, *Hizzoner Big Bill Thompson* (New York, 1930).

128. Hutchison, *Lowden of Illinois* I, 278–79; *Illinois Blue Book, 1917–18*, p. 526.

129. Joseph Tumulty, *Woodrow Wilson as I Knew Him* (New York, 1921), pp. 182–89, 191, 193–94; Ickes, *Autobiography of a Curmudgeon*, p. 237.

130. *Chicago Herald*, Oct. 6, 1916, p. 8; Oct. 17, 1916, p. 3; Oct. 20, 1916, p. 7.

131. *Chicago Tribune*, Nov. 2, 1916, p. 6; Nov. 8, 1916, p. 7; Nov. 9, 1917, pp. 2, 6; *Chicago Record Herald*, Oct. 4, 1916, p. 1.

132. *Chicago Tribune*, Nov. 5, 1916, p. 9; *Chicago Record Herald*, Oct. 4, 1916, p. 5; Oct. 7, 1916, p. 1; Oct. 14, 1916, p. 7; Oct. 15, 1916, p. 5; Oct. 22, 1916, p. 3; Oct. 29, 1916, p. 7.

133. *Chicago Tribune*, Nov. 2, 1916, pp. 6, 10–11; Nov. 4, 1916, p.6; Nov. 5, 1916, sec. 8, p. 4; Nov. 6, 1916, p. 18; *Chicago Record Herald*, Oct. 27, 1916, p. 1.

134. *Chicago Record Herald*, Oct. 29, 1916, p. 7.

135. *Chicago Tribune*, Nov. 6, 1916, p. 10; Nov. 9, 1916, p. 8; Dunne, *Illinois*, II, 368; *Illinois Blue Book, 1917–18,* pp. 578, 579.

136. Hutchison, *Lowden of Illinois* I, 295–97.

137. Ibid., I, 301–2; *Laws of the State of Illinois Enacted by the Fiftieth General Assembly* (Springfield, 1917), pp. 2–36.

138. *Illinois Blue Book 1925–26,* p. 276; Hutchison, *Lowden of Illinois* I, 322–24.

139. *Illinois Blue Book, 1927–28,* p. 789.

7

World War I and the Red Scare

World War I wrought havoc in the lives of Illinois citizens. As in the history of the nation, the "Great War" forms a watershed in the history of the state. Life and man's thought and outlook never again would achieve the freedom, confidence, optimism, and enthusiasm of the period of 1900–17. When Congress declared war on Germany on April 6, 1917, it set off a chain of events that altered the face of the nation and consequently of Illinois. The people of Illinois found themselves organized, taxed, regulated, and regimented in unprecendented fashion; their eyes, ears, and minds were assaulted constantly with patriotic slogans. Social, economic, and population changes of massive proportions resulted, but more important in the long run, World War I, as war always does, set off waves of intolerance and bigotry. Because of the establishment of the first organized governmental propaganda machine, most Americans accepted all of this without protest as a necessity to make the world "safe for democracy."

Europe, in the decades since 1870, had deteriorated into a cancerous mass of jealousy, fear, and discontent. The problems included territorial ambitions, both European and colonial, ethnic fear and hatred, and economic and military rivalry. Europe had tried to avoid war through a balance of power achieved by a system of military alliances. The blow that broke open the festering sore was the assassination, in Bosnia in the summer of 1914, of the Archduke Francis Ferdinand, heir apparent to the Austrian throne. This event set in motion the commitments of the balance of power so that one nation after another was drawn into the conflict, which quickly involved every major European power. World War I was characterized by the application of modern technology to war: the machine gun, tanks, aircraft, and poison gas. Despite the lethal and mobile character of the new weapons, however, by 1917 the war had reached a stalemate characterized by dreary trench warfare.[1]

As World War I began, Americans took the view that it was just another European quarrel which would not affect them. President Woodrow Wilson called upon Americans to be "impartial in thought as well as in action." Probably most Americans hoped to achieve this, but the mixed ethnic background of the citizens made it an impossible goal. Although many persons of German origin sympathized with the Central Powers, a majority of citizens favored the cause of England and France. The United States had ethnic, linguistic, cultural, and historic ties with England, as well as a sentimental feeling toward France dating from her aid in the Revolution. English propaganda was more effective than the heavy-handed efforts of the Germans. It quickly became apparent that the United States could not remain aloof from the war in the face of repeated violations of its neutrality. President Wilson insisted U.S. citizens should be free to travel or trade wherever they chose, but both sides interfered with the trade of the United States, and the Germans caused loss of American life when their submarines, another of the new weapons of war, sank such ships as the *Lusitania* and *Sussex*. Americans, already prejudiced in favor of England, would tolerate British interference with trade and property but became increasingly angry with the Germans for causing American deaths. When the Germans, renewing unrestricted submarine warfare, sank the *Sussex,* President Wilson, on April 19, 1916, threatened to break off diplomatic relations with Germany. After much diplomatic bickering, this was done on February 3, 1917, and on April 2, 1917, after three more American merchant ships had been sunk, President Wilson asked for a declaration of war against Germany. Congress complied four days later.[2] As the United States drew closer to war, it had the backing of the executive branch of Illinois. Although the government of Illinois was in the hands of the Republican party, Democrat Woodrow Wilson had its support. In a burst of patriotic ardor, Governor Lowden laid aside political considerations as he proclaimed, "If the President of the United States were a Prohibitionist or a Socialist, I would consider myself a traitor to my country if I did not support him with the same ardor and energy and enthusiasm . . . which I am showing the President now. There is only one test of patriotism in a war like this. Either we are for the government or we are against it."[3]

In this spirit, Lowden, when the United States broke diplomatic relations with Germany, telegraphed his support to Wilson, and a few days later a joint resolution of both houses of the general assembly pledged "to support the Government of the United States in maintaining the honor and dignity of our country. . . ." Lowden had the support of the fiftieth general assembly, which met from January to July, 1917. During the remainder of the war the legislature did not meet, leaving Lowden virtually a one-man government devoted almost solely to the war effort.[4]

Not all elected officials supported the war as totally as Lowden. When President Wilson called the special session of Congress to make the declaration of war, five Illinois congressmen voted against the resolution. The leader of the antiwar group in Congress, Fred A. Britten of Chicago, sponsored an amendment specifying that only those who volunteered should fight overseas. Britten argued that the American people did not support the war and that all of the wrongs of Germany and England did not justify the killing of untold thousands of Americans.[5]

Congressman William E. Mason, consistently pacifist and libertarian, spoke vigorously against the resolution. Mason held that Germany had acted within the limits of international law and had given no cause for war. He warned that the United States was unprepared for war and that the people of Illinois were not in favor of war. He insisted the war was wrong: "It is a dollar war. . . . It is a war between kings for money and for territory. It does not involve a single human life that interests a great republican democracy like the United States." Mason opposed the war because "it means an entrance on our part into European war and European politics, the dangers of which were foreshadowed by Washington and are familiar to every student of the history of the United States." Mason closed with the warning: "We will be tied to a treaty that we can not break without dishonor to a hundred million people, and your peace and your war and the destiny of your Republic hangs in the balance and in the caprice of a few crowned heads in the Old World."[6]

Senator Lewis, Democratic whip in the Senate, supported Wilson's policies with vigor and became a spokesman for the war. Senator Sherman, Republican, supported the war but criticized Wilson's handling of it, especially the lack of preparedness prior to involvement of the United States. Mayor William Hale Thompson of Chicago vigorously opposed the war at every turn.[7]

There was little wartime legislation in Illinois. Most governmental action originated by executive order or by the authority of the State Council of Defense (SCD), which was created by statute at the beginning of a war. The SCD consisted of fifteen persons appointed by the governor for a term to coincide with the duration of the war. Qualifications of members included specialized knowledge in industry, labor, transportation, or development of natural resources. The council had power of subpoena and the legislature mandated its cooperation with national and other state groups in promoting the war. Lowden appointed Chairman Samuel Insull (utilities magnate), J. Ogden Armour (meat-packer), John Walker (president of the Illinois Federation of Labor), Victor Olander (secretary of the IFL), B. F. Harris (Champaign businessman), John P. Hopkins (Democratic politician, succeeded by Roger Sullivan in October, 1918), Dr. Frank Billings (physician), Mrs. Joseph T. Bowen (social worker), John H. Harrison (Danville newspaper publisher), Levy Mayer (attorney), John G. Oglesby (lieutenant governor), David E. Shanahan (real estate and banking), John A. Spoor (railroads and banking), Frederick W. Upham (businessman in coal and lumber), and Charles H. Wacker (capitalist). Most of these people, except Walker and Olander, came from the business community. Appointment of labor leaders of such prominence was unprecedented, and when a confrontation between the industrialists and labor representatives threatened at the first meeting, Lowden exclaimed: "This war can be won by neither labor nor capital alone. Gentlemen, you have got to work together."[8]

When the war began, Illinois National Guard units were called to service almost immediately. By August the guard had reached 18,619 men and officers in strength. Subsequent additions brought the total to 25,000. The various branches of the armed services stepped up their recruiting efforts with a notable lack of success. In twenty days in April only 2,427 young men of Illinois enlisted, but with this meager number Illinois led all the states. One day recruiting officers stationed themselves outside the Cub ball park, solicited 18,000 men, and got no recruits. Enthusiasm for the war had to be manufactured.[9]

Faced with this kind of massive indifference, Congress passed the Selective Service Act on May 18, 1917. The first registration applied to all males age twenty-one to thirty. This registration, carried out by local election boards, was the first time a military draft had operated in the United States since the Civil War. Ultimately the federal government established draft boards under the direction of the governor. Governor Lowden believed completely in the draft and that it should be continued after the war as a reminder that all young men had obligations to the country. Lowden, who liked to be called Colonel as a tribute to his service in the National Guard, proclaimed, "Our citizenship has been too cheap. We have acquired the habit of looking to the government for everything expecting it to be a fairy godmother to whom nothing needs to be returned." Three successive registrations totaled 1,154,877 men; of these, 193,338 were inducted into military service. Illinois was third among the states in the number of draftees. In the first call for induction more than 10 percent failed to appear and more than 50 percent filed claims for exemption by reason of marriage, occupation, religion, or conscience.[10]

The federal government established several military installations in Illinois. The Naval Training Station at Great Lakes was expanded to become the world's biggest "jackie school," accommodating as many as 50,000 seamen. This involved land acquisition and the building of housing. The Great Lakes band, under the direction of Lieutenant John Philip Sousa, became nationally famous. Fort Sheridan was turned into an officer-training installation. Camp Grant, near Rockford, was established as a training center for the Army. It occupied more than 5,000 acres. Construction of Scott Field, near Belleville, was carried out quickly. Here early-day aviators were trained. A total of fourteen sqadrons originated at Scott Field. The Army established Chanute Field at Rantoul in July, 1917. The field boasted eleven wooden hangars, each with a capacity of eight aircraft, a ground school, and a flying school. A total of twenty-two squadrons had some of their training at Chanute. Contractors built the base at Chanute in six weeks. The training aircraft consisted of twenty-two Curtiss biplanes sporting 100-horsepower engines. The *Chicago Tribune* referred to the base as "a far-flung challenge to the Teuton nations."[11]

The federal government established broad and unprecedented controls over the economic life of the nation, and there were parallel controls in Illinois, set forth by gubernatorial proclamation and through the activities of the State Council of Defense. Greater production of food and its conservation were believed essential to the war. The SCD established a Food Production Committee and a

Farm Labor Administration to promote food production. The "War Garden Advisory Committee" urged citizens to grow gardens, and a "Boy's Working Reserve" was established to provide farm labor. When a seed-corn shortage threatened, the SCD established a "Seed Corn Administration" to inventory available stock and raise money to buy supplementary supplies. A food production conference sponsored by the SCD and the University of Illinois College of Agriculture was held in Urbana to explore ways of increasing production. A "Patriotic Food Show Committee," established to hold a meeting at the Coliseum in Chicago, posed the problem "What to eat and how to cook it." Farmers were urged to increase meat production, and restaurants and bakeries were carefully controlled to prevent waste and hoarding, as well as to find substitutes for flour. Food production increased substantially in most areas and dramatically in some, as Illinois farmers responded to the pleas of the new bureaucracy that it was the patriotic thing to do.[12]

Fuel production created similar problems. In August, 1917, Congress enacted the Federal Food and Fuel Control Act, which gave the president almost absolute control over mines, even to the extent of nationalizing them. Governor Lowden appointed Orrin Carter, chief justice of the Illinois Supreme Court, as fuel czar in Illinois. Justice Carter fixed state fuel prices after consulting with representatives of the miners and mine operators. Some effort was made to prevent hoarding of coal supplies by improving the distribution system.[13]

Although Illinois industry found itself regulated, it benefited from war contracts with both the United States and the allied powers. The SCD established the "Commercial Economy Administration" to promote economy in business. Local chairmen oversaw its operation. The regulations curtailed deliveries, restricted the privilege of returning merchandise, and made Christmas shopping unpatriotic in 1917. The Illinois Manufacturers Association established a War Industries Bureau in Washington to bring contracts to Illinois, and the SCD established the War Business Committee for the same purpose. These organizations brought some $510,000,000 worth of business to the state. Among the Illinois companies benefiting from war contracts were Western Cartridge, Deere and Company, Armour, Swift, American Steel Foundries, and the Northwestern Barb Wire Company. The U.S. arsenal at Rock Island was enlarged and a proving ground of 13,000 acres was established near Savannah.[14]

The SCD believed in retrospect that the greatest factor in the Illinois contribution to the war was the "uninterrupted social and industrial peace." With the exception of a few isolated disasters, among them the 1917 riot in East St. Louis, fewer strikes than normal occurred during this period. The SCD appointed a Labor Committee consisting of Walker, Dr. Frank Billings, and John H. Harrison which investigated the East St. Louis riot and came to the conclusion that it had resulted from the great influx of Blacks recruited by parties unknown. Walker served on President Wilson's Mediation Council, which helped to avert a strike among packing-house workers. The SCD appointed the Civilian Personnel Committee under the chairmanship of Charles A. Munroe for the purpose of cooperating with the U.S. Employment Service to find workers for war industries. The Labor Committee, under the chairmanship of Walker, whom Senator Lawrence Y. Sherman characterized as a "firebrand," was empowered to act as mediator of labor disputes. The free employment offices organized under the Illinois Department of Labor placed workers in war industries.[15]

Labor gained many benefits during the war, some by legislation such as the Adamson Act, which granted the eight-hour day to railway workers. Such benefits irritated employers. The operator of a brick factory protested to Senator Sherman about a proposal to shorten the hours of miners: "If miners' hours of labor are reduced, it will only be a question of time until the working hours in all industries will have to be adjusted to the same standard. If America is to keep her place as a leader among commercial nations of the world, she must increase her production rather than decrease it." Senator Sherman, always antilabor, agreed with the position and to constituents referred to the "weak-kneed" attitude of Congress toward labor. Sherman advocated the conscription of labor to thwart strikes.[16]

Partly because of advances in pay and working conditions, there were fewer strikes. Labor accepted to some degree the idea that they were partners in the war effort and accepted the patriotic propaganda aimed in their direction. Governor Lowden, at a luncheon honoring Theodore Roosevelt, said, "This is not a war of capital; it is not a war of labor; it is a war of all the people against autocracy in government. Surely, when our very future as a nation is at stake, there must be hearty cooperation between those who employ, on the one hand, and those who are employed, on the other." Barney Cohen, director of the Department of Labor, said,

"We must resist, as a single man, any attempt to saddle the Germanic system of labor economics upon free and enlightened America." Samuel Gompers, president of the American Federation of Labor, in a speech in Chicago called for citizens "to stand by our cause and our gallant Allies until the world has been made safe for freedom, for justice, for democracy, for humanity."[17]

Citizens of Illinois were bombarded with pleas to buy government bonds during this period. There were four separate "liberty loan" campaigns during the war and a victory loan after it was over. These bond issues, most tax-exempt, were oversubscribed. As another device to raise money, "thrift stamps" were sold. These were designed for people who were too poor to buy bonds. By calling them "thrift stamps" it was possible to appeal to the puritan ethic, and political leaders constantly labored to achieve total involvement of all citizens in the war effort. Governor Lowden spoke of the desirability of forming "habits of thrift" and closed his statement with the remark that this was "the people's war" in which the lowliest person could help by the purchase of the "thrift stamps." These constituted the political and patriotic equivalent of the "widow's mite" of the churches. No effort was spared to involve every citizen in the war.[18]

The SCD created a Women's Committee to provide women with "an opportunity for patriotic service at home or abroad." Some real benefits grew out of this, such as the move for day-care centers for the use of increasing numbers of mothers in industry. The committee also lobbied for a child labor law and aided in the placement of women who wished to work. The committee's Americanization Department endeavored to "awaken" in immigrant people the desire for conformity in American speech and principles, and its subcommittee on Colored Women placed black women in industry and worked to improve their efficiency and establish day-care nurseries for their children.[19]

The Women's Committee also conducted a recreation program, promoted community singing and the "Liberty Chorus," and organized a Speakers' Bureau, under the chairmanship of Janet Kellogg Fairbank. Some 315 women enrolled to tell women's groups how they could help win the war. The speeches were patriotic in nature, some interpreting the war. Speakers also told their audiences of various functions of the Women's Committee, how to conserve fuel, clothing, and food, and discussed the role of movies, art, and posters in the war effort. Several speeches promoted the bond issue and thrift.[20]

The SCD developed a number of programs for the welfare of soldiers, including the War Recreation Board, which maintained a clubhouse in Chicago for dances and theatrical entertainment. In addition, it cooperated with other organizations in their own wartime endeavors. The War Service Committee of the American Library Association supplied reading material to soldiers in the various training camps as well as overseas. The Salvation Army maintained canteen service at railway stations, and their Army-Navy Club provided sleeping quarters for servicemen. The Jewish Welfare Board showed motion pictures, organized recreational activities, and supplied stationary and newspapers. The YWCA boasted club and recreation facilities for servicemen. The Knights of Columbus provided recreational facilities, as did the YMCA. Many of these organizations, especially the Red Cross, provided facilities for women volunteers to make surgical dressings and supply other war needs. There were relief organizations for Lithuanians, French, Belgians, and Persians in Chicago.[21]

World War I marked the first massive, organized, official propaganda machine in the United States. Shortly after the declaration of war, President Wilson, by executive order, created the Committee on Public Information, under the chairmanship of the controversial George Creel, a veteran journalist. Creel became a very powerful man, recruiting top newspapermen (Lincoln Steffens, Irvin S. Cobb, Ray Stannard Baker, Ida Tarbell) literary people (including Booth Tarkington, Owen Wister, William Dean Howells, Fannie Hurst, Edna Ferber), and historians (led by Guy Stanton Ford) to develop propaganda for dissemination in schools and to the public. Artists also became involved, among them Charles Dana Gibson, who recruited still others to make posters and various visual representations. The Creel Committee went into the motion picture business as well, portraying the horrors of the alleged German militarism in theaters throughout the country. Some 75 million pamphlets, countless posters, and several full-length movies were distributed.[22]

President Wilson took the view that the war was the "grim business of the whole people." Thus, in the words of the Secretary of the Navy, Josephus Daniels, the purpose of the Creel Committee was the "mobilization of the mind of America." Efforts were made to present the American point of view and even to get antiwar materials into Germany, sometimes floating the leaflets in by balloons. George Creel denied that his agency engaged in censorship and asserted that it only sought to get truth to the people.[23]

In Illinois, as in the nation, authorities demanded conformity to the official view of the war. They represented the Allied cause as a holy one, designed to save freedom in the world, and the Germans as barbarians who were intent on bringing all people under the heel of military despotism. Several elder statesmen came to Illinois to promote the war, including Theodore Roosevelt, who came twice. Roosevelt reduced the issues to moralistic personal ones, and in Chicago urged the United States to do the "manly" thing. He believed that if a "ruffian" slapped a man's wife, the man must fight back and not expect someone else to avenge the insult. So as a nation, the United States must behave in the same fashion.[24] Later in the war Roosevelt, speaking in Springfield, attacked those who took an internationalist view, saying that just as no man could love another woman as he loved his wife, so the true patriot could not be an internationalist.[25] Former President Taft came to Springfield and proclaimed that an "evangel" ought to be preached proving the rightness of our position in the war. Taft described the Germans as "obsessed" and referred to the "cancer of militarism" and the "sin of Germany." Elihu Root, in Chicago, denied the right of discussion of the issues of the war. He asserted that once the proper authorities had made the decision for war, any opposing view was out of order.[26]

In the spirit of these pronouncements by national leaders, patriotic citizens of Illinois moved to bring the "message" to all citizens. One group so motivated was the "Four Minute Men," the brainchild of Donald Ryerson of the Chicago steel family. Ryerson presented his idea to a group of Chicagoans on April 2, 1917. The Four Minute Men, composed of volunteers and chartered by Illinois, delivered brief patriotic addresses at motion picture theaters throuthout the state. This was done with the support of the SCD, although the Four Minute Men were not a part of the official structure. Later the speeches were presented in church services and to fraternal groups and labor unions. The Four Minute Men promoted bond issues and aided in recruiting and, most important, urged the rightness of the cause. In Chicago some 451 speakers were enrolled, and similar records were made in some downstate cities.[27]

Another of the private groups that figured in the propaganda scene in Illinois was the National Security League, which dealt in an especially lurid kind of propaganda. The SDC thought well of the Chicago branch of the group and had its cooperation, but George Creel included it in his autobiography in a chapter entitled "High Priests of Hate." He noted, "A all times their patriotism was a thing of screams, violence and extremes and their savage intolerances had the burn of acid. From the first they leveled attacks against the foreign language groups, and were chiefly responsible for the development of a mob spirit in many sections. . . . They worked, of course in fertile ground, for there is a simplicity about hate that makes it attractive to a certain type of mind. It makes no demand on the mental processes, it does not require reading, estimate, or analysis, and by reason of its removal of doubt gives an effect of decision, a sense of well-being."[28]

The State Council of Defense promoted a massive patriotic propaganda campaign through its branches. Its Neighborhood Committees, headed by Harold Ickes, held mass meetings and distributed 220,000 pieces of patriotic literature and posters. Marguerite Jenison Pease, the historian of World War I in Illinois, described the most important function of the SCD: "To make the state a unit in the realization of the gravity of the situation and in the determination to prosecute the war to a successful conclusion." In 1917 the SCD urged universal public observation of the Fourth of July, and most communities added, to the usual patriotic observance, speeches on citizenship in time of war and on the causes of the war as seen by the Allies. The effort was broadened in 1918, when the goal was to change "the annual observance of the Fourth of July from an occasion of noise, frivolity and dissipation to one of high patriotic significance."[29]

In 1918 a war exposition was held in Grant Park featuring exhibits of fourteen carloads of captured war materials, as well as American war materials and exhibits by the Red Cross and various allied nations. Nearly 2 million people visited the exposition, which attempted to impart to the people the magnitude of the war.[30]

The SCD promoted a respectful attitude toward the national anthem and, urged on by citizens, discouraged the use of German in schools and churches. This last activity nearly ended the formal teaching of German. Governor Lowden, in a particularly chauvinistic statement, told the National Education Association, "The idea and the printed word are closely allied. You do not get the true American spirit if you are educated in a foreign tongue. The English tongue is the language of liberty, of self government and of orderly progress under the law."[31]

Authorities held a conference of newspaper editors to urge their cooperation, patriotism was made a part of the school curriculum, and the University of Illinois was mobilized to teach a course called "War Issues" in which the history, political science, economics, and

English departments participated to show "the moral superiority of the Allies." Traveling representatives of the French, British, Rumanian, Belgian, and other national groups made their way through Illinois, wined and dined to the echo of uplifting speeches on the rightness of the cause. The net result of the massive propaganda campaign was the greatest outburst of patriotism that the United States had ever known. Doubtless a massive effort was necessary to win the war, but it must be recognized that much of this was misdirected and resulted in an oppressive atmosphere. In retrospect it is tempting to say with Ralph Waldo Emerson: "When a whole nation is roaring patriotism at the top of its voice, I am fain to explore the cleanness of its hands and purity of its heart."[32]

In spite of all of this pro-Allied propanganda, opinion in Illinois was less than unanimous. Many German-Americans believed the German cause was one of survival and that Germany was a peace-loving nation victimized by the false propaganda of the Allies. This view was pronounced widely in the German-language press in Illinois, and just before the declaration of war, a delegation of twenty-five prominent German-Americans from Chicago went to Washington to persuade President Wilson not to take the side of the Allies.[33]

Others opposed the war as a matter of conscience, believing the taking of human life wrong under any circumstances. Jane Addams frequently delivered an address entitled "Patriotism and Pacifists in War Time" in which she asserted the right to speak against killing in time of war as in time of peace. It was difficult for the Establishment to attack the genteel Addams, but the fear and loathing that was directed at radical groups for their economic view made them desirable targets on any ground. The socialists and Internation Workers of the World traditionally believed that war was the chief curse of capitalism and one of its tools in the plot against workers. Mayor William H. Thompson opposed the war, presumably to woo the German-American voters who were his regular supporters. Congressman William E. Mason opposed the war as a pacifist of long standing.[34]

Several pieces of federal legislation dealt with the question of criticism of the war effort and the government of the United States. The Selective Service Act provided penalties for interference with the draft and arrests were made under this provision throughout the country. On June 15, 1917, Congress passed the Sedition Act, which provided for heavy penalties for interfering with the war effort or troup recruiting, or inciting mutiny or disloyalty. The

Congress strengthened this law on May 16, 1918, in the Espionage Act, which prohibited "uttering, printing, writing, or publishing any disloyal, profane, scurrilous, or abusive language or language intended to cause contempt, scorn, contumely or disrepute as regards the form of government of the United States," the Constitution, the flag, the uniform of the Army and Navy, or "any language intended to incite resistance to the United States or promote the cause of its enemies."[35]

Many states passed their own laws against sedition or advocating the overthrow of the government. In Illinois, the general assembly passed such an act after the war was over. By 1919 the fear of radical groups had fed on the intolerance bred during the war, and on June 28 of that year the Illinois law was approved, by which it became illegal "by word of mouth or writing" to advocate reformation or overthrow of the government, or to publish any book, or join any organization that did so. It became a crime to be present at any meeting or provide a meeting place for any group that so advocated. Displaying any flag or symbol of such a movement also became a crime. The law provided penalties of one to ten years in prison for the sections of the act deemed to be a felony and fines of $500 to $1,000 and up to a year in jail for those sections that were misdemeanors. The problem with such laws was that no matter what the intent of the legislation, enforcement in a judicial and equitable fashion was difficult in a time of national hysteria. The national legislation could be excused on grounds of national interest during wartime, although there were many injustices committed, but the Illinois law was enacted seven months after the Armistice. This seems to indicate that the legislature sought to capitalize on the hate and fear engendered by the war to eliminate the dissenting voices of the radicals, who posed a threat to established interests.[36]

Radical political groups, never numerous, aroused distaste but little violence prior to the war. The Socialist party, founded in 1901 by Eugene Debs and others, consisted of Marxists who believed the elimination of capitalism was the only way to end monopoly and the inequities of American democracy. The party reached its peak in membership and influence from 1910 to 1912. Like most radical groups, it was plagued with factionalism between those who wanted to avoid extreme measures and those who thought the demands were too mild. Leaders such as Morris Hillquit regarded the movement as evolutionary and believed there was no place in it for revolutionaries, stating that "Socialism has come to build, not to destroy." Members were expected to spend time promoting the party by distributing literature or conducting street-corner meetings. The party was always impoverished. Seymour Stedman, a Chicago attorney, borrowed money to help, and Theodore Debs once pawned his watch to aid the cause. The editor of the *Social Democratic Herald* moved the paper to Belleville to save money.[37]

The Industrial Workers of the World was founded in Chicago, seedbed of radical groups in the early years of the twentieth century. The IWW frightened the established interests more than any other group. The founding convention met in Brand's Hall on Chicago's Near North Side on June 27, 1905, and included 200 workers who represented forty trades or industries. Among the leaders were Daniel De Leon, Eugene Debs, and William D. Haywood. Haywood, who had gone to work in the mines at age nine, represented the Western Federation of Miners and was given the honor of the convention chairmanship. Using a piece of board for a gavel, Haywood opened the convention with the greeting "Fellow Workers." Many Illinois figures were prominent in the convention. When Eugene Debs rose to speak, he was flanked on one side by Lucy Parsons and on the other by Mary "Mother" Jones.[38]

The *Record Herald* called the meeting "Eugene V. Deb's convention" and headed their editorial "The Class Yawp." It insisted that the true way was through trade unionism rather than industrial unionism and proclaimed, "The class yawp will not be approved even by the sane socialists." The *Tribune* reported that Debs rejected the trade union concept and called for an organization "based on the class struggle." The convention noisily applauded A. M. Simons, editor of the *International Socialist Review*, as he said: "The proletariat of America stands ready to grasp any weapon, the ballot, the strike, the boycott, and the bullet, if necessary." By such rhetoric, the IWW was born in an atmosphere calculated to inspire the fear and hatred of industrialists and governments who were sensitive to the demands of business interests. By 1908 the IWW had borrowed words such as "sabotage" from the French syndicalist movement. These words inflamed the passions of the propertied classes as their fear for their possessions grew.[39]

Radical groups opposed war in general, and their methods seemed to impede the war effort. Thus it was easy during wartime to cloak repressive measures in patriotic fervor. Congress passed the conscription law with many misgivings because there had been no draft since the Civil War, and Americans had boasted that one of her freedoms was the absence of a conscription law. Many immigrants had fled Europe to escape military service in countries that were counted as monarchical despotisms by Americans. Jane Addams, watching Hull House immigrants register for the draft, wrote that these people faced "the final frontier of the hopes of their kind, the traditional belief in America as a refuge had come to an end. . . . All that had been told them of American freedom, which they had hoped to secure for themselves and their children, had turned to ashes." Many immigrants, counting on American freedom, had joined radical labor or political groups. Now they seemed threatened by the very thing that had caused them to immigrate, and some resisted the draft. Thus, even though these labor and political groups had taken no official stand on the war or the draft, it was easy for those who wanted to destroy a group such as the IWW to make the claim that such groups were disloyal to the United States.[40]

The first massive arrests came in Rockford as a group of men, alleged to be members of the IWW, marched and demonstrated against the draft, outraging the town's patriots. Upon instructions of the U.S. district attorney, the police arrested Clyde Hough, secretary of the IWW local, and Eric Swenson and Otto Pearson, both reputed to be IWW members. By the following day mass arrests of more than 100 had been made on charges of refusing to register. Women besieged the jails to seek information about their missing husbands. The *Rockford Register Gazette* proclaimed: "Every man who is not on the side of the government is against it. The demands of loyalty call for prompt compliance with whatever is necessary to win this war and to drive it with utmost efficiency and force. The plain truth is that there is no place in Rockford for traitors or slackers. If any young man has so far failed to comprehend the crisis the time for doing so is here. Line up or take the penalty."[41]

Ultimately the jails in Rockford and nearby Belvidere and Freeport were filled. Investigations were carried out by local police, District Attorney Charles F. Clyne, U.S. marshals, and Commissioner Lewis F. Mason. Some of those arrested were found to be registered, some too old or too young for the draft. These were released or fined for disorderly conduct for their part in the parade. A federal grand jury met in Freeport to investigate antidraft activity. The *Rockford Register Gazette* reported insults to the American flag, the waving of a red flag, and the singing of IWW songs in the jails. Eventually the grand jury indicted 134 "slackers." Bond for Clyde Hough, Emil Strom, and Earl Cully, charged with conspiracy, was set at $25,000, while the others were held on $1,000 bond. The Rockford police took advantage of the disarray to run several characters out of town, thereby "cleansing the city of representatives of the loafer class." Tension mounted as a tin box containing thirty-five sticks of dynamite was found in an alley.[42]

Judge Kenesaw Mountain Landis presided over the U.S. district court in the mass trial of the accused draft evaders. Referring to the defendants as "whining, belly-aching puppies," Judge Landis sentenced 117 men, 62 of them aliens, to a year and a day at hard labor in the Chicago House of Correction with the provision that they were subject to the draft upon release. Subsequently when their sentences had been served, 37 of the aliens were deported on grounds that they were guilty of "moral turpitude." The immigration bureau said failure to register was a "vicious and grave" offense.[43]

The enforcement of the Selective Service Act, and the allied problems of handling conscientious objectors and hunting for deserters, was a major problem throughout the war. The American Protective League, working with state and federal authorities, constituted a secret police. Asa M. Briggs, a Chicago figure, proposed the idea to Hinton Clabaugh, chief of the Federal Bureau of Investigation in Chicago. Approved by the FBI in Washington, many communities organized branches of the APL to look into draft evasion, desertion, espionage, and other unpatriotic acts. As Secretary of the Treasury McAdoo doubtfully pointed out, anyone with the price of dues in the organization could become an "operative." After the war, Emerson Hough, a Chicago-based professional writer, described the purpose of the APL as dealing with "Bolseviki, socialists, incendiaries, I. W. W.'s, Lutheran treason-talkers, Russellites, Bergerites, all the other-ites, religious and social fanatics, third-sex agitators, long haired visionaries and work haters from every race in the world." "Operatives" of the APL participated in most investigations of violations of war legislation, gathering information and presenting evidence in many of the cases. There was also a committee of the SCD in each county. As the military reported desertions in a given county, these groups would watch the deserters' homes to make sure that they did not return and report them if they did. Conscientious objectors were held at Camp Grant in what was popularly called "the leper colony."[44]

It was not long until the Socialist party felt the sting of antiwar hysteria. On September 5, 1917, the Department of Justice raided their headquarters in Chicago, seized records and literature, sent the office force home, and refused them the right to send out their mail. The mailing privilege of the *American Socialist* had already been canceled and the September raid forced cancellation of publication. The mailing privilege was canceled because postal officials objected to an advertisement for an antiwar pamphlet entitled "The Price We Pay." Adolph Germer, executive secretary of the party, wired Senator Lawrence Y. Sherman, reporting the raid and pleading, "In the name of Justice and the Democracy and Liberty for which the administration claims to be conducting this war, we appeal to you to bring this Rape of Americanism to the attention of Congress." Sherman unsympathetically suggested resort to the courts.[45]

Subsequently authorities in Chicago arrested and brought to trial Adolph Germer, Louis Engdahl, Reverend Irwin St. John Tucker, and Victor Berger on charges of conspiracy to obstruct the war under the Espionage Act. The *Tribune* referred to the guilty verdict, arrived at after the end of the war, as "a sweeping victory for the government in its fight against the 'red flag' and the seditious propagandists." The jury listened to the evidence for five weeks and took three ballots to convict. Engdahl edited the *American Socialist,* Tucker was a socialist clergyman, and Berger, a Milwaukee politician, had just been elected to Congress. Berger remarked, "It seems to be the historic fate of every ruling class to dig its own grave." U.S. Attorney Clyne, on the other hand, declared: "This verdict is but America's voice speaking. It is a verdict of this country's people. It is a death blow to Bolshevism which this five advocated, and to the 'red flag.' This jury has said that there can be but one flag in this country, the red, white, and blue, and that those who are not with this country are against it." Debs was arrested and tried for an antiwar speech made in Canton, Ohio. Debs, refusing to defend himself on technicalities, was sentenced to ten years in prison, but the others arrested with him, although convicted, had their sentences set aside on appeal because of technicalities.[46]

Similarly on September 5, 1917, authorities raided the headquarters of the IWW in Rockford and other cities around the country, seizing papers, books, reports, and even office furniture.

On September 28, Clyne obtained an indictment from the grand jury charging 166 leaders of the IWW with various crimes, notably of "felonious conspiracy" by sabotage and otherwise to prevent manufacturers from producing materials of war, by encouraging members to resist entry into the armed forces, of depriving manufacturers of their constitutional rights by preventing them from selling arms to the United States, of causing insubordination, disloyalty and refusal of duty in the armed forces, by cheating their employers by receiving money as wages while having the secret purpose "to render inefficient service, and to purposely assist in producing bad and unmarketable products and intentionally to retard, slacken and reduce production whenever employed, and intentionally to restrict and decrease the profits of said employers and interfere with and injure their trade and business, and secretly and covertly to injure, break up and destroy the property of said employers; and that they would teach, incite, induct, aid and abet other members so to do." The IWW achieved these ends, according to the indictment, by distribution through the post office of newspapers like *Solidarity* and books like Elizabeth Gurley Flynn's *Sabotage.*[47]

Although a minority of the membership favored action opposing the war, the IWW never took an official stand against it. Of the general executive board, only Frank Little stood for opposition to the war, and he was murdered four months after it began. Haywood believed opposition would bring persecution and divert the workers from the class struggle which he held paramount. But in carrying out their traditional program with the usual weapons —strike, boycott, and sabotage—they could hinder the war effort, and doubtless most citizens believed the IWW was antiwar and hence, in the popular mind, pro-German. Officially the IWW regarded the indictments as part of a "general reign of terror" whose goal was "to enslave the working class with the interest of a profit-mad coterie of industrial pirates."[48]

In substance the charges involved alleged conspiracy to violate the Selective Service Act, Espionage Act, and to use the mails to defraud. Judge Landis presided over the trial and threw out the count which had to do with using the mails to defraud. John Reed portrayed Judge Landis: "Small on the huge bench sits a wasted man with untidy white hair, and emaciated face in which two burning eyes are set like jewels, parchment-like skin split by a crack for a mouth; the face of Andrew Jackson three years dead." Choosing a jury was difficult because the prosecution wanted to make sure that no one of socialist leaning got on the jury. In the midst of the jury selection process, the prosecution charged jury tampering, Judge Landis discharged the whole panel, and they started over. Bond for Haywood was set at $25,000 initially but was later reduced to $15,000, which was guaranteed by William Bross Lloyd, Jacob Brunning, and George Kohler. Bond for the others was set at lesser amounts.[49]

The IWW charged harassment throughout the trial. They alleged their mail was being held up and quoted Senator King of Utah as saying this was done to prevent contributions for the defense from reaching them. In the trial, attorneys for the IWW tried to show that the union and its methods were the products of a dislocated social system that brought low wages, long hours, and hard working conditions. Judge Landis rejected this evidence, saying the American system was not on trial. Attorney George Vanderveer managed to elicit such information from many of the witnesses. Haywood cited contrasts of wealth and poverty and the "wage slavery" in mines and mills. Defense attorneys produced evidence to show that the IWW literature which could be construed as antiwar had not been circulated after the war began, and that, at worst, Haywood's attitude was that the war was no concern of the IWW. They brought out that sons of IWW members were fighting in France, and that many members worked in munition factories or loaded munitions on ships. Other witnesses testified to the general good character of the membership. Walter Nef testified that 80 percent of the freight handled at the Philadelphia docks consisted of war materials for the Allies and that there had been no strikes, fires, or other trouble. Haywood testified that sabotage did not always mean destruction of property but could consist of withholding of labor. The prosecution sought to break down this line of attack by insisting that the IWW promoted violence, revolution, destruction of property, and lessening of patriotism and that it aided antiwar activities.[50]

The trial dragged on for over four months, but the jury took only fifty-five minutes to find the defendants guilty. Haywood said Landis had conducted a fair trial and praised his bail policy in letting the defendants free on recognizance bonds. Landis sentenced the defendants to prison terms of up to twenty years and imposed fines of $5,000 to $20,000. Total fines levied amounted to $2,500,000, more than the defendants would earn in their working lives. The IWW leaders lost their appeals. A great psychological blow to the IWW occurred when Haywood, their trusted and beloved leader, jumped bail and fled to Russia. Money had to be raised to pay his bond, and although opinion was divided, there was bitterness toward Haywood, who, drunk and lonely, died in

1928 in Moscow.[51] The trial brought decline to the IWW because of the loss of leadership. In June, 1923, President Harding offered to commute the sentences of those still in jail but under circumstances which some could not accept because acceptance would imply guilt. Near the end of 1923, however, President Coolidge granted unconditional commutation for all wartime prisoners.[52]

The authorities were also concerned about an organization known as the Peoples Council of America for Democracy and Peace, a loose coalition of various pacifist forces. Founded by Louis P. Lochner, the group included a number of well-known radicals such as Scott Nearing, Morris Hillquit, and former Senator John D. Works. Nearing, chairman of the executive committee, said that by the time of the declaration of war by the United States, the People's Council represented 800,000 citizens (although this figure seems high). In any case, the membership had grown and become vocal enough to worry the administration. George Creel is supposed to have described the group as composed of "traitors and fools" and to have said, "we are fighting it to the death."[53]

In Chicago, the Peoples Council included such people as Seymour Stedman, socialist, Alderman John Kennedy, the Reverend Irwin St. John Tucker, Congressman William E. Mason, Professor Robert Morss Lovett of the University of Chicago, Arthur Fisher, son of President Taft's Secretary of War, Jane Addams and Mary McDowell, settlement-house workers, and the Reverend Jenkin Lloyd-Jones. Lovett reported that as the press became more hostile, their support and leadership evaporated. The group scheduled a meeting for May 27, 1917, in the Auditorium Theater. Almost by default Lovett was designated chairman of the meeting. He made every effort to insist that the meeting only called for a clarification of peace aims. The organization demanded a democratic peace which included no annexations, no indemnities, free development of all nationalities, an international organization for maintenance of world peace, a statement of peace goals, repeal of the Selective Service Act, and safeguard of the interests of labor. The meeting at the Auditorium was packed and the overflow crowd spread across Michigan Avenue into Grant Park. After the meeting Chicago police cracked heads in Grant Park and arrested several persons, none of them in the leadership of the meeting. Although the demands of the group sounded remarkably like President Wilson's Fourteen Points, the meeting was denounced and its participants were labeled traitors.

Lovett, whose son would soon die fighting in France, was singled out for special ridicule and hanged in effigy in front of his apartment house. The Reverend Frank Gunsaulus, preacher to the rich, speaking earlier in the day at the Auditorium, proclaimed, "If you approve of the shooting of Edith Cavell, the English nurse, attend the meeting. If you disapprove the sinking of the *Lusitania*, stay away. If you prefer to have the Hohenzollerns dictate terms at Washington instead of having President Wilson dictate, attend the meeting. As for me, I will promise to have this house fumigated before we hold services here next Sunday morning. The meeting this afternoon is as unpatriotic as a meeting in 1776 would have been to ask terms of peace in place of reading the Declaration of Independence."[54]

In late 1917 the Peoples Council scheduled a great national meeting in Minneapolis. Forbidden to meet in Minnesota by the governor, the group turned to Chicago, where Mayor Thompson said, "Pacifists are law-abiding citizens. I shall not have it spread broadcast that Chicago denies free speech to anyone." The meeting of the council (called "a society of antiwar cranks" by Mrs. Lowden) was scheduled for September 1. Governor Lowden, notified of the meeting by the National Security League, called the chief of police in Chicago and ordered him to break up the meeting. The executive committee of the council met and was dispersed. Seymour Stedman and others demanded to be arrested as a test case, but the police refused. Lowden had no legal right to give orders to the Chicago police and Mayor Thompson protested, only to be denounced by the Chicago press and to be hanged in effigy by the Veterans of Foreign Wars. Lowden, cheered by the crowds for his actions, proclaimed, "The People's Council is a treasonable conspiracy which must not find refuge under the guarantee of freedom of speech. If we lose this war, all of us will be lost. Freedom of speech in Illinois can not be used as a cloak for treason."

The principal session of the meeting was held the following day, September 2, in Chicago's West Side Auditorium. With Mayor Thompson back in control of his police, Governor Lowden sent four companies of the National Guard to break up the meeting. Rabbi Judah L. Magnes of New York addressed the council, and they also listened to Congressman Mason as he said, "No worse thing ever happened in the history of the United States than is happening now when people like you are branded as criminals and denied the right of free assembly." The council hurriedly adopted a platform calling for disarmament, repeal of the draft law, a statement of war aims, and peace without annexation or indemnity. The meeting adjourned before Lowden's troops arrived, avoiding a confrontation.[55]

Like organized groups that did not agree with the official view of the war, individuals were also attacked. One such victim was John L. Metzen, an IWW attorney from Chicago, who was tarred and feathered by agents of the American Protective League in downstate Staunton. The *Tribune* took the view that the act was one of "zealous Americanism" which was wrong only in that it would give Metzen "the opportunity to pose as a martyr." Near Havana a party of fifteen armed men attacked the home of Edmund Speckman, a former high school athlete of German parentage who was reported to have said in a poolroom that he would avoid the draft and to have made other unpatriotic remarks. Marie Klein, a nurse and enemy alien, was held on $2,000 bond in Chicago because she said that "the United States Liberty Bonds will be no good after the war."[56]

Enemy aliens also had a bad time. Authorities kept a close watch on German churches and organizations. In some cases, Germans suspected of disloyalty were required to keep an American flag flying outside their homes to avoid prosecution and German children were singled out to salute the flag. In East St. Louis, Judge Daniel Maddox of Litchfield kicked a hole in the bass drum of a German band because he disapproved of the way they played the national anthem. Perhaps the most shameful episode was the lynching of Robert Paul Praeger in Collinsville. Praeger, a German, had had difficulty with the United Mine Workers; when he was taken into protective custody by the police to save him from the miners, the rumor spread that the police had arrested a spy. A mob hanged Praeger, and although the identity of the leaders was known, none were convicted. Praeger apparently was not a spy, and the incident was denounced by many, including Governor Lowden.[57]

The Armistice ending the fighting in Europe finally arrived in the early morning hours of November 11, 1918, in Illinois. Citizens rang bells, blew whistles, and paraded in their job. This was followed by speechmaking and parading of returning military units. The Arts Club of Chicago, under the leadership of Janet Kellogg Fairbank and Mrs. John Alden Carpenter, put on a pageant celebrating the end of the war. Included in the pageant was Russia, represented by Mrs. Carpenter. Russia was recognized in the pageant by the society ladies of Chicago but was not much welcomed anywhere else. The Russian Revolution had taken place in the winter of 1917–18, and already conservatives were beginning to fret about this new "red" threat. Most citizens made little distinction between one left-wing group and another, seeing no difference between the IWW the Socialists, the communists of Russia, or the recent enemy, the Germans. Gradually the intolerance born of the war blossomed into a new kind of hatred, commonly called the great red scare. This transition happened so casually that most citizens were probably unaware that the momentum of war patriotism was now redirected at the new fear, the new threat to the well being of the rich and the comfortable.[58]

One of the organizations which fed on the red scare was the American Legion, created in 1919 by veterans of the war. Representatives of military units met in Paris in March, 1919, to lay plans for a veterans' organization. Another group met in St. Louis in May, and 112 delegates from Illinois met to set up a state group. The first state convention was held in Peoria on October 17–18, 1919. Illinois was divided into eleven districts. The intention of the group was to "kill radicalism by spreading Americanism." This was to be accomplished by a massive program of lectures by prominent citizens, historical pageants and exhibits, publication of books, motion pictures, patriotic sermons, and newspaper editorials. The campaign was directed "not only among the foreign-born but among all classes." The group was endorsed by both houses of the general assembly.[59]

Reference has been made elsewhere to the connection between the Farm Bureau and the red scare, but the group that capitalized most on the intolerance of the red scare was the Ku Klux Klan. The Klan, revived in 1915, flourished on whatever the local bigots would pay for. In some areas the Klan was anti-Semitic and in others anti-Black. In downstate Illinois it pushed hardest on the anti-Catholic theme and proclaimed its super-patriotism, supporting Protestant church groups, which they viewed as native American and untainted by "foreign" Catholicism. A common tactic of the Klan was to interrupt a church service by marching down the center aisle in full regàlia and hand the clergyman a donation—often $30—with a note of approval for the church activity. On December 3, 1922, a group of local Klansmen carried out this charade at the West Side Church of the Nazarene in Chicago, closing their note with "Yours for God, our country, our homes and each other." A district church official stood and said,

"We as a church do not oppose the Ku Klux Klan. As far as I know, it is a patriotic organization and has a good place in this day and age. The Nazarines fight only sin and the devil." On May 20, 1923, a similar episode occurred in the First Christian Church of Marion. There the letter of the Klan described the belief of the organization as "the tenets of the Christian religion; protection of pure womanhood; just law and liberty; absolute upholding of the Constitution of the United States; free public schools; free speech; free press and law and order." The clergyman said, "That tells you whether they are all right. They stand for something good."[60]

It is hard to attack a group who noisily proclaims such principles, but thoughtful persons questioned why the Klansman chose to appear robed and masked. While some politicians and clergymen quaked before the Klan, some citizens noted that lynching, murder, arson, beating, and mutilation were often cloaked in worthy principles as the reign of terror spread across the nation. In Illinois the Klan became a power in politics as they organized on the precinct level in East St. Louis and elected mayors in Paris and Decatur. In time the Klan established 287 local organizations, or Klaverns. One of the largest was in Urbana, where they were permitted to hold a huge meeting in the armory at the University of Illinois when the "Imperial Wizard" came to town. In Chicago twenty organizations claimed 100,000 members and another 100,000 in the suburbs. The Chicago Klan published a periodical entitled: *Dawn: A Journal for True American Patriots.*[61]

By 1919, with the IWW and the Socialist party leadership under fire and with many in jail or exile, the radical movement was in disarray. Many persons, disillusioned with the lack of progress in human and economic conditions, turned from earlier positions to support the brand of communism that had come to the fore in Russia in the Revolution of 1917–18. Lincoln Steffens, disillusioned with progressivism and the prospect for reform by the middle class, made two trips to Russia and came back a convert. Steffens provided an epigram that was converted into a propaganda phrase by the communists. To his friend, sculptor Jo Davidson, Steffens said of his trip to Russia, "I have been over into the future and it works." Corrupted into "I have seen the future and it works," the phrase served the communist cause for years.[62]

John Reed, Harvard-educated journalist, and Robert Minor, newspaper cartoonist of old native stock, became promoters of the cause. Trade unionists such as Chicago leader William Z. Foster became disenchanted with traditional labor methods and became communists. So did Max Eastman and Floyd Dell, the literary critic. Many immigrants like Benjamin Gitlow, William Wolf Weinstone, and Jay Lovestone brought European traditions into the movement. Among the Illinois leaders were William Bross Lloyd, Isaac Ferguson (lawyer), Abraham Stoklitsky (of the Russian Federation), and trade unionists such as painters Arne Swabeck and Jack Johnstone, steamfitter Charles Krumbein, machinist Andrew Overgaard, and Earl Browder, editor of the *Labor Herald*.[63]

The Socialist party held their convention in Chicago in August, 1919. The radicals divided on the question of whether to try to take over the old group or to separate and form a new one. The group desiring to take over the old organization, led by John Reed and Benjamin Gitlow, faced a massive security system set up by the moderates. The group caucused at Machinist Hall and agreed to force their way into the convention. They were seated in the hall the following morning when Adolph Germer, executive secretary of the Socialist party, had them ejected by the police amid cries that Germer was using the capitalist police against Socialists. The radicals, including most of the native American communists, moved to IWW Hall to form the Communist Labor party, electing Alfred Wagenknect as secretary.[64]

At the same time, the separatist group was meeting in Chicago at the Smolny Institute at 1221 Blue Island Avenue to form the Communist party. This group elected Charles Ruthenberg executive secretary and Louis Fraina as editor of publications. Chicago was the national headquarters of the party until 1927, when it was moved to New York. The official party paper was the *Communist*, edited by Fraina. The Communist party, favored by the eastern European ethnic groups, claimed to represent 58,000 persons, while the Communist Labor party claimed 30,000 members. Government agents closely watched the new organizations, and during the organizational meeting police broke in to tear down the radical decorations, including pictures of Lenin, Marx, and Trotsky, to the strains of the "Internationale" played by a brass band. Photographs were taken and agents made notes of the happenings of the convention.[65]

As fear of radical doctrines grew, most people identified these ideas with foreigners. The remedy consisted of deportation of aliens under the Alien Act or trial on grounds of sedition under federal or state law. The most spectacular deportation came with the eviction of 249 Russians transported on the *Buford* to Russia on December 21, 1919. President Wilson's attorney general, A. Mitchell Palmer, began plans for a wider operation. By late 1919, about half of the effort of the Federal Bureau of Investigation was directed at radical activities. Recently promoted from file clerk in the Library to Congress, J. Edgar Hoover got his start in investigation as head of the antiradical bureau of the FBI. Palmer conceived the idea of a nationwide, concerted, swift raid on all known radicals in their meeting places and homes. In cooperation with the Labor Department and the Commissioner of Immigration, the Department of Justice instructed agents to move at 8:30 P.M. on January 2, 1920, in all districts to arrest all known members of the Communist party and the Communist Labor party. The instructions called for the arrest of members and seizure of membership cards, charters of local groups, literature, books, papers, and pictures. Agents were instructed to sound walls but not to take money or jewelry from suspects. "Reasonable care and judgment" were mandated, but there was no mention of the use of search or arrest warrants.[66]

In Chicago the operation did not go according to the scenario. The state's attorney of Cook County, McClay Hoyne, could not abide letting A. Mitchell Palmer get all of the glory and credit as the chief enemy of the reds. Said to have been subsidized by the chamber of commerce or State Street merchants, Hoyne broadened the effort and included the IWW for another round of arrests. Claiming lack of cooperation of the federal authorities and noisily alleging that radicals were tipped off by federal agents, Hoyne moved a day early, sending out police and private detectives on January 1, 1920, at 4 P.M. Hoyne described the Justice Department as "petty, pusillanimous, and pussyfoot."[67]

Hoyne's agents raided the Communist party headquarters, the Communist Labor Hall, the IWW Hall, the German IWW, the North Side Syndicalist Club, the headquarters of the Russian Anarchists, and as many as 300 other meeting places, radical bookstores, and homes. Press estimates of the number arrested ranged from 150 to 200. Quantities of literature were seized at various headquarters, bookstores, and print shops. The Justice Department replied to Hoyne's charge of a tip-off as preposterous.[68]

The federal raids, under the direction of Edward J. Brennan, FBI superintendent, and John T. Creighton, special assistant attorney general sent out from Washington, began in Illinois as scheduled on January 2. Another group of 200 radicals was rounded up in Chicago by federal authorities. Some aliens were turned over to immigration authorities, while citizens were held for grand jury action. Raids also took place in Rockford, Moline, and East St. Louis. Eventually 183 were arrested in Rockford, 1 in Moline, and 6 in East St. Louis. Most of those arrested had names that were obviously eastern European, with a sprinkling of Scandanavians included. In Rockford, great attention was focused on the arrest of Alice Beal Parson, "prominent club woman and social leader," along with an alderman and a local physician. In Moline, authorities arrested Edgar Ownes, alleged to be the secretary of the Communist party in Illinois. In Chicago attention was focused on a few big names. William D. Haywood was arrested again, as was William Bross Lloyd. The usual bales of literature and correspondence were seized.[69]

Reaction was mixed. The *Rockford Register Gazette* wrote approvingly of the deportation proceedings: "There is no place in Rockford or anywhere else to this nation for the disgruntled subject of a foreign flag who seeks to spread his anarchistic doctrines through America. If they don't like this country and are not willing to give honest effort in return for the opportunities they find here, the sooner they go back across the waters, the better it will be for all concerned." The *Chicago Tribune* believed deportation of a few would be ineffectual, "like drawing off pus from an infection." The *Decatur Herald* saw the whole movement as a "plank in the platform of a number of aspiring statesmen," appealing to citizens who "find talking with their mouths far easier than thinking with their heads." The *Herald* concluded their editorial, "Fool notions can be taken out of the heads of 'Reds' by hanging them or by educating them. Why not give education a chance?"[70]

Nationally the "Palmer Raids" were among the most disgraceful episodes of American history. In May, 1920, twelve distinguished attorneys, including Roscoe Pound, Felix Frankfurter, and Ernst Freund, reported to the American people upon this assault on civil liberty. They described the illegal methods of the attorney general, including arrest without a warrant or other legal process, holding prisoners without access to friends, family, or counsel, entering homes and seizing property without search warrants. Further, they noted, "the Department of Justice has also constituted itself a propaganda bureau, and has sent to the newspapers and magazines of this country quantities of material designed to excite public opinion against radicals, all at the expense of the government and outside the scope of the Attorney General's duties." The lawyers went on to detail and document their case. They charged that both aliens and citizens had "been threatened, beaten with blackjacks, struck with fists, jailed under abominable conditions, or actually tortured." In Detroit, authorities held 130 to 140 prisoners in a room twenty-four by thirty feet for a week. The lawyers also protested the use of undercover agents and mass arrests without warrants. The lawyers closed their statement by noting that America has always boasted that it is a government of laws, not men, and noting that revolutions are caused by suppression and ruthlessness, not by the "simple rules of American law and American decency."[71]

In the midst of the fear, hatred, and intolerance of the Palmer Raids, twenty members of the Communist Labor party were indicted in Chicago on charges of violation of the Illinois Sedition Act. The trial lasted from June until August, 1920. The prosecution insisted that mere membership in the party was sufficient evidence of intent to carry out violent overthrow of the government. Included in the evidence was the text of the song "Red Flag" and a speech made by William Bross Lloyd before the act was passed. Clarence Darrow defended the radicals, but the conviction was almost a certainty when prosecutor Frank Comerford closed his lengthy and emotional summation by reciting all of the verses of the "Star Spangled Banner."[72]

The judge sentenced Lloyd and six others to the Joliet Penitentiary for from one to five years. Nine others were sentenced to one year in the Cook County Jail. The Illinois Supreme Court upheld the sentences with only Justice Orrin Carter dissenting. The U.S. Supreme Court refused to review the case. Lloyd and others began their sentences on November 21, 1922, but a week later were pardoned by Governor Len Small. Small cited the dissenting opinion of Justice Carter and commented that the provisions of the Sedition Act "were designed not so much, perhaps, to punish those who commit violent acts to overthrow the government, but rather it was drafted for the purpose of forbidding any person who held opinions distasteful to the majority of our citizens to express those opinions."[73]

Opinion varied widely as to the wisdom of Governor Small's action. Lloyd was part owner of the *Chicago Tribune,* which headed its story "Rich Red and 15 of his Pals Freed by Small." The *Decatur Herald* approved Small's pardon, saying, "It was not proved that these men had committed a single act of violence, violent as their opinions were. In this country, mere opinions, however much mistaken they may be, are not evidence of criminality." Small's mail was about equally divided on the issue.[74]

Dudley Field Malone complimented Small on his courage: ". . . every leader in these days who believes in free speech and free assembly as necessary to the functioning of our democracy, is bound to experience what you are going through now." Seymour Stedman approved the pardon, and one correspondent compared Small to Altgeld. The president of a building and loan company wrote, "I have been thinking for several days that I would write you a letter as a 100% American, free of this fanciful flub-dub and tyranny that is in the brains of a few prominent pukes of this country, for pardoning William Bross Lloyd and some other men. We have a few officials in this country who think they are the law, and that they should do the thinking for the people and trample down the constitution." Another wrote approvingly, "Americanism still lives." Most of the newly created American Legion posts passed resolutions condemning Small. The Oak Park Post 115 wrote that the pardon was an "insult to each and every man who served this country during the great war." The *Iowa Legionaire* said, "Governor Small has spit in the face of every veteran who has served."[75]

In World War I, Illinois responded well to the national crisis in service in the armed forces and production of food and war materials needed in the fight. Many made great sacrifices in life, health, and wealth. Few doubted or questioned the rightness of the cause. Illinois citizens illustrated all of the best qualities of the American people: loyalty, sacrifice for principle, purposefulness, tenacity, toughness of mind, and moral direction. On the other hand, the war set off waves of biogotry and intolerance never seen before. This element of the period illustrates the worst side of the American nation: fear, hatred, insecurity, violence, and materialism.

1. For the origins of the war, see S. B. Fay, *The Origins of the World War* (New York, 1928), or the more recent Laurence Lafore, *The Long Fuse: An Interpretation of the Origins of World War I* (Philadelphia, 1965). For the military developments see Cyril Falls, *The Great War* (New York, 1959).

2. A good short account of American involvement in the war is Daniel M. Smith, *The Great Departure* (New York, 1956).

3. William T. Hutchison, *Lowden of Illinois: The Life of Frank O. Lowden*, 2 vols. (Chicago, 1957), I, 328.

4. Marguerite Jenison, *The War-time Organization of Illinois* (Springfield, 1923), p. 1; *Laws of the State of Illinois Enacted by the Fiftieth General Assembly* (Springfield, 1917), p. 811; Ernest Ludlow Bogart and John Mabry Matthews, *The Modern Commonwealth 1893–1918* (Springfield, Ill., 1920), p. 457; Hutchison, *Lowden of Illinois*, I, 328.

5. *Congressional Record,* 65th Cong., 1 ses., part 1, vol. 3, (1917), p. 317.

6. Bogart and Matthews, *The Modern Commonwealth,* pp. 459, 474; *Congressional Record,* 65th Congressional, 1 ses., vol. 52, part 1 (1917), pp. 326–28.

7. Bogart and Matthews, *The Modern Commonwealth,* p. 474; Lloyd Wendt and Herman Kogan, *Big Bill of Chicago* (Indianapolis, 1953), pp. 149–60.

8. Jenison, *War Time-Organization,* pp. 29–34; Hutchison, *Lowden of Illinois,* I. 329. There are six boxes of papers relating to the State Council of Defense in the papers of John G. Oglesby in the Illinois State Historical Library.

9. Bogart and Matthews, *The Modern Commonwealth,* p. 461; Jenison, *War-Time Organization,* pp. 3, 82.

10. Jenison, *War-Time Organization,* pp. 4, 93, 99.

11. Ibid., pp. 31, 62, 117–42; *Chicago Tribune,* May 29, 1917, p. 7; July 12, 1917, p. 5.

12. *Final Report of the State Council of Defense of Illinois 1917–1918–1919* (Chicago, 1919), pp. 32, 38, 40–41 (referred to hereafter as *Final Report); Jenison, War-Time Organization,* pp. 224–29, 246–48.

13. Hutchison, *Lowden of Illinois,* I, 336; Jenison, *War-Time Organization,* p. 2.

14. *Final Report,* p. 65; Jenison, *War Time-Organization,* pp. 37, 289, 291, 310, 316, 320.

15. *Final Report,* p. 1; Laurence Y. Sherman to J. B. Berryman, Nov. 1, 1919, box 139, Sherman Papers, Illinois State Historical Library; Jenison, *War Time Organization,* p. 284.

16. E. F. Plumb to Sherman, Streator, Ill., Oct. 23, 1917, Sherman to Plumb, Oct. 27, 1919, and Sherman to W. A. Atkins, Oct. 22, 1919, box 139, Sherman Papers; Gordon S. Watkins, *Labor Problems and Administration during the World War* (Urbana, Ill., 1919), pp. 41–42.

17. Marguerite Jenison, *War Documents and Addresses* (Springfield, Ill., 1923), pp. 78, 121, 231.

18. Jenison, *War-Time Organization,* pp. 187–89, 209; Jenison, *War Documents and Addresses,* p. 213.

19. Jenison, *War-Time Organization,* pp. 22, 56, 66; *Final Report,* p. 146.

20. Jenison, *War-Time Organization,* pp. 49, 64, 119.

21. Ibid., pp. 325–55; *Final Report,* p. 64.

22. George Creel, *Rebel at Large, Recollections of Fifty Crowded Years* (New York, 1957), pp. 156–94.

23. Josephus Daniels, *The Wilson Era: Years of War and after 1917–1923* (Chapel Hill, N.C., 1946), pp. 224–26; Creel, *Rebel at Large,* p. 157.

24. Jenison, *War Documents and Addresses,* p. 24.

25. Ibid., p. 409.

26. Ibid., pp. 60, 82.

27. Jenison, *War-Time Organization,* p. 44; *Final Report,* p. 164. Ryerson took his plan to Washington and presented it to Creel, who was taken by this "rosy-cheeked youth" and his proposal. The Four Minute Men became a national group with a roster of 150,000 speakers. Creel, *Rebel at Large,* p. 162; *Final Report,* p. 30. Material for the speeches came from the national office and involved such topics as "Unmasking German Propaganda," and "What Our Enemy Really Is." Jenison, *War-Time Organization,* p. 44.

28. *Final Report,* p. 34; Creel, *Rebel at Large,* pp. 196–97; H. C. Peterson and Gilbert Fite, *Opponents of War 1917–1918* (Seattle, 1957), p. 18.

29. Jenison, *War-Time Organization,* p. 30; *Final Report,* p. 27.

30. *Final Report,* p. 32.

31. Ibid., pp. 73, 930; Hutchison, *Lowden of Illinois,* I, 376.

32. Harold Ickes, *The Autobiography of a Curmudgeon* (Chicago, 1969), pp. 190–91; Jacob Zeitling and Homer Woodbridge, ed., *Life and Letters of Stuart Pratt Sherman* (New York, 1919), I, 362; *Final Report,* pp. 31, 32, 34; William H. Gilman, Alfred R. Ferguson, and Merrell R. Davis, *The Journals and Miscellaneous Notebooks of Ralph Waldo Emerson, 1822–1826* (Cambridge, Mass., 1961), p. 302.

33. Bogart and Matthews, *The Modern Commonwealth,* p. 454.

34. Joseph G. Rayback, *A History of American Labor* (New York, 1959), p. 282; John C. Farrell, *Beloved Lady: A History of Jane Addams' Ideas on Reform and Peace* (Baltimore, 1967), pp. 172–73; Bogart and Matthews, *The Modern Commonwealth,* pp. 476, 483, 486; Hutchison, *Lowden of Illinois,* I, 379.

35. Peterson and Fite, *Opponents of War,* pp. 17–19, 23–29, 208–20.

36. *Laws of the State of Illinois Enacted by the Fifty-first General Assembly* (Springfield, 1919), pp. 420–21.

37. Ira Kipnis. *The American Socialist Movement 1897–1912* (New York, 1952), pp. 58, 97, 243, 335, 370, 421, 425.

38. Patrick Renshaw, *The Wobblies: The Story of Syndicalism in the United States* (Garden City, N.Y., 1968), pp. 37, 41, 43, 49, 70; Paul F. Brissenden, *The I.W.W.: A Study of American Syndicalism* (New York, 1957), pp. 67, 79; See also Melvin Dubofsky, *We Shall Be All: A History of the Industrial Workers of the World* (Chicago, 1969).

39. *Chicago Record-Herald,* July 6, 1905, p. 8; *Chicago Tribune,* June 20, 1905, p. 3; June 30, 1905, p. 5; Brissenden, *The I.W.W.,* p. 53.

40. Peterson and Fite, *Opponents of War,* pp. 21–29; Farrell, *Beloved Lady,* p. 176.

41. *Rockford Register-Gazette,* June 6, 1917, p. 10; June 7, 1917, pp. 2, 4.

42. Ibid., June 11, 1917, p. 1; June 13, 1917, p. 8; June 25, 1917, p. 2; July 2, 1917, p. 2. Curiously, Commissioner Mason was the son of Congressman William E. Mason, one of the most outspoken critics of the war.

43. *Rockford Register-Gazette,* July 6, 1917, p. 11; William Preston, Jr., *Aliens and Dissenters: Federal Suppression of Radicals, 1903–1933* (Cambridge, Mass., 1963), pp. 252–53.

44. Bogart and Matthews, *The Modern Commonwealth,* p. 484; *Final Report,* pp. 61, 95, 99, 101; Jenison, *War Time-Organization,* p. 76; Farrell, *Beloved Lady,* p. 174.

45. Adolph Germer to Sherman, Chicago, Sept. 5, 1917, and Sherman to Germer, Sept. 7, 1917, box 119, Sherman Papers; Bogart and Matthews, *The Modern Commonwealth,* p. 478; Hutchison, *Lowden of Illinois,* I, 377; *Chicago Tribune,* July 1, 1917, p. 12.

46. Ray Ginger, *The Bending Cross: A Biography of Eugene Victor Debs* (New Brunswick, N.J., 1949), pp. 353–76; Rayback, *History of American Labor,* p. 281; *Chicago Herald and Examiner,* July 1, 1918, p. 1; *Chicago Tribune,* Jan. 9, 1919, p. 1.

47. *Defense News Bulletin,* Nov. 10, 1917, pp. 1, 3–4; Jan. 19, 1918, p. 2; Feb. 16, 1918, p. 4; Bogart and Matthews, *The Modern Commonwealth,* p. 480.

48. Renshaw, *Wobblies,* pp. 169, 172, 174; *Defense News Bulletin,* Nov. 10, 1917, p. 3.

49. *Defense News Bulletin,* Aug. 24, 1918, p. 3; Renshaw, *Wobblies,* p. 177; *Chicago Tribune,* Feb. 13, 1918, p. 5; Apr. 7, 1918, p. 7; Apr. 16, 1918, p. 5; Feb. 16, 1918, p. 5.

50. *Defense News Bulletin,* Oct. 5, 1918, p. 3; Apr. 17, 1918, p. 1; *Chicago Herald and Examiner,* July 3, 1918, p. 1; Renshaw, *Wobblies,* pp. 181–86.

51. *Defense News Bulletin,* Aug. 24, 1918, p. 1; Renshaw, *Wobblies,* p. 193; Bogart and Matthews, *The Modern Commonwealth,* p. 480.

52. Dubofsky, *We Shall Be All,* pp. 461–62.

53. Peterson and Fite, *Opponents of War,* pp. 76–78; Scott Nearing, *The Making of a Radical: A Political Autobiography* (New York, 1972), p. 110.

54. *Chicago Tribune,* May 26, 1917, p. 7; May 27, 1917, part 1, p. 9; May 28, 1917, pp. 1, 4; May 29, 1917, p. 2; June 25, 1917, p. 7; Robert Morss Lovett, *All Our Years* (New York, 1948), pp. 140–50.

55. Hutchison, *Lowden of Illinois,* I, 378–79; Bogart and Matthews, *The Modern Commonwealth,* pp. 455, 485, 487; Peterson and Fite, *Opponents of War,* pp. 76–78.

56. *Defense News Bulletin,* Feb. 16, 1918, p. 6; *Chicago Tribune,* Feb. 16, 1918, p. 6; Apr. 7, 1918, p. 7; *Chicago Herald and Examiner,* June 30, 1918, p. 4.

57. *Chicago Tribune,* Feb. 23, 1918, p. 3; Apr. 7, 1918, p. 7; Apr. 26, 1918, p. 7. The best account of the Praeger lynching is in Frank Glenn Adams, "Anti-German Sentiment in Madison and St. Clair Counties: 1916–1919" (thesis, Eastern Illinois University, Charleston, 1966), pp. 47–69. See also pp. 14, 35–36, 37; Hutchison, *Lowden of Illinois,* I, 376; Jenison, *War-Time Organization,* p. 6; Donald R. Hickey, "The Praeger Affair: A Study in Wartime Hysteria," *Journal of the Illinois State Historical Society,* 62 (Summer, 1969), pp. 117–34.

58. *Chicago Tribune,* Dec. 6, 1918, p. 3; Hutchison *Lowden of Illinois,* II, 390–92; Jenison, *War-Time Organization,* p. 9.

59. *Chicago Daily Journal,* Jan. 6, 1920, p. 20; Jenison, *War-Time Organization,* pp. 27, 84. See also Robert K. Murray, *Red Scare, a Study in National Hysteria* (New York, 1964).

60. Paul Angle, *Bloody Williamson: A Chapter in American Lawlessness* (New York, 1952), pp. 134, 137–38; *Decatur Herald,* Dec. 4, 1922, p. 1.

61. David M. Chalmers, *Hooded Americanism: The History of the Ku Klux Klan* (Chicago, 1968), pp. 100–118, 183–89; Kenneth T. Jackson, *The Ku Klux Klan in the City 1915–1930* (New York, 1967), pp. 93–126. For a statement of Klan principles see the statement of Imperial Wizard Hiram Wesley Evans, "The KKK," in Loren Baritz, *The Culture of the Twenties* (Indianapolis, 1970), pp. 86–108. For a full history of the Klan, see William Pierce Randel, *The Ku Klux Klan, a Century of Infamy* (New York, 1965).

62. Theodore Draper, *The Roots of American Communism* (New York, 1957), pp. 115, 117.

63. Draper, *Roots of American Communism,* pp. 24, 61, 63, 117, 121, 126, 140, 141; Theodore Draper, *American Communism and Soviet Russia* (New York, 1960), p. 39; Irving Howe and Lewis Coser, *The American Communist Party: A Critical History (1919–1957)* (Boston, 1957), p. 65. These are three good biographies of John Reed. The most scholarly is Granville Hicks, *John Reed, the Making of a Revolutionary* (New York, 1968). See also Richard O'Connor and Dale Walker, *The Lost Revolutionary: A Biography of John Reed* (New York, 1968) and Barbara Gelb, *So Short a Time: A Biography of John Reed and Louise Bryant* (New York, 1973).

64. Draper, *Roots of American Communism,* pp. 176, 178; James Weinstein, *The Decline of Socialism in America 1912–1925* (New York, 1967), p. 209; Hicks, *John Reed,* pp. 335–64; O'Connor and Walker, *Lost Revolutionary,* pp. 251–53; Draper, *American Communism and Soviet Russia,* p. 19.

65. Draper, *Roots of American Communism,* pp. 173–84; Howe and Coser, *American Communist Party,* pp. 65, '6, 161.

66. Murray B. Levin, *Political Hysteria In America* (New York, 1971), p. 41; Zechariah Chafee, Jr., *Free Speech in the United States* (Cambridge, 1954), pp. 209–11.

67. Robert Morss Lovett, "The Trial of the Communists," *Nation* (Aug. 14, 1920), p. 185; Draper, *Roots of American Communism,* p. 204; *Chicago Tribune,* Jan. 2, 1920, p.1.

68. *Chicago Tribune*, Jan. 2, 1920, pp. 1, 2; *Chicago Daily Journal*, Jan. 2, 1920, p. 1; *Chicago Herald and Examiner*, Jan. 2, 1920, pp. 1, 2.

69. *Chicago Tribune*, Jan. 3, 1920, p. 1; Jan. 4, 1920, p. 1; Jan. 5, 1920, p. 1; Jan. 6, 1920, p. 1; Jan. 7, 1920, p. 1; Jan. 12, 1920, p. 5; *Rockford Register-Gazette*, Jan. 3, 1920, p. 1; *East St. Louis Daily Journal*, Jan. 3, 1920, p. 1; Jan. 4, 1920, pp. 1, 15; Jan. 9, 1920, p. 12; *Chicago Daily Journal*, Jan. 3, 1920, p. 1; *Chicago Herald and Examiner*, Jan. 3, 1920, p. 1; Jan. 4, 1920, p. 1.

70. *Rockford Register-Gazette*, Jan. 3, 1920, p. 6; *Chicago Tribune*, Jan. 6, 1920, p. 8; *Decatur Herald*, Jan. 3, 1920, p. 5.

71. *Report upon the Illegal Practices of the United States Department of Justice* (Washington, D.C., 1920), pp. 3, 4–5, 8, 22.

72. Howe and Coser, *American Communist Party*, p. 58; Lovett, "The Trial of the Communists," pp. 185–86; *The Nation*, Aug. 14, 1920, p. 174.

73. *Chicago Tribune*, Nov. 30, 1922, pp. 1, 2; *Decatur Herald*, Nov. 22, 1922, p. 2; ibid., Nov. 30, 1922, p. 1.

74. *Chicago Tribune*, Nov. 30, 1922, p. 1; *Decatur Herald*, Dec. 1, 1922, p. 6.

75. Dudley Field Malone to Small, New York, Dec. 16, 1922, box 125, Small Papers, Illinois State Historical Library; Seymour Stedman to Small, Chicago, Dec. 6, 1922, Erling H. Lind to Small, Chicago, Nov. 30, 1922, Daniel Kiefer to Small, Washington, D.C., n.d., and Elmon Armstrong to Small, Kansas City, Mo., Dec. 9, 1922, all in box 124, Small Papers. See also Resolutions of Hinsdale Post 250, Riverside Post 488, Walter Craig Post 60, Sycamore Post 99, Oak Park Post 115, and Norwood Post 740, all in box 124, Small Papers; *Iowa Legionaire*, Dec. 15, 1922, p. 5.

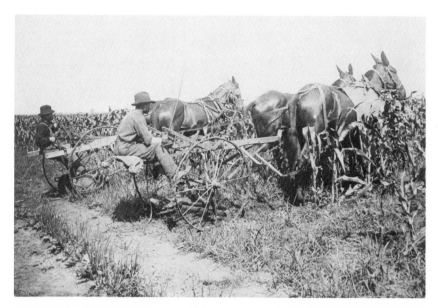

Cultivating corn with a one-row cultivator

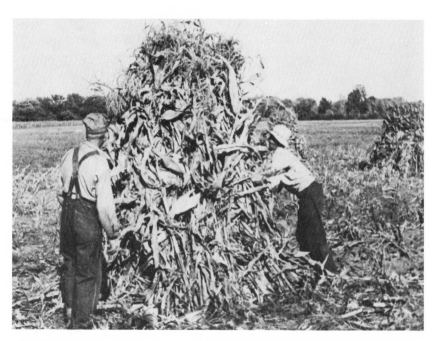

Shocking corn

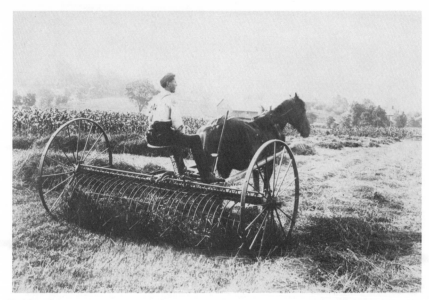

Raking hay

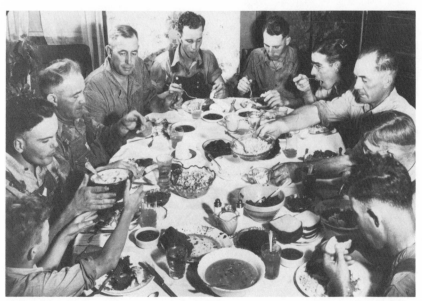

A threshing crew

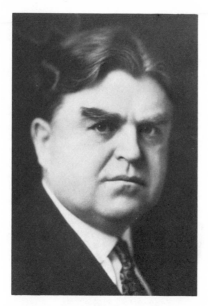

John L. Lewis, United Mine
Workers

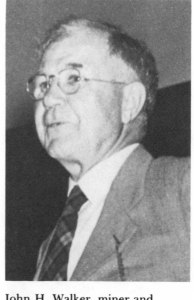

John H. Walker, miner and
president of the Illinois
Federation of Labor

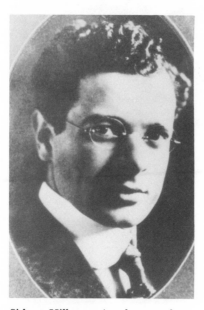

Sidney Hillman, Amalgamated
Garment Workers

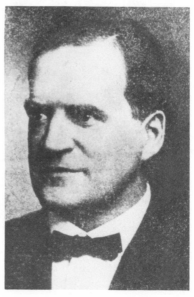

John Fitzpatrick, Chicago
Federation of Labor

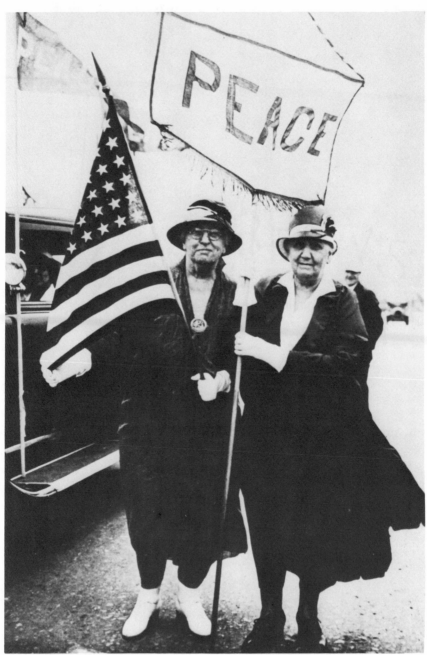

Jane Addams, right, founder of Hull House, and a friend, circa World War I

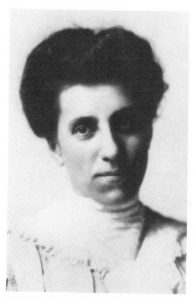

Julia Lathrop of Hull House

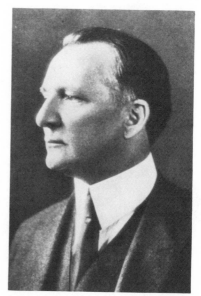

Raymond Robbins of the Chicago
Commons settlement house

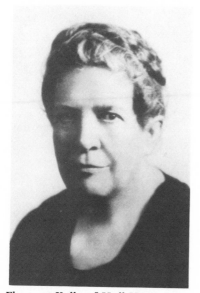

Florence Kelly of Hull House

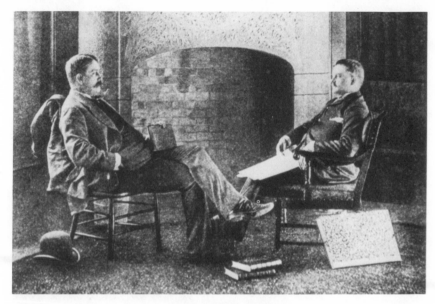

Daniel Burnham and John Wellborn Root, architects

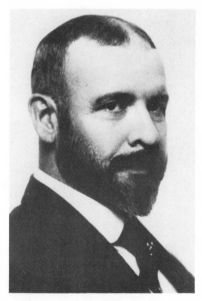

Louis Sullivan, designer of the
Chicago Carson, Pirie, Scott store
and Wright's teacher

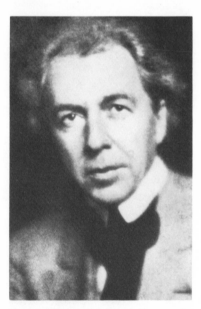

Frank Lloyd Wright, designer of
the "prairie house"

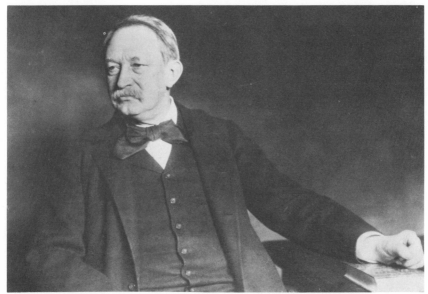

Theodore Thomas, first conductor of the Chicago Symphony Orchestra

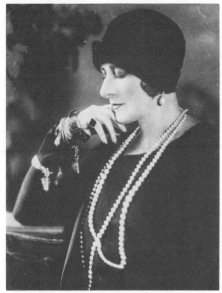

Mary Garden, star of the Chicago
Opera Company

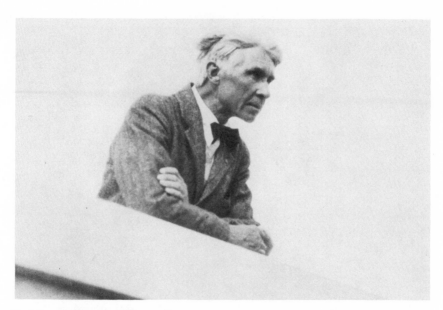

Carl Sandburg, journalist and poet

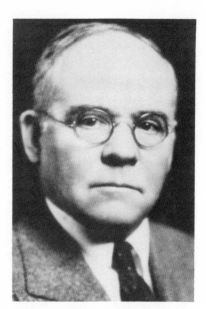

Edgar Lee Masters, poet and
novelist, author of *Spoon River
Anthology*

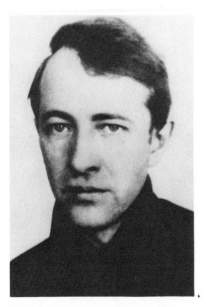

Floyd Dell, editor of the *Friday Review of Literature*

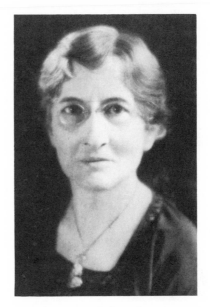

Harriet Monroe, founder of *Poetry* magazine

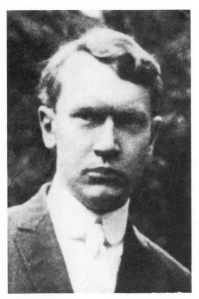

Vachel Lindsay, poet

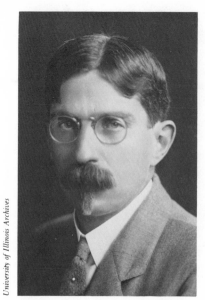

William A. Oldfather, classicist
and editor of the University of
Illinois *Studies in Language and
Literature*

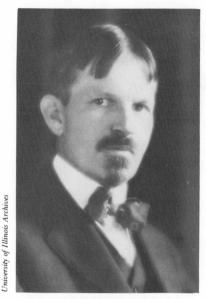

Clarence Alvord, historian at the
University of Illinois

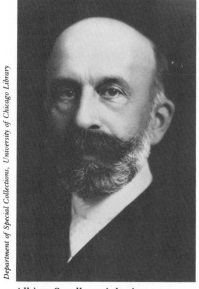

Albion Small, sociologist,
University of Chicago

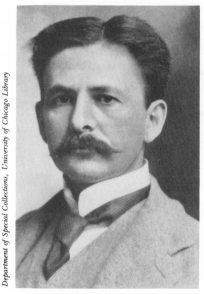

Albert Michelson, physicist,
University of Chicago

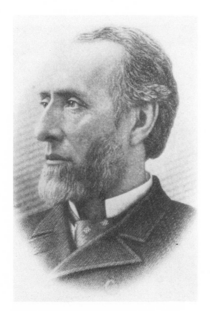

Shelby M. Cullom, U.S. Senator
1883–1913, U.S. Congressman
1865–71, Governor of Illinois
1877–83

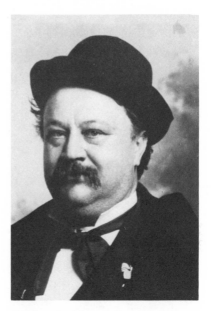

William E. Mason, U.S. Senator
1897–1903, U.S. Congressman
1887–91, 1917–21

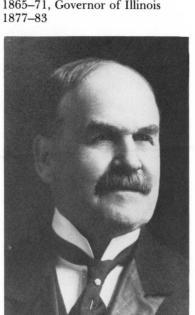

Albert J. Hopkins, U.S. Senator
1903–9, U.S. Congressman
1885–1903

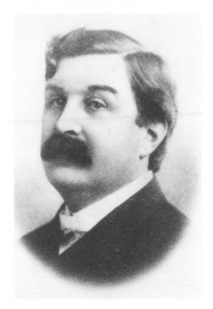

William Lorimer, U.S. Senator
1909–12, U.S. Congressman
1895–1901, 1903–9

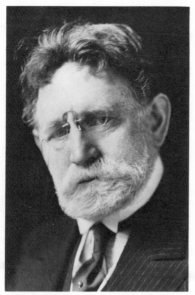

James Hamilton Lewis, U.S. Senator 1913–19, 1931–39

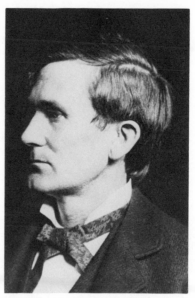

Lawrence Y. Sherman, U.S. Senator 1913–21

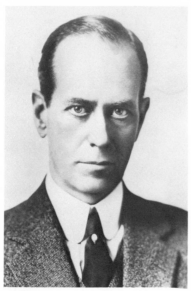

Medill McCormick, U.S. Senator 1919–25, U.S. Congressman 1917–19

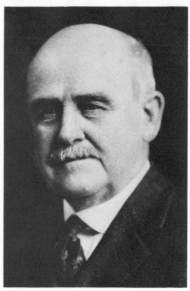

William B. McKinley, U.S. Senator 1921–26, U.S. Congressman 1905–13, 1915–21

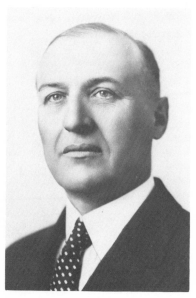

Otis F. Glenn, U.S. Senator
1928–33

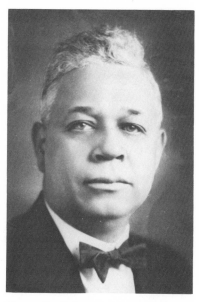

Oscar De Priest, U.S. Congressman
1929–35

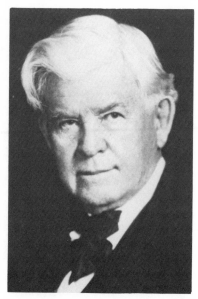

Henry T. Rainey, U.S. Congressman 1903–21, 1923–34

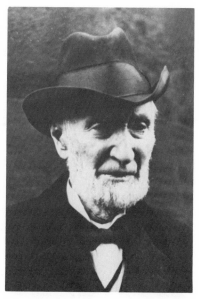

Joseph G. Cannon, U.S. Congressman 1873–91, 1893–1913, 1915–23

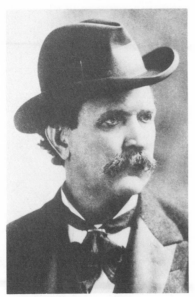

John R. Tanner, Governor
1897–1901

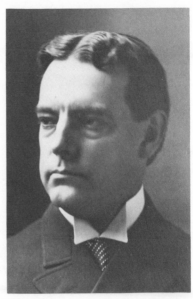

Richard Yates, Governor 1901–5,
U.S. Congressman 1919–33

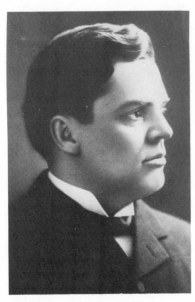

Charles S. Deneen, Governor
1905–13, U.S. Senator 1925–31

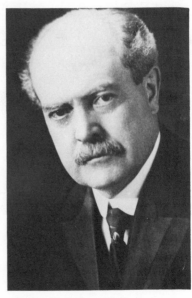

Edward F. Dunne, Governor
1913–17

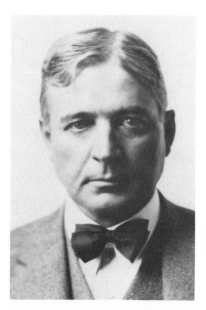

Frank O. Lowden, Governor
1917–21

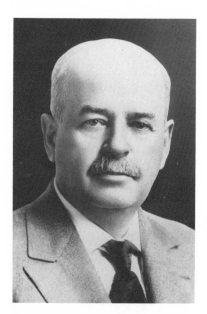

Len Small, Governor 1921–29

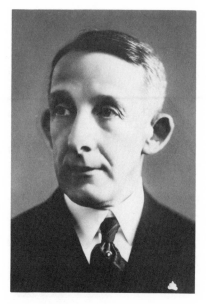

Louis F. Emmerson, Governor
1929–33

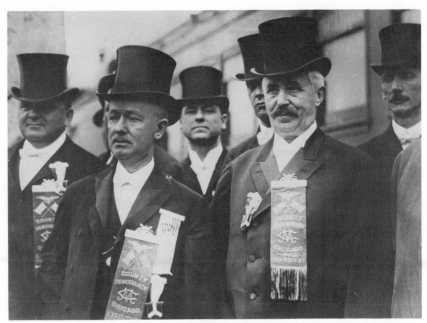

Michael "Hinky Dink" Kenna (front left) and John Powers

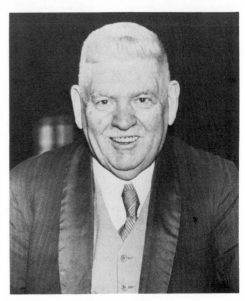

"Bathhouse" John Coughlin

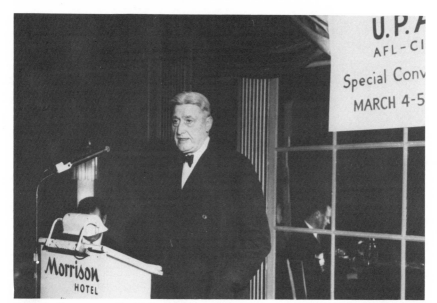

Adolph Germer, radical labor leader

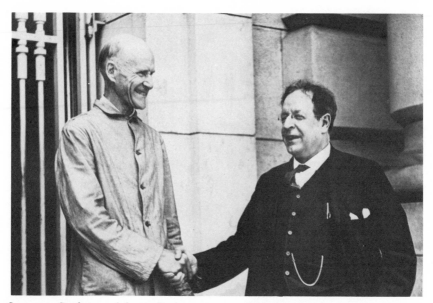

Seymour Stedman, right, radical attorney, and Eugene Debs, serving a sentence in Atlanta Prison, 1920

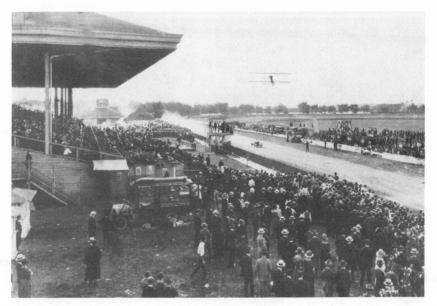

Lincoln Beachy (in the biplane) racing Barney Oldfield at a state fair

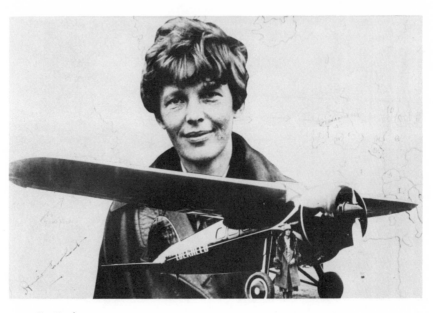

Amelia Earhart

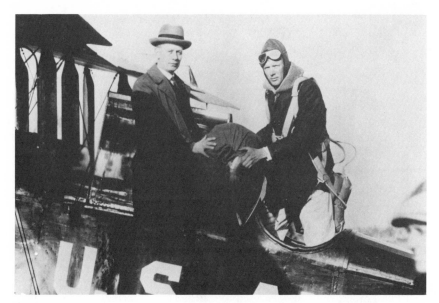

Charles Lindberg in Springfield, on a mail run between St. Louis and Chicago

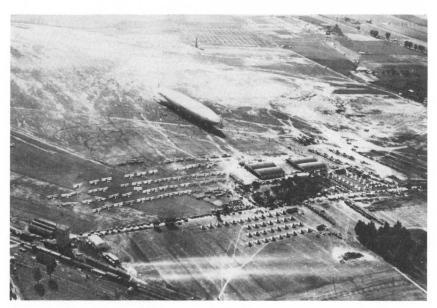

An early view of Scott Air Base near Belleville

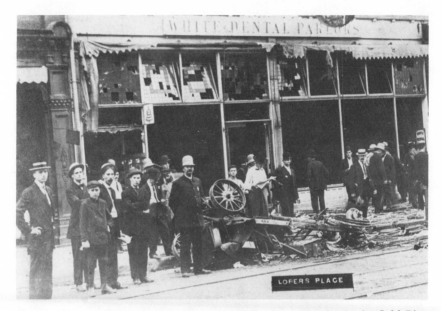

The remains of Harry Loper's cafe and car, destroyed in the Springfield Riot of 1908. Loper's car had been used to transport black prisoners away from a mob

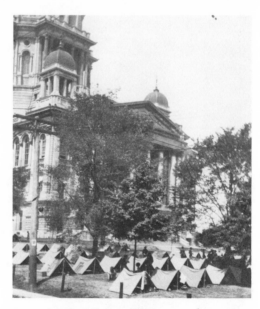

National Guard encampment on the statehouse lawn during the Springfield Riot, 1908

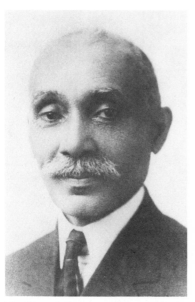

Ferdinand Barnett, lawyer, black
leader, and husband of Ida O.
Wells

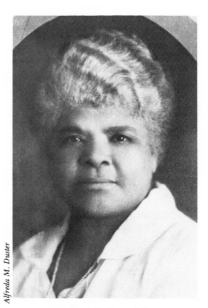

Alfreda M. Duster

Ida B. Wells, black activist

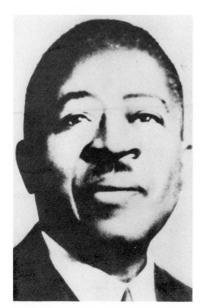

Robert Abbott, publisher of the
Chicago Defender

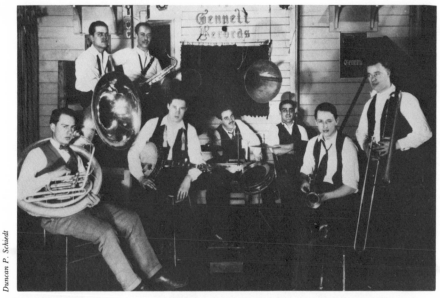

The Wolverines, 1924 (Bix Beiderbeck, trumpet; Vic Moore, drums; Dick Voynow, piano; Bob Gillette, banjo; Jimmy Hartwell, clarinet; George Johnson, tenor sax; Min Librook, bass; and Al Gandee, trombone)

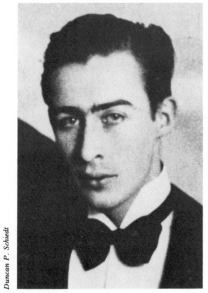

Dave Tough, jazz drummer

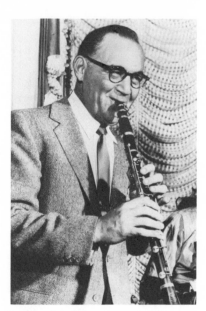

Benny Goodman, jazz musician, born near Hull House

8

Transportation

Nature blessed Illinois with a bounty of natural resources. Man superimposed on this a massive industrial system and magnificent farms to supply the needs of the nation. Illinois could not have achieved this without an equally effective transportation system. Illinois had a natural system of waterways: the Great Lakes and the Mississippi, Ohio, Illinois, and Wabash rivers. Through the foresight of men of early Illinois such as Stephen A. Douglas and William B. Ogden, Chicago became the terminal for both the eastern and western railroads, as well as for lines to New Orleans and Florida. One writer claimed that the switching yards of Chicago had an area larger than Rhode Island. This transportation system gave Illinois access to the raw materials of the nation, bringing cattle and hogs to the meat-packing industry and iron ore and coal to the steel mills.[1]

American railroads have a romantic mystique that in American folklore may be equaled only by the cowboy of the Old West. Generations of nostalgic Americans, yearning for the unhurried lives of the past, have sung:

> Come all you rounders, for I want you to hear,
> The story of a brave engineer.
> Casey Jones was the rounder's name.
> On a big eight wheeler of a mighty fame.

The ballad describes the legendary engineer of the Illinois Central who went to his death with his favorite engine rather than jumping to safety as the locomotive raced to disaster. "He stuck to his duty day and night" goes this song. Many others had to do with rail disasters, such as, "Mama, Mama, Mama have you heard the news? Daddy got killed on the C-B and Q's." Another song went, "There's many a man killed on the railroad, an' cast in a lonely grave."[2]

One old song celebrated the Wabash Cannonball, which ran to "Memphis, Mattoon, and Mexico." Another sang the glories of the Rock Island line, which was "the road to ride." Steve Goodman, a Chicago songwriter, immortalized an Illinois Central train with "The City of New Orleans." Referring to the "disappearing railroad blues" and "magic carpets made of steel," Goodman described the last days of a great train:

> Riding on the City of New Orleans
> Illinois Central, Monday Morning rail,
> Fifteen cars and fifteen restless riders,
> Three conductors and twenty five sacks of mail.

Many could identify with the nostalgia of a song by J. Clement called "I've got a thing about Trains":

> I get a sad kind of feeling
> When I see a passenger train.
> In this fast-moving world we live in,
> Nobody rides them much these days.[3]

The depot served as a social center and source of news and gossip in small-town America. The blast of the engineer's whistle announced the arrival of the train and brought to the station all of the town that was idle. The station was the club of the elderly men, loafers, and small boys. All looked down the shining ribbons of steel and romanticized about where they went. To many the rails represented an avenue to some future freedom, an escape from the humdrum of small-town life. One railroad historian described the fascination of trains, things of "beauty and wonder" which cheered the lonely, as a release from drudgery, the hours measured by the passage of the trains. Never would the automobile, the bus, the truck, or the airliner be able to match the romance of the trains in their days of glory.[4]

In 1900 steam railroads operated 11,003 miles of track within the boundaries of the state. The peak of mileage was reached in 1920 with 12,188 miles. Some track was abandoned later, however, and most of the increase after 1900 represented spurs, small feeder lines, and double-tracking of some of the line.[5] In 1925, 38 railroads entered Chicago; twenty-three of these were truck lines. The railroads moved 30,000 freight cars in and out of Chicago each day, and 1,376 passenger trains entered and left the city. Centralia, the major rail center in the southern part of the state, boasted thirty passenger trains a day, while Peoria had 137, as well as 158 freight trains, on the 13 steam and electric lines that entered the city.[6]

It is impossible to chronicle all of the railroads, but a few stand out as distinctly connected with Illinois. Among these the Illinois Central operated lines from Chicago to Cairo and Galena to Cairo as well as branch and feeder lines. Chartered in 1851, the Illinois Central operated 5,000 miles of track by 1900, making it one of the largest railroads in the country. In 1900, the line employed 32,000 workers and owed 918 locomotives and other rolling stock in proportion. The Central was closely related to Chicago, and under pressure from enviromentalist groups, in 1919 relinquished all rights to the Lakefront, making possible the building of the Field Museum, Shedd Aquarium, Adler Planetarium, and Soldiers Field. From 1921 to 1926, the Central electrified its suburban trains to lessen air pollution. New equipment was purchased, and in 1928 suburban trains carried 32,932,799 passengers.[7]

The Chicago, Burlington and Quincy Railroad grew from a small feeder line founded in 1849. By 1901 the road was brought into the Hill-Morgan empire as part of the Northern Securities Company. In that year the CB&Q operated 7,993 miles of track connecting Illinois with the northwestern part of the United States. The Northern Securities Company was dissolved by order of the Supreme Court in 1904 but by 1915 the line operated 9,366 miles of track.[8]

The Chicago and Eastern Illinois Railroad was chartered in 1894. By several consolidations the line was expanded so that by 1929 the line operated 945 miles of track and provided a second line to Florida. The Milwaukee Line was founded as a Wisconsin company, but by the beginning of the twentieth century it was essentially an Illinois company, counting among its directors Philip D. Armour, George M. Pullman, Norman B. Ream, and Marshall Field. By 1910 the line extended from Chicago to the Pacific, with nearly 10,000 miles of track, 1,199 locomotives, 518 passenger cars, and thousands of freight cars of various types.[9]

The Chicago and Rock Island, which built the first railroad bridge across the Mississippi at Rock Island in 1856, had expanded to operate 7,566 miles of track by 1928. The line operated north to Minneapolis, west to Denver, and south through Texas to Galveston and the Gulf.[10]

The trunk lines which terminated in Chicago were also important to Illinois. Among the larger ones, the Pennsylvania Railroad ran to Chicago, Peoria, and St. Louis from New York connecting

Illinois to the eastern markets. Similarly, the New York Central connected with some of the same cities and had a feeder line which ran from Chicago to Cairo via Danville, Paris, and Marshall. The Nickel Plate linked St. Louis, Peoria, and Chicago with Toledo, Cleveland, Erie, and Wheeling.[11] Illinois also had service to the West Coast through lines that terminated in Chicago. The Atchison, Topeka, and Sante Fe linked Chicago and Galesburg with Texas and with California via Albuquerque and the Grand Canyon, terminating in Los Angeles and San Francisco.[12]

Most of the railroads competed with the establishment of trains that provided remarkable luxury. In 1922 the Illinois Central, responding to the Florida boom, established the Floridian, a through train from Chicago to Miami. The Seminole, a slower train, traveled the same route. These trains used Illinois Central tracks to Birmingham, Central of Georgia tracks to Albany, and from there went to Miami via the Atlantic Coast line. In 1929 the Illinois Central advertised that on the St. Louis section of the Floridian it was possible to leave at 6:20 P.M. and arrive in Florida before breakfast in an all-steel, all-Pullman train. The Chicago and Eastern Illinois established the Dixie Limited to Miami in 1923. The Illinois Central's Panama Limited, all Pullman, left Chicago for New Orleans at 12:30 P.M. and arrived at 10:30 A.M. the following day.[13]

To the east, the Twentieth Century Limited, established by the New York Central in 1902, made the 961-mile trip from New York to Chicago in twenty hours, pulled by a ten-wheel locomotive. Among the services were a barbershop, maid and valet service, and train secretary. The diner served a meal for a dollar. The train carried twenty-seven passengers on the first run. On January 7, 1923, the Century left Chicago in five sections carrying 700 passengers. Similarly, in 1928 the Pennsylvania operated the Broadway Limited between Chicago and New York and the Spirit of St. Louis between St. Louis and New York. The Baltimore and Ohio operated the Capitol Limited from Chicago to Washington. To the West Coast, the Sante Fe's Chief was a favorite of the movie crowd. The Northwestern had its Northwestern Limited to Minneapolis and Corn King Limited to Omaha. The Corn King Limited featured all-steel cars, bedrooms, observation cars, a solarium, a soda fountain (during prohibition days), a luncheonette, ice-cube machine, electric cigar lighters, and a lounge for ladies. The Rock Island's Golden Gate Limited connected with the West Coast via the Southern Pacific.[14]

The railroads vied with each other in the quality of the food and appointments of the dining and sleeping cars. The first sleeping cars and diners dated from the Civil War period, and after 1899 Pullman had no competitors in their design. Steam heat was applied to railroad cars prior to 1900 but air conditioning had to wait until the end of the '20s. Pullman based his concept of the sleeping car on the model of a good hotel. He emphasized cleanliness as well as comfort. Some of the Pullman porters and dining-car stewards became famous. Dan Healy presided over the diner on the Chicago to Milwaukee segment of the Pioneer Limited of the Milwaukee line from 1899 to 1922. The meal on Healy's diner cost one dollar, with extra portions on request. The menu consisted of anchovies on toast, celery, tomatoes, olives, cucumbers, and salted almonds; mulligatawny soup or clear consommé; broiled salmon in egg sauce; sweetbread patties, roast beef or turkey; choice of several vegetable dishes; lobster salad; mince pie, strawberries, plum pudding in brandy sauce, tutti-frutti ice cream, assorted cake; Camembert, Rocquefort, or cream cheese; coffee, tea, or chocolate topped off with mint patties and Benedictine.[15]

The railroads provided service for small communitites as well. In 1926 the Illinois Central operated seven trains a day, each way, between Chicago and Carbondale. It also operated a feeder line between Leroy and Rantoul, with one passenger and one freight train each way each day. The passenger train stopped in Sabina, Glen Avon, Laurette, Lotus, Dickerson, Fisher, Dewey, Tomlinson, and Prospect. This enabled the citizens of these villages to connect with the Illinois Central main line at Rantoul.[16]

The Nickel Plate entered Illinois at Ridge Farm and crossed the state via Charleston. Six passenger trains a day traversed this route. In Coles County one of these trains arrived at Oakland (population 1,210) at 11:10 A.M. From there it stopped at Rardin (population 262) at 11:20 A.M., at Bushton (population 127) at 11:25, at Fairgrange (population 114) at 11:30, and arrived at Charleston (county seat, population 6,615) at 11:42 A.M. The distance from Oakland to Charleston was fourteen miles, and the traveling time in 1926 was thirty-two minutes. Thus, a small boy could, for a few pennies, travel to the county seat for a movie or chautauqua performance, a housewife could visit a larger city for shopping, or a farmer could visit the courthouse for legal business.[17]

The technology of railroading improved greatly in the twentieth century. By 1900 the Illinois Central had automatic couplers and airbrakes on all cars and steam heating and electric fans in passenger cars. The use of Timken roller bearings beginning in 1923 enhanced speed, reduced starting friction, and made maintenance easier. Railroads used a super heater to make steam hotter for more efficient engines by reducing premature condensation as the steam entered the cylinders. This in turn allowed for more efficient use of fuel and made possible larger and more powerful engines. Prior to 1930 almost all trains were pulled by steam engines, built heavier each year to meet the demands for speed and power. Between 1920 and 1929 the average load of freight carried per train increased from 708 to 804 tons. The average speed of freight trains in the same period increased from 10.3 to 13.2 miles per hour. In 1928 there were only fourteen diesels on the rails in the United States.[18]

During World War I the railroads lost control of their destiny in the face of nationalization. This situation lasted for sixteen months. The railroads charged mismanagement of the lines, alleging that the roads were returned to their owners in 1920 in poor condition. In spite of the anger of the railroads at nationalization, they seem to have made money during the time that they were operated by the government. The CB&Q, for example, had per-share earnings of $25.27 in 1918, as compared with $11.12 in 1923.[19]

Although the railroads did all they could to attract business by improving equipment and schedules, they faced increased pressure from the interurban in the early decades of the century and from the automobile during the '20s. Passenger traffic fell regularly throughout the '20s. Passenger miles in the United States totalled over 38 billion in 1923 but had fallen to 34 billion in 1927. In 1926 some 70,000 motor busses were rolling on the highways, half of them in interstate traffic. By that time regular bus schedules operated from Chicago to Detroit and St. Louis. The busses charged a fare of $7 from Chicago to St. Louis, while the train fare was $10.31. Motor bus operators could boast of several advantages besides cheaper fares. They stopped for passengers anywhere along the highway, in residential districts, or at hotels. Operation of a bus line required little capital, was subject to little regulation, and busses operated on highways built and maintained with tax dollars. The privately owned automobile caused much of the problem for shorter distances. The railroads complained of the onerous federal regulations, which the busses and trucks did not have to contend with.[20]

Railway Age, reflecting the panic of the railroads, called for federal regulation of busses. Pointing to the rapid growth of the bus lines, the magazine criticized the competition in areas where adequate train service existed and the difficulty of competition with an unregulated business.[21] In some instances railroad or interurban companies started bus lines to supplement their own operation. In 1928 the Chicago, South Shore and South Bend Railroad purchased busses to extend their service between South Bend and Detroit. Running on an eight-and-a-half-hour schedule, these "Golden Arrow Motor Coaches" seated twenty-five passengers and featured blue leather and plush upholstery, nickel-plated racks for parcels, an observatory bay, smoking lounge, lavatory, and drinking fountains, and carried heavy luggage in a rack on top of the bus.[22]

In the same manner, trucks cut into the freight revenue of the railroads, although this was not as disastrous as the decline of passenger fares. In 1925 more than 2 million trucks were registered in the United States. In 1926, 278,800 motor truck fleets operated two or more trucks, and of these 9,660 fleets operated ten or more trucks. The railroads attempted to meet the competition by improving schedules and service. The CB&Q, for example, set up a twenty-four-hour freight schedule between Chicago and Omaha and Chicago and Minneapolis, but it did not help.[23]

From 1900 to 1930, the electric railway constituted an important factor in the economic life of Illinois. The technology for the interurbans had existed for two decades prior to 1900. Thomas A. Edison and others had perfected this technology for streetcars, which operated in most major cities. By 1906 the two principal streetcar companies in Chicago operated over 700 miles of track, and by 1926 forty-six Illinois cities had local streetcar service.[24]

The interurban, usually an electric railway, drew most of its business from carrying passengers between cities. Most of the interurbans consisted of single-car trains, multiple cars being used only in rush hours and on the suburban trains of the larger cities. Having a low labor cost, the interurban was able to maintain low fares. Early interurbans looked much like city streetcars: wooden cars featuring clerestory windows and ornamented with stained glass and bright paint, usually orange. These gave way in the '20s to heavier, more powerful steel cars designed for speed. In the open countryside these cars could reach a speed of eighty miles per hour. The swaying of the cars gave the illusion of even greater speed in an age unaccustomed to a fast pace. The interurbans started the decline of the rural village, a process later hastened by the automobile. The interurban made short-range travel to schools, markets, and entertainment possible. Chautauqua grounds were often located on an interurban line between two cities. Excursion trips to amusemant parks and resorts were featured. The interurbans cut into the short-distance passenger business of the steam railroads but had little effect on long-distance travel because of lack of integration of the interurban lines and because on longer trips they were slower than steam railroads. Generally there was little cooperation between steam and electric railroads. Interurban freight business brought less revenue than did the passenger business, but a few lines, such as Illinois Traction, had substantial freight revenue.[25]

Some interurban lines were built prior to 1900, but expansion was rapid after that until World War I, when further building was halted. In 1907 Illinois had 2,754 miles of electric railroad track and the lines carried 703,494,000 revenue passengers. By 1912 the total trackage had expanded to 3,186 miles and the companies served 932,668,000 passengers. By 1917 Illinois contained 3,441 miles of track and over a billion passengers rode the cars. By 1932 the miles of track operated had declined to 2,456 and passengers carried dropped to 821,250,000.[26]

The interurban left behind a corps of nostalgia buffs much like those of steam railroads. One writer, speaking of "exhilarating speed" and "windows flung open against the warmth of a summers day scoop[ing] up the rich odors of the country side," described the interurban as "everyone's conveyance in the day before the family car," Yearning for those bygone days when trips were leisurely, "unhurried," and "unsophisticated," the historian of the inter-urban described the hissing of the wires, the clatter of the wheels, and the wail of the air horn which signaled the coming of the interurban.[27]

Among the unintegrated system of interurbans in Illinois were two major empires. Samuel Insull owned one; William B. McKin-ley, the other. These traction magnates distrusted each other, and each produced his own electricity. Insull controlled the Chicago, North Shore, and Milwaukee. The North Shore began operating in 1895. Insull bought the system in 1916 after it had fallen into difficulties, expanded and modernized the line, and gained entry to the Chicago Loop along the elevated tracks. The line provided high-speed commuter service and handled freight. In 1927 the North Shore carried over 10 million passengers and handled 843,000 tons of freight. It was possible to travel from Chicago to

Milwaukee in two hours and ten minutes on the North Shore. By 1924 the line operated 295 trains daily. Insull acquired the Chicago, South Shore and South Bend Railroad in 1925, just as the road was about to be sold for scrap. The Insull company renovated the line, purchased new steel cars, and arranged for entry into the city via the Illinois Central tracks, giving high-speed access to the Loop. Insull also controlled the Chicago, Aurora, and Elgin, providing service to the western suburbs of Chicago, and operated, through Middle West Utilities, other smaller lines, such as the Central Illinois Traction Company, which operated cars between Mattoon and Charleston, and the Southern Illinois Railway and Power Company, which operated an interurban line between Eldorado and Carrier Mills via Harrisburg.[28]

William B. McKinley, congressman and senator from Illinois, put together the second major interurban empire in the state. Originating in Danville in 1901, the system built lines radiating to Westville, Georgetown, Catlin, Ridge Farm, and St. Joseph. By 1903 McKinley completed the line to Champaign. By 1907 the line extended to Decatur, Springfield, and Clinton. By 1910 the line entered St. Louis, via Carlinville and Edwardsville, over the newly-completed McKinley Bridge. In the meantime McKinley built a line north to Bloomington and Peoria. With all of its branches the line operated some 400 miles of track and was one of the largest interurban systems in the United States. The company also owned the Illinois Power and Light Company, which supplied electricity to the railroad. Illinois Traction, carrying a number of parlor cars and sleepers, featured high-speed passenger service, considerable freight business, and unlike most interurbans, encouraged interchange with steam railroads. Although business fell off during the '20s and some of the less profitable lines were abandoned, in 1929 there were still twelve passenger trains a day operating each way from Springfield to St. Louis and Peoria.[29]

McKinley also operated streetcar lines in nineteen Illinois cities and various shorter interurban lines, some of which were part of a dream of linking his central Illinois line with Chicago and northern Illinois. Among these interurban lines were the Kewanee and Galva, the Chicago, Harvard and Geneva, and the Chicago, Ottawa, and Peoria. The dream was never realized; in the '20s McKinley gave up control of the company, and though for a time Insull had an interest in it, integration of the interurban networks was by then not feasible.[30]

Amid dreams of becoming another Insull or McKinley, many

promoters established interurban lines with names such as the Sterling, Dixon, and Eastern; the Springfield, Clear Lake, and Rochester; the Corn Belt Electric Railway; and the Fruit Growers Refrigeration and Power Company. Many of these ended in bankruptcy and few made a profit. Some ended like the Kankakee and Eastern, which ate up the inadequate resources of Dr. C. A. Van Doren, father of Carl and Mark Van Doren. Carl Van Doren wrote of the venture that it cost his father much sleep as others began to lose their savings in the "slow, dismal disaster."[31]

The interurban lines and steam railroads met the same fate, but the decline of the former was as quick as their appearance on the countryside. The reasons for the decline were much the same, all involving competition with the internal combustion engine in automobiles, trucks, and busses riding on ever-improving, tax-built, concrete highways. The automobile provided in greater degree the advantages that the interurban had over the steam trains in the short-fare business. The family automobile cut into passenger revenue, busses could handle the remainder of the passenger business easily, and the freight business of the interurban, involving few carload lots, was mostly short-distance so that it was well suited to truck transport. As business fell off in this unequal competition, the interurbans cut service and let the roadbed and cars deteriorate. There was little construction after 1915. By 1930 much of the passenger service had been abandoned, and in another thirty years all of it would disappear except for suburban commuter lines.[32]

The most spectacular Illinois development in transportation prior to 1930 was the construction of concrete highways. The increasing popularity of the automobile and the need for freight transport such as trucks could provide demanded this development, and Illinois government responded with unprecedented dispatch. Before 1900, prior to the common use of the automobile, bicyclists had mounted a propaganda campaign for improvement. Yet as David Wrone, the principal historian of the "hard roads" movement points out, the roads of Illinois were little better in 1910 than in 1818, and their condition discouraged prospective purchasers of automobiles. Early automobiles were fragile machines with little dependable power, and none were enclosed. From the time fall rains set in until good weather in the spring, the driver could not use his vehicle. The mud was so deep that even a horse drawing a high-wheeled, light buggy sometimes had difficulty picking his way through the mire. Most automobile. pioneers stored their machines in the barn until spring. In the summer the mud turned into dust almost as deep. The automobile churned this into a cloud, so that after a spin, the driver emerged from his toy wearing a layer of the Illinois countryside.[33]

Gradually, other groups took up the fight for good roads. By 1905 popular opinion supported action. In that year the general assembly, in the fashion of a legislative body not yet ready to move, provided for a state highway engineer and a three-man, unpaid commission to study the problem, carry on experiments, and give advice to local communities. Governor Deneen appointed to the commission Dr. Edmund J. James, of the University of Illinois, Lafayette Funk, of the seed-corn family, and Joseph Fulkerson of Jerseyville. The commission promoted dragging unimproved roads but did little to stimulate an integrated building program. It lingered on however, until a new law in 1913 made it obsolete.[34]

In the meantime, the University of Illinois established a road-testing laboratory. Efforts were made to determine whether concrete, brick, or macadam was the best building material. Citizens began to form "good roads associations," and by proclamation the governor established a "Good Roads Day" each year. A "Good Roads Congress" was held in Chicago on June 15, 1908. The *Tribune* supported the movement editorially, speaking of the benefits of good roads for mail carriers, farmers, railroads, markets, and merchants. The *Tribune* thought chauffeurs should be licensed, assuring proficiency in running the machine. In 1912 the *Tribune* noted the "Good Roads Day" and entitled their editorial "Pulling Illinois out of the Mud." Prior to 1910 only local governmental agencies licensed autos. In that year the general assembly passed a law requiring state licensing and provided that licensing fees were to be used for building roads.[35]

Governor Dunne made real progress toward the building of a highway system. During his campaign for the governorship, when he toured the state, Dunne realized that the condition of the roads had not been improved since he was a boy. In his inaugural address he described the imperative need for a highway system. Noting that in the forty-eight states Illinois ranked twenty-fourth in road improvement, Dunne asserted to the legislature that the problem touched the "agricultural, commercial, educational, social, religious, and economic welfare of Illinois." He took special note of the plight of rural Illinois. "Bad roads contribute to the unattractiveness, the isolation and monotony of country life that are responsible for the desertion of rural pursuits, especially by the young.

Experts in mental ailments agree that women in remote sections are the chief sufferers from the restriction of communications and social intercourse, which bad roads impose."[36]

Governor Dunne recommended legislation to promote roads by cooperation with the towns and counties, proper maintenance of roads once they were built, compulsory dragging of dirt roads, and the use of the automobile tax to pay the bill. Opinion about building hard roads was not all favorable. Some thought the building of the interurban lines would suffice and cost the tax payers nothing. Local road commissioners did not want to give up any of their prerogatives. Many farmers thought some improvement of the existing dirt roads would serve their purposes. Taxpayers were fearful of the enormous cost. Under the leadership of the Chicago Motor Club, the statewide Illinois Highway Improvement Association was organized to combat these opposing views.[37]

Responding to the plea of Governor Dunne, the general assembly passed the Tice Road Law of 1913. The new law reorganized the State Highway Department and provided for state assistance to any county which was willing, through a bond issue, to build and maintain the roads within their boundary. The law authorized the use of convict labor on the highways. The new highway department made an attempt to establish an integrated system so that roads to market towns would be connected with through highways. The legislature appropriated $400,000 to run the department and $400,000 for county aid in 1914 and $700,000 in 1915. Automobile license fees were to provide part of the money. Building of state-aid roads began in 1914 when Governor Dunne turned the first spadeful of dirt on the Aurora-Elgin highway. In that year the highway department let contracts for 91.97 miles of highway. About three-fourths of this was for concrete, which cost $10,320 per mile for a ten-foot-wide highway. The remainder was brick, which cost slightly more. It became apparent that the process of building all-weather roads would be expensive, with estimates ranging up to $140,000,000 to build 15,000 miles. Thus the state aid plan could hardly suffice.[38]

In 1916 the movement for better roads got encouragement from the federal government. The Federal Aid Road Act provided matching funds and appropriated $75,000,000 over a period of five years for improvement of any rural road used in mail delivery. The law prohibited the use of the money in towns of more than 2,500 in population. The federal government participated to the extent of 50 percent of the cost, provided the highway did not cost more than $10,000 per mile. Of this sum, Illinois was slated to get about $3,000,000. The plan was to go into effect in 1917. In Illinois the money was earmarked for the Cumberland Road (later designated U. S. Highway 40), running east and west, and the Dixie Highway (U. S. Highway 54), running north and south.[39]

As Governor Frank Lowden took office, the number of registered automobiles had increased and their owners were growing impatient with the condition of the roads. During Lowden's administration, voters approved a $60,000,000 bond issue designed to build 4,800 miles of road. As soon as the bond issue passed, the price of cement rose by 80 percent. Lowden accused the cement industry of rigging prices and refused to build roads or sell bonds until the price went down. Therefore only about 550 miles of road were built during his administration, mostly federal aid roads. The most important development in the Lowden years was the building of the Bates Experimental Road west of Springfield for testing various materials. On the basis of these tests, concrete became the standard highway paving material. Under Lowden the highway department acquired right-of-way for about 3,000 miles of road, and the Civil Administrative Code of 1917 created the Department of Public Works and Buildings, which took over the state highways. Thus, a groundwork was laid for feverish building during the administration of Governor Len Small.[40]

Armed with 1918 bond issue money and a growing public clamor for improved roads, Small began a massive building program. When he entered office in 1921, only a few miles of highway had been built with the bond issue money. With the cost up to $30,000 per mile, 409 miles were built in 1921, 741 in 1922, 1,085 in 1923, and 1,240 in 1924. At the peak of construction, contractors built 63 miles per week, employing 12,000 laborers and 3,000 teams of horses. One contractor completed 2,669 feet in one working day. With the money from the 1918 bond issue being rapidly depleted, Small recommended that a referendum be held in the 1924 election for a highway bond issue of $100,000,000 to provide an additional 3,000 miles of construction. The voters approved the issue. Small also recommended that a tax be put on gasoline, the proceeds to be used for highways. The general Assembly passed the tax on gasoline but the oil companies protested in the courts on the grounds that the tax violated the Fourteenth Amendment by denying due process and equal protection of the laws. The Supreme Court found the law to be unconstitutional.[41]

In 1925 another 906 miles of highway were built, and the Small administration boasted that it was possible to travel from Beloit, Wisconsin, to Cairo, Illinois, on a highway that was 95 percent concrete. By 1928 the Small administration had completed 4,793 miles of concrete highway, making a total in the state of 6,689 miles. During 1927 the first contracts were let under the 1924 bond issue.[42]

Politics were paramount in the building of roads. David Wrone notes that Small often built roads on the basis of whether a given county elected Small's candidates to the legislature. Wrone recounts that La Salle County got virtually no highway contracts after defeating Small's senatorial candidate. The situation in Clark County illustrates the political pressure that was brought. Most of Highway 1 from Chicago to Marshall had been built by the time Small was elected governor. In the election of 1920, Small, through a local politician from Marshall, B. M. Davison, promised that the road would be pushed on to West Union if Small were elected. One citizen wrote to Small that William Hollenbeck, local attorney, farmer, and former legislator, who had supported Oglesby in the primary, was trying to get the route changed to go near his farm. Similarly, just before the primary of 1928, Walter Cork, a Marshall insurance agent and state representative, after he had met with Casey businessmen, urged that plans be made to extend Route 49 south of Casey. A few days after the primary, Representative Cork wrote Governor Small urging that this route be abandoned because "our contractor friends in Casey proved to be our enemies the day of the Primary and defeated both of us in every precinct in the town." The Small papers are filled with pleas such as "You cannot afford to overlook your friends in La Motte Township."[43]

The improvement of the highways brought new problems, among them how to control speeds and how to prevent overloading of trucks, both of which could endanger life or break up the highway. In 1921 the general assembly passed an act providing for employment of 100 state highway police. In 1923 the legislature provided specifically for 100 policemen with the mental and physical qualifications required for a private in the Army. The state highway police were instructed to cooperate with local police, prevent breaking or destruction of the highways, collect delinquent license fees, and prevent overloading of trucks.[44]

In 1919 the legislature set speed limits for the state. Cars could travel at twenty-five miles per hour if they had pneumatic tires or twenty if they had solid tires. Light trucks were limited to fifteen or twenty miles per hour and heavier trucks to twelve or fifteen miles per hour. In this first law, enforcement was left to local officials, but after the creation of the highway patrol, enforcement of speed limits fell to them. The new highway police, patronage appointees all, were equipped with army-surplus motorcycles and sent out to enforce the motor vehicle law. The highway policeman was instructed to be courteous and firm and to aid travelers with information as to conditions of roads, nearest garages, or telephones. In particular he was to enforce the law concerning the overloading of trucks. The maximum load was 16,000 pounds on either axle. If a truck was overloaded, the officer was instructed to require the driver to unload a sufficient amount of the cargo to get down to the limit. This was the penalty for the first offense. For subsequent offenses, the driver was arrested and fined. Patrolmen inspected tires and kept metal-tired vehicles off the highway. They were instructed to enforce speed limits with judgment, noting whether the speed was dangerous to life. Jurisdiction was limited to paved roads outside corporate limits of towns. Officers could use a firearm only to protect their lives and were forbidden to accept cash bonds or other money. Officers were expected to direct traffic on special occasions and to prevent parking on highways.[45]

During September, 1923, the highway patrol made 140 arrests. Of these, 51 were for speeding and 63 for overloaded trucks. Other offenses included no license plates, no lights, drunken driving, careless driving, and bright lights or failure to dim. In the same month the highway patrol reported twenty-nine accidents, with thirty-eight persons injured and five fatalities. Causes of the accidents included being struck by a train, drunkenness, bad driving, speeding, no lights, broken wheels, broken steering rods, and vehicles with no lights parked on pavement.[46]

In time, aviation would be an equally important part of the transportation system of Illinois, and although it played a minor role in the economic life of the state prior to 1930, Illinois citizens contributed heavily to the pioneering efforts in the field. Prior to 1900, Illinoisians had to satisfy themselves with the observation of balloon ascensions. Then few impractical designs for heavier-than-air vehicles came forth, such as those of Dr. Arthur De Baisset in Chicago in 1884 and Edward Joel Pennington in Mt. Carmel in 1890; but the exaggerated claims of some inventors precluded raising money to finance the inventions. Historians agree the first flight of an airplane in Illinois came in 1909, when Glenn Curtiss piloted an airplane in three short flights at the Hawthorne Race

Track. The flights of Curtiss were hardly spectacular, but they aroused interest and dispelled doubt. Also few engineers such as Octave Chanute had been giving serious thought and study to the problem of flight. Chanute had long been collecting material and in 1901 had even brought Wilbur Wright to Chicago to lecture. So by 1910 the stage was set for a rapid expansion of activity.[47]

The most productive event in the early history of Illinois aviation came with the formation of the Illinois Aeroplane Club in Chicago in 1910. About 100 Chicagoans attended the meeting, bringing together would-be designers, aviators, and Chicago businessmen with money. The first officers were Octave Chanute, president, James E. Plew and Harold Fowler McCormick, vice-presidents, Robert M. Culling, secretary, and Charles F. Bartley, treasurer. The consulting engineer was Victor Lockheed. Harold Fowler McCormick gave $18,500 to the Aero Club to buy the site for Cicero Field and another $10,000 to prepare the field for use. Cicero Field consisted of 180 acres bounded by second streets and boasted a turf landing strip, sheet metal and wooden hangars, and maintenance and service for airplanes. The field became the headquarters for inventors, manufacturers, barnstormers, and flying schools, including that of Swedish-born Max Lilly, a student of the Wrights, who taught many fledgling pilots including Kathie Stinson, who got her license in 1912. Another woman pilot, Ruth "Angel Face" Law, trained at Cicero Field in 1911, bought her own Wright biplane at Dayton, and set several records including a nonstop flight from Chicago to New York in 1916.[48]

In 1911 the Aero Club held an international meet in Chicago financed primarily by Harold Fowler McCormick, with the support of Albert Lambert, of the St. Louis Aero Club, and Carl Fisher, the owner of the Indianapolis Speedway. The program took place in Grant Park and the prize money was so lucrative that the most famous aviators appeared in contests of endurance, speed, altitude, cross-country, and flying. The thrilling events included an altitude record of 11,642 feet set by Lincoln Beachey in a Curtiss airplane. Two pilots died in the meet. About a month later, Vandalia held an aviation meet featuring the Benoist flyers of St. Louis. The Benoist flyers represented the Benoist School of Aviation and the Benoist Aircraft Company, which manufactured airplanes. The Benoist company featured four models and advertised that "Benoist Planes Fly: Because they are constructed right."[49]

In 1911, *Aero* carried ads for a number of aviation activities in Illinois. The Curzon Aviators of East St. Louis offered Farman biplanes and flew out of the Washington Park Aviation Field. Alto W. Brodie of Chicago featured Farman and Blériot planes. The Webster Aeroplane Manufacturing Company in Chicago were builders of "Curtiss-type" biplanes and were agents for Curtiss engines. Mills and Mills Aviators Exchange advertised jobs for aviators. The International Aeroplane Manufacturing Company and School proclaimed "YOU CAN FLY" and boasted about "Vandie Lodvik, our latest graduate filling well-paying engagements." The whole idea of flight was so new that *Aero* ran a column called "The Diary of Flight," which listed recent events. For example, in Villa Grove on September 18, 1911, "Mr. G. Adams flew in a monoplane of his own building. The machine was wrecked and Adams suffered several severe injuries. The flyer was wrecked through one wheel sinking into a hole while he was driving the machine over the ground." Three days later Nils J. Nelson flew in Aledo, and on September 19, Louis Rosenbaum of Chicago was killed in a crash in Dewitt, Iowa. In many of the early biplanes the engine was mounted on the upper wing above the pilot. Rosenbaum died from the engine falling on him, a common hazard of the times.[50]

In 1912 Chicago hosted the Second International Aviation Meet and, immediately before the meet, the Gordon-Bennett Aviation Cup Race. Pilots offered airmail demonstrations in Illinois during 1912. In May, Farnum Fish piloted his plane from Chicago to Milwaukee carrying letters and materials for the Boston Store. The Aero Club of Illinois sponsored similar flights between Cicero, Elmhurst, and Wheaton. The Illinois State Fair had a mail-carrying stunt from Springfield to Williamsville, featuring Fish, Edward A. Korn, and "Sure Shot" Kearney.[51]

These pioneers demonstrated the feasibility of air travel and pointed the way to commercial uses, so that by World War I the doubters were fewer and the supporters of aviation were growing. World War I improved technology and trained pilots. Most of the aviation ventures of World War I centered around Chanute Field at Rantoul and Scott Field near Belleville, both built for training purposes. The veterans of the army flying service created a surplus of trained and experienced personnel available for commercial aviation.[52]

Thus at the end of World War I, all of the components for successful commercial flight were present. The technology had advanced sufficiently to promise success; now capital and leadership were needed to improve on this foundation and provide the necessary speed, comfort, safety, and economy of flight. An aviation magazine editorialized on the subject in 1920: "The world is waiting for great men to come who will be the great builders of airways, of transcontinental truck lines, of huge fleets of transatlantic air ships, bridging the new world with the old each day. The world is waiting for the Harrimans, Huntingtons, and Vanderbilts of the air."[53]

Many early pilots engaged in barnstorming or flying exhibitions, stunt flying, or carrying passengers for pay, though the living a pilot could derive from this life was meager. Itinerant flyers also suffered a high incidence of accidents, but they brought a knowledge of aviation to all parts of the country. Landing fields through the first half of the '20s were likely to be vacant fields, parks, or golf courses. Besides Cicero Field of the Aero Club of Illinois, Ashburn Field was opened in 1915, and Checkerboard Field at Maywood and Grant Park Air Mail Field were operating in 1919. Curtiss planes represented 75 percent of the total output in 1920. Other planes such as the JLG were being advertised by 1920. This all-metal monoplane featured a 185-horsepower engine, and carried six passengers and eighty gallons of fuel. An advertisement for this plane boasted that it had made the 130-mile trip from Atlantic City to Philadelphia in fifty-nine minutes and thirty-four seconds.

Pilots constantly set new records. In 1920 Irvin S. Amberg flew 440 miles from Omaha to Chicago in 3 hours and 26 minutes. In 1924 Lieutenant Russell Maugham flew from New York to San Francisco in 21 hours and 48 minutes, of which only 18 hours and 20 minutes was actual flying time. Many were looking forward to fast airmail service. The first airmail flight from New York to Chicago was in 1918. Service from Chicago to Cleveland came in 1919 and to Kansas City in 1922. A mail flight from St. Louis to Chicago, via Rantoul, came in 1920. By that time the *Chicago Tribune* carried a regular aviation column.[54]

Until 1926 there was no regulation of the aviation industry. Anyone could buy an airplane and fly it when and where he pleased. But mounting numbers of accidents and fatalities brought increasing demands for federal action. When the Goodyear blimp "Wing Foot" fell through the skylight of the Illinois Trust and Savings Bank in Chicago in 1919, killing thirteen persons, Senator Sherman demanded federal regulation, but this and similar demands failed until 1926, when the Air Commerce Act was signed into law. The law placed regulation under the Department of Commerce, and President Coolidge appointed Chicago attorney

William J. McCracken, Jr. to the post of assistant secretary of commerce for aeronautics. The law provided for licensing of pilots and aircraft and for traffic rules along the federal airways.[55]

In the last half of the '20s aviation came of age. Charles A. Lindbergh barnstormed through Illinois on a number of occasions and in 1926 was instrumental in helping set up regular airmail flights between St. Louis and Chicago via Springfield and Peoria. Peoria established a field of 70 acres in preparation for the flights. Robertson Aircraft Corporation of St. Louis, for whom Lindbergh flew, promoted the airmail run. Robertson requested a permanent field at Springfield of 100 acres, a hangar of sixty by twenty feet, facilities for gasoline, oil, electricity, a telephone, and night landing facilities. In February, 1926, Lindbergh made the test flight, requiring forty minutes to fly to Springfield from St. Louis and making the return trip in fifty minutes. Robertson warned the postal officials that 250 pounds of mail per day was needed to keep the flight going because it cost $1.01½ per mile for the flight. Lindbergh and other pilots flew the route five days a week, barely paying the cost of the flights. Postal officials promoted the service, urging other cities to send airmail via Springfield.[56]

In 1927, when Lindbergh flew the Atlantic in a little more than 23 hours, he was a well-known figure in Illinois aviation. As a result of his flight, he became a national hero in an era short on heroic figures. On August 15, 1927, Lindbergh came to Springfield as a part of his national tour and the local field was named for him. A year later Amelia Earhart, who graduated from Chicago's Hyde Park High School, became the first woman to fly the Atlantic, making a 2,000-mile trip from Newfoundland to Wales. Although Earhart's residence in Chicago had been brief, the *Chicago Tribune* identified her as a Chicago girl and dubbed her "Lady Lindy." Hardly more than a courageous extension of the stunt flying of an earlier age, these exploits provided authentic heroes and demonstrated that aviation was here to stay.[57]

By 1928, 5,000 landing fields operated in the United States; of these, 58 were located in Illinois. The Chicago Municipal Airport, opened in 1927, consisted of 640 acres bounded by Fifty-fifth and Sixty-third streets and Central and Cicero avenues. The runways were cinder at first. Lindbergh Field, located five miles west of Springfield, had only 57 acres. When Robertson Aircraft began flying trimotor passenger planes to Chicago in 1927, the city field was too short and they used a field operated by the Lock-Isbell Company on Chatham Road. By 1928 the National Air Transport of Chicago was the "country's largest air transport." Its planes flew 5,000 miles every twenty-four hours. A typical flight left Chicago at 8 A.M. and arrived in New York at 4:45 P.M. Yet in spite of the growth of aviation, when Julian Farwell, son of Arthur L. Farwell, socially prominent Chicagoan, was killed on a flight to Rantoul, the *Chicago Tribune,* reflecting the attitude of many toward aviation, commented, "He was one of the first of Chicago's wealthy young men to take up the sport."[58]

As the '20s closed, Illinois was poised on the edge of extensive commercial flight. From 1900 to 1930 the state had progressed from the horse and buggy to the automobile and from the train to the eve of air transportation. The pace of life had changed drastically, and with it the life-style of the people. Most families now spent much of their time in cars. Shopping for family staples, recreation, entertainment, and indeed the whole way of life had changed.

1. Stewart H. Holbrook, *The Story of American Railroads* (New York, 1941), p. 133.

2. Carl Sandburg, *The American Songbag* (New York, 1927), pp. 366–67, 368–69, 371. For a narrative account of Casey Jones, see Carlton J. Corliss, *Main Line of Mid-America: The Story of the Illinois Central* (New York, 1950), pp. 301–11. See also John Lomax and Alan Lomax, *American Ballads and Folk Songs* (New York, 1934), pp. 36–39. There are several versions of the ballad and a number of similar ones about other engineers and other wrecks. Another version of the story of Casey Jones can be found in *The Building of Mid-America: 20 Railroad Stories as Told by a Fifth Generation of an Illinois Central Family* (n.p., n.d.). A copy is in the Illinois Historical Survey, Urbana, Ill.

3. Alan Lomax, *The Folk Songs of North America in the English Language* (New York, 1960); Sun Records, 127, "Original Golden Hits," vol. 3 sung by Johnny Cash; Columbia Records, KCS 9943, "Hello, I'm Johnny Cash" sung by Johnny Cash; Warner Brothers Records, MS 2060. "Hobo's Lullaby," sung by Arlo Guthrie.

4. August Derleth, *The Milwaukee Road: Its First Hundred Years* (New York, 1948), pp. 2–5; Mary McCarthy, "The Man in the Brooks Brothers Shirt," in *The Company She Keeps* (New York, 1942), pp. 81–134.

5. U.S. Bureau of the Census, *Statistical Abstract of the United States 1929* (Washington, D.C. 1929), p. 394

6. *Official Directory of Classified Industries for the Buyers and Shippers of the Illinois Central Railroad, Yazoo, and Mississippi Valley Railroad* (Chicago, 1925), pp. 59, 69, 172.

7. Corliss, *Main Line of Mid-America,* pp. 312, 365–67, 373; *Poor's Manual of Railroads: 1924* (New York, 1924), pp. 1197–98.

8. Richard C. Overton, *Burlington Route: A History of the Burlington Lines* (New York, 1965), p. 3.

9. Ernest Ludlow Bogart and John Mabry Mathews, *The Modern Commonwealth 1893–1918* (Springfield, 1920), p. 132; *Statistical Abstract of the United States: 1929,* p. 412; Derleth, *Milwaukee Road,* pp. 137, 143, 194–95.

10. Holbrook, *The Story of American Railroads,* p. 136; *Statistical Abstract of the United States: 1929* p. 412; Robert G. Lewis, *Handbook of American Railroads* (New York, 1951), pp. 64–65.

11. Lewis, *Handbook of American Railroads*, pp. 152–54, 158, 176–78; Pennsylvania Railroad Company, 1846—*One Hundred Years of Transportation Progress—1946: A Brief History of the Pennsylvania Railroad* (n.p., 1945), pp. 4–5; Alvin F. Harlow, *The Road of the Century: The Story of the New York Central* (New York, 1947), pp. 388–89; Taylor Hampton, *The Nickel Plate Road: The History of a Great Railroad* (New York, 1947), pp. 191, 219, 230–31.

12. Lewis, *Handbook of Railroads*, pp. 3–5

13. *Railway Age*, Mar. 31, 1928, p. 749; *Central States Guide to Railroad, Traction, Motor Bus, and Hotels* (Nov., 1926), p. 81; *Illinois State Journal*, Jan. 3, 1929, p. 2.

14. John W. Starr, *One Hundred Years of American Railroading* (New York, 128), pp. 291–93; *Railway Age*, Sept. 1, 1928, p. 413; S. Kip Farrington, *Railroads of Today* (New York, 1949), pp. 21–23, 46–47.

15. The Pullman Company, *"No. 9": The Story of the First Pullman Car and the Evolution of Travel Comfort in 65 Years* (Chicago, 1924), p. 2; August Mencken, *The Railroad Passenger Car: An Illustrated History of the First Hundred Years with Accounts by Contemporary Passengers* (Baltimore, 1957), pp. 78–80; Joseph Husband, *The Story of the Pullman Car* (Chicago, 1917), p. 104; Association of American Railroads, *A Chronicle of American Railroads, including Mileage by States and Years* (Washington, D.C. 1957), p. 7; Derleth, *Milwaukee Road*, pp. 159–60.

16. *Central States Guide*, p. 88.

17. Ibid., p. 123.

18. Corliss, *Main Line of Mid-America*, p. 313; Farrington, *Railroads of Today*, pp. 210–11; Kenneth W. Downing, *With a Cinder in My Eye: A Layman's Memory and Sketches of American Trains* (Moline, Ill., 1951), pp. 27–28; *Railway Age*, Jan. 7, 1928, p. 17; Mar. 17, 1928, p. 625; Mencken, *Railroad Passenger Car*, pp. 52–53; *A Yearbook of Railroad Information* (New York, 1930), pp. 66–69.

19. Slason Thompson, *A Short History of American Railways* (Freeport, N.Y. 1925), pp. 357–77. For the effect on the Illinois Central, see Corliss, *Main Line of Mid-America*, pp. 359–60; Derleth, *Milwaukee Road*, pp. 203–5; I. Leo Sharfman, *The American Railroad Problem, Study in War and Reconstruction* (New York, 1921), pp. 65–99.

20. John B. Rae, *American Automobile Manufacturers: The First Forty Years* (Philadelphia, 1959), p. 91; *Railway Age*, Jan. 7, 1928, pp. 24–25, 80–81; January 28, 1928, p. 270.

21. *Railway Age*, Sept. 1, 1928, p. 399.

22. Ibid., Jan. 28, 1928, p. 286.

23. Ibid., p. 271; Overton, *Burlington Route*, pp. 344–45.

24. John F. Due, "The Life Cycle of an Industry: The Electric Interurban Railway," *Current Economic Comment*, Feb., 1960, p. 26; Ralph E. Heilman, "Chicago Traction, A Study in the Efforts of the Public to Secure Good Service," *American Economic Quarterly*, third series, 9, (1908), pp. 44, 48; *Illinois Blue Book, 1925–26*, pp. 558–59.

25. Due, "Life Cycle of an Industry," pp. 25, 29, 36, 45–47.

26. *Statistical Abstract of the United States: 1929*, p. 434; Ibid., *1934*, pp. 372–73.

27. William D. Middleton, *The Interurban* (Milwaukee, 1961), pp. 8, 12, 32.

28. George W. Hilton and John F. Due, *The Electric Interurban Railway in America* (Stanford, Calif., 1960), pp. 335–37, 351, 352; *Railway Age*, Mar. 17, 1928, p. 611; James D. Johnson, *Aurora Elgin, Being a Compendium of Word and Picture Recalling the Everyday Operations of the Chicago, Aurora and Elgin Railroad* (Wheaton, Ill., 1965), unpaged.

29. Hilton and Due, *The Electric Interurban*, pp. 346–49; Middleton, *Interurban*, p. 192; *Illinois State Journal*, Jan. 2, 1929, p. 14.

30. Hilton and Due, *The Electric Interurban*, pp. 342, 344, 346; John F. Due, "The Rise and Decline of the Midwest Interurban," *Current Economic Comment* 14 (Aug., 1952), p. 37; Middleton, *Interurban*, p. 192.

31. Hilton and Due, *The Electric Interurban*, pp. 250, 344, 346, 349, 351, 352.

32. Ibid., pp. 208–9, 237–38, 244–45; Middleton, *Interurban*, pp. 8, 316; Due, "Rise and Decline of the Midwest Interurban," p. 49; Due, "Life Cycle of an Industry,'" pp. 30–39.

33. The best account of the "hard roads" movement is David Wrone, "Illinois Pulls out of the Mud," *Journal of the Illinois State Historical Society* 58 (Spring, 1965), pp. 54–76. For early propaganda of the movement see Charles A. Taff, *Commercial Motor Transportation* (Homewood, Ill., 1961), p. 16.

34. Bogart and Matthews, *The Modern Commonwealth*, pp. 148–49.

35. *Chicago Tribune*, May 23, 1908, p. 10; Apr. 12, 1912, p. 9; Bogart and Matthews, *The Modern Commonwealth*, p. 148; Wrone, "Illinois Pulls out of the Mud," pp. 54–55.

36. Edward F. Dunne, *History of Illinois* 5 vols. (Chicago 1933), II, 330–31.

37. Ibid., II, 331; Bogart and Matthews, *The Modern Commonwealth*, p. 148; Wrone, "Illinois Pulls out of the Mud," p. 57.

38. Dunne, *History of Illinois*, II, 331–32; William T. Hutchinson, *Lowden of Illinois: The Life of Frank O. Lowden* 2 vols. (Chicago, 1957), I, 335; Bogart and Matthews, *The Modern Commonwealth*, p. 152; Wrone, "Illinois Pulls out of the Mud," p. 60.

39. Taff, *Commercial Motor Transportation*, p. 19; Bogart and Matthews, *The Modern Commonwealth*, p. 154; Hutchison, *Lowden of Illinois*, I, 356.

40. Bogart and Matthew, *The Modern Commonwealth*, p. 153; Wrone, "Illinois Pulls out of the Mud," pp. 70–71; Hutchison, *Lowden of Illinois*, I, 357–59; *Illinois Blue Book, 1925–1926*, pp. 342 ff: Len Small, *Illinois Progress* (Springfield, Ill., 1928), p. 128.

41. Small, *Illinois Progress*, pp. 105, 108, 128–32, 138; Wrone, "Illinois Pulls out of the Mud," p. 73; Dunne, *History of Illinois*, II 414; typescript of complaint of Standard Oil of Indiana *vs* State of Illinois, box 141, Small Papers, Illinois State Historical Library.

42. *Illinois Blue Book, 1925–26*, p. 1; Small, *Illinois Progress*, pp. 136–38.

43. Emanuel Diehl to Small, West Union, Ill., Dec. 30, 1920, and George D. Sutton to Small, Springfield, May 3, 1927, box 171, Small Papers; Walter Cork to Small, Marshall, Ill., Mar. 4, 1928, and Apr. 10, 1928, box 172, Small Papers; O. C. Seeders to Small, Palestine, Ill., June 22, 1922, box 171, Small Papers.

44. *Laws of the State of Illinois Enacted by the Fifty-second General Assembly* (Springfield, 1921), p. 572; *Laws of the State of Illinois Enacted by the Fifty-third General Assembly* (Springfield, 1923), pp. 562–64.

45. *Laws of the State of Illinois Enacted by the Fifty-first General Assembly* (Springfield, 1919), p. 678; William Hale Thompson to Leslie Small, Chicago, Nov. 16, 1922, box 224, Small Papers. Thompson recommended Excelsior motorcycles, the only motorcycle manufactured in Illinois. Fred Tarrant to Excelsior Motor Manufacturing and Supply Company, Chicago, Dec. 13, 1922, and Rules for State Highway Police Officers, issued by Division of Highways, Department of Public Works and Buildings, box 224, Small Papers.

46. Roster of Arrests, typescript, and Tabulation of Accidents on State Highways, box 224, Small Papers.

47. The principal work on the history of aviation in Illinois is Howard L.

Scamehorn, *From Balloons to Jets* (Chicago, 1957). For the early development see pp. 11–50. Also important is Leslie Orear, *A History of Aviation in Illinois*, MSS, Federal Writers Project, box 292, Illinois State Historical Library.

48. Scamehorn, *From Balloons to Jets*, pp. 53, 55, 69; Orear, *History of Aviation*, pp. 11, 33; Richard Paul Doherty, *"Origin and Development of Chicago O'Hare International Airport,"* (dissertation, Ball State University, Munice, Ind., 1971), p. 3.

49. Scamehorn, *From Balloons to Jets*, p. 81; Orear, *History of Aviation*, pp 16–20; *Aero: America's Aviation Weekly*, Sept. 30, 1911, pp. 560–71.

50. Ibid., pp. 556, 570–71.

51. Scamehorn, *From Balloons to Jets*, pp. 86, 95–97.

52. Ibid., pp. 114, 116, 119, 122, 124.

53. *Flying*, Oct., 1920, p. 593.

54. Scamehorn, *From Balloons to Jets*, pp. 104, 107, 109, 167, 169; *Chicago Tribune*, Sept. 26, 1920, p. 5; June 24, 1924, p. 1; Orear, *History of Aviation*, pp. 43, 50; Doherty, *Origin of O'Hare*, p. 4; *Flying*, July, 1029, pp. 357, 377.

55. Scamehorn, *From Balloons to Jets*, pp. 233–39.

56. Ibid., p. 205; R. M. Field to C. E. Jenks, Peoria, Jan. 29, 1926, William B. Robertson to C. E. Jenks, Anglum, Mo., Jan. 14, 1926, Robertson to Jenks, Feb. 15, 1926, and Robertson to President of Association of Commerce and Industry, Feb. 12, 1926, all in box 12, Papers of the Springfield Association of Commerce and Industry, Illinois State Historical Library; Charles A. Lindbergh, *We* (New York, 1927), pp. 80, 153–97.

57. Scamehorn, *From Balloons to Jets*, p. 207; Lindbergh, *We* pp. 213–20; *Postmark*, Springfield, July 10, 1927, pamphlet in box 12, Papers of Springfield Association of Commerce and Industry, Illinois State Historical Society Fred Goermer, *The Search for Amelia Earhart* (New York, 1966), p. 13; *Chicago Tribune*, June 24, 1928, picture section, p. 3.

58. *Chicago Tribune*, Apr. 7, 1928, p. 16; Nov. 2, 1928, p. 1; Orear, *History of Aviation*, pp. 54–55; Postal Affairs Committee to President, Sept. 11, 1928, box 12, Papers of Springfield Association of Commerce and Industry; *Railway Age*, Jan. 14, 1928, p. 149.

9

The Hard Sell:
Economic Change in the 1920s

The face and voice of Illinois changed further because of new business methods and attitudes during the 1920s, and despite the claims of advertising, the average person lost a little of his freedom of choice. During the '20s America became a nation of consumers, assaulted by the pleas of advertising and salesmanship aimed at causing them to purchase goods they had never before known they needed or wanted. New products appeared regularly to satisfy needs that did not exist. The consumption of goods became a status symbol of the middle class, previously a luxury reserved for the rich. It was the era of the high-pressure salesman, and the successful ones were elevated to sainthood during the era. Indeed, Bruce Barton wrote that Christ had been a salesman. Packaging became the most important part of the manufacture and sale of a product. The custom of buying by a brand name came into its own. "Keeping up with the Joneses" became a household phrase.[1]

Advertising, although a force in the first decade ot the twentieth century, really came into its own with World War I. The federal governmant used hard-sell techniques to promote patriotic ardor, to insure conformity, and to dispose of war bonds. As prosperity returned after the war and the nation lurched along the bumpy economic roads of the '20s advertising pointed the real direction of the business world. If the '20s generation elevated the salesmen of the country to sainthood, that materialistic generation worshiped the advertising man as the god of the economic world. Deprived of products and pleasures during the war, the citizenry now had money and was willing to spend it. Advertising agencies were prepared to make the most of this seller's market. National advertising expenditures rose from $1,400,000,000 in 1918 to $4,000,000,000 in 1929. Correspondence schools in advertising techniques were established by 1900, and soon major universities were establishing programs in marketing and advertising as schools of business appeared in most universities. New techniques of manufacture and new products caused production to soar, and the contents of the bulging warehouses had to be sold. The "ad men" stood by to achieve this end.[2]

Advertising agencies learned to play on feelings of inadequacy, guilt, shame, and fear, as well as to promote patriotism and nostalgia and to assert kindly attitudes toward motherhood, dogs, children, and apple pie. In this age of conformity which worshiped "the bitch-goddess SUCCESS" to use the phrase of William James, advertising preyed on the insecurity of those who feared failure. Mothers taught their children to be popular by avoiding offense and by conforming to middle-class standards. Taught that their ultimate goal was material success in the business world, young men believed that one avenue to success involved grooming and conforming to standards of fashion.[3]

The advertising business developed a mystique that made huckstering respectable. N. W. Ayer, one of the largest ad agencies, proclaimed in an advertisement for itself that "Modern advertising does more than appeal to the old simple instinct of possession. It opens new roads to freedom and leisure." Albert Lasker, "the father of modern advertising," regarded his trade as essentially education of the public. Noting that advertising raised the cost of goods to the consumer, Lasker wrote philosophically, "If the public is to be educated to the use of goods, it must pay the cost of its education." Lasker expressed no concern as to whether the public chose to be educated.[4]

Advertising based many of its claims on the success complex, and some ads were less than subtle. Post Bran Flakes proclaimed to the housewife, "How You Can Help Him Win! The very food you serve at the table can aid him in avoiding a condition that holds men back. A wife, in a sense, is custodian of her husband's health. The food she selects can help him in his daily battle for success."[5] Physical appearance was all-important in the success mystique. Consider the following dialogue between a husband and wife in an ad for the Arrow Starched Collar:

So that good looking Jones man got promoted, did he?

Yes; boys at the bank say he is the type.

Well, I'll say he has the clothes. Perhaps if you were more careful about your clothes, and wore nice-looking, comfortable starched collars, you might be enrolled in the battallion of bank vice-presidents.[6]

Advertising made the public keenly aware of bacteria, particularly their odor-causing properties, which could be socially disastrous. Good taste of the past was thrown aside to discuss all manner of bodily functions in the effort to peddle dentifrices, soap, sanitary napkins, deodorants, and beauty aids. Listerine proclaimed, "Not until the last vestige of dandruff is gone, can you be considered a fastidious person, acceptable socially." They warned that children could bring home from school a case of dandruff which could lead to baldness. Needless to say, Listerine could prevent this. May Breath, "a purifying deodorant for mouth and stomach," warned, "A few years ago bad breath was condoned as an unavoidable misfortune. Today it is judged one of the greatest social offenses."[7]
Kotex provided "correct appearance and hygienic comfort" while it deodorized. Modess provided a coupon to be clipped and handed to a sales person. The coupon read, "One Box of Modess, Please." This avoided embarrassment in crowded stores. Zonite proved that infection had succumbed to science. Fleishman's yeast aided in problems of complexion, constipation, colds, and boils. NUJOL provided "internal cleanliness" which made for "Health, Happiness and Success." It overcame "faulty elimination" without laxatives, which "leading physicians testify only aggravate the condition and often lead to permanent injury." Formament offered a "Germ-Killing Throat Tablet," while Ovaltine promised to banish "wakeful nerves and sleepless nights and store up lasting all-day energy." Williams Aqua-Velva "keeps your face like velvet all day," with a "man-style fragrance." Doctors tell you that "inferior toilet paper is harmful" so "see that your bathroom paper is safe," by using Scot Tissue. Old Dutch Cleanser "chase[d] dirt" and provided "healthful cleanliness." Lifebuoy discovered "B. O." and warned of the horrible fate of being ostracized if you did not use their product. Ipana warned of "pink toothbrush" as the first evidence of pyorrhea, and Listerine shifted its interest from dandruff when it discovered "halitosis" was a more severe problem.[8] Toothpaste sold well. Colgate "washed your teeth,"

Pepsodent removed the film, Pebeca prevented your mouth glands from drying up, Squibbs dental cream prevented "acid decay at the danger line," Forhams was the "most effective agent" against pyorrhea, and Dr. West's toothbrush fought the "mortal enemy of your smile—tooth decay."[9]

Advertising saw its main goal as creating an identity for a product through a brand name. The advertisement must do more than educate the public to the need to use soap, toothpaste, sanitary napkins, and deodorants or to create a desire for an automobile or cigarettes. This might lead to the purchase of a competitor's product, which was, as one historian put it, "as corrosive an idea as a businessman's mind can entertain." Thus advertising had to provide a slogan which would stick in the mind of the potential buyer to make him want to drive not just a car but a Buick; smoke not just any cigarette but a Lucky Strike; use not just any toothpaste but Colgate's. The advertising agencies achieved this by making claims, sometimes outrageous and rarely subtle, for the merits of a product and by packaging the product in an attractive, eye-catching exterior. The agencies took advantage of all the new technology in creating images. Radio provided one of the new outlets. Later, Dr. Lee De Forest, one of inventors of radio, would ask, "What have you done with my child?" Aircraft were used for advertising by skywriting, and motion picture theaters were also used to advertise. A new era was born when Dodge Brothers put $65,000 into an hour-long radio broadcast in 1928. New techniques in printing were also utilized, including high-speed, four-color presses.[10]

Among the advertising agencies of national prominence, the Chicago-based firm of Lord and Thomas quickly rose to a position of eminence. Just before the turn of the century, Lord and Thomas did a gross business of about $800,000 per annum with clients which included Armour and Anheuser-Busch. In 1898, Albert Lasker joined Lord and Thomas as a $10-a-week employee. Born in Germany of American parents, Lasker worked as a journalist before going into advertising at the age of eighteen. By 1904, Lord and Thomas had made Lasker a partner at a salary of $52,000 a year. By 1912 he owned the firm. In 1904, Lasker brought another advertising genius, John Kennedy, into the company, and three years later Claude Hopkins joined them. Great copywriters and super-salesmen, these men engaged primarily in selling themselves, Lord and Thomas, and advertising to prospective clients. As one historian described their methods, they would grasp prospective clients "by the corporate lapels . . . explaining, charming and persuading them into employing Lord and Thomas." Claude Hopkins said of Lasker: "So far as I know, no ordinary human being has ever resisted Albert Lasker."[11]

When Lasker came to Lord and Thomas, the firm employed one copywriter who earned $40 per week and one staff artist who got $35 per week. When, six years later, Lasker hired John Kennedy, he paid him $28,000 per year. Kennedy, an ex-member of the Royal Canadian Mounted Police, had gotten his advertising experience in patent medicines. He provided Lord and Thomas with their slogan, "Advertising is Salesmanship on Paper." Lasker made the most of the high salaries his firm paid. In a house publication in 1911, Lord and Thomas boasted, "One man in our Copy Department receives as much as the President of the United States Steel Corporation. Others are paid in proportion." Obviously the client who retained Lord and Thomas was getting the best. Another Lord and Thomas slogan proclaimed: "Salesmanship is mainly strategy." They referred to "That Modern Aladdin's Lamp—Called Advertising" which could make people buy things and put out money that they did not want to part with. Their view of the ad man was that "the able practitioner of true Advertising possesses nothing *less* than this splendid capacity and opportunity to *change* the *minds of millions,* at will, through a kind of literature which *compels Action.*"[12]

Lasker's greatest triumph came as he elevated Lucky Strikes into one of the three best-selling brands of cigarettes. Eventually the American Tobacco Company carried a $20,000,000 advertising budget with Lord and Thomas. One of Lasker's campaigns promoted smoking among women. To do this, prejudice had to be overcome, in part by selling the concept that women who smoked were thin while those who did not were fat. To the dismay of the candy industry, Lasker coined the slogan "Reach for a Lucky instead of a sweet." Lasker also persuaded stars of the Metropolitan Opera to do testimonials saying, "My living is dependent on my being able to sing, and I protect my precious voice by smoking Lucky Strike." Subsequently Lasker used movie stars in the same way.[13]

Hopkins and Lasker built Puffed Wheat and Puffed Rice into major sellers by emphasizing the process by which they were manufactured. They advertised the two cereals with the meaningless phrase, "the food shot from guns." Quaker Oats had to raise the price of the cereal to pay for the advertising. Hopkins built the sales of Schlitz beer by visiting the plant in Milwaukee. At one stage he came to a steam room where bottles were sterilized. He developed the idea that because of the sterilization process Schlitz was pure and free from germs. The Schlitz people pointed out that all breweries did this step to avoid spoilage. Hopkins replied that the public would not recognize this; furthermore the advertisements did not say that only Schlitz had this process. Schlitz sales grew, said Lasker, "as if a magic wand had been put over the firm."[14]

A major shift in business practice came with the upsurge of installment buying in the '20s. The Singer Sewing Machine Company had used this procedure for many years, but the automobile industry brought it to full use. In 1916, Maxwell instituted a credit plan with a 50 percent down payment and used the slogan "Pay as you Ride" in its advertising. In self-defense other auto makers were forced into similar plans. Ultimately the plan was used for household appliances, furniture, jewelry, clothing, and farm equipment. Observers estimated consumer credit in the United States at $4,357,000,000 in 1923. By 1929 estimates had soared to $8,183,000,000. Economists believed that 13.5 percent of retail sales in 1929 were by time-payment plan.[15]

In 1919, General Motors established the General Motors Acceptance Corporation to finance sales of their cars. Other motor companies followed with the "Dodge Plan," the "Paige-Jewett Plan," and the "Nash Plan." The usual contract called for a third of the purchase price as a down payment, with interest of 12 percent and twelve months to pay. By the end of the '20s, 75 percent of the automobiles sold were on some kind of installment plan. Unquestionably installment buying stimulated sales of new and used cars. A. R. Erskine, president of Studebaker Corporation, believed the elimination of installment buying would be disastrous. He believed that 65 percent of the people who bought cars would have to do without them if they could not buy on credit. The General Motors Acceptance Corporation lost only about one-fifth of 1 percent in default of loans.[16]

Gradually other industries became dependent on the installment system. It was estimated that in 1925 90 percent of the pianos, washing machines, and sewing machines, 80 percent of the trucks and phonographs, 75 percent of the tractors, and 70 percent of the furniture and gas stoves were sold on an installment plan. Until 1910 cash constituted the chief medium in the exchange of goods. But, as one writer put it, by the end of the '20s, "The Simple Simons of our day do not have to contend with any unprogressive

Pie-man. 'Show me first your penny' is not the slogan of the most rapidly expanding new industries."[17]

Those who questioned the widespread use of consumer credit noted that personal savings increased little during the 1920s. Some insisted the system was unhealthy because the power to purchase by installments was not used in a productive way but almost solely for luxury items. It was argued that the automobile was destructive to human life and, in a sense, to wealth. Supporters replied that the automobile had become necessary to business and had the advantage of forcing the improvement of roads. Others pointed out that installment buying caused the buyer's judgment to deteriorate because some clearly bought more than they could afford. Loss of employment caused loss of both the item purchased and the investment in it. It was further argued that the system caused overproduction and overpricing of goods. Many merchants advertised "no charge for credit," but as an increasing percentage of all goods was purchased on installment, the charge for credit was built into the purchase price. Unquestionably the consumer paid more for the product whether the "carrying charges" were concealed or not and whether he paid cash or not. Some made the claim that the poor were sucked into deeper debt by the system.[18]

The advantages of installment buying to the business community were obvious. It created a market. But with great expansion of plant facilities for the production of expensive consumer goods, the business community boarded a treadmill. The more they produced or could produce, the greater the need for new markets. Installment buying created a new market or demand for goods, or at least moved up the time when demand was effective. Through salesmanship and advertising, business created the idea that newer and bigger was better, and installment buying made it possible for more and more people to indulge themselves in this fantasy. Without arguing the issue of whether the standard of living was improved, the system created jobs and satisfied the desires of consumers. Merchants benefited from the fact that debts were paid in regular installments, which brought the customer back into the store, making more sales possible.[19]

The rapid growth of chain stores in retail business constituted another phenomenon of the business world. Chain stores caused consternation and dislocation in the business community. They put the individual store owner, formerly the backbone of the retail trade, at a disadvantage, changed the pricing structure, increased the use of advertising, and promoted name brands. The chain stores hit their peak around 1929. In Illinois independent retailers outnumbered the chain stores in that year. Of 96,900 retail stores, 76,838 were independent. Although 80 percent of the total were independent merchants, they did only 60 percent of the total dollar business.[20]

The growth of chain stores came about, in part, because of the urbanization of the population and the changed character of life in the cities. The automobile made it possible for rural people who had shopped in nearby villages to go to a larger population center to buy at a chain store. The chain stores gave, or seemed to give, lower prices, which attracted many. Several aspects of this system led to a change in family life. Where the housewife in an urban area had gone to several separate stores to buy meat, dairy goods, vegetables, or staple groceries, the chain stores provided all of these at one location, a throwback to the old general store. The chain stores provided less service, however. They did not deliver or provide credit. Many staple items were now sold in packages, often by brand name. The chain stores were impersonal and devoted to the profit motive, whereas many of the individual merchants were family friends, who provided extra service and made shopping a modest social event. As one writer commented, "It is . . . the aim of the chain stores to attract the customer, secure his money, and get him out as rapidly as possible." By volume sales, the chains could take a lower unit profit, thus driving the small merchant to the wall.[21]

Opponents of chain stores argued that they fostered unemployment by curtailing services, that they paid lower wages to their help, and that they bought insurance, employed lawyers, and purchased their stock elsewhere. It was said that they tended to be monopolistic and were controlled by absentee owners. More important, chain stores standardized communities, destroyed small businesses, and took money out of local communities. Undoubtedly the chains lessened the opportunity for individuals to own their own businesses. There is always a large mortality rate in retail businesses, but the competition of the chain stores increased the number of closures in groceries, meat markets, dry goods stores, and clothing stores. In 1925, in the five largest cities in Illinois, there were forty-three grocery stores per 10,000 population; by 1929 this figure had decreased to thirty-seven.

In a study in 1928, the Marketing Department of the College of Commerce at the University of Illinois surveyed forty-five villages in nineteen counties. The survey found that sales held steady in convenience products but fell in staples. Seventy-three percent of the general stores reported losses. Some of this was attributed to inefficiency and a smaller selection of goods. In addition to the mobility afforded by the automobile, some merchants attributed lower sales to the fact that farmers were spending money on autos that normally would have been spent on other retail products.[22]

The advantages of the chain store included a wider selection of products. And chains cut costs by group advertising, elimination of middlemen, less expensive warehousing, cheaper accounting procedures, and lower labor cost. The chain stores made the claim that they eliminated waste by experience, large-scale buying, and better-trained personnel. Whether or not these savings were passed on to the consumer is questionable, however.[23]

Of all the chain stores, those selling food products were the most important to families. By 1912, a few self-service stores had been established. By the early 1920s the combination stores, which sold meat, dairy products, fresh vegetables, and groceries, had appeared. By 1930, the supermarket concept had broadened. The prototype of the food chain was the Great Atlantic and Pacific Tea Company, commonly known as A&P. This chain started in the 1870s with a few stores, two of them in Chicago. By 1920, A&P operated 4,621 stores nationally, with $235,000,000 in gross sales. By 1928, the store had 15,177 stores, with gross sales of $973,000,000. It had eleven stores in Decatur alone in 1926. Kroger, the second largest national food chain, was founded in Ohio in 1902. By 1928, it had 3,749 grocery stores and 1,565 meat stores, mostly in the Midwest. It also owned seven bread bakeries, four cracker bakeries, seven cake bakeries, a slaughterhouse, a meat-packing plant, and full warehousing facilities.[24]

There were some Illinois-based food chains which could lay claim to being regional if not national operations. Among these was the Jewel Tea Company of Melrose Park, which, like many food companies, started as a home-delivery service. In 1899, Frank Vernon Skiff started the first route. In 1901, Skiff and his brother-in-law, F. P. Ross, opened a store on East Forty-third Street in Chicago. They incorporated in Illinois in 1904 and in New York in 1916. Their business was largely cash, direct to customers. Typically their salesmen, driving Ford trucks, carrying wire baskets full of staples, came to each door on their route. They carried coffee, tea, cereals, extracts, soap flakes and chips, graham crackers, spices, condiments, peanut butter, egg noodles, cosmetics, rice, spaghetti, and macaroni. For each purchase, the customer got credit toward premiums which included sweepers, coffee grinders, kitchen utensils, Haviland china, silverware, and towels. Although the stores increased in number, the routes continued to be the most important part of the business, grossing $16,800,000 in 1929. The 2,100 employees of Jewel Tea serviced some 600,000 customers.[25]

Another Illinois company, the National Tea Company, was incorporated in 1902. By 1920, the company had 163 stores grossing $18,700,000. By 1929, they had 1,627 stores with a gross of $90,200,000. They had a warehouse and bakery in Chicago and the India Tea Company operating wagon routes. There were other, smaller chains such as Piggly Wiggly, which advertised in 1926 that it "keeps 2,000,000 hens busy to supply the daily egg needs of Piggly Wiggly." These eggs could be bought for 28 cents per dozen in cartons.[26]

A study of pricing in Champaign-Urbana at the end of the '20s showed that all food products were 8.4 percent lower in all chains and 11.5 percent lower in sectional chains. The investigator found that the greatest consumer advantage was in staple, nonperishable items, while the least advantage was in meat, milk, and butter. The investigator found that a twenty-four-ounce loaf of bread cost 10 cents in downtown service stores, and 9.8 cents in neighborhood-service stores compared with 7.5 cents in national and sectional chains. In contrast, a slice of center-cut ham cost 48.3 cents per pound in downtown service stores, 39.8 cents in neighborhood service stores, and 41.7 cents in national and sectional chains. The survey of customers found that 28 percent of families had their groceries delivered, while 39.8 percent bought groceries on credit. Customers who patronized the chain stores listed price, store location, and wider selection as the major reasons for shopping there. Those who patronized local stores listed location, merchant personality, credit, delivery, and price as major factors in their buying habits.[27]

A large percentage of the variety store business was carried on by chain stores. The giant among these was F. W. Woolworth and Company. Unitl 1905, F. W. Woolworth owned all of the stores outright. In 1905 he incorporated, and by 1911 the company had 318 stores. At that time mergers brought in five other similar companies with 278 more stores. In 1928, Woolworth had 1,725 stores and gross sales of around $300,000,000. Other familiar names in the field were Kresge, Kress, Grand, Grant, and McCrory. Woolworth's and other "dime stores" were seen in most

Illinois cities; these variety stores grossed about 2 percent of the total retail sales of the nation.[28]

Department store chains also played an important part in Illinois life. Montgomery Ward and Company was founded in Chicago in 1872 as a mail-order house. The company continued as such until the post–World War I depression forced them to turn to retail outlets to bolster their profits. In 1926 they established their first ten stores, all in the Midwest. Among these were stores at Woodstock, Clinton, and Kankakee. By 1929, they had 532 retail stores with gross sales, both mail and store, totaling $267,000,000. Ward's manufactured part of the goods they sold, notably farm implements, cream separators, gasoline engines, harness, paint, wallpaper, and clothing. They adopted the installment plan during the 1920s.[29]

Sears, Roebuck and Company, which also originated in Chicago, followed a similar pattern. The company began as a modest business selling watches by mail, and continued to do business only by mail until 1925. The current name was adopted in 1893, and in 1895 Julius Rosenwald joined the firm. Rosenwald established the policy of keeping prices low by buying for less and keeping the overhead cost of sales down. In 1924 General Robert E. Wood, who had worked for Montgomery Ward and was enthusiastic about retail stores, moved to Sears. He was able to convince the management to move in the direction of the department store. In 1925 Sears opened eight stores, seven of them near the mail-order warehouses, three in Chicago, and one each in Seattle, Dallas, Kansas City, Philadelphia, and Evansville, Indiana. By 1929, Sears was operating 324 stores. Their gross sales totaled $415,000,000, of which $168,000,000 came through the stores.

Sears owned several manufacturing plants in Illinois by 1929. Among these was the David Bradley Farm Implement Works at Bradley, lumber yards at Cairo, EZ Stove Works at Kankakee, and the Bent Piano, Music and Phonograph Company, Illinois Wall Paper Mills, Illinois Paint Works, Wood and Fiber Box Company, and John A. Stain Varnish Company, all in Chicago. Sears manufactured other products outside the state. They also began using the installment plan in the 1920s.[30]

Also of interest in Illinois was the Spiegel, May, Stern and Company of Chicago (now Spiegel, Inc.). The company started as a single furniture store owned by Joseph Spiegel, who subsequently opened several more stores and in 1908 established a mail-order branch. By 1929, the company had built up a gross sales of $24,000,000, and the mail-order branch far outdistanced the retail outlets, the latter accounting for only $3,340,000 of the sales. The company relied on a small down payment and low interest rate. Its slogan became "no charge for credit."[31]

The drug business also became dominated by the chain store concept. One of the largest of these was Walgreen, an Illinois company. As late as 1908, C. R. Walgreen was operating a single drugstore at 4134 Cottage Grove Avenue in Chicago. By 1916 he had seven stores and incorporated the company. By 1928 he owned 330 stores, with gross sales of $32,400,000.[32]

No aspect of business activity touched so many lives as the automobile. When Hinky Dink Kenna bought an $8,000 automobile in 1905, the *Tribune* gave it a front-page headline, "Honk Honk for Hinky Dink," and had this comment about the bright-red vehicle: "When it is at full speed it looks like a streak of crimson." The Jackson Street bridge-tender commented, "The little fellow's machine has got 'em all skinned." By the '20s nearly every family had an automobile. Economically the automobile occupied the time of many and consumed natural resources at an unprecedented rate. It changed the shopping habits of the housewife, enhanced the operation of the chain stores, and put the rural villages out of business. It made suburban living possible for many who sought to escape the city. The railroads and interurbans suffered from it, and the horse began to disappear. By 1929, Robert and Helen Lynd in their sociological stucy of Muncie, Indiana, found that "ownership of an automobile has now reached the point of being an accepted essential part of normal living." Book publishing declined as people drove to the movies and gave up reading, and the shoe industry changed as people gave up walking.[33]

In 1919 Illinois licensed 478,438 automobiles; in 1929 the number had increased to 1,630,816. The difficulties created by the automobile were almost as great as the benefits derived from it. As early as 1904 speeding autos had caused problems; in that year five were arrested for "scorching" in Lincoln Park, and an auto "driven at high speed—said to be thirty miles an hour" ran into the Chicago River because the Rush Street bridge was open. Speeding was a special problem in the suburbs as rich Chicagoans drove their cars to summer homes. On July 8, 1908, an Evanston detective on a bicycle caught ten speeders, some of them going twenty-three miles per hour. Nationally nearly 15,000 persons died in auto-related accidents in 1923. The following year in Illinois, automobiles caused the deaths of 1,254 persons, more than half of them pedestrians.[34]

The prophets of doom expressed concern over the social

implications of the automobile. It was causing people to avoid church on Sunday, they said, many preferring to drive to the golf course, to a favorite fishing spot, to another city for lunch, or on a sight-seeing trip, as a "Sunday driver." The automobile was breaking down family life by making it easy for every member of the family to pursue his own interest, thus scattering the group. More important, the automobile was providing privacy for the amorous adventures of the youth of America. Doubtless motion pictures contributed to the concern about the morality of the "speed-crazy" generation as they portrayed drunken youth driving at top speed on their way to an orgy. The phrases "mad money" and "walking back" became commonplace in the vocabulary, as did the cliché about a "flat tire."[35]

The *Chicago Tribune* was concerned about the deterioration of "the manners, habits, and morals of youth." As one writer saw the problem, the automobile was detrimental in that it freed young people from parental surveillance. When they were out of sight of relatives and friends, they might do all sorts of immoral things. The automobile, said the *Tribune,* had provided a "luxurious, high-geared, speed-loving" generation which lacked the maturity to cope with temptation.[36]

The economic value of the automobile was obvious to those who feared its social consequences. Weighing the benefits and the liabilities of the new machine, most came to the conclusion that the automobile could not be done away with. The *Tribune* said, ". . . we should be foolish indeed, to give up an agency which brings so much which is wholesome and helpful into our society." The *Tribune* saw the solution in the "home where good habits and standards are honored" and "the pulpit whence comes inspiration to right living."[37]

The automobile quickly became the most important single industry in the nation. One writer estimated that it consumed 90 percent of the petroleum output, 80 percent of the rubber, 20 percent of the steel, 75 percent of the plate glass, and 25 percent of the machine tools. The manufacturing of the product was only the beginning of its influence. Concrete highways had to be built and repaired, retail businesses flourished and began selling automotive accessories, the housing industry changed, and resorts and tourist camps prospered.[38]

The great expansion in sales of automobiles became possible because of the widespread adoption of the installment credit system, the relative prosperity of the postwar period and the constantly decreasing price of automobiles as volume increased. By 1929 there were 2,477 dealers in new automobiles and 218 purveyors of used cars in Illinois. New car dealers sold automobiles worth $391,576,738 in that year. There also were 656 tire and battery stores, 415 brake, battery, and ignition shops, 552 tire shops, 3,967 filling stations, 1,120 filling stations combined with other stores, 153 body and fender shops, 39 parking garages or lots, and 30 radiator shops. In all of these categories there were 13,197 proprietors employing over 40,000 persons. Truly the automobile had come into its own.[39]

By any standard the automobile was a new industry. Apparently the first gasoline-powered car in the United States was a Benz brought to the Chicago World's Fair in 1893. Some electric cars came into use that same year, and gasoline automobiles could be bought by 1895. Two magazines, *Horseless Age* and *Motorcycle*, began publication in New York and Chicago in 1895. *Motor Age* began publication in 1899, and the American Automobile Association was founded in Chicago in 1902. In 1895 the *Chicago Times Herald* sponsored two automobile races. The first was on November 2, but none of the four cars finished. In the second the winner was J. Frank Duryea in his Duryea Motor Wagon, at an average speed of seven and a half miles per hour. Duryea manufactured automobiles in Peoria during the '20s.[40]

The industry grew fast, and familiar names began to appear in the advertisements. In 1908, the Illinois auto fan could purchase a Cadillac Thirty, advertised as "an all-steel masterpiece of mechanical simplicity and service," for $1,400. The car featured a thirty-horsepower, four-cylinder engine, three-speed and reverse transmission, 32-by-3½-inch tires, and seated five comfortably. By 1920 the customer could buy an Auburn five-passenger touring car for $1,895 or, from the same company, the Oakland Sensible Six for $1,395. By 1926 the Chicago buyer could get a Ford runabout for $250, an Auburn eight-cylinder roadster for $1,695, a Chevrolet touring car for $495 (balloon tires $25 extra), or a Moon sedan for $1,075. The Willys Knight Six could be bought for $1,750 to $2,495, with "an engine you will never wear out" so you could "count on keeping it years longer than other cars." The Flint Sixty ($1,525 FOB Flint, Michigan) provided "safety wherever you go." Also among the boasts: "A bad stretch of heavy mud road looms up ahead—you go through ruts, mud with only slightly slackened speed." Regardless of the merits of the car, it was a graphic description of driving conditions of the period. The eighteen Buick dealers of Chicago were already proclaiming "when better automobiles are built, Buick will build them."[41]

By 1928 Willys Overland announced that the new Whippet Six would sell for $695, the "lowest price in history for a six-cylinder automobile." In Chicago the purchaser could buy a Pontiac Cabriolet with a rumble seat for $795. In Springfield he could buy a Hupmobile eight-cylinder car for between $1,825 and $2,125. A Dodge Senior Six sport coupe with a rumble seat had a price tag of $1,795.[42]

Auto-related businesses grew rapidly. As roads improved and automobiles became more reliable, the citizenry ventured farther from home, making more filling stations necessary. In Decatur, "Elliot's Rotary Lift Station" advertised that the motorist desiring service could drive in at ground level and have his car lifted automatically. The owner made the claim: "It's as big an improvement over the old way of servicing cars as the gasoline pump is over the bucket and hose." Roadside restaurants became commonplace and the term "roadhouse" became a euphemism for the place that sold illicit liquor in the days of prohibition. In the smaller towns, citizens rented extra rooms to tourists and built cabins on the outskirts of towns for the use of motorists.[43]

Advertisements advised the tidy motorist that "motorists wise, Simonize" Decatur residents were urged to buy the Denker Battery (which was manufactured in Decatur), while competing ads offered "no more cranking" if you bought a Philco Battery, which had "surplus power in reserve." Those who patronized the Raybestos Brake Service could "absolutely rely on your brakes.'" Gebhart Motorist Supply offered Dayton Balloon Tires for twenty-, twenty-one-, and twenty-three-inch, rims. Gradually the tire industry was concentrated in the hands of a few companies such as Firestone, Goodyear, and the U.S. Rubber Company. These brand names became familiar as the companies competed both in advertising claims and in improvement of tires. There was gradual improvement in the quality of the rubber for longer life and in tread design for traction. Manufacturers adopted a safer cord design. By the mid-'20s it was possible to buy a low-pressure "balloon" tire which required thirty pounds of pressure as opposed to the sixty which had formerly been required. This made for more comfort. In 1926 in Decatur the driver who had a car with thirty-inch rims could buy a fabric tire from Federal for $8.25 or a cord balloon for $24.50. By 1928 Firestone was offering "gum-dipped tires" to "meet every motoring need" and assuring the motorist that "there is a Firestone dealer in your vicinity." "The Thinking Fellow" who did not own a car called a Yellow Cab, which would take him anywhere in Decatur for 50 cents. It was necessary to house the new auto. In Chicago the motorist could buy an "Ideal" garage for nothing down and two years to pay, or a brick or stucco garage to match his home for $10 down and two years to pay.[44]

Manufacturing in general in the 1920s underwent changes in technique and management procedures. Just as the salesmen and ad men dominated one end of the mercantile process, the '20s ushered in the industrial engineer and slide rule on the other end. Efficiency and more production for less labor cost were the keys to the new methodology. The automobile industry inaugurated the assembly line, following the lead of Henry Ford. Ford secured the loyalty of his workers by instituting a wage of $5 per day. The wage was high for the time, but Ford expected his workers to earn it. Ford's labor policy represented not only his desire for a stable and efficient labor force but also his flair for public relations, bringing world wide publicity. Prior to 1913, assembly of the Ford chassis required twelve hours and twenty-eight minutes. The first conveyor belt operation cut the time in half and by early 1914 to ninety minutes. Ford achieved this by making all cars nearly identical. As Ford once told an associate "The way to make automobiles is to make one automobile just like another automobile—just like one pin is like another pin when it comes out of the pin factory." Ford is also supposed to have said, "The customer can have a Ford any color he wants—so long as it is black." By the economy this achieved, Ford was able to sell one model of his car for $250.[45]

Frederick D. Taylor wrote extensively on the subject of scientific management. He proposed that employers hire only the most competent worker and then require that man to produce at the fastest rate possible by paying him a bonus for producing above the average of his class of workmen. He wrote, "And this means *high wages* and *low labor cost*. These conditions not only serve the best interests of the employer but they tend to raise each workman to the highest level which he is fitted to attain by making him use his best faculties, forcing him to remain ambitious and energetic, and giving him sufficient pay to live better than in the past." Engineers determined the standard by which men were paid by time and motion studies. Taylor believed that most workers were naturally lazy and that most employers had no idea of the time a job ought to take. By the time and motion study, the employer could set a standard time for a job and induce the worker to give up "soldiering" by giving him a reward for doing more or punishing him for doing less.[46]

Machine-made interchangeable parts became common in most industries. Secretary of Commerce Herbert Hoover, himself an engineer, promoted standardization in both parts and products. World War I brought mass production of war materials using processes which were later applied to consumer goods. Electric motors replaced the old steam plants which had provided the power to turn long shafts and systems of belts and pulleys. Harder tool steel made of carbide alloys made the manufacturing process more efficient. Mechanical loading devices replaced the unskilled worker, while new technical advances, such as glass-blowing and cigar-making machines, replaced the skilled worker. Unfortunately pride of craft also began to disappear as many workers were relegated to the production line.[47]

The consolidation of industry continued apace. By 1919 corporations owned all of the iron and steel rolling mills, 97.9 percent of the meat-packing industry, 86.1 percent of the automobile manufacturing, and 99.4 percent of the production of electrical manufacturing. Illinois continued to rank high in the basic industries. In 1919 there were 18,593 manufacturing plants with a production of $5,425,244,694. By 1929 the number of plants had declined to 15,333 but the value of products had increased. By 1929 only New York and Pennsylvania outdistanced Illinois in industrial production.[48]

In iron production, Illinois ranked third in the nation behind Pennsylvania and Ohio. In steel production, the state produced 4,763,789 tons in 1929. In the production of agricultural implements, Illinois ranked first in the nation throughout the decade. In 1919 the value of the product of sixty-eight plants was $128,284,716, while in 1929, forty-two plants produced $143,678,378. Notable among the companies were International Harvester at Chicago, John Deere at Moline, J. I. Case at Rockford and Rock Island, and Minneapolis-Moline at Moline. International Harvester had its tractor works, the Weber Wagon Company, and the McCormick Works at Chicago; manufactured threshers at West Pullman, harvesters and threshers, corn pickers, and engines at Deering Company works at Chicago, corn shellers, harrows, and hay loaders at Rock Falls, and plows in Canton; and owned steel mills at South Chicago. John Deere manufactured corn and cotton planters, disc harrows, beet tools, stalk cutters, plows, and wagons at Moline, and maintained a timber operation at Moline and an iron works at East Moline. Although not strictly farm machinery, the crawler tractor business came into its own in the 1920s. In 1909 the Holt Tractor Comapny established a plant at Peoria and in 1925 merged with the C. L. Best Gas Tractor Company to form Caterpillar Corporation, with headquarters at Peoria. In 1928 Allis Chalmers purchased the Monarch Tractor Company of Spring-field and began the manufacture of crawler tractors. International Harvester also added the tracked vehicles to their line in 1928.[49]

The changing technology of farming caused much of the production increase in the implement industry. In 1927 Illinois and Indiana combined produced tractors worth $46,332,515, while only two years later Illinois alone manufactured $93,529,912 worth of tractors. The purchase of a tractor required the farmers to buy other implements, and the sales of plows, cultivators, planters, and harvesters increased. Doubtless many farmers got caught in the "keeping-up-with-the Joneses" syndrome, in this case competition for biggest and equipment in the area.[50]

Illinois ranked first in the nation in meat-packing, but by 1929 the dollar value of the product declined. Business machines became important in Illinois industry with a product value of over $9,000,000. Confectionary items totaled $70,606,127 in 1929. Among the candy companies were the Paul F. Beiche Company of Bloomington and the Cracker Jack Company and Bunte Brothers in Chicago. This industry used quantities of corn syrup from companies like A. E. Staley of Decatur, thus providing an important market for farmers.[51]

Several companies produced passenger cars in the state over the years, but of these, only the Velie Motor Vehicle Company of Moline, incorporated in 1908, was still producing cars in 1928. The Velie Company, controlled by the Velie family, included on its board of directors George Peek, O. E. Masur, and C. C. Webber of the farm machinery industry, and in 1914 had a capacity of 3,000 vehicles per year. By 1928 it could produce 100 cars per day. In 1920 an advertisement for the Velie Thirty-four touring car boasted: "A car of snappy new 1920 design with deep, genuine leather upholstery and all the adornments and equipment you expect at a higher cost." The Velie Thirty-four sold for $1,585. In 1924 Velie was advertising the "largest six in the world for the price." The car had a wheelbase of 118 inches and a fifty-horsepower, valve-in-head engine. The five-passenger phaeton sold for $1,095 and the five-passenger sedan for $1,545. The Velie lasted until the depression drove it out of business.[52]

There were several other automobile companies formed in
Illinois. The Rayfield was manufactured in Springfield around
1912. In Chicago the Bush Motor Company manufactured a
four-cylinder car called the Bush which sold for $725. Also
Chicago-made were the Classic, the Coey Flyer, the Drexel, the
Elgin, the Ogren Six, the Portin-Palmer, and the Woods Electric.
The Bartholomew Motor Car Company produced a vehicle in
Peoria called the Glide, while the Roamer and the Halladay were
built in Streator and the Moline-Knight in East Moline. The New
Era was produced in Joliet. Most of these were four-cylinder cars,
but a few had six cylinders. Prices ranged from $495 for the
cheapest Portin-Palmer to $2,500 for the Ogren Six. Perhaps
the most expensive automobile manufactured in Illinois was the
Standard Eight sedan made by the Standard Steel Automobile
Company which in 1920 sold for $5,000.

The question arises as to why none of these auto manufacturers
survived. The answer may be found in the inability of small
companies to adapt to assembly-line, mass-production techniques,
due perhaps to an inadequate capital structure or lack of vision in
management. A more likely answer probably lies in the difficulty
of competing with rising giants like General Motors, Ford, and
Chrysler in promotion and the inability to go into national advertising. Henry Ford had the means to make his name a household word while the Coey Flyer or Portin-Palmer remained a
local product.[53]

Illinois fared better in the manufacture of trucks and commercial vehicles. In 1920 the *Tribune* proclaimed that Chicago was
"destined to becoming the greatest truck manufacturing and
distributing city in the world." The *Tribune* conceded that Detroit
was the center for passenger cars, but the same "conditions of labor
and supply" would, they predicted, make Chicago premier in
trucks. By 1927 Illinois could indeed boast that it was the first in the
nation in the production of commercial vehicles, including trucks,
busses, taxicabs, and hearses. Of those manufacturers that survived, Diamond T, a Chicago company, was important. The
company was incorporated in Illinois in 1915, and by 1917 they
were making trucks ranging from one to five tons and selling from
$1,485 to $4,100. International Harvester moved into the truck
line prior to 1920, making smaller three-quarter and one-ton
trucks that sold for $1,225 to $1,500. General Motors owned the
Yellow Truck and Coach Manufacturing Company, with plants at
Chicago and Moline. Among the trucks that were manufactured
early and disappeared from sight were the Coey, Dekalb, Fargo,

Harvey, Koeig and Luhrs, Lawson, Little Giant, Mercury, Nelson-LeMoon, Old Reliable, and Sandow.[54]

The spectacular growth in the use of the automobile required a greater production of gasoline, and as engines became more sophisticated, the quality of fuel had to be improved. The expansion and mechanization of industry also brought increased demand for lubricants. Illinois had been producing crude oil for many years, but as the refining of oil increased, it became necessary to build pipelines from Oklahoma. The refineries transported some crude by tank car, but the pipeline became essential. Operators regularly improved the pipeline operation. By 1916 diesel engines had replaced steam as a source of power for pumping oil, and by 1930 the diesels had been replaced by electric motors. By the end of the '20s pipe was being welded together rather than bolted into couplings. The quality of the pipe was improved through the use of high-carbon steel.[55]

In 1918 the first crude oil was delivered to Chicago from Oklahoma over a 670-mile pipeline built by Sinclair. This eight-inch line had a capacity of 20,000 barrels a day. In the same year Shell built a ten-inch pipeline to Wood River, where a new refinery was projected. Later Shell extended this line to East Chicago to another Shell refinery.[56]

In 1914 Standard Oil Company of Indiana was operating a refinery at Wood River; Texaco built another at Lockport. In that same year Indian Refining Company, a Maine corporation, was operating a refinery at Lawrenceville. Richmond Levering developed the company but lost control of it during World War I. Indian suffered growing financial trouble but in 1921 it boasted not only the refinery, but oil wells in Illinois, a small pipeline, 1,900 tank cars, 166 company-owned filling stations, and a world-famous brand of lubricating oil (Havoline). The company struggled through the '20s and in 1931 was purchased by Texaco.[57]

The Lincoln Oil and Refining Company at Robinson boasted a rated capacity of 1,000 barrels per day but by 1924 was so run-down it rarely produced that much. In 1924 the Ohio Oil Company purchased the refinery and its marketing outlets. James Donnell, president of Ohio Oil, visited the plant and ordered superintendent Ray Luton to rebuild. In two years a modern plant with a capacity of 5,000 barrels was in operation. Lincoln had a few stations that sold gasoline under the brand name of LINCO. All of these dealers were within a single day's tank-truck drive from the refinery.[58]

Shell built a new refinery near Wood River which began

production on September 23, 1918. Shell located the plant there because of the nearness to water and rail transportation and because Standard of Indiana already had a refinery there. During the first year of operation the Shell refinery processed 2,200,000 barrels of crude oil, manufacturing from it 66,000,000 gallons of fuel oil, 11,000,000 gallons of gasoline, and 13,000,000 gallons of kerosene. Until Shell established its own marketing system all of this was sold at wholesale. As Shell moved into retailing, the operation was expanded to include lubricating oils.[59]

Illinois ranked ninth in the nation in the refining of petroleum products in 1919 and by 1929 moved up to seventh place (behind California, Texas, New Jersey, Pennsylvania, Oklahoma, and Kansas). In 1929 Illinois had thirteen refineries which manufactured products worth $104,130,272. This included 789,440,843 gallons of gasoline, 319,962,929 gallons of fuel oil, and 46,465,951 gallons of lubricating oil.[60]

The problem of engine knock caused both automobile manufacturers and petroleum refineries to look for ways to effect a smoother performance. Charles F. Kettering of General Motors instituted research to show that General Motors engines were not responsible. In 1923 General Motors and Standard Oil of New Jersey combined to offer Ethyl, a tetraethyl lead additive to reduce engine knocks. General Motors and Standard Oil, later accused of being responsible for air pollution, licensed the product to other producers. Kettering pioneered in the production of quick-dry finish for autos and, about the same time, introduced an antifreeze solution which would not boil out. In 1926 Graham Edgar introduced octane ratings for gasoline.[61]

In the early years of the automobile the motorist purchased his gasoline at a grocery store, general store, or hardware store, where the dealers kept the product in a barrel at the rear of the store. The dealer drew off a bucket of gasoline from the barrel and poured it into the tank through a chamois-lined funnel to keep out impurities. In 1909 grocery stores sold 39 percent of the gasoline purchased, general stores accounted for 29 percent, and hardware stores for 29 percent; filling stations sold only 3 percent of the gasoline. By 1919 filling stations sold 47 percent of the gasoline, grocery stores declined to 29 percent, general stores to 18 percent, and hardware stores to 12 percent. By 1929 91.7 percent of the gasoline was sold by filling stations.[62]

In 1905 Harry Grenner and Clem Laessig, both formerly with Standard Oil, founded the Automobile Gasoline Company in St.

Louis and are credited with establishing the first drive-in filling stations. This initiated a major new retail business. By the end of the '20s garish filling stations, advertising the products of the oil companies, were seen everywhere. In the early '20s the station typically had one pump. Free air and water might be furnished but, if so, by self-service. By the end of the '20s the stations were more elaborately equipped with powered pumps, underground storage, compressed air, grease and oil service, and some with hydraulic lifts. The sale of accessories, fan belts, spark plugs, tires, tubes, batteries, and antifreeze became commonplace.[63]

The chemicals and plastics industries provided another facet of the economy which added considerable value during the '20s and foreshadowed greater impact in the decades to come. Inventors devised celluloid, the first synthetic plastic, in 1869 as a substitute for ivory in billiard balls. Forty years later promoters put forth a new product called Bakelite. By the end of the '20s, the petroleum industry had developed the field of petrochemicals to produce alcohol, glycols, ketones, and chlorinated hydrocarbons. The prohibition era fostered the Eighteenth Amendment to the Constitution, which forbade the use and sale of alcoholic beverages. When the Eighteenth Amendment put the Peoria distilleries out of the liquor business, they turned much of their productive capacity during the war to making the components of smokeless gunpowder. Later they manufactured celluloid and butanol. Derivatives of these were made into solvents and lacquers.[64]

Much of the new industry depended on increasing the generation of electric power and production of natural gas. The interurbans and street railways consumed electricity, and much of the hard consumer goods, especially household appliances, depended upon the availability of electric power. With the rapidly expanding availability of goods came their increasing use, causing pollution of the environment through uncontrolled belching smokestacks and indiscriminate dumping of waste materials into rivers and lakes. In Illinois the production of electricity increased to 3 billion kilowatt-hours in 1920. Nationally the production of natural gas doubled during the period; the production of electricity tripled. Steam plants accounted for about two-thirds of this production and water power for most of the rest.[65]

The career of Samuel Insull illustrates the growth of electrical power in Illinois. Born in 1859 in England, Insull migrated to the United States to become private secretary to Thomas A. Edison. Insull's drive and talent for organization were apparent, and he became a force in Edison's operations, learning about the production of electric power at the same time. Insull helped create the General Electric Company, which by 1892 had become a multimillion-dollar corporation. In that year J. P. Morgan and other bankers forced Edison and Insull out of the management of the company. Insull refused a subordinate position and accepted the presidency of the Chicago Edison Company. As the firm grew, so did Insull's fame, wealth, and power. His ability to raise capital for his ever-expanding empire also grew. His biographer describes his position before the structure collapsed: "In the hero-worshipping postwar decade, Insull became the Babe Ruth, the Jack Dempsey, the Red Grange of the business world. The people—butchers, bakers, and candle-stick makers who invested their all in his stocks—fairly idolized him, and even titans viewed him with awe."[66]

At the peak of his power Insull controlled Commonwealth Edison, which supplied electricity to the Chicago area, Peoples Gas Company, which provided natural gas to the city, the Public Service Company of Northern Illinois, Midland Utilities Company, which supplied electricity to 700 communities in Indiana, the elevated railways in Chicago, three interurban lines to suburban areas, North American Light and Power in the St. Louis area, and Middle West Utilities Company. This last, a gigantic holding company, supplied gas and electricity to 5,000 communities in thirty-two states.[67]

Typical of his operation was his acquisition of Central Illinois Public Service Company, which became the nucleus of the Middle West Utilities Company. Insull bought the company in 1912 when it had generating plants in Mattoon, Charleston, and the village of Kansas, with a total of 15,000 customers. It owned a streetcar line in Mattoon and an interurban line between Charleston and Matoon, a distance of ten miles. He added plants in several small communities and began building lines to others. In a dozen years CIPS furnished streetcar service, ice, gas, and water to many towns. Through consolidation Insull also reduced the price of electricity to communities.[68]

In 1919 Illinois ranked fourth in the nation in the production of electrical equipment, including batteries, electrical motors, and telephone and telegraph equipment, grossing $36,809,805. Much of this production came from the Hawthorne Works of Western Electric, the manufacturing unit of Bell Telephone. In 1926 Hawthorne Works employed some 30,000 workers. Chicago firms

Automatic Electric Company of Northlake, Kellog Switchboard and Supply, Cook Electric, Reliable Electric, and Leich Electric at Genoa produced similar equipment. In 1919 Illinois was contributing 79.7 percent of the total production of telephone equipment in the United States. By 1929 the value of the product of the electrical industry had nearly quadrupled, reaching a total of $435,021,917 in Illinois, which still ranked first in the nation.[69]

The gadget-conscious people of the United States took to the new products made possible by electricity. By 1926 Illinois had one telephone for each 4.4 persons. There were 1,372,601 telephones in the state that year, more than half of them in Chicago. Service for these was provided by some 600 telephone companies.[70]

Of equal importance was the development of radio. In 1900 Dr. Lee De Forest, an employee of Western Electric, invented the audion tube, giving Chicago claim to being the birthplace of the electronics industry. By 1929, 55 percent of Illinois families owned a radio. Generally the percentage was higher in urban areas. More than 63 percent of Chicago families had radios in 1929. Among the many companies that made radio receiving sets and parts was the Zenith Radio Corporation, which was incorporated in Illinois in 1923, superceding the Chicago Radio Laboratory founded five years earlier. The company manufactured radios for the home and promoted their product by advertising on their own station, WJAZ in Chicago. The company maintained an extensive research and development laboratory. Motorola and Admiral were also among the large producers of radios in Chicago, and a multitude of smaller companies produced parts for the industry.[71]

Ownership of a radio in the '20s could be an adventure requiring considerable skill and knowledge. For example, in 1926 it was possible to buy an "Operadio Consolette" for $79, but for $99.89 the purchaser also got six Cunningham tubes, two large Burgess 22½-volt B batteries, three 45-volt B. batteries, six Burgess Dry Cell A batteries, one loop, and an instruction book. In 1928 advertisements offered the "Freshman Equaphase Electric Radio" for $113 without tubes. By this time, however, the radio would operate "from any light socket" for less than 1 cent per hour. The radio had become a piece of furniture with the cabinet "paneled in genuine mahogany." In 1929 nearly 900 combination radio and electrical shops employing 2,503 persons sold radios, parts, and service. Also common was the combination of radio and musical instrument stores which, in 1929, employed 1,664 persons.[72]

Mechanical household appliances also became common in the

'20s. The first all-electric kitchen, exhibited at the Columbian Exposition in Chicago in 1893, was a marvel available to very few. In 1906 the Hurley Machine Company in Chicago designed the first electric washing machine for the home.[73]

In 1914 Maytag devised the first washing machine powered by gasoline engine, making this device available to farm women. In 1924 Sperlich and Uhlig invented the first ironers, a forerunner of a product marketed under the trade name Ironrite. In 1909 Silas and A. W. Altorfer designed a power washer under the brand name of ABC. This laid the groundwork for the Altorfer Brothers Company, incorporated in Illinois in 1916, which later became a part of the Nash-Kelvinator Corporation. The plant at Peoria made washing machines, ironers, and wringers and had a capacity of 50,000 machines a day.[74]

The household appliance industry depended on advertising and installment sales to dispose of their ever-increasing production. In 1929, 582 stores sold a general line of household appliances and another 34 sold and serviced refrigerators, both electric and gas-operated. The advertising for the products played on the fetish of cleanliness and the new appetite for leisure. The advertisement for the Hoover Vacuum Cleaner warned that "DIRT—dangerous destructive dirt!—is being found in rugs that were once thought to be clean." This problem could be solved simply by allowing "your authorized Hoover Dealer" to deliver a vacuum cleaner for $6.25 down.[75]

The happy owner of an Easy Washer, promised the advertisement, "washes most of the morning . . . then dances half the night." The Maytag Company boasted that their aluminum washer accounted for one out of every three sales of washers. The Maytag was, they said, "The Washer that Glorified Washday." The Thor Washer could be had in Decatur in 1926 for $89, on a contract which required $5 down and year to pay. The Thor consisted of a copper tub, steel frame, swinging metal wringer with rubber cushion rolls. In Chicago in the same year the housewife could buy a rebuilt Thor for $1 down and $1 a week and get a year's supply of soap to go with it.[76]

Domestic refrigeration was largely unknown prior to World War I. For many years the ice man, first with a horse-drawn wagon and later with a truck, was a familiar sight in every city. Householders were provided with a cardboard sign which told him how big a piece of ice to bring into the house and place in the massive wooden icebox. Small boys followed his vehicle on hot summer days, hoping to pick up a cooling chip of ice. Gradually the mechanical refrigerator became essential in households that could afford the device. Again, ownership was made easy by the install-ment plan. Kelvinator had a unit that could be installed in the old icebox and Frigidaire promised "ice cubes in generous quantities" and said, "Food is kept fresh and wholesome—health is safe-guarded." In 1928 a Zerozone refrigerator sold for $190.[77]

Even the most casual observer must look upon the economic development of the '20s with ambivalence. Many new products added to the comfort and leisure of Americans. These products created new jobs and added to the affluence of American workers. Much of this however, was achieved by an appeal to the baser side of human nature and by playing on a fear of disease or social ostracism. In a material sense progress was made, but a high price in the depletion of natural resources paid for that progress.

1. James P. Wood, *The Story of Advertising* (New York, 1958), hp. 365–66.

2. Ibid., pp. 363–64; Frank Presby, *The History and Development of Advertising* (Garden City, N.Y., 1929), p. 582.

3. William James to H. G. Wells, Sept. 11, 1906 in Henry James, *The Letters of William James*, 2 vols. (Boston, 1920), II, 260.

4. *Literary Digest*, Mar. 21, 1925, p. 80; Albert Lasker, "The Personal Reminis-cences of Albert Lasker," *American Heritage*, 6, Dec., 1954, p. 81.

5. *Good Housekeeping*, June, 1928, p. 276.

6. Ibid., p. 342.

7. Frank Rowsome, *They Laughed When I Sat Down, an Informal History of Advertising* (New York, 1959), p. 127; *Literary Digest*, Mar. 14, 1925, p. 69; *Good Housekeeping*, May, 1928, p. 155.

8. *Literary Digest*, March 14, 1925, p. 75; Mar. 27, 1925, p. 77; Mar. 28, 1925, pp. 50, 52, 73; *Good Housekeeping*, May, 1928, pp. 115, 190; June, 1928, pp. 1, 271; Wood, *Story of Advertising*, pp. 381, 383, 384.

9. *Literary Digest*, Mar. 7, 1925, pp. 61, 70; Mar. 14, 1925, p. 70; Mar. 21, 1925, pp. 58, 61; Mar. 28, 1925, p. 66.

10. Wood, *Story of Advertising, pp. 367, 403, 414;* Presby, *History and Development of Advertising*, pp. 578, 579; Rowsome, *They Laughed When I Sat Down*, p. 90.

11. Rowsome, *They Laughed When I Sat Down*, pp. 132–35; "Reminiscences of Albert Lasker," pp. 74–76.

12. "Reminiscences of Albert Lasker," pp. 78–79; Lord and Thomas, *Real Salesmanship in Print: Strategy in Advertising* (Chicago, 1911), p. 23; Lord and Thomas, *Book of Advertising Tests: Articles That Actually Say Something about Advertising* (Chicago, n.d.), p. 19; Lord and Thomas, *Concerning a Literature Which Compels Action: Altruism in Advertising* (Chicago, 1911), pp. 11–12, 16–17. See also Claude C. Hopkins, *My Life in Advertising* (Chicago, 1966).

13. "Reminiscences of Albert Lasker," pp. 82–84; Wood, *Story of Advertising*, pp. 374, 377.

14. *Advertising*, pp. 374, 377.

15. John Rovensky, "The Relation of Installment Selling to the Credit Structure," *Proceedings of the Academy of Political Science* 12 (1926–1928), p. 596; *The Economic*

Almanac for 1941–1942 (New York, 1941), p. 351; Edwin R. A. Seligman, *The Economics of Installment Selling: A Study in Consumer Credit with Special Reference to the Automobile,* 2 vols. (New York, 1927), I, 16, 17.

16. Harold E. Wright, *Financing of Automobile Installment Sales* (Chicago, 1927), pp. 20, 23, 75; Seligman, *Economics of Installment Selling,* I, 27, 28; William A. Grimes, *Financing Automobile Sales by the Time Payment Plan* (Chicago, 1926), p. 58.

17. William Trufant Foster, "The Basic Meaning of the Growth of Installment Selling," *Proceedings of the American Academy of Political Science* 12 (July 1926–1928), p. 613; Seligman, *Economics of Installment Selling,* I, 30, 100–101.

18. Lawson Purdy, "Installment Purchasing and Installment Saving in Relation to Family Welfare," *Proceedings of the American Academy of Political Science* 12 (1926–1928), p. 609; Milton Ayres, "Installment Selling and Finance Companies," *Annals of the American Academy of Political and Social Science* 196 (Mar. 1938), pp. 123–25; Harvey W. Huegy, *Economics of Installment Credit* (Urbana, Ill., 1934), p. 5; Seligman, *Economics of Installment Selling,* I, 214, 218, 223, 235, 236, 237, 249.

19. Foster, "Growth of Installment Selling," p. 612; Ayres, "Installment Selling," p. 126.

20. Godfrey M. Lebhar, *Chain Stores in America, 1859–1950* (New York, 1952), p. 5; *Fifteenth Census of the United States, 1930: Distribution, Retail Change* (Washington, D.C., 1933), p. 605.

21. Daniel Bloomfield, *Chain Stores* (New York, 1931), p. 50; Theodore Beckman and Herman C. Nolen, *The Chain Store Problem: A Critical Analysis* (New York, 1938), pp. 217–20, 223.

22. "The Automobile and the Village Merchant," *Bureau of Business Research Bulletin 19* (Urbana, Ill., 1928), pp. 9–17; Paul D. Converse, "Business Mortality of Illinois Retail Stores from 1925–1930," *Bureau of Business Research Bulletin 41* (Urbana, Ill., 1932), pp. 30–35; Beckman and Nolen, *The Chain Store Problem,* p. 234.

23. Beckman and Nolen, *The Chain Store Problem,* pp. 204, 212; Bloomfield, *Chain Stores,* pp. 105–23.

24. *Poor's Manual of Industrials, 1928,* pp. 2861, 3600; Lebhar, *Chain Stores in America,* p. 365; Edwin P. Hoyt, *That Wonderful A&P* (New York, 1969); *Decatur Herald,* Apr. 3, 1926, p. 2.

25. Lebhar, *Chain Stores in America,* p. 336; *Poor's Manual of Industrials, 1928,* pp. 1039–40; Jewel Tea Company, *Working for Jewel* (Chicago, 1927), pp. 10–11, 13, 16, 18, 19, 27, 50.

26. *Poor's Manual of Industrials, 1929,* pp. 1180–81; Lebhar, *Chain Stores in America,* p. 336; "Food Chains," *Illinois Business Review* 15 (May, 1955), p. 3; *Decatur Herald,* Apr. 3, 1926.

27. Paul D. Converse, "Price and Services of Chain and Independent Stores in Champaign-Urbana," *Natma Bulletins,* 1931 series, pp. 11–14, 18, 19, 23.

28. Lebhar, *Chain Stores in America,* p. 32; Bloomfield, *Chain Stores,* p. 46.

29. Lebhar, *Chain Stores in America,* p. 379; Boris Emmett and John E. Jenck, *Catalogs and Counters, a History of Sears, Roebuck and Company* (Chicago, 1950), p. 343; *Poor's Manual of Industrials, 1928,* p. 570; Orange A. Smalley and Frederick D. Sturdevant, *The Credit Merchants, a History of Spiegel, Inc.* (Carbondale, Ill., 1973).

30. Emmett and Jenck, *Catalogs and Counters,* pp. 680–81; Lebhar, *Chain Stores in America,* pp. 39, 44–45, 379; Bloomfield, *Chain Stores,* pp. 39, 48; *Poor's Manual of Industrials, 1928,* p. 522; Smalley and Sturdevant, *The Credit Merchants,* p. 302.

31. Smalley and Sturdevant, *The Credit Merchants,* p. 302; Lebhar, *Chain Stores in America,* p. 42.

32. "Drug Stores," *Illinois Business Review* (Jan., 1955), p. 3; Bloomfield, *Chain Stores*, pp. 39–46; Lebhar, *Chain Stores in America*, pp. 20–22, 378.

33. George Soule, *Prosperity Decade: From War to Depression, 1917–1929* (New York, 1947), pp. 168–69; Robert V. Mitchell, "Trends in Rural Retailing in Illinois, 1926–1938" *Bulletin of the Bureau of Business Research* 59 (Urbana, Ill., 1939), pp. 7–8; John B. Rae, *The American Automobile* (Chicago, 1965), p. 94; *Chicago Tribune*, July 16, 1908, p. 1.

34. *Chicago Tribune*, July 8, 1904, p. 4; Aug. 18, 1904, p. 1; Oct. 22, 1924, p. 2; *Illinois Blue Book 1925–26*, p. 373; *Illinois Blue Book, 1929–30*, p. 458.

35. Richard Griffith and Arthur Mayer, *The Movies* (New York, 1970), p. 195; Rae, *The American Automobile*, p. 94; Soule, *Prosperity Decade*, p. 168.

36. *Chicago Tribune*, June 8, 1924, part 1, p. 8.

37. Ibid.

38. Rae, *The American Automobile*, p. 88.

39. *Fifteenth Census, 1930: Distribution*, p. 591; Soule, *Prosperity Decade*, pp. 164–65.

40. Victor S. Clark, *History of Manufactures in the United States*, 3 vols. (New York, 1929), III, 157; Robert F. Karloevitz, *This Was Trucking: Pictoral History of the First Quarter Century of Commercial Motor Vehicles* (Seattle, 1966), pp. 35–36; Romeo B. Garrett, "The Role of the Duryea Brothers in the Development of the Gasoline Automobile," *Journal of the Illinois State Historical Society* 68 (Apr., 1975), pp. 174–80.

41. *Chicago Tribune*, May 30, 1908, section 2, part 1, p. 4; Sept. 5, 1920, part 3, p. 4; *Chicago Herald and Examiner*, Apr. 2, 1926, p. 23; Apr. 4, 1926, part 1, pp. 8, 14, 15, 25.

42. *Chicago Tribune*, Apr. 12, 1928, p. 14; Oct. 24, 1928, p. 30; *Illinois State Register*, Nov. 4, 1928, part 4, p. 4.

43. Rae, *The American Automobile*, p. 93; *Decatur Herald*, Apr. 4, 1926, p. 19.

44. *Literary Digest*, Mar. 21, 1928, p. 74; *Decatur Herald*, Apr. 3, 1926, p. 8; Apr. 4, 1926, p. 26; Apr. 4, 1928, pp. 12, 15, 18, 25; *Chicago Herald and Examiner*, Apr. 21, 1926, part 1, p. 4; Rae, *The American Automobile*, p. 90; *Chicago Tribune*, June 10, 1928, part 2, p. 12.

45. Soule, *Prosperity Decade*, p. 169; Rae, *The American Automobile*, pp. 58, 59, 62.

46. Frederick W. Taylor, *The Principles of Scientific Management* (New York, 1939), pp. 28–29, 45–47. See also Sudhir Kakir, *Frederick Taylor; A Study in Personality and Innovation* (Cambridge, Mass., 1970).

47. Thomas C. Cochran, *The American Business System: A Historical Perspective 1900–1955* (New York, 1957), pp. 15–20; Soule, *Prosperity Decade*, pp. 127–29.

48. *Fourteenth Census of the United States, 1920: Manufacturers* (Washington, D.C., 1924), pp. 310, 329–30; *Fifteenth Census of the United States, 1930: Manufacturers* (Washington, D.C., 1933), pp. 16–19.

49. *Poor's Manual of Industrials, 1928*, pp. 552, 1340; "Crawler Tractors," *Illinois Business Review*, Sept., 1954, p. 3.

50. *Fifteenth Census of the United States, 1929: Manufactures: Reports by Industries*, (Washington, D.C., 1933), p. 1119.

51. Ibid., pp. 174, 1123, 1346; "Candy," *Illinois Business Review*, Apr., 1953, p. 3; *Poor's Manual of Industrials, 1928*, p. 851.

52. *Poor's Manual of Industrials, 1914*, p. 1691; *Poor's Manual of Industrials, 1928*, pp. 3149–50; *Chicago Tribune*, Sept. 19, 1920, part 9, p. 1; June 8, 1924, part 2, p. 10.

53. H. L. Barber, *Story of the Automobile* (Chicago, 1917), pp. 221–29; Ralph C. Epstein, *The Automobile Industry* (New York, 1928), pp. 337–38; Newton Bateman

and Paul Selby, *History of Sangamon County,* 2 vols. (Chicago, 1912), II, part I, p. 785; *Chicago Tribune,* Oct. 17, 1920, part 3, p. 14.

54. Barber, *Automobile,* pp. 231–39; Epstein, *Automobile Industry,* pp. 377–84; *Poor's Manual of Industrials, 1928,·* pp. 1960, 2313; U.S. Bureau of the Census, *Biennial Census of Manufacturing: 1927* (Washington, D.C., 1930), p. 1153.

55. Harold F. Williamson et al., *The American Petroleum Industry: The Age of Energy 1899–1959* (Evanston, Ill., 1963), pp. 72, 192–95, 196–98, 362.

56. Ibid, pp. 70, 91, 100–101; Kendall Beaton, *Enterprise in Oil* (New York, 1957), p. 339.

57. Raymond Foss Bacon and William Allen Hamor, *The American Petroleum Industry,* 2 vols. (New York, 1916), I, 262–70; Beaton, *Enterprise in Oil,* pp. 298–99; Williamson, *American Petroleum Industry,* p. 431.

58. Hartzell Spence, *Portrait in Oil: How the Ohio Oil Company Grew to Become Marathon* (New York, 1962), pp. 235–38; *Poor's Manual of Industrials, 1928,* p. 1364.

59. Beaton, *Enterprise in Oil,* pp. 142–47.

60. *Fifteenth Census, 1929: Manufactures,* pp. 771, 773.

61. Rae, *The American Automobile,* p. 90; Williamson, *American Petroleum Industry,* pp. 501–02.

62. Williamson, *American Petroleum Industry,* pp. 217, 227, 469.

63. Beaton, *Enterprise in Oil,* p. 143; Williamson, *American Petroleum Industry,* pp. 470–71.

64. Bernard E. Schaar, "The Origins of the Plastics Industry," *Chemistry* 40 Nov., 1967, pp. 19–20; Williamson, *American Petroleum Industry,* p. 429; Clark, *History of Manufacturing,* 111, 331.

65. Bureau of the Census, *Statistical Abstract of the United States* (Washington, D.C., 1929), p. 368; Soule, *Prosperity Decade,* p. 182.

66. For a sympathetic biography see Forrest McDonald, *Insull* (Chicago, 1962). The quotation is on p. 237.

67. Ibid., p. 275.

68. Ibid., p. 153–54.

69. *Fourteenth Census, 1920: Manufacturers,* p. 337; *Fifteenth Census, 1930: Manufacturers,* p. 1123; *Illinois Blue Book, 1925–26,* p. 559; "Telephone and Telegraph Equipment," *Illinois Business Review,* Sept., 1950, p. 3; *Poor's Manual of Industrials, 1928,* pp. 2184, 3043.

70. *Illinois Blue Book, 1925–26,* p. 559.

71. *Illinois Business Review,* Jan., 1950, p. 3; *Abstract of the Fifteenth Census of the United States* (Washington, D.C., 1933), pp. 431, 432, 449.

72. *Chicago Herald and Examiner,* Apr. 4, 1926, part 5, p. 4; *Chicago Tribune,* Apr. 15, 1928, part 1, p. 27; *Fifteenth Census 1930: Distribution,* p. 592.

73. Earl Lifshey, *The Housewares Story* (Chicago, 1973), p. 128; *Poor's Industrials, 1928,* p. 1675; "Home Laundry," *Illinois Business Review,* July, 1956, p. 3.

74. *Poor's Manual of Industrials, 1928,* pp. 815–16; "Home Laundry," *Illinois Business Review,* July, 1956, p. 3.

75. *Fifteenth Census, 1930: Distribution,* p. 592; *Literary Digest,* Mar. 28, 1925, p. 68.

76. *Good Housekeeping,* Mar., 1928, p. 307; May, 1928, p. 245; *Chicago Tribune,* June 10, 1928, part 1, p. 25; *Decatur Herald,* Apr. 3, 1926, p. 12; *Chicago Herald and Examiner,* Apr. 4, 1926, part 1, p. 7.

77. *Illinois Business Review,* Aug., 1957; p. 3; *Decatur Herald,* Apr. 4, 1926, p. 12; *Chicago Tribune,* Apr. 12, 1928, p. 15; June 10, 1928, part 1, p. 15.

10

Blacks in Illinois:
Contributions and Problems

Black persons constituted a growing percentage of the population of Illinois during the first thirty years of the twentieth century. In 1900, 85,078 Blacks lived in Illinois, representing 1.8 percent of the total population (4,819,951.) By 1910 the number of Blacks had grown to 109,049, but as white population had increased at about the same rate, the percentage of Blacks in Illinois was then 1.9 percent. World War I changed the scene; in 1920 there were 182,274 black citizens and the percentage had increased to 2.8 percent as large numbers of Blacks emigrated from the South. The exodus from the South continued through the 1920s. Nearly quadrupling in three decades, the black population numbered 328,972 in 1930, representing 4.3 percent of the total Illinois population of 7,630,654. By 1930, ninety-six counties had one or more black citizens (only Calhoun, Cass, Cumberland, Hamilton, and Mason had none).[1]

Several factors stimulated the black migration to the North. World War I brought increased job opportunities because many young men were drafted, and wartime demands on industry created a need for increased productivity. European immigrants had provided a continuing cheap labor supply for industry, but the war and the nativism of the '20s brought a decline in immigration, and Blacks moved north to fill the void. Wages and working conditions in northern industry were better than in the South, although Blacks may have improved their finances since the cost of living was also higher. Blacks in the North could command only substandard housing, but this was better than the plantation shacks of the South. Blacks also came seeking better educational opportunities for their children, and in spite of increasing numbers of lynchings in the North, they suffered less violence than in the South. There was a decline in the need for plantation workers when the boll weevil swept through the South, bringing crop failures. Many Blacks suffered from the evils inherent in the sharecrop and credit system of the South. For all these reasons Blacks began to look upon the North as a land of opportunity.[2]

Newspapers such as the Chicago *Defender* encouraged southern Blacks in this belief and urged them to migrate to the North. Illinois was a natural destination for them because good railway connections on the Illinois Central and the Chicago and Eastern Illinois railroads were available. Most towns along these lines received some immigrants, but Chicago got the largest share. Centralia had 1,108 Blacks in 1930, Springfield 3,324, Champaign 1,598, East St. Louis 11,226, but Chicago had 233,903 black people within its limits by 1930. Thus 71 percent of the black citizens of Illinois lived in Chicago. Numerous companies recruited black labor by circulating rumors through the South of the labor needs of industries, and railroads offered club rates to groups which made it possible for families to come North. Because of the nature of the industries to which the Blacks came, they congregated in already overpopulated areas such as the south side of Chicago, the packinghouse area of East St. Louis, or the east side of Springfield.[3]

Black citizens experienced difficult times during the late nineteenth and early twentieth centuries, and Illinois mirrored these conditions. Blacks had been relieved of the burden of slavery a generation earlier only to find that freedom did not mean equality. Former slaves were freed physically in the sense that they could move from place to place and leave a job if they chose, but gradually the establishment chipped away at the legal equality of Blacks, until, culminating in the case of Plessy *vs.* Ferguson in 1896, the Supreme Court made segregation legal.[4]

Stimulated by the proslavery defense of the pre–Civil War South, a racist ideology developed which seeped into the consciousness of nearly every white American—belief of the biological and hereditary inferiority of Blacks. Armed with this deep-seated prejudice, racists generated a long list of stereotypes about the character, capacities, and propensities of Afro-American citizens. Perhaps the most difficult problem for Blacks was generated by the widespread belief of Whites in the immense sexual desire and capacity of black males. Racists alleged that black males had immense sex organs, that they were exceedingly lustful for women, particularly white women, and that their most common crime was rape. This facet of racism generated great emotional fervor in those who hated and feared Blacks. Black men were never able to escape this charge, and their greatest fear was an accusation of rape or even sexual activity by consent with a white woman. The great boxer, Jack Johnson, who had twice married white women, faced charges under the Mann Act and had to close his "Cabaret de Champion" in Chicago because of accusations that he had amorous relationships with white women and because the clientele in his cafe was mixed. The black man who was accused of rape might be lynched without a trial or, if tried, sent to the gallows without much of a hearing. The legend grew that most lynchings were the result of the rape of white women by black men, although in less than one-fourth of the lynchings investigated by the NAACP was rape alleged. Studies in Chicago showed the rate of sexual criminality among Blacks was about equal to their proportion of the population.

The press had a major responsibility in the allegations about the criminality of Blacks. One study showed that nearly half of the news articles about Blacks had to do with crime, and most newspapers commonly identified the ethnic background of black criminals.[5]

Most Whites viewed Blacks with contempt. Whites believed their middle-class social practices were the norm and judged standards of beauty and behavior by white models. Whites viewed Blacks as physically unattractive, and it was commonly said that all Blacks looked alike; Edgar Lee Masters recalled a song, "All Coons look alike to me." Among common racist views were the stereotypes that Blacks had an offensive body odor and that black denoted evil and ugliness. It was commonly said that Blacks dressed in a flashy manner, that they were boisterous, loud, coarse, and inclined to shove Whites about in public places, that they had an exaggerated sense of self-importance, and that they lacked civic consciousness and pride. Whites also accused Blacks of being improvident and lazy, saying that they did not save their money or buy homes, and that if they did own a home, they felt no pride in ownership and failed to keep the place in good repair. Whites believed Blacks were not interested in holding jobs, that they were fond of gambling, and that vice and criminality were their life, with rape their specialty, murder their sport, and razors their usual instrument of mayhem.[6] Most white males, the opinion makers of society for the first three decades of the twentieth century, had been reared in the essentially sexist and racist Puritan ethic compounded by Victorianism, and in this climate conflict was inevitable.[7]

Blacks responded to white racism in a variety of ways. One wing of black leadership, headed by W. E. B. Du Bois, urged resistance, while another, led by Booker T. Washington, urged accommodation. Many Blacks suffered a loss of pride and attemptd to become as much like Whites as possible, discarding racial identity in the process. The conflict is illustrated by the fact that in a single issue of the *Chicago Defender,* there were thirty-four advertisements for hair straighteners and skin whiteners. The *Defender* tried editorially to instill racial pride and solidarity, but their advertisements measured the depth of their failure.[8]

Many emigrant Blacks came from agricultural pursuits in the South, yet few became farmers in Illinois. In fact, the number of black farmers steadily declined between 1900 and 1930. In 1900 there were 1,486 black farmers in Illinois. By 1930 there were only 893, and most of these were in the extreme southern portion of the state. Why there were so few farmers among the black population is hard to assess. They may have wanted to escape agriculture, and farming in Illinois would have been different from that in Mississippi or Alabama. It would have taken more money to get adequate equipment and stock for the typical corn or hog operation, and they may have encountered white prejudice which precluded their renting land or getting loans. Furthermore, most black farmers were none too prosperous. The average size of their farms was 51.4 acres. Nearly half were on dirt roads, only seventeen had water in the house, ninety-seven had telephones, and only six had an electric motor for farm use.[9]

Likewise relatively few Illinois Blacks were able to go into business for themselves. In 1930 Blacks owned 1,058 stores, more than half of which were groceries, restaurants, and drugstores, and the average sales per store amounted to only $6,112, indicating that they were mostly small neighborhood operations. Aside from the proprietors, these stores employed only 696 people, less than one per store on the average.

The professions also were largely closed to Blacks. The black population of Illinois in 1930 contained only 331 physicians, 795 teachers, 159 dentists, and 192 lawyers, judges, and justices. Of the 854 black musicians, most could perform only in houses of prostitution, black-and-tan cabarets, and bootleg saloons.[10]

Most employers hired Blacks only for menial jobs, and few

pursued skilled occupations. In 1901 two-thirds of all female black wage-earners in Chicago worked as domestics. Black girls had to compete for jobs as domestics with immigrant girls, and immigrant girls were often more adequately prepared. Whites were less prejudiced against Blacks in this work, however, and black females could command better wages as domestics than in other jobs. The head of the Chicago Colored Women's Business Club advised black girls to train themselves as domestics because their wages were better than those of clerks, and as late as 1930 half of the black female wage-earners in the state worked as domestics. Laundries employed another substantial group. Black males had wider opportunities by 1930, but most worked as laborers, servants, waiters, or at other unskilled jobs.[11]

Transportation provided jobs for many black males. They had almost a monopoly as porters and waiters on Pullmans. There were a few skilled black workers on the railroads, but white workers were prejudiced against Blacks, and in some cases seniority rights were denied to black switchmen or brakemen. There were some black teamsters, partly because black strikebreakers had been used in the Chicago teamsters' strike of 1906 and then kept on. The automobile gave employment to many Blacks as car washers and greasers, but they could rarely command jobs as taxicab drivers until after World War I, when Blacks owned some cab companies in Chicago and employed black drivers. Considerable numbers worked in the rapidly multiplying gasoline stations. Opportunities expanded for blacks in manufacturing: some 6,000 Blacks worked in the packinghouses of Chicago in 1920, and 150 worked for International Harvester in the farm implement business. Sears, Roebuck and Company employed nearly as many in the mail order business, and Blacks had long worked in the coal mines of Illinois.[12]

The attitude of labor unions drastically affected the position of black workers. White workers were frightened of competition with Blacks, despite the paradoxical racist allegations that Blacks were lazy, would not work, and were incapable of learning skills. Fear of competition generated much of the prejudice, in part because Blacks were often brought to Illinois as strikebreakers. Mine operators of Illinois used Blacks in the coal mines in this capacity, bringing about the Virden and Pana riots in 1898. Black strikebreakers helped break the packinghouse strikes of 1894 and 1904 and a teamsters strike against Montgomery Ward in 1905. Governor Altgeld had recommended a law prohibiting the importation of strikebreakers, and after the riots at Virden and Pana such a law was passed during the Tanner administration.[13]

Some unions took the attitude that it was best to recruit black members to avoid having them used as strikebreakers. John Fitzpatrick of the Illinois Federation of Labor made this point, but some unions overtly prohibited black membership. The Brotherhoods of Locomotive Firemen, Engineers, Trainmen, Conductors, and Clerks all had constitutional provisions which prohibited Blacks from joining. The union of Masters, Mates, and Pilots likewise excluded black members as did the Machinists, Railway Mail Association, Telegraphers, and Wire Weavers. Theoretically Blacks could join most of the unions in the American Federation of Labor, but in practice many of the trade unions had no black members, often eliminating them by the apprentice system. The Hod Carriers' and Janitors' unions accepted Blacks without prejudice. The UMW accepted Blacks in good faith, and in 1900 nearly two-thirds of the black unionists were miners. The memberships of some unions, such as the Sleeping Car Porters, were all black.[14]

Because of outright barriers such as that of the Machinists or de facto elimination by careful selection of apprentices, the avenues to skilled trades were largely closed to Blacks. In some instances a trade learned in the South where there was no union could not be used in the North because of control by a union. This sometimes caused a black man to hold a lower position after migration. Greene and Woodson, careful students of black labor, give the example of a black bricklayer who earned $5 to $6 a day in Mississippi but could only work as a stockyard laborer for $2.50 to $2.75 a day in Chicago.[15]

As time went on, conditions changed so that traditional jobs held by Blacks became less available. As urban, upper-class families moved into apartments, fewer domestic positions were available because apartment houses were designed to cut servant costs, family units were smaller, and increased use of kitchen appliances made it possible for housewives to do more of their own work. Immigrants provided competition in various areas. German and Italian barbers took the business of Blacks, partly because Whites preferred to patronize white barbershops. Blacks were replaced as janitors and waiters for the same reason. Some occupations became unionized, which also tended to eliminate Blacks.[16]

Generally, employers of Blacks were satisfied with their work. A survey after the Chicago race riot in 1919 showed that employers of Blacks found them to be less guilty of absenteeism and to require no more supervision than white laborers; some employers found that immigrant labor required more supervision. Nonetheless many employers paid their black workers less than Whites doing the same job and refused promotions to Blacks. In plants using the piecework system, Blacks were usually placed in jobs where the return was lower.

For their part, Blacks tended to be distrustful of unions, believing they discriminated and did not give equal benefits. Older black residents in industrial areas were more amenable to union recruitment than new arrivals from the South, since Blacks from that area had little familiarity with unions. Generally from rural areas, southern Blacks had less experience in dealing with Whites, so union organizers, usually white, aroused their suspicions.

Customarily the most recent immigrants were hired for the heaviest and dirtiest work. This had been true of the successive waves of new Americans from central, southern, and eastern Europe, but with each of these groups there was an "upward occupational mobility" which allowed them to move out of these jobs. This was not the case with Blacks however. They continued, generation after generation, to sweep floors and dig ditches.[17]

Segregation, prejudice of Whites, exploitation by greedy landlords, and poverty forced Blacks to live in substandard housing. Carl Sandburg, reporting on the Chicago race riot of 1919, listed housing as a primary cause of racial problems. In most cities some kind of de facto segregation existed which kept Blacks out of white neighborhoods. As increasing numbers of Blacks moved into other areas, however, conditions became congested, rents rose, and neighborhoods declined. Then, as more affluent Blacks moved out of the old neighborhoods into the periphery of white areas, white residents became frightened by real estate operators who convinced property owners that values would go down if Blacks moved in.[18]

Generally, Blacks were less likely to own their homes and were subject to crowding. In 1920 there were twenty-two persons per owned home for Blacks while there were ten persons per owned home for Whites, and in that year the median value of black-owned homes amounted to $2,928. By 1930 only 10.5 percent of black families in Chicago owned their homes; in East St. Louis the percentage was 29.1. For the state, the percentage declined until about 1930. In 1900, 23.3 percent of the Blacks in Illinois owned their homes but the figure declined to 18.2 percent in 1920 and then rose slightly in 1930 to 19.5 percent. Generally, black homes lacked the conveniences of the times. Only about one-third of the black homes in Illinois had a radio in 1930, while more than half of the white homes had one.[19]

The congestion in Chicago reached intolerable levels in the twentieth century. The Hull House district illustrates the problem as successive waves of migrants moved into what had been a native white neighborhood. The native Americans gave way in turn to Irish, Germans, Russian Jews, Italians, Greeks, and eventually Blacks and Mexicans, the last groups arriving during World War I. With each successive group, the area became more crowded and run-down. Edith Abbott spoke of "rickety porches, stairs and sheds, rotting clapboards and shingles, grimy smoke covered, and dingy from lack of paint." Abbott reported that some families, with as many as six to a room, slept with guns under the bed to shoot rats. Plumbing was lacking or broken.[20]

Black ghettos were often in or next to areas of prostitution and vice, which bolstered the claim that Blacks were addicted to vice, but most new arrivals, hard pressed to find homes anywhere, could not pick their location. In spite of the decrepit dwellings rents soared, often increasing 50 percent as black families, who always paid more than Whites for comparable quarters, moved in. In 1917 the Urban League found that on a given day there were 664 Blacks applying to rent houses in Chicago from agents who had fifty houses available.[21]

When the migration from the South started, most Chicago Blacks lived between Twenty-second and Thirty-ninth streets with State Street the chief artery of the black district. Soon this area had doubled in population and people were spilling into other areas. Blacks could not spread to the north because of the Loop or to the west because of railroad yards and industry, so they had to expand south and east, often into areas that had been upper-class. The process of blockbusting had already begun as real estate agents caused panic among property owners. Carl Sandburg told of a "club woman" who, on the advice of such an agent, sold a $26,000 apartment building for $14,000, but as Blacks moved into the building, rents increased from $35 to $50 per month. Panic and tension caused friction in many neighborhoods. "Neighborhood Improvement Associations," often hastily devised, tried to keep neighborhoods white by using violence, pressure, and offers to buy property purchased by Blacks.[22]

In Springfield conditions were the same. Housing was run-down; sanitary facilities and water supply were poor. Blacks were segregated by custom if not by law, and they had little choice but to pay the higher rents charged for substandard homes. Investigators in 1914, finding black homes in poor neighborhoods that were clean and orderly, were convinced that Blacks wanted better homes. Landlords were blamed for the policy of "give less and charge more than for white tenants." In East St. Louis, Blacks crowded around the periphery of the industrial area, living in wooden shacks. Elliott Rudwick describes that area of the city as an industrial slum. Blacks, segregated in all areas of life—schools, lunchrooms, and work—lived in an unhealthy and ugly environment, filled with grime, odors, and noise.[23]

As early as 1874 Illinois law prohibited exclusion of a child from school because of race. The law was loosely drawn, however, and in practice many schools segregated black children, and many districts maintained all-black schools. School boards achieved segregation by drawing school district lines according to population distribution. School officials used segregation to avoid contact between the races because it was argued that the best way to avoid violence was to keep the races apart. By 1920 ten elementary schools and Wendell Phillips High School in Chicago were predominately black. School administrators favored segregation, although there was little racial problem in the schools. In spite of segregation, however, black children attended school in about the same proportion as white children. In 1920, 61.8 percent of the Blacks in the state between ages five and twenty were in school. By 1930 the percentage had climbed to 68.6 percent. In Springfield in 1910, 83.4 percent of black children age six to nine attended school. This compared to 78.6 percent of white children of the same age group. In the age group ten to fourteen, 89.8 percent of the black children were enrolled in school compared to 90.3 percent of the white children. In the age group fifteen to twenty, 23.5 percent of the Blacks and 23.1 percent of the Whites were in school.[24]

Blacks also met segregation in recreational facilities, and more racial incidents occurred in parks and playgrounds than in the schools. Much of the segregation arose from voluntary racial grouping, with Blacks staying out of recreational facilities understood to be white territory. Whites intimidated Blacks if they tried to use public facilities dominated by Whites. In Chicago, white street gangs such as "Ragan's Colts," a notorious gang of Irish hoodlums, enforced such segregation. For example, it was understood that Blacks could use only the Twenty-sixth Street Beach on the South side.[25]

Discrimination in public businesses was extralegal, but by intimidation and embarrassment Blacks were kept out of some facilities. Store owners instructed clerks to give slow or bad service to Blacks, while restaurant owners instructed waiters to ignore black customers, overcharge them, or serve spoiled food. Theater managers segregated restrooms and refused tickets to Blacks or relegated them to poorer seats. Because of fear of humiliation, Blacks stayed out of such places. Some saloons on Chicago's South Side attracted a mixed clientele, which scandalized the blue-nosed establishment of Chicago.[26]

Perhaps the most fearful thing to Blacks in the United States was the possibility of lynching or injury at the hands of a mob. The NAACP listed twelve lynchings in Illinois between 1900 and 1915. Every black man knew that if he committed a crime or was accused falsely of a crime, he might die at the hands of a mob. Such incidents were born out of white fear, racist resentment of Blacks, and distrust of the normal processes of law and its enforcement in the courts. Lynch law was the extreme manifestation of the racist attitude, which enforced segregation and insisted on discrimination in employment, social status, and political disfranchisement. Many mobs, not satisfied with the deaths of their victims, tortured and mutilated them first. Police officials, often sympathetic to the mob, offered little or no protection as the victim was dragged from his cell.[27]

A few examples of lynching in Illinois will suffice to illustrate mob action. The citizens of Belleville carried out a lynching on June 6, 1903. Local newspapers generally took the attitude that mob action constituted justice. The account of the *Belleville Advocate* began: "A black spot on the brick pavement of the public square is the only vestige of a sign left which marks the place where David Wyatt, the fiend who attempted to take the life of County Superintendent of Schools, Charles Hertel, expiated his crime last Saturday night."[28]

David Wyatt, a black teacher, came to the office of Superintendent Hertel to get his teacher's certificate renewed. Hertel refused the renewal and later Wyatt returned, renewed his plea, and, again refused, drew a revolver and shot Hertel. Police arrested Wyatt and a mob gathered. Police dispersed the mob three times, once with fire hoses, but later the mob entered the jail and removed Wyatt. In the town square they erected a pole from which Wyatt was hanged; kerosene was poured over him and lighted, "producing an odor of burning flesh which was entirely in keeping with the rest of the awful spectacle. Not satisfied with burning their victim, the ringleaders produced knives and in a short time the man's body was horribly mutilated and the assailants danced about the swinging corpse in ghoulish glee." Later the mob cut down the body and placed it on a bonfire to finish the burning.[29]

Later in the summer of 1903, a similar incident occurred in Danville. On July 24, James Wilson, a black man, allegedly attempted to assault Mrs. Thomas Burgess, the wife of a section hand, in Alvin, north of Danville. The authorities arrested Wilson and placed him in the Vermilion County jail. The following day, John D. Metcalf, a black man, allegedly murdered Henry Galterman. Metcalf was arrested and placed in the Danville City jail, where a mob gathered and overpowered the city police. The mob hanged Metcalf at the site where he had allegedly killed Galterman. As his body swung from a telephone pole, the mob fired shots at his body. One bullet cut the rope, and when he fell to the ground, the mob dragged Metcalf to the county jail, where his body was burned.[30] The mob then turned their attention to James Wilson. Here Sheriff Whitlock provided stronger resistance. Crying "Let's get the nigger who assaulted the woman at Alvin," the mob got a sixty-foot railroad rail to batter down the jail door. Sheriff Whitlock's deputies fired their shotguns down the length of the rail, killing at least one man and creating what came to be known in Danville as the "sore finger brigade." The mob dispersed. Subsequently Governor Yates sent the Illinois National Guard to keep order for a few days.[31]

The most gruesome lynching in Illinois took place in Cairo in 1909. In November the nude body of Anna Pelley, a Cairo shopgirl, was found in an alley. Cairo was "overwhelmed" by the story of outrage and murder of Pelley, aged twenty-four, a native of nearby Anna. Bloodhounds led pursuers to the city jail, where William James, a coal driver, was being held in a cell. Just how he committed rape and murder in an alley some distance away while he was in jail was never explained.[32]

James did not admit the crime even after intense "sweating" by the sheriff. As a mob gathered, the sheriff took James from the jail and started north with him to escape the mob, but it caught up with the sheriff and his prisoner near Belknap and forced the return of James to Cairo. An abortive attempt to hang him was made and several members of the mob shot him, after which his body was dragged to the scene of the crime, where his heart was cut out, cut up in pieces, and carried away for souvenirs. Then a woman applied a torch to his body. After the corpse had been consumed in the flames, James's skull was placed on a stick and displayed in a park overnight. Unsated, the mob then broke into the jail and lynched Harry Solzner, who was accused of murdering his wife. A coroner's jury viewed the body of James and came to the conclusion that he had met death at the "hands of parties unknown." The headline in the *Cairo Bulletin* was "Cairo Reaps Fruit of Many Murders Unpunished, Rope, Fire and Shot the Means of an Avenging Mob."[33]

In August, 1908, the Springfield police were holding Joe James, a young black drifter, on charges of having murdered Clergy Ballard, a stationary engineer, white and respectable. James had been in Springfield since June, when, on his second day in town, he had been jailed for vagrancy. He had become a trusty in the jail, and on July 4 the jailer had sent him out to do an errand. Instead of returning, James had gone into an area east of the square which contained houses of prostitution, saloons, and run-down boarding-houses adjoining the black district. Enjoying himself, James played the piano in "Dandy Jim" Smith's saloon, shot dice, and became very drunk.[34]

Around midnight, Blanche, Ballard's sixteen-year-old daughter, returned from White City, an amusement park, where she had celebrated the national birthday. After going to bed, she became aware that someone was in her room. Her screams awakened the family and frightened off the intruder. Outside the house, Ballard encountered the intruder, was stabbed several times, and subsequently died. Some of the family saw the fleeing assailant well enough to report that he was black and wore a dark coat and light trousers.[35]

The following morning James was found sleeping in Reservoir Park a few blocks away. After being badly beaten by Ballard's sons before the police arrived, James was put in jail again, now charged with murder. The local newspapers fanned the anger of the local populace. The *Illinois State Journal* commented, "Battling in the defense of his home, a humble working man fell under the cruel knife thrusts of a black midnight prowler who had invaded the sleeping room of his defenseless daughter." There was talk of lynching, but anger had cooled by August.[36]

Then, on August 14, Mrs. Mabel Hallam, twenty-one-year-old wife of a streetcar conductor, reported that she had been raped by a black man, a "black viper" as the *Illinois State Register* put it. According to her story, she was awakened while her husband was at work and dragged from her bed to the garden in the rear, where she was raped. Police arrested George Richardson, a black laborer, for the crime. Hallam made positive identification of Richardson.[37]

With both James and Richardson in jail and accused of crimes of monstrous proportion, crowds gathered around the jail, and the sheriff and chief of police concocted a plan to get the prisoners out of Springfield. A false fire alarm brought the fire engines to the jail, and as the attention of the crowd was diverted momentarily, the police put the prisoners in an automobile in the alley and, unnoticed, drove them rapidly away. They were taken north and put on a train to Bloomington, where they were again placed in jail.[38]

When the mob found that their prey had escaped, anger grew. The prisoners had been spirited away in an automobile belonging to Harry Loper, local cafe owner. Urged on by leaders, the mob moved to Loper's cafe, destroying the furnishings, wrecking the place, and burning the auto which had been used in the transfer of the prisoners. One man died at the scene. It was never clear whether his death was accidental or caused by Loper or the mob. Having sated their anger at Loper, the mob moved east of the courthouse to the black district. A large area was burned and three Whites sustained wounds which resulted in their deaths. By 2:30 A.M. the mob had progressed about six blocks east of the courthouse. They had burned and looted; now they would perpetrate a lynching. The mob dragged a black barber named Scott Burton from his home, hanged him, shot some forty bullets into his body, and committed repeated atrocities on his body with knives, amid shouts of "Look at the nigger swing."[39]

In the meantime Governor Charles Deneen had called out the National Guard, and by 3:30 A.M. enough units had arrived to disperse the mob. Eventually, seven troops of cavalry and four regiments of infantry arrived in Springfield. The guard performed well but was unable to cover the city adequately. The following night a mob gathered and before being dispersed lynched William Donnegan at the corner of Spring and Edwards streets, a block from the capitol. Donnegan was an eighty-year-old black man whose only offense seemed to be that he had a white wife. There were sporadic outbreaks after this, but no more lives were lost.[40]

Subsequently James was brought back to Springfield and stood trial for the murder of Clergy Ballard. He was convicted, largely on circumstantial evidence, and hanged in the county jail. In the case of George Richardson, Mrs. Hallam appeared after the riot and signed a statement that Richardson was not the man who had raped her. The authorities had discovered that she had a venereal disease, and when it was found that Richardson did not have the disease, the authorities concluded that Hallam was lying.[41]

Investigation of the deaths of several people in the riot was hampered by the reluctance of witnesses to testify. Coroner's juries came to the conclusion that each of the men had met his death at the hands of "parties unknown." At the request of State's Attorney Frank Hatch, a grand jury, all white, was convened. Investigation was made by the police, the National Guard, and the state's attorney. The grand jury returned 117 indictments relating to the riot. Of these, six were for murder, the others for malicious mischief, rioting, burglary, larceny, arson, and inciting a riot. The grand jury also reported to the judge "the cowardly, contemptuous action" of some members of the Springfield police.[42]

Of those indicted, almost none paid any penalty for their part in the riot. An exception was Kate Howard, operator of a notorious hotel in Springfield, who, when arrested for urging on the mob, committed suicide by swallowing cyanide on the steps of the jail. Another was a youth named Roy Young, who pleaded guilty on charges of larceny and rioting and was sentenced to the state reformatory. But police accused Abe Raymer, a young Zionist, of being one of the principal leaders of the mob, and although there was substantial evidence against him, he was acquitted. So also were Ernest "Slim" Humphrey, Madge Clark, and William "Fingers" Lothrington, all believed to be heavily involved. Dismayed by the reluctance of the jury to bring in a verdict of guilty, the state's attorney allowed a few to enter guilty pleas with a fine of $1. In most instances he did not bring those indicted to trial.[43]

Generally, white reaction to the riot was indifferent or approving. Kate Howard was dubbed "Springfield's Joan of Arc." Some blamed the riot on the liquor traffic or on politics. Springfield newspapers emphasized the criminality of Blacks and attempted to shift the blame to them. Most alleged that the lynchings would not have happened if Burton and Donnegan had not fired guns at the mob, thus angering them and provoking them to violence. Black reaction split between those who sought accommodation in the manner of Booker T. Washington and those who were more militant in the demand for equal treatment. The former generally took the position that the riot had been caused by lawless elements of both races. The Pleasant Grove Baptist Church adopted a statement: "We are American citizens who love order and obey the laws, spurn with contempt the low and vicious among all races, without regard to color and nationality, and agree to see that every effort within our power be exerted to rid our city of that class among us." *The Forum,* Springfield's black newspaper, at first took a conservative stand but became bitter about the wholesale acquittals of the rioters, calling the trial a "farce" and a "travesty." *The Broadax,* a black newspaper in Chicago, took an angrier stance, referring in its headlines to anarchy and lynch law, lawless bands of white Christians, and the cowardice and racial prejudice of Governor Deneen. The editor, Julius Taylor, proclaimed, "The negro needs a second Toussaint L'Ouverture, Christophe or Dessalines to teach him bravery and heroism. That it is far nobler and holier to die fighting to protect his loved ones at home than figuring on occupying front seats in heaven."[44]

Because of widespread publicity, the Springfield riot had far-reaching consequences. The incident seeped into the national consciousness because it had occurred in the hometown of Abraham Lincoln. By 1908 lynching had become epidemic, and the Springfield riot served as a capstone to these episodes of horror. Many people, black and white, were so repelled by what happened in Springfield that they were determined to form an organization that would help end lynching and other injustices. The founding of the National Association for the Advancement of Colored People in 1909 and 1910 resulted from dismay at the Springfield riot. By chance a man named William Walling had arrived in Springfield during the riot. Walling, born in the South, was a humanitarian and socialist, and he wrote a strong article about the riot for *The Independent.* Mary White Ovington read Walling's article and wrote to him. Ovington, a Radcliffe graduate, had given up the life of a socialite to become a practicing radical, and Blacks regarded her as a friend. She, Walling, and Henry Moscovitz met and issued a call for organization. They were able to draw into the organization W. E. B. Du Bois, whose Niagara Movement was crumbling. Also present was Oswald Garrison Villard, Charles Edward Russell, William Monroe Trotter, and Ida Wells-Barnett, distinguished black leader from Chicago. The new organization was biracial and for many years was the most militant group promoting the welfare of Blacks. Du Bois joined the staff as director of publications and research. Walling believed the presence of Du Bois made the organization viable. The NAACP constituted the only positive good that grew out of the Spring-field riot.[45]

In the summer of 1917 another race riot occurred in East St. Louis, which liked to call itself the "Pittsburgh of the West." East St. Louis had developed rapidly into an industrial town, counting all the great meat-packers, the Aluminum Ore Company, and the Missouri Malleable Iron Company among the plants there. Because most major rail lines going into St. Louis passed through the city, dismal switching yards marred the waterfront on the east side of the Mississippi. Unregulated growth of the industries and railroads created a dirty, smelly town in which the workers were crowded into ghettos. Between 1900 and 1910 the population of East St. Louis doubled, and one-tenth of the population of 59,000 was black. These black people lived in oppressive situations, seg-regated in washrooms, locker rooms, lunchrooms, schools, and even the jail. As long as there was no challenge of this, there was peace, but with the approach of World War I there was a new influx of black migrants which drastically altered the situation.[46]

Several factors increased tension in East St. Louis. At the time of the national election of 1916, local Democratic leaders had accused the Republicans of colonization of Blacks for their votes. There seems to have been little evidence to support this, but the Wilson administration bolstered the charge by ordering an investigation. The tension caused by economic fear of Whites that Blacks might take their jobs also contributed to the potential for violence. In the spring of 1917 workers formed a union at Aluminum Ore. To break the union, the company imported southern Blacks. The work force had been all white until 1913, but by 1916 the company had 280 black production workers. The union, called the Alumi-num Ore Employees Protective Association, made some effort to recruit Blacks. On April 18, 1917, a strike was called. The company imported strikebreakers, employed Pinkerton detectives, borrowed guns from the U.S. government, and barred union members from the plant. Amid rumors of new arrivals of Blacks from the South, Aluminum Ore broke the strike and refused to reemploy the strikers.[47]

The packing industry faced similar but less severe problems. When workers went on strike, the packers used fewer strikebreak-ers. and unionists got their jobs back. Against the background of the labor disputes, rumors circulated constantly of new arrivals of Blacks from the South. Local newspapers fed their readers a reg-ular diet of such rumors and created a stereotype of the vicious,

Many Blacks were unwilling to accept second-class citizenship and a vocational education. Du Bois insisted that Blacks should demand full equality, including voting rights and an education commensurate with ability. He promoted the best kind of education for the "talented tenth" and remarked of Washington: "So far as Mr. Washington preaches Thrift, Patience, Industrial Training for the masses, we must hold up his hands and strive with him. . . . But so far as Mr. Washington apologizes for injustice, North or South, does not rightly value the privilege and duty of voting, belittles the emasculating effects of caste distinctions, and opposes the higher training and ambition of our brighter minds,—so far as he, the South or the Nation, does this—we must increasingly and firmly oppose them."[75] Thus the lines were drawn and the black community split about evenly on the issues of accommodation versus militant demands for equality.

More militant Chicago leaders, who supported the Du Bois attitudes, organized the Equal Opportunity League in 1903 to ward off legal segregation in the schools. The Chicago leaders in this movement were Edward Morris, Charles Bentley, James Madden, Ferdinand Barnett, Edward Wilson, and John G. Jones. This group met in Springfield to create a statewide organization. Although the Chicago group dominated, they were unable to get sanction of an anti-Tuskegee statement because of the conservatism of downstate Blacks. In 1905 Charles Bentley and James Madden established a Chicago branch of the Niagara Movement after going to the first meeting of the group in Canada. This was an elitist group of Blacks fostered by Du Bois. The first meeting was held in Canada because they were refused meeting space in Buffalo. The group, militant in fighting school segregation, worked to get a Black appointed to the New Chicago Charter Commission and protested the showing of *The Clansman* in Chicago. The organization lasted until 1908, when its remnants joined the NAACP.[76]

Several organizations in Illinois aimed at improvement of the black minority's situation. Some of the settlement houses included Blacks in their programs, but many believed the presence of Blacks would discourage participation of deprived white populations. Moreover, the settlement houses were devoted to the principle of upgrading a neighborhood and were rarely found in black areas. The Wendell Phillips settlement in Chicago, an offshoot of Hull House, was biracial. In Chicago in 1904 Celia Parker Wooley, who devoted herself to the cause of equal opportunity, founded the

Frederick Douglass Center, which was limited to the improvement of Blacks. The Douglass Center was distinguished by the fact that its facility was designed by Frank Lloyd Wright. In 1908 the Phillis Wheatley Club founded a home in Chicago for the protection of black girls emigrating from the South. The Phillis Wheatley Club was a black organization aimed at neighborhood improvement in the area of Fifty-first and Dearborn streets. The home provided a haven for rural girls who found their way to the city and aided them in coping with urban conditions. Room and board were provided for $1.25 per week.[77]

The NAACP movement in Chicago was sponsored by Jane Addams, Rabbi Emil Hirsch, and black leaders such as George Hall and Charles Bentley. The organization was biracial, and the first president was Judge Edward O. Brown, a white man. The organization interested itself in achieving equal rights through the courts and legislature. This biracial group sometimes found itself at odds with the new black emphasis on self-help and racial solidarity because many Blacks were suspicious of help by Whites. Both the *Broadax* and the *Defender* editorially looked with doubt on the new organization. Some good was accomplished, however, and the NAACP led the fight against showing the film *Birth of a Nation* in Chicago. Unfortunately the Chicago chapter of the NAACP suffered from lack of leadership and money, although Julius Rosenwald pledged one-fourth of the budget until 1914.[78]

The National Urban League was founded in 1911 by a coalition of earlier black improvement organizations. Eugene Kinckle Jones, a well-educated black teacher, became the League's first director. Operating primarily in industrial areas, the league provided travelers' and social aid, as well as promoting job opportunities for Blacks and aiding in their integration into the industrial scene. In 1915–16 Jones and T. Arnold Hill began organization in Chicago. Robert E. Polk, professor of sociology at the University of Chicago, became the first president of the Chicago Urban League, and Horace Bridges of the Chicago Ethical Culture Society became its second. An office was opened in 1917 and T. Arnold Hill stayed on as executive secretary. The new organization promised to work for better race relations, recreation, and to aid the delinquent and the impoverished. During World War I it faced massive problems with the influx of Blacks from the south. The branch founded in East St. Louis after the riot lasted only about three years.[79]

During the period after World War I there was a new era of black consciousness and pride. Among the promoters of this feeling was Jamaican-born Marcus Garvey, a confident black man who glorified black culture. Crying "let my people go," Garvey proclaimed that "the black man needs his own government, with his own president in the Black House and a black God in Heaven." Garvey hoped to establish black business activities through his Universal Negro Improvement Association. A key to this operation was the Black Star Steamship Line, which Garvey hoped would link black people from all parts of the world in business activity. In Chicago Garvey made a UNIA organization effort but was opposed by Robert S. Abbott, the publisher of the *Chicago Defender*. Garvey won a libel suit against Abbott and later Abbott won a libel suit against Garvey; each claimed he had been maligned in the speeches or writings of the other. In spite of Abbott's opposition, the UNIA made progress in Chicago. Even after the steamship line had been lost, there were still some 9,000 members in the city. Though Garvey's efforts at improving the economic life of black people were unsuccessful, he was an important figure who, as one black spokesman put it, "had performed a spiritual miracle in getting colored people together and inculcating race pride."[80]

Crucial to growing black awareness were the black newspapers in Illinois after 1900. The best known of these was the *Defender*, published in Chicago after 1905. The publisher, Robert Abbott, was born on St. Simons Island, off the coast of Georgia. Abbott grew up in Savannah and learned the printer's craft at Hampton Institute, the same school that produced Booker T. Washington. Abbott came to Chicago, studied law, and founded the *Defender* on a shoestring. He supported Washington's views on many things but was far more militant in demanding equal rights for Blacks. He disliked Du Bois and denounced the NAACP for being biracial. By the end of World War I, the *Defender* had a circulation of 250,000. Widely distributed in the South, it contained pleas for southern Blacks to migrate to the North.[81]

Perhaps the most colorful black newspaper in Illinois was the *Broadax*, published in Chicago by Julius F. Taylor. Unlike most Blacks of his time, Taylor was a Bryan Democrat. He was sharply critical of black clergy and churches and disliked Washington, whom he called the "white man's Nigger" and "The Great Beggar of Tuskegee." The outspoken Taylor agitated the black community constantly from the time he arrived in Chicago until the closing of his paper in 1931, although he let up on Washington after 1910. After the Springfield riot of 1908 he described one of the leaders of the riot, Kate Howard, as "a highly respectable fast lady of the town, who has for some time conducted a free and easy bawdy house in the capitol city." Governor Charles Deneen operated by "cowardice and trembling fear of racial prejudice," while Mayor Roy Reece "ran up the white feather" and the National Guardsmen were "tin horn soldiers."[82]

The *Chicago Whip* began publication during the summer of 1919 as the most militant of the Chicago black papers. Founded concurrently with the 1919 race riot, the *Whip* urged Blacks to fight back. Denouncing all Whites indiscriminately, the *Whip* was published until 1922. Downstate the *Forum* was published in Springfield from 1904 to 1917. An eight-page weekly, the *Forum* was edited by B. L. Rogers and Will H. Barbour. Cautious and conservative, the paper urged the Tuskegee virtues of hard work, thrift, and accommodation, and urged Blacks to be inconspicuous, undemanding, and inoffensive in all things. In the view of the editors, respectability and Republicanism were the keys to everything. Unlike Julius Taylor, the editors viewed Governor Deneen as "magnanimous executive and a fearless man."[83]

A great number of individuals contributed to the leadership of the black communities in Illinois. Many were professional people, but perhaps preeminent among the militants was Ida Wells-Barnett. Born in Mississippi, Ida Wells taught school and edited a militant newspaper in Memphis. She came to the Columbian Exposition in Chicago in 1893 and stayed to marry Ferdinand Barnett. Uncompromising in her stand against the Tuskegee group, Wells-Barnett bitterly attacked the concept of accommodation. Active in antilynching movements, woman suffrage, and settlement work, she maintained a close relationship with Jane Addams and was the only Chicago Black to participate in the founding of the NAACP.[84]

Dr. Daniel Hale Williams also occupied a preeminent place in the black elite of Chicago. Born in Pennsylvania of a good family, Williams received a solid medical education and founded Provident Hospital in Chicago. Although preoccupied with professional concerns, Williams became involved in matters of race. Always insisting that the staff at Provident be highly qualified regardless of race, he organized the National Medical Association for black physicians, who were excluded from white organizations. Early in his career Williams supported Washington, but broke with him and moved to the Du Bois camp and into the Niagara Movement, as did the eminent black dentist Charles Bentley. Williams identified his own demand for professional excellence with the concept of the "talented tenth" which Du Bois espoused.[85]

Opposed to Williams personally, professionally, and philosophically, Dr. George Cleveland Hall was a follower of Booker T. Washington. Dr. Williams sought to have Dr. Hall barred from Provident Hospital on the grounds that his training was inadequate. Hall charged that Williams preferred white physicians to black ones, and the feud reached into all segments of the black community. It is said that the black female elite, led by Mrs. Williams and Mrs. Bentley, ostracized Mrs. Hall, "whose laughter and clothes were both apt to be a little loud." Dr. Hall, a close friend of Washington, accepted the presidency of the Chicago chapter of the National Negro Business League.[86]

Several black attorneys had great influence. Edward E. Wilson, educated at Oberlin and Williams, was admitted to the bar in Chicago where he became assistant state's attorney. He attacked accommodation and segregation in all forms, including a plan for a black YMCA, calling it an avenue "for travelling to heaven by a back alley." Edward H. Morris, another successful black lawyer, became nationally known in his opposition to Washington, whom he blamed for much of the lynching in the United States. Ferdinand Barnett, lawyer and assistant state's attorney for a time, also opposed Washington.[87]

Perhaps the most devoted supporter of Booker T. Washington was S. Laing Williams, also an attorney. Williams, well educated and a leader of the social elite, operated as an agent for Washington, keeping him informed of developments in the Niagara Movement and the NAACP. Allan Spear suggests that Williams supported Washington because of his desire for public office, which for many years was impossible without the help of Tuskegee. Williams' wife, Fannie Barrier Williams, wrote for the New York *Age,* one of Booker T. Washington's newspapers.[88]

In communities downstate, black leaders exhibited little militance. In Springfield in 1908 Dr. S. A. Ware was described as "an intense race man at all times, a genial good fellow to meet, charitable in impulses, of broad and liberal views." Attorney Charles Gibbs, at the same time, was described as "one of those men capable of real leadership in the great task of leading the race out of Egypt into the promised land." Mrs. Gibbs was a musician and president of the Springfield Colored Women's Club. The Gibbs children, Leota and Charles, Jr., were musicians. Daniel Neal was described as "a true champion of the race."[89] Many other Blacks were successful in a social or economic way without having much to do with the various black ideologies. An example is a black businessman named Troy Porter who lived in Paris, Illinois. Porter ran a store, a plumbing shop, and a contracting business and operated a prosperous farm. A prosperous Black in a small town was a rarity. The only hint of any alignment with the broader forces of black ideology was Porter's membership in the National Negro Business League.[90]

In Chicago the richest Black was Jesse Binga, a poorly educated barber who set up in real estate, opened a bank, and married Eudora Johnson, a sister of John "Mushmouth" Johnson, a gambling lord of Chicago's South Side. Mrs. Binga inherited a fortune from her brother, thus increasing Binga's wealth. Binga joined the National Negro Business League but contributed little to the organization.[91]

With a few exceptions, established and educated Blacks who had social pretensions identified with Du Bois, his militant position, the Niagara Movement, and the NAACP. Doubtless they could see themselves as part of the "talented tenth," deserving of equality with the Whites and capable of the first-rate education advocated by Du Bois. On the other hand, the newly arrived with less education tended to accept the idea of accommodation put forth by Washington.[92]

Black citizens quickly gained importance in the political life of Illinois. Prior to 1932, Blacks traditionally voted the Republican ticket because they associated Lincoln and the Republicans with emancipation. Harold Gosnell, careful historian of black politicians, quotes Major John R. Lynch, a black congressman from Mississippi in Reconstruction days, as saying, "The colored voters cannot help but feel that in voting the Democratic ticket in national elections they will be voting to give their endorsement and their approval to every wrong of which they are the victims, every right of which they are deprived, and every injustice of which they suffer." Some political leaders, notably Mayor Thompson, Governor Deneen, and Senator Lorimer, regularly courted the black vote. In 1916 and 1920, 80 percent of black voters supported Hughes and Harding over their Democratic opponents. After this the percentage of black votes that the Republicans could command began to fall off. Although radical groups such as the Socialists and Communists made overtures, Blacks remained unresponsive and unrevolutionary throughout the period.[93]

Political organizations easily reached the Blacks, because in all cities they were segregated by one device or another and demonstrated a political solidarity. Gosnell notes that Blacks who came North, unlike immigrant people, were eligible to vote immediately, and it was often charged that black votes were for sale. When the race riots occurred in Springfield, East St. Louis, and Chicago, the press charged that much of the blame lay with the politicians, who had corrupted Blacks by buying votes and by turning their backs on vice in black communities. In Chicago and Cook County, Blacks elected representatives to city, county, and state offices. In East St. Louis part of the tension leading to the riot of 1917 arose from Democratic charges that Republicans were colonizing black voters in the area.[94]

The early years of the twentieth century were the halcyon days of the political clubs. In Chicago the most prestigious white Republican organization was the Hamilton Club. Its counterpart among Blacks was the Sumner Club, organized in 1898 as a social and political group. Among the leaders in the organization were Edward H. Morris, distinguished black lawyer, and Robert L. Taylor, who got his start in politics as a page for Congressman John A. Logan. Two years later Edward H. Wright founded the Appomattox Club for similar purposes. This club maintained impressive quarters and counted many of the black elite of Chicago among its members.[95]

Many black leaders used military position as a springboard to a political career. This was particularly true of the Eighth Illinois Regiment of the National Guard. The regiment had a distinguished record in both the Spanish-American War and World War I. Colonel John R. Marshall of this regiment held a variety of appointive posts, as did his successor, Colonel Franklin A. Dennison. Major Robert R. Jackson also held a number of elective posts.[96]

Edward H. Wright ran for the city council in 1915 and became the first black alderman. Wright had previously served on the county commission and was elected ward committeeman in 1920. Edward H. Morris was elected to the Illinois House in 1890 and 1902. Dr. Alexander Lane was elected to the House of Representatives in 1906 and 1908, as was Edward D. Green in 1910. In 1912 Major Robert R. Jackson was elected to the House and was reelected for four terms. A postal employee, Jackson capitalized on his military record and his membership in a number of fraternal organizations. Besides his popularity with Blacks, Jackson had the support of Congressman Madden. In 1914 Sheadrick Bond Turner joined Jackson in the legislature and served four terms. In 1918 Warren B. Douglas, an attorney, was elected to the legislature, making a total of three Blacks there. In 1918 Adelbert H.

Roberts replaced Jackson. In 1928 Roberts became the first Black elected to the Illinois Senate. In 1924 the first district sent Sheadrick Bond Turner and Charles H. Griffin to the State House of Representatives, while Warren B. Douglas and George T. Kersey went from the third district. With Senator Roberts, this put five Blacks in the general assembly. Griffin was a well-known insurance and real estate operator. The same five men were reelected in 1926. In 1928 the legislature contained six Blacks: Harris B. Gaines and George W. Blackwell from the first district, George T. Kersey and William E. King from the third district, William J. Warfield from the fifth district, and Senator Roberts.[97]

The best-known black politician prior to 1930 was Oscar De Priest. Born in Florence, Alabama, in 1871, De Priest, the son of an independent-minded ex-slave, was a large man with a shock of white hair which gave him a striking appearance. The family emigrated to Kansas in the great exodus of 1878. De Priest, an aggressive youngster, attended a normal school in Kansas which gave him his limited education. Always adverturesome, De Priest ran away from home at age seventeen and in 1889 arrived in Chicago, where he built a real estate business and helped organize the Negro Business League. He was elected to the Chicago City Council in 1915 but did not stand for reelection, having been indicted for graft. In 1928, after building a political following, De Priest secured the Republican nomination and election to the U.S. Congress, the first black man elected from Illinois. De Priest was a ward committeeman and delegate to the Republican National convention that year. Always controversial, many newspapers attacked De Priest as being only a cheap politician, but among the rank and file he always had support.[98]

On the state scene, black voters supported a wide variety of candidates, and Mayor Thompson was one of those who benefited. In one political rally the mayor embraced a black child and was attacked by his opposition with a flyer which contained a drawing of Thompson kissing a black child accompanied by the caption: "Do you want Negroes or White Men to Run Chicago? Bye, Bye, Blackbirds." Thompson exhibited the flyer at black political meetings and turned the attack to his advantage. He posed as the champion of the people, and although Thompsonism became the synonym for graft and corruption, he derived wide support on Chicago's South Side. Senator Lorimer played the same game with Blacks until he was removed from the Senate in 1912 for election fraud. After his removal, Lorimer returned to Chicago for a hero's welcome which included a reception at Orchestra Hall, where Bishop Archibald Carey of the Abyssinean Baptist Church gave the invocation. Governor Deneen courted the black vote, and while he was a cold individual, Blacks respected him for his support of an antilynching bill and for his vigorous action in several lynchings and in the Springfield race riot of 1908.[99]

Some of the richest Blacks derived their wealth from vice. Among those in Chicago in this category was John "Mushmouth" Johnson, who ran a gambling house on the South Side for many years. Henry "Teenan" Jones was involved in a saloon and gambling business in which he made a great deal of money. Daniel M. Johnson combined gambling with the mortician's trade to make a fortune.[100]

Although Blacks have been largely ignored in Illinois history, they played an increasingly important part in the state. They suffered injuries ranging from discrimination in employment, housing, and education to lynching, but they provided important leadership in various areas. From John "Mushmouth" Jackson to the eminent physician Dr. Daniel Hale Williams, many success stories can be told. The contributions of Blacks to the professions, music, and the economy of the state are massive. They performed much of the labor and provided a sizeable market for the economy.

1. Charles E. Hall, *Negroes in the United States 1920–1932* (Washington, D.C., 1935), pp. 10–11; *Fifteenth Census of the United States, 1930: Population,* vol. III, part I (Washington, D.C., 1932), pp. 591, 600–608.

2. Allan H. Spear, *Black Chicago: The Making of a Negro Ghetto 1890–1920* (Chicago, 1970), p. 129; Chicago Commission on Race Relations, *The Negro in Chicago* (Chicago, 1922), pp. 80–84 (hereafter referred as *The Negro in Chicago*).

3. *Fifteenth Census, 1930: Population,* vol. III, part I, pp. 608–813; *The Negro in Chicago,* p. 87; Spear, *Black Chicago,* p. 11.

4. *The Negro in Chicago,* p. 87; Plessy *vs.* Ferguson, 165 U.S. 537 (1896). For the development of racist ideas see Donald F. Tingley, "The Rise of Racialistic Thinking in the United States in the Nineteenth Century" (dissertation, University of Illinois, Urbana, 1952).

5. Tingley, "Rise of Racialistic Thinking," pp. 32–70, 175–211; *Chicago Tribune,* Nov. 1, 1912, p. 11; Nov. 2, 1912, p. 8; Nov. 8, 1912, p. 1; *Chicago Record-Herald,* Oct. 30, 1912, p. 3; Oct. 31, 1912, p. 11; Nov. 1, 1912, p. 8; Nov. 17, 1912, p. 5; Nov. 20, 1912, p. 11; Jack Johnson, *Jack Johnson Is a Dandy: An Autobiography* (New York, 1969), pp. 47–48; National Association for the Advancement of Colored People, *Thirty Years of Lynching in the United States 1889–1918* (New York, 1969), pp. 9–10; Walter White, *Rope and Faggot: A Biography of Judge Lynch* (New York, 1929), pp. 54–63.

6. Edgar Lee Masters, *Vachel Lindsay, a Poet in America* (New York, 1935), p. 238; *The Negro in Chicago,* pp. 440–43.

7. Arnold Rose, *The Negro in America* (New York, 1944), p. 24.

8. *Chicago Defender,* June 2, 1917, passim.

9. Hall, *Negroes in the United States,* pp. 583, 590.

10. Ibid. pp. 293, 304, 500–504; Harold F. Gosnell, *Negro Politicians, the Rise of Negro Politics in Chicago* (Chicago, 1935), p. 120.

11. Lorenzo Greene and Carter G. Woodson, *The Negro Wage Earner* (Washington, D.C., 1930), p. 93.

12. Ibid., pp. 103, 110–11, 266, 310–11; *The Negro in Chicago,* p. 361.

13. Green and Woodson, *The Negro Wage Earner,* pp. 132–33, 252–53; Earl R. Beckner, *A History of Labor Legislation in Illinois* (Chicago, 1929), pp. 68–69; Selig Perlman and Philip Taft, *Labor Movements,* Vol. 4 of *History of Labor in the United States, 1896–1932,* (New York, 1935), p. 67; John H. Keiser, "Black Strikebreakers and Racism in Illinois, 1865–1900," *Journal of the Illinois State Historical Society* 65 (Autumn, 1972), pp. 313–26.

14. John H. Keiser, "John Fitzpatrick and Progressive Unionism 1915–1925" (dissertation, Northwestern University Evanston, Ill., 1965), pp. 165, 166–67; *The Negro in Chicago,* pp. 406, 408; Greene and Woodson, *The Negro Wage Earner,* pp. 346–47, 350–51; Philip A Taft, *The A.F.L. in the Time of Gompers* (New York, 1957), pp. 308–9, 315.

15. Greene and Woodson, *The Negro Wage Earner,* p. 316.

16. *The Negro in Chicago,* p. 357; Greene and Woodson, *The Negro Wage Earner,* pp. 95, 96, 98, 227, 238–39.

17. *The Negro in Chicago,* pp. 365, 373, 377, 399, 403.

18. Carl Sandburg, *The Chicago Race Riots: July, 1919* (New York, 1919), p. 4; *The Negro in Chicago,* pp. 93, 341.

19. Hall, *Negroes in the United States,* pp. 259, 261, 262, 263, 264, 265, 268.

20. Edith Abbott, *The Tenements of Chicago, 1908–1935* (Chicago, 1936), pp. 93, 189.

21. *The Negro in Chicago,* p. 92.

22. Sandburg, *The Chicago Race Riots,* pp. 45–47; Spear, *Black Chicago,* pp. 23–25.

23. John Ihder, "Housing in Springfield, Illinois," in Shelby Harrison, ed. *The Springfield Survey,* 3 vols. (Springfield, Ill., 1918), I. 16–17, 117–18; Elliott M. Rudwick, *Race Riot at East St. Louis, July 2, 1917* (Carbondale, Ill., 1964), p. 5.

24. Spear, *Black Chicago,* pp. 51, 203–5; U.S. Bureau of the Census, *The Negro Population of the United States, 1790–1915* (New York, 1969), pp. 402, 806; *Fifteenth Census, 1930: Population,* vol. III, part I, p. 595.

25. Spear, *Black Chicago,* pp. 205–6; *The Negro in Chicago,* pp. 285, 341.

26. Spear, *Black Chicago,* pp. 206–7; *The Negro in Chicago,* pp. 299, 321, 323, 325.

27. NAACP, *Thirty Years of Lynching,* pp. iii, 83; Arthur F. Raper, *The Tragedy of Lynching* (New York, 1970), pp. 1–45; Arnold Rose, *The Negro in America* (New York, 1944), pp. 184–86; Benjamin Brawley, *A Social History of the American Negro* (New York, 1921), p. 318.

28. *Belleville Advocate,* June 12, 1903, p. 2.

29. Ibid., Sept. 4, 1903, p. 1.

30. *Champaign Daily News,* July 27, 1903, pp. 4, 7; July 28, 1903, p. 1; July 29, 1903, pp. 1, 7; *Belleville Advocate,* July 31, 1903, p. 3.

31. Ibid.

32. *Cairo Bulletin,* Nov. 10, 1909, p. 1; *Chicago Tribune,* Nov. 10, 1909, p. 7; *Illinois State Register* (Springfield), Nov. 10, 1909, p. 1.

33. *Cairo Bulletin,* Nov. 11, 1909, p. 1; Nov. 12, 1909, p. 1; Nov. 13, 1909, p. 1; *Chicago Tribune,* Nov. 11, 1908, p. 2, Nov. 13, 1909, p. 1; *Illinois State Register,* Nov. 12, 1909, p. 1.

34. *Illinois State Journal*, (Springfield), Oct. 24, 1908, p. 2; *Illinois State Register*, Sept. 17, 1908, p. 1; *Springfield Record*, Sept. 18, 1908, p. 1. The best published account of the Springfield riot is James L. Crouthamel, "The Springfield Race Riot of 1908," *Journal of Negro History* 45 (July, 1960), pp. 164–81. Crouthamel's article has some minor inaccuracies but is generally good.

35. *Illinois State Register*, Sept. 16, 1908, p. 7.

36. *Illibois State Journal*, July 5, 1908, p. 1, July 6, 1908, p. 4.

37. *Illinois State Register*, Aug. 14, 1908, p. 1.

38. *Illinois State Journal*, Aug. 15, 1908, p. 1.

39. Ibid.

40. *Chicago Tribune*, Aug. 16, 1908, p. 1; *Springfield Record*, Aug. 17, 1908, p. 1; *Illinois State Register*, Aug. 16, 1908, p. 1.

41. *Illinois State Register*, Sept. 2, 1908, p. 1; Sept. 19, 1908, p. 5; *Springfield Record*, Sept. 1, 1908, p. 2; *Illinois State Journal*, Oct. 24, 1908, p. 1.

42. *Illinois State Register*, Aug. 20, 1908, p. 1; *Illinois State Journal*, Aug. 18, 1908, p. 1; Aug. 20, 1908, p. 6; *Springfield Record*, Sept. 4, 1908, pp. 4, 6; Sept. 6, 1908, p. 2.

43. *Illinois State Register*, Aug. 18, 1908, p. 1; Aug. 20, 1908, p. 1; Aug. 22, 1908, p. 1; Aug. 27, 1908, p. 5; Aug. 29, 1908, p. 6; Sept. 24, 1908, p. 1; Sept. 25, 1908, p. 4; Nov. 20, 1908, p. 5; Nov. 29, 1908, p. 22; *Springfield Record*, Aug. 27, 1908, p. 8; Sept. 24, 1908, p. 1; Oct. 11, 1908, p. 1; *Illinois State Journal*, Aug. 19, 1908, p. 1; Sept. 5, 1908, p. 10; Oct. 8, 1908, p. 10; *Chicago Tribune*, Oct. 11, 1908, p. 4.

44. *Illinois State Journal*, Aug. 16, 1908, pp. 1, 3, 5; *Illinois State Register*, Aug. 15, 1908, p. 1; Aug. 16, 1908, p. 3. For the pro-Washington view see *Forum (Springfield)*, Sept. 5, 1908, p. 2, in which the editor advises the black people of Springfield to "cast down your bucket where you are." See also *Forum*, Sept. 26, 1908, p. 1; *Broadax*, Aug. 22, 1908, p. 1.

45. William Walling, "Race War in the North," *Independent*, 65, Sept. 3, 1908, pp. 529–34; Mary White Ovington, "Beginnings of the N.A.A.C.P.," *Crisis*, 32, June, 1926, pp. 76–77; Mary White Ovington, *The Walls Came Tumbling Down* (New York, 1947), pp. 100–115.

46. The definitive work on the East St. Louis riot is Rudwick's *Race Riot at East St. Louis*. For a description of East St. Louis, see pp. 4–6, 219. *East St. Louis Daily Journal*, May 27, 1917, p. 7.

47. Rudwick, *Race Riot*, pp. 7–15, 16–20, 24–26.

48. Ibid., pp. 24–26, 27–37.

49. Ibid., pp. 27–37.

50. Hutchison, William T. *Lowden of Illinois: The Life of Frank O. Lowden*, 2 vols. (Chicago, 1957), I, 338; *East St. Louis Daily Journal*, July 13, 1917, p. 4.

51. Rudwick, *Race Riot*, pp. 38–54.

52. *Chicago Defender*, July 14, 1917, p. 4.

53. *East St. Louis Daily Journal*, July 13, 1917, p. 4.

54. Ibid., June 4, 1917, p. 1.

55. Rudwick, *Race Riot*, pp. 52–53; *East St. Louis Daily Journal*, July 12, 1917, p. 1.

56. Rudwick, *Race Riot*, p. 154, 155.

57. Ibid., pp. 91–94; *East St. Louis Daily Journal*, July 5, 1917, p. 1; July 6, 1917, p. 1; July 8, 1917, p. 1; July 9, 1917, p. 1, July 11, 1917, p. 1; July 12, 1917, p. 1; July 15, 1917, p. 1: July 19, 1917, p. 1; Rudwick, *Race Riot*, pp. 160–62.

58. *East St. Louis Daily Journal*, July 8, 1917, p. 1; *Final Report of the State Council of Defense of Illinois 1917–1918–1919* (Chicago, 1919), p. 1.

59. Rudwick, *Race Riot,* pp. 91, 94–116; *Chicago Defender,* Aug. 18, 1917, p. 1; Oct. 13, 1918, p. 1.

60. Rudwick, *Race Riot,* pp. 118–31; *East St. Louis Daily Journal,* July 12, 1917, p. 1; *Chicago Defender,* Dec. 1, 1917, p. 3.

61. The definitive work on the Chicago race riot of 1919 is William M. Tuttle, Jr., *Race Riot: Chicago in the Red Summer of 1919* (New York, 1970). See pp. 3–10 for the origins of the Chicago riot. *Chicago Defender,* Aug. 2, 1919, p. 1.

62. Tuttle, *Race Riot: Chicago,* pp. 64, 242; *The Negro in Chicago* (Chicago, 1922), p. 1.

63. Tuttle, *Race Riot: Chicago,* pp. 53, 207; *The Negro in Chicago,* p. 40; *Chicago Tribune,* July 29, 1919, pp. 1, 3.

64. *The Negro in Chicago,* pp. xvi–xvii, xxiii.

65. Tuttle, *Race Riot: Chicago,* pp. 75, 79–80, 82, 84–87, 89, 92–95, 101, 103, 215.

66. Carl Sandburg, *The Chicago Race Riots,* p. 21; Tuttle, *Race Riot: Chicago,* pp. 104, 109, 113, 123, 129, 155.

67. Tuttle, *Race Riot: Chicago,* p. 32; *The Negro in Chicago,* pp. 11–15, 55.

68. *Chicago Defender,* Aug. 2, 1919, p. 4.

69. *The Chicago Whip,* Aug. 9, 1919, p. 10.

70. *The Chicago Tribune,* July 20, 1919, p. 8; July 31, 1919, p. 6.

71. *Chicago Defender,* Aug. 9, 1919, p. 9.

72. Tuttle, *Race Riot: Chicago,* pp. 249–50.

73. W. E. B. Du Bois, *The Souls of Black Folks* (Chicago, 1903), p. 41; Booker T. Washington, *Up from Slavery* (New York, 1901), p. 219.

74. Spear, *Black Chicago,* p. 86.

75. Du Bois, *The Souls of Black Folks,* pp. 58–59; see also W. E. B. Du Bois, "The Talented Tenth," in Booker T. Washington, ed., *The Negro Problem: A Series of Articles by Representative Negroes of Today* (New York, 1903), pp. 33–75.

76. Spear, *Black Chicago,* p. 85.

77. Allen F. Davis, *Spearheads for Reform: The Social Settlements and the Progressive Movement 1890–1914* (New York, 1967), pp. 94–95; *Chicago Tribune,* June 1, 1908, p. 9.

78. Spear, *Black Chicago,* pp. 87, 89.

79. Arvarh E. Strickland, *History of the Chicago Urban League* (Urbana, Ill., 1966), pp. 12, 24, 26, 27, 34, 36, 39.

80. Marcus H. Boulware, *The Oratory of Negro Leaders 1900–1968* (Westport, Conn., 1969), pp. 55–56, 59; Gosnell, *Negro Politicians,* p. 113; Edmund D. Cronon, *Black Moses: The Story of Marcus Garvey and the Universal Negro Improvement Association* (Madison, Wis., 1955), pp. 3–4, 50, 60, 75, 206, 211.

81. See Metz T. P. Lochard, "The Negro Press in Illinois," *Journal of the Illinois State Historical Society* 56 (Autumn, 1963), pp. 570–91. His discussion of Robert Abbott and the *Defender* is on pp. 572–73.

82. Spear, *Black Chicago,* p. 82; *Broadax,* Aug. 22, 1908, p. 1.

83. Lochard, "The Negro Press in Illinois," pp. 575–76; *Chicago Whip,* Aug. 9, 1919, p. 10. See the masthead of *Forum,* Jan. 11, 1908.

84. Gosnell, *Negro Politicians,* p. 25; Spear, *Black Chicago,* p. 58. See also Alfreda M. Duster, ed., *Crusade for Justice: The Autobiography of Ida B. Wells* (Chicago, 1970).

85. Spear, *Black Chicago,* p. 53. For a full biography of Dr. Williams, see Helen Buckler, *Daniel Hale Williams, Negro Surgeon* (New York, 1968).

86. Ibid., p. 72.

87. Ibid., p. 61.

88. Spear, *Black Chicago*, pp. 66, 69. See the letters of Fannie Barrier Williams to the *New York Age*, Aug. 27, 1908, p. 1; Sept. 17, 1908, p. 11.

89. *Directory of Sangamon County's Colored Citizens: A History of the Negro in Sangamon County: A Directory of Lodges, Churches, Parks, Amusements, Mechanics, Business Firms, and Citizens* (Springfield, Ill., 1926), unpaged.

90. *New York Age*, Nov. 12, 1908, p. 1.

91. Spear, *Black Chicago*, p. 74.

92. Ibid., pp. 56, 71.

93. Gosnell, *Negro Politicians*, pp. 23, 27–29; Sterling D. Spero and Abram L. Harris, *The Black Worker, the Negro and the Labor Movement* (Port Washington, N.Y., 1931), pp. 402–29.

94. Gosnell, *Negro Politicians*, pp. 15, 23.

95. *Sunday Chicago Inter-Ocean*, Jan. 14, 1908, p. 28; Spear, *Black Chicago*, p. 109.

96. Gosnell, *Negro Politicians*, p. 111.

97. Spear, *Black Chicago*, p. 78; *Illinois Blue Book*, 1909, 1911, 1912–13, 1915–16, 1917–18, 1919–20, 1921–2, 1923–24, 1925–26, 1927–28.

98. Gosnell, *Negro Politicians*, pp. 75, 163–65, 167, 181; Spear, *Black Chicago*, p. 78. In 1916 De Priest was indicted on charges of conspiring to protect gambling in his aldermanic district. He was acquitted of the charge. *Chicago Record-Herald*, Oct. 15, 1916, part 1, p. 1; *Chicago Tribune*, June 9, 1917, p. 1.

99. Gosnell, *Negro Politicians*, pp. 37, 38, 39–40; Lloyd Wendt and Herman Kogan, *Big Bill of Chicago* (Indianapolis, 1953), p. 256; Joel A. Tarr, *A Study in Boss Politics: William Lorimer of Chicago* (Urbana, Ill., 1971), p. 308.

100. Gosnell, *Negro Politicians*, pp. 118, 122, 126, 128, 130.

11

The Popular Culture of the 1920s

The increased industrialization of the twentieth century created more leisure time for more people. Pressure from labor unions, a humanitarian outlook, and efficient industrial techniques contributed to this phenomenon. Many people now possessed free time and increased income. A popular culture developed to satisfy the blue- and white-collar workers, the mechanics and clerks of the nation. The rich or well-to-do always had leisure and ways to enjoy it, but before the end of the '20s it was necessary to create new outlets to fill the idle time of the less affluent and the less well-educated. As one reporter put it, "Millions learned to play where only thousands played before." The reporter, approving the new way of life, wrote, "The right to play is the final clause in the charter of democracy. The people are king—*et le roi s'amuse.*" The rich had frivolous amusements, but they also supported the operas, the symphonies, the legitimate theater, the art galleries, the poets, the little magazines, and the novelists. The less affluent did not have the educationally derived intellectual resources to support these enterprises, and popular culture was sometimes transitory, commercial, shallow, and elusive. Coupled with a growing rebellion against Victorianism, the new culture created a revolution in manners and morals. Some of it, such as jazz, came from the people, but much of it emerged from commercial ventures. Illinoisians participated in these pleasures with the same enthusiasm as the rest of the nation.[1]

Abel Green and Joe Laurie, writing a history of show business, described the 1920s as "a gigantic playground." They believed prohibition was the "last gasp of the dying old order" which spurred on a "glorious 10-year bat" in which sex was rediscovered and the heroes were as diverse as Al Capone and Charles A. Lindbergh.[2] It was a shallow period and the heroes were often celluloid. People tired of the rigors of progressive era liberalism and wearied of the demands of an all-out effort to make the world safe for democracy. The people engaged in irresponsible play for a decade; only the depression slowed their play.

During the first twenty years of the twentieth century, vaudeville constituted the people's theater. One historian of vaudeville describes this theater as "America in motley, the national relaxation." He saw vaudeville as "a dig in the nation's ribs, its simplicity as naive as the circus."[3]

Vaudeville was a variety show of magic acts, songs, dances, and animal acts, all centering around the comedian who was the headliner, and it provided a training ground for actors, including many who later succeeded in movies and radio. Important circuits of vaudeville theaters, such as the Keith-Albee-Orpheum circuit, covered all the major cities from New York to San Francisco. For a time after 1907, Klaw and Erlanger merged with the Schuberts to produce a second large circuit. Many small circuits, such as Kohl and Castle, operated in the Midwest. Playing the big houses brought relative wealth to the entertainers. An opportunity to play the Palace Theater in New York (which continued a two-a-day schedule until 1931) constituted success for the vaudeville performer.[4]

Comedians used topical materials designed to appeal to the unsophisticated. As early as 1902 Ed Wynn poked fun at college boys, and the Marx brothers put on an act called "Fun in Hi Skule." The nature of the audience made it possible to denigrate education. Many performers, including W. C. Fields, started as jugglers, and animal acts served as fillers for the bills. Audiences responded to ethnic humor. Al Jolson got his start in blackface, and comics stereotyped Irish, German, Jewish, and Italian immigrants. Comedians used racy jokes and double entendre to liven up their acts. As the medium declined, comedians injected more suggestive material into their acts; earlier comics used a minimum of sexual allusion. From time to time managers tried to dignify vaudeville by bringing in performers from the legitimate theater. Figures such as David Belasco, Ethel Barrymore, and Sarah Bernhardt made forays onto the vaudeville stage.[5]

Vaudeville rose to such heights that many song titles, catch phrases, and comic lines became household words. "Mr. Gallagher and Mr. Sheen," the theme song of Ed Sheen and Al Gallagher, who met in Chicago in 1910, became a part of the vocabulary. Many stars in movies, radio, and stage rose from vaudeville. Eva Tanguay, Nora Bayes, Fred Astaire, Al Jolson, Lily Langtry, and Will Rogers all started in vaudeville. By 1905 Bill "Bojangles" Robinson was dancing in vaudeville, while Buster Keaton and Charlie Chaplin were bringing roars of laughter from audiences all over the country. Eddie Cantor and Fannie Brice had achieved stardom by 1910. Mae West appeared in vaudeville as early as 1912, as did Texas Guinan, an institution into the 1920s.[6]

Chicago became a center of vaudeville, both in performance and in management and booking, and several impresarios operated in and around the city. One firm, Jones, Linck, and Schafer, started in the slot machine business and built a small vaudeville circuit centering around their biggest theater, the Colonial. The firm sold tickets at the Boston Store in Chicago for 1 cent in order to attract attention to the opening of the theater. Ten thousand people showed up to see four shows on the first day. Another Chicago impresario, John Jay Murdock, booked many vaudeville headliners into his theater, the Masonic Temple Roof, which in its best days had a prestige almost equal to that of New York City's Palace.[7]

The firm of Kohl and Castle controlled much of the booking throughout the Midwest. Charles F. Kohl, the senior partner of the organization, died in 1910, leaving an estate of some $7,000,000 illustrating the lucrative nature of the business. After operating independently for years, Kohl and Castle merged with the Orpheum circuit, which added to their prestige. They also maintained connections to the West Coast in cooperation with Meyerfield and Lehman, booking acts from Chicago to San Francisco.[8]

Most towns of some size had vaudeville theaters. In 1924 the Majestic in Springfield, part of the Orpheum circuit, ran six acts, three performances a day combined with a Pathe news movie. A large number of small neighborhood theaters also sprang to life. Many of these theaters offered entertainment for as little as 25 cents in 1912. Opened in 1908, the Bijou Theater in Quincy had the first of the small-town storefront shows. Agents booked 150 to 200 of these out of Chicago each week. The smaller towns unable to support a regular vaudeville theater sometimes had similar but inferior entertainment through medicine and tent shows which traveled the countryside. Some of these presented a vaudeville show, others a play. In addition to performing, between acts the tent-show personnel sold patent medicines guaranteed to cure anything. Many theatrical figures learned their craft in the medicine or tent shows.[9]

By World War I vaudeville was beginning to decline, a trend that accelerated during the 1920s. By the end of the '20s vaudeville was dead. Historians and vaudeville buffs have speculated about the causes of its demise, but the rising popularity of movies and radio provided the final blow. At first many vaudeville managers saw no danger in motion pictures and often showed one-reel firms with their acts. Gradually, however, as the manufacturing techniques became smoother, motion pictures became major competitors of vaudeville. Then radio appeared, a form of free entertainment that could be enjoyed at home.[10]

One historian cites other reasons for the rapid decline of vaudeville. As it began to fade, promoters desperately increased the size of the bills, putting on perhaps five bills a day instead of the standard two. This bled the performer physically and made it impossible to come up with new material for gags and songs. The public tired of the old jokes, and as performers ran out of material they used more vulgarity, for which much of the public was not ready. Also, the old comedians had produced laughter with unsophisticated slapstick and exaggerated costumes. In an effort to make vaudeville more sophisticated, promoters required performers to wear dinner jackets or evening gowns, thus destroying its earlier simple appeal.[11]

Edward Albee, of the Keith-Albee-Orpheum circuit, got much of the blame for the decline; Albee brought increased sophistication and eliminated simple slapstick. One historian believes the death of vaudeville came because low comedy gave way to sophisticated acts, grotesque costumes gave way to formal wear, and chorus lines replaced the old dance routines. In short, when it was no longer the theater of the people, vaudeville died.[12]

Motion pictures created the chief area of competition for vaudeville in the entertainment world. As early as the 1880s, Thomas Edison had conceived the idea of combining motion pictures with the phonograph. He organized a department of his laboratory for further experiments, resulting, in 1889, in the Kinetoscope, a device combining music with an animated picture. As the technique was improved, competitors appeared. Edison, always jealous of patent rights, brought suits against many of these. Of the competitors, Biograph Studios and Vitagraph Studios produced more films than Edison. D. W. Griffith, a young man from Kentucky who had been both an actor and reporter before he drifted into filmmaking, directed most of the Biograph films.[13]

Chicago flourished briefly as the chief center of moviemaking when William Selig, a pioneer in the field, led the industry there. Selig excelled with adventure movies, using cowboys, Indians, and other Wild West subjects. Selig made Tom Mix, with his horse Tony, one of the early stars. Mix, a ranch foreman and town marshal in Oklahoma, brought some knowledge of the western frontier to the screen under Selig's direction. Selig also created thrilling pictures involving lions, tigers, and beautiful girls who often risked their lives to make the movies.[14]

As early as 1905 observers called moving pictures "the poor man's amusement." These varied from little more than slide-illustrated songs to actual moving pictures featuring a spectacular event such as an automobile race. By 1910 two production companies in Chicago were turning out ten films a week at a cost of about $1,000 each. Gradually the moviemakers moved into more dramatic productions. Sherlock Holmes stories, for example, made popular movies. By 1907 10-cent moviehouses were reaping a profit. Many were family-operated storefront theaters. One family member sold tickets, another ran the projector, while another played the piano to accompany the silent movies. Moralists protested that movies were bad for the lower classes. Soon vaudeville began to complain about the competition, bringing demands to license movie theaters. The distribution and showing of films grew rapidly in Chicago, perhaps because of the availability of locally made films. It is estimated that there were fewer than a hundred theaters in Chicago in 1906, but by 1910 there were some 12,000, mostly in converted stores.[15]

Some firsts were recorded in early Chicago productions. As early as 1907 a film was made that coordinated sound with visual image. This was an operation called camera-phone. The presentation used three projectors and employed fifty people for special stage effects. The bill included a travelogue, entitled "Around the World," and a fire-fighting spectacle in which the audience could hear the sounds of water, the crackling of fire, and ringing bells. Many difficulties arose with this—talking movies were years in the future. Eventually Edison's lawyers turned their attention to the Chicago movie producers. Selig had traveled in the West, so when Edison brought suits against him, he thought of Los Angeles as a desirable area for moviemaking. Selig had popularized the cowboy movie, and the romantic cowboy, wearing buckskins, a ten-gallon hat, and carrying a Winchester rifle or a Colt revolver had become a stock character. The standard plot involved a chase with horses, cowboys, Indians, stagecoaches, and wagon trains, and Selig decided southern California was the best place to make this kind of movie. The climate made it possible to make movies the year around, and there was clear air for good lighting, which made for minimum investment in studios. Any building could be used for dressing rooms and offices. The main advantage of California, however, was that it was some 3,000 miles from Edison's lawyers. Vitagraph, Biograph, and other filmmakers followed Selig to California, and Los Angeles succeeded Chicago as the movie capital of the world.[16]

The important change in moviemaking during the 1920s was the development of the star system. In the early years of movies, the actors and actresses were not identified. With the advent of the new system, however, people went to see favorite actors, highly touted by publicity, without much consideration of the merit of the show. Immediately people such as Charlie Chaplin, Mary Pickford, and Theda Bara became stars. Most Americans developed an intense interest in the private lives of the performers, and producers found it necessary to create stars with great personal appeal. Fox portrayed Theda Bara as the world's most desirable woman, and Metro made Francis X. Bushman the first matinee idol.

Some actresses became early-day sex symbols. In 1926 Clara Bow was billed as "the hottest jazz baby in films." Promoters gave the same treatment to Gloria Swanson, Colleen Moore, Lillian Gish, and Mary Pickford.

An adoring public also paid rapt attention to Hollywood marriages. In 1920, for example, when Douglas Fairbanks and Mary Pickford were married, the publicity surrounding the event created enormous audiences for their pictures.[17]

Among those who became very important in movies was Charlie Chaplin. Chaplin emerged from vaudeville, in which he had worked after emigrating from England, and soon he became a favorite in comedy. In 1916, for example, his movie *Floor Walker* broke all records, earning some $10,000 a day. Chaplin drew a salary of $125,000 a year, with another $10,000 for each movie released. People also flocked to one-reel movies with all-children casts. Among the first of these was one called *Kids of the Movies*.[18]

By the end of World War I, movies had developed into big business, and actors and actresses had acquired a keen sense of their ability to earn money. In 1919 Chaplin, Pickford, William S. Hart, Douglas Fairbanks, and D. W. Griffith organized United

Artists and hired William Gibbs McAdoo as legal counsel for $100,000 a year. Subsequently stars began commanding breathtaking salaries. In 1919 Adolph Zukor signed Mary Miles Mintor to a three-year contract at $1,300,000 per year. Norma Shearer drew a similar salary. John Gilbert, the highest paid star of the '20s, received $10,000 a week as a result of his success in a film called *The Big Parade*.[19] Many great comedians acted in the movies. In addition to Chaplin there was Harold Lloyd, who after the 1925 movie *The Freshman* earned more money than Chaplin. In addition Buster Keaton, Harry Langdon, Will Rogers, and W. C. Fields brought roars of laughter from audiences. By the end of the '20s the public was rushing to see movies starring Eddie Cantor, George Jessel, and Joe E. Brown.[20]

By 1920 a new group of western stars, including William S. Hart, William Farnam, and Gary Cooper, had appeared, and Tom Mix had passed his peak. The studios also had to produce a new group of sex symbols as earlier stars aged. Lupe Velez, Mary Noland, Doris Costello, Irene Rich, Billy Dove, Norma Talmadge, and Constance Talmadge emerged during this period, and among leading men Gilbert Roland, Richard Arlen, Gary Cooper, Jimmy Gleeson, John Barrymore, Richard Barthelmess, and Adolph Menjou rose to the top. Al Jolson became the most famous actor of the period as his *Jazz Singer* became a classic.[21]

The movies enriched a number of show business figures. Most of the big money went to producers and exhibitors of movies, but Harold Lloyd was reputed to be worth $15,000,000. In addition to the cost of the film stars, production costs also soared. Story properties cost more as studios began to use best-selling novels and successful plays. Expensive settings and costumes, although they could be used over and over, added to costs. Movie lots included whole cities, villages, wharfs, and railroad stations which could be redesigned for any kind of movie. Some studios acquired ranches close to Los Angeles where they could keep horses, cattle, and props needed for western movies. Some producers, among them Adolph Zukor, William Fox, and Louis B. Mayer, became as well known as the stars they produced.[22]

As interest in the private affairs of the stars increased, movie magazines and gossip columnists came to prominence. Some of the stories about the stars' dissolute lives were exaggerated for publicity purposes but many were true. Some stars went into an early decline as a result of bootleg whisky or drugs, and some were addicted to high-powered cars and expensive women. By the early

'20s Hollywood had gained the reputation of being the sin capital of the world. The stars, many of whom regarded themselves as above the law or the restraint of conventional society, were the new idols. They basked in the adulation of an adoring middle class, people who vicariously participated in episodes that they could not or dared not involve themselves in personally. World War I had relaxed sexual morality, and motion pictures reflected this change in mores. Many included drinking scenes in spite of prohibition. Although divorce was frowned upon in middle-class life, motion pictures portrayed divorce, seduction, and the use of drugs and liquor as symbols of fashionable living. Many in the Bible Belt were shocked by the movies but still went to see them.[23]

Some stars got into serious trouble. Fatty Arbuckle, a famous comic, was accused of rape. Others were accused of equally serious offenses. As a result, in 1922 the major studios organized a group called the Motion Picture Producers and Distributors of America. They pledged themselves to self-censorship and appointed Will H. Hays of Indiana, postmaster general under Harding, to be the custodian of the nations's morals. The Hays office became the sole judge of decency and cut the racier parts of some movies. The Motion Picture Producers and Distributors of America was a trade association which smoothed the way for foreign concessions and watched for unfavorable legislation on the national or state level. The Hays office caused movies to become less realistic. The early westerns had portrayed frontier life realistically. William S. Hart had played a hard-drinking, hard-riding, fast-shooting character, often an outlaw. As the new morality hit the movie industry this version of the Old West changed. The new hero appeared on the side of law and order, bringing outlaws to justice, and did not drink, smoke, or use his pistols except when forced to in the interest of justice.[24]

During the 1920s the movie industry built large movie houses in major cities. Seating 2,000 to 6,000, these theaters cut into the revenues of vaudeville, the legitimate theater, and lesser forms of show business such as the circus and the chatauqua. In Chicago, Balaban and Katz built the first of the great theaters, the Central Park. Seating 2,200 people, it featured a garish decor of crimson velvet and marble, uniformed ushers, and walls filled with paintings. By 1921 Balaban and Katz owned four theaters, and by 1928 they had created twelve, bringing in 30,000,000 admissions per year. Small towns soon had smaller imitations of the big theaters. Lloyd Lewis, writing in 1929 about this phenomenon, believed that 75 percent of the patrons of these theaters were women and children. He alleged that the plush interiors gave housewives a momentary escape from boredom and an erotic thrill.[25]

By 1916 the *Chicago Tribune* was printing a regular column by "Mae Tinee," called "Right off the Reel," carrying bits of gossip about the stars and notices and reviews of movies. In 1916 dozens of movie ads appeared in Chicago papers. Then showing at the Colonial Theater was *The Birth of a Nation*, whose racist overtones would later bring about the passage of a law forbidding showings of any performance derogatory to a particular ethnic group. Also appearing at that time was John Barrymore, in *Justice* at the Powers, while his brother Lionel was playing in *The Brand of Cowardice* at the Orpheum. Douglas Fairbanks and the Keystone Cops were at the Kenmore, and Mary Pickford had two movies going at the same time. Dorothy Gish was playing at the Gold. At the Crawford, Bryant Washburn and Margaret Clayton were playing in *The Prince of Graustark* by George Barr McCutcheon, a local writer.[26]

Among the listings in a random issue of the *Tribune* in 1920 were Constance Talmadge playing in D. W. Griffith's million-dollar spectacle *Fall of Babylon*, and Wallace Reid in his latest "zippie" picture, *What's Your Hurry?* Also playing in Chicago was Will Rogers in *Cupid and the Cowpuncher* and Charlie Chaplin and Marie Dressler in *Tillie's Punctured Romance*. In 1924 the selections were even more formidable. Marion Davies was playing in *Eulanda* at the Roosevelt Theater, Tom Mix was in *O You Tony* at the Monroe, and at the Senate, Cecil B. DeMille's *Feet of Clay* was playing, combined with a stage show containing thirty saxophone artists. At the Kimbark, Rudolph Valentino was playing in *Monsieur Beaucaire*, while the Plaisance presented Lon Chaney in *The Hunchback of Notre Dame*. On one date in 1928 a moviegoer could see Pickford in *My Best Girl*, Jolson in *The Jazz Singer*, and Chaney in *The Hunchback of Notre Dame*. Harold Lloyd appeared in *Speeding* and Clara Bow in *Red Hair*. Later that year audiences saw Jolson in *Singing Fool* at the McVickers, Rin Tin Tin in *Land of the Silver Fox* at the Orpheum, and John Barrymore in *Tempest* at the Uptown—with sound. In the first mention of talking pictures, John Barrymore was advertised as appearing in "Vitaphone talkies." Once the talking picture arrived, only the silent stars who had adequate speaking voices managed to hang on.[27]

The movie industry brought concern from the upper class of

most cities, and there was always talk of censorship or a board to pass on the fitness of movies. As early as 1913 Mayor Harrison announced the creation of a Chicago censorship board, suggesting that it consist of twenty-five men and women, two or three of whom could be called upon at any time to sit in judgment with policemen on the propriety of the films. The *Chicago Inter-Ocean* reported, "Besides suggestive pictures, the Mayor believes that portrayals of hold-ups, murders, and other forms of crime should be eliminated. It is proposed that the board be under the direction of Major Funkhouser, to whom has been delegated the supervision of the city's morals." In spite of the concern of those who would censor or curtail the movies, the industry continued to grow.[28]

It was estimated in 1922 that 20,000,000 Americans attended the movies daily. The previous year the American people had paid $800,000,000 for admissions to movies and theaters, in addition chewing $44,000,000 worth of gum, eating $408,000,000 worth of candy, drinking $448,000,000 worth of soft drinks, and smoking $1,700,000,000 worth of tobacco. It was assumed that the consumption of these products was related to the holiday air of the times, when all kinds of recreational diversions were sought.[29]

Radio also added a new dimension to the popular culture and contributed heavily to the economy by providing new jobs in industry, sales, and service. Radio brought standardized speech to America, provided access to popular clichés, informed the public instantaneously in politics and sports, and supplied entertainment. People in the remotest village of Illinois heard popular songs almost as soon as they came out. The latest lines of comedians entered the public domain. Radio enabled people in rural areas and villages to keep up on sports events, contributing to the development of the 1920s as the "golden age of sports." Radio had a great impact on the political life of the nation, and Illinoisians could hear their favorite politicians in their living rooms. The medium provided for a more informed electorate as news events, political issues, and developments around the world became readily known. Radio could also be used for spreading misinformation and propaganda, and such charges were made from time to time.

Westinghouse began operation of the first commercial radio station in America. The station, KDKA of Pittsburgh, began broadcasting on November 2, 1920. On that day Warren Harding defeated James Cox for the presidency and KDKA broadcast the results. The following year, 1921, Westinghouse opened station

KYW in Chicago with the songs of Mary Garden from the Chicago Opera. Opera made up nearly the entire KYW broadcast schedule during its first season. A little later the station broadcast the World Series.

Much early broadcasing in Illinois provided services for farmers. Editors of farm papers began to tell their readers that radio would be a great boon to farmers. Farm wives could listen to the radio while doing their work and the farmer could hear market and weather reports.[30] By 1925 Illinois had thirty-seven radio stations in operation. Many of these broadcast livestock, grain, dairy, and vegetable prices as well as weather reports.

As radio stations flourished, radio receiving sets became common. By 1925 the census showed that 12 percent of farm homes had receivers. Most small-town banks kept a radio and posted changes in livestock and grain prices for farm clients. Clubs, churches, schools, and county Farm Bureau offices installed radio sets for the entertainment of members and information on markets and weather. The early sets, ranging in price up to $250, were battery-powered; not until 1927 was it possible to operate radios with household current. After that nearly all city users had sets powered by household current, although few farm homes had electricity during the '20s. Nevertheless, by 1930 more than half the farm homes in Illinois were equipped with radio receivers. Many of the early sets were home-made devices put together by people intrigued with the new toys.[31]

Sears, Roebuck and Company operated one of the early stations in Chicago. Catering largely to a farm audience, it broadcast first under the call letters WBBX. In 1924 the station changed to WES for "World's Economy Store." Still later the call letters were changed to WLS for "World's Largest Store." WGN in Chicago was considered a highbrow station because it broadcast educational programs. The *Chicago Tribune*, under the direction of Colonel Robert R. McCormick, got into radio to furnish sports, market news, and summaries of current events. By 1923, using the call letters WGN for "World's Greatest Newspaper," the station broadcast music from the Drake Hotel. In the early twenties, WGN interrupted programs to broadcast police calls. The Chicago police force had no communication system of its own, so WGN would call squad cars which had been equipped with receivers to inform them of a robbery or the route taken by fleeing criminals. This practice made programs exciting but destroyed continuity. The medium was so new that listeners accepted whatever came along without complaint.[32]

Many of the Chicago stations developed stars that became households names throughout Illinois. At WGN an announcer named Quin Ryan, the mainstay of the station, broadcast all kinds of programs and doubled as a character named Uncle Walt, telling bedtime stories to children. WBBM specialized in jazz music, which was not quite respectable in the minds of many, so their programming was thought to be exceedingly daring. As the broadcasting day lengthened and receivers became more common, most Chicago stations broadcast popular music from the hotels. KYW, which had a staff of thirty by 1925, broadcast the dance music of the "Night Hawks" each evening from the Congress Hotel. WLS sponsored the Isham Jones orchestra, which broadcast from the College Inn in the Sherman Hotel. WLS also had a popular announcer, George D. Hay, who was known to listeners as "the solemn old judge," and a popular children's program called the "Woodshed Theater," put on by Ford Rush and Glen Rowl. The station was especially noted for the "National Barn Dance," standard listening each Saturday night for the farmers of Illinois.[33]

Many stations continued farm service programs. WLS cooperated with the American Farm Bureau Federation and the National Livestock Producers of Illinois. KYW presented a weekly program for the Farm Bureau Federation called the "Voice of the Farmer." Over its station WDAP the Chicago Board of Trade broadcast grain prices at half-hour intervals. The Union Stockyards started a station called WAAF which broadcast regular market reports. The *Daily Drovers Journal,* one of the state farm magazines, purchased WAAF a little later. In 1928 Sears and Roebuck decided to sell WLS, and it was purchased by the *Prairie Farmer*. The *Prairie Farmer* was published by Burridge Butler, who saw radio as a service to farmers. For many years, WLS was dedicated to programming for the farmer.[34]

The profusion of stations brought regulation. There was considerable confusion as stations sought to gain audiences by increasing their power illegally and sometimes shifting channels, and a landmark court case came out of Illinois in an effort to remedy these problems. Colonel McCormick, disturbed because other stations infringed on the frequency of WGN, brought suit in the case of the *Tribune* Company *vs.* Oak Leaves Broadcasting Station. The decision in this case brought about a standard by which U.S. broadcasting was regulated. Partly as a result of this case, Congress, in 1927, created the Federal Radio Commission, which regulated broadcasting in radio. In 1934 the commission was renamed the Federal Communications Commission.[35]

Ultimately the entrepreneurs of radio established the network system of stations. In 1924 a group of stations headed by WXYZ (Detroit) joined with WGN (Chicago), WOR (New York), and WLW (Cincinnati) to form the nucleus of the Mutual Broadcasting System. These were high-powered stations whose audiences covered many states. In 1926 the National Broadcasting Company was established by Radio Corporation of America, the largest distributor of radio receivers in the world. One of New York's major stations, WEAF, was purchased from American Telephone and Telegraph Company for $1,000,000, and NBC was built around it, with an agreement in the purchase from A T and T to use their lines for transmitting programs from city to city. Subsequently the Columbia Phonograph Broadcasting System went into operation in 1927 as the third major network. The American Broadcasting Company was part of NBC and did not become an independent network until 1942.[36]

With the advent of the networks, a star system developed in radio. The names, themes, and lines of the stars became known to everybody. Some of these acts originated in Chicago, and one of the most famous was "Amos 'n' Andy." Created by Freeman Gosden, who played Amos, and Charles Correll, who played Andy, the act was first broadcast on WGN under the name of "Sam 'n' Henry," but two years later it went on WMAQ under the new name of "Amos 'n' Andy," which continued for decades. Situation comedy may have had its origin in 1925 when Marion and Jim Jordan, a pair of old vaudevillians, became famous as Fibber McGee and Molly. This led to dozens of similar programs humorously describing what was assumed to be a typical American household.[37]

Announcers such as Graham McNamee, Milton Cross, Ted Husing, Norman Brokenshire, and Norman Pierce were famous for their broadcasts of sports and special news events. These individuals, capable of extensive ad-lib chatter, usually worked without a script. Some of the musical groups, such as Harry Horlick's "A & P Gypsies," the "Ipana Troubadors," and Harry Reser's "Cliquot Club Eskimos" achieved fame. Many who made their debut in other aspects of show business became famous through radio. Will Rogers, an important vaudevillian figure, was one of these. In some cases stars like Mary Garden from the Chicago Opera added to their national fame through radio.

Many newscasters also became well known. H. V. Kaltenborn, one of the most famous, was broadcasting as early as 1925 over

WEAF in New York. More picturesque than the German-born Kaltenborn was Floyd Gibbons, who became the prototype of the war correspondent. He cultivated the image of a swashbuckling reporter. He wore a white patch over the eye he had lost during World War I, a trench coat, and a rakish hat. Although people sometimes doubted his stories, he had engaged in many adventurous episodes. Gibbons was a native of Chicago, although he wandered all over the world for years.[38]

Despite the disgust of old-time politicians, radio provided a new outlet in politics. In 1924 listeners heard the national nominating conventions by radio. Quin Ryan broadcast the 1924 Republican convention and the 1928 Democratic convention for WGN. Al Smith at first had great disdain for radio, saying, "When I talk to people, I want to see the whites of their eyes, I don't want 'em to be ten miles away." Later Smith broadcast extensively in his 1928 campaign.

Perhaps nothing got so much impetus from radio as sports. In July, 1921, eighty stations broadcast the Dempsey-Carpentier heavyweight championship fight. Radio also carried baseball games. Graham McNamee and Ted Husing were among the leading sports announcers. Interest grew so much in boxing, particularly in the heavyweight class, that by the time Dempsey fought Tunney in 1926, radio broadcasts carried the event in detail.[39]

An idea of the variety of early broadcasting can be gained from the radio column of the *Chicago Tribune*. On October 20, 1924, there was an extensive listing of activities at WGN. It was taking an election poll and broadcasting from the Drake Hotel. Quin Ryan was the chief sports announcer. Board of Trade reports were broadcast every half-hour from 9:35 A.M. to 1:25 P.M. From 1:10 to 2:30 there was a luncheon concert by the Drake Concert Ensemble and the Blackstone String Quartet. From 2:30 to 3:00 there was the Lyon and Healey Artist Series and from 3:00 to 3:30 "rocking chair time." The half-hour between 5:00 and 5:30 was devoted to the Board of Trade summary and Stock Exchange quotation. The next half-hour carried "Skeezix" with Uncle Walt. WMAQ at that time was broadcasting only two hours a day.[40]

Jazz music, at first thought immoral by the staid, came into its own during the '20s. Essentially a music of the people, particularly black people, jazz has its roots in spirituals and in Africa. Almost undefinable, jazz involves improvisation and feel of the musician for his musical language. It is, perhaps, to use a later phrase, the true "soul" music. The great Louis Armstrong, when asked what jazz is, said, "My idea of how a tune should go." Fats Waller, in reply to a similar question, said, "Madam, if you don't know by now, don't mess with it!"[41]

For all practical purposes, jazz started in New Orleans, where it was played at funerals and in the houses of prostitution in the flamboyant Storyville. Many of the musicians had taught themselves to play various instruments—cornet, clarinet, trombone, and tuba. They marched for weddings and political rallies, and played for fraternal organizations, picnics, and election campaigns, but they were at their best at funerals. Many worked in houses of prostitution, cabarets, and dance halls.[42]

In 1917 during World War I, the Navy, in an effort to stamp out prostitution, closed Storyville. Seeking employment, many of the musicians came up the river to Memphis and Chicago. Some played on the riverboats en route. Among the early jazz artists from New Orleans were Joe "King" Oliver, Louis Armstrong, Jimmy Noone, Ferdinand Joseph "Jelly Roll" Morton, Johnny Dodds and his brother Warren "Baby" Dodds, Edward "Kid" Ory, and Earl Hines. Chicago jazz started with the arrival of "King" Oliver and his band. The "King" left New Orleans in 1918 and soon was playing in Chicago.[43] Louis Armstrong came to Chicago in 1922 to join the Oliver band, and from then on the story of jazz in America coincides with the story of Louis Armstrong. Born in New Orleans in 1900, Armstrong had acquired a cornet in the orphanage where he lived. He played for funerals, picnics, and in honky-tonks, making a few dollars wherever he could.

Armstrong described his arrival in Chicago on July 8, 1922, at the Twelfth Street station. Taking a cab to the South Side, where Oliver was playing in the Lincoln Gardens Cafe, he recounted that as he got out of the cab, he could hear Oliver's band playing and said to himself, "My God, I wonder if I'm good enough to play in that band." He went inside to join the band, which consisted at that time of "King" Oliver (trumpet), Johnny Dodds (clarinet), Honor Neutre (trombone), "Baby" Dodds (drums), Bill Johnson (bass), and Lillian Hardin (piano). "Lil" Hardin later became Armstrong's first wife. Armstrong played second trumpet.[44]

Preston Jackson later said that Lil Hardin deserved great credit for Armstrong's fame. Hardin, who always remembered Armstrong with fondness, recalled that when he appeared in Chicago, they called him "Little Louis" because he already weighed 226 pounds. Hardin could read and write music and she was able to write down the music that Armstrong composed. She was a fine pianist and had graduated with honors from Fisk University.[45]

About a year after Armstrong arrived in Chicago, Hoagie Carmichael and Bix Beiderbeck went to the South Side to hear the King Oliver band. Carmichael described the effect of Armstrong's music:

> It's the summer of 1923. We took two quarts of bathtub gin, a package of muggles, and headed for the black and tan joint where King Oliver's band was playing. The King featured two trumpets, piano, and bass fiddle and the clarinet. As I sat down to light my first muggle, Bix gave the sign to a big black fellow, playing second trumpet for Oliver, and he slashed into Bugle Call Rag.
>
> I dropped my cigarette and gulped my drink. Bix was on his feet, his eyes popping. For taking the first chorus was that second trumpet, Louis Armstrong. Louis was taking it fast. Bob Gillette slid off his chair and under the table. He was excitable that way. "Why," I moaned. "Why isn't everybody in the world here to hear that?" I meant it. Something as unutterably stirring as that deserved to be heard by the world. Then the muggles took effect and my body got light. Every note Louis hit was perfection. I ran to the piano and took the place of Louie's wife. They swung into Royal Garden Blues. I had never heard the tune before, but somehow I knew every note. I couldn't miss. I was floating in a strange deep blue whirlpool of jazz. It wasn't the marijuana. The muggles and the gin were, in a way, stage props. It was the music. The music took me and it had me and it made me right.[46]

Louis Armstrong was happy playing with his old friend King Oliver and the Dodds brothers and Lil Hardin. He said that when he began to play, it felt like old times. Armstrong and Oliver were so attuned to each other that each supported the other without writing down any of the music. Armstrong recalled that he had "lived so closely with his [Oliver's] music that I could follow his lead in a split second." Armstrong thought all of his dreams had come true as he played with his idol. Hardin did what she could to get Armstrong away from Oliver because she thought Armstrong's growth as a musician would stop if he only followed Oliver's lead. But for nearly half a century the name and music of Louis Armstrong would be known the world around.[47]

King Oliver and Louis Armstrong and others brought jazz from New Orleans to the South Side of Chicago, and from this grew a Chicago-style jazz played by white musicians as well as black. It is conceded that among white jazz musicians, Bix Beiderbeck has to be considered first. Louis Armstrong said that Bix was "a man as serious about his music as I am." Another musician said that Bix had an ear that was so good that "he can tell you the pitch of a belch!" The tragic life of Bix Beiderbeck began in 1903 in Iowa. Beiderbeck early showed an extraordinary musical ear. He took piano lessons and his family had dreams of his becoming a concert pianist. When he was in high school, however, Beiderbeck acquired a cornet and began to imitate jazz music on records. Subsequently his family, hoping to improve his academic life, which had suffered from his devotion to music, sent him to Lake Forest Academy near Chicago. But he spent more time with music than was good for his studies, and in 1922 was dismissed for academic failure. In the meantime, however, he had formed a small orchestra and was playing engagements in towns near Lake Forest.[48]

Beiderbeck spent time listening to musicians such as the New Orleans "Rhythm Kings," who were playing at Chicago Friar's Inn, and other groups such as King Oliver's band. Gradually he gained experience and began to improvise a style of his own, which caused some musicians to rank him as the top jazz trumpeter of all time. His technique shows in records that he made with a group called the "Wolverines," playing such tunes as "Tiger Rag." His music, like that of all jazz artists, became a highly personal thing. He did not play jazz as the Blacks did, although he was influenced by Louis Armstrong and some of the other great black musicians.

Ultimately, drinking and the irregular life of a jazz musician destroyed Bix Beiderbeck. In 1931, his health already ruined, he insisted on playing an engagement at Princeton when he was quite ill; he developed pneumonia and died on August 7, 1931. In the meantime he had played with a number of important bands, including those of Jean Goldkette, and Paul Whiteman, who said of him, "Bix was not only the greatest musician I've ever known, but also the greatest gentleman I've ever known."[49]

Many young Chicagoans, intrigued by the New Orleans jazz artists, made the rounds to the Friar's Inn, Lincoln Gardens Inn, or Dreamland Cafe to hear Louis Armstrong, King Oliver, or the Dodds brothers. Some of these young men had prior training in music, which they coupled with a great enthusiasm for jazz to create the Chicago style. Among these was Dave Tough, a drummer born in Oak Park in 1907. He patterned his early technique after Baby Dodds but went on to develop a style that made him one of the great jazz drummers of all time, playing with some of the big bands such as Ray Noble and Tommy Dorsey.

Unfortunately he, like Beiderbeck, became a victim of alcohol. He died in 1948 in New York as a result of a fall.[50]

Dave Tough became acquainted in the post–World War I era with a group of aspiring young jazz artists called the "Austin High School Gang," students at Austin High School, located at Washington Boulevard and Central Avenue. Among them were clarinetist Frank Teschmacher, bassist Jim Lannigan, saxophonist Bud Freeman, and brothers Jimmy and Dick McPartland. As boys they went regularly to an ice cream parlor called the Spoon 'n' Straw which had a phonograph and jazz records. Tough, a little older, began taking them to hear jazz. By 1925, with Tough on drums and Bix Beiderbeck on trumpet, they had organized as the "Wolverines." They made a number of impressive recordings, but they eventually split up and went their separate ways, seeking more individual approaches.

Others contributed to the Chicago sound as well. Francis "Muggsy" Spanier, who as a boy sneaked into the Dreamland Cafe to hear Louis Armstrong, later developed as one of the great jazz cornetists. Charles "Pee Wee" Russell, clarinet, once a student at the Western Military Academy in Alton, was also associated with Chicago, although he was only there for a brief time. Other musicians active in Chicago jazz were Earl Hines, Jess Stacy, "Mezz" Mezzrow, and George Wettling.[51]

No discussion of jazz musicians, in Chicago or the nation, would be complete without mention of Benny Goodman. Born in the ghetto around Hull House, Goodman studied with Franz Schoepp of the Chicago Musical College. At the age of thirteen Goodman was playing well, and he released his first recording in 1926 at the age of seventeen. In addition to formal training with Schoepp, Goodman listened to many jazz artists and was influenced by Frank Teschmacher and "Pee Wee" Russell. He was not an imitator, but developed a style of his own.

Although many of the New Orleans greats could not read music, the individualistic improvisation they gave their tunes caused the soul to soar. To the Blacks and an increasing number of Whites it was inspiring, although it was a people's music and represented a lower-class immorality to those who had "arrived." The young white musicians of Chicago, however, seized upon its freedom and gave it a new personality, and by the mid-1920s some of the big bands, including Paul Whiteman's, Fletcher Henderson's, and Jean Goldkette's, had made it respectable.[52]

Among those who enjoyed jazz were Chicago's gangsters. Al

Capone and his gang frequently showed up at the Friar's Club, the Dreamland Cafe, Tancils, the Grand Terrace, or the Pekin Cafe. Musicians were generally glad to see Capone, who handed out generous tips for playing his favorite tunes. On the other hand, a slight misunderstanding could bring gunplay. Muggsy Spanier recalled, as a boy, sitting on the curb outside the Pekin Cafe listening to the music and then running home as pistols rang out while their owners tried to keep the beat of the music with their guns. Although the gangsters might bring extra pay, they were an occupational hazard.[53]

Other forms of popular music began to appear, with the songs of such writers as Irving Berlin and George M. Cohan. Cohan introduced "Over There" in 1917, followed by a great outpouring of war songs, including "I'm in the Army Now" and "Say a Prayer for the Boys over There." After the war people were still singing Gus Edwards's "In My Merry Oldsmobile," and an accordion craze appeared, with songs of improbable titles such as "Yacky Hacky Wicky Wacky Woo" and "Yacka Foola Hicky Doola." New dances such as the Shimmy, the Charleston, and the Black Bottom made their appearance during the early and mid-'20s, but by the end of the 1920s this craze had passed in favor of a slower, smoother, sweeter music represented by the songs of Bing Crosby, Rudy Vallee, and Guy Lombardo and his Royal Canadians. This music led to the creation of the great ballrooms, many featuring the dime-a-dance hostess. Chicago was at the forefront of this movement with the establishment of the Trianon, opened in 1922 at a cost of $1,000,000. The Trianon paid $5,000 for a six-day engagement of a dance band.[54]

By 1930 athletics had become a major part of the popular culture. In an age when real heroes were few, the names of Bobby Jones, Babe Ruth, Red Grange, and Jack Dempsey became familiar to all. School boys memorized the batting averages of their favorite baseball team, and the heavyweight boxing champion of the world seemed more important than the president of the United States. Illinois produced a number of these heroes and was the scene of many thrilling contests that became more real to the fans through radio broadcasts. Announcers such as Quin Ryan, Ted Husing, and Graham McNamee brought excitement to the most lackluster contest.[55]

Although the '20s produced more interest in athletics, many sports dated back prior to 1920. Both the University of Illinois and the University of Chicago became powers in college football soon after the turn of the century. In 1900 it was announced that the University of Illinois was to have the best athletic field in the nation, with a grandstand that would seat 1,500 spectators. George Huff came to Illinois in 1895 and the following year was appointed athletic director and varsity baseball coach. He continued as athletic director until 1935, although he gave up coaching in 1919. Under his guidance Illinois finished no worse than second in the Western Conference in baseball for twenty-three of twenty-four years.[56]

In varsity football, Coach Robert Zuppke dominated the scene at Illinois from 1913 to 1941. Born in Germany in 1879, Zuppke majored in philosophy at the University of Wisconsin and hoped to achieve fame in the art world with his painting. One of the few coaches who had never played varsity football, Zuppke coached at Muskegon, Michigan, and Oak Park High School. At the latter school he was undefeated for three seasons. The resultant publicity caused George Huff to offer him employment. When Zuppke came to Urbana, Illinois had been competing in the Big Ten for seventeen years and had never won a championship. In the following sixteen years, Zuppke won the championship seven times and produced national champions in 1914, 1923, and 1927. The Illinois clubs compiled a record of 137-79-12 under his guidance.[57]

Zuppke once said, "I dislike the obvious." Therein lay the key to his success. Using speed and deception, he developed plays called the "Flying Trapeze," the "Whoa Backs," and the "Flea Flicker." A luckless opposing coach once said that to deal with a Zuppke team it was necessary "to determine one of two things—whether Illinois was using two balls or none at all." Zuppke invented the spiral snap from center, the screen pass, and the huddle (also attributed to Amos Alonzo Stagg). Even in a losing season Zuppke could produce at least one spectacular win over a favored team. It was after such a win over Ohio State in 1921 that the name "Fighting Illini" was conferred on the team.[58]

Many football stars came from the Illinois teams, among them George Halas, Harold Pogue, Chuck Carney (the first man to make All-American in two sports—football and basketball), Russ Crain, Al Nowack, and Jud Timm. Most fans, however, remember the Red Grange era. The son of a deputy sheriff, Grange attended Wheaton High School, where he was an outstanding athlete. In a game against Downers Grove he scored six touchdowns and kicked nine field goals.

At Illinois Grange showed equal brilliance. The University

dedicated Memorial Stadium on October 18, 1924, before 67,000 fans. On that day, as Quin Ryan of WGN broadcast the game, the 175-member band marched in new blue-and-orange uniforms and ten cheerleaders urged on the crowd. It was necessary to turn away thousands of spectators as Grange ran for five touchdowns to beat a tough Michigan team by a score of 39 to 14. During his athletic career, Grange played 237 games, carried the ball 4,013 times, gained 32,820 yards, and scored 531 touchdowns. This was a hero for the '20s. Offers of employment poured in. In the new age of advertising Grange endorsed products, and four years after leaving the University he was appearing at two Chicago theaters "In person on the stage doing his football stuff." He was also in court answering a paternity charge in 1928.[59]

The University of Chicago produced similarly great football teams under the leadership of Amos Alonzo Stagg. Born in New Jersey in 1862, Stagg graduated from Yale Divinity School. He played baseball as an undergraduate and took up football only after he was in graduate school, and excelled in both sports. He found that he was not cut out for the ministry and accepted an offer from William Rainey Harper to coach at the University of Chicago in 1892. In those days of few rules, the first game of the season was with Hyde Park High School and Coach Stagg played end on the university team. Stagg coached at Chicago until 1931, when mandatory retirement caused him to leave Chicago for a coaching job at the College of the Pacific. In 1914 the University of Chicago named their new football stadium for him. The first to use numbers on his player's jerseys, Stagg invented the T-formation, the quick kick, the man-in-motion, the flanker, and cross-blocking.[60]

During his forty years at the University of Chicago, Stagg's teams won 229, lost 108, and tied 27. Stagg won conference championships in 1896, 1899, 1905, 1907, 1908, 1913, and 1924. Stagg also coached baseball and won five conference championships before he gave up that sport in 1909. He also coached four champion track teams. Stagg coached many stars but, by reputation, Walter Eckersall was the greatest. A star at Hyde Park High School, Eckersall weighed only 145 pounds, but he was All-American quarterback from Stagg's 1905 team. Among the other greats for the Chicago Maroons were Clarence Herschberger, Wally Staffen, Hugo Bezdek, Andy Wynant, Harlan Page, Fritz Crisler, Austin McCarty, and Joe Pondelik.[61]

In professional sports, baseball achieved the most public attention. The year 1901 might be regarded as the beginning of professional baseball in Illinois. The Three-I league was founded in that year, the first Class B league. After 1901 Chicago had two professional teams, the White Sox and the Cubs. The White Sox won the American League pennant in 1901, 1906, 1917, and 1919. The Cubs won the National League pennant in 1906, 1907, 1908, 1910, 1918, and 1929. The 1906 World Series was the only one involving both Chicago teams. The Cubs, with the famous "Tinker to Evers to Chance" combination, won 116 games during the season. The Sox won 93 games but batted only .228 and thus were regarded as sure losers in the series. Nonetheless, the Sox won four games out of six.[62]

In 1907 the Cubs beat the Detroit Tigers in the World Series, winning four straight games. Joe Tinker, John Evers, and Frank Chance led the Cubs in this victory, while Ty Cobb played for the Tigers. Chance was manager in 1908, and Mordecai "Three Fingers" Brown achieved fame as a relief pitcher. In 1908 the same teams played in the series. The Cubs, winning four games out of five, clinched the series for the second year in a row. Franklin P. Adams, writing in the *New York World* during the 1908 season, was moved to poetry:

> These are the saddest of possible words—
> Tinker to Evers to Chance;
> Trio of beartraps and fleeter than birds
> Tinker to Evers to Chance.
> Thoughtlessly pricking our gonfalon bubble—
> Making a Giant hit into a double—
> Words that are weighty with nothing but trouble—
> Tinker to Evers to Chance.[63]

In 1910 the Cubs won the National League pennant again. In the World Series they played the Philadelphia Athletics with Evers out of the games because of a broken leg. Mordecai Brown paced the Cub pitchers, but they lost the series in five games. In 1917 the White Sox came back to win the pennant and beat McGraw's Giants in six games. In 1918 the White Sox, expected to repeat their victory of 1917, were so badly split that they lost out during the regular season. The Cubs, however, won the National League pennant again. The series opponents of the Cubs in 1918 were the Boston Red Sox, and in the first game of the series, Cub fans first saw George Herman "Babe" Ruth in action. Ruth was a pitcher at this time, and the series ended with the Red Sox winning four of six games.[64]

The 1919 season represents one of the black moments of sports—the infamous "Black Sox" scandal. In 1919 the Chicago White Sox won the American League championship and opposed the Cincinnati Reds in the World Series. Impressive during the regular season, the White Sox were heavily favored to win. The Cincinnati Reds won the series, which might have ended as mere statistics in the record book except that rumors of bribery persisted. It turned out that many people were victims of a series of rigged games. George M. Cohan lost $30,000 betting on the White Sox, while Mont Tennes, a Chicago gambler, lost some $80,000. Near the end of the 1920 season, Charles Comiskey suspended eight of his top players on charges of conniving with gamblers to throw the 1919 World Series. The players were indicted in Cook County court but were acquitted in 1921. The accused players were never allowed to play baseball again, however, and the whole episode shocked the country.[65]

As a result of the scandal, organized baseball appointed Judge Kenesaw Mountain Landis as commissioner of baseball. Judge Landis, a puritanical type, lent an image of respectability to the game and tended to allay fears that people might have. One historian, David Voigt, believes that the appointment was window dressing and that the concept of "baseball's single sin" is a myth. He believes there may have been other rigged games and that Landis only found enough scapegoats to reassure the public.[66]

In 1929, with Joe McCarthy as manager, the Chicago Cubs again won the National League pennant. The Cubs then had such stars as Rogers Hornsby and Hack Wilson. The opponents of the Cubs were the Philadelphia Athletics, coached by Connie Mack. The Athletics won the series in five games.[67]

No account of baseball in Illinois would be complete without mention of the Three-I League. It was organized at Peoria on January 30, 1901, and the cities of Cedar Rapids, Davenport, Rock Island, Rockford, Peoria, Decatur, Bloomington, and Terre Haute had teams. Before play started the first year, Evansville replaced Peoria in the league. There was a 110-game schedule, and salaries were fixed at $750 per month. Many who were unable to see major league games could cheer on the Three-I League teams. Many players, including Carl Hubbell and Birdie Tebbetts, went on to major league fame. Illinois teams won the league championship twenty times in thirty years, dominating the Iowa and Indiana teams.[68]

On the sports pages the *Chicago Tribune* carried articles dealing with boxing, bowling, cycling, horse racing, billiards, track, curling, poker, whist, chess, and golf, as well as college athletics and professional baseball. There was also some effort to play polo around Chicago. The Onwentsia Country Club had a team, as did Lake Forest. This was the sport of rich men; in 1920, when Onwentsia beat Lake Forest 16 to 4, the star of the game was Lawrence Armour.

Track was also becoming important. The big stimulus for track came from Northwestern when an alumnus, James Patten, a grain broker, gave the money to build Patten Gymnasium. It was the first indoor track-and-field facility in the Midwest and brought new interest to track events.[69]

During the 1920s millions of people bought tickets to college football and big-league baseball games and even more listened to these contests on radio. More people were also participating in sports. Golf had been a sport of the rich, but by the 1920s golf courses were becoming so common that anyone who could afford balls and a few clubs could play. By 1924 eighty-nine cities had municipal golf courses and white- and blue-collar workers were playing. Most cities built tennis courts in municipal parks, and swimming pools, campgrounds, and summer camps became common. By 1924 there were 2,000,000 golfers and 500,000 tennis players.[70]

As popular music and recreation developed, popular literature appeared in the comic strips and the Sunday supplements of newspapers. The mammoth Sunday newspaper arrived at the beginning of the twentieth century. The *Chicago Tribune* pioneered the Sunday edition. By 1900 it was publishing sixty-page Sunday papers, and by 1914 it was issuing seventy-two pages, including comic strips, a magazine section, and sections devoted to theater, household hints, sports, and a society page. By 1914 the Sunday *Tribune* had a circulation of 550,000, as usual larger than the daily circulation, for the Sunday paper had become an American institution, each family member turning to a favorite part of the paper for Sunday morning reading.[71]

The first daily comic strip, "Mutt and Jeff," appeared in the *San Francisco Chronicle* in 1907. This strip, drawn by Bud Fisher, was featured at first on the sports page because Mutt was a racetrack tout. Later Fisher syndicated the strip. George Herman drew a strip called "Krazy Kat," which also came out of California. R. F. Outcault created Buster Brown and the adventures of his brindle bull pup. George McManus produced a number of strips; among the earliest were "The Newlyweds" and "The Newlyweds and Their Baby." In 1912 he brought out "Bringing Up Father," the story of Maggie and Jiggs. Several familiar cartoons of the twenties originated in Chicago. The *Chicago Tribune*, always a pioneer, was the source of Sydney Smith's "Andy Gump" in 1917. Frank King's "Gasoline Alley" started in that newspaper two years later. Frank Willard's "Moon Mullen" began in 1923, and Harold Gray's "Little Orphan Annie" appeared in the *Tribune* in 1924. Illinoisians eagerly awaited the next episode in the adventures of Maggie and Jiggs, Happy Hooligan, and Harold Teen, and daily papers carried comic strips as regular offering.[72]

At first these strips devoted themselves to a particular humorous incident in the life of the hero. Later, cartoonists created a continuing series, and some of the columns, such as "Little Orphan Annie," continued for many years. The comics represented the prejudices of the times. The creator of "Harold Teen" poked fun at youth, and various ethnic groups were the butt of other cartoonists. "The Katzenjammer Kids," drawn by Rudolph Dirks, portrayed the Germans in a derogatory fashion. Maggie and Jiggs stereotyped the new-rich "lace-curtain" Irish. The *Inter-Ocean* in 1906 carried a strip entitled "Sven Swenson, Son of Sweden and Misfortune." In 1908, just before the Springfield riot, the *Illinois State Register* carried a comic strip involving a black watermelon thief named Rastus who was referred to often as "that derned coon." In 1912, the *Tribune* carried a strip entitled "Sambo Remo Rastus Brown," and the Rock Island *Argus* had one entitled "Rastus."[73]

The comics also reflected social conditions of the time. "Gasoline Alley" was a tribute to the automobile age, and "Winnie Winkle the Bread Winner" was a reflection of the new status of women in the business world. One of the popular early comic strips was George McManus's "Newlyweds." In a strip in the *Tribune* in 1908, the "Newlyweds" planned a picnic for their son Napoleon. They forgot to bring along the son's milk, the father ran home for it, they missed the train, the baby broke the milk bottle, and it rained. This was slapstick humor to which most families could relate. "Toots and Casper," appearing in smaller newspapers such as the *Decatur Herald* by 1924, presented a similar picture of a young married couple with children.[74]

Perhaps the most striking feature of the 1920s was national prohibition. The Eighteenth Amendment to the Constitution, prohibiting the sale or consumption of alcoholic beverages, went into effect January 16, 1920. In Congress, Senator Sherman, Republican of Illinois, voted for the amendment, while Senator Lewis, Democrat, voted against it. Illinois became the twenty-sixth state to ratify it in January, 1919. By the end of that month enough states had ratified the amendment to make it a part of the Constitution.[75]

Reaction to this amendment varied. Supporters of prohibition labeled the amendment the "noble experiment." In Norfolk, Virginia, Billy Sunday preached a mock funeral service for John Barleycorn in which he said, "Good-bye John, you were God's worst enemy. You were hell's best friend. I hate you with a perfect hatred." On the other hand, there was the angry statement of H. L. Mencken, "All the great villanies of history have been perpetrated by sober men, and chiefly by teetotalers," and another by Bernard De Voto: "In the heroic age our forefathers invented self-government, the Constitution, and Bourbon, and on their way to them they invented rye. Our political institutions were shaped by our whiskies, would be inconceivable without them, and share their nature."[76]

The prohibition movement reached formidable proportions before World War I, and the war contributed to the cause. It was made to seem unpatriotic to use grain for beer and liquor when it was needed for food. Prohibitionists said beer was unpatriotic because it was a German drink. The war also accustomed people to wider governmental control of all aspects of life. But whatever motives may have entered into prohibition, the people of the United States did not take well to the whole thing. Lager beer went up from 10 cents a quart to 80 cents a quart, rye whiskey from $1.70 to $7 a quart, and gin from 95 cents to $5.95 per quart. It soon became evident that most people were drinking as much as before. It was estimated that at the end of the prohibition period Americans were drinking 790,000,000 gallons of beer, 110,000,000 gallons of wine, and spirits totaling 200,000,000 gallons. People spent $2,888,000,000 a year on liquor which put this illegal business in the same category as automobiles, steel, and other major industries. It seems that almost everybody drank in homes, private clubs, hotels, speakeasies, and barely disguised saloons.[77]

The prohibition amendment brought contempt for law, particularly among young people, who thought prohibition was only one more attempt of the older generation to prevent them from living life as they chose. The upper classes, pillars of the community, engaged in illicit drinking as much as others. The passing of the neighborhood saloon was a blow to the working man because this had been his club, and a form of entertainment compensated only partially by radio and the movies.[78]

Bootleggers imported liquor from abroad; it was not difficult to bring in Canadian or Scotch whiskey or French wine, avoiding the Coast Guard ships. The manufacture of industrial alcohol increased, and much of this was diverted into domestic uses. There were thousands of illegal stills. Some of these provided a family supply, while others were capable of turning out thousands of gallons of liquor. Many families brewed beer for home consumption or sale. Neighborhoods of largely immigrant families made wine. Medicinal alcohol was diverted into more sociable uses; during the first year of prohibition some 300,000 illegal prescriptions were filled by druggists in Chicago. Even sacramental wine set aside for churches was put into traffic.[79]

The government worked valiantly to enforce the law but without much success. Attempts to dry up a city of any size were increasingly difficult. As early as June of 1920 District Attorney Clyne reported that the dockets of the federal courts in Chicago were congested with 500 or 600 prohibition-related cases pending. By 1921 the *Tribune* found that at least 4,000 illegal saloons were operating in the city, selling beer, wine, and whiskey. Anyone could buy liquor in Chicago without resorting to deviousness. The *Tribune* revelations brought a renewed effort to enforce the laws, but it was only modestly and temporarily successful.[80]

In 1923 Chicago elected a reform mayor, William E. Dever, who made every effort to clean up the liquor traffic, but his efforts were wrecked by the pressures of gangsters. The Prohibition Bureau had only 134 agents working out of its Chicago headquarters. These men would have had trouble taking care of the city of Chicago alone, but they also had to cover Iowa, Illinois, and part of Wisconsin. In addition there was little desire of officials or citizens to enforce the law, and judges tended to let offenders off with minor sentences.[81]

The prohibition amendment opened up new lines of endeavor for the underworld. During the early part of the twentieth century, vice was rampant in Chicago, but much of it was run by small operators. Mont Tennes, for instance, controlled the gambling. Tennes operated bookmaking and wire services to various racetracks from a cigar store at 121 North Clark Street, and he had agents and runners all over the city. James "Big Jim" Colosimo controlled prostitution. Colosimo owned several resorts, the most important presided over by his wife at 2106 Armour Avenue. Colisimo was the big man in vice until 1920. Important in politics, he cooperated with Hinky Dink Kenna and Bathhouse John Coughlin and was able to deliver the Italian vote of the first ward to these two politicians.[82]

Johnny Torrio succeeded Colosimo, who had brought him from New York in 1918 to serve as a bodyguard and gunman. Torrio, who had been a member of a Brooklyn gang called the "Five Points Gang," had recruited Al Capone from the same gang to work for Colosimo; Capone later became Torrio's senior lieutenant. In 1920, just as prohibition came into effect, rivals killed Colosimo. His death was marked by one of the first spectacular gangster funerals. Among those following Colosimo to Oakwood Cemetery were a thousand members of the first ward Democratic club, headed by Coughlin and Kenna. The crowd sang hymns, and Colosimo's attorney, Rocco De Stephano, delivered the eulogy.[83]

Johnny Torrio then turned the already massive resources of the syndicate to bootlegging. Born in Italy in 1877, Torrio had gained the attention of Chicago police long before Colosimo's death. Torrio was the boss of the suburban town of Burnham, where he owned the Burnham Inn. In 1923 he "took possession" of Cicero and Stickney. Although Torrio found opposition in the suburbs, he was able to overcome it, using intrigue, bribery, and corruption of elections to gain control. Police and municipal officials cooperated with Torrio both in Chicago and in the suburbs. When federal officials raided, they found his places had been tipped off. When corruption failed, Torrio, ably aided by Capone, used the submachine gun and sawed-off shotgun to enforce his authority. Dividing the city among leaders of the syndicate, he maintained order until individual gangsters chafed under the restraint and sought to move into new areas. These rebellions brought a series of gang wars in which many gangsters were killed. Dion O'Bannon, who ruled part of the North Side, was killed in the flower shop which he used as a cover. His funeral was another spectacular gangland affair. O'Bannon lay in state in a $10,000 coffin, and twenty-four automobiles full of flowers and 122 funeral cars, as well as many private cars, followed the hearse to the cemetery.[84]

In Chicago, Torrio grossed $4,000,000 a year from beer, $3,000,000 from gambling, and $2,000,000 from prostitution. He took another $4,000,000 from similar operations in the suburbs. The illegal liquor was sold through 12,000 speakeasies and brothels. Torrio had a good relationship with Governor Small, as well as with Chicago officials. He was able to persuade Small to issue a pardon for Harry Cusick and his wife, Alma, who were convicted of being white slavers for the Torrio organization.[85]

Eventually Torrio was severely wounded in one of the gang wars. Frightened by his narrow escape, he turned over the rackets in Chicago to Capone, who had previously been in charge of prostitution in Cicero. Just as Torrio had increased the wealth and power of the syndicate over what it was in the days of Colosimo, Capone pushed the organization to new heights. By the end of the '20s Capone had an armed gang of 700 men working for him, and he rode in an armored car, escorted by bodyguards with pistols and submachine guns. In 1927 it was estimated that Capone's syndicate grossed $60,000,000 from liquor and beer, $25,000,000 from gambling and dog tracks, and $10,000,000 from vice. Although Capone was guilty of the most atrocious crimes in the law books, the government was never able to convict him of any of these. The best they could do was to send him to federal prison on charges of income tax violation. He was released from prison in 1939 and died in 1940 at the age of forty-two with his mind wrecked by syphilis. Unlike his flamboyant predecessors, Capone was buried quietly.[86]

Chicago was the most notorious city in Illinois for gangland activities, but by no means the only one. Downstate operations, though smaller, were just as efficient. Uncertain law enforcement in rural Illinois contributed to the success of these operations. County sheriffs, deputies, constables, and small-town police were not noted for their efficiency in crime detection or law enforcement. The Illinois highway police were political appointees. And all were as subject to corruption as their counterparts in Chicago. The rapid extension of paved highways in the state also made it possible for gangs to operate over a wide area. As automobiles became more efficient and faster, outlying areas became just as prone to criminality, particularly bootlegging, as the cities.[87]

Among the most notorious downstate gangs were the Sheltons. Of the five brothers, sons of a sober dirt farmer in Wayne County, three—Carl, Earl, and Bernie—were involved in the rackets. Carl, the eldest, born in 1888, was the brains; he engaged in whatever negotiation was necessary to corrupt authority. Bernie, the youngest, born in 1899, provided the muscle for the organization. The Sheltons served prison terms at various times for a number of minor offenses.

With the coming of prohibition every community had its bootlegger, and the Sheltons brought them into a syndicate offering protection and providing outlets for the liquor. Numerous small operations were also involved in slot machines and prostitution as a part of the Shelton federation. The Sheltons became notorious for waging a bloody battle against the Ku Klux Klan, which made the pretense of promoting law and order. After the decline of the Klan, the Sheltons controlled crime in an area south from Fairfield to Carbondale and west to East St. Louis.[89]

A second faction grew under the leadership of Charlie Birger. Born in New York, Birger had served in the cavalry of the U.S. Army and still operated with military dash. He carried himself erect, wore puttees, two pistols in holsters, and often carried a submachine gun. Birger had worked for the Sheltons, but after a quarrel he formed his own gang. He and the Sheltons carried on a running battle, using armored cars and an airplane for aerial bombing on one occasion, which caused a number of deaths of gangland and public figures. Birger eventually ran into trouble when he was accused of killing a highway patrolman. He was hanged on April 19, 1928, on the lawn of the Benton jail, the last public hanging in Illinois. The Birger and the Shelton gangs were so bold that they were willing to pose for pictures with fast cars, submachine guns, and sawed-off shotguns.[90]

Sometimes gangsters were able to acquire Robin Hood images for themselves. Capone, for instance, was a popular figure, and many chose to look on Birger and Carl Shelton as community benefactors. And young men growing up in slum areas, seeing that those outside the law seemed to have the most powerful cars and the flashiest clothes—goals of many youngsters of the time —provided a ready-made source of manpower for the gangs.

Gangsters flourished in defiance of the law because the public did not care. Capone pointed out that when he sold liquor to some fashionable individual on the Gold Coast it was called bootlegging, but when the purchaser served this liquor, his act was described as hospitality. No law in the United States was ever ignored as much as the prohibition law, and since many people drank bootleg liquor, they were unlikely to demand that public officials move aggressively against the gangsters.[91]

In 1929 John Gunther wrote about the problem of hoodlums in an article in *Harper's Magazine*. Gunther noted that although he had lived in Chicago for years, he had never seen a murder. Gangland murders occurred almost daily in Chicago, but few ordinary people were in danger since gangsters only killed each other. He said gangsters did cost the average citizen substantial amounts of money, however, beyond what he may have paid for alcohol or prostitution, through payment of "protection" money. It was estimated that some sixty rackets, taking $136,000,000 a year out of the pockets of Chicago citizenry, were in operation in 1929. Gunther listed small retail businesses, including bakeries, fish markets, filling stations, and florists, that paid tribute to gangland people.[92]

The revolution in manners and morals disturbed the serenity of those who held to Victorian standards, and by 1920 many were concerned about the dress and attitude of young women. Increased feminist pressure had brought women the right to vote, and World War I had opened up new employment opportunities which seemed to free women from their traditional role in the kitchen, but the new and more daring costume, as well as other superficial rebellions, was a reaction against Victorianism. To demonstrate their new status, women cast off their petticoats. Style dictated that hemlines should rise, first to the ankle and later above the kneecap. One writer who believed that modesty and chivalry were dead, Mr. Grundy, described the young women of the day as "ill bred young hoydens whose well aimed blows give society its black eye." He believed young females had lost the gentle charm of a bygone era, and attributing the decline to a lack of parental authority, and recommended a reassertion of parental authority— by force if necessary.[93]

This article was answered by several people who were a part of the generation being condemned. One young man blamed the older generation for the problems of youth, saying that the elders had given them the world "knocked to pieces, leaky, red-hot, threatening to blow up." He proclaimed that the younger generation could not accept it, and insisted that the chief difference between the younger generation and the older was that the former were more honest and frank. Angrily referring to "tin-pot ideals," the young man said to Mr. Grundy, "Our music is distinctly barbaric, our girls are distinctly not a mixture of arbutus and barbed wire. We drink when we can and what we can, we gamble, we are extravagant—but we work, and that's about all that we can be expected to do; for, after all, we have just discovered that we are all very near to the Stone Age."[94]

The older generation pointed with alarm at the free and easy character of the modern scene. They worried about the dances young people were doing as the toddle and the shimmy passed on to the Black Bottom and the Charleston. The editor of the *Hobart College Herald,* in Geneva, New York, saw danger in the new dancing: "The dance and its process of degradation has passed from slight impropriety to indencency and now threatens to become brazenly shameless. From graceful coordination of movement it has become a syncopated embrace." The student paper at the New Mexico College of Agricultural and Mechanical Arts wrote that the modern way of dancing was an "offense against common decency."[95]

Dubbed the "flapper," the girl of the 1920s wore shorter and shorter dresses, cut low at the top and short at the bottom, and rolled her silk hosiery below the knee. Frightened for the future, older people sought to explain why morality had degenerated. Some thought that the increased mobility and relative privacy of automobiles contributed to the decline. Others worried about commercial dance halls, modern fashions, pocket flasks, unclean movies, and the abdication of parental authority. Not all observers saw the generation as immoral, however. President David Felmley of Illinois State Normal University found that "the problem of indecent dancing is as old as dancing itself." He went on to say that he believed young people of the '20s were "morally sound as a class."

Inevitably the flapper, in her long-waisted, short-skirted dress and cloche hat, became the subject of movies and comic strips, and thus did the manners and morals of the urban rich quickly reach the villages. The flapper did everything she could to attract attention, smoking cigarettes in public, often conspicuously in the streets, and being seen in the thousands of speakeasies that had sprung up. The heavy drinking, sexual freedom, and smoking of cigarettes touched the rural areas less, but even there young women were wearing shorter skirts and hair and doing things their grandmothers would never have dreamed of.[96]

The prohibition era—the "age of flaming youth"—brought with it a contempt for convention as well as for law. But society did not, contrary to the fears of the older generation, deteriorate, nor was civilization destroyed, during the decade of the "roaring '20s."

1. Robert L. Duffus, "The Age of Play," *Independent,* 113, Dec. 20, 1924, p. 557.
2. Abel Green and Joe Laurie, Jr., *Show Biz from Vaude to Video* (New York, 1951), p. 230.

3. Douglas Gilbert, *American Vaudeville: Its Life and Times* (New York, 1940), p. 3.

4. Joseph Laurie, *Vaudeville: From the Honky Tonk to the Palace* (New York, 1953), p. 361; Gilbert, *American Vaudeville*, pp. 84, 201, 213, 238, 385; Green and Laurie, *Show Biz*, p. 46.

5. Green and Laurie, *Show Biz*, pp. 7, 47, 58, 60; Gilbert, *American Vaudeville*, pp. 251, 260.

6. Green and Laurie, *Show Biz*, pp. 24, 25, 26, 28, 29; Gilbert, *American Vaudeville*, pp. 187, 327–28, 331–33.

7. Laurie, *Vaudeville*, pp. 244, 246; Gilbert, *American Vaudeville*, pp. 208, 220.

8. Gilbert, *American Vaudeville*, p. 210; Laurie, *Vaudeville*, p. 361; Green and Laurie, *Show Biz*, p. 4.

9. Green and Laurie, *Show Biz*, pp. 69, 71; Gilbert, *American Vaudeville*, p. 186; Laurie, *Vaudeville*, p. 241; *Illinois State Register*, Nov. 2, 1924, part 2, p. 8.

10. Gilbert, *American Vaudeville*, pp. 5, 392.

11. Ibid., p. 392.

12. Ibid.

13. Benjamin B. Hampton, *A History of the Movies* (New York, 1931), pp. 6, 34, 49.

14. Ibid., p. 34.

15. Green and Laurie, *Show Biz*, pp. 48–50.

16. Albert R. Fulton, *Motion Pictures: The Development of An Art from Silent Films to the Age of Television* (Norman, Okla., 1960), pp. 73, 81; Hampton, *History of the Movies*, pp. 34, 49, 77.

17. Green and Laurie, *Show Biz*, pp. 141, 146.

18. Ibid., pp. 147, 153.

19. Ibid., p. 257.

20. Arthur Knight, *The Liveliest Art: A Panoramic History of the Movies* (New York, 1957), p. 126; Green and Laurie, *Show Biz*, p. 261.

21. Green and Laurie, *Show Biz*, pp. 112, 124.

22. Ibid., p. 350; Knight, *The Liveliest Art*, p. 110.

23. Knight, *The Liveliest Art*, p. 114.

24. Ibid.; Hampton, *History of the Movies*, p. 297.

25. Lloyd Lewis, "The Deluxe Picture Palace," *New Republic*, 58, Mar. 27, 1929, p. 297.

26. *Chicago Tribune*, Nov. 2, 1916, pp. 11, 17; Nov. 4, 1916, pp. 16–17.

27. Ibid., Sept. 1, 1920, p. 22; Apr. 1, 1924, p. 25; Oct. 16, 1924, p. 22; Apr. 3, 1928, p. 42; Apr. 4, 1928, p. 5; Apr. 12, 1928, p. 30; Oct. 19, 1928, p. 36.

28. *Chicago Daily Inter-Ocean*, Apr. 15, 1913, p. 1.

29. Duffus, "Age of Play," p. 540.

30. Green and Laurie, *Show Biz*, p. 231; Ben Gross, *I Looked and I Listened: Informal Recollections of Radio and T.V.* (New York, 1970), pp. 52–53.

31. James F. Evans, *Prairie Farmer and WLS: The Burridge D. Butler Years* (Urbana, Ill., 1969), pp. 155–56, 158.

32. Gross, *I Looked and I Listened*, p. 25; Evans, *Prairie Farmer*, p. 162.

33. Evans, *Prairie Farmer*, p. 162.

34. Ibid., pp. 163–64.

35. Frank C. Waldrop, *McCormick of Chicago, an Unconventional Portrait of a Controversial Figure* (Englewood Cliffs, N.J., 1966), p. 200; Gross, *I Looked and I Listened*, p. 84.

36. Gross, *I Looked and I Listened*, pp. 99, 107, 110.

37. Green and Laurie, *Show Biz*, p. 241; Gross, *I Looked and I Listened*, pp. 153, 156.

38. Gross, *I Looked and I Listened*, pp. 85, 166.

39. *Chicago Tribune*, June 26, 1928, p. 1; Gross, *I Looked and I Listened*, pp. 63, 89.

40. *Chicago Tribune*, Oct. 20, 1924, p. 10.

41. Martin Williams, *The Jazz Tradition* (New York, 1970), pp. 15, 20; Barry Ulanov, *A History of Jazz in America* (New York, 1957), p. 5; Marshall Winslow Stearns, *The Story of Jazz* (New York, 1956), p. 3.

42. Ulanov, *A History of Jazz*, pp. 35, 46, 63.

43. Ibid., pp. 50, 58, 61, 64, 68.

44. Louis Armstrong, *Satchmo* (New York, 1954), pp. 179, 182–84, 188; Ulanov, *A History of Jazz*, pp. 71–72; Nat Shapiro and Nat Hentoff, *Hear Me Talkin' to Ya: The Story of Jazz by the Men Who Made It* (New York, 1955), pp. 64, 103.

45. Shapiro and Hentoff, *Hear Me Talkin'*, pp. 101, 102.

46. Ibid., p. 141; Stearns, *The Story of Jazz*, p. 175.

47. Armstrong, *Satchmo*, p. 190.

48. Shapiro and Hentoff, *Hear Me Talkin'*, pp. 148, 158; Richard Hadlock, *Jazz Masters of the Twenties* (New York, 1965), pp. 76–77.

49. Ulanov, *A History of Jazz*, pp. 133, 138; Shapiro and Hentoff, *Hear Me Talkin'*, p. 162; Williams, *The Jazz Tradition*, pp. 56, 59, 63; Hadlock, *Jazz Masters*, p. 78.

50. Hadlock, *Jazz Masters*, pp. 131, 134, 137; Shapiro and Hentoff, *Hear Me Talkin'*, p. 121.

51. Hadlock, *Jazz Masters*, pp. 107, 110, 115, 116, 118, 128; Stearns, *The Story of Jazz*, p. 176; Shapiro and Hentoff, *Hear Me Talkin'*, p. 118; Nat Shapiro and Nat Hentoff, *The Jazz Makers* (New York, 1957), p. 108.

52. Hadlock, *Jazz Masters*, pp. 108, 116, 137; Stearns, *The Story of Jazz*, p. 165.

53. Shapiro and Hentoff, *Hear Me Talkin'*, pp. 104, 116, 122, 129, 130.

54. Gross, *I Looked and I Listened*, p. 178; Green and Laurie, *Show Biz*, pp. 98, 125, 129, 135, 227–29, 230, 291, 314.

55. George Mowry, *The Twenties: Fords, Flappers and Fanatics* (Englewood Cliffs, N.J. 1963), p. 82.

56. *Illinois State Journal*, Jan. 8, 1900, p. 6; Kenneth L. Wilson and Jerry Brondfield, *The Big Ten* (Englewood Cliffs, N.J. 1967), p. 58.

57. Wilson and Brondfield, *The Big Ten*, pp. 90–91.

58. Ibid., pp. 43, 92–93; Robert E. Burnes, *50 Golden Years of Sports* (St. Louis, 1948), p. 43.

59. Wilson and Brondfield, *The Big Ten*, pp. 89, 117, 119–21; Burnes, *50 Golden Years of Sports*, pp. 87, 93; Mowry, *The Twenties*, p. 83; *Chicago Tribune*, Oct. 19, 1924, part 2, p. 1; Oct. 26, 1928, p. 19.

60. Burnes, *50 Golden Years of Sports*, p. 11; Wilson and Brondfield, *The Big Ten*, p. 69.

61. Wilson and Brondfield, *The Big Ten*, pp. 67, 70.

62. Burnes, *50 Golden Years of Sports*, p. 18; Lee Allen, *The World Series: The Story of Baseball's Annual Championship* (New York, 1969), pp. 58–59; Frank Mencke, *The Encyclopedia of Sports* (New York, 1963), pp. 97, 98.

63. Allen, *The World Series*, pp. 61, 62, 63–64; Burnes, *50 Golden Years of Sports*, pp. 21, 25; *Record-Herald*, Oct. 11, 1908, p. 1; Oct. 15, 1908, p. 1; *Chicago Tribune*, Oct. 9, 1908, pp. 1–2; Federal Writers Project, *Baseball in Old Chicago* (Chicago, 1939), p. 42.

64. Allen, *The World Series,* pp. 84, 87, 88; Burnes, *50 Golden Years of Sports,* pp. 31, 60.

65. Allen, *The World Series,* pp. 92, 96; Burnes, *50 Golden Years of Sports,* p. 4; *Chicago Tribune,* Sept. 23, 1920, p. 1; Sept. 24, 1920, p. 1.

66. David Quentin Voigt, "The Chicago Black Sox and the Myth of Baseball's Single Sin," *Journal of the Illinois State Historical Society* 62 (Autumn, 1969), pp. 293–306.

67. Allen, *The World Series,* pp. 122–25.

68. Hy Turkin and S. C. Thompson, *The Official Encyclopedia of Baseball* (New York, 1963); Norman M. Paulsen, comp. and ed., *Three-I League Record Book* (Waterloo, Iowa, 1950), p. 2.

69. *Chicago Tribune,* Jan. 7, 1900, pp. 17–20; Sept. 5, 1924, part 2, p. 4; Wilson and Brondfield, *The Big Ten,* p. 79.

70. Duffus, "Age of Play," pp. 539–40.

71. Frank Luther Mott, *American Journalism—a History: 1690–1960* (New York, 1969), p. 584.

72. Thomas Craven, ed. *Cartoon Cavalcade* (New York, 1943), pp. 16–17; Mott, *American Journalism,* p. 595.

73. Craven, *Cartoon Cavalcade,* pp. 16, 101; Mott, *American Journalism,* p. 585; *Inter-Ocean,* Jan. 7, 1906, comics section, p. 3; *Illinois State Register,* July 5, 1908, comics section, p. 2; *Rock Island Argus,* Nov. 3, 1912, part 4, p. 1.

74. *Chicago Tribune,* June 14, 1908, comics section, p. 1; Sept. 1, 1920, p. 18; Sept. 25, 1920, p. 15; *Decatur Herald,* Jan. 1, 1924, p. 15.

75. Charles Merz, *The Dry Decade* (Seattle, 1930), pp. 1, 309, 310, 316.

76. Merz, *Dry Decade,* p. 210; Henry Lee, *How Dry We Were* (Englewood Cliffs, N.J., 1963), pp. 150, 210.

77. Irving Fisher, *The Noble Experiment* (New York, 1930), p. 115; Lee, *How Dry We Were,* p. 205; Merz, *Dry Decade,* p. 25.

78. *Report on the Enforcement of the Prohibition Laws of the United States,* House Document no. 722, 71st Congress, 3rd session (Washington, D.C., 1931), p. 21.

79. Merz, *Dry Decade,* pp. 59, 112–15.

80. Ibid., pp. 59, 138.

81. Ibid., p. 155; Herbert Asbury, *The Great Illusion: An Informal History of Prohibition* (Garden City, N.Y., 1950), p. 296.

82. John Landesco, *Organized Crime in Chicago* (Chicago, 1968), pp. 27–37, 45–83. This was originally published in 1929 as Part III of the Illinois Crime Survey.

83. Landesco, *Organized Crime in Chicago,* pp. 25, 85–86, 191–92.

84. Ibid., pp. 189, 194–95.

85. Lloyd Wendt and Herman Kogan, *Big Bill of Chicago* (Indianapolis, 1953), p. 237.

86. Landesco, *Organized Crime in Chicago,* p. 94; Lee, *How Dry We Were,* p. 128.

87. Illinois Association for Criminal Justice, *The Illinois Crime Survey* (Chicago, 1929), p. 337.

88. Paul Angle, *Bloody Williamson: A Chapter in American Lawlessness* (New York, 1952), p. 215; John Bartlow Martin, "The Sheltons: America's Bloodiest Gang," *Saturday Evening Post,* 222 Mar. 18, 1950, p. 25.

89. Ibid., pp. 52, 54.

90. Angle, *Bloody Williamson,* pp. 212, 254–55; Martin, "The Sheltons," pp. 25–26.

91. Landesco, *Organized Crime in Chicago,* pp. 207–21; Asbury, *The Great Illusion,* p. 29.

92. John Gunther, "The High Cost of Hoodlums," *Harpers Monthly Magazine,* 159 Oct. 1929, pp. 529–30, 540.

93. Mr. Grundy, "Polite Society," *Atlantic Monthly,* 125 May, 1920, pp. 608, 609.

94. John F. Carter, Jr., "These Wild Young People: By One of Them," *Atlantic Monthly,* 126 Sept., 1920, pp. 302, 304.

95. "Is the Younger Generation in Peril?" *Literary Digest,* 69, May 14, 1921, pp. 11–12.

96. Ibid., pp. 61, 68; "The Battle of the Skirts," *Outlook,* 132 Oct. 18, 1922, pp. 275–76.

12

Politics in the 1920s

During the administrations of Governors Deneen, Dunne, and Lowden, Illinois could lay claim to a degree of political progressivism. In Illinois as in the nation, however, progressivism constituted a minority force from 1920 to 1930, which was one of the most sordid periods of American political life. The scandals of the Harding administration were unmatched for forty years. During this period of highly materialistic attitudes, men measured progress by buildings and dollars, rarely by improvement of the lot of less fortunate people. Laboring men lost much of the gain made during World War I, and the farmer's economic position steadily declined as the nature of his business changed. Politicians, seeking ways to get their vote, demonstrated little interest in really doing anything for minority groups.

State administrations were characterized by what H. L. Mencken called "'the hogpen mores' that prevail in American politics."[1] Most disheartening of all, voters in Illinois did not seem to care. Tired of progressivism and Wilson's idealism, most preferred to sit back in apathy and let things drift. When superior candidates were offered, the voters usually rejected them.

Many new forces entered the political scene during the 1920s, some beyond the control of politicians. The Eighteenth Amendment prohibiting the manufacture, sale, or transportation of liquor, brought the rise of gangsterism and promoted a lack of respect for the law. In Illinois gangsters exerted political influence, and politicians found it necessary (or thought they did) to cater to the wishes of the gangster element.[2]

Before prohibition the question of Sunday closing of saloons and other problems associated with liquor traffic had long agitated state politics. Anton J. "Tony" Cermak, one of the political bosses in Illinois, got his start in politics through the United Societies, an organization of immigrant groups. interested in the "personal liberty laws" designed to keep taverns open on Sunday, the traditional day of leisure for working men. Their crusade changed emphasis as prohibition went into effect. There was cleavage between Chicago and downstate on the question of liquor and its sale; generally, downstate was dry while Chicago was wet.[3]

When prohibition came, gangsters took over the multimillion-dollar illicit liquor traffic in Illinois. Because of the magnitude of this business, gangsters attempted to gather influence in local and state government. It was believed that Mayor Thompson of Chicago had connections with organized crime. When Thompson was deposed in 1923 by William Dever, gangsters moved to destroy any progress that Chicago might have made under Dever. Al Capone intimidated Michael Hinky Dink Kenna and his friend Bathhouse John Coughlin in Chicago's first ward as he moved into the graft that Kenna and Coughlin had formerly kept for themselves. Len Small, governor during much of the '20s, was also accused of having connections with organized crime. Among the honorary pallbearers at Big Jim Colosimo's funeral were eight aldermen, two congressmen, two judges, and important political figures such as Democrat Michael Igoe and Republican "Diamond Joe" Esposito. Among the active pallbearers were Alderman John Coughlin and state Senator John Griffin.[4]

On August 26, 1920, the Nineteenth Amendment to the Constitution went into effect. This amendment guaranteed women the right to vote, creating a new element in American politics. Generally speaking, the women's vote changed politics very little. Indeed, it has been pointed out that women began voting in an election which marked the beginning of one of the most corrupt periods of American history, although one of the pleas for woman suffrage had been that they would clean up American politics if allowed to vote. There were women reformers who kept constant watch on politicians, however, and many became active in politics, to the discomfort of old-school political bosses.

Increasingly, politicians found it necessary to pay attention to the black vote and to give Blacks some recognition in political organization. In areas where there was a large black population, both the Republican and Democratic parties had black precinct committeemen to get out the black vote on election day. The Republicans gave lip service to support of the Blacks, although they

did not do very much to aid them. But particularly after Blacks
began to elect black officials to the legislature and city and county
offices in Chicago and Cook County, party leaders could not afford
to ignore them.[5]

Other ethnic groups were important in urban politics. A Polish
or Czech name might appear among party officials in areas of
heavy concentration of those groups. One Chicago political
historian has noted that Italian political figures were sometimes
members of the notorious Unione Sicilione, a group that had
connections with gangsters as well as politicians. In the Italian
sections of the city, committeemen were likely to bear names such
as Serritella, Pacelli, Vignola, or Porcaro. Generally, Jewish names
predominated in areas populated by Jews. Irish leaders had long
held posts in the committees of both parties, particularly in the
Democratic party. About one-fourth of the political leaders in
Chicago were Irish. The Republicans drew strong support from
Swedish, German, and Italian people, while the Democrats held
power in Irish, Polish, and Czech wards. Many local political
leaders were born abroad and still more were second generation.[6]

In 1920 Chicago could lay claim to being the third most foreign
city in the United States (after New York and Boston). Seventy-two
percent of the people of Chicago were first- or second-generation
foreign stock. Less than one-fourth of Chicago's population were
native Americans, and some of these were third-generation
immigrants who voted with their ethnic group. Chicago contained
more Scandinavians, Poles, Czechs, Serbo-Croatians, and Lithuanians than any other city in the nation. It also had the second
largest German, Greek, Slovak, Jewish, and Negro populations and
the third largest Italian population in the country. All these ethnic
groups tended to vote in what they regarded as their best interest,
and sometimes in what seemed to be the best interest of their
fatherland. Germans in Illinois favored Hughes over Wilson in
1916 because they regarded Wilson as pro-British. Italians were
inclined the same way, as were Swedes, who went along with
Hughes because of their distrust of England and Russia. Czechs
tended to be anti-German, while Poles supported Wilson because
they regarded him as a friend of an independent Poland. But in
most cases, after the declaration of war, ethnic groups supported
the war effort. After the war, Germans and Italians voted
Republican because they regarded the Treaty of Versailles as an
injustice to their respective fatherlands. Blacks took little interest in
either the war or the League of Nations and continued their
Republican support. Jews supported the League of Nations.[7]

The question of prohibition aroused great interest among ethnic groups. Their leader, Tony Cermak, led a hands-off policy toward the liquor trade. Immigrants, most of whom drank, opposed restrictive laws and stood for what they called personal liberty. The questions of immigration restriction and the reorganized Ku Klux Klan also posed dilemmas for ethnic groups. On one hand, the Republicans had been responsible for immigration restriction; on the other, the Ku Klux Klan was associated with the Democratic party.[8]

Between 1920 and 1932 Chicago ethnic groups slowly switched from Republican to Democratic. There were variations among the groups, but almost all tended to undergo some voting change. By 1928 the Irish, Czechs, Poles, Lithuanians, and Yugoslavs were mostly Democratic. Germans and Jews were on somewhat the same path. Swedes stayed with their traditional Republican leadership, however. Blacks underwent the least change and generally remained Republican until the '30s. Politicians promoted block voting and emphasized the separateness of the ethnic groups. According to Fred Lundin, Swedish-descended Republican political boss, "The party that eliminated the hyphen would eliminate itself from politics."[9]

The political picture in Illinois underwent leadership change in the 1920s. Some of the old figures were still around, but new leaders had made their appearance. The 1920s was the most dismal period in the history of the Democratic party, as Republicans covered Democratic candidates with an avalanche of ballots at every level of government in Illinois. The only major exception was the election of William Dever as mayor of Chicago in 1923.

The Republican party had as many factions as ever. The old leadership of Fred Busse, on the North Side of Chicago, passed into the hands of Edward Brundage, twice elected attorney general, and Medill McCormick. On the South Side of Chicago, Charles S. Deneen, former governor, still had a respectable following, attracting support in the outlying areas and from the better elements of the city. He possessed a reputation as an honest reformer and progressive, and even after his defeat by Dunne in 1912, held considerable political influence. The West Side of Chicago had, in the early years of the twentieth century, been in the hands of William Lorimer, the prototype of the political boss. Lorimer's star was in eclipse after he was kicked out of the Senate for a fraudulent election in 1911, but his political weight showed up from time to time in Illinois. In his later years Lorimer was wealthy and could not be discounted.[10]

Fred Lundin took over the active manipulation of Lorimer's political machine. The self-effacing Lundin came to the United States at the age of eleven. He referred to himself as "insignificant me," but contemporary politicians were more likely to call him "foxy Fred." The "Poor-Swede," as Lundin liked to be called, was colorful. One historian described him in this way: "His long black frock coat was tight at the waist and it flared around his thighs. On his head was a black plainsman's hat. He wore a black windsor tie and a black low-cut waistcoat, ornamented with an enormous gold watch chain. His round eyes hid behind amber spectacles." Lundin worked as a newsboy, bootblack, and branched out into his own business. Raising a little money, he invented a soft drink called "Juniper Ade" which he peddled from street corners, wearing his outlandish garb while two Blacks strummed guitars. His business brought affluence, and he ventured into politics. At first a disciple of Lorimer, Lundin emerged as the real leader as his mentor moved into the shadows. To "Juniper Ade" Lundin added a line of patent medicines and grew rich. In spite of his pretense that he had no political influence, he was powerful in patronage politics.[11]

These Chicago factions moved from alliance to alliance with various other factions. After the defeat of Lorimer, the West Side group was closely tied to Thompson, who controlled the mayor's office from 1915 until the end of the '20s (with the exception of Dever's term). The state offices were in the hands of downstate politicians after 1920, but even Len Small and Louis Emmerson were able to reach the governor's chair only with the aid of the Chicago political factions. It should be noted that downstate Republicans were hardly less corrupt than their Chicago contemporaries.[12]

The Democratic party continued in the hands of various political bosses. After 1916 the Harrison-Dunne faction of the party lost its potency. Roger Sullivan was the undisputed boss of the Democratic party from then until his death in 1920. When Sullivan died, George Brennan, another of the Irish contingent, took over the leadership. Harold Ickes, the old progressive turned Democrat, was a close friend of Brennan and referred to him as "Wily George Brennan."[13]

Born in New York, Brennan, the son of a coal miner, worked in the mines in Illinois until an accident cost him a leg. After that he taught school for a time before coming to Chicago, where he got involved in politics. Brennan was white-haired, impressive, forceful, full of Irish charm, but devoted to the patronage system. He loved intrigue and was capable of making a deal with any faction of the Democratic party, not to mention with Republicans if it suited his purposes. Brennan could get along with such diverse characters as Tony Cermak and Michael Igoe or industrial manipulators like Samuel Insull or Janet Kellogg Fairbank. While Roger Sullivan had made little effort to placate other ethnic groups such as the Czechs, Brennan was able to win the support of Cermak. He brought, at least temporarily, the Harrison-Dunne faction into working alliance by supporting the reform candidate for mayor, William Dever, in 1923.

Brennan died in 1928, and Harold Ickes believed it was his intent that Michael Igoe would be his successor. However, the new king was Cermak.[14] Born in Czechoslovakia in 1873, Anton J. Cermak came to the United States a year later. His family settled in Braidwood, Illinois, where, as a young man, Cermak worked in the mines. Later a brakeman on the Elgin, Joliet and Eastern Railroad, he worked on street railways and gained a reputation as a drinker and brawler. Married in 1894, he moved to Lawndale, where he became a joiner, frequenting various lodges and fraternal organizations. He eventually became spokesman for the Czechs of his neighborhood. From 1902 until 1910 Cermak served as a representative in the general assembly, a post he won without help from either Sullivan or Harrison. Generally, Cermak voted with the Sullivan faction on state matters, although he remained close to Harrison politically. He voted for many progressive laws, such as direct election of senators, the use of voting machines, and strengthening civil service requirements.[15]

Cermak formed the organization called United Societies for Local Self-government to fight enforcement of Sunday closing laws, and he served as secretary of this organization until the end of prohibition. He was an alderman in Chicago by 1909, and had then become influential in banking, building and loan companies, and real estate, as well as owning the firewood business which had been his first enterprise. Cermak held a number of appointive posts throughout his career. He returned to the city council in 1919, succeeding Otto Kerner, also a Czech and father of the man who was later to marry Cermak's daughter and be governor of Illinois. Cermak counted among his friends another Czech leader, A. J. Sabath, a Bohemian Jew who served many years in Congress.

Cermak continued as a secondary figure throughout the '20s until the death of Brennan brought him into the leadership of the Democratic party—important since Chicago was the second largest

Bohemian city in the world—and in 1931 he was elected mayor. He was shot by an assassin early in 1933.[16]

Illinois politics during the '20s was built on the spoils system, with patronage the chief interest of most political leaders. The Democratic party was the minority party throughout the decade, but its politicians were beginning to create a power base during this period. Many Democratic leaders were important vote getters, and although most could not be listed as members of "high society" in any part of the state, some of them became quite wealthy. Patrick Nash, of the Irish contingent, was listed among those with the highest incomes received in Chicago in 1925. Several others, such as Roger Sullivan, had become wealthy through a combination of business and politics.[17]

Charles Merriam, a political science professor who also worked in politics, wrote of the chaos of formal government, pointing out that many elements of informal government were important in carrying on the business of the state. Among these he listed political parties and factions, civic societies, business, labor, racial groups, religious groups, regional groups, professional groups, women's groups, the press, and the underworld.

Not all of the leaders came from the lower classes. The McCormicks were important in politics, Medill in actual participation and Robert, his brother, through the *Tribune*. Some of the old progressives such as Raymond Robins, Harold Ickes, and Janet Kellogg Fairbank joined the Democratic party. Many of these figures, not interested in a personal venture into politics, worked behind the scenes.[18]

The campaign of 1920 brought forth new contenders for high elected offices at both the state and national levels, many possessing less ability than those who had gone before. The Republican national convention, meeting in Chicago, excited Illinoisians because, for the first time in many years, they had a serious contender for the presidential nomination. Governor Lowden had support for the nomination, and during the last years of his gubernatorial term he looked like a man running for president. Lowden, always plagued by his connections with the Pullman Company, selected Louis L. Emmerson, the Illinois secretary of state, as his campaign manager. Emmerson lived in Mt. Vernon, and Lowden took every opportunity to identify himself with downstate Illinois and as a farmer by virtue of his magnificent farm.[19]

Harold Ickes tried to convince Lowden that Emmerson knew

little about national politics and had no influence with national leaders. Ickes said of Emmerson, "He was just a back-country crackerbox politician with neither aptitude for such a job nor imagination." In spite of this advice, Lowden insisted on keeping Emmerson. Although Lowden had the support of most Illinois Republicans, Mayor Thompson opposed him. When it developed that Lowden had thirty-eight votes in the Illinois delegation to Thompson's seventeen, the mayor dramatically resigned from the delegation because of "the moral issue" of Lowden's large expenditures in the campaign.[20]

In the preconvention days, charges of excessive expenditures by Lowden persisted. Eventually Emmerson admitted large expenditures in Missouri. He insisted that he did not know what the money was for, but the revelation brought fears of bribery, and Lowden later thought this incident may have defeated him in the convention. Emmerson had paid out $32,000 to the Lowden manager in Missouri. Of this, $17,000 went to Jake Babler, the Republican national committeeman, who in turn had paid $2,500 to each of two uncommitted St. Louis delegates.[21]

Among the other major contenders for the nomination was General Leonard Wood. His managers were Frank Hitchcock of Nebraska, Taft's manager in 1912 and postmaster general, and William C. Proctor, the soap king from Cincinnati. As the convention approached, General Wood set up his headquarters in Peacock Alley in the Congress Hotel. Most candidates tried to identify themselves with Theodore Roosevelt and his wing of the party, and Wood was no exception. In his headquarters was a large bust of Roosevelt near which Wood stood in his olive-drab field uniform decorated with the Congressional Medal of Honor to emphasize his military career and his friendship with Roosevelt.[22]

Also important in the convention was Senator Hiram Johnson of California, whose chief managers were William Wrigley, Jr., Chicago chewing gum magnate, and Albert D. Lasker, Chicago advertising man and assistant chairman of the Republican National Committee. Wrigley, of the Hamilton Club, leaving nothing to chance in his desire to be a kingmaker, ran for delegate to the convention as a Lowden man and contributed money to Wood's campaign. Johnson posed as the successor to Roosevelt's progressivism, and there were many pictures of Roosevelt in his campaign headquarters in the Auditorium Hotel. An almost religious fervor permeated the Johnson campaign, much like the emotion that attended Theodore Roosevelt's campaigns.[23]

At the beginning of the convention there was talk of Senator Warren Harding of Ohio, but most political observers did not take his candidacy seriously. Harding had not distinguished himself as a senator and he had serious personal handicaps. Whatever chance he had came because of the manipulations of Harry Daugherty, an old Ohio friend who promoted the Harding presidential boom from obscurity. Harding had been carrying on an affair with Nan Britton, a girl from his hometown of Marion, Ohio. Nan had borne an illegitimate daughter to Harding and at the time of the 1920 Republican national convention was living in Chicago with her sister and brother-in-law, Mr. and Mrs. Scott Willits. Willits, a musician with the Chicago Opera, lived on the South Side. The baby was boarded out, and Nan had taken a job as a secretary. Harding had hardly arrived in Chicago when he rushed to the Willits apartment to see Nan; he also met her several other times during the convention. Nan tried to persuade Harding to meet his daughter, but he refused, although he continued financial support for both Nan and the child. Much of this was unknown to other politicians and the delegates.[24]

Herbert Hoover, who had made a reputation for himself during World War I as a humanitarian and a bureaucrat in the Wilson administration, was also a contender for the nomination. One historian has said that his headquarters in the Auditorium Hotel looked more like a college seminar than a political room. Older men like Oscar Straus and fledgling politicians like Robert Taft, son of the former president, debated the issues of the day there.[25]

As the convention opened, half of the 984 delegates were uncommitted. This unusual situation created the appearance of an open convention. National Chairman Will Hays opened the convention, and Henry Cabot Lodge, the senator from Massachusetts who had been responsible for the defeat of the League of Nations, was elected temporary and permanent convention chairman. On the fourth ballot, General Leonard Wood had 314½ votes, Lowden had 289, Hiram Johnson had 140½, and Harding had 61½.[26]

At this point the convention adjourned, and Harding was discouraged. William Allen White described how in a hotel elevator he met Harding, slightly drunk, with bloodshot eyes, unshaven, and looking very rocky. His optimistic manager, Harry Daugherty, exhilarated by the tension, went on talking to key figures and promoting the Harding fortunes. That night the party elders congregated in the famous smoked-filled room, actually a suite, on the fourth floor of the Blackstone Hotel. The dominant figures among the group who gathered that night to decide who was to be the candidate were old-guard senators, among them Medill McCormick.[27]

After discussing the possibilities, the group agreed that the choice should be Harding. Senator Frank Brandegee of Connecticut said, "There ain't any first-raters this year. This ain't 1880 or any 1904; we haven't any John Shermans or Theodore Roosevelts; we got a lot of second-raters and Warren Harding is the best of the second-raters." The next day, on the tenth ballot, Harding was nominated. Harding, an experienced poker player, is said to have remarked, "We drew to a pair of deuces and filled." After seeing Nan once more, Harding went back to Marion, Ohio, to conduct a front-porch campaign. He traveled little in the campaign, sitting at home making speeches, often confusing, to visiting delegations of the Republican faithful.[28]

The Democratic national convention met in San Francisco on July 5. Among the leading presidential contenders were A. Mitchell Palmer, Wilson's attorney general, and William G. McAdoo, Wilson's son-in-law. Ultimately the convention was deadlocked in the same manner as the Republicans'. McAdoo's handicap was his relationship to Wilson. Many were apathetic toward the Wilsonian liberalism, and many, including Senators McCormick and Sherman, were antagonistic to the League of Nations as a result of the fulminations of the irreconcilables. Eventually James M. Cox, governor of Ohio, emerged with the nomination. Cox had a background similar to Harding's. Both were publishers of small-town newspapers, both had spent some time in Congress, and just as Harding was senator from Ohio, Cox was governor of that state. But although the backgrounds of Harding and Cox were similar, there was no question that the latter was superior to Harding in personal as well as political morals, not to mention intellectual capacity. The Democrats nominated Franklin Delano Roosevelt, who had distinguished himself as assistant secretary of the Navy during the Wilson administration, to run with Cox.[29]

The primary election for state offices in Illinois was held on September 15, 1920. Governor Lowden was undecided whether to run for governor again after his defeat in the Republican national convention. On June 23, 1920, Len Small of Kankakee, the state treasurer, announced his candidacy. After conferring with Senators McCormick and Sherman, former Governor Deneen, and his attorney general, Edward Brundage, representing the more respectable factions of the Republican party, Lowden announced that he would not run for reelection. He then worked with other Republican leaders to put together a slate headed by Lieutenant Governor John G. Oglesby, the son of the Civil War governor of Illinois and a highly competen individual. Fred Sterling stood for lieutenant governor, Louis Emmerson for reelection as secretary of state, and Edward Brundage for reelection as attorney general.[30]

For U.S. senator, Lowden supported William B. McKinley of Champaign, a banker and traction magnate, Senator Sherman having announced that he would not be a candidate for reelection. Frank L. Smith of Dwight, chairman of the Republican state committee, wanted not only reelection as chairman, but also Sherman's seat in the Senate. The Deneen-West faction refused to support Smith on either count, so he had to court the Lundin-Thompson faction in Chicago. Smith worked to aid the candidacy of Lowden in the national convention because he hoped for Lowden's support, but he was also working hand in glove with Thompson. On May 9, 1920, at the Republican state convention, Thompson and Smith combined to reelect the latter chairman of the Republican state committee. Thompson supported Small in his bid for the gubernatorial nomination.[31] In addition to Smith and McKinley contending for the senatorial nomination, B. M. Chipperfield of Pekin entered the race.

The race for the gubernatorial nomination was complicated by four candidates. In addition to Small and Oglesby, Oscar Carlstrom and Edward Woodruff entered the primary, a bitter race which brought forth charges of corruption. Oglesby spoke in ninety-eight counties in twenty-six days and topped off his campaign with a speaking tour of Cook County to fight the Thompson-Lundin faction. Thompson made Lowden the issue with personal attacks on the governor, shouting that Lowden was a liar and that since Oglesby was Lowden's candidate, the people should support Small. Smith conducted his campaign in company with Thompson and Lundin. In the primary, Oglesby carried eighty-two downstate counties by such narrow margins that, with Thompson's support, Small overcame him in Cook County. Small won by 8,000 votes in the state total. McKinley beat Smith in the contest for senator, and Sterling, Emmerson, and Brundage were nominated.[32]

In the Democratic primary, J. Hamilton Lewis defeated Barrett O'Hara, lieutenant governor in the Dunne administration and a congressman, by an overwhelming majority. Peter Waller ran ahead of Robert Emmet Burke by some 4,000 votes to capture the Democratic nomination for senator.[33]

Republican gubernatorial candidate Len Small, son of a country physician, had achieved considerable local prominence in Kankakee County, and in 1904 had been elected state treasurer. President Taft later had appointed him assistant U.S. treasurer in charge of the subtreasury in Chicago, and he became state treasurer again in 1916, but this was hardly a distinguished record to bring to the candidacy for the state's highest office.[34]

Small's opponent, Lewis, was colorful. He attended Houghton College in Georgia and the University of Virginia and later studied law, coming to Chicago in 1903, after service in the Spanish-American War. During the mayorality of Edward F. Dunne he was city attorney and corporation council, and in 1912 he was elected for a term in the U.S. Senate, where he had the honor of being elected the first Democratic whip in its history.[35]

The national campaign made relatively little impact on Illinois. Harding motored around the edge of Chicago and visited Fort Sheridan but made no speeches in the city or state. Cox came to Chicago for a major speech on October 30, 1920, and events gave him an opportunity to seek the Irish vote. It happened that at the time, the Chicago Irish were mourning Terrence McSwiney, the mayor of Cork who had just died after a seventy-four-day hunger strike in a British prison. Cox, taking note of this incident, promised help to the Irish by taking the problem of Irish independence to the League of Nations if he were elected. Cox stood fast in his devotion to Wilsonian policy, charging that those who opposed the league were essentially pro-German. He lashed out at the corruption of the Thompson administration, saying, "You are driving a knife blade into your own heart when you allow that machine to be perpetuated which is making your city, your state a stench in the nostrils of mankind." His major speech was in the Colliseum, but he also spoke at Carter Harrison High School on the South Side and at St. Stanislaus Auditorium in the Polish district, and ended with a midnight reception at the South Shore Country Club. He then spoke at Patten Gymnasium in Evanston. All of this was carried off with flamboyance, parades, and red fire.[36]

Although the *Tribune* held that the nomination of Harding was engineered by the eastern "Pocketbook Gang," Colonel McCormick supported Harding in the campaign. And when Hiram

Johnson came to Chicago on behalf of Harding, he proclaimed that a vote for Harding was a vote against the league, saying that it was becoming "respectable to preach Americanism again." The *Tribune* believed that Cox harped too much on corruption and that his campaign really boiled down to one point—that if the Americans elected Harding, they would be considered corrupt.[37]

In the state campaign, Lewis provided good copy for the newspapers. He set forth a platform which involved protection of tenants from profiteering landlords, tax reform, home rule for Chicago, a better deal for labor, legislation to lower the high cost of living, and industrial peace through arbitration of labor disputes. Lewis emphasized that all interest earned on public funds must be promptly paid into the treasury. This was preliminary to later attacks on Small for his conduct of the state treasury. Lewis promisted better roads, improvement of waterways, humanization of state institutions, welfare for children, justice to women, a larger inheritance tax, protection for farmers, and a program for veterans of World War I. He carried on a vigorous campaign, attacking Thompsonism and linking Small to the corrupt Thompson machine. He said that the state was "becoming a cesspool of American politics." This condition was getting such that "missionaries should be brought into Illinois to rescue it from heathenism," and pointed out that the Republican *Chicago Tribune* editorially proclaimed that Small was Thompson's puppet.[38]

Of Small's handling of the treasury Lewis said, "If I am elected, then the nefarious practice of making millionaires of state treasurers through their loaning state funds privately will be stopped. As I have declared to the people of Mr. Small's hometown, his election would be a stain on the state and an insult to the honor of Illinois." In the middle of October, Lewis announced that his campaign was so strenuous, with two speeches a day, that even his famous whiskers were going untrimmed. His personality brought many colorful descriptions from reporters. As he spoke at Decatur, one reporter noted, "Upon the high school rostrum there stood J. Hamilton Lewis, Democratic candidate for governor, tonight, in his buttonhole there bloomed a pair of baby rosebuds, surrounded by a bit of fern. His face, decked with the golden whiskers which rival even the beards of the Smith Brothers for fame was agleam with a quiet smile. He had just been introduced as the next governor of Illinois. In the next few minutes the speaker explained the Tammany tiger and convinced at least 300 persons that the next occupant of the gubernatorial chair should wear pink whiskers and speak like a Shakespearian."[39]

An incident in Litchfield caused further comment. Lewis, always flowery in his speech, was having lunch in a Litchfield restaurant and said to a waitress, Ruby Lynn, "Ah, my dear, when I gaze upon your wealth of chestnut hair which the rays of beneficient and salubrious sun have kissed into a delicate gold; when I observe the little dimple nesting so coyly in that shapely chin, I rejoice that the committee whose work it was to pick my itinerary should place the town of Litchfield on the list. Ruby, you may bring me a cup of coffee, if you please." According to the reporter, Miss Lynn giggled and said, "You know, Senator, I've been kidded by experts."[40]

Lewis, always quick with a quip about Len Small, came up with quotable quotes at nearly every whistle-stop. In Litchfield, saying that Thompson had picked Small as the governor of Illinois, he remarked, "Some fruit is picked green, some is picked ripe, while some is just picked rotten." Later he commented that he thought it was appropriate that Thompson had gone to a town where there was an insane asylum to get his political servant; another time he suggested that the governor's chair is "too big for Small."[41]

Unfortunately Lewis was a racist. Speaking at the soldiers' home in Danville, Lewis, a colonel in the Spanish-American War, said that he would not ask them to vote for him, but "if a soldier hasn't a sufficient sense of patriotism in him to know what to do at the ballot box to save his country from political debauchery and degradation, I'll not tell him. You fought for a principle of what is right and not for a party name. You fought for a free ballot and a fair count. Then, after all your sacrifice, you have seen yonder in Chicago one of the greatest political crimes in the history of the union, the stealing of a nomination for governor by a set of corrupt black and white men."[42] Near the end of the campaign, as the Black issue kept cropping up, Lewis on one occasion commented, "I want a just community here, but before God this is a white man's government. While I want no white man's government that will misgovern any Negro or any white man, I will have no criminal Negro misgovern any white man by crooked manipulation of the ballots."[43]

Small spent much of his campaign answering charges made against him by Lewis and John Maynard Harlan, the son of the former justice of the U.S. Supreme Court who was running for governor on the Harding-Coolidge Republican ticket. The main thrust of the Republican campaign was a special train that took off from Chicago during the middle of October to run for two weeks through the state. The train carried Smith, McKinley, Brundage, Sterling, and Emmerson, as well as other leaders of the Republican party. Small charged that Lewis, as senator, had violated his oath of office by helping to appropriate millions of dollars which were squandered. Small spoke of his own platform of hard roads, a more liberal policy for education, and better salaries for teachers. Small denied the charges of Harlan and Lewis that he had withheld funds from the state while he was treasurer, saying, "The mountain labored and brought forth a mouse, and John Harlan thundered in the index and whispered in the appendix." He asked who was financing Harlan's independent campaign.[44]

Small charged Lewis with profiteering from contracts that were given to friends and clients during World War I. He spoke of the bonds which had been sold during the war which then were worth less than par. He asserted that Lewis was a friend of the public utilities. Medill McCormick, cured of his earlier progressivism, supported the Republicans, announcing that he was going to vote a straight Republican ticket. Small answered the charges that he was a tool of Thompson and other political bosses, saying that he was proud of his Republican associates, and he invoked the memory of Theodore Roosevelt in saying that even this great man had once been attacked by Lewis.[45]

William E. Mason, the former senator and congressman from Illinois, took the stump for the Republican ticket. Speaking in Mattoon, Mason, whose powers of vituperation matched those of Lewis, spoke of Lewis's exchange with the pretty waitress in Litchfield: "Somehow, somewhere, in the state, perhaps in front of the little Litchfield restaurant, there should be erected a stone with an inscription something like this: Here rests the gubernatorial aspirations of James Hamilton Lewis, stilled forever November 2 by the cryptic challenge of Ruby Lynn, a demure waitress of Litchfield, who speaking the verdict of Illinoisians said to the senator, 'You know, Senator, I have been kidded by experts.'"[46] Small, as did all Republicans in 1920, spent much of his rhetoric on national topics, particularly taking issue with Wilson. It was said that Lewis sometimes avoided being linked with Wilson, but Small did his best to link both him and Cox to Wilson.[47]

Lewis had support from various intellectuals of the state, mostly professors from the University of Chicago such as William E. Dodge, James McLaughlin, Shaler Matthews, and Horace Bridges. The *Chicago Tribune* came out for Lewis in spite of its usual Republican leaning. The newspaper always found Thompson and his political backer, Lundin, distasteful, and since it was obvious that Small was linked with these men, the *Tribune* could not support him:

> We do not see how a Republican who was convinced before the

primaries that the nomination of Len Small, protege of William Hale Thompson and Fred Lundin, would be an extraordinarily bad thing for the state, can be reconciled to the election of Len Small. Mr. Small has not changed. His backing and the purposes of his backing are the same. They were opposed before as bad. They must be opposed now as bad. The nomination of Small was the necessary preliminary. But it gains nothing for his Chicago Tammany backing unless he is elected. The state does not lose anything through this Tammany unless Small is elected. . . . We do not like Lewis's national politics. We could not support him for a federal office at this time because we think his national principles and ideas are hurtful. But the administration of the state of Illinois does not involve Lewis's national party tendencies and principles. As a state administrator, he will be better than Len Small and he will not carry Len Small's crowd into office. A voter who is soundly Republican on national issues is perfectly free to choose the best administrator he can get in the tickets presented to the state and Lewis is better than Small.[48]

The *Illinois State Register* reprinted the *Tribune* editorial and also supported Lewis, saying that the principle issue was "Thompson Tammanyism," and pointed out that Lowden had warned against this corrupt alliance. The *Tribune* said that a vote for Harding was a vote for the nation and a vote for Lewis was a vote for Illinois. The *Decatur Herald,* also normally Republican, hoped Small would be beaten, although they supported the rest of the Republican ticket.[49]

When the votes were counted on November 2, 1920, Senator Harding had defeated Governor Cox by almost a three to one majority in Illinois. On the state ticket, Small ran considerably behind the national ticket but beat Lewis by 500,000 votes. McKinley won the senate seat of Sherman by 800,000 votes. It was a dark day for the Democrats. In the congressional delegation elected, the Republicans outnumbered the Democrats by twenty-five to three. Henry T. Rainey lost his seat, and the three Democrats elected were from Chicago, among them Adolph Sabath. Former governor Yates and former senator Mason were elected at large. Mason died on November 7, 1922, and his daughter, Winifred Mason Huck, was appointed to fill out his term, the first woman to serve in Congress from Illinois. Among the Republican notables in the delegation were James Mann of Chicago, Frank Funk of Bloomington, and Joseph Cannon of Danville, serving his last term. Unquestionably involved in the victory was a rejection of Wilsonian policies and the liberalism of the progressives.[50]

Conservatism, apathy, and corruption had triumphed in Illinois as in the nation, and subsequently the Small administration became deeply involved in nepotism and corruption. When the general assembly created the Department of Purchases and Construction, which had control of building highways, Small appointed his son, Leslie, as director of the department. His son-in-law, A. E. Inglesh, was the administrative auditor of the Department of Finance. Almost immediately after Small took office, events developed which seemed to lend substance to the charges of Small's misuse of public funds during his term as state treasurer.[51]

Soon after coming into office, Small vetoed appropriations made for the office of Attorney General Edward J. Brundage. Brundage was, in Small's view, from the wrong faction of Chicago politics, and the cut of some $700,000 would seriously handicap Brundage's office. Aided by the *Chicago Tribune*, Brundage began an investigation of Small's handling of funds. It had long been customary for the state treasurer to be the recipient of state funds and to lend these out at interest and keep the interest for himself, causing the post of state treasurer to become one of the most lucrative positions in state government. By the time Small became treasurer, the law had been changed somewhat and he had turned in some $450,000 of the interest money. According to the testimony of Harry C. Luehrs, a seventeen-year employee of the state treasurer's office, one of the largest recipients of state funds was the First Trust and Savings Bank of Kankakee. The letterhead of this bank listed Len Small as president and his son-in-law, Inglesh, as assistant cashier.[52]

It then developed that Small, together with brothers Edward and Vernon Curtis, had established a fictitious bank in Grant Park, the home of the Curtises. Small had deposited state funds in this bank, which paid the minimum rate of interest allowed by law to the state. Actually they had been lending money to Chicago industrialists at inflationary wartime rates. The difference between the minimum interest and the actual interest was alleged to have gone into the pockets of the three conspirators.

Brundage got a criminal indictment against Small in the Sangamon County court in July, 1921. On a change of venue the trial was held in Waukegan, and it resulted in acquittal for Small and his associates, although many believed that he was guilty. Eventually the story came out that manipulation had been used in the selection of the jury that heard the Small case. Solicitors were sent around the Waukegan area, offering as a premium to the householders upon whom they called a choice between a picture of

President Harding or one of Governor Small. By the reaction they got to Small's picture, the sympathies of the household were determined, and with this information in advance, it was easy to get a sympathetic jury. Subsequently, four of the jurors received state patronage jobs. Two became state highway policemen, one a game warden, and one a foreman at a penitentiary.[53]

Despite the acquittal, Brundage instituted civil proceedings in circuit court in Sangamon County and got a judgment against Small for a sum of over $1,000,000. The case was appealed to the Supreme Court of Illinois and was eventually settled, with Small being required to give the state an additional $650,000. This was done in 1927, after he had been reelected for a second term. One careful historian of the period described the Small administration in this way: "Now followed an administration which for waste, mismanagement, inefficiency, intrigue, manipulation, and downright disregard for public interest has few parallels in the history of the United States."[54]

The Small administration was characterized by the greatest patronage machine the state had ever known. Small first came into the limelight in 1902 when an investigation was made of the operation of the Kankakee State Hospital. Small had been president of the institution's board of trustees for eight years, and during this period from 5 to 10 percent of employees' wages had been appropriated to build up the political funds of Small and Governor Yates. The Yates administration tried unsuccessfully to cover up this scandal. Small was now in a position to apply this same technique on a state-wide basis. The integrated administrative organization which started in the reforms of the Lowden administration actually made it easier for the Small administration to set up a patronage machine.[55]

It is notable that the Illinois Constitution of 1922 was defeated during the Small administration by a vote of about five to one. Thompson and Small were against the constitution, but so also were exgovernor Dunne, Harold Ickes, Clarence Darrow, Charles Merriam, Victor Olander, Seymour Stedman, and other liberal and radical political figures. The constitution was also opposed by the Hearst papers, the Chicago Federation of Labor, and the Illinois Federation of Labor. Chicagoans generally felt that the new document gave too little representation to Cook County. There was opposition to a provision for a state income tax and some felt it was too favorable to the utility companies.[56]

On a more constructive side, the Small administration was noted for building concrete highways. The movement for the building of hard roads had started during the Dunne administration, and under Lowden's administration, $60,000,000 in road-building bonds were issued. By the end of the first Small administration, 2,982 miles of concrete highway had been built.

The Small administration also promoted recreation areas, including Starved Rock State Park and the Lincoln homestead in Springfield. New Salem State Park was dedicated on May 19, 1921. The Metamora courthouse and Cahokia Mounds were acquired in 1920. Also acquired by the state as recreation areas were Black Hawk Watchtower Park in Rock Island, the White Pine Forest in Ogle County, Giant City Park in Union and Jackson counties, and the Pierre Menard Home.[57]

The Small administration could also boast of improvements on the lakes-to-gulf waterway. Five locks, each 110 feet wide and 600 feet long, at Lockport, where the Chicago sanitary canal came into the Illinois River, at Brandon Road, two miles south of Joliet, at Dresden Island, fourteen miles downstream from there, at Marseilles, and at Starved Rock between Ottawa and Utica. The total distance involved was some sixty-three miles, taking care of a fall of 140 feet in the Illinois River. All of this construction redounded to Small's credit.

Both the improved highways and development of state parks were results of the popularity of the automobile. It was now no longer necessary to travel on mud roads, and easier to visit the park. All of this building was looked upon with pride and was an important element of progress, but it was a period of great materialism, when people were more impressed with the construction than with whether or not taxpayers were paying too much through graft and kickbacks. Small, even in the face of charges of the most serious kinds of corruption, could weather the political storm because of his claims to being a "builder."[58]

In the off-year elections of 1922, the Republicans won twenty seats in the congressional delegation, and the Democrats captured seven. Richard Yates and Henry R. Rathbone, both Republicans, were elected at large. Democrats won five seats in Chicago, among them that of Adolph Sabath. Henry T. Rainey regained his seat, and J. Earl Major from Hillsboro made his first appearance in the Congress. Frank Funk was elected for another term, but James R. Mann did not seek reelection and died on November 30, 1922.[59]

In 1924 the party primaries in Illinois were moved to April, and late in 1923 Governor Small announced that he would be a candidate for renomination. He had the support of Thompson, who went to Springfield to demonstrate his support. Small's wife had died in 1922 and Thompson implied that her death was caused by Brundage's attack on Small and swore to avenge her by defeating Brundage. In the meantime, the reform group of the Republican party, headed by Lowden, picked a slate headed by Thurlow G. Essington. A state senator of good reputation, Essington was a Phi Beta Kappa from the University of Illinois and held a J.D. degree from the University of Chicago Law School, where he had graduated cum laude. Running with Essington was Edward J. Brundage, Small's old enemy. Medill McCormick was seeking renomination with this faction. The *Chicago Tribune,* on the eve of the primary, supported this slate, endorsing Essington and editorializing that his nomination would "insure the state of Illinois honesty, economy, efficiency, and progressivism of government."[60]

Of Small the *Tribune* said, "Small is an astonishing character. He is by instinct a man of low cunning. He is inclined by nature to short-changing rather than to high seas piracy. He was in his proper place when he was making his bit off of the coal sold to the Kankakee insane asylum by O'Gara, King and Company of Chicago." The *Chicago Herald and Examiner* endorsed Small, saying that Essington was the tool of the Brundage faction. In the presidential preferential primary, Calvin Coolidge contended with Hiram Johnson of California for the Republican delegates to the national convention. Small defeated Essington by some 60,000 votes, while Coolidge outpointed Johnson by 150,000. Oscar Carlstrom, Small's candidate for attorney general, beat Brundage, illustrating how little the charges against Small had aroused the voters.[61]

In the Democratic primary, William G. McAdoo contested for presidential delegates in Illinois. His forces were led by the Harrison-Dunne faction, and the opposition was led by Mayor Dever and George Brennan. McAdoo lost, so the Illinois delegates went to the convention uncommitted. Colonel A. A. Sprague won the nomination for senator in the Democratic primary. For governor, the contest was between Judge Norman Jones, Lee O'Neil Browne, and several other minor contenders. Jones overwhelmed Browne (who had been involved in the Lorimer case years earlier) by almost a two to one margin.[62]

The Republican national convention of 1924 opened in Cleveland, Ohio, on June 10. President Harding had died a year earlier in San Francisco's Palace Hotel. As the convention opened, Senator

Thomas Walsh of Montana was working his way through the tangle of testimony about Teapot Dome and the other scandals of the Harding administration, but Chicagoans were interested as much in the trial of Leopold and Loeb for the murder of Bobby Franks as they were in the convention. The convention promised little excitement because Calvin Coolidge was in control. Arthur Brisbane, writing for the *Chicago Herald and Examiner,* sized it up this way, "Presently Mr. Coolidge's convention will tell us who is to be the candidate for vice-president. No news until then. The platform will be an elaborate simplification of the American sentence: 'We are sitting pretty.' Republicans count on Democrats, their wet-and-dry, Klan-or-no-Klan troubles to make the certainty of Republican victory doubly sure."[63]

Not even the side issues of the convention created much excitement. Feminists gathered at Cleveland to demand an equal-rights-for-women law. Several Illinois figures were mentioned as possibilities for the vice-presidency, including former governor Lowden, former governor Deneen, William S. Wrigley, Jr., Secretary of State Emmerson, and Charles Dawes. Lowden insisted that he would not accept the nomination, but the talk went on. As the convention opened, Andrew Mellon, industrialist, banker, and Secretary of the Treasury under Harding, Coolidge, and Hoover, got more vigorous applause than Calvin Coolidge, testifying to the materialism of the time. William Randolph Hearst commented that this was a banker's convention and the money interest would be served. Hearst thought the Democrats had a good opportunity to win in 1924 if they remembered the principles of Jefferson and Jackson.[64]

On the first ballot, Coolidge had a majority, La Follette got 34 votes, and Hiram Johnson only 10 out of more than 1,100 votes cast. There was considerable interest in who was to be Coolidge's vice-presidential candidate, and in spite of his protests, Lowden was nominated, getting a majority of the votes on the second ballot. Sixty of the sixty-one delegates from Illinois voted for Lowden; William Wrigley, Jr., got a single vote. But Lowden refused the nomination. The convention then turned to another Illinois figure, General Charles G. "Hell and Maria" Dawes, a Chicago banker.[65]

The Democratic national convention met in Madison Square Garden in New York on June 24. There was more interest in this convention because even before it met, the Democrats were feuding over the issues of prohibition and the Ku Klux Klan. William Jennings Bryan announced that he thought the nominee should be a dry progressive, but among the contenders Alfred E. Smith, the governor of New York, was wet and anti-Klan. The McAdoo forces said they could control the convention, but the delegation had been elected on a no-preference basis and included the usual diverse group of Illinois Democrats. Mayor Dever brought Kenna, Igoe, and Cermak with him, while Janet Kellogg Fairbank, leader of Chicago society, and Anna L. Smith, from downstate, represented the newly enfranchised women of the Illinois democracy. The delegation, for the most part, agreed with Al Smith on his position on the issues, and a majority voted for him at the convention.[66]

Brennan, now well established as the boss of the Democratic party, was instrumental in the effort to stop the candidacy of McAdoo, whose position was unclear on the issues of the Klan and prohibition. Brennan and Cermak, representing their ethnic constituencies, were against the Klan and for the right of people to drink alcoholic beverages when and where they pleased. Brennan was elected national committeeman and Kellogg Fairbank was elected national committeewoman. Several Illinois figures were mentioned as vice-presidential candidates, among them Lewis, the party's candidate for governor in 1920. Carter Harrison supported McAdoo, and several delegates wore "Dever For President" badges on the convention floor.

Fistfights and riots broke out between the McAdoo and Smith partisans as the convention opened, and it grew more confused by the hour as a number of minor candidates appeared. Lewis G. Stevenson, son of the former vice-president, nominated David S. Houston, former secretary of agriculture and treasury. Franklin Roosevelt, on crutches after his bout with polio, nominated Al Smith. Igoe seconded the Smith nomination in a speech in which he linked McAdoo to the oil scandals of the Harding administration. As tempers flared, the convention refused, by a single vote, to adopt an anti-Klan plank. The ever-present split between the northern and southern Illinoisans was apparent in this vote. Thirteen Illinois delegates voted against the anti-Klan plank, all of them from downstate.[67] The convention, deadlocked between Smith and McAdoo after days of anger and controversy, nominated dark horse John W. Davis of West Virginia. To run with him they nominated Charles Bryan, the brother of William Jennings Bryan.

There was dissatisfaction with the candidates on the part of progressives of both parties, and on July 18 the Progressive party was revived. Their convention nominated Senator La Follette for the presidency and Senator Burton K. Wheeler, Democrat from Montana, for the vice-presidency.[68]

The Democrats nominated Judge Norman L. Jones of Carrolton for governor. A successful lawyer, Jones was the partner of Henry Rainey, one of the most progressive members of Congress. Jones served two terms in the general assembly and was a circuit judge from 1914 to 1929. After his defeat for the governorship, he was elected to the Illinois Supreme Court and eventually became chief justice. Judge Jones was an eminently respectable if somewhat colorless political figure, and he had the editorial endorsement of the *Illinois State Register*, the *Chicago Tribune*, and the *Chicago Daily News*. The *Tribune* said of Small:

> In our opinion he is not a Republican. In this campaign he is a syndicate candidate, supported by some Republicans, and as the straw votes show, by Democrats and La Follettes. Len Small is not a Republican. His platform is contrary to the Republican national platform and to the principles of Republicanism.
>
> In our opinion, far from its being the duty of any Republican to vote for Len Small, it is the duty of all Republicans to vote against him because they are Republicans. He is a discredit to the Republican party of Illinois and, as his platform shows, a renegade from it and a traitor to Republican principles.
>
> Good citizens, regardless of party, should vote for Norman L. Jones, the Democractic candidate for governor.[69]

The *State Register* quoted the editorial of the *Chicago Daily News* endorsing Jones. The *Daily News* commented that "a patriotic, purposeful people should not let their state by engulfed in a mere partisan wave, whether it be Republican, Democratic, or Progressive. In a clear cut contest between Small and Jones the latter would win hands down. Let's make it such!" Jones had impressive support, led by Mrs. Arthur Meeker, from the Women's Roosevelt Republican League. At a party at the home of Mrs. Potter Palmer, a campaign was opened to promote Jones's candidacy. Mrs. Walter Dodd said at the meeting, "Although I have always been a Republican, I feel that the issue this fall has been made by Mr. Small between personal integrity as represented by Mr. Jones, the Democratic candidate, and misuse of public funds and of a public office, represented by Governor Small."[70]

Small spent the campaign on the defensive as the Democrats took advantage of every opportunity to uncover his record of the previous four years. The Democrats had hopes of a Republican bolt, and the *Tribune* had a column to explain to the voters how they could scratch their ticket in order to vote for Jones and still support the Republican national ticket. Democrats linked Small with the Ku Klux Klan, which had endorsed him in the primary, and with the La Follette progressive campaign. The implication was that Small preferred to ignore Coolidge and seek support from the liberals. V. Y. Dallman, in a signed column in the *Illinois State Register,* charged that Small never mentioned Coolidge or Dawes in his speeches.[71]

Small spoke of his record of roads and a five-cent streetcar fare for Chicagoans. Jones hammered away at Small's bad record. Speaking to Republicans in Rock Island, he said, "To you Republicans who glory in traditions and ideals of your party I say, join with me in restoring Illinois to the glory that was hers from Lincoln to Lowden." Jones charged that Small was trying to make hard roads the only issue, and that his record was not as good as it might have been even in that. Jones alleged that there was waste and graft in road building. The *Tribune* editorialized that the way to get hard roads was to elect Jones, and it advocated the use of license fees instead of a hundred-million-dollar bond issue that Small was promoting.

Several times during the campaign, efforts were made to link Small with the Ku Klux Klan. It was charged that horses of the National Guard were used in a Klan parade in Springfield. Democrats also brought up the old charges that Small had misused public funds as state treasurer and that he had been acquitted by fraudulent means.[72]

The Democrats proclaimed that Small had created a monstrous bureaucracy, raising state expenditures to unprecedented levels. Small's opponents also hit hard at his use of the governor's pardoning power, particularly his pardon of Harry and Alma Cusick on pandering charges. George Brennan, referring to the Cusick case, said, "In God's name, men and women, do you mean to say in the face of this damning evidence that you are going to stand idly by and let that beast continue as governor of the state of Illinois?" Following up these attacks, Jones's supporters distributed a vicious pamphlet entitled "Sex Pardons and Paroles by Governor Len Small." The gist of the pamphlet was that Small had pardoned individuals convicted of such sex crimes as rape, incest, and indecent liberties and asked the question, "What is the matter with Small?" Jones closed his campaign hammering at the Small record, urging "rebuke Small and plunder."[73]

There was little interest in the presidential race in Illinois. Coolidge did not come to the state, although Davis spoke three times in Illinois. He charged that Republicans were extravagant and wasteful of public funds, and during a speech in Chicago he denounced the Ku Klux Klan, saying, "I . . . declare that, whether it is called the Ku Klux Klan or any other name, any organization that challenges the doctrine of religious toleration does violence to American ideals and cannot be approved by those who believe, like myself, in those principles." The most significant issue was illustrated when, as Davis was speaking in Chicago, the gallery began to yell, "Give us beer!" Since Coolidge did not come to Illinois, the national campaign for the Republicans was taken care of by Dawes, who proposed that Coolidge thrift was the best reason to elect him, saying that Coolidge would save the nickels of the country.[74]

Just as four years earlier, the Republicans made a clean sweep in Illinois in 1924, and Coolidge had a clear majority over all the other candidates. He mustered 1,453,321 votes in the state and carried eighty-eight counties. Davis got 576,975 votes. La Follette mustered 432,027, testifying to a revolt against the major parties. La Follette took as many votes from Davis as from Coolidge.

In the gubernatorial election the results were closer but decisive for Small, who ran behind Coolidge, collecting 1,366,436 votes, but easily beat Jones, who got 1,021,408. Deneen, who beat McCormick in the primary, polled 1,449,180 votes for senator, while Sprague got 806,702. Also winning was Omer Custer of Galesburg, who was elected to the position of state treasurer, starting a considerable political career. Carlstrom, Small's candidate for attorney general, was elected too. As the results came in, Small cried, "I am vindicated." On February 24, 1925, Senator McCormick died in Washington, and Small appointed Deneen to fill out his term.[75] In the Sixty-ninth Congress, elected in 1924, Republicans won twenty-two of the twenty-seven seats in the Illinois delegation. Among the familiar Republican names were Richard Yates and Frank Funk. The Democrats held three Chicago seats, including Sabath's, and two downstate, one of which was Rainey's.

Soon after the 1924 election, the political alliance of Len Small and Big Bill Thompson came to an end, and Lundin became the principal Chicago backer of Small and dispenser of patronage in the city.

The road-building program continued in the second Small administration. A million-dollar bond issue for further building of roads was approved by the voters in the general election of 1924, and during the last four years of Small's administration some 3,331 miles of concrete highway were built, making a total of 7,777 miles in service by 1928. Most of this had been built during Small's administration, although as his detractors pointed out, the costs were sometimes exorbitantly high, and the foundation for the "hard roads" movement had been laid in the Lowden administration, when the first bond issue of $60,000,000 had been floated. The charges of corruption against the Small administration continued through the second four years, and before Small was out of office, his son, Leslie, director of the Department of Purchases and Construction, was ordered to stand trial on charges of rigging contracts in highway building. It was charged that Leslie Small had given road contracts in return for campaign contributions.[76]

Perhaps the most shocking scandal of the decade involved Senator-elect Frank L. Smith. Smith had been in Illinois Republican politics for many years. Born in Dwight in 1867, he was orphaned at an early age. Starting from humble origins, Smith taught school briefly, became a telegrapher, real estate operator, and important in local politics. He served a term in Congress and in 1921 was appointed to the Illinois Public Utilities Commission by Len Small. The commission was a political plum of importance because it regulated public utilities, including those controlled by Samuel Insull, and the possibility of graft was unlimited. Smith had been a Republican national committeeman and had held several minor elective and appointive posts, but he had larger ambitions.[77]

In 1926, Smith contended in the primary with Senator McKinley for the senate seat and won by 44,000 votes. George Brennan won the Democratic primary. In the fall, Smith defeated Brennan and independent Republican Hugh McGill for the post, getting more than 842,000 votes to Brennan's 774,000, while McGill trailed with 156,000 votes.[78]

Following rumors of large campaign expenditures, an investigating committee of the U.S. Senate, presided over by Senator James A. Reed of Missouri, found that Smith had spent more than $250,000 on his campaign. Insull contributed $125,000 of this sum, and since Smith was chairman of the utilities commission, it was obvious that the relationship was improper. On December 7, 1926, Senator McKinley died, and Governor Small appointed Smith to fill the unexpired term. He was refused both seats, however, that of McKinley's unexpired term and the one to which he had been elected. But the political sting was lessened when it developed that Insull had also contributed to Brennan's campaign fund. There was some question about whether Insull had contributed the money himself or had taken it illegally from his company. Insull insisted there was nothing wrong with either his making the contribution or the manner in which he paid it to the candidates.

In the off-year election for the Seventieth Congress, the Republicans lost one seat but controlled the delegation twenty-one to six. The seat lost by the Republicans was in Chicago, where James T. Igoe won back the seat he had won two years earlier.[79] The scandal in the senatorial race did nothing to enhance the political reputation of Illinois. In less than twenty years, Illinois had one senator removed from the Senate, another denied his seat on grounds of fraud, and a governor indicted for fraud. The Springfield, Massachusetts, *Republican* described Chicago as the "rottenest city in the rottenest state in the union." William Allen White, writing in his *Emporia Gazette,* commented that "under primary, under convention, under a despotism or under a pure democracy Illinois would be corrupt and crooked. . . . it has been that way for two generations. It is in the blood of the people."[80]

The 1928 primaries were held on April 10. Governor Small announced his candidacy for renomination, and it seemed for a time that he was sure to win a third disgraceful term as chief executive of the state. His political ally Smith, in spite of being twice rejected by the Senate, was a candidate for renomination, trying to vindicate his reputation, and it looked for a time as though he too might win another try at the senatorship. Soon, however, a roadblock was placed in their way. Louis Emmerson, political manager for Lowden, announced his candidacy in opposition to Small. At the same time Otis Glenn, one of the prosecutors in the Herrin massacre trials, announced for the senatorship in opposition to Smith. Uniting behind those two men, Small's foes put forth a great effort to overcome Small and Smith.[81]

In the Democratic primary, Chief Justice Floyd E. Thompson of the Illinois Supreme Court was unopposed for governor. The Democrats had two contenders for senator, Cermak and James O. Monroe. This primary developed into another notorious and disgraceful political episode in Illinois history. During the campaign, a Republican figure, "Diamond Joe" Esposito, was found dead with fifty-eight machine-gun bullets in his body. Esposito had been killed in gangland fashion, and it was widely assumed that his assassins were gangsters who were behind the Small-Smith-

Thompson faction. Senator Deneen, who was among those opposing the corruptionists, attended Esposito's funeral and that night his house was bombed, as was that of Judge John Swanson, candidate for state's attorney in Cook County, who narrowly escaped death in the episode. Senator Deneen said that this was an attempt by the syndicate to seek a dictatorship in the state and blamed incumbent State's Attorney Crowe for the crime. The story put out by Crowe, that the bombing had probably been perpetrated by Deneen and Swanson for publicity purposes, impressed no one. Thus, using the slang of the gangster era of the '20s, this primary became known as the "pineapple primary" ("pineapple" being a slang term for a bomb).[82]

Small's opponents in the primary of 1928 again accused him of being connected with the Ku Klux Klan. Small denied any connection, but Emmerson made note of the fact that Small had had the endorsement of the Klan in 1924. There were also many accusations of connections with gangsterism through Thompson, and Glenn complained that Insull had money invested in the Small-Smith campaign and brought up the charge of Small's embezzlement of funds.

The *Chicago Tribune* endorsed Emmerson and Glenn in the state races and Lowden for president, four days before the primary commenting, "A Republican who cares at all for his party or his state cannot vote for Small. He will want to break the back of the present control and in the primaries Emmerson gives him the chance to do that. Governor Small is a calamity to Illinois and his attitude towards Chicago makes his continuance in office a threat to the city. Emmerson's success would eliminate him."[83]

The *Tribune* pointed out that Small had been forced to pay back more than $500,000 to the treasury, that he pushed franchise bills in the legislature for Insull, and that he had promised a gasoline tax that was unconstitutional. The editorial accused Small of creating a spoils system, noting that his son and son-in-law were on the state payroll, and of using the road-building program for political purposes. On the other hand, they said that Emmerson's record was a good one. Following up this editorial, the *Tribune* published another, entitled "Pineapples and Plunder," in which they linked Small with the gangsters through his control of law enforcement and the power of pardon.[84]

Moderate Republicans made an effort to connect Thompson and Long with Small and Smith. Hence the campaign was directed as much at Thompson as Small. Ed Litsinger, candidate for the Cook

County Board of Review, said that Big Bill Thompson had the "carcass of a rhinoceros and a brain of a baboon." The *Tribune* commented, "That hurt his feelings."

There was one further act of violence on primary day. Octavious C. Grenady, candidate for ward committeeman of the "bloody twentieth" ward, was machine-gunned to death. Grenady, a black veteran of World War I, was an ally of Deneen.[85]

Glenn beat Smith in the senatorial race by a vote of 855,356 to 611,897. Emmerson beat Small by the sizeable margin of 1,051,556 to 611,764. In the Democratic primaries, Floyd E. Thompson, unopposed, won the right to oppose Emmerson. Cermak defeated Monroe by a vote of 176,750 to 71,068. The day after the primary the *Tribune* was joyful in victory. They said editorially, "Small has been repudiated. Frank Smith will never again bring disgrace to Illinois, standing hat in hand at the door of the Senate begging for the seat he would dishonor. Illinois has purged herself of her shame."[86]

Subsequently there were threats of grand jury investigations of the violence attending the primary. The evidence showed that the murders of Grenady and Esposito and the attempts on the lives of Deneen and Swanson resulted from the close connection between gangsters and politicians. The *Tribune* alleged that Capone had toured Chicago on primary day on behalf of certain candidates that the gang wanted elected.[87]

Emmerson, dubbed "lop-eared Lou" by Thompson, was born in Albion in 1863. He had held a number of local and appointive offices, and his reputation was decidedly better than Small's. Born in Roodhouse, Floyd Thompson was only forty-one at the time he made the race for governor. He had been an editor, publisher, schoolteacher, and successful lawyer. Glenn was a man of unblemished reputation. Born in Mattoon, he had graduated from the University of Illinois and had been a state senator and state's attorney.[88]

The Republican national convention of 1928 opened in Kansas City on June 10. There had been interest in the convention in Illinois since Calvin Coolidge had announced the previous autumn that he did not "choose to run for president in 1928," and Thompson had sponsored a "draft Coolidge" boom, hoping to thwart the ambitions of Lowden, who was a prime contender for the Republican presidential nomination. But forty of the fifty districts had elected pro-Lowden delegates, and Lowden picked up ten at-large delegates in the state convention. Lowden's showing represented a defeat for Small and Thompson.

Several dissatisfied groups put in an appearance during the pre-convention activities, among them a cavalcade of Republican farmers near mutiny over the economy. Farmers faced increasingly difficult circumstances throughout the 1920s. The prices they paid for goods were kept artificially high, while the prices they received for produce were low. Lowden was more acceptable to farmers than Hoover, and President Coolidge had just vetoed the McNary-Haugen Bill, which it was hoped would bring some relief to farmers. So Lowden supported the farmers, particularly the plan for an equalization fee to bring up farm prices. The inevitable delegation of Pullman porters also showed up at the convention with signs demanding a higher wage and pointing up the Lowden connection with the Pullman Company.[89]

With most of the Illinois delegation supporting Lowden, senatorial candidate Glenn put Lowden's name in nomination. Thompson was still supporting Coolidge, and Wrigley favored Hoover. The Deneen forces, supporting Lowden, carried the day at the convention and managed to keep control of the delegation. Roy O. West, the long-time supporter and confidant of Deneen, was the principal strategist. Lowden announced that he would not be a candidate for president on the Republican ticket if the platform did not contain the Midwest farm plank. But as the convention opened, the farm plank was defeated and Lowden withdrew from the race. Then there was an argument over the liquor question, but the dries won this battle handily. There was also an unsuccessful "stop Hoover" movement in the preconvention activity of the farm-belt group, but after Andrew Mellon brought word that Coolidge would not accept the draft, the convention nominated Hoover on the first ballot. There was some struggle for the vice-presidency: General Dawes did not want to be renominated, so the convention turned to Charles Curtis of Kansas in an effort to reconcile the Midwesterners to the Hoover candidacy.[90]

The Democratic national convention opened in Houston later in June. The *Tribune* reported that "Houston's heat is like hell fire," and in this steaming atmosphere the rhetoric became even hotter. Most of the Illinois delegation, led by George Brennan, supported Al Smith, governor of New York. As the convention opened, Brennan and other Smith backers tried to keep the floor fights from getting out of hand. Many of the Illinois Democrats, who arrived in Houston on special trains, wore little bells in their lapels with the slogan "Ring it again with Al Smith." Among the Illinois delegation were J. Hamilton Lewis, former mayor Dever, Lewis

Stevenson, Michael Kenna, Tony Cermak, Adolph Sabath, F. X. Busch, Jacob Arvey, and T. J. Courtney.[91]

Farmers demanded a strong farm plank in the platform, but the great question before the convention opened was to what degree the convention would support repeal of the Eighteenth Amendment. Many people in the convention, including Smith and Brennan, favored immediate repeal, but not all delegates agreed. The *Tribune* suggested that the theme song of the convention should be "How Dry I Am."[92]

The keynote speaker was Claude Bowers, New York editor and sometime diplomat. Bowers laid on the Republicans in the harshest tones, proclaiming, "We battle for the honor of the nation, besmirched, and bedraggled by the most brazen and shameless carnival of corruption that ever blackened the reputation of the decent and self-respecting people." Hitting at the Republican record and using the new advertising terminology of the time, Bowers referred to "pillage and plunder—the gold dust twins of normalcy." Henry T. Rainey promised the convention that the corn belt would go to the Democrats if they had a strong farm plank. [93]

The name of Alfred E. Smith was put into nomination by Franklin Roosevelt, who was to run for governor of New York. In his speech for Smith, Roosevelt said, "We offer one who has the will to win—who not only deserves success but commands it. Victory is his habit—the happy warrior, Alfred E. Smith." The convention nominated Smith on the first ballot. To balance the ticket with Smith, a big city man who was for the repeal of prohibition, the convention nominated Senator Joseph Robinson of Arkansas for vice-president. Robinson was from a rural state and was a dry.[94]

As it turned out, the convention was dry indeed. It rejected the wet plank that Brennan and Cermak wanted, but it was made quite clear that Al Smith would work for the repeal of prohibition, so the dry delegates were rather sullen. In spite of their views on prohibition, though, the Illinois delegation stuck with Smith for the most part.

An additional antagonism at the convention involved religion. Southern delegates were not pleased with the nomination of a Roman Catholic for president, and there were fistfights on the floor as Southerners debated the issue of party loyalty versus religious or social principles.[95]

In the campaign for governor in 1928, Thompson pledged a reform administration. He promised legislation compelling publication of state payrolls, accounts of the use of public funds, and where public moneys were deposited. He called for election law reform, revision of the criminal code and judicial system, a more effective civil service law, revision of revenue and tax laws, better care for the mentally ill, better financing of highways, and laws for the protection of workers.

Emmerson pledged a businesslike administration in which efficiency would be the key. He promised to appoint good men to governmental posts, continued construction of roads through bond issues, a sound and just tax system, improvement of the condition of the farmer, a helpful attitude toward industry, protection of wage earners, help for the coal-mining industry, charitable institutions free from spoils politics, and progress in building the lakes-to-gulf waterway.

The *Tribune* held that Thompson was sounder on the good roads issue than were the Republican candidates headed by Emmerson, and in an editorial the newspaper endorsed Thompson, pointing up his good record and the fact that he had resigned his post of chief justice of the Supreme Court to run for governor, hoping to bring about the reformation of state politics. The *Tribune* felt Emmerson had been in state politics too long. It was noted that Thompson had made a sacrifice to run for the office, and it was hoped he would be a better man in the office than would Emmerson.[96]

Both Thompson and Emmerson pledged a more judicious use of the pardon power. Thompson promised to submit written opinions telling of his reasons for pardon. Emmerson said that he would not allow partisan politics to sway him in such matters.

The *Decatur Herald* and *Illinois State Register* endorsed Thompson as the best man to carry out the political house-cleaning so long overdue in Illinois, the latter in these words: "Young, vigorous and personifying the finest idealism in public and private life, Judge Thompson has conducted a brilliant campaign. He has carried the fight to the enemy and, win or lose, they will know they have been in a real contest. He has challenged the constitutional right of his opponent to hold the office of governor even if he shall be elected, and he has issued challenges to joint debate on vital issues. All these challenges have been rejected. His fight has not been a negative one. It has been positive and constructive.[97]

The senatorial race in Illinois was spirited. Tony Cermak promoted not only his own candidacy but also repeal of the Eighteenth Amendment, demanding that the states be allowed to decide their own liquor policy. He charged that the election of Hoover would spell the end of liberty and that the Republican party had sold out to the Anti-Saloon League. Cermak pointed to the increase of crime, insanity, hypocrisy, and corruption under prohibition. He closed his campaign with an attack on the dry forces and charged that Glenn was an alcoholic, producing a hospital chart which purported to show that Glenn had been hospitalized on three separate occasions for alcoholism. Glenn denied this, saying he had been in the hospital for a nervous ailment. Glenn admitted that he liked a bottle of beer now and then but insisted that he was not an alcoholic. He maintained that he was not pledged to any group, dry or wet, and denied not only the charge of alcoholism but also the implication that he was a hypocrite as well.[98]

Hoover did not come to Illinois to campaign, but he had plenty of support. Although Governor Lowden refused to endorse either candidate, Hoover got the endorsement of Jane Addams, Graham Taylor, Julia Lathrop, and Edith Abbott from the liberal social workers. Charles Evans Hughes came to Chicago to speak for Hoover and to say that Smith's speeches were claptrap. The *Decatur Herald* endorsed Hoover, as did the *Tribune*. Although it said that Smith was right on the wet issue, the *Tribune* endorsed Hoover editorially: "In his knowledge of international policies and interests throughout the markets of the globe, in his grasp of the economic laws effecting our industrial development and our commercial expansion, in his true conception of the relation of tariff protection and of immigration restriction to the continued prosperity of our industries and of our wage earning and agricultural classes, Mr. Hoover, both in official action and in public discussion, has demonstrated the soundness of his judgment and of his theories of public policy."[99]

Smith did come to Illinois, speaking in Alton, Bloomington, Springfield, Joliet, and Chicago. He had an audience of 10,000 in Springfield and 5,000 at Alton. Chicago gave Smith the full political treatment during his stay there. He had an auto tour of the city, spoke in the Armory, and watched a fireworks display in Grant Park across from the Congress Hotel, where he was staying. Mrs. Smith accompanied her husband to Illinois, went to a movie, and then had lunch at the home of Mrs. Kellogg Fairbank. Included among the guests were Mrs. Potter Palmer and Mrs. J. Hamilton Lewis.

In his speech in Chicago, Smith called the Republicans a

do-nothing party. He hit at the oil scandals, said that prohibition was a fiasco, and devoted himself to the farm problem. He noted that Lowden had ripped into the Coolidge farm policy and spoke appreciatively of Lowden. Of the Coolidge administration on prohibition he said, "Its record is one of double-dealing and double-crossing. The poor, weak, vacillating, broken-down Republican machine is unable to offer a constructive suggestion for the relief of the present intolerable situation." Smith maintained that the record of Coolidge was a guarantee of what might be expected of Hoover. Commenting further on prohibition Smith said, "As far as the fundamentals of relief from the situation, or scientific study of it, are concerned, the Republican party has played the old ostrich trick of sticking its head down in the sand because it neither hears nor sees anything, believes that everything is alright."

Smith had the endorsement of Senator George Norris and Senator Robert La Follette, both former Republican progressives. Smith supporters founded an organization called the Alfred E. Smith Independent League of Illinois, which included Mrs. Kellogg Fairbank, Mrs. Dorothy Aldus, Robert Allerton, Harold Fowler McCormick, Franklin MacVeagh, Agnes Nestor, Mrs. Joseph Ryerson, and Albert A. Sprague. Some of these, notably MacVeagh, were Republicans.[100]

Although the Democrats slated good candidates on both the national and state level, they were unable to achieve a victory. Hoover defeated Smith in Illinois by a vote of 1,769,141 to 1,313,817. Emmerson had 1,709,818 to Thompson's 1,284,879. In the senatorial race Glenn got 1,594,031 votes while Cermak got 1,315,338.

In the Illinois delegation to the Seventy-first Congress, the Republicans held their usual edge of twenty-one to six. Richard Yates continued in one of the at-large seats. The other was won by Ruth Hanna McCormick, widow of Medill McCormick and daughter of Marcus Alonzo Hanna. McCormick was the first woman to be elected to Congress from Illinois, and in this election Oscar De Priest, from the first district, became the first black person elected to Congress from Illinois. The election of these two testified to the changing importance of both women and Blacks.[101]

So ended the politics of the 1920s. It was an unappetizing period filled with corrupt politicians, gangsters, violence, and boodle. It was a dismal era for Illinois and even more dismal for the Democratic party. It was largely because of this period, because of the Smalls, the Frank Smiths, and the Big Bill Thompsons, that

Illinois came to be regarded as one of the most corrupt states. But with the election of Emmerson in 1928 Illinois made a modest beginning toward a better day.

1. H. L. Mencken, *On Politics; A Carnival of Buncombe*, ed. Malcolm Moos (New York, 1960), p. 149.

2. For a discussion of various forces in Chicago Politics, see Charles E. Merriam, *Chicago, a More Intimate View of Urban Politics* (New York, 1929), pp. 92–93.

3. Alex Gottfried, *Boss Cermak of Chicago: A Study in Political Leadership* (Seattle, 1962), pp. 52–56.

4. John Landesco, *Organized Crime in Chicago* (Chicago, 1968), pp. 42n, 87–88, 199; Lloyd Wendt and Herman Kogan, *Bosses in Lusty Chicago: The Story of Bathhouse John and Hinky Dink* (Bloomington, Ind., 1967), pp. 344–45.

5. Nine black representatives served at various times in the House of Representatives from 1900–1928. All were Republicans and all were elected from either the first or third districts. They were Edward H. Morris, Alexander Love, Robert Jackson, Edward D. Green, Sheadrick Bond Turner, Benjamin H. Lucas, B. Douglas, Adelbert H. Roberts, William F. King, George T. Kersy, and Charles H. Griffin. Short biographical sketches of each may be found in the *Illinois Blue Books*. See also Harold F.Gosnell, *Negro Politicians,the Rise of Negro Politics in Chicago* (Chicago, 1966), pp. 63–92. For Thompson's standing with Blacks see pp. 37–62. Harold Gosnell, *Machine Politics: Chicago Model* (Chicago, 1937), pp. 44–45. John Myers Allswang, *The Political Behavior of Chicago's Ethnic Groups, 1918–1932* (dissertation, University of Pittsburgh, 1957), p. 57. See also John M. Allswang, "The Chicago Negro Voter and the Democratic Consensus: A Case Study, 1918–1936." *Journal of the Illinois State Historical Society* (Summer, 1967), pp. 145–75.

6. Gosnell, *Machine Politics*, pp. 44–45.

7. Allswang, *Political Behavior*, pp. 122–62.

8. Ibid., pp. 86–107.

9. Ibid., pp. 54, 108–11, 264.

10. Merriam, *Chicago*, pp. 94–96.

11. Lloyd Wendt and Herman Kogan, *Big Bill of Chicago* (Indianapolis, 1953), pp. 81–86.

12. Merriam, *Chicago*, p. 95.

13. Harold Ickes, *The Autobiography of a Curmudgeon* (Chicago, 1969), pp. 240; Gottfried, *Cermak*, pp. 122–24.

14. Merriam, *Chicago*, pp. 178–79; Ickes, *Autobiography*, pp. 254–55.

15. Edward F. Dunne, *Illinois: The Heart of the Nation*, 5 vols. (Chicago, 1933), V, 12; Gottfried, *Cermak*, pp. 15–25.

16. Gottfried, *Cermak*, pp. 52–56; Gosnell, *Machine Politics*, p. 13.

17. Gosnell, *Machine Politics*, p. 12.

18. Merriam, *Chicago*, pp. 92–93.

19. Hutchison, *Lowden of Illinois: The Life of Frank O. Lowden*, 2 vols. (Chicago, 1957), II, 408–28.

20. Ickes, *Autobiography*, pp. 228–29.

21. Hutchison, *Lowden of Illinois*, II, 452–53; Francis Russell, *The Shadow of Blooming Grove: Warren G. Harding and His Times* (New York, 1968), p. 352.

22. Russell, *Shadow of Blooming Grove*, pp. 356–57.

23. Ibid., pp. 340, 357.

24. Ibid., pp. 344, 357–58.

25. Ibid., p. 357.

26. Ibid., pp. 356, 365.

27. Ibid., p. 365.

28. Ibid., pp. 379–80.

29. Mark Sullivan, *Our Times: The United States 1900–1925*, 6 vols. (New York, 1936), VI, 109.

30. Wendt and Kogan, *Big Bill*, pp. 184–87; Hutchison, *Lowden*, II, 471–72.

31. Hutchison, *Lowden*, II, 444–47.

32. Ibid., pp. 471–77; *Illinois Blue Book, 1921–22*, pp. 690, 692–93.

33. *Illinois Blue Book, 1921–22*, pp. 690, 692–93.

34. Dunne,*Illinois*, III, 33.

35. Ibid., III, 4; *Chicago Tribune*, Oct. 19, 1920, p. 2.

36. *Chicago Tribune*, Sept. 6, 1920,p. 5; Oct. 30, 1920, pp. 2, 6; Oct. 31,1920, p. 1; Nov. 1, 1920, p. 1.

37. Ibid., Oct. 17, 1920, part 1, p. 7; Frank Waldrop, *McCormick of Chicago, an Unconventional Portrait of a Controversial Figure* (Englewood Cliffs, N.J., 1966), p. 196.

38. *Chicago Tribune*, Oct. 16, 1920, p. 5; Oct. 17, 1920, part 1, p. 5.

39. Ibid., Oct. 17, 1920, part 1, p. 5, 6; Oct. 19, 1920, p. 2.

40. Ibid., Oct. 20, 1920, p. 2.

41. Ibid., Oct. 20, 1920, p. 2; Oct. 21, 1920, p. 4; Oct. 23, 1920, p. 5.

42. Ibid., Oct. 24, 1920, part 1, p. 4.

43. Ibid., Oct. 27, 1920, p. 4.

44. Ibid., Oct. 17, 1920, part 1, p. 5; Oct. 19, 1920, pp. 2, 12.

45. Ibid., Oct. 19, 1920, p. 12; Oct. 20, 1920, p. 2; Oct. 30, 1920, p. 6.

46. Ibid., Oct. 27, 1920, p. 7.

47. Ibid., Oct. 27, 1920, p. 4.

48. Ibid., Oct. 18, 1920, p. 8; Oct. 22, 1920, pp. 5, 8.

49. *Illinois State Register*, Nov. 1, 1920, pp. 1, 4; *Decatur Herald*, Nov. 2, 1920, p. 6.

50. *Illinois Blue Book, 1921–22*, pp. 768–71, 772–73, 790; Dunne, *Illinois*, II, p. 404.

51 *Illinois Blue Book, 1925–26*, pp. 1, 21–22; Len Small, *Illinois: Progress 1921–1928* (Springfield, Ill., 1928), p. 8.

52. Dunne, *Illinois*, II, 404–10; C. R. Miller to W. W. Murphy, Kankakee, Aug. 21, 1920, box 11, and typescript of testimony of Harry C. Leuhrs in folder 18, box 403, Small Papers, Illinois State Historical Library.

53. Dunne, *Illinois*, II, 404–10; Wendt and Kogan, *Big Bill*, pp. 204–5; Affadavits of Walter Repbow, Frank Reardon, John B. Felds, and Alex Smith, folder 16, box 403, Small Papers. See also *Chicago Tribune*, Apr. 6, 1924, part 1, p. 8. The *Tribune* reported that eight of the jurors received state jobs and that the sheriff who took care of the jury also was rewarded with a patronage job.

54. Dunne, *Illinois*, II, 404–10; Carroll H. Wooddy, *The Case of Frank L. Smith, A Study in Representative Government* (Chicago, 1931), p. 154.

55. Wendt and Kogan, *Big Bill*, p. 62.

56. *Illinois Blue Book, 1925–26*, p. 257; Hutchinson, *Lowden of Illinois*, II, 530; Dunne, *Illinois*, II, 424–54.

57. *Illinois: Progress 1921–1928*, pp. 140–51.

58. Ibid., pp. 3–4, 5, 269–79.

59. *Illinois Blue Book, 1927–28*, p. 790.

60. Wendt and Kogan, *Big Bill*, pp. 215–16; Hutchinson, *Lowden of Illinois*, II, 531–36; *Chicago Tribune*, Apr. 5, 1924, p. 8; Apr. 6, 1924, p. 25; Thurbow G. Essington Political leaflet, box 20, Small Papers.

61. *Chicago Tribune*, Apr. 6, 1924, part 1, p. 8; *Chicago Herald and Examiner*, Apr. 7, 1924, p. 8; *Illinois Blue Book, 1925–26*, pp. 870–71, 911–12.

62. *Chicago Tribune*, Apr. 6, 1924; part 1, p. 8; Apr. 9, 1924, p. 1; *Illinois Blue Book, 1925–26*, pp. 870–71, 911–12.

63. *Chicago Herald and Examiner*, June 9, 1924, p. 6; June 11, 1924, part 1, p. 1; Mark Sullivan, *Our Times*, pp. 247–52; *Chicago Tribune*, Apr. 2, 1924, p. 3; Apr. 8, 1924, p. 5; June 1, 1924, p. 1.

64. *Chicago Tribune*, June 9, 1924, pp. 2, 3; *Chicago Herald and Examiner*, June 9, 1924, p. 1; June 11, 1924, part 1, p. 1; June 12, 1924, part 2, p. 8.

65. *Chicago Tribune*, June 9, 1924, p. 1; June 11, 1924, p. 1; June 13, 1924, p. 1; *Chicago Herald and Examiner*, June 10, 1924, part 1, p. 1, June 13, 1924, part 1, p. 1.

66. *Chicago Tribune*, June 24, 1924, p. 1; *Chicago Herald and Examiner*, June 8, 1924, part 1, p. 1; June 26, 1924, part 1, p. 1; June 27, 1924, part 1, p. 2.

67. *Chicago Tribune*, Apr. 9, 1924, p. 5; June 8, 1924, part 1, p. 18, June 23, 1924, pp. 1, 2; June 26, 1924, p. 3; June 29, 1924, part 1, p. 1; *Chicago Herald and Examiner*, June 9, 1924, p. 7; June 24, 1924, part 1, p. 1; June 27, 1924, part 1, p. 1.

68. Belle LaFollette and Fola LaFollette, *Robert M. LaFollette*, 2 vols. (New York, 1953), pp. 1110–14.

69. W. A. Townsend and C. Boeschenstein, *Illinois Democracy: A History of the Party and Its Representative Members, Past and Present*, 4 vols. (Springfield, 1935), II, 58; *Chicago Tribune*, Apr. 2, 1924, p. 3; April 8, 1924, p. 5; June 1, 1924, p. 1.

70. *Illinois State Register*, Nov. 1, 1924, p. 5; *Chicago Tribune*, Oct. 16, 1924, p. 11; Oct. 22, 1924, p. 14.

71. *Chicago Tribune*, Oct. 28, 1924, p. 8; Oct. 29, 1924, p. 6; *Illinois State Register*, Nov. 1, 1924, p. 1.

72. *Chicago Tribune*, Oct. 21, 1924, p. 5; Oct. 23, 1924, p. 16; Oct. 29, 1924, p. 8; Nov. 1, 1924, p. 1; campaign speeches of Len Small, box 11 and 20, Small Papers.

73. *Chicago Tribune*, Oct. 23, 1924, p. 4; Nov. 2, 1924, part 1, p. 3. A copy of the pamphlet "Sex Pardons and Paroles by Governor Len Small" is in box 20, Small Papers.

74. *Chicago Tribune*, Oct. 17, 1924, p. 1.

75. *Illinois Blue Book, 1925–26*, pp. 809–13; *Illinois Blue Book, 1927–1928*, p. 790; Carrol H. Wooddy, *The Case of Frank L. Smith, a Study in Representative Government* (Chicago, 1931), p. 142; Ickes, *The Autobiography of a Curmudgeon*, p. 239.

76. *Illinois State Register*, Nov. 3, 1928, p. 3; Dunne, *History of Illinois*, II, 410–13; Wendt and Kogan, *Big Bill*, pp. 218–19, 267.

77. Wooddy, *Case of Frank L. Smith*, pp. 71–103.

78. Dunne, *Illinois*, II, 420–23.

79. Ibid., pp. 422–23. *Blue Book of Illinois, 1927–28*, p. 790.

80. Wooddy, *Case of Frank L. Smith*, p. 293.

81. Merriam, *Chicago* pp. 292–93.

82. Merriam, *Chicago* pp. 294–95.

83. *Chicago Tribune*, Apr. 3, 1928, p. 10; Apr. 4, 1928, p. 5; Apr. 5, 1928, pp. 1, 2, 7; Apr. 6, 1928, p. 10.

84. Ibid., Apr. 6, 1928, p. 10; Apr. 7, 1928, p. 10.

85. Ibid., Apr. 9, 1928, p. 1; Apr. 11, 1928, p. 1.

86. *Illinois Blue Book, 1928–29*, pp. 929, 931; *Chicago Tribune*, Apr. 11, 1928, p. 10.

87. *Chicago Tribune*, Apr. 12, 1928, p. 1.

88. Wendt and Kogan, *Big Bill*, p. 308; Dunne, *History of Illinois*, III, 18, 224–25; *Illinois Blue Book, 1929–30*, p. 122.

89. Hutchison, *Lowden of Illinois,* II, 580–83; *Chicago Tribune,* June 10, 1928, part 1, p. 10.

90. Hutchison, *Lowden of Illinois,* II, 584–601; *Chicago Tribune,* June 10, 1928, part 1, p. 3; June 11, 1928, p. 1; June 12, 1928, p. 1; June 15, 1928, p. 1; June 16, 1928, p. 1.

91. *Chicago Tribune,* June 24, 1928, part 1, p. 1; June 27, 1928, p. 1.

92. Ibid., June 25, 1928, p. 10.

93. Ibid., June 28, 1928, pp. 2, 6, 7.

94. Ibid., June 28, 1928, pp. 1, 2; June 29, 1928, p. 1; June 30, 1928, p. 1.

95. Ibid., June 28, 1928, p. 1.

96. *Illinois State Register,* Nov. 1, 1928, p. 9; *Chicago Tribune,* Oct. 7, 1928, p. 12; Oct. 26, 1928, pp. 14, 20; Oct. 28, 1928, part 1, p. 10; Nov. 2, 1928, p. 12.

97. *Illinois State Register,* Nov. 2, 1928, p. 4; Nov. 4, 1928, p. 4; Nov. 5, 1928, p. 5; *Chicago Tribune,* Oct. 17, 1928, p. 2; Oct. 26, 1928, p. 4; Oct. 27, 1928, p. 8.

98. *Decatur Herald,* Nov. 5, 1928, p. 1; *Illinois State Register,* Nov. 2, 1928, p. 1; Nov. 3, 1928, p. 1; *Chicago Tribune,* Apr. 8, 1928, part 1, p. 3; Oct. 26, 1928, p. 14; Oct. 27, 1928, p. 5; Oct. 30, 1928, p. 6; Nov. 2, 1928, p. 20.

99. *Chicago Tribune,* Nov. 1, 1928, p. 15; Nov. 4, 1928, part 1, p. 12; Oct. 25, 1928, p. 1; Oct. 31, 1928, p. 5; Nov. 1, 1928, p. 15; Nov. 4, 1928, part 1, p. 12; *Decatur Herald,* Nov. 4, 1928, p. 4.

100. *Chicago Tribune,* Oct. 16, 1928, p. 5; Oct. 17, 1928, p. 2; Oct. 18, 1928, pp. 1, 1; Oct. 19, 1928, p. 1.

101. *Illinois Blue Book, 1929–30,* pp. 740–43, 853.

13

The Structured Society: Illinois in 1928

Although poised on the brink of the Great Depression, Illinois, by 1928, had made great material strides. Population increased from 4,821,550 in 1900 to 7,630,654 in 1929. The state had literally passed from the horse-and-buggy age into the age of heavier-than-air flight. New products and labor-saving devices had made life easier for most citizens. Travel was faster and more convenient. As families acquired automobiles, new jobs were created in sales and maintenance of the novel machines. Wages increased and the workweek shortened. In 1913 a laborer in a blast furnace worked an average week of 72.5 hours for 17 cents per hour. In 1929 the workweek had been cut to 63.8 hours and the same laborer received an average of 37 cents per hour.[1]

The decrease in the length of the workweek was a real gain, but the increase in wages was deceptive. Using 1913 prices as a base for a cost-of-living index of 100, the cost-of-living index in 1928 was 171.3. In other words, the dollar in 1928 was worth about 65 cents in terms of its purchasing power.

Factory workers produced an astounding quantity of goods by 1930 and farmers an equally astounding abundance of food products. Yet most did not receive a fair share of their production.

Illinois contributed heavily to the intellectual life of the nation through the great universities and institutions such as the Art Institute, Chicago Symphony, and Chicago Opera, as well as deriving talent and genius from its sons and daughters who became writers, composers, and performers. The shorter workweek and general increase in affluence brought the need for a popular culture, fulfilled through radio, motion pictures, and a popular literature.

Illinois progressed in providing rights and opportunities for women, who gained the right to vote and provided a symbolic rebellion against Victorianism through drastic changes in dress and behavior. Partly because of World War I, new job opportunities for women opened up, and when the war ended, women did not give up their newfound freedom.

Not all was progress, however. Robert Cowley has noted that the '20s were beset by problems that are usually identified with the 1970s. These problems, acquired in the name of progress, included urban decay, traffic, crime, pollution of air and water, and political corruption. Cowley notes that in the '20s these problems were still manageable, but no solutions were sought.[3]

The period brought other changes. The life-style of Illinoisians became more frenetic as transportation, communications, and the pressure to produce speeded up life. And there was a new impersonality: citizens began to feel like cogs in machines.

Perhaps the most striking feature of the new style was the way in which society was structured. In politics, for example, there was an increasing ability of machine organizations to control and manipulate. Industry was controlled more and more by combinations of business under the influence of bankers and lawyers. Although labor organization was not yet as strong as it would become, the destiny of workers was more in the hands of unions. Cities began to find it necessary to organize recreation through municipal playgrounds and programs. Sports became big business.

Nearly everything was controlled and structured so that individuality was hampered. World War I hastened this process in the name of patriotism. But freedom that is surrendered, however temporarily, can never be wholly regained, and somehow the confidence, optimism, and self-reliance of the people were lost. Only the farmer was an exception, and his world was more precarious and circumscribed in 1928 than in 1900 because of his increased dependence on outside forces for his livelihood.

The citizens of Illinois were the beneficiaries of the industrialized society but were its victims as well. Material progress was inevitable and irreversible. Illinoisians, by and large, lived a more comfortable life in 1928 than in 1900. But they also lost a little.

1. U.S. Bureau of the Census, *Abstract of the Fifteenth Census of the United States* (Washington, D. ., 1933), pp. 55, 336; *Statistical Abstract of the United States, 1900* (New York, 1964), p. 6.

2. U.S. Bureau of the Census, *Statistical Abstract of the United States, 1929* (Washington, D. ., 1929), pp. 329, 347; *Abstract of the Fifteenth Census of the United States* (Washington, D.C., 1933), pp. 792–93.

3. Robert Cowley, "The Jazz Age: A Shadow on the Seventies," *Saturday Review,* N.S., 2, May 17, 1975, p. 13.

Bibliography

PRIMARY SOURCES

MANUSCRIPT COLLECTIONS

Federal Writers Project. A collection of historical manuscripts and materials gathered under the auspices of the Works Progress Administration.

Oglesby Papers. Letters and documents of Lieutenant Governor John G. Oglesby. Illinois State Historical Library.

Papers of the Springfield Association of Commerce and Industry. Illinois State Historical Library.

Sherman Papers. Letters and documents of Senator Lawrence Y. Sherman. Illinois State Historical Library.

Small Papers. Letters and documents relating to Governor Len Small. Illinois State Historical Library.

NEWSPAPERS

Chicago:

Broadax
Chicago Daily Inter-Ocean
Chicago Daily Journal
Chicago Daily News
Chicago Defender
Chicago Evening Post
Chicago Herald and Examiner
Chicago Record
Chicago Record-Herald
Chicago Tribune
Chicago Whip

Downstate Illinois:

Belleville Advocate
Cairo Bulletin

Centralia Sentinel
Champaign Daily News
Decatur Herald
East St. Louis Daily Journal
Evening Citizen (Cairo)
Forum (Springfield)
Illinois State Journal (Springfield)
Illinois State Register (Springfield)
Quincy Daily Whig
Rockford Register-Gazette
Rock Island Argus
Springfield Record

Out-of-state:

New York Age

Printed Memoirs and Autobiographies

Anderson, Margaret. *My Thirty Years War*. New York, 1930.

Anderson, Sherwood. *Sherwood Anderson's Memoirs*. New York, 1942.

Armstrong, Louis. *Satchmo*. New York, 1954.

Carnevali, Emanuel. *The Autobiography of Emanuel Carnevali*. Compiled and prefaced by Kay Boyle. New York, 1968.

Cullom, Shelby M. *Fifty Years of Public Service*. Chicago, 1911.

Dawes, Charles G. *The First Year of the Budget of the United States*. New York, 1923.

———. *Journal as Ambassador to Great Britain*. New York, 1939.

———. *A Journal of the Great War*. New York, 1923.

———. *A Journal of the McKinley Years*. Chicago, 1959.

———. *A Journal of Reparations*. New York, 1939.

———. *Notes as Vice President*. Boston, 1935.

Dell, Floyd. *Homecoming*. New York, 1933.

Duster, Alfreda M., ed. *Crusade for Justice: The Autobiography of Ida B. Wells*. Chicago, 1970.

Garden, Mary, and Louis Biancoli. *Mary Garden's Story*. New York, 1951.

Hansen, Harry. *Midwest Portraits: A Book of Memories and Friendships*. New York, 1923.

Harrison, Carter H. *Growing up with Chicago*. Chicago, 1944.

———. *Stormy Years*. Indianapolis, 1938.

Hopkins, Claude C. *My Life in Advertising*. Chicago, 1966.

Ickes, Harold. *Autobiography of a Curmudgeon*. Chicago, 1969.

James, Henry, ed. *The Letters of William James*. 2 vols. Boston, 1920.

Johnson, Jack. *Jack Johnson Is a Dandy: An Autobiography*. New York, 1969.

Jones, Mary H. *Autobiography of Mother Jones*. Chicago, 1925.

Lovett, Robert Morss. *All Our Years*. New York, 1948.

Masters, Edgar Lee. *Across Spoon River*. New York, 1936.

Monroe, Harriet. *A Poet's Life: Seventy Years in a Changing World*. New York, 1938.

Nearing, Scott. *The Making of a Radical: A Political Autobiography*. New York, 1972.

Thomas, Rose Fay. *Memoirs of Theodore Thomas*. New York, 1911.

Thomas, Theodore. *A Musical Autobiography*. 2 vols. Chicago, 1905.

Washington, Booker T. *Up from Slavery*. New York, 1901.

Wright, Frank Lloyd. *An Autobiography*. New York, 1943.

Zeitling, Jacob, and Horner Woodbridge, eds. *Life and Letters of Stuart Pratt Sherman*. New York, 1919.

Illinois Documents

Andros, S. O. "Coal Mining Practice in District II." *Illinois State Geological Survey Bulletin* 7. Urbana, 1914.

———. "Coal Mining Practice in District III." *Illinois State Geological Survey Bulletin* 9. Urbana, 1915.

———. "Coal Mining Practice in District IV." *Illinois State Geological Survey Bulletin* 12. Urbana, 1915.

———. "Coal Mining Practice in District V." *Illinois State Geological Survey Bulletin* 6. Urbana, 1914.

———. "Coal Mining Practice in District VI." *Illinois State Geological Survey Bulletin* 8. Urbana, 1914.

———. "Coal Mining Practice in District VII." *Illinois State Geological Survey Bulletin* 4. Urbana, 1914.

"The Automobile and the Village Merchant." *Bureau of Business Research Bulletin* 41. Urbana, 1928.

Blatchley, Raymond S. "Petoleum in Illinois in 1912 and 1913." *Illinois State Geological Survey Circular* 8. Urbana, n.d.

Burlinson, W. L. and O. M. Allyn. "Soybeans and Cowpeas in Illinois." *University of Illinois Agricultural Experiment Station Bulletin* 198. Urbana, 1917.

Cady, Gilbert H. "Coal Resources of District I." *Illinois State Geological Survey Bulletin* 10. Urbana, 1915.

"A Compilation of the Reports of the Mining Industry of Illinois from the Earliest Records to 1954."

Converse, Paul D. "The Automobile and the Village Merchants." *Bureau of Business Research Bulletin* 19. Urbana, 1928.

———. "Business Mortality of Illinois Retail Stores from 1925 to 1930." *Bureau of Business Research Bulletin* 41. Urbana, 1932.

———. "Price and Services of Chain and Independent Stores in Champaign-Urbana." *Natma Bulletin*. Urbana, Ill., 1931.

DeTurk, E. E., F. C. Bauer, and L. H. Smith. "Lessons from the Morrow Plots." *University of Illinois Agricultural Experiment Station Bulletin* 300. Urbana, 1927. Ewing, J. A., comp. *Illinois Agricultural Statistics*. Illinois Department of Agriculture, Springifield, 1948.

Ewert, Arthur F. "Early History of Education in Illinois—The Three Oldest Colleges." *Illinois Blue Book 1928–1929*. Springfield, 1929, pp. 301–04.

Final Report of the State Council of Defense of Illinois 1917–1918–1919. Chicago, 1919.

Garcia, John A. "A Mining Engineer's View of the Future of the Illinois Coal Industry from the Standpoint of Recovery." *Illinois State Geological Survey Bulletin* 60. Urbana, 1931.

Graham, Herman D. "The Economics of Strip Coal Mining with Special Reference to Knox and Fulton Counties, Illinois." *Bulletin of Bureau of Economic and Business Research* 60. Urbana, 1948.

Handschin, W. F., J. B. Andrews, and E. Rauchenstein. "The Horse and the Tractor: An Economic Study of Their Use on Farms in Central Illinois." *University of Illinois Agricultural Experiment Station Bulletin* 231. Urbana, 1921.

Illinois Agricultural Statistics Circular 445. Springfield, 1949.

Illinois Blue Book, 1903, 1905, 1907, 1909, 1911, 1912–13, 1913–14, 1915–16, 1917–18, 1919–20, 1921–22, 1923–24, 1925–26, 1927–28,

1928–29, 1929–30.

Jenison, Marguerite. *War Documents and Addresses.* Springfield, 1923.

Johnston, P. E., and K. H. Myers. "Harvesting the Corn Crop in Illinois: An Economic Study of Methods and Relative Costs." *University of Illinois Agricultural Experiment Station Bulletin* 373. Urbana, 1931.

Laws of the State of Illinois Passed by the Forty-first General Assembly. Chicago, 1899.

Laws of the State of Illinois Passed by the Forty-fourth General Assembly. Springfield, 1905.

Laws of the State of Illinois Passed by the Forty-fifth General Assembly. Springfield, 1907.

Laws of the State of Illinois Passed by the Forty-sixth General Assembly. Springfield, 1909.

Laws of the State of Illinois Passed by the Forty-seventh General Assembly. Springfield, 1911.

Laws of the State of Illinois Passed by the Forty-seventh General Assembly at the Third Special Session. Springfield, 1912.

Laws of the State of Illinois Passed by the Forty-eighth General Assembly. Springfield, 1913.

Laws of the State of Illinois Passed by the Fiftieth General Assembly. Springfield, 1917.

Laws of the State of Illinois Passed by the Fifty-first General Assembly. Springfield, 1919.

Laws of the State of Illinois Passed by the Fifty-second General Assembly. Springfield, 1921.

Laws of the State of Illinois Passed by the Fifty-third General Assembly. Springfield, 1923.

Mitchell, Robert V. "Trends in Rural Retailing in Illinois, 1926 to 1938." *Bulletin of the Bureau of Business Research* 59. Urbana, 1939.

Norton, L. J., and B. B. Wilson. "Prices of Illinois Farm Products from 1886 to 1929." *University of Illinois Agricultural Experiment Station Bulletin* 351. Urbana, 1930.

O'Hara, Barratt. *Report of the Senate Vice Committee Created under the Authority of the Senate of the Forty-ninth General Assembly as a Continuation of the Committee Created under the Authority of the Senate of the Forty-eighth General Assembly, State of Illinois.* Chicago, 1916.

Report of Illinois Department of Mines and Minerals 1955. Springfield, 1955.

U.S. DOCUMENTS

Biographical Directory of the American Congress 1774–1961. Washington, D.C., 1961.

Congressional Record, 65th Congress, 1 session, 1917, part 1, vols. 3, 12, and 52.

Money Trust Investigations before a Subcommittee of the Committee on Banking and Currency: Interlocking Directorates. 3 vols. Washington, D.C., 1913.

Plessy *vs.* Ferguson, 165 U.S. 537, 1896.

Report on the Enforcement of the Prohibition Laws of the United States. House Document no. 722, 71st Congress, 3rd session. Washington, D.C., 1931.

Report upon the Illegal Practices of the United States Department of Justice. Washington, D.C., 1931.

Swift and Company *vs.* United States, 196 U.S. 375, 1905.

Tolley, H. R., and L. M. Church. "The Standard Day's Work in Central Illinois. Performance of Implements and Crews as Indicated by Reports from 600 Farmers in a Typical Corn-Belt Area." *U.S. Department of Agriculture Bulletin* 814. Washington, D.C., 1920.

U.S. Bureau of the Census. *Abstract of the Census of Manufacturing, 1914.* Washington, D.C., 1917.

————. *Abstract of the Twelfth Census of the United States.* Washington, D.C., 1900.

————. *Biennial Census of Manufacturing, 1927.* Washington, D.C., 1930.

————. *Fifteenth Census of the United States, 1930.* Washington, D.C., 1932.

————. *Fifteenth Census of the United States, 1930: Abstract.* Washington, D.C., 1933.

————. *Fifteenth Census of the United States, 1930: Agriculture.* Washington, D.C., 1932.

————. *Fifteenth Census of the United States, 1930: Manufacturers.* Washington, D.C., 1933.

————. *Fifteenth Census of the United States, 1929: Manufacturers: Reports by Industries.* Washington, D.C., 1933.

————. *Fifteenth Census of the United States, 1930: Population.* Washington, D.C., 1932.

————. *Fifteenth Census of the United States, 1930: Distribution: Retail Change.* Washington, D.C., 1933.

————. *Fourteenth Census of the United States, 1920: Manufacturers.* Washington, D.C., 1924.

————. *Fourteenth Census of the United States, 1920: State Compendium: Illinois.* Washington, D.C., 1924.

————. *The Negro Population of the United States, 1790–1915.* New York, 1969.

————. *Statistical Abstract of the United States, 1900.* New York, 1964.

————. *Statistical Abstract of the United States, 1929.* Washington, D.C., 1929.

————. *Thirteenth Census of the United States: Agriculture.* Washington, D.C., 1912.

————. *Thirteenth Census of the United States Taken in the Year 1910: Manufacturers, Reports by States.* Washington, D.C., 1912.

————. *Twelfth Census of the United States: Manufacturers.* Washington, D.C., 1900.

————. *Twelfth Census of the United States: Occupations.* Washington, D.C., 1900.

————. *Twelfth Census of the United States: Population*. Washington, D.C., 1900.

United States *vs.* International Harvester Company, 24 U.S. 693, 1927.

MISCELLANEOUS REPORTS, DIRECTORIES, AND ANNUALS

Art Institute of Chicago. *Annual Report for 1910–11, 1911–12, 1913–14, 1918, 1922, 1924.*

————. *Annual Report for the Year Ending June 1, 1907*. Chicago, 1907.

————. *Annual Report for the Year Ending June 1, 1909*. Chicago, 1909.

————. *Twenty-First Annual Report of the Trustees for the Year Ending June 1, 1900*. Chicago, 1900.

Central States Guide to Railroad, Traction, Motor Bus, and Hotels. Nov., 1926.

Defense News Bulletin. 1917, 1918.

Directory of Sangamon County's Colored Citizens: A History of the Negro in Sangamon County: A Director of Lodges, Churches, Parks, Amusements, Mechanics, Business Firms, and Citizens. Springfield, Ill., 1926.

The Economic Almanac for 1941–1942. New York, 1941.

Lewis, Robert G. *The Handbooks of American Railroads*. New York, 1951.

Marquis, Albert Nelson, ed. *Who's Who in America, 1940–1941*. Chicago, 1940.

Official Directory of Classified Industries for the Buyers and Shippers on the Illinois Central Railroad, Yazoo, and Mississippi Valley Railroad. Chicago, 1925.

Poor's Manual of Industrials. 1914, 1928.

Poor's Manual of Railroads. New York, 1924.

The Springfield Survey. 3 vols. Springfield, 1918.

University of Illinois Studies in Language and Literature. Urbana, 1915.

A Yearbook of Railroad Information. New York, 1930.

MISCELLANEOUS CONTEMPORARY MAGAZINES, ADVERTISEMENTS, AND COMMENTARY

Aero: America's Aviation Weekly
Chemistry
Chicago Banker
Flying
Good Housekeeping
Illinois Business Review
Literary Digest
Railway Age
Saturday Evening Post

SECONDARY SOURCES

BOOKS

Abbott, Edith. *Women in Industry: A Study in American Economic History*. New York, 1910.

————. *The Tenements of Chicago, 1908–1935.* Chicago, 1936.

Alinsky, Saul, *John L. Lewis: An Unauthorized Biography.* New York, 1949.

Allen, John W. *Legends and Lore of Southern Illinois.* Carbondale, Ill., 1963.

Allen, Lee. *The World Series: The Story of Baseball's Annual Championship.* New York, 1969.

Alvord, Clarence Walworth. *The Illinois Country 1673–1818.* Springfield, Ill., 1920.

Anderson, Sherwood. *Winesburg, Ohio.* John H. Ferres, ed. New York, 1966.

Angle, Paul. *Bloody Williamson: A Chapter in American Lawlessness.* New York, 1952.

Armour, J. Ogden. *The Packers, the Private Car Lines and the People.* Philadelphia, 1906.

Asbury, Herbert. *The Great Illusion: An Informal History of Prohibition.* Garden City, N.Y., 1950.

Association of American Railroads. *A Chronicle of American Railroads, Including Mileage by States and Years.* Washington, D.C., 1957.

Bacon, Raymond Foss, and William Allen Hamor. *The American Petroleum Industry.* 2 vols. New York, 1916.

Barber, H. L. *Story of the Automobile.* Chicago, 1917.

Baritz, Loren. *The Culture of the Twenties.* Indianapolis, 1970.

Bateman, Newton, and Paul Selby. *History of Sangamon County.* 2 vols. Chicago, 1912.

Bauer, Marion. *Twentieth Century Music, How It Developed, How to Listen to It.* New York, 1933.

Beaton, Kendall. *Enterprise in Oil.* New York, 1957.

Beckman, Theodore, and Herman C. Nolen. *The Chain Store Problem: A Critical Analysis.* New York, 1938.

Beckner, Earl R. *A History of Labor Legislation in Illinois.* Chicago, 1929.

Berstein, Irving. *The Lean Years: A History of the American Worker 1920–1933.* Baltimore, 1966.

Best, R. B. *We Are What We Have To Be.* New York, 1965.

Bloomfield, Daniel. *Chain Stores.* New York, 1931.

Bogart, Ernest Ludlow, and John Mabry Matthews. *The Modern Commonwealth 1893–1918.* Springfield, Ill., 1920.

Bolles, Blair. *Tyrant from Illinois.* New York, 1951.

The Book of Chicagoans, 1917. Chicago, 1917.

Boulware, Marcus H. *The Oratory of Negro Leaders 1900–1968.* Westport, Conn., 1969.

Brawley, Benjamen. *A Social History of the American Negro.* New York, 1921.

Bridges, Roger D. *New Salem: A Memorial to Abraham Lincoln.* Springfield, Ill., 1934.

Bright, John. *Hizzoner Big Bill Thompson.* New York, 1930.

Brissenden, Paul F. *Earnings of Factory Workers 1899–1927.* Washington, D.C., 1929.

————. *The I.W.W.: A Study of American Syndicalism.* New York, 1957.

Brody, David. *The Butcher Workmen, a Study of Unionization.* Cambridge, Mass., 1964.

————. *Labor in Crisis: The Steel Strike of 1919.* New York, 1965.

Buckler, Helen. *Daniel Hale Williams, Negro Surgeon.* New York, 1968.

Buder, Stanley. *Pullman: An Experiment in Industrial Order and Community Planning.* New York, 1967.

The Building of Mid-America: 20 Railroad Stories as Told by a Fifth Generation of an Illinois Central Family. n.p., n.d. (A copy is in the Illinois Historical Survey, Urbana.)

Burnes, Robert E. *50 Golden Years of Sports.* St. Louis, 1948.

Chafee, Zechariah, Jr. *Free Speech in the United States.* Cambridge, Mass., 1954.

Chalmers, David M. *Hooded Americanism: The History of the Ku Klux Klan.* Chicago, 1968.

Chicago Commission on Race Relations. *The Negro in Chicago.* Chicago, 1922.

Church, Charles A. *History of the Republican Party in Illinois 1854–1912.* Rockford, Ill., 1912.

Clark, Victor S. *History of Manufactures in the United States.* 3 vols. New York, 1929.

Cochran, Thomas C. *The American Business System: A Historical Perspective 1900–1955.* New York, 1957.

Coleman, Charles H. *Eastern Illinois State College: Fifty Years of Public Service.* Charleston, Ill., 1950.

Corliss, Carlton J. *Main Line of Mid-America: The Story of the Illinois Central.* New York, 1950.

Crampton, John A. *The National Farmers Union: Ideology of a Pressure Group.* Lincoln, Nebr., 1965.

Craven, Thomas, ed. *Cartoon Cavalcade.* New York, 1943.

Creel, George. *Rebel at Large, Recollections of Fifty Crowded Years.* New York, 1957.

Cronin, Edmund David. *Black Moses: The Story of Marcus Garvey and the Universal Negro Improvement Association.* Madison, Wis., 1955.

Daniels, Josephus. *The Wilson Era: Years of War and after 1917–1923.* Chapel Hill, N.C., 1946.

Davis, Allen F. *Spearheads for Reform: The Social Settlements and the Progressive Movement 1890–1914.* New York, 1967.

Davis, J. McCan. *The Breaking of the Deadlock.* Springfield, Ill., 1904.

Davis, Ronald L. *A History of Opera in the American West.* Englewood Cliffs, N.J., 1965.

————. *Opera in Chicago.* New York, 1966.

Derleth, August. *The Milwaukee Road: Its First Hundred Years.* New York, 1948.

Douglas, Paul H. *Real Wages in the United States 1890–1926.* New York, 1966.

————, and Aaron Director. *The Problem of Unemployment.* New York, 1934.

————, Curtice N. Hitchcock, and Wilfred E. Adkins. *The Worker in Modern Society.* Chicago, 1923.

Downing, Kenneth W. *With a Cinder in My Eye: A Layman's Memory and Sketches of American Trains.* Moline, Ill., 1951.

Draper, Theodore. *American Communism and Soviet Russia.* New York, 1960.

————. *The Roots of American Communism.* New York, 1957.

Dreiser, Theodore. *Jennie Gerhart.* New York, 1911.

————. *Sister Carrie.* New York, 1965.

Dubofsky, Melvin. *We Shall Be All: A History of the Industrial Workers of the World,* Chicago, 1969.

Du Bois, W. E. B. *The Souls of Black Folk.* Chicago, 1903.

Duffey, Bernard, *The Chicago Renaissance in American Letters: A Critical History.* Lansing, Mich., 1954.

Dunne, Edward F. *Illinois: The Heart of the Nation.* 5 vols. Chicago 1933.

Emmett, Boris, and John E. Jenck. *Catalogs and Counters, a History of Sears, Roebuck and Company.* Chicago, 1950.

Epstein, Ralph C. *The Automobile Industry.* Chicago, 1928.

Evans, James F. *Prairie Farmer and WLS: The Burridge D. Butler Years.* Urbana, Ill., 1969.

Falls, Cyril. *The Great War.* New York, 1959.

Farrell, John C. *Beloved Lady: A History of Jane Addams' Ideas on Reform and Peace.* Baltimore, 1967.

Farrington, S. Kip. *Railroads of Today.* New York, 1949.

Faulkner, Harold U. *The Decline of Laissez Faire 1897–1917.* New York, 1951.

Fay, S. B. *The Origins of the World War.* New York, 1928.

Fisher, Irving. *The Noble Experiment.* New York, 1930.

Fite, Gilbert C. *George N. Peek and the Fight for Farm Parity.* Norman, Okla., 1954.

Fulton, Albert R. *Motion Pictures; The Development of an Art from Silent Films to the Age of Television.* Norman, Okla., 1960.

Gelb, Barbara. *So Short a Time: A Biography of John Reed and Louise Bryant.* New York, 1973.

Gilbert, Douglas. *American Vaudeville: Its Life and Times.* New York, 1940.

Gilman, William H., Alfred R. Ferguson, and Merrell R. Davis. *The Journals and Miscellaneous Notebooks of Ralph Waldo Emerson, 1822–1826.* Cambridge, Mass., 1961.

Ginger, Ray. *The Bending Cross: A Biography of Eugene Victor Debs.* New Brunswick, N.J., 1949.

Glaab, Charles N. *The American City.* Homewood, Ill., 1963.

Goermer, Fred. *The Search for Amelia Earhart.* New York, 1966.

Gosnell, Harold F. *Machine Politics: Chicago Model.* Chicago, 1937.

————. *Negro Politicians, the Rise of Negro Politics in Chicago.* Chicago, 1935.

Gottfried, Alex. *Boss Cermak of Chicago: A Study in Political Leadership.* Seattle, 1962.

Green, Abel, and Joe Laurie, Jr. *Show Biz from Vaude to Video.* New York, 1951.

Greene, Lorenzo, and Carter G. Woodson. *The Negro Wage Earner.* Washington, D.C., 1930.

Griffith, Richard, and Arthur Mayer. *The Movies.* New York, 1970.

Grimes, William A. *Financing Automobile Sales by the Time Payment Plan.* Chicago, 1926.

Gross, Ben. *I Looked and I Listened: Informal Recollections of Radio and T.V.* New York, 1970.

Hadlock, Richard. *Jazz Masters of the Twenties.* New York, 1965.

Hall, Charles E. *Negroes in the United States 1920–1932.* Washington, D.C., 1935.

Hampton, Benjamen B. *A History of the Movies.* New York, 1931.

Hampton, Taylor. *The Nickel Plate Road: The History of a Great Railroad.* New York, 1947.

Harlow, Alvin F. *The Road of the Century: The Story of the New York Central.* New York,1947.

Harrison, Shelby, ed. *The Springfield Survey.* 3 vols. Springfield, Ill., 1918.

Hayter, Earl W. *Education in Transition: The History of Northern Illinois University.* De Kalb, 1974.

Hecht, Ben. *A Child of the Century.* New York, 1954.

Hicken, Victor. *The Purple and the Gold: The Story of Western Illinois University.* Macomb, Ill., 1970.

Hicks, Granville. *John Reed, The Making of a Revolutionary.* New York, 1968.

Hilton, George W., and John F. Due. *The Electric Interurban Railway in America.* Stanford, Calif., 1960.

Hofstadter, Richard. *The Age of Reform.* New York, 1955.

Holbrook, Stewart. *The Age of Moguls.* Garden City, N.Y., 1953.

———. *The Story of American Railroads.* New York, 1941.

Howard, John Tasker. *Our American Music: Three Hundred Years of It.* New York, 1939.

———, and George Kent Bellows. *A Short History of Music in America.* New York, 1957.

Howe, Irving. *Sherwood Anderson.* New York, 1951.

———, and Lewis Coser. *The American Communist Party: A Critical History (1919–1957).* Boston, 1957.

Hoxie, Robert Franklin. *Trade Unionism in the United States.* New York, 1921.

Hoyt, Edwin P. *That Wonderful A & P.* New York, 1969.

Huegy, Harvey W. *Economics of Installment Credit.* Urbana, Ill., 1934.

Husband, Joseph. *The Story of the Pullman Car.* Chicago, 1917.

Hutchison, William T. *Lowden of Illinois: The Life of Frank O. Lowden.* 2 vols. Chicago, 1957.

Illinois Association for Criminal Justice. *The Illinois Crime Survey.* Chicago, 1929.

Jackson, Kenneth T. *The Ku Klux Klan in the City 1915–1930.* New York, 1967.

Jenison, Marguerite. *The War-time Organization of Illinois.* Springfield, Ill., 1923.

Jewel Tea Co. *Working for Jewel*. Chicago, 1927.

Johnson, Henry. *The Other Side of Main Street*. New York, 1943.

Johnson, James D. *Aurora 'n' Elgin, Being a Compendium of Word and Picture Recalling the Everyday operations of the Chicago, Aurora and Elgin Railroad*. Wheaton, Ill., 1965.

Kakir, Sudhir. *Frederick Taylor: A Study in Personality and Innovation*. Cambridge, Mass., 1970.

Karolvitz, Robert F. *This Was Trucking: Pictorial History of the First Quarter Century of Commercial Motor Vehicles*. Seattle, 1966.

Kile, Orville Merton. *The Farm Bureau through Three Decades*. Baltimore, 1948.

Kipnis, Ira. *The American Socialist Movement 1897–1912*. New York, 1952.

Knight, Arthur. *The Liveliest Art: A Panoramic History of the Movies*. New York, 1957.

Kolko, Gabriel. *The Triumph of Conservatism: A Reinterpretation of American History, 1900–1916*. Chicago, 1963.

La Follette, Bela. *Robert M. La Follette*. 2 vols. New York, 1953.

Lafore, Lawrence. *The Long Fuse: An Interpretation of the Origins of World War I*. New York, 1965.

Landesco, John. *Organized Crime in Chicago*. Chicago, 1968.

Laurie, Joseph. *Vaudeville: From the Honky Tonks to the Palace*. New York, 1953.

Lebhar, Godfrey M. *Chain Stores in America, 1859–1950*. New York, 1952.

Lee, Henry. *How Dry We Were*. Englewood Cliffs, NJ., 1963.

Le Massena, C. E. *Galli-Curci's Life of Song*. New York, 1945.

Lentz, Eli G. *Seventy-five Years in Retrospect: Southern Illinois University, 1874–1949*. Carbondale, Ill., 1955.

Levin, Murray B. *Political Hysteria in America*. New York, 1971.

Lifshey, Earl. *The Housewares Story*. Chicago, 1973.

Lindbergh, Charles A. *We*. New York, 1927.

Lindsey, Almont. *The Pullman Strike*. Chicago, 1942.

Lomax, Alan. *The Folk Songs of North America in the English Language*. New York, 1960.

Lomax, John, and Alan Lomax. *American Ballads and Folk Songs*. New York, 1934.

Lord and Thomas. *Book of Advertising Tests: Articles That Actually Say Something about Advertising*. Chicago, n.d.

———. *Concerning a Literature Which Compels Action: Altruism in Advertising*. Chicago, 1911.

———. *Real Salesmanship in Print: Strategy in Advertising*. Chicago, 1911.

Madison, Charles A. *American Labor Leaders*. New York, 1950.

Marshall, Helen E. *Grandest of Enterprises: Illinois State Normal University, 1857–1874*. Normal, Ill., 1956.

Masters, Edgar Lee. *Vachel Lindsay, a Poet in America*. New York, 1935.

McCarthy, Mary. *The Company She Keeps*. New York, 1942.

McCormick, Cyrus. *The Century of the Reaper*. New York, 1931.

McDonald, Forest. *Insull*. Chicago, 1962.

McKinney, Isabel. *Mr. Lord: The Life and Words of Livingston C. Lord.* Urbana, Ill., 1937.

Meeker, Arthur. *Chicago with Love: A Polite and Personal History.* New York, 1955.

Mencke, Frank. *The Encyclopedia of Sports.* New York, 1963.

Mencken, August. *The Railroad Passenger Car: An Illustrated History of the First Hundred Years with Accounts by Contemporary Passengers.* Baltimore, 1957.

Mencken, H. L. *On Politics; A Carnival of Buncombe.* Malcolm Moos, ed. New York, 1960.

Mendalowitz, David H. *A History of American Art.* New York, 1964.

Merriam, Charles. *Chicago, a More Intimate View of Urban Politics.* New York, 1929.

Merz, Charles. *The Dry Decade.* Seattle, 1930.

Middleton, William D. *The Interurban.* Milwaukee, 1961.

Mitchell, John. *Organized Labor, Its Problems, Purposes and Ideals and the Present Future of American Wage Earners.* Philadelphia, 1903.

Mott, Frank Luther. *American Journalism—a History: 1690–1960.* New York, 1969.

Mowry, George. *The Era of Theodore Roosevelt.* New York, 1958.

———. *The Twenties: Fords, Flappers, and Fanatics.* Englewood Cliffs, N.J., 1963.

Mueller, John H. *The American Symphony Orchestra: A Social History of Musical Taste.* Bloomington, Ind., 1951.

Murray, Robert K. *Red Scare, a Study in National Hysteria.* New York, 1964.

National Association for the Advancement of Colored People. *Thirty Years of Lynching in the United States 1889–1918.* New York, 1969.

Nevins, Allan. *Illinois.* New York, 1917.

Nowlan, James D., comp. *Illinois Major Party Platforms 1900–1964.* Urbana, Ill., 1966.

O'Connor, Richard, and Dale Walker. *The Lost Revolutionary: A Biography of John Reed.* New York, 1968.

Overton, Richard C. *Burlington Route: A History of the Burlington Lines.* New York, 1965.

Ovington, Mary White. *The Walls Came Tumbling Down.* New York, 1947.

Patterson, Joseph Medill. *A Little Brother of the Rich.* New York, 1908.

Paulsen, Norman M., comp. and ed. *Three-I League Record Book.* Waterloo, Iowa, 1950.

Peisch, Mark L. *The Chicago School of Architecture: Early Followers of Sullivan and Wright.* New York, 1964.

Pennsylvania Railroad Company. *1846—One Hundred Years of Transportation Progress—1946: A Brief History of the Pennsylvania Railroad.* n.p., 1945.

Perlman, Selig, and Philip Taft. *Labor Movements.* Vol. 4 of *History of Labor in the United States, 1896–1932.* New York, 1935.

Peterson, Florence. *Strikes in the United States, 1880–1936.* Washington, D.C., 1938.

Peterson, H. C., and Gilbert Fite. *Opponents of War 1917–1918*. Seattle, 1957.

Plochman, George K. *The Ordeal of Southern Illinois University*. Carbondale, Ill., 1957.

Presby, Frank. *The History and Development of Advertising*. Garden City, N.Y., 1929.

Preston, William, Jr. *Aliens and Dissenters: Federal Suppression of Radicals 1903–1933*. Cambridge, Mass., 1963.

Pullman Company. *"No. 9": The Story of the First Pullman Car and the Evolution of Travel Comfort in 65 Years*. Chicago, 1924.

Rae, John B. *The American Automobile*. Chicago, 1965.

———. *American Automobile Manufacturers: The First Forty Years*. Philadelphia, 1959.

Rammelkamp, Charles H. *Illinois College: A Centennial History, 1829–1929*. New Haven, Conn., 1929.

Randall, Frank A. *History of the Development of Building Construction in Chicago*. Urbana, Ill., 1949.

Randel, William Pierce. *The Ku Klux Klan, a Century of Infamy*. New York, 1965.

Raper, Arthur F. *The Tragedy of Lynching*. New York, 1970.

Rayback, Joseph G. *A History of American Labor*. New York, 1959.

Reck, Franklin M. *The 4-H Story: A History of 4-H Club Work*. Ames, Iowa, 1951.

Renshaw, Patrick. *The Wobblies: The Story of Syndicalism in the United States*. Garden City, N.Y., 1968.

Republicans of Illinois, a Portrait and Chronological Record of Members of the Republican Party. Chicago, 1905.

Rice, James M. *Peoria: City and County, Illinois*. Chicago, 1912.

Rogers, W. G. *Ladies Bountiful*. New York, 1968.

Rose, Arnold. *The Negro in America*. New York, 1944.

Rowsome, Frank. *They Laughed When I Sat Down, an Informal History of Advertising in Words and Pictures*. New York, 1959.

Rudwick, Elliott M. *Race Riot at East St. Louis, July 2, 1917*. Carbondale. Ill., 1964.

Russell, Francis. *The Shadow of Blooming Grove: Warren G. Harding and His Times*. New York, 1968.

Saloutos, Theodore, and John D. Hicks. *Twentieth Century Populsm: Agricultural Discontent in the Middle West 1900–1913*. Lincoln, Nebr., n.d.

Sandburg, Carl. *The American Songbag*. New York, 1927.

———. *The Chicago Race Riots: July, 1919*. New York, 1919.

Scamehorn, Howard L. *From Balloons to Jets*. Chicago, 1957.

Seligman, Edwin R. A. *The Economics of Installment Selling: A Study in Consumer Credit with Special Reference to the Automobile*. 2 vols. New York, 1927.

Serof, Victor I. *Debussy, Musician of France*. New York, 1956.

Shapiro, Nat, and Nat Hentoff. *Hear Me Talkin' to Ya: The Story of Jazz by the Men Who Made It.* New York, 1955.

Sharfman, I. Leo. *The American Railroad Problem, a Study in War and Reconstruction.* New York, 1921.

Shean, Vincent. *Oscar Hammerstein I: The Life and Exploits of an Impressario.* New York, 1956.

Sinclair, Upton. *The Jungle.* New York, 1965.

Small, Len. *Illinois Progress 1921–1928.* Springfield, Ill., 1928.

Smalley, Orange A., and Frederick D. Sturdevant. *The Credit Merchants, a History of Spiegel, Inc.* Carbondale, Ill., 1973.

Smtith, Daniel M. *The Great Departure.* New York, 1956.

Soule, George. *Prosperity Decade: From War to Depression, 1917–1929.* New York, 1947.

Spear, Allen H. *Black Chicago: The Making of a Negro Ghetto 1890–1920.* Chicago, 1970.

Spence, Hartzell. *Portrait in Oil: How the Ohio Oil Company Grew to Become Marathon.* New York, 1962.

Spencer, A. P. *Centennial History of Highland, Illinois, 1837–1937.* Highland, Ill., 1937.

Spero, Sterling D., and Abram L. Harris, *The Black Worker, the Negro and the Labor Movement.* Port Washington, N.Y., 1931.

Staley, Eugene. *History of the Illinois State Federation of Labor.* Chicago, 1930.

Starr, John W. *One Hundred Years of American Railroading.* New York, 1928.

Stearns, Marshall Winslow. *The Story of Jazz.* New York, 1956.

Strickland, Arvarh E. *History of the Chicago Urban League.* Urbana, Ill., 1966.

Sullivan, Louis H. *The Autobiography of an Idea.* New York, 1924.

Sullivan, Mark. *Our Times: The United States 1900–1925.* 6 vols. New York, 1936.

Swanberg, W. A. *Dreiser.* New York, 1965.

Swift, Louis Franklin. *The Yankee of the Yards: Biography of Gustavus Franklin Swift.* Chicago, 1927.

Swisher, Carl Brent. *American Constitutional Development.* New York, 1943.

Taff, Charles A. *Commercial Motor Transportation.* Homewood, Ill., 1961.

Taft, Phillip A. *The A.F.L. in the Time of Gompers.* New York, 1957.

Tallmadge, Thomas E. *The Story of Architecture in America.* New York, 1927.

Tarbell, Ida M. *The Life of Elbert H. Gary: The Story of Steel.* New York, 1925.

Tarr, Joel A. *A Study in Boss Politics: William Lorimer of Chicago.* Urbana, Ill., 1971.

Tate, H. Clay. *The Way It Was in McClean County, 1972–1822.* Bloomington, Ill., 1972.

Taylor, Albion G. *Labor Policies of the National Association of Manufacturers.* Urbana, Ill., 1928.

Taylor, Frederick W. *The Principles of Scientific Management.* New York, 1939.

Thompson, Slason. *A Short History of American Railways.* Freeport, N.Y., 1925.

Tingley, Donald F., ed. *Essays in Illinois History*. Carbondale, Ill., 1968.

Townsend, W. A., and C. Boeschenstein. *Illinois Democracy: A History of the Party and Its Representative Members, Past and Present*. 4 vols. Springfield, Ill., 1935.

Tumulty, Joseph. *Woodrow Wilson as I Knew Him*. New York, 1921.

Turkin, Hy, and S. C. Thompson. *The Official Encyclopedia of Baseball*. New York, 1963.

Tuttle, William M., Jr. *Race Riot: Chicago in the Red Summer of 1919*. New York, 1970.

Ulanov, Barry. *A History of Jazz in America*. New York, 1957.

Waldrop, Frank C. *McCormick of Chicago, an Unconventional Portrait of a Controversial Figure*. Englewood Cliffs, N.J., 1966.

Waller, Robert A. *Rainey of Illinois, a Political Biography, 1903–34*. Urbana, Ill., 1977.

Watkins, Damon D. *Keep the Home Fires Burning, a Book about the Coal Mines*. Columbus, Ohio, 1937.

Watkins, Gordon S. *Labor Problems and Administration during the World War*. Urbana, Ill., 1919.

Webster, Martha F. *The Story of Knox College, 1837–1912*. Galesburg, Ill., 1912.

Weinstein, James. *The Decline of Socialism in America 1912–1925*. New York, 1967.

Wendt, Lloyd and Herman Kogan. *Big Bill of Chicago*. Indianapolis, 1953.
———. *Bosses in Lusty Chicago: The Story of Bathhouse John and Hinky Dink*. Bloomington, Ind., 1967.

White, Walter. *Rope and Faggot: A Biography of Judge Lynch*. New York, 1929.

Wiebe, Robert H. *Business Men and Reform: A Study of the Progressive Movement*. Chicago, 1962.

Williams, Martin. *The Jazz Tradition*. New York, 1970.

Williamson, Harold F., Ralph L. Andreane, Arnold R. Daum, and Gilbert C. Klose. *The American Petroleum Industry: The Age of Energy 1899–1959*. Evanston, Ill., 1963.

Wilson, Kenneth L., and Jerry Brondfield. *The Big Ten*. Englewood Cliffs, N.J., 1967.

Wood, James P. *The Story of Advertising*. New York, 1958.

Wooddy, Carroll H. *The Case of Frank L. Smith, a Study in Representative Government*. Chicago, 1931.

Wright, Harold E. *Financing of Automobile Installment Sales*. Chicago, 1927.

MAGAZINE AND JOURNAL ARTICLES

Allswang, John M. "The Chicago Negro Voter and the Democratic Concensus: A Case Study, 1918–1936." *Journal of the Illinois State Historical Society* (summer, 1967): 145–75.

Ayres, Milton. "Installment Selling and Finance Companies." *Annals of the American Academy of Political and Social Science* 196 (Mar., 1938): 121–29.

"The Battle of the Skirts." *Outlook* 132 (Oct. 18, 1922): 275–76.

Bridges, Roger D. "The Origins and Early Years of the Illinois State Historical Society." *Journal of the Illinois State Historical Society* 68 (Apr., 1975).

Buenker, John. "Edward F. Dunne: The Urban New Stock Democrat as Progressive." *Mid-America* 50 (Jan., 1968): 3–21.

Carter, John F., Jr. "'These Wild Young People': By One of Them." *Atlantic Monthly* 126 (Sept., 1920): 301–4.

Cole, Arthus C. "Illinois and the Great War." In Bogart and Matthews, *The Modern Commonwealth 1893–1918.* pp. 452–91.

Cowley, Robert. "The Jazz Age: A Shadow on the Seventies." *Saturday Review,* N.S. 2 (May 17, 1975): 12–18.

Crouthamel, James L. "The Springfield Race Riot of 1908." *Journal of Negro History* 45 (July, 1960): 164–81.

Dilliard, Irving. "When Woodrow Wilson Was Invited to Head the University of Illinois." *Journal of the Illinois State Historical Society* 60 (winter, 1967): 370–76.

Du Bois, W. E. B. "The Talented Tenth." In Booker T. Washington, ed., *The Negro Problem: A Series of Articles by Representative Negroes of Today,* New York, 1903, pp. 31–75.

Due, John F. "The Life Cycle of an Industry: The Electric Interurban Railway." *Current Economic Comment* 22 (Feb., 1960): 25–42.

———. "The Rise and Decline of the Midwest Interurban." *Current Economic Comment* 14 (Aug., 1952): 36–51.

Duffus, Robert L. "The Age of Play." *Independent* 113 (Dec. 20, 1924): 539–40, 556.

Foster, William Trufant. "The Basic Meaning of the Growth of Installment Selling." *Proceedings of the American Academy of Political Science* 12 (1926–28): 612–18.

Garrett, Romeo B. "The Role of the Duryea Brothers in the Development of the Gasoline Automobile." *Journal of the Illinois State Historical Society* 68 (Apr., 1975): 174–80.

Grundy, Mr. "Polite Society."*Atlantic Monthly* 125 (May, 1920): 606–12.

Gunther, John. "The High Cost of Hoodlums." *Harper's Monthly Magazine* 159 (Oct., 1929): 529–40.

Heilman, Ralph E. "Chicago Traction, a Study in the Efforts of the Public to Secure Good Service." *American Economic Quarterly,* third series, 9, 1908.

Hickey, Donald R. "The Praeger Affair: A Study in Wartime Hysteria." *Journal of the Illinois State Historical Society* 62 (summer, 1969): 117–34.

Hodge, John E. "The Chicago Civic Opera Company, Its Rise and Fall." *Journal of the Illinois State Historical Society* 55 (spring, 1962): 5–30.

Hough, Clarence A. "The Art Institute of Chicago." *Art and Archaeology* 12 (Sept.-Oct., 1921): 144–53.

Ihder, John. "Housing in Springfield, Illinois." In Harrison, *The Springfield Survey,* vol. 1, pp. 16–17.

"Is the Younger Generation in Peril." *Literary Digest* 69 (May 14, 1921): 9–12, 58.

Keiser, John H. "Black Strikebreakers and Racism in Illinois, 1865–1900." *Journal of the Illinois State Historical Society* 65 (autumn, 1972): 313–26.

————. "John H. Walker: Labor Leader from Illinois." In Tingley, ed., *Essays in Illinois History,* pp. 75–100.

Lambert, Belle Short. "The Women's Club Movement in Illinois." *Transactions of the Illinois State Historical Society* 9, 1904.

Lasker, Albert. "The Personal Reminiscences of Albert Lasker." *American Heritage* 6 (Dec., 1954): 73–89.

Lewis, Lloyd. "The De Luxe Picture Palace." *New Republic* 58 (Mar. 27, 1929): 175–76.

Lochard, Metz T. P. "The Negro Press in Illinois." *Journal of the Illinois State Historical Society* 56 (autumn, 1963): 570–91.

Lovett, Robert Morss. "The Trial of the Communists." *Nation* 111 (Aug. 14, 1920): 185–86.

Martin, John Bartlow. "The Sheltons: America's Bloodiest Gang." *Saturday Evening Post* 222 (Mar. 18, 1950): 24–25, 48–70.

McCauley, Lena M. "Friends of American Art." *Art and Archaeology* 12 (Sept.-Oct., 1921): 173–78.

————. "Some Collectors of Paintings." *Art and Archaelogy* 12 (Sept.-Oct., 1921): 154–72.

Ovington, Mary White. "Beginnings of the NAACP." *Crisis* 32 (June, 1926): 76–77.

Poole, Ernest. "The Meat Strike." *Independent* 57 (July 28, 1904): 179–84.

Purdy, Lawson. "Installment Purchasing and Installment Saving in Relation to Family Welfare." *Proceedings of the Academy of Political Science* 12 (1926–28): 608–11.

Rammelkamp, Charles H. "Four Historic Societies of Jacksonville, Illinois." *Journal of the Illinois State Historical Society* 18 (Apr., 1925).

Rovensky, John. "The Relation of Installment Selling to the Credit Structure." *Proceedings of the Academy of Political Science* 12 (1926–28): 595–99.

Scharr, Bernard E. "The Origins of the Plastics Industry.'" *Chemistry* 40 (Nov., 1967): 19–20.

Scott, Roy V. "John Patterson Stelle: Agrarian Crusader from Southern Illinois." *Journal of the Illinois State Historical Society* 55 (autumn, 1962): 229–49.

Voigt, David Quentin. "The Chicago Black Sox and the Myth of Baseball's Single sin." *Journal of the Illinois State Historical Society* 62 (autumn, 1969): 293–306.

Walling, William. "Race War in the North." *Independent* 65 (Sept. 3, 1908): 529–34.

Wrone, David. "Illinois Pulls Out of the Mud." *Journal of the Illinois State Historical Society* 58 (spring, 1965): 54–76.

Theses and Dissertations

Adams, Frank Glenn. "Anti-German Sentiment in Madison and St. Clair Counties: 1916–1919." Thesis, Eastern Illinois University, Charleston, Ill., 1966.

Allswang, John Myers. "The Political Behavior of Chicago's Ethnic Groups, 1918–1932." Dissertation, University of Pittsburgh, 1957.

Davenport, Cora Lillian. "The Rise of the Armours, an American Industrial Family." Thesis, University of Chicago, 1930.

Doherty, Richard Paul. "Origin and Development of Chicago O'Hare International Airport." Dissertation, Ball State University, Muncie, Ind., 1971.

Keiser, John H. "John Fitzpatrick and Progressive Unionism 1915–1925. Dissertation, Northwestern University, Evanston, Ill., 1965.

Lilly, Samuel Alvin. "The Political Career of Roger C. Sullivan." Thesis, Eastern Illinois University, Charleston, Ill., 1964.

Tingley, Donald F. "The Rise of Racialistic Thinking in the United States in the Nineteenth Century." Dissertation, University of Illinois, Urbana, Ill., 1952.

Recordings

Columbia Records, KCS 9943, "Hello, I'm Johnny Cash." Sung by Johnny Cash.

Sun Records, #127, "Original Golden Hits," vol. 3. Sung by Johnny Cash.

Warner Brothers Records, MS 2060, "Hobo's Lullaby." Sung by Arlo Guthrie.

Index

HANDBOOK OF HEALTH PSYCHOLOGY
AND BEHAVIORAL MEDICINE

Handbook of
Health Psychology
and Behavioral Medicine

Jerry M. Suls
Karina W. Davidson
Robert M. Kaplan

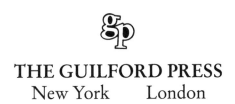

New York   London

Library of Congress Cataloging-in-Publication Data

Handbook of health psychology and behavioral medicine / edited by Jerry M. Suls, Karina W. Davidson, Robert M. Kaplan.
      p. ; cm.
   Includes bibliographical references and index.
   ISBN 978-1-60623-895-0 (hardcover: alk. paper)
   1. Clinical health psychology—Handbooks, manuals, etc.   2. Medicine and psychology—Handbooks, manuals, etc.   I. Suls, Jerry M.   II. Davidson, Karina W.   III. Kaplan, Robert M.
   [DNLM: 1. Behavioral Medicine. 2. Psychological Theory. 3. Psychology, Medical. WB 103 H2365 2010]
   R726.7.H365 2010
   616.001′9—dc22

                                        2010009373

About the Editors

Jerry M. Suls, PhD, is Professor of Psychology and Collegiate Fellow at the University of Iowa and also an affiliate of its College of Public Health. Dr. Suls has published over 150 articles and chapters and edited over 10 volumes. He has also served as Chair of the National Institutes of Health Behavioral Medicine Interventions and Outcomes Study Section and as President of Division 38 (Health Psychology) of the American Psychological Association. His research focuses on psychological risk factors for cardiovascular disease, symptom perception, and social norms about health behaviors.

Karina W. Davidson, PhD, is the Herbert Irving Associate Professor of Behavioral Medicine in Medicine and Psychiatry and Director of the Center for Behavioral and Cardiovascular Health at Columbia University. She has published over 120 articles, chapters, and monographs. Dr. Davidson's research focuses on interventions for, and the biopsychosocial mechanisms implicated in, anger and depression as predictors of worse outcomes for patients with cardiovascular disease. She has been the recipient of service awards from the Society of Behavioral Medicine and the American Psychological Association and is also the Founding Convener of the Cochrane Behavioral Medicine Field.

Robert M. Kaplan, PhD, is Distinguished Professor of Health Services at the University of California, Los Angeles, and Distinguished Professor of Medicine at the University's David Geffen School of Medicine. He is an elected member of the Institute of Medicine of the National Academy of Sciences and past president of several organizations, including Division 38 (Health Psychology) of the American Psychological Association, the Society of Behavioral Medicine, and the Academy of Behavioral Medicine Research. Dr. Kaplan is Editor-in-Chief of *Health Psychology* and former Editor-in-Chief of the *Annals of Behavioral Medicine*. He is the author, coauthor, or editor of more than 18 books and approximately 450 articles or chapters.

Contributors

Dennis Abraham, MD, Division of Cardiovascular Medicine, Duke University Medical Center, Durham, North Carolina

Austin S. Baldwin, PhD, Department of Psychology, Southern Methodist University, Dallas, Texas

Estela Blanco, MPH, Division of Global Public Health, Department of Medicine, University of California, San Diego, La Jolla, California

Ulrike Boehmer, PhD, School of Public Health, Boston University, Boston, Massachusetts

Hayden B. Bosworth, PhD, Center for Health Services Research in Primary Care, Health Services Research and Development Service, Durham Veterans Administration Medical Center, Durham, North Carolina

Deborah Bowen, PhD, Department of Community Health Science, School of Public Health, Boston University, Boston, Massachusetts

Jonathan B. Bricker, PhD, Division of Public Health Sciences, Fred Hutchinson Cancer Research Center, and Department of Psychology, University of Washington, Seattle, Washington

Jose L. Burgos, MD, MPH, Department of Medicine, University of California, San Diego, La Jolla, California

Alan J. Christensen, PhD, Department of Psychology, University of Iowa, Iowa City, Iowa

Christopher L. Coe, PhD, Harlow Center for Biological Psychology, University of Wisconsin, Madison, Wisconsin

Karina W. Davidson, PhD, Center for Behavioral Cardiovascular Health, Division of General Medicine, Columbia University, New York, New York

Maximilian de Courten, MD, MPH, Department of Epidemiology and Preventive Medicine, Monash University, Melbourne, Australia

Catherine S. Diefenbach, MD, Clinical Cancer Center, Department of Medicine, New York University, New York, New York

Michael A. Diefenbach, PhD, Department of Urology and Oncological Sciences, Mount Sinai School of Medicine, New York, New York

William W. Dressler, PhD, Department of Anthropology, University of Alabama, Tuscaloosa, Alabama

Merrill F. Elias, PhD, MPH, Department of Psychology and Graduate School of Biomedical Sciences, University of Maine, Orono, Maine

Angela Fagerlin, PhD, Center for Behavioral and Decision Sciences in Medicine, Division of General Medicine, University of Michigan, and Ann Arbor VA Health Services Research and Development, Ann Arbor, Michigan

Lucy F. Faulconbridge, PhD, Center for Weight and Eating Disorders, Department of Psychiatry, University of Pennsylvania, Philadelphia, Pennsylvania

Emma Frean, MPH, Department of Epidemiology and Preventive Medicine, Monash University, Melbourne, Australia

Howard S. Friedman, PhD, Department of Psychology, University of California Riverside, Riverside, California

Melanie A. Greenberg, PhD, Veterans Affairs Medical Center, San Diego, California

Yaniv Hanoch, PhD, School of Psychology, University of Plymouth, Plymouth, Devon, United Kingdom

Manjunath Harlapur, MD, Center for Behavioral Cardiovascular Health, Division of General Medicine, Columbia University, New York, New York

Alison K. Herrmann, MS, Division of Cancer Prevention and Control Research, School of Public Health, University of California, Los Angeles, Los Angeles, California

Laura Higginbotham, BA, School of Medicine, University of Virginia, Charlottesville, Virginia

Karen Hooker, PhD, Center for Healthy Aging Research, Department of Human Development and Family Sciences, Oregon State University, Corvallis, Oregon

Padmini Iyer, BS, Center for Behavioral Cardiovascular Health, Division of General Medicine, Columbia University, New York, New York

Jean E. Johnson, PhD, RN, FAAN, School of Nursing, University of Wisconsin, Madison, Wisconsin, and School of Nursing, University of Rochester, Rochester, New York

Robert M. Kaplan, PhD, Department of Health Services, School of Public Health, University of California, Los Angeles, Los Angeles, California

Quinn D. Kellerman, MA, Department of Psychology, University of Iowa, Iowa City, Iowa

Friederike Kendel, PhD, Institute for Medical Psychology, Charité–Universitätsmedizin Berlin, Berlin, Germany

Margaret L. Kern, PhD, Department of Psychology, University of California, Riverside, Riverside, California

Marc T. Kiviniemi, PhD, Department of Health Behavior, University at Buffalo, Buffalo, New York

Maya Rom Korin, PhD, Center for Behavioral Cardiovascular Health, Division of General Medicine, Columbia University, New York, New York

Ian M. Kronish, MD, Division of General Internal Medicine, Mount Sinai School of Medicine, New York, New York

Diane Lauver, PhD, RN, FNP-BC, FAAN, School of Nursing, University of Wisconsin, Madison, Madison, Wisconsin

Madeline Li, MD, PhD, Department of Psychosocial Oncology and Palliative Care, Princess Margaret Hospital, Toronto, Ontario, Canada

William R. Lovallo, PhD, Behavioral Sciences Labs, Veterans Affairs Medical Center, Oklahoma City, Oklahoma

Tana Luger, MA, Department of Psychology, University of Iowa, Iowa City, Iowa

Devin Mann, MD, Division of General Internal Medicine, Mount Sinai School of Medicine, New York, New York

René Martin, PhD, RN, Center for Research in the Implementation of Innovative Strategies in Practice, Veterans Affairs Medical Center, and College of Nursing, University of Iowa, Iowa City, Iowa

Philip M. McCabe, PhD, Department of Psychology, University of Miami, Coral Gables, Florida

Jeanne M. McCaffery, PhD, Weight Control and Diabetes Research Center, Department of Psychiatry and Human Behavior, Miriam Hospital, Brown Medical School, Providence, Rhode Island

John Mirowsky, PhD, Population Research Center and Department of Sociology, University of Texas at Austin, Austin, Texas

Nihal E. Mohamed, PhD, Department of Urology, Mount Sinai School of Medicine, New York, New York

Sarosh J. Motivala, PhD, Cousins Center for Psychoneuroimmunology, Semel Institute, Department of Psychiatry and Biobehavioral Sciences, University of California, Los Angeles, Los Angeles, California

Daniel A. Nation, PhD, Department of Psychiatry, University of California, San Diego, La Jolla, California

Perry M. Nicassio, PhD, Cousins Center for Psychoneuroimmunology, Semel Institute, Department of Psychiatry and Biobehavioral Sciences, University of California, Los Angeles, Los Angeles, California

Brian Oldenburg, PhD, Department of Epidemiology and Preventive Medicine, Monash University, Melbourne, Victoria, Australia

JoEllen Patterson, PhD, Marriage and Family Therapy Program and Department of Family Medicine, University of San Diego, San Diego, California

Thomas L. Patterson, PhD, Department of Psychiatry, University of California, San Diego, La Jolla, California

Kenneth A. Perkins, PhD, Department of Psychiatry, Western Psychiatric Institute and Clinic, University of Pittsburgh, Pittsburgh, Pennsylvania

Ellen Peters, PhD, Decision Research, Eugene, Oregon

Thomas Rice, PhD, Vice Chancellor's Office, University of California, Los Angeles, Los Angeles, California

Dylan Habeeb Roby, PhD, Department of Health Services and Center for Health Policy Research, School of Public Health, University of California, Los Angeles, Los Angeles, California

Gary Rodin, MD, Department of Psychosocial Oncology and Palliative Care, Princess Margaret Hospital, Toronto, Ontario, Canada

Catherine E. Ross, PhD, Population Research Center and Department of Sociology, University of Texas at Austin, Austin, Texas

Alexander J. Rothman, PhD, Department of Psychology, University of Minnesota, Minneapolis, Minnesota

Amy M. Sawyer, PhD, RN, School of Nursing, University of Pennsylvania, and Philadelphia Veterans Affairs Medical Center, Philadelphia, Pennsylvania

Joseph E. Scherger, MD, MPH, Department of Family Medicine, University of California, San Diego, San Diego, California, and Eisenhower Medical Center, Rancho Mirage, California

Neil Schneiderman, PhD, Department of Psychology, University of Miami, Coral Gables, Florida

Alan Schwartz, PhD, Department of Medical Education, University of Illinois at Chicago, Chicago, Illinois

Daichi Shimbo, MD, Center for Behavioral Cardiovascular Health, Division of General Medicine, New York, New York

Ilene C. Siegler, PhD, Department of Psychiatry and Behavioral Sciences, Duke University Medical Center, Durham, North Carolina

Ann Marie Smith, MA, Department of Family Medicine, University of San Diego, San Diego, California

Avron Spiro, PhD, Department of Epidemiology, Boston University and Massachusetts Veterans Epidemiology Research and Information Center, VA Boston Healthcare System, Boston, Massachusetts

Sara M. St. George, MA, Department of Psychology, University of South Carolina, Columbia, South Carolina

Steffanie A. Strathdee, PhD, Division of Global Public Health, Department of Medicine, University of California, San Diego, La Jolla, California

Jerry M. Suls, PhD, Department of Psychology, University of Iowa, Iowa City, Iowa

Gina Turner, PhD, Division of Humanities and Social Sciences, Northampton Community College, Bethlehem, Pennsylvania

Thomas A. Wadden, PhD, Center for Weight and Eating Disorders, Department of Psychiatry, University of Pennsylvania, Philadelphia, Pennsylvania

Terri E. Weaver, PhD, RN, School of Nursing and Center for Sleep and Respiratory Neurobiology, Division of Sleep Medicine, University of Pennsylvania School of Medicine, Philadelphia, Pennsylvania

Gerdi Weidner, PhD, Department of Biology, San Francisco State University, San Francisco, California

Rebecca West, MS, RN, FNP-BC, School of Nursing, University of Wisconsin, Madison, Madison, Wisconsin

David A. Williams, PhD, Departments of Anesthesiology, Internal Medicine/Rheumatology, Psychiatry, and Psychology, University of Michigan School of Medicine, Ann Arbor, Michigan

Dawn K. Wilson, PhD, Department of Psychology, University of South Carolina, Columbia, South Carolina

Nicole Zarrett, PhD, Department of Psychology, University of South Carolina, Columbia, South Carolina

Brian J. Zikmund-Fisher, PhD, Center for Behavioral and Decision Sciences in Medicine, Division of General Medicine, University of Michigan, and Ann Arbor VA Health Services Research and Development, Ann Arbor, Michigan

María Luisa Zúñiga, PhD, Division of Child Development and Community Health, Department of Medicine, University of California, San Diego, La Jolla, California

of diseases, including cancer, heart disease, infection, hypertension, psoriasis, and other conditions. The critiques were quite conventional and focused largely on methodology. For example, Relman and Angell argued that the studies did not apply traditional statistical techniques, such as the intention-to-treat principle. When patients are randomly assigned to treatment or to placebo groups, it is not uncommon for some patients to cross over and gain the treatment to which they were not assigned. Statisticians have concluded that the least bias occurs when patients are analyzed as though they got the treatment to which they were assigned, even though they crossed over. They use the expression "once randomized, always analyzed" (Hollis & Campbell, 1999).

It was argued that some of the better-known results, such as Spiegel, Bloom, Kraemer, and Gottheil's (1989) classic study on the effects of psychotherapy for breast cancer patients, could not be replicated by other investigators (Coyne, Hanisch, & Palmer, 2007). Similar criticisms were leveled at studies of interventions to reduce heart disease through modifications of Type A behavior (Friedman et al., 1986). We discuss the issue of Type A behavior later in the chapter. Relman and Angell (2002) also argued that the observational studies on psychosocial effects had serious methodological flaws, including confounding, weak effects, and overinterpretation of data because of multiple comparisons. Few of the studies were systematic clinical trials, and many of the inferences were based on correlational evidence. The critics argued that the psychosocial literature had failed to establish causal relationships and that investigators had often overinterpreted their results (Relman & Angell, 2002).

Williams and Schneiderman countered that virtually all studies have methodological problems (Williams et al., 2002). To dismiss an entire area because there are some methodological flaws in specific studies, according to their argument, was unreasonable. Furthermore, they presented persuasive arguments that most epidemiological studies have the same methodological problems identified in the psychosocial studies. Few evaluations of surgical techniques, for example, are based on randomized clinical trials. Furthermore, it was never clear what Angell

meant by "mental state." Later, she attempted to exclude mood and sense of physical well-being from the definition. She claimed to be challenging "the view that mental state can *directly* cause or substantially modify organic disease independent of personal habits such as smoking, drinking alcohol, or overeating" (Relman & Angell, 2002, p. 560).

Differences in Interpretations

How could distinguished scientists, looking at the same evidence, come to such different conclusions? Some of the difference might just be disciplinary bias. Some might suggest that traditional medical scientists are inherently suspicious of or do not respect evidence from the behavioral sciences. However, many of the differences in interpretation reflect different methodological traditions, including the weight given to observational studies, differences in the sophistication of trial design, and attention and effort expended to obtain "gold-standard," clinical-to-outcome variables.

Causal Interpretation

Many of the studies supporting the importance of psychosocial variables are observational in nature. Although much of epidemiology is based on observational studies, traditional biomedical scientists place greatest credence on blinded randomized clinical trials. They regard observational studies as being weaker designs and are often concerned about "confounding variables," or factors that may have affected the outcome independently of the postulated causal factor (Greenland & Morgenstern, 1989, 1991, 2001). Statistical adjustment is often regarded as insufficient to correct for third-variable explanations (Greenland & Morgenstern, 2001). There are many good examples demonstrating that experimental studies and observational studies come to different conclusions (Barrett-Connor, 2004). For example, it was widely believed that hormone replacement therapy was associated with decreases in cardiovascular disease (Barrett-Connor & Bush, 1991; Barrett-Connor & Miller, 1993), osteoporosis (Barrett-Connor, Grady, & Stefanick, 2005), and some breast cancers (Grady et al., 2008). However, a randomized

The Great Debate
on the Contribution
of Behavioral Interventions

Robert M. Kaplan
Karina W. Davidson

Although health psychology (or "behavioral medicine") has evolved as a legitimate area of medical intervention, there are still some skeptics. A major controversy was initiated by a 1985 editorial in the *New England Journal of Medicine* titled "Disease as a Reflection of the Psyche" (Angell, 1985). In the editorial, Angell argued that "the literature contains very few scientifically sound studies of the relation, if there is one, between mental state and disease" (cited in Relman & Angell, 2002, p. 1570). Angell made it clear that she excluded the effects of personal habits, such as tobacco use, alcohol consumption, and overeating. Instead, she focused on a poorly defined construct of "mental state."

Angell and colleague, *New England Journal of Medicine* editor Arnold Relman, were later invited to the meeting of the Psychosomatic Society to participate in a debate about the value of behavioral interventions. Relman and Angell (2002) debated with Drs. Neil Schneiderman and Redford Williams (Williams, Schneiderman, Relman, & Angell, 2002), and the contest came to be known as "The Great Debate." Both Schneiderman and Williams are major figures in the behavioral medicine field. Schneiderman developed the behavioral medicine program at the University of Miami and is a former president of the International Society of Behavioral Medicine and a former editor of *Health Psychology*. Williams is a psychiatrist and Head of the Division of Psychiatry and Behavioral Science at Duke University. He is a former president of the Society of Behavioral Medicine and the International Society of Behavioral Medicine.

Content of the Great Debate

Relman and Angell asked their opponents to provide the best examples of the benefits of psychosocial interventions. Willimans and Schneiderman offered 21 articles, and Relman and Angell contributed an additional two. The 23 articles were then systematically evaluated. After considering the 23 articles, Relman and Angell (2002) concluded that none offered evidence that psychosocial interventions had meaningful effects on health outcomes. The articles covered a wide variety project would not have reached fruition. We are also grateful to the funding agencies that supported our research while this project was progressing. Jerry M. Suls was partly supported by the National Institute on Aging (NIA; Grant No. AG024159) and by the National Science Foundation (Grant No. BCS-SGER 0634901). Karina W. Davidson was supported by the National Heart, Lung and Blood Institute (Grant Nos. HL-088117, HC-25197, HL-076857, HL-080665, HL-101663, and HL-084034); by the National Center for Research Resources, a component of the National Institutes of Health (NIH) and the NIH Roadmap for Medical Research (Grant No. UL1 RR024156); and by an unrestricted research grant from the Hinduja Foundation. Robert M. Kaplan was partially supported by the NIH (Grant Nos. RC2 HL 101811, California Center for Comparative Effectiveness and Outcomes Improvement; P01 AG020679-01A2, UCLA Claude D. Pepper Older Americans Independence Center; and NIH/NIA 5P30AG028748) and by the Centers for Disease Control and Prevention UCLA/RAND Prevention Research Center (Grant No. UL1 RR024156).

Preface

We began the process of developing this book with a special vision and purpose. Besides exposing the reader to health psychology theory, research, and practice, we wanted to provide health psychologists with constructs, methods, and findings from related health fields. Hence, the *Handbook* considers important mainstream health psychology/ behavioral medicine topics, such as stress and illness; psychological risk factors; the role of personality and psychopathology; behavioral approaches to prevention, intervention, and coping; social psychology; decision making; and psychoneuroimmunology. Yet it also presents coverage of topics that the health psychology/behavioral medicine student, researcher, or practitioner typically will not find in the literature of our field. In this volume, readers will obtain grounding in health economics, health services research, epidemiology, genetics, medical sociology, medical anthropology, global issues, nursing science, and animal models of disease. We assembled leading experts from psychology and related sciences, public health, and medicine to provide succinct, accessible introductions to critical concepts and contemporary issues in their respective disciplines. As a result, this book has developed into a transdisciplinary venue for the theory, science, and practice of health psychology and the related health fields that provide significant input and interactions.

Written for advanced students, researchers, and clinical practitioners, the 36 chapters are organized into five major sections: Health Psychology in the Context of Medicine and Theory; Psychological Foundations of Health Psychology; Contributions of Other Sciences to Health Psychology; Health Psychology, Public Health, and Prevention; and Health Psychology and the Medical Specialties. To ensure that the volume is providing cutting-edge material, we recruited established research scientists and psychological and medical clinicians as well as "next-generation" professionals to offer original contributions. We hope the *Handbook* will serve as a primary text in graduate health psychology/behavioral medicine courses and as a reference work for researchers, practitioners, and health policy professionals. If we can help to create a milieu in which the basic scientist, clinical practitioner, public health interventionist, and policymaker can sit down and "break bread together," then we will have accomplished our aim.

We would like to thank Jim Nageotte of The Guilford Press for his insights, support, counsel, and patience, and Jane Keislar for keeping us on task. Without them, this

Contents

PART I

HEALTH PSYCHOLOGY IN THE CONTEXT OF MEDICINE AND THEORY

clinical trial demonstrated that hormone replacement therapy actually increased the risk of breast cancer and may have slightly increased the risk of some cardiovascular outcomes, including stroke (Prentice, 2008; Prentice & Anderson, 2008). When there is a conflict between the results of randomized trials and observational studies, it is typically assumed that the randomized trial is correct and the observational study, incorrect. One concern is that few psychosocial studies are true randomized clinical trials that clearly demonstrate the causal benefit of treatment.

Trial Design

Over the course of the last 20 years, strict sets of rules have evolved for large-scale randomized clinical trials. Traditional biomedical researchers put the greatest weight on randomized trials that follow these very strict protocols. Furthermore, they like to see multiple identical or very similar trials in the same area of investigation, and they prefer large-scale trials with heterogeneous subject populations. Several rules for conducting and reporting clinical trials have evolved. These are best outlined in the Consolidated Standard of Reporting Trials (CONSORT) guidelines for reporting the results of randomized clinical trials (Moher, Schulz, & Altman, 2001). For example, there are specific protocols for participant randomization. Large trials often have rules for the specification of the primary specific outcome measures. This protects against investigators evaluating many different outcomes after the trial is complete and reporting only those outcomes that are statistically significant. There are also rules about how to handle participants who are randomly assigned to one treatment but ultimately decide to use an alternative treatment. Relman and Angell (2002) pointed out that many of the behavioral trials have not followed the execution and reporting rules required to ensure minimal bias.

Outcome Measures

Another component of the debate concerned choice of the primary definition of outcome variables. Many variables evaluated in behavioral studies might not be considered to be appropriate, clinically relevant outcome measures. The most persuasive evidence includes randomized studies in which the outcomes are disease events or death. Blood pressure, for example, is important because it is related to myocardial infarction (MI), stroke, and premature death. However, change in blood pressure, is not necessarily a clinically-relevant outcome. Instead, it is an intermediate outcome. In large epidemiological studies, investigators have been forced to demonstrate the meaning of these intermediate variables by showing that reductions in these variables ultimately result in changes in outcomes, such as significant disease events or death. For example, the Hypertension Detection and Follow-Up Program (HDFP) was a significant milestone because it showed that lowering blood pressure results in fewer deaths from heart attack and stroke (Hypertension Detection and Follow-Up Program Cooperative Group, 1979, 1982). There have been other examples in which changes in the intermediate factor did not result in the expected changes in outcome. Perhaps the best example is the Cardiac Arrhythmia Suppression Trial (CAST). Previous observational studies had documented an association between increased cardiac arrhythmias and death. Several drugs suppress arrhythmia, and it was assumed that these drugs would also lower the death rate from heart disease. Thus, clinical practice drifted to regularly using these drugs in people with cardiac arrhythmias. In CAST, despite usual clinical practice, patients were randomly assigned to take cardiac arrhythmia suppression drugs or a placebo. The study demonstrated that patients assigned to the drug actually had a higher death rate than those assigned to placebo, and the trial was stopped early because of clear harm to patients in the treatment arm (Cardiac Arrhythmia Suppression Trial [CAST] Investigators, 1989). A similar, unexpected finding emerged in a trial on the control of Type 2 diabetes. High blood glucose is related to diabetic complications and to early death from heart disease. Thus, it was assumed that aggressive management of blood glucose would reduce complications and cardiovascular events. The Action to Control Cardiovascular Risk in Diabetes (ACCORD) trial randomly assigned 10,251 patients with Type 2 diabetes and other cardiovascular disease (CVD) risk factors to an intensive regimen of blood sugar control or to usual care. Those in the aggressive therapy arm achieved significantly lower blood sugar levels. However, there were significantly more deaths in the intensive treatment group (Gerstein et al., 2008). Aggressive treatment of blood sugar achieves the goal of lowing blood sugar but does not achieve the goal of therapy—to extend life expectancy.

In the next section we review several major CVD trials that show the relationship between behavioral interventions and heart disease outcomes.

A Brief Review of the Psychosocial Evidence

Since "The Great Debate" considered only a limited number of articles, it may be worthwhile to provide a general overview. The argument that psychosocial factors affect health outcomes has been in the literature for at least 80 years. Canon (1936) in discussing homeostasis, argued that psychological stress provokes changes in the cardiovascular, respiratory, muscular, metabolic, immune, and central nervous systems. McEwen (2007, 2008a, 2008b) advanced the concept of allostasis and allostatic load. "Allostasis" literally means maintaining stability or homeostasis. Threats cause adjustments in the cardiovascular system to adapt to challenges. Continual exposure to these threats results in physiological changes, ultimately resulting in changes in immune function and health outcomes.

Although it is widely believed that stress can cause serious problems, such as coronary heart disease (CHD), the evidence has been mixed. The Institute of Medicine, as part of a systematic review, found results to be inconsistent across studies (Institute of Medicine (U.S.). Committee on Health and Behavior: Research Practice and Policy, 2001). The reason the literature appears to be so complicated is that stress clearly affects mediators of health outcome. For example, systematic research shows that stress can affect adrenal steroids and catecholamines, dehydroepiandrosterone, prolactin, growth hormones, and cytokines (McEwen, 2008a). There has been wide speculation that responses to stress in some personality types are associated with hypertension (Smith, 1992). There is little doubt that acute stressors cause blood pressure fluctuation (Smith, Ruiz, & Uchino, 2004). The critical issue is whether stress results in permanent changes and ultimately in increases in the chance of death or disability from heart attack or stroke (Smith et al., 2004). Large epidemiological studies tend not to support the belief that hypertension is related to personality. For example, the Coronary Artery Risk Development in Young Adults (CARDIA) study found that depression predicted the incidence of hypertension (Davidson, Jonas, Dixon, & Markovitz, 2000), although this finding was not replicated in a later reanalysis over a 10-year follow-up. However, in some subgroups, there were trends in this direction. In particular, there was a suggestive trend in white men (but not black men, black women, or white women) between depression and the development of hypertension. There was also a nonsignificant trend between anxiety and the development of hypertension in white men. The one variable in which there was better evidence for the 10-year follow-up was hostility, as measured by the Cook–Medley Hostility subscale of the Minnesota Multiphasic Personality Inventory (MMPI). However, the trend was only statistically significant for black women. There was a nonsignificant trend in the same direction for white men, white women, and black men (Yan et al., 2003).

The research on hostility grew out of a long-standing interest in Type A behavior. Over a half-century, more than a thousand scientific papers on Type A behavior were published. However, systematic reviews were not able to show that Type A behavior reliably predicted outcomes for CHD (Institute of Medicine [U.S.], Committee on Health and Behavior: Research Practice and Policy, 2001). Friedman and Adler (2007) noted that chronic anxiety, chronic anger, and depression may be better predictors. For many years, investigators were able to show systematic relationships between Type A behavior and mediator variables, including heart rate, blood pressure, lipids, and neuroendocrine functioning. Nevertheless, the real importance of mediating intermediate variables is the final expression through changes in disability or death. The Type A behavior studies were simply unable to document effects on important, clinically relevant health outcomes.

Clinical Trials

A variety of clinical trials have evaluated the effects of psychosocial interventions on health outcomes. The trials are summarized in Table 1.1. The Recurrent Coronary Prevention Project (RCPP), conducted between 1977 and 1985 (Friedman et al., 1986), was designed to determine whether Type A behavior can be altered, and if so, whether the altered Type A behavior results in a reduction of coronary disease. Eight hundred sixty-two white male patients were randomly assigned to a special behavioral treatment plus cardiac counseling or to a control group that got cardiac counseling without the special behavioral component. Over the course of 4.5 years, those in the behavioral plus cardiac counseling treatment group had significantly lower scores on Type A behavior questionnaires than those assigned to a cardiac counseling group. More importantly, there was a reduction in recurrence of MIs. After 4.5 years, 89% of those in the special behavioral cardiac counseling group had survived without recurrence of their heart attacks, in comparison to 80.2% in those who got counseling alone. After nearly 10 years, there was still a survival advantage for those in the special behavioral cardiac

TABLE 1.1. Summary of Major Behavioral Clinical Trials Relevant to Heart Disease

Trial	Reference	Subjects	Length of follow-up	Intermediate outcome	Outcome
Recurrent Coronary Prevention Project (RCPP)	Friedman et al. (1986)	592 special behavioral cardiac plus counseling (treatment); 270 counseling control; predominantly white male	4.5 years and 8.5 years	Reduction in Type A behavior in treatment group	Significant reduction in survival without cardiac recurrence in treatment group, maintained to 8.5 years
Ischemic Heart Disease Stress Monitoring Trial	Frasure-Smith et al. (1993)	397 psychosocial support; 372 control; all white and male; after dropout, 232 treatment, 229 control	7 years	Reduction in general distress in treatment	Mortality lower in treated group at 3 years, but not different by 6 years; reduction in recurrent myocardial infarction maintained
Montreal Heart Attack Readjustment Trial (M-HART)	Frasure-Smith et al. (1997)	692 treatment; 684 control; white males and females	1 year	Change in depression nonsignificant; change in anxiety nonsignificant	No effect on mortality, but borderline harm for women ($p = .06$)
Sertraline Antidepresant Heart Attack Trial (SADHART)	Glassman et al. (2002)	186 sertraline; 183 placebo; mixed ethnicity and gender	Varied—up to 3 years	Significant reduction in depression in sertraline group	No effect on left ventricular ejection fraction or mortality
Enhancing Recovery In Coronary Heart Disease (ENRICHD)	Berkman et al. (2003)	1,238 cognitive-behavioral; 1,243 control; good representation of black and white, male and female	3.5 years	Significant reduction in depression, increase in social support in cognitive-behavioral group	No effect on mortality or coronary heart disease events

group (77.2 vs. 71.0%). Analysis of intermediate variables showed that those in the special cardiac intervention group scored lower on Type A behavior, hostility, anger, impatience, life satisfaction, self-efficacy, social support, and depression. However, among these variables, only self-efficacy and depression changes predicted subsequent CHD events.

Perhaps the most influential study was the Ischemic Heart Disease Life Stress Monitoring Program was conducted between 1983 and 1986. The study led by Nancy Frasure-Smith was designed to determine whether emotional support during a time when people are highly vulnerable could reduce the rate of nonfatal MI or coronary death. The study involved random assignment of 769 white male subjects. The dropout rate in this study was relatively high. Among 397 men assigned to the treatment group, 58% completed the trial. In the control group, the dropout rate for 372 participants was equivalent (62%). The study authors were not allowed to use full randomization; instead the Institutional Review Board (IRB) instructed them to inform participants about the arm of the assignment, then see if they would consent. The study demonstrated that those exposed to the psychosocial treatment experienced a greater benefit in self-reported health. Furthermore, there was a reduction in cardiac mortality in the treatment group 3–4 years after the intervention. However, the treatment and control groups had comparable cumulative mortality rates about 6 years after the trial began. Considering cumulative MI occurrences, the results favored the intervention group (Frasure-Smith, Lespérance, & Talajic, 1993).

The Montreal Heart Attack Readjustment Trial (M-HEART) was designed to replicate the finding that emotional support at a time of high vulnerability can reduce the incidence of cardiac death and nonfatal MI. However, the study was designed to improve upon the earlier Frasure-Smith study by including both male and female participants, and usual randomization was employed. The study was conducted in Montreal between 1992 and 1997. White men and women (1,376 participants) were randomly assigned to emotional support treatment or to a control group, and follow-up to the primary outcome was almost 100%

in both arms of the trial. The intervention did not have a significant effect on either depression or anxiety. Although there was no overall effect of treatment, one surprising result emerged from the study. There was a near significant ($p = .064$) higher mortality rate among women who had received the intervention. This effect was not apparent for men (Frasure-Smith et al., 1997).

Despite the inconsistent results from early trials, a variety of related results stimulated interest in treating depression among those with CHD. In the Sertraline Antidepressant Heart Attack Randomized Trial (SADHART; Glassman et al., 2002), patients who had experienced heart attacks and who met the criteria for a major depressive disorder were randomly assigned to take the antidepressant sertraline or placebo. Evidence from the study clearly demonstrated that sertraline was effective in lowering depression, particularly among those who experienced more than one major depressive episode. However, the intervention was not powered to examine major health outcomes, so it did not have significant effects for the major health outcomes, including death, MI, heart failure, stroke, angina, or a composite endpoint.

Perhaps the most important intervention trial conducted thus far is Enhancing Recovery in Coronary Heart Disease (ENRICHD) (Berkman et al., 2003). The goal of the study conducted between 1996 and 2004 was to determine whether 6-month treatment for depression and/or low social support shortly after an MI would result in a reduction in mortality or fatal heart disease. This carefully conducted study randomly assigned 2,481 subjects to either treatment or usual care. The treatment was cognitive-behavior modification, preferably in a group, and with antidepressant medication for those who were severely depressed. The intervention resulted in a statistically significant but clinically negligible reduction in depression, as assessed by the Beck Depression Inventory. Those in the intervention group, which included a social support component, also experienced significant improvements in a social support index. Figure 1.1 summarizes the cumulative proportion of deaths in the intervention and usual care groups for the 42 months following enrollment. As shown in Figure 1.1, there was no evidence that the

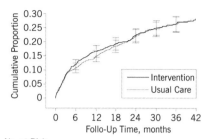

FIGURE 1.1. Cumulative mortality in intervention and control arms of ENRICHD. From Berkman et al. (2003, p. 3111).

intervention resulted in better health outcomes. Figure 1.2 summarizes hazard of death ratios for specific subgroups. Overall, none of the subgrouping factors resulted in changes in the hazard ratios. However, the near significant trend for women was in the unexpected direction; women in the usual care group had lower (although not statistically significant) chances of dying than did those in the intervention group. These results are similar to those reported in the Frasure-Smith M-HEART study (Frasure-Smith et al., 1997).

In summary, we remain uncertain about the potential benefits of psychosocial inter-

vention for patients with heart disease. In 2005, the National Heart, Lung and Blood Institute convened a working group on the assessment and treatment of depression for patients with CVD. The group noted that a significant number of patients with heart disease meet the criteria for major depression (15–20%). Despite the inconsistent results from randomized clinical trials, the group recommended pharmacological or behavioral intervention immediately after MI for patients at risk. The group also concluded that the ENRICHD trial was too short to establish the benefit of treatment and argued that treatment should be extended for longer than 6 months. Finally, the group suggested that a new randomized controlled trial (RCT) involving patients with moderate depression be conducted (Davidson et al., 2006).

By way of summary, observational evidence consistently does show relationships between time urgency, anger, depression, and heart disease. However, RCTs evaluating the causal status of these psychosocial risk marker interventions have produced mixed results. The trials with the strongest experimental designs tend to challenge the benefits of psychological interventions for clinical health outcomes. Thus, we need significantly more investigation to determine the benefits of psychosocial intervention.

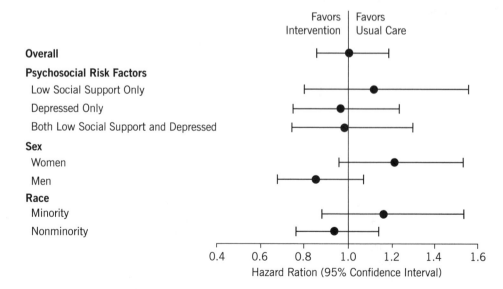

FIGURE 1.2. Effect of ENRICHD intervention on risk of death on nonfatal myocardial infarction. From Berkman et al. (2003, p. 3112).

Resolution of the Great Debate

"The Great Debate" lingered for years. However, by 2006, some of these issues had been resolved. One of the problems was that the entire debate focused on just 23 research studies. Many of these were nonexperimental, epidemiological investigations. The studies often included intermediate outcomes rather than real clinical outcomes, and they excluded from the debate studies on health behaviors, such as adherence, diet, and exercise.

Over time, it was acknowledged that some of the standards required by Relman and Angell (2002) were unrealistic. For example, they argued that many of the psychosocial effects were weak, and that stronger science would require odds ratios of more than 3 or 4 for psychological risk factors. This is an unusual standard that would require increases in risks of 300–400%. These odds ratios are larger than those for the effects of elevated low-density lipoprotein (LDL) cholesterol or blood pressure on heart disease outcomes, including those effects found in RCTs.

A related concern was the argument that good science requires an absolute understanding of the mechanisms of action. Although the mechanisms underlying effective psychosocial interventions have been difficult to elucidate, the same can be said about the mechanisms for many successful medical and pharmaceutical interventions.

Another issue was the relatively few large-scale RCTs on psychosocial interventions. One of the most important RCTs was the RCPP, mentioned earlier, in which 862 post-MI patients were randomly assigned to either regular counseling or specialized cardiac counseling. Those who received the specialized cardiac counseling had a 50% decrease in the recurrence of coronary events over an interval of 4.5 years. Although Relman and Angell (2002) acknowledged that this was an impressive effect, they dismissed some of the results, suggesting that the benefits of the cardiac counseling might be attributed to unmeasured indirect effects, such as changes in lifestyle or diet. This seemed like a weak argument because assignment to the treatment group, independent of what happened afterward, did result in better patient outcomes (Williams et al., 2002). More importantly, changes in lifestyle and diet are behavioral efforts. The positive outcomes should be regarded as a benefit of behavioral intervention, not as evidence against behavioral approaches.

Ultimately, both sides felt that they had prevailed in "The Great Debate." However, several years later, there is growing consensus that the debate stimulated better research and more critical thinking about the role of psychosocial interventions (Freedland, Miller, & Sheps, 2006).

What Was Left Out of the Debate?

Perhaps the most difficult problem in "The Great Debate" is what was left out. Relman and Angell (2002) systemically excluded the effects of health behavior on health outcome. Furthermore, they attempted to exclude everything other than what they referred to as "mental state." A careful look at the relationship between health behavior and health outcome reveals substantial evidence supporting the value of behavioral intervention. In this section we review a few examples. More detailed reviews may be found elsewhere (Fisher et al., 2010).

Tobacco

Cigarette smoking is the leading cause of premature death in the United States and soon will be the leading cause of death in the entire world (multiple references and datasets are available at *www.cdc.gov/tobacco*). Cigarette smoking is associated with most of the major causes of death, including cancer, cardiovascular disease, lung disease, and stroke (U.S. Public Health Service, Office of the Surgeon General, and National Center for Chronic Disease Prevention and Health Promotion, 2004). There is substantial evidence that behavioral programs can successfully reduce the rate of smoking in committed smokers, and that community interventions can prevent the use of tobacco in susceptible youths (Biglan, Ary, Smolkowski, Duncan, & Black, 2000). Furthermore, smoking interventions can reduce the burden of disease and death (Anthonisen et al., 2005). Health promotion strategies successfully reduce the use of tobacco in the United States and many other countries

(Hyland, Travers, Dresler, Higbee, & Cummings, 2008; Hyland, Wakefield, Higbee, Szczypka, & Cummings, 2006). These interventions were regarded as one of the most important public health accomplishments of the 21st century. In countries where tobacco use has declined, there have been significant reductions in CVD, lung cancer, and chronic obstructive pulmonary disease (Barzi et al., 2008).

Diet

The percentage of the U.S. population that is overweight or obese has systematically increased over the last 30 years (Wang & Beydoun, 2007; Wang, Beydoun, Liang, Caballero, & Kumanyika, 2008). Obesity is clearly related to diseases of the heart and gall bladder, to cancer, and to diabetes (Murphy et al., 2006).

The increase in obesity is related to the consumption of high-fat foods, sugar-sweetened beverages, and massive introduction of high-fructose corn syrup sweeteners (Bray, Nielsen, & Popkin, 2004). Many studies show that behavioral interventions can successfully control weight, although evidence for long-term control of weight outcomes has been inconsistent (Mann et al., 2007). Intervention studies using peer education techniques have been successful in a variety of communities (Perez-Escamilla, Hromi-Fiedler, Vega-Lopez, Bermudez-Millan, & Segura-Perez, 2008). Furthermore, RCTs have shown that cognitive-behavioral modification is associated with improvements in LDL cholesterol, blood glucose, and triglycerides (Epstein, Valoski, Wing, & McCurley, 1994; Kuller, Simkin-Silverman, Wing, Meilahn, & Ives, 2001). Dietary fat modification has been associated with better weight control in both adults and children. Ultimately, individual and community interventions have been successful. However, considerably more research and dissemination of information are necessary to conquer the American obesity epidemic.

Physical Inactivity

The obesity epidemic is also associated with physical inactivity. Evidence suggests that moderate activity is associated with decreases in all causes of mortality (Warbur-

ton, Nicol, & Bredin, 2006). Furthermore, physical activity lowers the risk of diabetes, heart disease, and other disabilities (Boule, Haddad, Kenny, Wells, & Sigal, 2001). Physical activity is also related to long-term weight control (Hawley & Dunstan, 2008). Physical activity may also be associated with lower levels of depression (Penedo & Dahn, 2005).

Systematic RCTs show that physical activity may reduce the chances of transition from prediabetes to diabetes (Knowler et al., 2002; Lindstrom et al., 2006), and may successfully moderate blood glucose levels in those with diabetes. A cost-effectiveness analysis of the trial showed that diet and physical activity were more effective and cost-effective in slowing the transition to diabetes than was metformin, the most commonly used medicine in this field (Herman et al., 2005).

Conclusions

"The Great Debate" achieved considerable attention. It considered whether psychosocial factors are important in biomedical and clinical science. That debate focused on 23 published articles, most of which dealt with psychological factors and personality.

Part of the difference of opinion highlighted in the debate is that biomedical scientists and behavioral researchers apply methodologies differently. Biomedical scientists are more focused on RCTs and outcomes, such as disease events or mortality. Greater concentration on these outcomes may help to advance behavioral science.

Perhaps the most important factor overlooked in "The Great Debate" is what was excluded. Systemically eliminated from the discussion were behaviors such as tobacco use, diet, and physical inactivity. When these factors are considered, it is clear that behavioral factors have a major impact on health outcomes.

Further Reading

Angell, M. (1985). Disease as a reflection of the psyche. *New England Journal of Medicine, 312*(24), 1570–1572.

Berkman, L. F., Blumenthal, J., Burg, M., Carney, R. M., Catellier, D., Cowan, M. J., et

al. (2003). Effects of treating depression and low perceived social support on clinical events after myocardial infarction: The Enhancing Recovery in Coronary Heart Disease Patients (ENRICHD) Randomized Trial. *Journal of the American Medical Association, 289*(23), 3106–3116.

Coyne, J. C., Hanisch, L. J., & Palmer, S. C. (2007). Psychotherapy does not promote survival (Kissane et al., 2007): Now what? *Psycho-Oncology, 16*(11), 1050–1052.

Davidson, K. W., Kupfer, D. J., Bigger, J. T., Califf, R. M., Carney, R. M., Coyne, J. C., et al. (2006). Assessment and treatment of depression in patients with cardiovascular disease: National Heart, Lung and Blood Institute Working Group Report. *Annals of Behavioral Medicine, 32*(2), 121–126.

Epstein, L. H., Valoski, A., Wing, R. R., & Mc-Curley, J. (1994). Ten-year outcomes of behavioral family-based treatment for childhood obesity. *Health Psychology, 13*(5), 373–383.

Fisher, E., Fitzgibbonm, M., Glasgow, R., Haire-Joshu, D., Hayman, L., & Kaplan, R. (2010). *Behavior matters.* Manuscript under view.

Frasure-Smith, N., Lespérance, F., Prince, R. H., Verrier, P., Garber, R. A., Juneau, M., et al. (1997). Randomised trial of home-based psychosocial nursing intervention for patients recovering from myocardial infarction. *Lancet, 350,* 473–479.

Freedland, K. E., Miller, G. E., & Sheps, D. S. (2006). The Great Debate, revisited. *Psychosomatic Medicine, 68*(2), 179–184.

Friedman, M., Thoresen, C. E., Gill, J. J., Ulmer, D., Powell, L. H., Price, V. A., et al. (1986). Alteration of Type A behavior and its effect on cardiac recurrences in post myocardial infarction patients: Summary results of the Recurrent Coronary Prevention Project. *American Heart Journal, 112*(4), 653–665.

Gerstein, H. C., Miller, M. E., Byington, R. P., Goff, D. C., Jr., Bigger, J. T., Buse, J. B., et al. (2008). Effects of intensive glucose lowering in Type 2 diabetes. *New England Journal of Medicine, 358*(24), 2545–2559.

Prentice, R. L., & Anderson, G. L. (2008). The Women's Health Initiative: Lessons learned. *Annual Review of Public Health, 29,* 131–150.

Relman, A. S., & Angell, M. (2002). Resolved: Psychosocial interventions can improve clinical outcomes in organic disease (Con). *Psychosomatic Medicine, 64*(4), 558–563.

References

Angell, M. (1985). Disease as a reflection of the psyche. *New England Journal of Medicine, 312*(24), 1570–1572.

Anthonisen, N. R., Skeans, M. A., Wise, R. A., Manfreda, J., Kanner, R. E., & Connett, J. E. (2005). The effects of a smoking cessation intervention on 14.5-year mortality: A randomized clinical trial. *Annals of Internal Medicine, 142*(4), 233–239.

Barrett-Connor, E. (2004). Commentary: Observation versus intervention—what's different? *International Journal of Epidemiology, 33*(3), 457–459.

Barrett-Connor, E., & Bush, T. L. (1991). Estrogen and coronary heart disease in women. *Journal of the American Medical Association, 265*(14), 1861–1867.

Barrett-Connor, E., Grady, D., & Stefanick, M. L. (2005). The rise and fall of menopausal hormone therapy. *Annual Review of Public Health, 26,* 115–140.

Barrett-Connor, E., & Miller, V. (1993). Estrogens, lipids, and heart disease. *Clincis in Geriatric Medicine, 9*(1), 57–67.

Barzi, F., Huxley, R., Jamrozik, K., Lam, T. H., Ueshima, H., Gu, D., et al. (2008). Association of smoking and smoking cessation with major causes of mortality in the Asia Pacific Region: The Asia Pacific Cohort Studies Collaboration. *Tobacco Control, 17*(3), 166–172.

Berkman, L. F., Blumenthal, J., Burg, M., Carney, R. M., Catellier, D., Cowan, M. J., et al. (2003). Effects of treating depression and low perceived social support on clinical events after myocardial infarction: The Enhancing Recovery in Coronary Heart Disease Patients (ENRICHD) randomized trial. *Journal of the American Medical Association, 289*(23), 3106–3116.

Biglan, A., Ary, D. V., Smolkowski, K., Duncan, T., & Black, C. (2000). A randomised controlled trial of a community intervention to prevent adolescent tobacco use. *Tobacco Control, 9*(1), 24–32.

Boule, N. G., Haddad, E., Kenny, G. P., Wells, G. A., & Sigal, R. J. (2001). Effects of exercise on glycemic control and body mass in Type 2 diabetes mellitus: A meta-analysis of controlled clinical trials. *Journal of the American Medical Association, 286*(10), 1218–1227.

Bray, G. A., Nielsen, S. J., & Popkin, B. M. (2004). Consumption of high-fructose corn syrup in beverages may play a role in the epidemic of obesity. *American Journal of Clinical Nutrition, 79*(4), 537–543.

Cannon, W. B. (1936). *Digestion and health.* New York: Norton.

Cardiac Arrhythmia Suppression Trial (CAST) Investigators. (1989). Preliminary report: Effect of encainide and flecainide on mortality in a randomized trial of arrhythmia suppression after myocardial infarction. *New England Journal of Medicine, 321*(6), 406–412.

Coyne, J. C., Hanisch, L. J., & Palmer, S. C.

(2007). Psychotherapy does not promote survival (Kissane et al., 2007): Now what? *Psycho-Oncology, 16*(11), 1050–1052.

Davidson, K., Jonas, B. S., Dixon, K. E., & Markovitz, J. H. (2000). Do depression symptoms predict early hypertension incidence in young adults in the CARDIA study?: Coronary Artery Risk Development in Young Adults. *Archives of Internal Medicine, 160*(10), 1495–1500.

Davidson, K. W., Kupfer, D. J., Bigger, J. T., Califf, R. M., Carney, R. M., Coyne, J. C., et al. (2006). Assessment and treatment of depression in patients with cardiovascular disease: National Heart, Lung and Blood Institute working group report. *Annals of Behavioral Medicine, 32*(2), 121–126.

Epstein, L. H., Valoski, A., Wing, R. R., & McCurley, J. (1994). Ten-year outcomes of behavioral family-based treatment for childhood obesity. *Health Psychology, 13*(5), 373–383.

Fisher, E., Fitzgibbon, M., Glasgow, R., Haire-Joshu, D., Hayman, L., & Kaplan, R. (2010). *Behavior matters.* Manuscript under review.

Frasure-Smith, N., Lespérance, F., Prince, R. H., Verrier, P., Garber, R. A., Juneau, M., et al. (1997). Randomised trial of home-based psychosocial nursing intervention for patients recovering from myocardial infarction. *Lancet, 350,* 473–479.

Frasure-Smith, N., Lespérance, F., & Talajic, M. (1993). Depression following myocardial infarction. Impact on 6-month survival. *Journal of the American Medical Association, 270*(15), 1819–1825.

Freedland, K. E., Miller, G. E., & Sheps, D. S. (2006). The Great Debate, revisited. *Psychosomatic Medicine, 68*(2), 179–184.

Friedman, H. S., & Adler, N. E. (2007). The history and background of health psychology. In H. S. Friedman & R. C. Silver (Eds.), *Foundations of health psychology* (pp. 3–18). New York: Oxford University Press.

Friedman, M., Thoresen, C. E., Gill, J. J., Ulmer, D., Powell, L. H., Price, V. A., et al. (1986). Alteration of Type A behavior and its effect on cardiac recurrences in post myocardial infarction patients: Summary results of the Recurrent Coronary Prevention Project. *American Heart Journal, 112*(4), 653–665.

Gerstein, H. C., Miller, M. E., Byington, R. P., Goff, D. C., Jr., Bigger, J. T., Buse, J. B., et al. (2008). Effects of intensive glucose lowering in Type 2 diabetes. *New England Journal of Medicine, 358*(24), 2545–2559.

Glassman, A. H., O'Connor, C. M., Califf, R. M., Swedberg, K., Schwartz, P., Bigger, J. T., Jr., et al. (2002). Sertraline treatment of major depression in patients with acute MI or unstable angina. *Journal of the American Medical Association, 288*(6), 701–709.

Grady, D., Cauley, J. A., Geiger, M. J., Korni-

tzer, M., Mosca, L., Collins, P., et al. (2008). Reduced incidence of invasive breast cancer with raloxifene among women at increased coronary risk. *Journal of the National Cancer Institute, 100*(12), 854–861.

Greenland, S., & Morgenstern, H. (1989). Ecological bias, confounding, and effect modification. *International Journal of Epidemiology, 18*(1), 269–274.

Greenland, S., & Morgenstern, H. (1991). Design versus directionality. *Journal of Clinical Epidemiology, 44*(2), 213–215.

Greenland, S., & Morgenstern, H. (2001). Confounding in health research. *Annual Review of Public Health, 22,* 189–212.

Hawley, J. A., & Dunstan, D. W. (2008). The battle against obesity-attacking physical inactivity as a primary means of defense. *Nature Clinical Practice Endocrinology and Metabolism, 4*(10), 548–549.

Herman, W. H., Hoerger, T. J., Brandle, M., Hicks, K., Sorensen, S., Zhang, P., et al. (2005). The cost-effectiveness of lifestyle modification or metformin in preventing type 2 diabetes in adults with impaired glucose tolerance. *Annals of Internal Medicine, 142*(5), 323–332.

Hollis, S., & Campbell, F. (1999). What is meant by intention to treat analysis?: Survey of published randomised controlled trials. *British Medical Journal, 319*(7211), 670–674.

Hyland, A., Travers, M. J., Dresler, C., Higbee, C., & Cummings, K. M. (2008). A 32-country comparison of tobacco smoke derived particle levels in indoor public places. *Tobacco Control, 17*(3), 159–165.

Hyland, A., Wakefield, M., Higbee, C., Szczypka, G., & Cummings, K. M. (2006). Anti-tobacco television advertising and indicators of smoking cessation in adults: A cohort study. *Health Education Research, 21*(3), 348–354.

Hypertension Detection and Follow-Up Program Cooperative Group. (1979). Five-year findings of the hypertension detection and follow-up program: I. Reduction in mortality of persons with high blood pressure, including mild hypertension. *Journal of the American Medical Association, 242*(23), 2562–2571.

Hypertension Detection and Follow-Up Program Cooperative Group. (1982). Five-year findings of the hypertension detection and follow-up program: III. Reduction in stroke incidence among persons with high blood pressure. *Journal of the American Medical Association, 247*(5), 633–638.

Institute of Medicine. (U.S.), Committee on Health and Behavior: Research Practice and Policy. (2001). *Health and behavior the interplay of biological, behavioral, and societal influences.* Washington, DC: National Academy Press.

Knowler, W. C., Barrett-Connor, E., Fowler, S.

E., Hamman, R. F., Lachin, J. M., Walker, E. A., et al. (2002). Reduction in the incidence of type 2 diabetes with lifestyle intervention or metformin. *New England Journal of Medicine, 346*(6), 393–403.

Kuller, L. H., Simkin-Silverman, L. R., Wing, R. R., Meilahn, E. N., & Ives, D. G. (2001). Women's Healthy Lifestyle Project: A randomized clinical trial: Results at 54 months. *Circulation, 103*(1), 32–37.

Lindstrom, J., Ilanne-Parikka, P., Peltonen, M., Aunola, S., Eriksson, J. G., Hemio, K., et al. (2006). Sustained reduction in the incidence of type 2 diabetes by lifestyle intervention: Follow-up of the Finnish Diabetes Prevention Study. *Lancet, 368,* 1673–1679.

Mann, T., Tomiyama, A. J., Westling, E., Lew, A. M., Samuels, B., & Chatman, J. (2007). Medicare's search for effective obesity treatments: Diets are not the answer. *American Psychologist, 62*(3), 220–233.

McEwen, B. S. (2007). Physiology and neurobiology of stress and adaptation: Central role of the brain. *Physiological Reviews, 87*(3), 873–904.

McEwen, B. S. (2008a). Central effects of stress hormones in health and disease: Understanding the protective and damaging effects of stress and stress mediators. *European Journal of Pharmacology, 583*(2–3), 174–185.

McEwen, B. S. (2008b). Understanding the potency of stressful early life experiences on brain and body function. *Metabolism, 57*(Suppl. 2), S11–S15.

Moher, D., Schulz, K. F., & Altman, D. (2001). The CONSORT statement: Revised recommendations for improving the quality of reports of parallel-group randomized trials. *Journal of the American Medical Association, 285*(15), 1987–1991.

Murphy, N. F., MacIntyre, K., Stewart, S., Hart, C. L., Hole, D., & McMurray, J. J. (2006). Long-term cardiovascular consequences of obesity: 20-year follow-up of more than 15 000 middle-aged men and women (the Renfrew–Paisley study). *European Heart Journal, 27*(1), 96–106.

Penedo, F. J., & Dahn, J. R. (2005). Exercise and well-being: A review of mental and physical health benefits associated with physical activity. *Current Opinion in Psychiatry, 18*(2), 189–193.

Perez-Escamilla, R., Hromi-Fiedler, A., Vega-Lopez, S., Bermudez-Millan, A., & Segura-Perez, S. (2008). Impact of peer nutrition education on dietary behaviors and health outcomes among Latinos: A systematic literature review. *Journal of Nutrition Education and Behavior, 40*(4), 208–225.

Prentice, R. L. (2008). Women's health initiative studies of postmenopausal breast cancer. *Advances in Experimental Medicine and Biology, 617,* 151–160.

Prentice, R. L., & Anderson, G. L. (2008). The Women's Health Initiative: Lessons learned. *Annual Review of Public Health, 29,* 131–150.

Relman, A. S., & Angell, M. (2002). Resolved: Psychosocial interventions can improve clinical outcomes in organic disease (Con). *Psychosomatic Medicine, 64*(4), 558–563.

Smith, T. W. (1992). Hostility and health: Current status of a psychosomatic hypothesis. *Health Psychology, 11*(3), 139–150.

Smith, T. W., Ruiz, J. M., & Uchino, B. N. (2004). Mental activation of supportive ties, hostility, and cardiovascular reactivity to laboratory stress in young men and women. *Health Psychology, 23*(5), 476–485.

Spiegel, D., Bloom, J. R., Kraemer, H. C., & Gottheil, E. (1989). Effect of psychosocial treatment on survival of patients with metastatic breast cancer. *Lancet, 2,* 888–891.

U.S. Public Health Service, Office of the Surgeon General, and National Center for Chronic Disease Prevention and Health Promotion. (2004). *The health consequences of smoking: A report of the Surgeon General.* Atlanta, GA: Author.

Wang, Y., & Beydoun, M. A. (2007). The obesity epidemic in the United States—gender, age, socioeconomic, racial/ethnic, and geographic characteristics: A systematic review and meta-regression analysis. *Epidemiologic Reviews, 29,* 6–28.

Wang, Y., Beydoun, M. A., Liang, L., Caballero, B., & Kumanyika, S. K. (2008). Will all Americans become overweight or obese?: Estimating the progression and cost of the U.S. obesity epidemic. *Obesity (Silver Spring), 16*(10), 2323–2330.

Warburton, D. E., Nicol, C. W., & Bredin, S. S. (2006). Health benefits of physical activity: The evidence. *Canadian Medical Association Journal, 174*(6), 801–809.

Williams, R., Schneiderman, N., Relman, A., & Angell, M. (2002). Resolved: Psychosocial interventions can improve clinical outcomes in organic disease—rebuttals and closing arguments. *Psychosomatic Medicine, 64*(4), 564–567.

Yan, L. L., Liu, K., Matthews, K. A., Daviglus, M. L., Ferguson, T. F., & Kiefe, C. I. (2003). Psychosocial factors and risk of hypertension: The Coronary Artery Risk Development in Young Adults (CARDIA) study. *Journal of the American Medical Association, 290*(16), 2138–2148.

CHAPTER 2

The Biopsychosocial Model and the Use of Theory in Health Psychology

Jerry M. Suls
Tana Luger
René Martin

Data without a model is just noise.
—CHRIS ANDERSON, Editor of *Wired*

The biopsychosocial model is a scientific model constructed to take into account the missing dimensions of the biomedical model.
—GEORGE ENGEL (1980, p. 525)

A few years ago, one of the authors (Suls) was having lunch with a new Health Psychology PhD who had arrived recently to take a postdoc at the university medical center. In response to "How are things going?" the postdoc reported that he was well but a bit frustrated about being unable to interest the physicians in one of his research ideas. He was especially disconcerted that they expressed no interest in a study's potential to test an important theory. Suls asked, "You didn't talk with them about *theory*?! Most physicians lose interest when they hear the 'T-word.' Why not discuss 'mechanisms of action' or the treatment implications the research might have?" While modern medicine has considerable respect for biological and biochemical theory, physicians tend to be quite skeptical about *behavioral* theories. Many are unaware of or have no ready access to efficacious, effective, and professionally relevant psychosocial interventions. Physicians are pragmatists who functionally

practice within the biomedical model, even if they have awareness of psychosocial factors.

But was the young postdoc misguided in wearing his theoretical premises on his sleeve as he attempted to initiate a collaborative relationship with physicians? In the basic sciences, if a student is trying to pitch a new research study, then it is normative and rigorous to start with the theory and predictions before speculating about potential practical applications. But to gain access to medical collaborators, patient samples, and extramural funding from the National Institutes of Health (NIH), health psychology researchers must adopt a data-driven stance and move as quickly as possible to the implications for public health. In fact, when reviewers evaluate a grant application, they are instructed to give special weight to the project's impact, defined in terms of the potential benefits for public health. "Theory" is not completely missing from NIH grant applications, but it tends to be presented in a low-key fashion—kept in the background and, arguably, serving as a kind of wallpaper. Articles published in medical journals have very brief introductions and discussion sections; theorizing is kept to a minimum. We think there is some evidence that health psychologists have followed the lead of medical researchers. This modus operandi has been successful. However, as we argue below, it may mean that health psychologists leave behind the behavioral theoretical frameworks that make them unique (see Epstein, 1992; Schneiderman, 1987). In fact, theory may represent one of the most distinctive contributions psychologists can bring to the health sciences and medical practice (methodological expertise is another).

The other characteristic that makes psychologists and other behavioral scientists unique is their reliance on and appreciation of the biopsychosocial model. As we argue below, behavioral theory development and the biopsychosocial model go together. Neither has received as gracious a reception from some parts of the medical establishment or from some health psychologists, as we think it should.

This chapter contrasts the traditional biomedical model with the biopsychosocial model and provides a survey of the reception and adoption of the latter perspective. Then we consider the role that both model and theory testing have played in contemporary health psychology and why theory has played a less than optimal role. Finally, we offer some suggestions about how this state of affairs might be improved.

A Brief Note about Scientific Medicine

"Medical science" is a common phrase, but it is often forgotten that a strong scientific research agenda in medicine is a relatively recent development. Lewis Thomas (1983), physician, experimental pathologist, policy advisory, and former administrator of the Memorial Sloan-Kettering Cancer Institute, described how medicine and medical education were principally about diagnosis and prognosis until the 1930s and 1940s, perhaps because that really was all it could accomplish. The introduction of effective medications for infectious diseases, medi-

cal technologies, and mechanism-based research changed that, but research still is not second nature to medical practice. Here is what Thomas said about medical education: "The M.D. program was not then, and still is not, very satisfactory training for research in biomedical science. Then, as now, the Ph.D. program provided a much more rigorous and profound experience in science, with a better grounding" (p. 154). He observed that the MD has the advantage in ensuring that physicians make connections between problems in biology and human disease. Thomas's focus on biology is appropriate because the dominant model of scientific medicine is molecular biology. However, Thomas did not acknowledge that this biological focus can cause physicians to give too little attention to the patient and the social context in which disease is manifested. Ironically, William Osler, one of pioneers of scientific medicine, is reported to have said, "It is sometimes more important to know what patient has a disease than what disease a patient has" (from Herman, 2005, p. 375).

Another contemporary feature of medicine and medical practice is its focus on specific diseases. This structure is most salient in the organization of the NIH into, for example, the National Heart, Lung and Blood Institute, the National Cancer Institute, and the National Institute of Diabetes and Digestive and Kidney Diseases. Writing about the modern scientific physician, Miettinen (2001) observed, "While countless ladies and gentlemen know the practices of their own specialties of medicine, they do not really know . . . the principles of medicine at all: the content is solely about particular illnesses" (p. 1327).

What is wrong about a focus on specific diseases? Kaplan (1990) has written about how the emphasis on a particular outcome can lead to spurious inferences. One of his examples is the Physicians' Health Study (Steering Committee of the Physician's Health Study Research Group, 1988), a large clinical trial, which demonstrated that taking an aspirin a day (vs. placebo) reduced the risk of heart attack. However, Kaplan pointed out that scrutiny of the results reported in the primary publication showed that the overall rate of mortality did not decrease; cardiac deaths were lower, but deaths from strokes actually were higher. Thus, Kaplan asked whether aspirin actually conferred a benefit or only shifted cause of death from one category to another. A disease-specific approach risks inflating the importance of intervention effects and may fail to recognize the importance of quality of life as an outcome.

Epstein (1992) also observed the tendency for health psychologists to adapt a "reductionist approach within the field to reduce mechanisms responsible for behavioral effects and disease to biological influences" (p. 493). This leads to an exclusive focus on biological processes and reluctance to emphasize top-down and behavioral factors.

A limited role for behavioral theory, a narrow focus on specific diseases, and lack of attention to factors that are not strictly biological hamper our understanding of the complex causes of physical disease, health care, and health policy. As we describe below, many of these trends stem from the dominant, albeit often implicit, model in medicine.

The Biopsychosocial Model

PROFESSOR X (a psychologist): We must learn to speak the language of medicine.

PROFESSOR Y: We should understand the language of medicine, but making it our primary language is another story.

—Overheard at a Society of
Behavioral Medicine meeting

The dominant model of disease among medical practitioners is biomedical, with molecular biology as its basic scientific discipline. The biomedical model holds that biological/physiological processes or mechanisms are sufficient to understand, prevent, and treat illness. The model is predicated on reductionism and mind–body dualism, and requires that explanations are reduced to physical–chemical terms before they have meaning (Engel, 1980).

The biomedical model also encourages so-called "magic bullet" solutions to health problems. These refer to prevention or treatment measures that "cure" a condition, usually with a surgical procedure, new medical technology, or medication. In the late 19th and 20th centuries, when infectious diseases were the predominant cause of death, the pursuit of magic bullets was very attractive, especially after the success of antibiotics (particularly, the sulfa drugs) and the polio vaccine. These successes and those of other medical technologies, such as insulin for treatment of Type 1 diabetes, created enormous support for the biomedical model. What is often forgotten is that the prevalence of infectious diseases actually dropped precipitously prior to the introduction of antibiotics, in large part as a consequence of public health measures, such as adequate sewage disposal, and improved nutrition and housing in the late 19th century (Friedman & Adler, 2007; McKeown, 1976). Even with these improvements, we currently live in an evolving public health environment, where infectious diseases are again major sources of mortality (e.g., AIDS, infant diarrhea, flu pandemics). Antibiotics and vaccines provided only a temporary and illusory magic bullet.

Public health measures had as much, if not more, to do with social and political reform as advances in biological science. As early as the 1840s, Rudolf Virchow, the father of cellular pathology who became a political and social reformer, declared medicine to be a social science after witnessing how the circumstances of Polish miners contributed to their health problems.

Nonetheless, proponents "of the biomedical model, claim that its achievements more than justify the expectation that in time all major problems will succumb to further refinements in biomedical research" (Engel, 1980, p. 536). The difficulty is that biomedicine's successes have been in areas for which the physical–chemical framework is appropriate, leaving other areas neglected (Engel, 1980). Susser and Susser (1996) provide an apt example:

> Peptic ulcer . . . illustrates the limitations of a narrow frame of reference for a chronic disease. The causal framework of the gastrophysiologist is likely to focus on the wall of the stomach and that of the neurophysiologist, on the autonomic nervous system. . . . The human geneticist considers familiality in blood groups and secretor status, and the microbiologist brings the recent discoveries about *Helicobacter pylori* to bear. The epidemiologist includes all the above and adds smoking as an individual risk factor. (p. 675)

However, even these factors are not sufficient explanations because ulcer prevalence rose mysteriously at the beginning of the 19th century and, no less mysteriously, began to decline in the 1950s. Susser and Susser observe that even if the explanation lies in the historical behavior of Helicobacter microorganisms, then the other levels of analysis are still important for diagnosis, explanation, and treatment.

The biopsychosocial model provides a framework to include physical–chemical factors *and* the areas neglected by biomedicine. George Engel (1977) was the first to articulate this approach to guide health researchers and practitioners in research, intervention, and practice (see also Matarazzo, 1980; Schwartz, 1982). The "biopsychosocial model" refers to the idea that biological, psychological, and social processes are integrally and interactively involved in physical illness and health, medical diagnosis, medical treatment, and recovery. The understanding of the full complement of influences at multiple levels of analysis was held as a goal by Engel. He observed that "while the bench scientist can with relative impunity single out and isolate for sequential study components of an organized whole, the physician does so at the risk of neglect of, if not injury to, the object of study" (1980, p. 536).

What does it mean to say that biological, psychological, and social factors are integrally involved in physical health? It means that single-factor, or even single-domain explanations are likely to be inadequate. Second, it argues that a change in one domain (e.g., the biological) necessarily results in changes in other domains (e.g., psychological and social). A third implication is medical diagnosis that considers the interaction of biological, psychological, and social factors should lead to improved diagnosis. Furthermore, interventions involving all of these elements should fare better than treatments grounded on any single class of variables (Schwartz, 1982; Suls & Rothman, 2004).

The biopsychosocial perspective advocates a multilevel approach to diagnose, explain, and treat any medical problem. Biological/physiological processes; cognition, emotion, and behavior; the immediate social context (family and friends); and macroprocesses (e.g., public health regulations) all play a role in the diagnosis, etiology, practice, and promotion of physical well-being. In short, the biomedical model directs the researcher and practitioner to look for a biological/physiological cause and curing agent, while the biopsychosocial model alerts the researcher, practitioner or policymaker to the need for multiple levels of analysis and appreciation of all potential domains that contribute to the problem and its "solution."

By insisting that a single level of analysis is probably insufficient, the biopsychosocial model can guide researchers and practitioners to the kinds of multiple variables that are potentially important. A more formal and systematic conceptual tool will be required, however, to direct the systematic search for relevant variables and possible relationships and/or mechanisms among them. That tool is "theory," by which we mean a consistent and well-defined framework to test a falsifiable hypothesis about the real world.

The Reception and Adoption of Health Psychology/Behavioral Medicine

The biopsychosocial model was formally introduced in the 1970s, but how has it fared since then (Schwartz & Weiss, 1978)? The field of health psychology certainly has made enormous progress in the last 40 years with the growth of new professional societies, such as Division 38 of American Psychological Association and the Society of Behavioral Medicine; the fuller integration of psychologists into older societies, such as the American Psychosomatic Society; and development of many special interest societies. A welcome by-product of the increasing number of societies hospitable to health psychologists is the increasing number of journals with which to disseminate research, such as the *Journal of Behavioral Medicine, Annals of Behavioral Medicine, Health Psychology, Psychology and Health,* and *Health Psychology Review.* Furthermore, already-existing journals, such as *Psychosomatic Medicine, Journal of Personality and Social Psychology,* and *Journal of Consulting and Clinical Psychology,* have also served as prestigious outlets. Similarly, graduate training programs have also multiplied, and the number of health psychologists serving on the faculties of universities or medical schools has increased markedly (Rodin & Stone, 1987).

The number of behavioral health-related grant proposals has also grown so large that at least four study sections are chartered at the NIH to evaluate health psychology/behavioral medicine research, and many more panels evaluate health psychological proposals. At one time physical health was a topic that received little attention from the American Psychological Association, but now mind–body interaction is a common topic, and the improvement of physical health has been included as one of the major missions of the organization (*www.apa.org/about*). The role of psychological and behavioral factors for physical health has been deemed so significant that in 1993 Congress established the Office of Behavioral and Social Sciences Research as a separate entity at the NIH to promote behavioral and social sciences, to integrate behavioral and biomedical knowledge, and to facilitate interdisciplinary research between social, behavioral, and biomedical scientists (Anderson, 1998). Finally, as the contents of this handbook attest, empirical advances by health psychologists have been made in disease etiology, health promotion, and treatment. But how significant have these changes been, and to what degree has the biopsychosocial model been received in other health-related fields?

The Biopsychosocial Model in Medical Education

Engel believed it was vital that an appreciation of patients and their social contexts be incorporated into the medical education of physicians. However, there are indications that not much has changed in medical education. A survey of medical school education indicated that about 50% of the schools queried offered less than 40 hours of instruction in psychosomatic medicine and health psychology (Waldstein, Neumann, Drossman, & Novack, 2001).

An Archival Inquiry

As a first approximation of the degree to which the medical establishment has adopted the biopsychosocial model, Suls and Rothman (2004) conducted MEDLINE searches of titles and abstracts from 1974 through 2001 for the terms "biomedical," "biopsychosocial," and "biobehavioral" (the latter is used almost synonymously with the second). The year 1974 was chosen as a starting point because Engel introduced the term "biopsychosocial" in 1977. Use of these terms does not mean that investigators or authors embraced this perspective, but at minimum, references to them indicate that the biopsychological model was recognized. An examination of Figure 2.1 shows an obvious increase in the use of the terms "biopsychosocial" and "biomedical" in the published literature, by a factor of five, but these terms were cited only once for every nine times that the term "biomedical" was mentioned.

Another index also was assessed in the archives: The number of times the word "behavior" appeared in the titles or abstracts of published articles was counted in four major medical journals—*New England Journal of Medicine, Lancet, Journal of the American Medical Association*, and *Annals of Internal Medicine*—from 1974 to 2001. *Behavior* was mentioned about 60 times from 1974 to 1977 but more than 100 times from 1998 to 2001. Although the count was doubled, the absolute number of appearances was small: The term "behavior" only appeared in 0.002% of articles in the early years and 0.004% in the years with its most frequent appearance (1990–1993). These indicators, however crude, suggest some acknowledg-

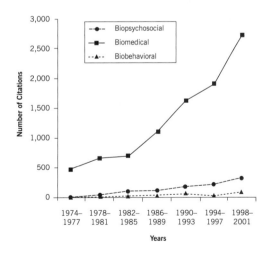

FIGURE 2.1. Frequency of citations of the terms "biopsychosocial," "biobehavioral," and "biomedical" in MEDLINE. From Suls and Rothman (2004). Copyright 2004 by the American Psychological Association. Adapted by permission.

ment of the biopsychosocial model by the medical establishment, but the perspective clearly has not been fully embraced.

The Biopsychosocial Model Instantiated in Research

Another, no less critical, index is whether health psychologists actually follow the biopsychosocial model. Suls and Rothman (2004) reasoned that one way to gauge research practices is to assess whether researchers actually measure the four kinds of variables (i.e., biological, psychological, social and macro [cultural, socioeconomic status, ethnicity]) in their studies. Accordingly, the authors read and coded the frequency with which each class of variables was measured and/or manipulated in all of the studies published in a year of the Division 38 journal, *Health Psychology*, between November 2001 and September 2002.

It comes as no surprise that psychological variables were represented in almost 95% of the papers. Social, biological/physiological, and macrovariables were each represented in about 50–55% of the papers. However, the macrovariables only referred to the sample, while the biological variables most often referred to a particular patient sample. Notably, only 26% of the studies included measures from all four domains. This means that most studies did not explore the interrelations and interactions across levels or classes of variables.

To summarize, while the biopsychosocial model has had an impact, it is modest with respect to impact on the medical establishment and has not yet been fully adopted even by health psychologists. Admittedly, Suls and Rothman (2004) only surveyed a single journal in a single year, so conclusions should be drawn cautiously. Also, in certain clinical literatures, such as family medicine or ambulatory pediatrics, behavior or behavioral issues are discussed more frequently, but the coverage in some areas of medicine is slight.

Theories in Health Psychology

In the preceding section, we presented archival data suggesting that only in a minority of instances do health psychologists measure variables that represent all of the levels of analysis assumed to be important in the biopsychosocial model. This has an implication for theory because the absence of one or more levels of analysis implies that missing levels are irrelevant, or it is acceptable to leave variables at the other levels free to vary.

Researchers often defend their decisions to narrow domains of inquiry by noting the conceptual, operational, and logistic difficulties associated with measuring variables at all levels. A similar difficulty is encountered in theory building and theory testing. The difficulty associated with conceptualizing how different levels interact discourages theorizing across levels and reinforces a narrow focus. However, lacking a theory, the investigator cannot identify those factors most plausibly related to the outcome of interest (Rothman, 2004).

Health Behavior as an Example

The area of health behavior is relevant because a number of scholars have examined the extent to which theory testing and development have been a concern there. An encouraging sign is Noar and Zimmerman's (2005) report that theoretically informed health behavior change programs tend to be more effective than those without a theoretical basis—supporting Lewin's (1943), "There is nothing so practical as a good theory" (p. 118). In another review of published studies on health behavior change, Painter, Borba, Hynes, Mays, and Glanz (2008) examined the proportion of published research that used no theory, was informed by theory, applied theory, tested theory, or built a new theory. "Theory" was only mentioned in 36% of the articles. The majority of those papers (68%) were informed by theory, that is, mentioned a theory or theoretical constructs, but none were actually measured. Eighteen percent of the sample applied the theory; that is, at least some of the constructs of the theory were operationalized in the study. Only about 4% of the research actually tested a theory or alternative theories, and only 9% involved the development of a new theory. Of the theories mentioned in this study sample, three dominated: transtheoretical model/stages of change (28%; Prochaska & Velicer, 1997), social cognitive theory (28%; Bandura, 1989), and the health belief model (20%; Becker, 1974; Rosenstock, 1966).

Painter and colleagues (2008) concluded that use of theory was limited, that only a few theoretical approaches were represented, and that testing and advancement of theory were rare in the empirical health behavior change literature. They also noted that community-level theories were scarcely represented.

The Dangers of Imitating Epidemiology

An issue that we believe is closely related to the less than optimal utilization of theory in health psychology is the field's relationship and imitation of epidemiology. Several areas of health psychology depend heavily on epidemiological findings. Disease risk factors, especially of a behavioral nature, that have been identified in large sample population studies using epidemiological methods comprise a major category of factors studied by health psychologists in promotion, intervention, and understanding of etiology. Specific examples are socioeconomic status (Adler et al., 1994), hostility (Smith, 1992), and social support (Cohen & Syme, 1985; House, Landis, & Umberson, 1988).

Although health psychologists rely on epidemiological research findings, a narrow focus on risk factors without understanding the role they play with other factors is an atheoretical endeavor. Epidemiological methods are correlational and usually require very large samples and brief survey instruments. Adding measures to assess possible mediating factors is a luxury in large-scale population studies. Not surprisingly, epidemiology does not typically test theories. When health psychologists adopt such an approach there are dangers. One such example is represented by the two-decades-long effort to document the effects of the Type A behavior pattern (Rosenman et al., 1964), a construct that has now faded from the research agenda. One reason we think it failed is that Type A behavior was narrowly defined and studied apart from the broader literature on personality, individual differences, and person–situation interactions. It was treated as an epidemiological risk factor, simply entered with traditional cardiac risk factors in risk equations. As this area of study increasingly borrowed from psy-

chological theory (Glass, 1977; Matthews, 1982), however, it became clear that Type A behavior did not comprise a single coherent construct, that only certain elements (i.e., hostility) were toxic, and that the latter conferred risk via plausible cognitive, social, and physiological mechanisms (Matthews, Gump, Harris, Haney, & Barefoot, 1994).

The reader might object that the steady decline in deaths from heart disease since the last 1970s results partly from a better understanding about the risk factors for cardiovascular disease and behavioral intervention (i.e., smoking cessation–prevention). These benefits partly occurred because of non-theory-driven identification of risk factors by epidemiologists. But we might ask whether the benefits would have been even greater if study of risk factors had been more theory driven.

Within the fields of epidemiology, there have been calls to incorporate theoretical frameworks. Krieger (2001) observed that epidemiologists tend to ignore the overarching question of what is the global factor or "spider" responsible for the particular pattern of factors. A lack of overarching theory in epidemiology or explanations of the current and changing health status of human societies results in a missed step in the research process because explanations of disease and etiology drive epidemiological hypotheses. In this light, imitating epidemiology in its traditional form seems like a poor strategy for health psychologists.

Translation

The NIH has placed great emphasis in the last decade on "translation." By this, policymakers mean the conversion of laboratory knowledge into new products, and the adoption of such products by providers into routine clinical practice (from bench to bedside). In this way, translational research can demonstrate a return on society's investment in basic science. In 2006, NIH initiated the Clinical and Translational Science Awards for support of centers to reduce the time it takes for laboratory discoveries to become treatments for patients, to engage communities in clinical research efforts, and to train clinical and translational researchers (see *www.ncrr. nih.gov/clinical_research_resources/clinical_and_translational_science_awards*).

Currently, 46 medical research institutions in 26 states have translation centers. One set of observers noted, however, that much of the work so far has been devoted to "finding surrogate biomarkers that can predict the outcome of new therapies" (Horig, Marincola, & Marincola, 2005, p. 706).

Translation can go in the opposite direction—using what is learned at the bedside to inform and to raise questions for bench science (see Lelford, 2008). However, Sonntag (2005) observed,

> So far, translational research/medicine has rather been a linear concept rooted in traditional (academic) approaches to provide therapies for diseases (from bench to bedside). . . . Little attention [has been paid] to patient-oriented research that involves understanding the underlying cause of disease and its treatments (from bedside to bench). (p. 1)

A promising exception is seen in implementation models, such as the RE-AIM (reach, efficacy, adoption, implementation, and maintenance) model and practical clinical trials (Glasgow, Davidson, Dobkin, Ockene, & Spring, 2006; Glasgow, Magid, Beck, Ritzwoller, & Estabrooks, 2005; Tunis, Stryer, & Clancy, 2003). Such models advocate attention to the implementation of interventions in real-world environments at the very earliest stages of research conceptualization and design. For example, an early consideration of the implementation environment influences the selection of dependent variables to make them maximally informative for practitioners and policymakers. The inclusion of such practical dependent variables has the potential to facilitate and improve the ultimate adoption of all sorts of health interventions.

A Clarification and Critique of Theory

Even when there is a commitment to behavioral theory (e.g., Painter et al., 2008; Suls & Rothman, 2004), some observe that "there is a growing concern that we are not tending to our theories as well as we ought" (Michie, Rothman, & Sheeran, 2007, p. 249; see also Brewer & Rimer, 2008). Some qualify as middle-range theories—the theory of reasoned action (Ajzen & Fishbein, 1980), self-regulation theory (Cameron & Leventhal, 2003; Carver & Scheier, 2001), or social

cognitive theory (Bandura, 1989)—because their level of specificity derives propositions and predictions that permit empirical testing (in contrast to "grand theories" using large, abstract constructs that often cannot be readily operationalized in precise and concrete ways). However, even in the case of well-specified theories, there are barriers for development, such as reliance on correlational methods that prevents the researcher from being able to infer causation ($X \rightarrow Y$) and address the mediating variables in the causal path ($X \rightarrow M \rightarrow Y$) (Michie et al., 2007).

Another problem is connected with the multiple levels of analysis that the biopsychosocial model requires. How feasible is it to include all relevant constructs and processes in a single study to develop theory (Michie et al., 2007)? The answer, of course, is that one researcher cannot. Furthermore, insistence on taking the "kitchen sink" approach likely produces work that fails to identify the exact mechanism causing the effect. The need for small-scale experiments that provide a "causal chain analysis" seems like a more appropriate strategy, with a focus on understanding the mechanisms behind each individual link in the chain to understand fully the entire process in the future. Ultimately, this must be a collaborative effort; it is not enough for one investigator in isolation to plan a detailed research program to advance theory. As Weinstein and Rothman (2005) argue, "It takes a village to raise a theory" (p. 296). But how does one engage the scientific village? In the next section, we describe an approach that health psychology, the other behavioral sciences, and medical science may be able to adapt for their purposes.

The Full-Cycle Approach

Health psychology has at least two masters; cognitive behavioral theory and clinical and public health practice. We are expected to contribute to theory by creating new models and adding to existent models of human behavior, and to contribute to improvements in health outcomes for the public.
—LEVENTHAL, MUSUMECI, AND CONTRADA (2007, p. 381)

A new approach is needed to overcome the obstacles that face the full implementation of the biopsychosocial model, and the development and testing of behavioral theory. In brief, the four major obstacles are (1) the dominant emphasis of practice-based solutions, which makes theory testing a subsidiary aim; (2) the conceptual and logistical difficulties for any single study to follow the biopsychosocial model's call to consider all relevant factors; (3) the contemporary political–economic climate which reinforces both biomedical "cures" and biomedical explanations; and (4) overemphasis on translation research that reinforces a one-way linear sequence, whereby better practice becomes the ultimate criterion of success and "curiosity-based" research is discouraged (see Weissmann, 2005).

We advocate the adaptation of the full-cycle approach developed by social psychologist Robert Cialdini and elaborated by sociologists Gary Alan Fine and Kimberly Elsbach, and organizational psychologists Jennifer Chatman and Francis Flynn. Because the full-cycle approach was developed exclusively for social behavioral topics, it is not a perfect match for the challenges in health psychology, but with some modifications (see below) it can be made appropriate.

Cialdini (1980) developed the full-cycle perspective in the context of experimental social psychological research. He was attracted to the virtues of laboratory experiments that can "(1) register even whisper-light effects and (2) allow no phenomenon but the one under direct study to produce the predicted data pattern" (p. 23). However, these appealing features have a downside because lab experiments "capture phenomena without regard for their importance in the course of naturally occurring human behavior" (p. 24). Stated differently, a theory speaks to the existence of effects it predicts, but "it does not speak to the ecological importance of those effects" (p. 24).

To compensate for these limitations, Cialdini argues that theory building should begin with hypothesis building through multiple real-world observations (i.e., induction). These observations, whether based on anecdotes, ethnography, surveys, archival sources, and so forth, provide hunches about both possible relationships between variables and indices of their ecological importance. These observations and hunches

should then lead to specific laboratory tests (deduction) of the refined hypotheses under controlled conditions. But the process does not end there because the researcher should then cycle back to further real-world observations for refinement. "Naturally occurring instances should be employed not only to identify effects suitable for experimental study but also to check on the validity of the findings from that experimentation" (p. 43). The recursive design is a critical feature of the full-cycle approach and corrects for the tendency whereby researchers develop theory based on one methodological approach, then return to the same methodological approach to test their new ideas. As Chatman and Flynn (2005) note, "Full-cycle research travels back and forth between the naturally occurring phenomenon and controlled settings. This bidirectional flow enables researchers to draw theoretical insights from one setting and apply them to another" (p. 243).

The full-cycle approach also recognizes the importance of knowledge based on exploring, observing, and assessing a phenomenon as it exists naturally, and on manipulating or controlling the phenomenon. Linking the two different ways of knowing recursively has the virtue that both induction and deduction are critical and dependent on each other. In fact, cycling between induction and deduction is important because each provides feedback on the adequacy of the other approach. Furthermore, inductive–deductive cycles help to determine which peripheral ideas strengthen the core and which constitute new branches of inquiry.

The full-cycle approach also has another implication. Besides naturalistic observation that helps in discovery of new phenomena, "there are also cases where the impetus for an important line of research may come from observing a *lack* of an effect in the natural environment where there should be one" (Mortensen & Cialdini, 2009, p. 18). Theory and experimentation can then learn why expected effects are missing or how to create those effects.

Adapting the Full-Cycle Approach to Health Psychology

Modifying this approach for the biopsychosocial model makes "bench to bedside" and "bedside to bench" part of the scientific cycle. It also reinforces the need for researchers and practitioners to be part of the same research team. Moreover, the vital roles that practice and medical outcomes play are clear as they serve as inputs and outputs in this dynamical approach.

Adapting this model to physical health requires an extra element. Cialdini thought only a single researcher would be sufficient to pursue the full cycle. In the field of social psychology, this may be feasible, but the biopsychosocial model embraces more levels of analysis, each with its own body of knowledge, measurement, and technology. Advancing the understanding of physical well-being demands not just interdisciplinary teams but scientist-practitioner teams whose members play various roles depending on the phase of the cycle.

With respect to theory development and testing, it is important to appreciate that it is probably impossible for a theory to be simultaneously general, accurate, and simple (Fine & Elsbach, 2000; see Thorngate, 1976). The more simple *and* accurate a theory is, for example, the less generalizable it is likely to be in a variety of contexts. The more generalizable *and* simple the theory, the less likely it is to be accurate. As Weick (1979) notes, the dilemma is that to maximize any two of the virtues of generality, accuracy, and simplicity, the researcher automatically has to sacrifice the third one. So bench research might be simple and accurate but questionable in its generalizability. Large-scale surveys may be simple and generalizable but accuracy may be quite limited. In summary, *any single method* of data collection results in trade-offs in the resulting theory's simplicity, generalizability, and accuracy.

A search for a method that combines all three elements—accuracy, simplicity, and generalizability—might be futile, but theory may be built by alternating among sets of data that provide one or more of these elements, or by incorporating the research of others with data that complement one's own (Weick, 1979). Nothing speaks better for the need for interdisciplinary teams. As noted earlier, in the case of behavioral medicine, those teams require scientists and practitioners engaged in the full cycle together. By adopting this approach, NIH-supported Clinical Translational Research Centers could be a real boon for behavioral health, but the mode of operation will have to take a full-cycle *and* recursive form to be maximally effective.

Obstacles

The essential components of a full-cycle approach are available. The biopsychosocial model also provides a viable guide to suggest the kinds of factors that should be explored; however, there are barriers to adoption of such an approach.

Chatman and Flynn (2005) acknowledge that academic journals tend to specialize in a limited set of methodologies. Editorial reviewers may be selected more on the basis of their expertise in a particular methodology but be less familiar with different methods (see Suls & Martin, 2009). Reviewers expect new results to be grounded in existing research findings, which usually means collecting data with the same conventional methodology. These are not intractable problems, but they can slow down the progress to a truly translational full-cycle approach.

Where Do We Go from Here?

It seems a universal characteristic of the scientific enterprise that the mining of any vein of research and theory, however enthusiastically initiated and however diligently prosecuted, tends to go deeper rather than broader and ultimately to become isolated unless diverted into new directions by outside influences.
—ESTES (1975, p. 15)

To avoid this predicament, we propose that collaboration between basic scientists and clinical practitioners be seen as not just a bonus but as a necessity, and we recommend the creation of a special NIH funding mechanism (e.g., a special kind of R01) to facilitate such collaborations. In action, persons desiring to be funded would be required to consult with researchers of different backgrounds than their own. For example, an applied application for funding would need to outline a budget to retain a basic researcher on salary, as well as the regular team of health psychologists, physicians, or public health researchers. This would aid the infusion of theory into the applied work. Similarly, an application addressing a basic research question would need to recruit a clinician or educator for consultation. As a result, the basic researcher would be advised of the practical reality of the health system. This should serve to produce work that is more feasible and more easily translated.

Another proposal is that clinical translational science centers encourage (if not require) scientists in the basic biological and behavioral sciences to spend structured time on medical wards or in the community and with practitioners and patients to learn about the real world of medical care. (This is being done at some clinical translational centers already.) Comparable experiences in the basic research setting should also be created for medical practitioners. This would encourage the kind of back-and-forth, recursive, and cyclical experiences that provide fuel for basic theory, research, and implementation.

Conclusions

The previous section offers some top-down, hierarchical strategies to encourage the adoption and dissemination of the full-cycle approach for health psychology and medical science/practice. But we are not so foolish as to think that great science, practice, or intervention requires a "road map." Great scientists and practitioners rarely follow road maps or bureaucratic rules (Weissmann, 2005). Curiosity, anecdote, careful observation, sustained thinking, hard work, serendipity, and a community of (heterogeneous) scholars (the "village" referred to earlier) are required. We would add that both the biopsychosocial model and the full-cycle perspective also need to be in the air. We end with another quotation from Lewis Thomas (1974, quoted in Weissman, 2005). What research and practice "need is for the air to be made right. If you want a bee to make honey, you do not issue protocols on solar navigation or carbohydrate chemistry, you put him together with other bees . . . and you do what you can to arrange the general environment around the hive. If the air is right, the science will come in its own season, like pure honey" (p. 1762)

Further Reading

Boyer, B. A. (2008). Theoretical models of health psychology and the model for integrating

medicine and psychology. In B. A. Boyer & M. I. Paharia (Eds.), *Comprehensive handbook of health psychology* (pp. 3–30). New York: Wiley.

Engel, G. (1977). The need for a new medical model: A challenge for biomedicine. *Science, 196*, 129–136.

Friedman, H., & Adler, N. (2007). The history and background of health psychology. In H. Friedman & R. Silver (Eds.), *Foundations of health psychology* (pp. 3–18). New York: Oxford University Press.

Glasgow, R. E., Magid, D. J., Beck, A., Ritzwoller, D., & Estabrooks, P. A. (2005). Practical clinical trials for translating research into practice: Design and measurement recommendations. *Medical Care, 43*, 551–557.

Matarazzo, J. (1980). Behavioral health and behavioral medicine: Frontiers of a new health psychology. *American Psychologist, 35*, 807–817.

Suls, J., & Rothman, A. (2004). Evolution of the biopsychosocial model: Prospects and challenges for health psychology. *Health Psychology, 23*, 119–125.

References

Adler, N. E., Boyce, T., Chesney, M. A., Cohen, S., Folkman, S., Kahn, R. L., et al. (1994). Socioeconomic status and health. The challenge of the gradient. *American Psychologist, 49*, 15–24.

Ajzen, I., & Fishbein, M. (1980). *Understanding attitudes and predicting behavior.* Englewood Cliffs, NJ: Prentice-Hall.

Anderson, N. B. (1998). Levels of analysis in health science: A framework for integrating sociobehavioral and biomedical research. *Annals of the New York Academy of Sciences, 840*, 563–576.

Bandura, A. (1989). Human agency in social cognitive theory. *American Psychologist, 44*, 1175–1184.

Becker, M. (1974). The health belief model and personal health behavior. *Health Education Monographs, 2*(4), 324–473.

Brewer, N. T., & Rimer, B. K. (2008). Perspectives on health behavior theories that focus on individuals. In K. Glanz, B. K. Rimer, & K. Viswanth (Eds.), *Health behavior and health education: Theory, research, and practice* (4th ed., pp. 149–165). San Francisco: Jossey-Bass.

Cameron, L., & Leventhal, H. (2003). Self-regulation, health and illness: An overview. In *The self-regulation of health and illness behavior* (pp. 1–13). New York: Routledge.

Carver, C. S., & Scheier, M. (2001). *On the self-regulation of behavior.* New York: Cambridge University Press.

Chatman, J. A., & Flynn, F. J. (2005). Full-cycle micro-organizational behavior research. *Organization Science, 16*, 434–447.

Cialdini, R. B. (1980). Full-cycle social psychology. In L. Bickman (Ed.), *Applied Social Psychology Annual* (Vol. 1, pp. 21–47). Beverly Hills, CA: Sage.

Cohen, S., & Syme, S. L. (Eds.). (1985). *Social support and health.* San Diego, CA: Academic Press.

Engel, G. L. (1977). The need for a new medical model: A challenge for biomedicine. *Science, 196*, 129–136.

Engel, G. L. (1980). The clinical application of the biopsychosocial model. *American Journal of Psychiatry, 137*, 535–544.

Epstein, L. H. (1992). Role of behavior theory in behavioral medicine. *Journal of Consulting and Clinical Psychology, 60*, 493–498.

Estes, W. (1975). The state of the field: General problems and issues of theory and metatheory. In W. Estes (Ed.), *Handbook of learning and cognitive processes* (pp. 1–24). Hillsdale, NJ: Erlbaum.

Fine, G. A., & Elsbach, K. (2000). Ethnography and experiment in social psychological theory building: Tactics for integrating qualitative field data with quantitative lab data. *Journal of Experimental Social Psychology 36*, 51–76.

Friedman, H. S., & Adler, N. E. (2007). The history and background of health psychology. In H. Friedman & R. Silver (Eds.), *Foundations of health psychology* (pp. 3–18). New York: Oxford University Press.

Glasgow, R. E., Davidson, K. W., Dobkin, P. L., Ockene, J., & Spring, B. (2006). Practical behavioral trials to advance evidence-based behavioral medicine. *Annals of Behavioral Medicine, 31*, 5–13.

Glasgow, R. E., Magid, D. J., Beck, A., Ritzwoller, D., & Estabrooks, P. A. (2005). Practical clinical trials for translating research into practice: Design and measurement recommendations. *Medical Care, 43*, 551–557.

Glass, D. C. (1977). *Behavior patterns, stress and coronary disease.* Hillsdale, NJ: Erlbaum.

Herman, J. (2005). The need for a transitional model: A challenge for biopsychosocial medicine? *Families, Systems, and Health, 23*, 372–376.

Horig, H., Marincola, E., & Marincola, F. M. (2005). Obstacles and opportunities in translational research. *Nature Medicine, 11*, 705–708.

House, J. S., Landis, K. R., & Umberson, D. (1988). Social relationships and health. *Science, 241*, 540–545.

Kaplan, R. M. (1990). Behavior as the central

outcome in health care. *American Psychologist, 45*, 1211–1220.

Krieger, N. (2001). Theories for social epidemiology in the 21st century: An ecosocial perspective. *International Journal of Epidemiology, 30*, 668–677.

Lelford, H. (2008). The full cycle. *Nature, 453*, 843–845.

Leventhal, H., Musumeci, T., & Contrada, R. (2007). Current issues and new directions in psychology and health: Theory, translation, and evidence-based practice. *Psychology and Health, 22*, 381–386.

Lewin, K. (1943). Psychology and the process of group living. *Journal of Social Psychology, SPSSI Bulletin, 17*, 113–131.

McKeown, T. (1976). *The modern rise of population.* London: Edward Arnold.

Matarazzo, J. (1980). Behavioral health and behavioral medicine: Frontiers of a new health psychology. *American Psychologist, 35*, 807–817.

Matthews, K. A. (1982). Psychological perspectives on the Type A behavior pattern. *Psychological Bulletin, 91*, 293–323.

Matthews, K. A., Gump, B. B., Harris, K. F., Haney, T. L., & Barefoot, J. C. (1994). Hostile behaviors predict cardiovascular mortality among men enrolled in the Multiple Risk Factor Intervention Trial. *Circulation, 109*, 66–70.

Michie, S., Rothman, A., & Sheeran, P. (2007). Advancing the science of behavior change. *Psychology and Health, 22*, 249–253.

Miettinen, O. S. (2001). The modern scientific physician: 7. Theory of medicine. *Canadian Medical Association Journal, 165*, 1327–1328.

Mortensen, C., & Cialdini, R. B. (2009). Full-cycle social psychology for theory and application. *Social and Personality Psychology Compass, 4*, 53–63.

Noar, S. M., & Zimmerman, R. S. (2005). Health behavior theory and cumulative knowledge regarding health behaviors: Are we moving in the right direction? *Health Education Research, 20*, 275–290.

Painter, J. E., Borba, C., Hynes, M., Mays, D., & Glanz, K. (2008). The use of theory in health behavior research from 2000 to 2005: A systematic review. *Annals of Behavioral Medicine, 35*, 358–362.

Prochaska, J. O., & Velicer, W.F. (1997). The transtheoretical model of health behavior change. *American Journal of Health Promotion, 12*, 38–48.

Rodin, J., & Stone, G. (1987). Historical highlights in the emergence of the field. In G. Stone, S. Weiss, J. Matarazzo, N. Miller, J. Rodin, C.

Belar, et al. (Eds.), *Health psychology: A discipline and a profession* (pp. 15–26). Chicago: University of Chicago Press.

Rosenman, R. H., Friedman, M., Straus, R., Wurm, M., Kositchek, R., Hahn, W., et al. (1964). A predictive study of coronary heart disease: The Western Collaborative Group Study. *Journal of the American Medical Association, 189,* 15–22.

Rosenstock, I. M. (1966). Why do people use health services? *Milbank Memorial Fund Quarterly, 44,* 94–124.

Rothman, A. J. (2004). Is there nothing more practical than a good theory?: Why innovations and advances in health behavior change will arise if interventions are used to test and refine theory. *International Journal of Behavioral Nutrition and Physical Activity, 1,* 11.

Schneiderman, N. (1987). Basic laboratory research in health psychology. In G. Stone, S. Weiss, J. Matarazzo, N. Miller, J. Rodin, C. Belar, et al. (Eds.), *Health psychology: A discipline and a profession* (pp. 77–90). Chicago: University of Chicago Press.

Schwartz, G. (1982). Testing the biopsychosocial model: The ultimate challenge facing behavioral medicine. *Journal of Consulting and Clinical Psychology, 50,* 1040–1053.

Schwartz, G., & Weiss, S. (1978). Yale Conference on Behavioral Medicine: A proposed definition and statement of goals. *Journal of Behavioral Medicine, 1,* 3–12.

Smith, T. (1992). Hostility and health: Current status of a psychosomatic hypothesis. *Health Psychology, 11,* 139–150.

Sonntag, K.-C. (2005). Implementations of translational medicine. *Journal of Translational Medicine, 3,* 1–3.

Steering Committee of the Physicians' Health Study Research Group. (1988). Preliminary report: Findings from the aspirin component of the ongoing Physicians' Health Study.

New England Journal of Medicine, 318, 262–264.

Suls, J., & Martin, R. (2009). The air we breath: A critical look at practices and alternatives to the traditional peer review process. *Perspectives on Psychological Science, 4,* 40–50.

Suls, J., & Rothman, A. (2004). Evolution of the biopsychosocial model: Prospects and challenges for health psychology. *Health Psychology, 23,* 119–125.

Susser, M., & Susser, E. (1996). Choosing a future for epidemiology: From black box to Chinese boxes and eco-epidemiology. *American Journal of Public Health, 86,* 674–677.

Thomas, L. (1974). The planning of science. In *The lives of a cell* (pp. 99–102). New York: Viking Press.

Thomas, L. (1983). *The youngest science: Notes of a medicine-watcher.* New York: Viking Press.

Thorngate, W. (1976). "In general" vs. "it depends": Some comments on the Gergen–Schlenker debate. *Personality and Social Psychology Bulletin, 2,* 404–410.

Tunis, S. R., Stryer, D. B., & Clancy, C. M. (2003). Practical clinical trials: Increasing the value of clinical research for decision making in clinical and health policy. *Journal of the American Medical Association, 290,* 1624–1632.

Waldstein, S. R., Neumann, S., Drossman, D., & Novack, D. (2001). Teaching psychosomatic (biopsychosocial) medicine in United States medical schools: Survey findings. *Psychosomatic Medicine, 63,* 335–343.

Weick, K. E. (1979). *The social psychology of organizing.* New York: McGraw-Hill.

Weinstein, N., & Rothman, A. (2005). Commentary: Revitalizing research on health behavior theories. *Health Education Research, 20,* 294–297.

Weissmann, G. (2005). Roadmaps, translational research, and childish curiosity. *FASEB Journal, 19,* 1762.

PART II

PSYCHOLOGICAL FOUNDATIONS OF HEALTH PSYCHOLOGY

CHAPTER 3

Emotions and Stress

William R. Lovallo

Behavioral Medicine and Psychological Factors in Health and Disease

Physicians and laypeople alike have long believed that a person's state of health is affected by his or her state of mind. Along with this belief is the idea that an emotional disposition and severe reactions to acute and chronic stressors can have a long-term negative impact on one's health. Although this belief is widely shared and intuitively compelling, the search for convincing evidence has not yielded simple answers or solid proof. However, evidence is accumulating in support of the idea that negative states of mind, negative emotions, and intense stress reactions can have deleterious effects on the well-being of our bodies. The flip side of this idea is that positive states of mind have beneficial effects on health and physical well-being. Proof that positive states of mind have positive effects on the body has been similarly, if not more, difficult to develop. This chapter is not exhaustive coverage of the literature supporting these positions on stress and health. Excellent reviews have been published (McEwen, 2006; Schwartz et al., 2003; Thrall, Lane, Carroll, & Lip,

2007; Treiber et al., 2003). This chapter is an overview of how we currently think about psychological dispositions and reactions to events, and how these may relate to physiological function from the brain down to the rest of the body. The study of emotions and stress reactions can enrich the study of behavioral medicine, and it can help to advance our understanding of how individual differences in emotional disposition may relate to disease and resistance to disease.

Behavioral and Psychological Tendencies Are Also Physiological Characteristics

In considering how emotional reactions and stress responses may affect health, it is essential to look at the connections between mind and body that support the relationship between behavior and health. To clarify, the term "behavior" is used here to include overt behaviors, as well as subjective experience, emotional states, and the brain states associated with them. In short, our inner life, including thoughts, emotions, and subjective reactions are as much part of our behavior as our overtly observable behavior. This effort to join our inner experience to our larger behavioral repertoire may improve ways of studying the relationships between emotions, stress, and health by reducing the disconnection sometimes thought to exist between mental processes and physiological outputs.

Understanding the connections between subjective states and our physiological processes has been greatly enhanced by the emerging field of "affective neuroscience," which is based on the idea that emotions are more than subjective phenomena and also more than bodily states. In this formulation, emotions are instantiated in brain activity, but they necessarily include subjective experience (affect) and cognitions (interpretations of the events we are encountering). In this chapter, I discuss ways to think about how emotional responses are related to external events, using the influential model of Richard Lazarus and Susan Folkman (1984). Next, I consider how this model, which is based on cognitive principles, may be translated into a physiological model based on brain function. In thinking about emotions, stress, health, and disease, it is perhaps important not only to develop general principles for this study but also to recognize that people differ in surprising and interesting ways with regard to their individual risk for disease. This consideration leads us to consider individual differences in emotional reactions and stress responses. Finally, I consider how studies of differences in stress reactivity can make use of this information by focusing most productively on the levels in the system that are relevant to health and disease for a given person.

Events Shape Emotional Reactions by Appraisals and Coping Resources

Following earlier observations by Walter Cannon that life events and our interpretations of them could produce physical symptoms (Cannon, 1928, 1957), Lazarus noted in the 1950s that persons could have powerful physiological responses to events they encountered, even when those events had no ability to harm persons who witnessed them (Lazarus, Baker, Broverman, & Mayer, 1957). The earliest and most striking example of this is a study Lazarus conducted, in which college-age volunteers watched a film made by a group of anthropologists who were studying a native African puberty transition rite involving the lengthwise cutting of the lower surface of the boys' penises, called a subincision procedure (Koriat, Melkman, Averill, & Lazarus, 1972). Not surprisingly, this caused significant anxiety in the viewers, and recordings of skin conductance changes indicated significant physiological reactions as well. Although we find this an expected and normal reaction to such a film, Lazarus was thoughtful enough to undertake the challenge of explaining this reaction. In the process of doing so, he also noted that not all audiences had such a reaction. Japanese students were far less reactive than Americans. It was clear from this that the emotional reaction of the Americans was not a necessary response to the film, but one based on personal experiences that could shape the interpretation of the filmed event and define the subjective experience of the viewer. This led Lazarus to formulate a hypothesis that stress reactions could result from events that are not actual physical encounters with danger in the world, but are instead purely psychological processes associated with emotional reactions (Lazarus, 1999; Lazarus & Folkman, 1984).

In this formulation, a two-stage appraisal process that evaluates the event in light of the available coping resources can lead to emotional reactions, including stress responses (see Figure 3.1). According to Lazarus and Folkman (1984), the first step, labeled the "primary appraisal," is intended to address whether the encountered event is a threat to well-being or may be safely ignored. Events we judge to be benign or irrelevant to our well-being are not processed further and accordingly have no further role to play in stress reactions. For example, a prospective college student who does badly on the Scholastic Aptitude Test may feel a sudden shock accompanied by feelings of hopelessness and anxiety, along with increases in heart rate and blood pressure. Lazarus and Folkman would say that news of the low score violated the student's belief in his or her qualification to attend college and posed a potential obstacle to a commitment to higher education and the self-fulfillment that it provides.

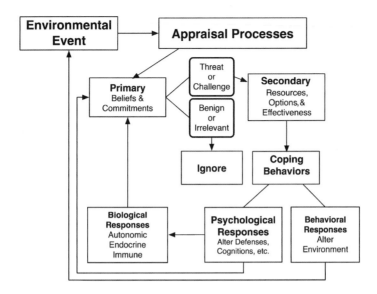

FIGURE 3.1. The Folkman and Lazarus (1988) model of psychological stress. Environmental events are appraised as to threat value (primary appraisals). If an event is judged potentially harmful, then a secondary appraisal process weighs the potential courses of action and their likelihood of successfully reducing the threat posed by the event. Such appraisal processes are thought to underlie emotional responses that underlie psychological stress responses.

This conflict with the student's beliefs and commitments becomes the basis of a threat appraisal that leads to the next set of steps in forming a psychological stress reaction. In contrast, a high school student who had no college aspirations might view the same test score as irrelevant and may consequently have no particular response.

Events that are evaluated as having real or potential harmful outcomes are then subjected to a secondary appraisal step. Here, the event is reassessed in light of the person's available coping options and characteristic coping style. Suppose it is still early in the college application cycle, and our student did badly on an entrance exam. In this case, the student could reappraise the event in light of the option to study a preparatory course and retake the test. This reappraisal might suffice to reduce the feeling of failure and the associated physiological reactions. This example also suggests that our student has a tendency to use a problem-focused coping style that assesses the problem itself (a low score) in light of possible strategies to address the core problem (study a specific preparatory course that would improve skills on the test). In contrast, an emotion-focused

student might cope by doing something to reduce the anxiety, such as going to a movie with friends, but he or she might not initially think of retaking the test after better preparation. Most people in fact might do a bit of both. The literature on appraisal and coping has been reviewed extensively (Suls, David, & Harvey, 1996; Taylor & Stanton, 2007).

A striking feature of this scenario is how a test score printed on a piece of paper can produce profound effects in the body, based on the interpretation of the meaning of the number and the extrapolation to its consequences for the person's future. This translation of an abstract piece of information into an interior reality and then to a bodily response is the core chain of events in the psychological stress process and the key point of departure in how events in our daily lives can come to affect health. Additionally, experience tells us that some people tend to react in a stressful manner, whereas others do not. This dimension of individual differences complements our thoughts on basic mechanisms and completes our basic theme of laying out the psychobiological model of emotions, stress, and disease.

Emotions Are Action Dispositions with Affect, Cognition, Behavior, and Visceral States

In describing the appraisal model of psychological stress, I noted without comment that the appraisal process underlies emotional reactions to the environment, and that emotions go hand in hand with behavioral motivations. It seems that negative emotions and behavioral motives to struggle or escape are essential to the formation of psychological stress reactions (Lovallo, 2005b). Emotions are therefore not only feeling states but they are also psychophysiological processes that underlie behavioral tendencies (Schulkin, Thompson, & Rosen, 2003). For purposes of this discussion, I define an "emotion" as a complex event that has four components: cognition, behavior, visceral outputs, and affect (Kagan, 1994). Emotions have cognitive underpinnings and interactions; they are shaped by our thoughts and in turn our emotional state can color our thoughts and interpretations of the world (Lazarus, 1991; Schulkin et al., 2003). Emotions are accompanied by more or less intense physiological reactions that have a degree of specificity to the emotion in question (al'Absi et al., 1997; Sinha, Lovallo, & Parsons, 1992). Emotions are associated with overt behaviors; specific facial expressions accompany basic emotions, such as fear, anger, and disgust (Ekman, 1993; Ekman & Friesen, 1971), and complex ones, such as pride (Tracy & Robins, 2004), and these expressions act as a means of social communication, indicating the internal state of the individual and also suggesting intentions and what actions are likely to occur next. In a similar fashion, emotion-related postures serve as modes of social communication and preparation for adaptive behavior (Appleton, 2006; Niedenthal, 2007). Finally, emotions carry distinct, unobservable subjective feelings that accompany their affective dimension. These four components work harmoniously to motivate us for the actions needed to cope with the environment, to obtain what we need, and to avoid what is harmful.

This motivational and emotional apparatus prepares us for coping efforts and supports these behaviors in response to demands for homeostasis (Cannon, 1928). This same set of systems is at work during periods of stress that call for more intense use of resources to meet extraordinary threats (Lovallo, 2005b). The value of examining stress states and their underlying emotional origins from a psychophysiological perspective is that stress effects on health can be reasonably deconstructed in ways that may help in testing the proposition that stress contributes to disease, and that positive states of mind may contribute to health. To illustrate one way to examine stress reactivity and disease, I have introduced a multilevel model that incorporates psychological processes and physiological outputs in the study of stress reactivity (Lovallo, 2005a). In this case I examine how three levels of organization associated with individual differences in brain function, bodily outputs, and peripheral stress mechanisms each can have different contributions to disease pathophysiology.

Individual Differences in Emotions and Stress Reactivity Underlie Differences between People in Risk for Disease

To make sense of the complexity of the human brain and its controls over bodily function, we have attempted to advance a model that addresses brain–body interactions at three levels of systems organization that are plausibly associated with individual differences in emotions and disease risk (Lovallo, 2005a; Lovallo & Gerin, 2003). These three levels take into account Lazarus's model of psychological stress and the primary role that conscious and unconscious appraisals have in shaping responses at the level of the hypothalamus and brainstem, and ultimately at the level of the periphery. The discussion indicates ways in which exaggerated reactivity may arise at each of these levels in the system and how these lead to different considerations of the relationship between exaggerated reactivity and disease causation.

Level I: Cognitions, Emotions, and Brain Activity

At the top level of our working model are the neural structures and their communications that form the basis for our cognitions and our affective responses. These are shown as Level I mechanisms in the upper portion of Figure 3.2. The key areas involved in these high-level processes are the parts of the prefrontal cortex involved in working memory,

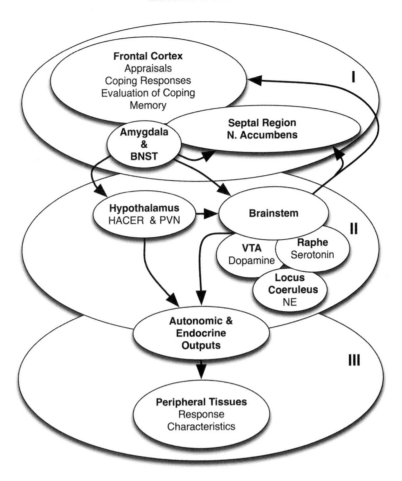

FIGURE 3.2. Three levels of brain organization and peripheral function that may be responsible for individual differences in cardiovascular and endocrine reactivity to stress. BNST, bed nuclei of the stria terminalis, an extension of the amygdala closely associated with the septal nuclei and the nucleus accumbens. The amygdala and BNST are therefore in extensive two-way contact with activity in the prefrontal cortex and are a determinant of output from these prefrontal–limbic processes and outputs to the hypothalamus and brainstem. HACER, hypothalamic areas controlling emotional responses, a term coined by Orville Smith et al. (1993) to describe lateral hypothalamic areas that determined autonomic outflow in primates during emotional episodes. VTA, ventral tegmental area, a region of the higher brainstem having the nuclei that give rise to mesolimbic dopaminergic neuronal projections to the prefrontal cortex, nucleus accumbens, and the limbic system. NE, norepinephrine. The locus coeruleus contains norepinephrine-producing cell bodies with axonal projections to most of the central nervous system.

in decision making from a cognitive perspective, and in weighing decisions based on their motivational and hedonic characteristics. These cognitive processes depend on several key prefrontal regions and interacting limbic system structures. For greater clarity these prefrontal and limbic areas are referenced in Figure 3.3. Environmental events that lead to emotional responses and perhaps re-

sult in stress reactions begin with external events and sensory information arriving at the amygdala. The primary outputs from the amygdala emerge via the central nucleus and are transmitted to the prefrontal cortex via the bed nuclei of the stria terminalis. This extension of the amygdala has extensive two-way interactions with the prefrontal cortex. At the same time, cognitive appraisals of the

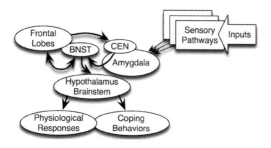

FIGURE 3.3. Pathways and structures underlying the formation of emotions and stress responses. CEN, central nucleus of the amygdala. BNST, bed nuclei of the stria terminalis, an extension of the amygdala closely associated with the septal nuclei and the nucleus accumbens. The amygdala and BNST are therefore in extensive two-way contact with activity in the prefrontal cortex and are a determinant of output from these prefrontal–limbic processes and outputs to the hypothalamus and brainstem.

environmental event depend on key prefrontal regions, including the dorsolateral and ventromedial prefrontal cortexes and the anterior cingulate gyrus. On the limbic side of the equation, the diagram focuses on the amygdala and bed nuclei of the stria terminalis because of their role as gateways for the initial affective and motivational tagging of incoming information. Incoming sensory information is processed in the amygdala in light of inborn and Pavlovian conditioned memories or, more simply, emotional memories. Together these prefrontal and limbic processing systems engage in a dialogue in the fashioning of appraisals and coping responses that may be referred to in short as prefrontal–limbic interactions.

In working together, these limbic and prefrontal structures permit conscious assessment of the events we face, evaluating their motivational characteristics, and helping us to make decisions about response alternatives and their consequences (Blair et al., 2006; Campbell, 2007). Activity in areas associated with cognition during stress responses can act to modify the development of physiological reactions, either reducing or enhancing them (Critchley, Mathias, & Dolan, 2002; Gianaros, May, Siegle, & Jennings, 2005). However, these strongly rational processes are only partly effective in evaluating the meaning of events we may en-

counter, forming emotional reactions, and choosing alternative ways to respond to potential threats. Pavlovian conditioned associations, along with feedback from the body, add motivational bias to the prefrontal–limbic dialogue that shapes our appraisals and coping responses. Work by Damasio (1994) and colleagues has shown that working memory alone is not sufficient to arrive at adaptive strategies for our lives. While current events may be processed in consciousness with the help of working memory, the limbic system is similarly active in evoking emotional and motivational memories associated with past occurrences of the same or similar events. In particular, the amygdala assesses inputs from external sensory modalities and draws on prior conditioning to begin to add affective weight to this complex stream of inputs (Rolls, 2000). At the same time, inputs from the viscera arrive at the amygdala by way of the insular cortex to provide a "gut feel" about the emerging picture of the ongoing event (Amaral, Price, Pitkanen, & Carmichael, 1992; Critchley, Wiens, Rotshtein, Ohman, & Dolan, 2004; Halgren, 1992). Outputs from the amygdala and insula reach areas that give rise to affective experience, and that have extensive two-way connections to the prefrontal cortex, including the anterior cingulate gyrus and the orbitofrontal cortex (Kosson et al., 2006).

The significance of this convergence of bodily sensations, inputs from the amygdala, and higher conscious processing of events is illustrated by neurological cases highlighting the degree of impairment caused by a loss of any of these sources of information. The famous case of Phineas Gage, whose head was penetrated by an iron tamping rod that entered the roof of the mouth, passed through the left eye socket, and exited at the midline of the top surface of the skull, was the first to illustrate the behavioral consequences of medial prefrontal damage (Harlow, 1868). Gage was apparently intact in terms of his cognitive abilities; he was able to talk and remembered well the circumstances of his injury, and he was able to maintain employment in a variety of menial jobs until his death 19 years later. What changed in Gage after his injury was that he became undependable in his behavior, was very altered in his social relations, and failed to follow through with long-range plans, and in fact his friends felt that he was not able to distinguish adequately between practical and impractical courses of action. Damasio (1994) reported on contemporary neurological cases that displayed similar deficits. Patients with strokes or traumatic injury to the ventromedial prefrontal cortex and adjacent orbitofrontal cortex were found to be cognitively intact but to have abnormal motivational and emotional behavior, and difficulty choosing between choices (Bechara, Damasio, Tranel, & Damasio, 1997). These deficits are increasingly severe in persons who sustain such damage very early in life (Anderson, Bechara, Damasio, Tranel, & Damasio, 1999) probably because these victims are deprived of a chance to develop a storehouse of experience on which to draw when confronted with events requiring adaptive decision making.

The foregoing discussion of these neurological cases suggests that damage to the ventromedial prefrontal cortex, the anterior cingulate gyrus, the amygdala, and related areas of the temporal lobe cause alterations in the processes specified in Lazarus's model of psychological stress. Persons with damage to these areas either fail to assess danger adequately or fail to make adequate plans to cope with challenges they face. Figure 3.2 is intended to reference these regions as forming the basis of appraisals, choices among coping strategies, and evaluation of their effectiveness. Damage to the relevant regions is likely to result in poorly calibrated assessments of safety versus threat, in particular when amygdalar inputs are disrupted. In one dramatic case, a woman with bilateral damage to the amygdala fails to recognize even obvious sources of danger, such as automobile traffic on city streets (Adolphs et al., 2005). It seems to follow that in such a person, choices among coping responses and subsequent assessments of their effectiveness would be highly impaired in the absence of normal amygdalar inputs. For this reason the top portion of Figure 3.2 makes reference to prefrontal–limbic interactions in shaping initial responses to ongoing events. This Level I process forms the basis of our ability to appraise the significance of events and prepare for adaptive responses to them.

A final consideration is the degree to which such prefrontal–limbic interactions are conscious and plan-driven or automatic and reflexive. The foregoing presentation would

suggest they are conscious ones, and in some cases this may be so. Certainly the studies of social modeling by Schachter and Singer (1962) strongly point to conscious, interpretive processes in shaping the emotions of persons being tested. However, much brain activity that underlies our emotional reactions and ensuing stress responses is highly automated and does not rely on conscious processing. A very likely explanation for this is that the amygdala is the critical point in the nervous system for the formation of Pavlovian conditioning. Starting with a core of inborn reflexes, such as a fear of snakes in primates (Halgren, 1992), unfolding experience elaborates on these reflexes with an increasing repertoire of associations formed by the convergence at the amygdala of bodily responses to external inputs (unconditioned reflexes) and attentional responses to external sensations (orienting responses), resulting in conditioned associations (Jones & Powell, 1970). If we consider Pavlovian conditioning as the basis for emotional memory formation, then it is likely that future encounters with similar events will evoke affective, visceral, and behavioral responses with little or no cognitive processing.

The description of brain systems associated with emotional experience and expression suggests that emotional response biases can arise as a result of cognitive processes that operate consciously. Similarly, unconscious processing of events, due to emotional memories associated with Pavlovian conditioning, can also result in differential emotional reactivity to events. As one example, persons who are high in trait hostility tend to have large cardiovascular and endocrine responses to stress, particularly when the situation elicits hostile reactions (Brondolo et al., 2003; Pope & Smith, 1991; Suarez & Williams, 1989). Regardless of the source, biases in emotional reactivity can cause altered responses to psychological stressors that may cause differential responsiveness in peripheral physiological systems. Closely tied to these cognitive–emotional response systems are regions of the medial and orbitoprefrontal cortex that interact with the hypothalamus to exert tonic and phasic inhibition of the outgoing expression of the emotions. Suspected individual differences in the degree of regulation exerted by these areas of the prefrontal cortex should therefore be considered as a factor in emotional responsivity and its ability to modulate outputs to the hypothalamus and brainstem (Hilz et al., 2006). It is a fundamental tenet of reactivity theory that persistent biases of these sorts can in principle lead to long-term dysregulation of physiological function. This in turn can act either as a cause of disease or as a contributor to disease progression in a preclinical condition.

Level II: Brain Activity Forming Emotions Can Shape Outputs to the Body

The term "emotion" derives from the word for "movement" and shares strong ties with the word "motivation." Emotions are fundamental to our preparation for and execution of actions to cope with the environment, to obtain what we need, and to avoid what is a danger to us. These motivationally driven behavioral responses require appropriate bodily adjustments to support the needed behaviors. As shown in Figure 3.2, Level II, outputs from the prefrontal–limbic interactions described earlier descend to the level of the hypothalamus and brainstem, where they are capable of significantly shaping the descending outputs that determine autonomic and endocrine activity patterns. The role of the hypothalamus in emotional expression was dramatically demonstrated in the work of Walter Cannon and Philip Bard (Bard, 1928). In this case, they studied cats whose entire brain had been removed above the level of the hypothalamus. However, two facts of considerable importance were revealed. First, the cats remained viable as long as food and water were provided to them, indicating that the hypothalamus possessed the necessary regulatory centers to maintain homeostasis. Second, the cats could easily be provoked to a state of rage by stroking of the fur. The rage response incorporated sympathetic outflow (the fur was erect), endocrine responses, and a full defensive posture. This showed that the hypothalamus possesses the necessary organization to integrate emotional displays, including visceral responses and complex behavioral adjustments. This conclusion was further established in early studies by Ranson (1934) of electrical stimulation of the hypothalamus, which also showed that sympathetic outflow, endocrine responses, and motor activity were integrat-

ed by systems of nuclei at this level (Swanson & Sawchenko, 1980). In attempting to cast Lazarus's model of psychological stress in physiological terms, we may view the hypothalamus as the highest structure at which prefrontal–limbic processes at Level I begin to find bodily expression and to have an impact at Level III in the periphery.

Along with the hypothalamus, specific sets of nuclei in the brainstem are important in regulating the outputs to the body and also in setting the state of the entire central nervous system. As indicated in Level II of Figure 3.2, the locus coeruleus sets the activational state of the brain and spinal cord through ascending and descending noradrenergic neurons (Aston-Jones, Ennis, Pieribone, Nickell, & Shipley, 1986; Grant, Aston-Jones, & Redmond, 1988). The ventral tegmental area contains dopaminergic cell bodies that provide ascending fibers that are active at the limbic system and prefrontal cortex in periods calling for attention to motivationally salient environmental events and also in establishing the subjective reward value of specific cues (Drevets et al., 2001; Koepp et al., 1998). This same system is involved in the prefrontal regulation of hypothalamic responses to stress (Spencer, Ebner, & Day, 2004). A third set of nuclei forms the raphe system that provides serotonergic inputs to these same prefrontal and limbic brain regions, and appears to be important in long-term regulation of emotional states. These systems are, not surprisingly, responsive to experience, and primates exposed to prolonged social stress show reduced levels of serotonin and serotonin metabolites in the prefrontal cortex, suggesting persistent effects on mood resulting from social stressors (Fontenot, Kaplan, Manuck, Arango, & Mann, 1995; Lesch & Mossner, 2006). These three sets of nuclei and their projections therefore work to establish global response patterns in relation to external events. Swanson refers to these systems as "state generators" (Swanson, 2000), and in the context of a cerebral model of stress reactivity, I have referred to these systems as the "central feedback subsystem" (Lovallo, 2005b). This phrase is intended to call attention to the role of higher decision-making processes served by prefrontal–limbic interactions, producing patterns of response in lower structures, but also using the state generators to bring together the activities of disparate regions to produce coordinated behaviors that have adaptive value.

From the perspective of physiological stress reactivity in the context of behavioral medicine, persistent biases in the operations of these output and state generation systems have implications for mood regulation, emotional responses, and ultimately, impact on the body. Here I introduce the phrase "hypothalamic gain factor" to describe how the hypothalamus treats inputs from Level I systems. If we think broadly about the hypothalamus as a transducer of the information from the prefrontal cortex and limbic system, it also becomes feasible to think of this transduction as an individual-difference factor in which the signals are amplified to a greater degree in some persons than in others. Alterations in the operation of hypothalamic and brainstem output pathways are therefore an important link in the chain of causality leading to heightened reactions to emotion producing stimuli and stressful experiences.

Evidence of greater hypothalamic activation during novelty and stress exposure in the spontaneously hypertensive rat and in hypertensive and prehypertensive humans suggest that there exists an elevated hypothalamic gain factor supplied to outgoing emotion-related signals from higher cortical centers (al'Absi & Lovallo, 1993; al'Absi, Lovallo, McKey, & Pincomb, 1994; Goncharuk, Van Heerikhuize, Swaab, & Buijs, 2002; Roman, Seres, Pometlova, & Jurcovicova, 2004). The endocrine component of stress responses is linked to the cardiovascular component at the level of the paraventricular nucleus of the hypothalamus (Lovallo, 2005b). Even in the case of a normal cognitive and affective response to external events, exaggerated outputs via the hypothalamus and brainstem will result in enhanced reactivity in peripheral systems, with potential consequences for their long-term regulation.

Level III: Responses by the Body May Alter the Progression of Disease States

Peripheral physiology is the third level in the model in which disease processes may be altered by individual differences in stress reactivity. Ultimately, whatever appraisals and coping responses are selected by the central nervous system, and whatever response biases might occur at the level of the hypothalamus and brainstem, no model of reactivity is complete without considering the effectors by which physiological change is made to occur. Autonomic and endocrine outputs act by signaling receptors on smooth muscles and endocrine cells of peripheral tissues. For any given output signal, responses may be enhanced or diminished by altered effector function. As a result, the possibility exists that altered peripheral physiology may contribute to development or progression of disease (Schwartz et al., 2003).

A complete discussion of the ways in which peripheral physiological response systems might contribute to elevated stress reactivity is beyond the scope of this chapter due to the range of tissues involved. However, a short discussion of the blood vessel and the heart in relation to hypertension illustrates some of the possibilities. Blood pressure is determined jointly by cardiac output, a measure of the volume of blood flow through the system in a given time unit, and by peripheral resistance, the resistance to blood flow created by restrictive elements in the blood vessels (Rushmer, 1989). Inborn and acquired features of the structure and function of the heart and blood vessels can affect the resting blood pressure and the response of the blood pressure to stress.

Consider the blood vessels and their contribution to vascular resistance. In particular, the small arterioles form a point in the vascular tree with particularly high flow resistance. This flow resistance is a desirable feature of the vascular system that allows a drop from high pressure in the arteries to low pressure flow in the fine capillaries, a point where most nutrient and metabolite exchange occurs with the tissues. To accomplish this pressure drop, the arterioles have especially thick walls for their small diameter, with the highest proportion of autonomically innervated smooth muscle cells of all blood vessel types (Berne & Levy, 1972). The richness of sympathetic nerve endings on the vascular smooth muscle, and the thickness of this muscle layer, both suggest that vascular response factors may be a significant source of differences in both resting blood pressure and its response to stress (Allen, Obrist, Sherwood, & Crowell, 1987;

Turner, Sherwood, & Light, 1992). These differences may arise as a result of genetic differences in intrinsic growth factors found in the vascular wall that can increase the thickness of the muscle layer more in some persons than in others. A thicker vascular wall could produce a higher resting pressure due to a narrowed internal diameter of the blood vessel. In addition, any given increase in sympathetic outflow would produce a greater constrictive response, leading to a greater increase in flow resistance and a larger systemic blood pressure rise in response to stress (Folkow, 1990). The combination of elevated resistance response and potentially enhanced secretion of smooth muscle growth factors together may contribute to the increasing resting pressure seen during the development of hypertension. In this case, the tendency toward increased pressure could occur even in the case of normal emotional responsivity and normal levels of hypothalamic gain, although both of these other factors may also play a role in essential hypertension.

The other side of the blood pressure response equation is the heart and its tendency to increase cardiac output during a wide range of behavioral and emotional stressors. Cardiac output in turn is a result of the frequency with which the heart beats and its force of contraction (Rushmer, 1989). Increased heart rate in most behavioral challenges is a result of reduced vagal outflow to the heart, resulting in an increase in rate toward the human heart's intrinsic rate of 105–120 beats per minute. Force of contraction is associated with beta-adrenoreceptors on cardiac muscle cells. Individual differences in receptor populations could have a substantial effect on cardiac responsiveness during stress, leading to large increases in blood flow, and thereby to large blood pressure responses. Peripheral beta-receptor densities are a significant source of individual differences in cardiovascular reactivity (Mills et al., 1994; Mills, Dimsdale, Ziegler, Berry, & Bain, 1990). Other evidence indicates that administration of nonselective and cardioselective beta-blocking agents reduces cardiac responsivity to stress in nonhuman primates and human volunteers (Ablad et al., 1988; Ades, Thomas, Hanson, Shapiro, & LaMountain, 1987; Cacioppo et al., 1994; Kaplan, Manuck, Adams, Weingand, & Clark-son, 1987; Trap-Jensen et al., 1982). It should be noted that such blockade does not abolish the response to mental stress, although it does attenuate it (Ablad et al., 1988). In addition to beta-adrenoreceptor function in the heart, prehypertensive states are often accompanied by increased thickness of the wall of the left ventricle (Folkow, 1990; Jokiniitty, Majahalme, Kahonen, Tuomisto, & Turjanmaa, 2001; Majahalme, Turjanmaa, Tuomisto, Kautiainen, & Uusitalo, 1997). This left ventricular wall thickening may be associated with elevated levels of peripheral muscle growth factors, as in the blood vessel, and this process is enhanced by elevated peripheral resistance, leading to greater work by the cardiac muscle needed to overcome the higher peripheral resistance (Palatini, 1999).

The foregoing discussion suggests that peripheral tissue factors and autonomic receptor densities are likely to be important factors in determining individual differences in stress reactivity and potentially in disease etiology. In studies of spontaneously hypertensive rats and related strains, stress increases the likelihood and progression of hypertension, and peripheral mechanisms are partly responsible for these effects (Brown, Li, Lawler, & Randall, 1999; Lawler, Barker, Hubbard, & Allen, 1980). The relationships among individual differences in stress reactivity, stressor exposure in daily life, and disease onset and progression are as yet unclear in humans. Research on animal models indicates that stress can enhance cardiovascular disease progression in predisposed animals, such as the spontaneously hypertensive rat. Some of this effect is due to enhanced central mechanisms governing stress reactivity, and some of it is a response in vulnerable peripheral tissues that are more readily altered by stress (Folkow, 1990; Okamoto, Nosaka, Yamori, & Matsumoto, 1967).

Evidence for Individual Differences in Reactivity at Different Levels in the System

In the previous discussion, I have singled out evidence from human and animal models to suggest that differences between individuals can arise at three levels of organization in the system: Level I is concerned with the formation of appraisals, and emotional reactions to those appraisals, due to individual differences in frontal–limbic processes. Level II is concerned with hypothalamic and brainstem mechanisms. Level III concerns peripheral differences in autonomic and endocrine effector systems. This evidence was summarized with little attention to the selectivity of the evidence to each of the specified levels of organization. Indeed, in the spontaneously hypertensive rat, there is good evidence that elevated basal function and reactions to stress are supported by strain differences found at all three of the levels discussed. This raises the practical question of whether it is possible to dissect out different levels of systems function in data obtained from human volunteers in studies of stress reactivity. In earlier presentations of this model, we provided examples, mostly from our own research, showing how self-report, endocrine, and other sources of data could be used to infer what level in the system was responsible for reactivity differences between defined groups of subjects (Lovallo, 2005a, 2005b; Lovallo & Gerin, 2003). This evidence is summarized here.

Level I Effects of Stress Reactivity

In considering Level I, we conducted a study of remitted alcoholics and healthy controls, and wanted to examine limbic system differences in response to public speaking as a social stressor (Panknin, Dickensheets, Nixon, & Lovallo, 2002). Because of the long-term drinking history of the alcoholics, we were interested in ruling out peripheral cardiac damage, along with possible changes in brainstem regulation of the heart, as causes of reduced stress responses. In this case we used a simple orthostatic challenge, having the subjects stand in place for 5 minutes while we made cardiovascular measurements. In this case, equivalent heart rate and blood pressure responses occurred in both groups, allowing us to have some confidence that reduced response to public speaking in the alcohol-dependent group was not a result of cardiac or autonomic damage because reflex regulation of the heart and blood vessels was intact in these individuals.

More often, the purpose is to identify subjects who have exaggerated emotional reactivity. Evidence from epidemiological studies shows that hostile individuals are at increased risk of myocardial infarction and sudden death (Dembroski & Costa, 1987; Dembroski, MacDougall, Costa, & Grandits, 1989; Everson et al., 1997). In a laboratory study, we concluded that the overriding factor supporting enhanced cardiovascular reactions in highly hostile young men was the action of frontal–limbic processes associated with hostile interpretations of the situation and a strong tendency to have angry responses following these interpretations (Everson, McKey, & Lovallo, 1995). Other colleagues had shown that subjects high in cynical hostility were likely to have large cardiovascular responses to harassment (Suarez & Williams, 1989, 1990). We were interested in knowing whether the reactions of hostile individuals were specific to their hostile tendencies. In this study we recruited healthy males in their early 20s and conducted a structured interview for Type A behavior and assessed the answers for hostile style and content (Dembroski & Costa, 1987). Persons high versus low in hostility were invited back to the lab for a study characterized as examining blood pressure responses during work on cognitive tasks. On this second visit, the hostility groups were tested on two mental arithmetic tasks separated by a rest period. A subset of high- and low-hostility subjects served as a control group that completed both tasks under neutral conditions with no provocation. In contrast, the remaining subjects were exposed to the following scenario: Toward the end of the rest interval, a new experimenter appeared in the testing room and claimed that the first one had forgotten an appointment and had to leave unexpectedly. She picked up the magazines provided for the subject just as a phone rang outside the lab. She answered the call, leaving the door open so the subject could hear her talking with an imagined friend about several trivial social topics while he waited with nothing to occupy his time. During the second task, this rude experimenter also interrupted the second task with several harshly spoken comments, telling the subject to hurry up, to speak louder, and saying that he got an answer wrong when in fact it was correct.

Data collection involved a range of cardiovascular parameters and structured self-reports of positive and negative moods, as well as an open-ended debriefing designed to elicit spontaneous reports of the subject's state of mind during the study. The control group proved useful in showing that the high- and low-hostility groups did not differ in any cardiovascular variables or self-reported moods in either phase of the study. Both high- and low-hostility control subjects had smaller cardiovascular responses to the repeated task, consistent with adapting to a familiar challenge. In the harassment groups, the low-hostility subjects had similar responses on both the first and the second task, indicating that they were not reactive to this challenge. In contrast, the hostile subjects who underwent provocation had larger heart rate, blood pressure, and rate–pressure product responses (a measure of myocardial oxygen demand) during the second task. They appeared to have responded to the harassment with increased responses to the mental arithmetic. Debriefing the harassed subjects revealed substantial differences in how the high-hostility subjects interpreted the situation and personalized the perceived slight. While the low-hostility group indicated that the new experimenter seemed a little brusque and even rude, they usually attributed this to her "having a bad day." On the other hand, the high-hostility subjects took this behavior as a personal offense, with one subject actually removing his electrodes and declaring that he would not participate in a study where people were treated like this. (He was debriefed and sheepishly expressed regret for spoiling his data.) Our interpretation of these findings was that the highly hostile subjects reacted in a rigidly fixed way to this situation, did not seek to find an alternative explanation for the experimenter's behavior, and reacted out of habit in an unreflective, hostile manner.

In addition, data from the control groups proved useful in ruling out alternative explanations. First, the high- and low-hostility subjects in the nonharassed condition reported similar mood states at all points in the experiment and also had equivalent cardiovascular responses to the two tasks. Other evidence indicates that under neutral circumstances, the cardiovascular responses to mental arithmetic are due to the expenditure of cognitive effort and to the nonspecific social challenge of being monitored for accuracy. Thus, the emotional content of the control task was equal for the two hostility subgroups. Since the cognitive effort involved in the neutral task did not cause any between-group differences in response, we concluded that the high-hostility subjects were not different from low-hostility subjects in hypothalamic or brainstem outputs, or in peripheral mechanisms governing their stress responses. This suggests that epidemiological findings of greater all-cause mortality among hostile individuals (Everson et al., 1997) may derive from differences in cognitive interpretations of events in daily life, and the subsequent emotional reactions to these events rather than specific alterations in response tendency at lower levels in the system.

Level II Effects of Stress Reactivity

There is also evidence that individual differences in hypothalamic reactivity can be identified under certain conditions in the lab, suggesting that some individual differences in stress response and disease risk depend on Level II differences in reactivity. In one study, we had normotensive and borderline hypertensive young men visit the lab on 4 separate days in a lengthy study of stress and caffeine responses. Testing the subjects each day for cardiovascular activity and cortisol output prior to any other manipulation made the days directly comparable. We found that cortisol output was elevated in the borderline hypertensive group on the first two lab visits, while the normotensives had a steady, lower level of output across all 4 days (al'Absi & Lovallo, 1993). Structured self-reports of positive and negative moods indicated that the risk groups were identical in their subjective states on all 4 days. We inferred that the increased hypothalamic activity in the borderline hypertensives was a nonspecific response to the general anticipation of a novel environment and being faced with unfamiliar tasks and study procedures. Under this logic, hypothalamic activity of the borderline hypertensives was exaggerated even though their self-reports indicated otherwise-similar cognitive and affective responses to the situation.

A related form of evidence was obtained during an epidemiological study of cardiovascular reactivity, and subsequent myocardial infarction and incidence of stroke in middle-aged men (Everson, Kaplan, Goldberg, & Salonen, 1996; Everson et al., 2001). In this case, a tendency toward a high level of reactivity was assessed from the degree of systolic blood pressure rise seen in anticipation of a bicycle ergometer exercise stress test. The group of volunteers with the largest responses had the worst disease outcomes. It is likely that these greater anticipatory responses depended on systemic gain factors and not specific emotional response differences, given the absence of any emotionally valenced provocation associated with the test. This interpretation admittedly involves some speculation because there were no self-reports to allow us to rule out differential cognitive interpretations and consequently biased emotional responses to the test in those with the largest systolic blood pressure responses. Nonetheless, the presence of anticipatory responses bears a resemblance to our earlier data on the anticipatory cortisol responses in the borderline hypertensive group.

Level III Effects of Stress Reactivity

Level III processes include those governed by peripheral response systems. Exaggerated stress responses that are due to altered response characteristics of peripheral tissues are usually taken as a sign of preclinical or clinical disease. To take one example, in the case of hypertension, blood vessel thickening might occur very early in the disease process, accompanied by exaggerated blood pressure responses to stress. Similarly, the elevated tonic and phasic blood pressure levels seen in hypertension development result in increased thickening of the left ventricular wall. In the spontaneously hypertensive rat, and perhaps in humans with essential hypertension, genetically determined differences in tissue growth factors may underlie the process of muscle cell growth that propels the blood vessels and heart toward hypertrophy, setting off a spiral that leads ultimately to heart failure and death. A question for reactivity researchers is how to separate peripheral mechanisms from mechanisms associated with Levels I and II in our model. First is to rule out altered evaluation of the situation and heightened emotional reactiv-

ity in the population under study. One way to do this is to make careful measures of how subjects are appraising the situation and what their affective state is during the stressor in question. While perhaps not an absolute proof that frontal–limbic processes are not at work, the absence of such a difference provides some confidence that appraisal processes are not the primary cause of group differences in reactivity. Second is to rule out mechanisms at Level II in the model. We have interpreted a lack of group differences in cortisol secretion to suggest that there is no differential responsivity at the level of the paraventricular nucleus of the hypothalamus, the nucleus responsible for generating cortisol responses, and also tying these to sympathetic outputs to the periphery (Swanson & Sawchenko, 1980). For this reason, it seems that equivalent cortisol response is a useful way of considering hypothalamic activation and sympathetic outputs to be comparable in the groups being tested. By this logic, any remaining group difference in cardiovascular response is likely to be due to peripheral response mechanisms.

However, specific tests of peripheral contributions to cardiovascular and endocrine components of the stress responses may require a combination of specific autonomic function tests and perhaps sympathetic outflow measurements (Anderson & Mark, 1989; Dunlap & Pfeifer, 1989). Although these may be technically demanding, there are some simple means for assessing the role of brainstem outputs as causes of reactivity differences. As noted earlier, a simple orthostatic challenge test may suffice to test for normal or abnormal sympathetic outflow to the heart and blood vessels, providing useful information about peripheral regulation (Panknin et al., 2002). In another case, we were able to examine vascular reactivity in borderline hypertensive young men by administering caffeine and measuring their blood pressure responses at rest (Pincomb et al., 1996). Prior work had shown that the blood pressure response to caffeine depends on enhanced smooth muscle activity causing increased peripheral resistance (Pincomb et al., 1985), allowing us to interpret the effect of caffeine in the borderline hypertensive group as being due to an increased vascular wall response.

Conclusions

The foregoing discussion draws our attention to the essential question of the nature of causality in the stress reactivity hypothesis: Can persistently exaggerated emotional and stress reactions cause disease in an otherwise healthy person? The evidence in humans that large stress responses can be a sole cause of disease is not convincing. In part this derives from the extensive background work needed to rule out subclincal disease in human volunteers and the necessarily lengthy follow-up necessary to observe the appearance of disease in the study population. Work with animal models suggests that healthy-appearing primates who have large cardiovascular responses to social stress may be at increased risk of coronary atherosclerosis (Kaplan et al., 1983; Manuck, Kaplan, Adams, & Clarkson, 1989). The same appears to be true for humans (Jennings et al., 2004), although the base of data is sketchier.

We might also ask why it is necessary to try to refine our systems view of factors contributing to stress reactivity in different groups. Much work in the field of epidemiology and in the laboratory focuses on single measures of reactivity, such as blood pressure rise, and views these as equivalent across groups and different studies. While this may suffice for some purposes, the discussion in this chapter is an attempt to dissect the nature of reactivity differences in response to emotionally relevant stressors to gain some leverage in understanding underlying mechanisms. Under this view, two groups with equivalently large blood pressure responses might not be seen as equivalent if one has a very large, negative emotional response to a stressor, while the other has larger peripheral responses. It seems important to make such distinctions if studies of reactivity are to contribute to a mechanistic understanding of psychological factors and health and disease.

Acknowledgments

Preparation of this chapter was supported by the National Institutes of Health (Grant Nos. AA12207 and HL32050) and by the Department of Veterans Affairs. I thank Noha Farag, MD, for her critical reading of an earlier version of this chapter.

Further Reading

Anderson, S. W., Bechara, A., Damasio, H., Tranel, D., & Damasio, A. R. (1999). Impairment of social and moral behavior related to early damage in human prefrontal cortex. *Nature Neuroscience, 2,* 1032–1037.

Cannon, W. B. (1928). The mechanism of emotional disturbance of bodily functions. *New England Journal of Medicine, 198,* 165–172.

Damasio, A. R. (1994). *Descartes' error: Emotion, reason, and the human brain.* New York: Putnam.

Everson, S. A., McKey, B. S., & Lovallo, W. R. (1995). Effect of trait hostility on cardiovascular responses to harassment in young men. *International Journal of Behavioral Medicine, 2,* 172–191.

Folkman, S., & Lazarus, R. S. (1988). Coping as a mediator of emotion. *Journal of Personality and Social Psychology, 54,* 466–475.

Gianaros, P. J., May, J. C., Siegle, G. J., & Jennings, J. R. (2005). Is there a functional neural correlate of individual differences in cardiovascular reactivity? *Psychosomatic Medicine, 67,* 31–39.

Schulkin, J., Thompson, B. L., & Rosen, J. B. (2003). Demythologizing the emotions: adaptation, cognition, and visceral representations of emotion in the nervous system. *Brain and Cognition, 52,* 15–23.

Schwartz, A. R., Gerin, W., Davidson, K. W., Pickering, T. G., Brosschot, J. F., Thayer, J. F., et al. (2003). Toward a causal model of cardiovascular responses to stress and the development of cardiovascular disease. *Psychosomatic Medicine, 65,* 22–35.

References

Ablad, B., Bjorkman, J. A., Gustafsson, D., Hansson, G., Ostlund-Lindqvist, A. M., & Pettersson, K. (1988). The role of sympathetic activity in atherogenesis: Effects of beta-blockade. *American Heart Journal, 116,* 322–327.

Ades, P. A., Thomas, J. D., Hanson, J. S., Shapiro, S. M., & LaMountain, J. (1987). Effect of metoprolol on the submaximal stress test performed early after acute myocardial infarction. *American Journal of Cardiology, 60,* 963–966.

Adolphs, R., Gosselin, F., Buchanan, T. W., Tranel, D., Schyns, P., & Damasio, A. R. (2005). A mechanism for impaired fear recognition after amygdala damage. *Nature, 433,* 68–72.

al'Absi, M., Bongard, S., Buchanan, T., Pincomb, G. A., Licinio, J., & Lovallo, W. R. (1997). Cardiovascular and neuroendocrine adjustment to public speaking and mental arithmetic stressors. *Psychophysiology, 34*, 266–275.

al'Absi, M., & Lovallo, W. R. (1993). Cortisol concentrations in serum of borderline hypertensive men exposed to a novel experimental setting. *Psychoneuroendocrinology, 18*, 355–363.

al'Absi, M., Lovallo, W. R., McKey, B. S., & Pincomb, G. A. (1994). Borderline hypertensives produce exaggerated adrenocortical responses to sustained mental stress. *Psychosomatic Medicine, 56*, 245–250.

Allen, M. T., Obrist, P. A., Sherwood, A., & Crowell, M. D. (1987). Evaluation of myocardial and peripheral vascular responses during reaction time, mental arithmetic and cold pressor. *Psychophysiology, 24*, 648–656.

Amaral, D. G., Price, J. L., Pitkanen, A., & Carmichael, S. T. (1992). Anatomical organization of the primate amygdaloid complex. In J. P. Aggleton (Ed.), *The amygdala: Neurobiological aspects of emotion, memory, and mental dysfunction* (pp. 1–66). New York: Wiley-Liss.

Anderson, E. A., & Mark, A. L. (1989). Microneruographic measurement of sympathetic nerve activity in humans. In N. Schneiderman, P. Kaufmann, & S. Weiss (Eds.), *Handbook of research methods in cardiovascular behavioral medicine* (pp. 107–115). New York: Plenum Press.

Anderson, S. W., Bechara, A., Damasio, H., Tranel, D., & Damasio, A. R. (1999). Impairment of social and moral behavior related to early damage in human prefrontal cortex. *Nature Neuroscience, 2*, 1032–1037.

Appleton, J. A. (2006). Postulating that our neurological models for musculoskeletal support, movement, and emotional expression come from archetypal forms in early organisms. *Medical Hypotheses, 66*, 1029–1035.

Aston-Jones, G., Ennis, M., Pieribone, R. A., Nickell, W. T., & Shipley, M. T. (1986). The brain nucleus locus coeruleus: Restricted afferent control of a broad efferent network. *Science, 234*, 734–737.

Bard, P. (1928). A diencephalic mechanism for the expression of rage with special reference to the sympathetic nervous system. *American Journal of Physiology, 84*, 490–515.

Bechara, A., Damasio, H., Tranel, D., & Damasio, A. R. (1997). Deciding advantageously before knowing the advantageous strategy. *Science, 275*, 293–294.

Berne, R. M., & Levy, M. N. (1972). *Cardiovascular physiology* (2nd ed.). St. Louis, MO: Mosby.

Blair, K., Marsh, A. A., Morton, J., Vythilingam, M., Jones, M., Mondillo, K., et al. (2006). Choosing the lesser of two evils, the better of two goods: Specifying the roles of ventromedial prefrontal cortex and dorsal anterior cingulate in object choice. *Journal of Neuroscience, 26*, 11379–11386.

Brondolo, E., Rieppi, R., Erickson, S. A., Bagiella, E., Shapiro, P. A., McKinley, P., et al. (2003). Hostility, interpersonal interactions, and ambulatory blood pressure. *Psychosomatic Medicine, 65*, 1003–1011.

Brown, D. R., Li, S. G., Lawler, J. E., & Randall, D. C. (1999). Sympathetic control of BP and BP variability in borderline hypertensive rats on high- vs. low-salt diet. *American Journal of Physiology, 277*, R650–R657.

Cacioppo, J. T., Berntson, G. G., Binkley, P. F., Quigley, K. S., Uchino, B. N., & Fieldstone, A. (1994). Autonomic cardiac control: II. Noninvasive indices and basal response as revealed by autonomic blockades. *Psychophysiology, 31*, 586–598.

Campbell, T. G. (2007). The best of a bad bunch: The ventromedial prefrontal cortex and dorsal anterior cingulate cortex in decision making. *Journal of Neuroscience, 27*, 447–448.

Cannon, W. B. (1928). The mechanism of emotional disturbance of bodily functions. *New England Journal of Medicine, 198*, 165–172.

Cannon, W. B. (1957). "Voodoo" death. *Psychosomatic Medicine, 19*, 182–190.

Critchley, H. D., Mathias, C. J., & Dolan, R. J. (2002). Fear conditioning in humans: The influence of awareness and autonomic arousal on functional neuroanatomy. *Neuron, 33*, 653–663.

Critchley, H. D., Wiens, S., Rotshtein, P., Ohman, A., & Dolan, R. J. (2004). Neural systems supporting interoceptive awareness. *Nature Neuroscience, 7*, 189–195.

Damasio, A. R. (1994). *Descartes' error: Emotion, reason, and the human brain.* New York: Putnam.

Dembroski, T. M., & Costa, P. T., Jr. (1987). Coronary prone behavior: Components of the type A pattern and hostility. *Journal of Personality, 55*, 211–235.

Dembroski, T. M., MacDougall, J. M., Costa, P. T., Jr., & Grandits, G. A. (1989). Components of hostility as predictors of sudden death and myocardial infarction in the Multiple Risk Factor Intervention Trial. *Psychosomatic Medicine, 51*, 514–522.

Drevets, W. C., Gautier, C., Price, J. C., Kupfer, D. J., Kinahan, P. E., Grace, A. A., et al. (2001). Amphetamine-induced dopamine release in human ventral striatum correlates with euphoria. *Biological Psychiatry, 49*, 81–96.

Dunlap, E. D., & Pfeifer, M. A. (1989). Autonomic function testing. In N. Schneiderman, P. Kaufmann, & S. Weiss (Eds.), *Handbook of research methods in cardiovascular behav-*

ioral medicine (pp. 91–106). New York: Plenum Press.

Ekman, P. (1993). Facial expression and emotion. *American Psychologist, 48,* 384–392.

Ekman, P., & Friesen, W. V. (1971). Constants across cultures in the face and emotion. *Journal of Personality and Social Psychology, 17,* 124–129.

Everson, S. A., Kaplan, G. A., Goldberg, D. E., & Salonen, J. T. (1996). Anticipatory blood pressure response to exercise predicts future high blood pressure in middle-aged men. *Hypertension, 27,* 1059–1064.

Everson, S. A., Kauhanen, J., Kaplan, G. A., Goldberg, D. E., Julkunen, J., Tuomilehto, J., et al. (1997). Hostility and increased risk of mortality and acute myocardial infarction: The mediating role of behavioral risk factors. *American Journal of Epidemiology, 146,* 142–152.

Everson, S. A., Lynch, J. W., Kaplan, G. A., Lakka, T. A., Sivenius, J., & Salonen, J. T. (2001). Stress-induced blood pressure reactivity and incident stroke in middle-aged men. *Stroke, 32,* 1263–1270.

Everson, S. A., McKey, B. S., & Lovallo, W. R. (1995). Effect of trait hostility on cardiovascular responses to harassment in young men. *International Journal of Behavioral Medicine, 2,* 172–191.

Folkman, S., & Lazarus, R. S. (1988). Coping as a mediator of emotion. *Journal of Personality and Social Psychology, 54,* 466–475.

Folkow, B. (1990). "Structural factor" in primary and secondary hypertension. *Hypertension, 16,* 89–101.

Fontenot, M. B., Kaplan, J. R., Manuck, S. B., Arango, V., & Mann, J. J. (1995). Long-term effects of chronic social stress on serotonergic indices in the prefrontal cortex of adult male cynomolgus macaques. *Brain Research, 705,* 105–108.

Gianaros, P. J., May, J. C., Siegle, G. J., & Jennings, J. R. (2005). Is there a functional neural correlate of individual differences in cardiovascular reactivity? *Psychosomatic Medicine, 67,* 31–39.

Goncharuk, V. D., Van Heerikhuize, J., Swaab, D. F., & Buijs, R. M. (2002). Paraventricular nucleus of the human hypothalamus in primary hypertension: Activation of corticotropin-releasing hormone neurons. *Journal of Comparative Neurology, 443,* 321–331.

Grant, S. J., Aston-Jones, G., & Redmond, D. E., Jr. (1988). Responses of primate locus coeruleus neurons to simple and complex sensory stimuli. *Brain Research Bulletin, 21,* 401–410.

Halgren, E. (1992). Emotional neurophysiology of the amygdala within the context of human cognition. In J. P. Aggleton (Ed.), *The amygdala: Neurobiological aspects of emotion, memory, and mental dysfunction* (pp. 191–228). New York: Wiley-Liss.

Harlow, J. M. (1868). Recovery from the passage of an iron bar through the head. *Journal of the Massachusetts Medical Society, 2,* 327–347.

Hilz, M. J., Devinsky, O., Szczepanska, H., Borod, J. C., Marthol, H., & Tutaj, M. (2006). Right ventromedial prefrontal lesions result in paradoxical cardiovascular activation with emotional stimuli. *Brain, 129,* 3343–3355.

Jennings, J. R., Kamarck, T. W., Everson-Rose, S. A., Kaplan, G. A., Manuck, S. B., & Salonen, J. T. (2004). Exaggerated blood pressure responses during mental stress are prospectively related to enhanced carotid atherosclerosis in middle-aged Finnish men. *Circulation, 110,* 2198–2203.

Jokiniitty, J. M., Majahalme, S. K., Kahonen, M. A., Tuomisto, M. T., & Turjanmaa, V. M. (2001). Pulse pressure is the best predictor of future left ventricular mass and change in left ventricular mass: 10 years of follow-up. *Journal of Hypertension, 19,* 2047–2054.

Jones, E. G., & Powell, T. P. S. (1970). An anatomical study on converging sensory pathways within the cerebral cortex of the monkey. *Brain Research, 83,* 793–820.

Kagan, J. (1994). On the nature of emotion. *Monographs of the Society for Research in Child Development, 59,* 7–24.

Kaplan, J. R., Manuck, S. B., Adams, M. R., Weingand, K. W., & Clarkson, T. B. (1987). Inhibition of coronary atherosclerosis by propranolol in behaviorally predisposed monkeys fed an atherogenic diet. *Circulation, 76,* 1364–1372.

Kaplan, J. R., Manuck, S. B., Clarkson, T. B., Lusso, F. M., Taub, D. M., & Miller, E. W. (1983). Social stress and atherosclerosis in normocholesterolemic monkeys. *Science, 220,* 733–735.

Koepp, M. J., Gunn, R. N., Lawrence, A. D., Cunningham, V. J., Dagher, A., Jones, T., et al. (1998). Evidence for striatal dopamine release during a video game. *Nature, 393,* 266–268.

Koriat, A., Melkman, R., Averill, J. R., & Lazarus, R. S. (1972). The self-control of emotional reactions to a stressful film. *Journal of Personality, 40,* 601–619.

Kosson, D. S., Budhani, S., Nakic, M., Chen, G., Saad, Z. S., Vythilingam, M., et al. (2006). The role of the amygdala and rostral anterior cingulate in encoding expected outcomes during learning. *NeuroImage, 29,* 1161–1172.

Lawler, J. E., Barker, G. F., Hubbard, J. W., & Allen, M. T. (1980). The effects of conflict on tonic levels of blood pressure in the genetically borderline hypertensive rat. *Psychophysiology, 17,* 363–370.

Lazarus, R. S. (1991). Cognition and motivation in emotion. *American Psychologist, 46,* 352–367.

Lazarus, R. S. (1999). *Stress and emotion: A new synthesis.* New York: Springer.

Lazarus, R. S., Baker, R. W., Broverman, D. M., & Mayer, J. (1957). Personality and psychological stress. *Journal of Personality, 25,* 559–577.

Lazarus, R. S., & Folkman, S. (1984). *Stress, appraisal and coping.* New York: Springer.

Lesch, K. P., & Mossner, R. (2006). Inactivation of 5HT transport in mice: Modeling altered 5HT homeostasis implicated in emotional dysfunction, affective disorders, and somatic syndromes. In F. B. Hoffmann (Ed.), *Handbook of Experimental Pharmacology* (pp. 417–456). Heidelberg: Springer.

Lovallo, W. R. (2005a). Cardiovascular reactivity: Mechanisms and pathways to cardiovascular disease. *International Journal of Psychophysiology, 58,* 119–132.

Lovallo, W. R. (2005b). *Stress and health: Biological and psychological interactions* (2nd ed.). Thousand Oaks, CA: Sage.

Lovallo, W. R., & Gerin, W. (2003). Psychophysiological reactivity: mechanisms and pathways to cardiovascular disease. *Psychosomatic Medicine, 65,* 36–45.

Majahalme, S., Turjanmaa, V., Tuomisto, M., Kautiainen, H., & Uusitalo, A. (1997). Intraarterial blood pressure during exercise and left ventricular indices in normotension and borderline and mild hypertension. *Blood Pressure, 6,* 5–12.

Manuck, S. B., Kaplan, J. R., Adams, M. R., & Clarkson, T. B. (1989). Behaviorally elicited heart rate reactivity and atherosclerosis in female cynomolgus monkeys (*Macaca fascicularis*). *Psychosomatic Medicine, 51,* 306–318.

McEwen, B. S. (2006). Protective and damaging effects of stress mediators: Central role of the brain. *Dialogues in Clinical Neuroscience, 8,* 367–381.

Mills, P. J., Dimsdale, J. E., Nelesen, R. A., Jasiewicz, J., Ziegler, M. G., & Kennedy, B. (1994). Patterns of adrenergic receptors and adrenergic agonists underlying cardiovascular responses to a psychological challenge. *Psychosomatic Medicine, 56,* 70–76.

Mills, P. J., Dimsdale, J. E., Ziegler, M. G., Berry, C. C., & Bain, R. D. (1990). Beta-adrenergic receptors predict heart rate reactivity to a psychosocial stressor. *Psychosomatic Medicine, 52,* 621–623.

Niedenthal, P. M. (2007). Embodying emotion. *Science, 316,* 1002–1005.

Okamoto, K., Nosaka, S., Yamori, Y., & Matsumoto, M. (1967). Participation of neural factor in the pathogenesis of hypertension in the spontaneously hypertensive rat. *Japanese Heart Journal, 8,* 168–180.

Palatini, P. (1999). Ambulatory blood pressure monitoring and borderline hypertension. *Blood Pressure Monitoring, 4,* 233–240.

Panknin, T. L., Dickensheets, S. L., Nixon, S. J., & Lovallo, W. R. (2002). Attenuated heart rate responses to public speaking in individuals with alcohol dependence. *Alcoholism: Clinical and Experimental Research, 26,* 841–847.

Pincomb, G. A., Lovallo, W. R., McKey, B. S., Sung, B. H., Passey, R. B., Everson, S. A., et al. (1996). Acute blood pressure elevations with caffeine in men with borderline systemic hypertension. *American Journal of Cardiology, 77,* 270–274.

Pincomb, G. A., Lovallo, W. R., Passey, R. B., Whitsett, T. L., Silverstein, S. M., & Wilson, M. F. (1985). Effects of caffeine on vascular resistance, cardiac output and myocardial contractility in young men. *American Journal of Cardiology, 56,* 119–122.

Pope, M. K., & Smith, T. W. (1991). Cortisol excretion in high and low cynically hostile men. *Psychosomatic Medicine, 53,* 386–392.

Ranson, S. W. (1934). The hypothalamus: Its significance for visceral innervation and emotional expression. *Transactions of the College of Physicians and Philadelphia, 4*(2), 222–242.

Rolls, E. T. (2000). Precis of *The brain and emotion. Behavior and Brain Science, 23,* 177–191; discussion 192–233.

Roman, O., Seres, J., Pometlova, M., & Jurcovicova, J. (2004). Neuroendocrine or behavioral effects of acute or chronic emotional stress in Wistar Kyoto (WKY) and spontaneously hypertensive (SHR) rats. *Endocrine Regulation, 38,* 151–155.

Rushmer, R. M. (1989). Structure and function of the cardiovascular system. In N. Schneiderman, P. Kaufmann, & S. Weiss (Eds.), *Handbook of research methods in cardiovascular behavioral medicine* (pp. 5–22). New York: Plenum Press.

Schachter, S., & Singer, J. E. (1962). Cognitive, social, and physiological determinants of emotional state. *Psychological Review, 69,* 379–399.

Schulkin, J., Thompson, B. L., & Rosen, J. B. (2003). Demythologizing the emotions: Adaptation, cognition, and visceral representations of emotion in the nervous system. *Brain and Cognition, 52,* 15–23.

Schwartz, A. R., Gerin, W., Davidson, K. W., Pickering, T. G., Brosschot, J. F., Thayer, J. F., et al. (2003). Toward a causal model of cardiovascular responses to stress and the development of cardiovascular disease. *Psychosomatic Medicine, 65,* 22–35.

Sinha, R., Lovallo, W. R., & Parsons, O. A.

(1992). Cardiovascular differentiation of emotions. *Psychosomatic Medicine, 54,* 422–435.

Smith, O. A., Astley, C. A., Spelman, F. A., Golanov, E. V., Chalyan, V. G., Bowden, D. M., et al. (1993). Integrating behavior and cardiovascular responses: Posture and locomotion: I. Static analysis. *American Journal of Physiology, 265,* R1458–R1468.

Spencer, S. J., Ebner, K., & Day, T. A. (2004). Differential involvement of rat medial prefrontal cortex dopamine receptors in modulation of hypothalamic–pituitary–adrenal axis responses to different stressors. *European Journal of Neuroscience, 20,* 1008–1016.

Suarez, E. C., & Williams, R. B., Jr. (1989). Situational determinants of cardiovascular and emotional reactivity in high and low hostile men. *Psychosomatic Medicine, 51,* 404–418.

Suarez, E. C., & Williams, R. B., Jr. (1990). The relationships between dimensions of hostility and cardiovascular reactivity as a function of task characteristics. *Psychosomatic Medicine, 52,* 558–570.

Suls, J., David, J. P., & Harvey, J. H. (1996). Personality and coping: Three generations of research. *Journal of Personality, 64,* 711–735.

Swanson, L. W. (2000). Cerebral hemisphere regulation of motivated behavior. *Brain Research, 886,* 113–164.

Swanson, L. W., & Sawchenko, P. E. (1980). Paraventricular nucleus: A site for the integration of neuroendocrine and autonomic mechanisms. *Neuroendocrinology, 31,* 410–417.

Taylor, S. E., & Stanton, A. L. (2007). Coping resources, coping processes, and mental health. *Annual Reviews of Clinical Psychology, 3,* 377–401.

Thrall, G., Lane, D., Carroll, D., & Lip, G. Y. (2007). A systematic review of the effects of acute psychological stress and physical activity on haemorheology, coagulation, fibrinolysis and platelet reactivity: Implications for the pathogenesis of acute coronary syndromes. *Thrombosis Research, 120,* 819–847.

Tracy, J. L., & Robins, R. W. (2004). Show your pride: Evidence for a discrete emotion expression. *Psychological Science, 15,* 194–197.

Trap-Jensen, J., Carlsen, J. E., Hartling, O. J., Svendsen, T. L., Tango, M., & Christensen, N. J. (1982). Beta-adrenoceptor blockade and psychic stress in man: A comparison of the acute effects of labetalol, metoprolol, pindolol and propranolol on plasma levels of adrenaline and noradrenaline. *British Journal of Clinical Pharmacology, 13,* 391S–395S.

Treiber, F. A., Kamarck, T., Schneiderman, N., Sheffield, D., Kapuku, G., & Taylor, T. (2003). Cardiovascular reactivity and development of preclinical and clinical disease states. *Psychosomatic Medicine, 65,* 46–62.

Turner, J. R., Sherwood, A., & Light, K. C. (1992). High cardiovascular reactivity to stress: A predictor of later hypertension development. In K. C. Light, A. Sherwood, & J. R. Turner (Eds.), *Individual differences in cardiovascular response to stress* (pp. 281–293). New York: Plenum Press.

CHAPTER 4

Cognitive and Affective Influences on Health Decisions

Angela Fagerlin
Ellen Peters
Alan Schwartz
Brian J. Zikmund-Fisher

People appear to comprehend and respond to information during decision making by using two separable but interacting modes of information processing (Epstein, 1994; Kahneman, 2003; Reyna, 2004). For instance, Epstein's (1994) model defines a deliberative[1] and an experiential system. The experiential system is intuitive, automatic, and nonverbal, whereas the deliberative system is an analytical system that functions by way of established rules of logic and evidence (e.g., probability theory). While everyone employs both of these information-processing systems to at least some degree, individuals may differ in the extent to which deliberative or experiential thinking influences their processing of information in decisions. For example, whereas a medical professional's understanding of risk as statistical probability may be more heavily influenced by the deliberative system, a layperson's understanding may rely on more experiential ways of knowing (Reventlow, Hvas, & Tulinius,

2001). Even within a single individual, different decision contexts or primes may lead to greater reliance on the deliberative versus experiential systems in decision making.

Under ideal conditions, patients making medical decisions would use the deliberative mode of information processing, with approaches such as subjective expected utility theory (SEUT; Savage, 1954), to decide on the best choice among their available options; that is, they would consider the probability of each possible event occurring and their perception of the utility or personal value of each outcome and then integrate both pieces to come up with a single aggregated valuation of each choice that could be used to find the personally best option. However, as shown in numerous studies by Kahneman and Tversky (Kahneman, Slovic, & Tversky, 1982; Kahneman & Tversky, 1973; Tversky & Kahneman, 1974), people's decisions frequently violate SEUT. These violations have been shown in a vast array of conditions, including many in the domain of medical decision making. Many of these violations occur because information processing also occurs in the experiential system and, in fact, this system may be the default mode with which

---

[1]Although Epstein uses the term "rational," we prefer to use the term "deliberative" for this mode of information processing because the experiential mode can also produce quite rational decisions.

people process information for decisions (Kahneman, 2003).

In this chapter, we begin by discussing a number of the most prevalent decision-making biases that emerged from the experiential system and were identified by Kahneman, Tversky, and others. We also suggest ways in which they are likely to influence people's medical decision making. A full discussion of health-care-relevant decision-making biases is, however, beyond the scope of this chapter.[2]

The influence of the experiential system is also demonstrated in the role that affect plays in decision making. SEUT is a pure information-processing model, without consideration of the decision maker's current affective state or anticipated affective reactions to outcomes except insofar as they are incorporated into utility estimates. Affect, however, has been shown to influence both perceptions of likelihood and valuations of outcomes, a set of effects dubbed the "affect heuristic" (Slovic, Finucane, Peters, & MacGregor, 2004). More generally, affect appears to function in multiple ways, guiding judgment and decision processes in health and other domains (Peters, Lipkus, & Diefenbach, 2006). The second part of the chapter focuses on the role of affect in decision making.

Finally, even in SEUT, people's decisions about their health care should be dependent on their understanding of the likelihood of different outcomes. Yet strong evidence exists that people's risk perceptions often diverge from the true level of risk, and that how risk information is presented to patients can have a significant effect on their understanding and reactions. We conclude our chapter by discussing how risk perceptions are formed and how they can be influenced by both affective and cognitive biases. Then, because quantitative information is becoming an increasingly important component of health decision making, we review the lit-

erature on optimal methods for presenting information to help patients make informed decisions.

Classic Decision Biases Relevant to Medical Decision Making

Framing

"Framing" is the term used to describe the fact that people make different decisions or have different preferences based on how the information is presented. It was first described in Tversky and Kahneman's (1981) classic experiment, the "Asian Flu Problem." In this study, two groups of people read scenarios about two possible public health plans for combating an Asian flu that otherwise was expected to kill 600 people. One group of participants was told that the first plan would result in the sure death of 400 people, whereas, in the second plan, there was a two-thirds probability that all 600 people would die (loss frame). The other group of subjects was told that the first plan would result in 200 people living; whereas the second plan would result in a one-third probability of all 600 people living (gain frame). Of course, the number of people who would live or die in each plan was equivalent across both frames. However, more individuals chose Plan 2 when the options were presented in a loss frame, and more individuals chose Plan 1 when the same options were presented in a gain frame.

This gain–loss sensitivity is reflected in prospect theory (Kahneman & Tversky, 1979), a generalization of SEUT that can be used to explain many decision biases. It hypothesizes that people evaluate gains and losses relative to a reference point (rather than to final outcomes) and further predicts that individuals are risk seekers when presented with information framed in terms of losses but are risk averse when the scenario is described in terms of gains. In terms of health care decisions, it would suggest that people's motivation to perform screening behaviors are stronger when the discussion emphasizes the losses (being less healthy than now) that can result from failing to act versus the gains (improvements in health or security) from acting. For example, decisions about mammography may be perceived as risky because there is a chance that cancer could be found

---

[2]For additional discussion of a number of other biases in health decision making, we recommend the excellent review by Chapman and Elstein (2000). In addition, we are unable to include other topics that may be of interest to readers, including methods to reduce cognitive effort (e.g., providing fewer options: Iyengar & Lepper, 2000; presenting less information: Peters, Dieckmann, Dixon, Hibbard, & Mertz, 2007; and support theory: Slovic, 2000).

as a result of undergoing the mammogram (Edwards, Elwyn, Covey, Matthews, & Pill, 2001). If the goal of a health message were to persuade women to undergo a mammogram, a loss-framed message (which would focus on the risks of "losing" by allowing an undetected cancer) would be expected to be more effective than a gain-framed message (e.g., emphasizing peace of mind, one of the benefits of mammography).

The framing effect has been tested in several medical domains with similar results. In one of the first examples of the framing effect in a medical scenario, McNeil, Pauker, Sox, and Tversky (1982) surveyed ambulatory patients, graduate students, and physicians. Members of all three groups were asked to imagine they had lung cancer and to make a treatment decision (surgery vs. radiation) based on cumulative probabilities and life-expectancy data. The authors manipulated whether this data was presented in a survival or mortality frame. In all three populations, more individuals chose surgery if the information was presented in a survival frame rather than if the same information was presented in a mortality frame. The survival frame seemed to induce more risk aversion as all patients would survive radiation treatment, but some patients would not survive surgery (i.e., 10 would die during surgery).

Furthermore, a review of the literature (Edwards et al., 2001) examining the effectiveness of loss- versus gain-framed messages for detection behaviors revealed that loss-framed messages were generally more effective than gain-framed messages, thus supporting prospect theory. When the target behavior is prevention (rather than detection), research has consistently shown that gain-framed messages are more effective in some situations (e.g., use of infant car restraints, regular physical exercise, and obtaining sunscreen) (Apanovitch, McCarthy, & Salovey, 2003; Rothman, Martino, Bedell, Detweiler, & Salovey, 1999). This finding is explained by the fact that gain-framed messages work better in situations where the outcomes are certain (e.g., using an infant car seat surely decreases injuries and deaths of children), whereas where there is uncertainty and risk (e.g., whether or not a mammogram will have a positive result), loss-framed messages are more effective in

promoting the desired behavior (Apanovitch et al., 2003).

Default or "Status Quo" Biases

A "default bias" occurs when people actively fail to choose an option and instead go with the default option, even if it is not in their best interest. As Kressel, Chapman, and Leventhal (2007) note, people will accept the default position (the choice implied by no response) "regardless of its implication" and thus accept (or reject) options they would not have accepted (or rejected) if the choice had not been the default option. The default bias is especially prevalent when people do not have strong preferences to influence their decisions or in situations with considerable barriers to choosing a new course of action (Halpern, Ubel, & Asch, 2007; Slovic, 1995).

The default bias has been shown to influence many domains of consumer choice (e.g., what stocks to invest in, water allocation plans; Samuelson & Zeckhauser, 1988), as well as health care decision making. Some specific health-related examples include organ donation (Johnson & Goldstein, 2003, 2004), flexible spending accounts (Halpern et al., 2007), mandated flu vaccinations for all health care workers (Halpern et al., 2007) and end-of-life care preferences as recorded in living wills (Kressel & Chapman, 2007; Kressel et al., 2007). We discuss two of these domains, organ donation and use of living wills, in more detail.

Johnson and Goldstein (2003, 2004) have conducted several studies examining the impact of default options in organ donation. In one study (2003), they randomized participants into one of three groups. In the first group, participants were told to imagine they had just moved to a new state, and the organ donation default was they were not willing to donate their organs (opt-in default). In the second group, participants were told that their new state's donation default was that they were willing to donate their organs (opt-out default). In the third group, there was no default and participants just had to choose whether to donate their organs. When they examined the number of people who effectively consented to organ donation, a remarkable outcome was observed: Only 42% of those in the opt-in consented to organ donation, compared to 82% of the opt-out subjects and 79% of those in the no-default condition. In a more ecologically valid study, Johnson and Goldstein (2004) examined consent to donate rates across European countries that differed in terms of whether they had opt-in or opt-out defaults for organ donation. The four countries that used opt-in defaults had significantly lower rates (range: 4.25–27.5%) than those countries that had opt-out defaults (range: 85.9–99.98).

The default bias can also be found in people's completion of living wills. Living wills are fraught with problems (Fagerlin & Schneider, 2004), and recent studies have shown that people's end-of-life treatment preferences, as outlined in living wills, may be strongly influenced by the default options present in the document (Kressel & Chapman, 2007; Kressel et al., 2007). In one study, older outpatients (65 years and older) were given living will forms that described 22 different care decisions (Kressel et al., 2007). The forms differed only in terms of whether a default option was provided and whether the default option, when provided, was to want treatment to be given or to be withheld. Individuals provided the give-treatment default option were more likely than those provided the withhold-treatment default option to indicate they wanted treatment. This finding held in 21 out of 22 decisions (and was significantly higher in seven of those decisions).

There have been a number of explanations for the default bias. Choosing the default option may minimize decisional conflict and reduce the cognitive effort required to make a choice (Chapman & Elstein, 2000). Additionally, many people view default options as recommendations made by a policymaker/authority figure (Halpern et al., 2007; Johnson & Goldstein, 2004) and thus attribute more validity to them. This would be particularly true in cases in which the authority is a trusted figure (Halpern et al., 2007).

Omission Biases

An "omission bias" is defined as perceiving bad outcomes caused by omissions (failures to act) as being more acceptable than equally severe outcomes caused by direct acts (commissions; Ritov & Baron, 1990; Spranca, Minsk, & Baron, 1991). This distinction may result from perceiving omissions as resulting from ignorance, whereas commissions may be the product of malicious intent and/or be due to more active behavior (Spranca et al., 1991). One of the earliest studies of the omission bias presented a scenario in which a disease would kill 10 out of 10,000 children (Ritov & Baron, 1990). A vaccine is available that can prevent the disease in all children, but it is accompanied by side effects that can result in the death of children receiving it. A significant number of individuals indicated they would reject the vaccine on behalf of their child even when the likelihood of dying from the vaccine was lower than the likelihood of dying from the disease. These participants revealed that they preferred to have their child die from the disease (which they did not cause) than to die from receiving the vaccine (which they would have ordered). Another study found a significant link between responses on such hypothetical scenarios and actual vaccination behavior among readers of *Mothering* magazine (Meszaros et al., 1996). In a more recent study, Wroe, Turner, and Salkovskis (2004) found that parents' worries about anticipated regret resulting from acts of omission or commission predicted their likelihood to vaccinate their children.

Yet harms of omission are not always preferred to harms of commission. Fagerlin, Zikmund-Fisher, and Ubel (2005a) found an opposite effect in which action was preferred for hypothetical cancer treatment decisions. In this study, participants who were asked to imagine they had been diagnosed with cancer chose between watchful waiting and surgery. Sixty-five percent of respondents indicated they would choose surgery over watchful waiting, even though the risk of death from watchful waiting was only 5%, whereas the risk of death from surgery was 10%. This discrepancy compared to previous studies may be due to the type of scenario used; that is, prevention decisions (e.g., vaccines) may be fundamentally different than treatment decisions from which people may derive particular solace or value by doing something rather than nothing.

Anchoring and Adjustment

When people have beliefs about how likely something is to occur (i.e., a probability estimate), those beliefs should logically be revised whenever new information suggests that the true probability is higher or lower than previously thought. However, people tend to place too much weight on their initial estimates and fail to adjust their estimates adequately, a bias known as "anchoring and adjustment" (Tversky & Kahneman, 1974) or "conservatism" (Edwards, 1968). Anchoring can occur even under conditions with no logical link between original and new information. For example, Ariely (2008) describes a study in which students were shown nice bottles of wine, imported chocolate, a cordless trackball, a cordless keyboard, and a graphic design book. Students were then asked to record the last two digits of their Social Security number and to write those numbers in the form of a dollar amount next to the names of the items previously shown. After indicating whether they would be willing to pay that amount for the item, students recorded the maximum price they would be for each item. Those whose Social Security numbers were in the upper 20% made bids that were between 216 and 346% higher than those whose Social Security numbers were in the lowest 20%—even though there is no logical reason why one's Social Security number should in any way be related to how much one values good food or computer accessories.

This effect has also been shown in several health psychology domains. For example, Poses, Bekes, Copare, and Scott (1990) asked physicians in a surgical intensive care unit (ICU) to estimate the probability of patients' survival until they were discharged from the hospital. Then, 48–72 hours later, they were asked to make a new set of estimates. Even with the introduction of considerable new information during the intervening 2–3 days, physicians' estimates varied very little from their initial estimates. Patients show similar effects in estimating their disease risk. In one study, participants were asked whether they believed their risk of colon cancer was higher or lower than 70%, or higher or lower than 30%. They were then asked to estimate their risk of colon cancer. Respondents who were asked whether their risk was higher or lower than 70% gave higher point estimates than those who were asked whether their risk was higher or lower than 30% (Klein & Stefanek, 2007).

Affect and Emotion in Assessments of Utility

A fundamental requirement of SEUT is that patients must be able to make accurate predictions about how they would feel if they experienced various outcomes (Ubel, Loewenstein, Schwarz, & Smith, 2005). Such assessments of quality of life define the outcome or "utility" values that are the direct inputs into SEUT calculations. Yet the utility (or disutility) that one experiences something (e.g., pain) may be very different than what one predicts based on prior experience (including earlier times when one was in pain).

To start, research in "affective forecasting" has shown that people have difficulty predicting their future feelings (Wilson & Gilbert, 2003). When making predictions about future feelings, people must make predictions about (1) the valence of their future feelings, (2) the type of emotions they will experience, (3) the initial intensity of those emotions, and (4) the duration of those emotions (Wilson & Gilbert, 2003). While errors in any of these four areas can occur, they are most common in people's predictions of the intensity and duration of their emotions.

Mispredictions can result through a number of mechanisms. First, people may misconstrue how an event will play out (Griffin & Ross, 1991). More specifically, by incorrectly imagining how an event will occur, people may mispredict how they will feel in that situation. For example, if a pregnant woman imagines an unmedicated childbirth that involves no unexpected complications (and the emotions that result from such a scenario) and then has an emergency Caesarean section, she likely will have misconstrued the valence of emotions experienced, the specific emotions she will feel, and the intensity and duration of those emotions (Wilson & Gilbert, 2003).

Second, people may make incorrect predictions about what parts of the experience will have the greatest impact on their emotional states (Dunn, Wilson, & Gilbert,

2003). For instance, Redelemeir and Kahneman (1996) asked patients to rate their level of pain (using a handheld computer) while undergoing a colonoscopy. Within an hour of the colonoscopy and again 1 month after the procedure, patients were asked to make a retrospective evaluation of the "total amount of pain experienced." Results showed that the retrospective judgments were significantly correlated with the peak intensity of pain and the pain that occurred in the final 3 minutes of the procedure. Longer procedures were not rated any more negatively than shorter procedures. Even more strikingly, the researchers later conducted a randomized clinical trial of normal versus extended colonoscopy (in which the procedure was artificially lengthened by leaving the scope in without moving it in order to end the experience with relatively less discomfort) and found that extended colonoscopy patients not only gave the procedure a better retrospective evaluation but also had higher rates of repeat colonoscopies in the future (Redelmeier, Katz, & Kahneman, 2003). Other research has found that duration matters during the experience, but that duration is not a significant predictor of the recall of that experience (whereas peak and final pain did influence recall; Ariely, 1998; Fredrickson & Kahneman, 1993). These results suggest significant discrepancies between people's actual experiences and their recall of those very same experiences. Since people make most decisions based on their recall, erroneous judgments likely result. Understanding these judgments, however, may help medical professionals design interventions that encourage healthy behaviors.

Third, people overestimate how much an event will affect their lives because they do not consider how the event fits into the broader context of their lives. This concept is referred to as "focalism" (Wilson, Wheatley, Meyers, Gilbert, & Axsom, 2000). For instance, when imagining what life would be like with a colostomy bag, people likely focus on images of plastic pouches and how their lives would be limited by having such a pouch (e.g., no more bikinis!) (Ubel et al., 2005), and although people might experience these types of feelings, they may fail to imagine all the events in their lives that will not be affected by the colostomy (e.g., enjoying dinner at their favorite restaurant,

watching their child do something especially adorable, going to an entertaining movie). Thus, people underestimate how all these other events will impact their happiness, and overestimate how much the focal event (i.e., having a colostomy bag) will influence their happiness.

Fourth, people have difficulty predicting how they will behave in a state that is different than their current state. Loewenstein (1999, 2005) called this the "hot–cold" empathy gap." In this situation, people who are in a "cold" state have difficulty predicting how they would feel in a "hot" state, and vice versa. For example, drug addicts underestimate how much would they would crave their drugs when in withdrawal; pregnant women, prior to labor, overestimate their desire to have an unmedicated birth compared with preferences during labor (Christensen-Szalanski, 1984); and sexually active individuals who are not in the "heat of the moment" overestimate their likelihood of using condoms during a sexual encounter. Conversely, when people are in a "hot" state, they underestimate the influence of that state and overestimate the stability of their preferences: For example, a person in drug withdrawal cannot imagine a state in which the craving does not exist.

There are numerous studies examining how affective forecasting can affect medical decision making, several of which are nicely described in Lowenstein's (2005) paper on the impact of hot–cold empathy gaps. Loewenstein argues that many medical decisions are made at times of duress—for instance, when people are in pain or have just received a dire diagnosis (thus causing considerable stress). In these cases the hot-to-cold empathy gap results in people overestimating the duration and intensity of these negative feelings. Furthermore, people underestimate the impact of these feelings on their medical decision making.

An interesting example of this is Chochinov, Tataryn, Clinch, and Dudgeon's 1999 study of terminal cancer patients. Patients were asked twice a day to rate their quality of life on a number of criteria, including the will to live. The results showed that patients' will to live fluctuated considerably—and the fluctuation was positively correlated to patients' ratings of negative emotions. As Loewenstein (2005, p. 552) argued, "Patients, it seems, did not base their will to live on a long-run average of their health and happiness, but, as hot-to-cold empathy gaps would predict, weighted their immediate feelings very heavily when assessing their own will to live." In another example, Ditto, Jacobson, Smucker, Danks, and Fagerlin (2006) asked older adults (age 65+) to indicate their end-of-life treatment preferences in a cold state (Time 1). A subset of individuals were hospitalized during the course of the study period. Participants who were hospitalized for 48+ hours were asked to again indicate their treatment preferences for a subset of those preferences (Time 2). Because these preferences were typically assessed within 7 days of hospitalization, the preferences were assessed in a hot state. Following this relatively serious hospitalization, people's desire for life-sustaining treatment declined significantly compared to their preferences when they were first assessed. Yet when preferences were assessed again (Time 3), approximately 6 months later, desire for life-sustaining treatment returned to their original "cold-state" preferences.

Several studies have shown the potential consequences of mispredicting one's affective responses to a major medical procedure. First, Smith and colleagues (2008) interviewed kidney patients on a waiting list for a renal or renal–pancreatic transplant. Patients were asked to estimate the magnitude of improvement in their lives following transplantation (e.g., how much more they would work and travel, and their overall quality of life). In each case, people significantly overestimated the benefits they would secure by receiving a transplant. In contrast, studies have shown that people overestimate how much their quality of life would be negatively affected by a colostomy and therefore having to defecate into a bag (Smith, Sherriff, Damschroder, Loewenstein, & Ubel, 2006). In both of these cases, people's inability to predict their actual future quality of life likely impaired their ability to make the best decision possible.

Cognitive and Affective Biases in Risk Perception

Risk perceptions play a significant role in people's health decision making, even when objective risk information is explicitly communicated. Furthermore, cognitive and emotional biases can distort people's perceptions of the value of different outcomes, as well as influence their subjective perceptions of likelihood.

Availability Bias

For instance, the "availability bias" (Tversky & Kahneman, 1973) describes people's tendency to estimate the likelihood of an event by searching their memory and deriving a sense of relative risk based on how easy or difficult it is to come up with relevant examples. As a result, the probabilities of rare, recent, or especially vivid events are consistently overestimated, whereas likelihood of ordinary, dated, or less memorable events is underestimated even if the events are common. An example of this bias in medical decision making has been documented in physicians' diagnoses. Detmer, Fryback, and Gassner (1978) asked surgeons to estimate in-hospital mortality rates for all surgical patients. Estimates made by surgeons from high-mortality specialties (in which patient deaths were more likely to have occurred recently) were more than double the estimates made by surgeons from low-mortality specialties for the identical patients.

Patients also poorly calibrate their quantitative estimates of health risks, such as the chance of developing cancer. For example, women asked to estimate their lifetime risk of breast cancer often provide figures that are 10–25% higher (and sometimes even more) than the true percentage (Croyle & Lerman, 1999; Fagerlin, Zikmund-Fisher, & Ubel, 2005b; Lerman et al., 1995). Such overestimates are likely due to the salience of cancer messages in the media and the visible impact of cancer on interpersonal relationships, two factors that increase the availability of cancer memories. Similarly, when celebrities develop cancer, people's risk perceptions and worry about that particular cancer may increase, especially when compared to other types of cancer and other diseases (Klein & Stefanek, 2007). Klein and Stefanek (2007) suggest that physicians can counteract availability biases by providing vivid counterexamples. For example, if a patient is reluctant to undergo a treatment because he or she knows of someone who has had a negative experience, the physician can provide alternative vivid or salient stories of patients who have benefited from it.

Risk as Feelings

Researchers have recently begun to examine links between risk perceptions and feelings. When patients are provided with specific risk information rather than estimating it themselves, the information presented is translated into intuitive "gist" representations that may include anxiety, worry, or distress about disease risks (Reyna, 2004; Rothman & Kiviniemi, 1999). These powerful emotions can have significant impacts on people's responses to their health conditions (Cameron, Leventhal, & Love, 1998; Lerman et al., 1991; Lofters, Juffs, Pond, & Tannock, 2002; McCaul & Tulloch, 1999; Rothman & Kiviniemi, 1999; Trask et al., 2001), yet it remains unclear whether emotional responses mediate cognitive risk perceptions, shape behavior independently, or both (Finucane, Alhakami, Slovic, & Johnson, 2000; Loewenstein, Weber, Hsee, & Welch, 2001). Resolving such questions is especially important given that perceptions of both value and likelihood may differ substantially when considering emotion-laden outcomes (e.g., as electric shocks) versus affect-poor outcomes (e.g., money) (Hsee & Rottenstreich, 2004; Rottenstreich & Hsee, 2001).

One important psychological perspective on these questions is the "affect heuristic" or "risk as feelings" hypothesis (Loewenstein et al., 2001; Slovic et al., 2004). This view recognizes the fact that affective reactions to risky situations can be different than cognitive evaluations, and the resulting behavior is likely to be driven more by affective reactions than by cognitive deliberations (Bechara, Damasio, Tranel, & Damasio, 1997; Damasio, 1994). A strong early proponent of the importance of affect in decision making was Zajonc (1980), who argued that affective reactions to stimuli are often the very first reactions, occurring automatically and subsequently guiding information processing and judgment. If Zajonc is correct, then affective reactions may serve as orienting mechanisms, helping us to navigate quickly and efficiently through a complex, uncertain, and sometimes dangerous world. Risk as feelings suggests that people use their emotional reaction to risky situations (e.g., feelings of fear or excitement) as information to make judgments about the probabilities of outcomes. Feelings about risk are not always sensitive to objective probability differences, and instead are determined by situational factors such as vividness of outcomes, temporal proximity to the outcome, and the feelings of others.

Researchers studying the affect heuristic have proposed that people consult or "sense" an affect pool in the process of making judgments (Finucane et al., 2000; Slovic & Peters, 2006). Just as imaginability, memorability, and similarity serve as cues for probability judgments (e.g., the availability and representativeness heuristics), affect may serve as a cue for many important judgments (including risk perceptions). Using an overall, readily available affective impression can be easier and more efficient than weighing the pros and cons of various reasons or retrieving relevant examples from memory, especially when the required judgment or decision is complex or mental resources are limited. This characterization of a mental shortcut has led to labeling the use of affect as a "heuristic" (Finucane et al., 2000).

The affect heuristic has been studied in risk perceptions in particular. Perceptions of risk and benefit are often negatively correlated in people's minds (and judgments). In reality, however, risks and benefits are typically positively correlated because things that are high in risk but low in benefit do not survive the marketplace. We think that individuals derive their perceptions of risk in part through their affective reactions to them. If one feels good about some treatment or risky activity, then one looks to one's affective reactions to it as a marker of both perceived risk ("I feel good about it; therefore, it must not be risky") and perceived benefit ("I feel good about it; therefore, it must be beneficial"). In other words, affect is used as information to guide perceptions of risk and benefit. Now, clearly individuals do not use their affective reactions only (other information counts, too), but the evidence suggests that affect matters in a causal way to guide these perceptions, at least in part.

Alhakami and Slovic (1994) found that the inverse relationship between perceived risk and benefit of an activity (e.g., using pesticides) was linked to the strength of positive or negative valence associated with that activity. This result implies that people base their judgments of an activity or a technology on not only what they think about it but also how they feel about it. If people like an activity, they are moved toward judging the risks as low and the benefits as high; if they dislike it, they tend to judge the opposite—high risk and low benefit. Under this model, affect comes prior to, and directs, judgments of risk and benefit, much as Zajonc (1980) proposed. This process, which is called "the affect heuristic," suggests that if a general affective view guides perceptions of risk and benefit, providing information about benefit should change perception of risk, and vice versa. For example, information stating that benefit is high for a technology such as nuclear power should lead to more positive overall affect, which in turn would decrease perceived risk. These predictions were confirmed (Finucane et al., 2000).

The Influence of Context on Risk Representations

Risk perceptions can also be inappropriately influenced by the contextual nature of the situation. More specifically, contextual information could shape patients' comprehension of and affective reaction to critical information, which could influence their subsequent choices. Single numerical probabilities or frequencies, such as "20%" or "14 out of 1,000," are rather pallid by themselves. As a result, people often have a difficult time knowing how to feel and react to such stand-alone probabilistic information (Teigen & Brun, 2000; Windschitl, Martin, & Flugstad, 2002) because they need additional information for those statistics to have personal meaning, prompt an affective reaction (e.g., concern, surprise, relief), and/or promote action (e.g., seeking prevention). Comparisons with contextual information facilitate meaning and affective responses. For example, research has shown that people's evaluations of medical options change significantly when they compare the numbers for two alternatives side by side versus consider each option singly (Hsee, 1996; Hsee, Blount, Lowenstein, & Bazerman, 1999). Furthermore, highly numerate people are more apt to make such comparisons than less numerate people (Peters et al., 2006).

In one example, subjects read about two infertility clinics that differed in their *in vitro* fertilization success rates and their distance from the patient (Zikmund-Fisher, Fagerlin, and Ubel, 2004). When each clinic was considered in isolation, study participants had little ability to judge whether clinic success rates (e.g., 28%) represented a positive or negative attribute; thus, they tended to favor the nearby clinic over the more distant one. When compared side by side, however, respondents had a strong preference for the higher success rate of the more distant clinic. This preference reversal demonstrated that the hard-to-evaluate attribute (success rates) was deemphasized in people's decision making because of the lack of context.

However, although context data can provide comparison numbers, sometimes the context is "loaded" and may push people's affective reactions in one direction. The end result can be a systematic bias in people's decisions. For example, Fagerlin, Zikmund-Fisher, and Ubel (2007) found that people's attitudes toward the risks and benefits of treatments were influenced by whether their own personal risk was presented as above or below average. Similarly, Windschitl and colleagues (2002) found that people perceived a female patient to be more at risk for a disease when the prevalence rate among men was lower versus higher, even though the stated risks for female patients remained exactly the same. These results highlight the discrepancy between people's objective knowledge about the risk of an event occurring and their "intuitive perceptions" about whether the event will occur.

Risk Communication: Providing Information to Support More Informed Choices

As more and more patients are expected to take an active role in their own medical decisions (Charles, Gafni, & Whelan, 1997; Laine et al., 1996), numerous educational materials and decision aids have been developed to help patients understand their medical diagnosis, and the risks and benefits of their treatment options. Such materials often must communicate significant amounts of risk and benefit information, since patients need to understand precisely the chances that a treatment may be successful, cause side effects, or reduce future disease risk to make preference-congruent decisions.

Due to the growing requirements to communicate numerical information to patients, there has recently been a significant push toward research that provides direct guidance regarding how best to present numerical information to increase the likelihood of patients making informed medical decisions. While several reviews cover such information in detail (Covey, 2007; Fagerlin, Ubel, Smith, & Zikmund-Fisher, 2007; Lipkus, 2007; Peters, Hibbard, Slovic, & Dieckmann, 2007), we review some of the most basic issues below.

Use of Frequencies versus Percentages

Research has consistently shown that both patients and physicians show better understanding of risk information (in terms of gross comparison and risk assessment tasks) if risks are presented in terms of frequencies (e.g., 5 out of 100 people experience a side effect) rather than percentages (5%; Hoffrage & Gigerenzer, 1998) or "1 in N" formats (Cuite, Weinstein, Emmons, & Colditz, 2008). The advantage of frequency over percentage formats, however, does not appear to hold when individuals need to perform calculations with the given numbers (e.g., divide a risk in half; Cuite et al., 2008; Waters, Weinstein, Colditz, & Emmons, 2006). People do, however, prefer to receive risk information in frequencies rather than proportions (Schapira, Nattinger, & McHorney, 2001).

Part of the justification for frequency formats comes from recent work suggesting that individual numeracy (ability to think about and work with probabilities, fractions, and ratios) mediates people's ability to transform proportions into percentages and vice versa (Peters et al., 2006). Study participants read a scenario about a psychiatric patient and were asked to assess the risk of violence if the patient were discharged. The risk of violence was presented as either 10% or 10 (out of 100). Although ratings by highly numerate individuals did not differ across conditions, less numerate individuals had a strong tendency to view 10% risk as less concerning than a 10 out of 100 risk.

Use of Absolute versus Relative Risks

Regardless of whether percentage or frequency formats are used, the feelings and perceptions evoked by changes in risk can be very different depending on whether the risk difference is presented in an absolute versus relative form. Although patients consistently report a preference to receive risk information in terms of a relative risk reduction format (Hux & Naylor, 1995; Sheridan, Pignone, & Lewis, 2003), research has consistently shown that changes in risks (e.g., an increase from 6 to 8%) are perceived as much larger when described in relative risk terms (33% more risk) rather than the absolute risk change (an increase of 2%). This inconsistency is well documented in both psychological and medical decision contexts (particularly when discussing risk reductions in which the absolute risk is low; Baron, 1997; Forrow, Taylor, & Arnold, 1992; Malenka, Baron, Johansen, Wahrenberger, & Ross, 1993).

An alternative approach to either absolute or relative risk presentations is to focus attention on the absolute increment or decrement in risk, without discussing the relative change. Such "incremental risk" approaches have been demonstrated to reduce worry about risks of medication side effects (Zikmund-Fisher, Fagerlin, Roberts, Derry, & Ubel, 2008), presumably because they highlight how much risk the patient faces regardless of whether the medication is taken. These approaches appear to be adequately comprehended by patients when supported by graphical displays (Zikmund-Fisher, Ubel, et al., 2008).

Formats Used to Present Numerical Risk and Benefit Information

Statistical information regarding the risks and benefits of treatment can be presented in many formats: verbally (e.g., the risk of incontinence following radical prostatectomy is "moderate"), numerically (e.g., 60 in 100), or graphically (e.g., in a pictograph). However, research has shown that using verbal labels only is the poorest method of communicating risk–benefit information (Burkell, 2004). The primary concern regarding use of verbal labels is that people vary widely in the numerical probabilities they assign to verbal labels. For example, although one individual may equate low risk of a side effect with a 10% risk, another may view low risk as a 1% risk.

Furthermore, other research has shown that presenting information in graphical formats can result in increased understanding and changes in decision making when compared with presenting statistics using solely numbers. One possible explanation for this finding is that graphical displays may facilitate more experiential processing that enables people to comprehend the gist of the graph without interpreting the details. Thus, while tabular presentations may only result in analytical learning, graphical formats (which often also include the raw numbers) may engage both analytical and gist types of processing (see also Reyna, 2004).

Several excellent reviews of graphical communication have explored the strengths, weaknesses, and overall effectiveness of a vast variety of graphs (Ancker & Kaufman, 2007; Lipkus, 2007; Lipkus & Hollands, 1999). These reviews highlight the importance of understanding the goals of risk communication and choosing graphs that achieve those goals. Is the goal to present single-risk numbers or to compare treatments or multiple risks? Alternatively, is the goal to show how risk changes over time, or to show the incremental risk that might be caused by a treatment? For instance, line graphs highlight trends (e.g., effectiveness of a drug over time), whereas bar graphs allow viewers to compare multiple options. A graph to show the differential rates of impotence following each type of prostate cancer treatment (e.g., surgery, external beam radiation brachy therapy), therefore, would be better structured as a bar graph than as a line graph.

Several studies have examined the effectiveness of various types of graphical formats (e.g., line graphs, bar graphs, pie graphs, pictographs). These studies have shown that not all graphical formats are equally effective in communicating risk information. In one study, participants viewing vertical bar graphs and pictographs (image matrices) had quicker reaction times and better comprehension than with other formats (Feldman-Stewart, Brundage, & Zotov, 2007). Another study compared five graphical formats and one table format regarding both verbatim

knowledge of the risk information presented (e.g., "Compared to people who did not take a pill, approximately how many fewer people would need bypass surgery if they took Pill B?") and gist knowledge (e.g., "Who is less likely to need bypass surgery: a person who took Pill A or a person who took Pill B?") (Hawley et al., 2008). Although tables appeared to result in the best verbatim knowledge, they were among the worst formats for communicating gist knowledge. However, pictographs performed well on both gist and verbatim knowledge measures. These results are consistent with dual-process theories, in that tables (a highly analytical format) tend not to engage the more experiential/associative learning process that often underlies our gist understandings of the world.

Conclusions

This review has highlighted the difficulties people face when trying to make health-related decisions. Numerous biases can affect the decision-making process, in terms of how people make decisions and how critical medical information is presented.

The study of the psychology of judgment and decision making has identified basic heuristics that contribute to biases in probability judgment, valuation of outcomes, and choices between alternative courses of action. In this review, we have traced most of these heuristics to the simultaneous operation of dual cognitive processes in judgment, and particularly to the experiential/intuitive judgment system, which highlights associations between events and offers rapid evaluations of decision situations.

Recent research has demonstrated that the responses of the intuitive system reflect not only cognitive strategies but also considerable input from the affective system. Emotions—experienced, anticipated, and remembered—play an important and increasingly well-recognized role in health decision making by patients and providers. Future study must consider cognitive and affective processes, and their influence on judgment and decision making, to improve both our understanding of how people make health choices and our ability to improve them.

Further Reading

Chapman, G. B., & Elstein, A. S. (2000). Cognitive processes and biases in medical decision making. In G. B. Chapman & F. A. Sonnenberg (Eds.), *Decision making in health care: Theory psychology and applications* (pp. 183–210). Cambridge, UK: Cambridge University Press.

Fagerlin, A., Ubel, P. A., Smith, D. M., & Zikmund-Fisher, B. J. (2007). Making numbers matter: Present and future research in risk communication. *American Journal of Health Behavior, 31*(Suppl. 1), S47–S56.

Lipkus, I. (2007). Numeric, verbal, and visual formats of conveying health risks: Suggested best practices and future recommendations. *Medical Decision Making, 27*(5), 696–713.

Peters, E., McCaul, K. D., Stefanek, M., & Nelson, W. (2006). Understanding cancer risk perceptions: Contributions from judgment and decision-making research. *Annals of Behavioral Medicine, 31*(1), 45–52.

Redelmeier, D. A., Rozin, P., & Kahneman, D. (1993). Understanding patients' decisions: Cognitive and emotional perspectives. *Journal of the American Medical Association, 270*(1), 72–76.

Reyna, V. F. (2004). How people make decisions that involve risk: A dual-processes approach. *Current Directions in Psychological Science, 13*(2), 60–66.

References

Alhakami, A., & Slovic, P. (1994). A psychological study of the inverse relationship between perceived risk and perceived benefit. *Risk Analysis, 14*(6), 1085–1096.

Ancker, J., & Kaufman, D. (2007). Rethinking health numeracy: A multidisciplinary literature review. *Journal of American Medical Informatics Association, 14,* 713–721.

Apanovitch, A., McCarthy, D., & Salovey, P. (2003). Using message framing to motivate HIV testing among low-income, ethnic minority women. *Health Psychology, 22*(1), 60–67.

Ariely, D. (1998). Combining experiences over time: The effects of duration, intensity changes and on-line measurements on retrospective pain evaluations. *Journal of Behavioral Decision Making, 11*(1), 19–45.

Ariely, D. (2008). *Predictably irrational*. New York: HarperCollins.

Baron, J. (1997). Confusion of relative and absolute risk in valuation. *Journal of Risk and Uncertainty, 14,* 301–309.

Bechara, A., Damasio, H., Tranel, D., & Damasio, A. (1997). Deciding advantageously before knowing the advantageous strategy. *Science, 275,* 1293–1295.

Burkell, J. (2004). What are the chances?: Evaluating risk and benefit information in consumer health materials. *Journal of the Medical Library Association, 92*(2), 200–208.

Cameron, L. D., Leventhal, H., & Love, R. R. (1998). Trait anxiety, symptom perceptions, and illness-related responses among women with breast cancer in remission during a tamoxifen clinical trial. *Health Psychology, 17*(5), 459–469.

Chapman, G. B., & Elstein, A. S. (2000). Cognitive processes and biases in medical decision making. In G. B. Chapman & F. A. Sonnenberg (Eds.), *Decision making in health care: Theory, psychology and applications* (pp. 183–210). Cambridge, UK: Cambridge University Press.

Charles, C., Gafni, A., & Whelan, T. (1997). Shared decision-making in the medical encounter: What does it mean? (or it takes at least two to tango). *Social Science and Medicine, 44*(5), 681–692.

Chochinov, H. M., Tataryn, D., Clinch, J. J., & Dudgeon, D. (1999). Will to live in the terminally ill. *Lancet, 354,* 816–819.

Christensen-Szalanski, J. J. (1984). Discount functions and the measurement of patients' values: Women's decisions during childbirth. *Medical Decision Making, 4*(1), 47–58.

Covey, J. (2007). A meta-analysis of the effects of presenting treatment benefits in different formats. *Medical Decision Making, 27*(5), 638–654.

Croyle, R. T., & Lerman, C. (1999). Risk communication in genetic testing for cancer susceptibility. *Journal of the National Cancer Institute Monographs, 25,* 59–66.

Cuite, C., Weinstein, N., Emmons, K., & Colditz, G. (2008). A test of numeric formats for communicating risk probabilities. *Medical Decision Making, 28,* 377–384.

Damasio, A. R. (1994). *Descartes' error: Emotion, reason, and the human brain*. New York: Putnam.

Detmer, D., Fryback, D., & Gassner, K. (1978). Heuristics and biases in medical decision making. *Journal of Medical Education, 53,* 682–683.

Ditto, P. H., Jacobson, J. A., Smucker, W. D., Danks, J. H., & Fagerlin, A. (2006). Context changes choices: A prospective study of the effects of hospitalization on life-sustaining treatment preferences. *Medical Decision Making, 26*(4), 313–322.

Dunn, E., Wilson, T., & Gilbert, D. (2003). Location, location, location: The misprediction of satisfaction in housing lotteries. *Personality and Social Psychology Bulletin, 29*(11), 1421–1432.

Edwards, A., Elwyn, G., Covey, J., Matthews, E., & Pill, R. (2001). Presenting risk information a review of the effects of framing and other manipulations on patient outcomes. *Journal of Health Communication, 6*(1), 61–82.

Edwards, W. (1968). Conservatism in human information processing. In B. Kleinmuntz (Ed.), *Formal representation of human judgment* (pp. 17–52). New York: Wiley.

Epstein, S. (1994). Integration of the cognitive and psychodynamic unconscious. *American Psychologist, 49*(8), 709–724.

Fagerlin, A., & Schneider, C. E. (2004). Enough: The failure of the living will. *Hastings Center Report, 34*(2), 30–42.

Fagerlin, A., Ubel, P. A., Smith, D. M., & Zikmund-Fisher, B. J. (2007). Making numbers matter: Present and future research in risk communication. *American Journal of Health Behavior, 31*(Suppl. 1.), S47–S56.

Fagerlin, A., Zikmund-Fisher, B. J., & Ubel, P. A. (2005a). Cure me even if it kills me: Preferences for invasive cancer treatment. *Medical Decision Making, 25*(6), 614–619.

Fagerlin, A., Zikmund-Fisher, B. J., & Ubel, P. (2005b). How making a risk estimate can change the feel of that risk: Shifting attitudes toward breast cancer risk in a general public survey. *Patient Education and Counseling, 57*(3), 294–299.

Fagerlin, A., Zikmund-Fisher, B. J., & Ubel, P. A. (2007). "If I'm better than average, then I'm ok?": Comparative information influences beliefs about risk and benefits. *Patient Education and Counseling, 69*, 140–144.

Feldman-Stewart, D., Brundage, M., & Zotov, V. (2007). Further insight into the perception of quantitative information: Judgments of gist in treatment decisions. *Medical Decision Making, 27*(1), 34–43.

Finucane, M. L., Alhakami, A., Slovic, P., & Johnson, S. M. (2000). The affect of heuristic judgments of risks and benefits. *Journal of Behavioral Decision Making, 13*, 1–17.

Forrow, L., Taylor, W. C., & Arnold, R. M. (1992). Absolutely relative: How research results are summarized can affect treatment decisions. *American Journal of Medicine, 92*, 121–124.

Fredrickson, B. L., & Kahneman, D. (1993). Duration neglect in retrospective evaluations of affective episodes. *Journal of Personality and Social Psychology, 65*(1), 45–55.

Griffin, D., & Ross, L. (1991). Subjective construal, social inference, and human misunderstanding. In M. P. Zanna (Ed.), *Advances in experimental social psychology* (Vol. 24, pp. 319–356). New York: Academic Press.

Halpern, S. D., Ubel, P. A., & Asch, D. A. (2007). Harnessing the power of default options to improve healthcare. *New England Journal of Medicine, 357*, 1340–1344.

Hawley, S. T., Zikmund-Fisher, B., Ubel, P.,

Jankovic, A., Lucas, T., & Fagerlin, A. (2008). The impact of the format of graphical presentation on health-related knowledge and treatment choices. *Patient Education and Counseling, 73*(3), 448–455.

Hoffrage, U., & Gigerenzer, G. (1998). Using natural frequencies to improve diagnostic inferences. *Academic Medicine, 73*(5), 538–540.

Hsee, C. K. (1996). The evaluability hypothesis: An explanation for preference reversals between joint and separate evaluations of alternatives. *Organizational Behavior and Human Decision Processes, 67*, 247–257.

Hsee, C. K., Blount, S., Lowenstein, G. F., & Bazerman, M. H. (1999). Preference reversals between joint and separate evaluations of options: A review and theoretical analysis. *Psychological Bulletin, 125*, 576–590.

Hsee, C. K., & Rottenstreich, Y. (2004). Music, pandas, and muggers: On the affective psychology of value. *Journal of Experimental Psychology: General, 133*(1), 23–30.

Hux, J. E., & Naylor, C. D. (1995). Communicating the benefits of chronic preventive therapy: Does the format of efficacy data determine patients' acceptance of treatment? *Medical Decision Making, 15*(2), 152–157.

Iyengar, S. S., & Lepper, M. R. (2000). When choice is demotivating: Can one desire too much of a good thing? *Journal of Personality and Social Psychology, 79*(6), 995–1006.

Johnson, E., & Goldstein, D. (2003). Do defaults save lives? *Science, 302*, 1338–1339.

Johnson, E., & Goldstein, D. (2004). Defaults and donation decisions. *Transplantation, 78*(12), 1713–1716.

Kahneman, D. (2003). A perspective on judgment and choice: Mapping bounded rationality. *American Psychologist, 58*(9), 697–720.

Kahneman, D., Slovic, P., & Tversky, A. (Eds.). (1982). *Judgment under uncertainty: Heuristics and biases.* Cambridge, UK: Cambridge University Press.

Kahneman, D., & Tversky, A. (1973). On the psychology of prediction. *Psychological Review, 80*, 237–251.

Kahneman, D., & Tversky, A. (1979). Prospect theory: An analysis of decision under risk. *Econometrica, 47*(2), 263–291.

Klein, W., & Stefanek, M. (2007). Cancer risk elicitation and communication: Lessons from the psychology of risk perception. *Cancer, 57*(3), 147–167.

Kressel, L., & Chapman, G. (2007). The default effect in end-of-life medical treatment preferences. *Medical Decision Making, 27*(3), 299–310.

Kressel, L., Chapman, G., & Leventhal, E. (2007). The influence of default options on the expression of end-of-life treatment preferences in advance directives. *Journal of General Internal Medicine, 22*(7), 1007–1010.

Laine, C., Davidoff, F., Lewis, C. E., Nelson, E. C., Nelson, E., Kessler, R. C., et al. (1996). Important elements of outpatient care: A comparison of patients' and physicians' opinions. *Annals of Internal Medicine, 125*(8), 640–645.

Lerman, C., Lustbader, E., Rimer, B., Daly, M., Miller, S., Sands, C., et al. (1995). Effects of individualized breast cancer risk counseling: A randomized trial. *Journal of the National Cancer Institute, 87*(4), 286–292.

Lerman, C., Trock, B., Rimer, B. K., Boyce, A., Jepson, C., & Engstrom, P. F. (1991). Psychological and behavioral implications of abnormal mammograms. *Annals of Internal Medicine, 114*(8), 657–661.

Lipkus, I. (2007). Numeric, verbal, and visual formats of conveying health risks: Suggested best practices and future recommendations. *Medical Decision Making, 27*(5), 696–713.

Lipkus, I. M., & Hollands, J. G. (1999). The visual communication of risk. *Journal of the National Cancer Institute Monographs, 25,* 149–163.

Loewenstein, G. (Ed.). (1999). *A visceral account of addiction.* Cambridge, UK: Cambridge University Press.

Loewenstein, G. (2005). Hot–cold empathy gaps and medical decision-making. *Health Psychology, 24*(4), S49–S56.

Loewenstein, G. F., Weber, E. U., Hsee, C. K., & Welch, N. (2001). Risk as feelings. *Psychological Bulletin, 127*(2), 267–286.

Lofters, A., Juffs, H. G., Pond, G. R., & Tannock, I. F. (2002). "PSA-itis": Knowledge of serum prostate specific antigen and other causes of anxiety in men with metastatic prostate cancer. *Journal of Urology, 168*(6), 2516–2520.

Malenka, D. J., Baron, J. A., Johansen, S., Wahrenberger, J. W., & Ross, J. M. (1993). The framing effect of relative and absolute risk. *Journal of General Internal Medicine, 8*(10), 543–548.

McCaul, K. D., & Tulloch, H. E. (1999). Cancer screening decisions. *Journal of the National Cancer Institute Monographs, 25,* 52–58.

McNeil, B. J., Pauker, S. G., Sox, H. C., Jr., & Tversky, A. (1982). On the elicitation of preferences for alternative therapies. *New England Journal of Medicine, 306*(21), 1259–1262.

Meszaros, J. R., Asch, D. A., Baron, J., Hershey, J. C., Kunreuther, H., & Schwartz-Buzaglo, J. (1996). Cognitive processes and the decisions of some parents to forego pertussis vaccination for their children. *Journal of Clinical Epidemiology, 49*(6), 697–703.

Peters, E., Dieckmann, N., Dixon, A., Hibbard, J., & Mertz, C. (2007). Less is more in presenting quality information to consumers. *Medical Care Research and Review, 64*(2), 169–190.

Peters, E., Hibbard, J. H., Slovic, P., & Dieckmann, N. F. (2007). Numeracy skill and the communication, comprehension, and use of risk and benefit information. *Health Affairs, 26*(3), 741–748.

Peters, E., Lipkus, I., & Diefenbach, M. (2006). The functions of affect in health communications and in the construction of health preferences. *Journal of Communication, 56*(Suppl. 1), S140–S162.

Peters, E., Vastfjall, D., Slovic, P., Mertz, C. K., Mazzocco, K., & Dickert, S. (2006). Numeracy and decision making. *Psychological Science, 17*(5), 407–413.

Poses, R. M., Bekes, C., Copare, F. J., & Scott, W. E. (1990). What difference do two days make?: The inertia of physicians' sequential prognostic judgments for critically ill patients. *Medical Decision Making, 10,* 6–14.

Redelmeier, D., Katz, J., & Kahneman, D. (2003). Memories of a colonoscopy: A randomized trial. *Pain, 104*(1–2), 187–194.

Redelmeier, D. A., & Kahneman, D. (1996). Patient's memories of painful medical treatments: Real-time and retrospective evaluations of two minimally invasive procedures. *Pain, 116,* 3–8.

Reventlow, S., Hvas, A., & Tulinius, C. (2001). "In really great danger . . . ": The concept of risk in general practice. *Scandinavian Journal of Primary Health Care, 19*(2), 71–75.

Reyna, V. (2004). How people make decisions that involve risk: A dual-processes approach. *Current Directions in Psychological Science, 13*(2), 60–66.

Ritov, I., & Baron, J. (1990). Reluctance to vaccinate: Omission bias and ambiguity. *Journal of Behavioral Decision Making, 3,* 263–277.

Rothman, A., Martino, S., Bedell, B., Detweiler, J., & Salovey, P. (1999). The systematic influence of gain- and loss-framed messages on interest in and use of different types of health behavior. *Personality and Social Psychology Bulletin, 25*(11), 1355–1369.

Rothman, A. J., & Kiviniemi, M. T. (1999). Treating people with information: An analysis and review of approaches to communicating health risk information. *Journal of the National Cancer Institute Monographs, 25,* 44–51.

Rottenstreich, Y., & Hsee, C. K. (2001). Money, kisses, and electric shocks: On the affective psychology of risk. *Psychological Science, 12*(3), 185–190.

Samuelson, W., & Zeckhauser, R. (1988). Status quo bias in decision making. *Journal of Risk and Uncertainty, 1,* 7–59.

Savage, L. J. (1954). *The foundations of statistics.* New York: Wiley.

Schapira, M. M., Nattinger, A. B., & McHorney, C. A. (2001). Frequency or probability?: A qualitative study of risk communication formats used in health care. *Medical Decision Making, 21*(6), 459–467.

Sheridan, S. L., Pignone, M. P., & Lewis, C. L. (2003). A randomized comparison of patients' understanding of number needed to treat and other common risk reduction formats. *Journal of General Internal Medicine, 18*(11), 884–892.

Slovic, P. (1995). The construction of preference. *American Psychologist, 50*(5), 364–371.

Slovic, P. (2000). What does it mean to know a cumulative risk?: Adolescents' perceptions of short-term and long-term consequences of smoking. *Journal of Behavioral Decision Making, 13*, 259–266.

Slovic, P., Finucane, M. L., Peters, E., & MacGregor, D. G. (2004). Risk as analysis and risk as feelings: Some thoughts about affect, reason, risk, and rationality. *Risk Analysis, 24*(2), 311–322.

Slovic, P., & Peters, E. (2006). Risk perception and affect. *Current Directions in Psychological Science, 15*(6), 322–325.

Smith, D., Loewenstein, G., Jankovich, S., Jepson, C., Feldman, H., & Ubel, P. (2008). Mispredicting and misremembering: Patients with renal failure overestimate improvements in quality of life after a kidney transplant. *Health Psychology, 27*(5), 653–658.

Smith, D. M., Sherriff, R. L., Damschroder, L., Loewenstein, G., & Ubel, P. A. (2006). Misremembering colostomies?: Former patients give lower utility ratings than do current patients. *Health Psychology, 25*(6), 688–695.

Spranca, M., Minsk, E., & Baron, J. (1991). Omission and commission in judgement and choice. *Journal of Experimental Social Psychology, 27*(1), 76–105.

Teigen, K. H., & Brun, W. (2000). Ambiguous probabilities: When does $p = 0.3$ reflect a possibility and when does it express a doubt? *Journal of Behavioral Decision Making, 13*(3), 345–362.

Trask, P. C., Paterson, A. G., Wang, C., Hayasaka, S., Milliron, K. J., Blumberg, L. R., et al. (2001). Cancer-specific worry interference in women attending a breast and ovarian cancer risk evaluation program: Impact on emotional distress and health functioning. *Psycho-Oncology, 10*, 349–360.

Tversky, A., & Kahneman, D. (1973). Availability: A heuristic for judging frequency and probability. *Cognitive Psychology, 5*(2), 207–232.

Tversky, A., & Kahneman, D. (1974). Judgment under uncertainty: Heuristics and biases. *Science, 185*, 1124–1131.

Tversky, A., & Kahneman, D. (1981). The framing of decisions and the psychology of choice. *Science, 211*, 453–458.

Ubel, P. A., Loewenstein, G., Schwarz, N., & Smith, D. (2005). Misimagining the unimaginable: The disability paradox and healthcare decision making. *Health Psychology, 24*(Suppl. 4), S57–S62.

Waters, E., Weinstein, N., Colditz, G., & Emmons, K. (2006). Formats for improving risk communication in medical tradeoff decisions. *Journal of Health Communication, 11*, 167–182.

Wilson, T. D., & Gilbert, D. T. (2003). Affective forecasting. In M. P. Zanna (Ed.), *Advances in experimental social psychology* (Vol. 35, pp. 345–411). San Diego, CA: Academic Press.

Wilson, T. D., Wheatley, T., Meyers, J. M., Gilbert, D. T., & Axsom, D. (2000). Focalism: A source of durability bias in affective forecasting. *Journal of Personality and Social Psychology, 78*(5), 821–836.

Windschitl, P. D., Martin, R., & Flugstad, A. R. (2002). Context and the interpretation of likelihood information: The role of intergroup comparisons on perceived vulnerability. *Journal of Personality and Social Psychology, 82*(5), 742–755.

Wroe, A. L., Turner, N., & Salkovskis, P. M. (2004). Understanding and predicting parental decisions about early childhood immunizations. *Health Psychology, 23*(1), 33–41.

Zajonc, R. B. (1980). Preferences need no inferences. *American Psychologist, 35*, 151–175.

Zikmund-Fisher, B., Fagerlin, A., Roberts, T., Derry, H., & Ubel, P. (2008). Alternate methods of framing information about medication side effects: Incremental risk versus total risk occurrence. *Journal of Health Communication, 13*(2), 107–124.

Zikmund-Fisher, B. J., Fagerlin, A., & Ubel, P. A. (2004). "Is 28% good or bad?": Evaluability and preference reversals in health care decisions. *Medical Decision Making, 24*(2), 142–148.

Zikmund-Fisher, B. J., Ubel, P. A., Smith, D. M., Derry, H. A., McClure, J. B., Stark, A., et al. (2008). Communicating side effect risks in a tamoxifen prophylaxis decision aid: The debiasing influence of pictographs. *Patient Education and Counseling, 73*(2), 209–214.

CHAPTER 5

Specifying the Determinants of People's Health Beliefs and Health Behavior

How a Social Psychological Perspective Can Inform Initiatives to Promote Health

Marc T. Kiviniemi
Alexander J. Rothman

Health is complex. At any moment in time, a person's health is influenced by a complicated interplay between biological, behavioral, psychological, and social systems. Thus, efforts to promote health might target all of these systems. For example, one might treat a person at risk for heart disease by prescribing drugs to address arteriosclerosis, by encouraging changes in diet and exercise behaviors, or by altering the social environment to reduce chronic stress triggers. The effectiveness of such efforts rests on an understanding of the basic principles that regulate these systems.

It is from research in psychology and, in particular, social psychology, that we have been able to specify how the social and physical environment in which people live shapes and is shaped by people's thoughts, feelings, and behaviors (Jones, 1985). At its core, social psychology can be said to have two take-home messages: First, people's perceptions of a situation or a behavior often matter far more in determining their thoughts, feelings, and behaviors than do the objective features of the situation. Second, people's behavior is powerfully influenced by their environment, including other people around them, and these influences often occur outside our awareness (Ross & Nisbett, 1991).

In this chapter we illustrate how a social psychological analysis can be used to understand how people manage their health and health practices. An exhaustive introduction to these issues is, of course, beyond the scope of this chapter. We have elected to focus on a set of core issues that not only illustrate basic principles in social psychology but also demonstrate how these principles have been used to develop strategies to promote health and to prevent or manage illness.

Why Social Psychology?

Why do social psychological perspectives matter in understanding health behavior? First, social psychologists have a long history of specifying the determinants of people's behavior, especially health behaviors that tap important personal and social values. For example, one of the earliest areas of social psychological inquiry was the relation between attitudes and behaviors (La Piere, 1934), and, in particular, when and why people act in ways inconsistent with their attitudes. This basic social psychological research laid the groundwork for development of the first generation of health intervention strategies derived from social psychological models (e.g., Janis, 1967; Leventhal, 1970). Given the variety of health issues in which knowledge of the importance of a given behavior does not always translate into behavior change, the social psychological tradition of examining multiple determinants of behavior informs the complexity of understanding health behavioral choices.

Second, in the past three decades an important shift has taken place in the nature and diversity of factors we consider as potential influences on health problems. The biopsychosocial approach (Engel, 1977) assumes that health problems are the result of far more than biological causes, and that determinants of health and health problems involve an interaction of factors at multiple levels of analysis, including biology, the individual person's psychological makeup, the person's relationships and social environment, and the broader cultural and environmental context in which the person exists (for an analysis of psychosocial influences on two common health issues, cancer and heart disease, see Andersen, 2002; Smith & Ruiz, 2002). Although it is not always clear that a biopsychosocial mindset has been fully integrated into medical research and practice, the approach is well integrated in health psychology (Suls & Rothman, 2004). Because social psychology examines the interplay between the individual and the social environment, it is well positioned to contribute to a biopsychosocial understanding of health behavior and health outcomes.

Our goal in this chapter is to provide an introduction to ways in which the principles of social psychology inform our understanding of how people think about, engage with, and respond to health issues. Specifically, we explore the use of basic principles from social psychology to understand health behavior and health outcomes in three domains: the relation between people's attitudes about health issues and their health behaviors, the use of persuasion techniques to encourage people to change behaviors, and the influence of other people on an individual's health behaviors and health outcomes. In each section, we present an introduction to relevant social psychological principles, a discussion of how those principles can be used to understand health behavior and health outcomes, and an exploration of ways those principles might be applied to change health behaviors or address health problems.

Attitudes and Health Behavior

The "antidrug" ads sponsored by the Office of National Drug Control Policy (Kelder, Maibach, Worden, Biglan, & Levitt, 2000) and the VERB campaign for the Centers for Disease Control and Prevention (Huhman et al., 2005) are two examples of widely disseminated public health campaigns designed to change health behavior practices. Health education messages such as these have long been designed to make individuals feel more positively or more negatively toward a particular health behavior. Communications that attempt to create or change beliefs, such as "Drugs are bad" or "Exercise is fun and good" are attempts to create or change individuals' attitudes about that particular behavior.

In social psychological terms, an "attitude" is evaluation of a particular thing (in this case, a health behavior) and, more specifically, an evaluation that indicates at least some degree of favor or disfavor (Eagly & Chaiken, 1993). Thus, believing that colorectal cancer screening is a good thing and that people should do it, feeling disgusted by the idea of eating green leafy vegetables, and holding negative views about contraception use are all examples of attitudes about different health behaviors.

Health campaigns attempt to change attitudes because attitude change is seen as a necessary, if not solely sufficient, route to changing behavior; thus, the person who has positive attitudes about colorectal cancer screening should be more likely to be compliant with screening recommendations than a person whose attitudes are more negative. Given the importance of attitudes, this section provides an introduction to what attitudes are, how and when they affect health-related behavior, and how this knowledge informs intervention strategies to change behavior. In a subsequent section, we address principles from social psychology that can guide efforts to change people's attitudes about health issues.

Properties of Attitudes

A substantial focus of social psychological research on attitudes has been to understand better how attitudes are structured and how differences in structure affect people's behavioral decisions. This area of research has revealed that attitudes can differ on dimensions well beyond their valenced evaluation, and that these dimensions can influence how attitudes affect and are affected by people's behavior. We focus our discussion on two important points about attitude properties, the components that make up one's attitudes about a particular issue and the strength of that attitude (for more in-depth introductions to theory and research on attitudes, see Eagly & Chaiken, 1998; Fabrigar, MacDonald, & Wegener, 2005; Pratkanis, Breckler, & Greenwald, 1989).

Health professionals are often frustrated by patients' failure to engage in preventive health behaviors, even when they believe that the behavior would have substantial health benefits. Although there are a variety of reasons why there might be a divergence between people's behavior and beliefs, one reason may rest in an understanding of how people's attitudes are structured. An important distinction is made in the attitudes literature between the "cognitive" component of one's attitudes—the information, beliefs, and thoughts one has about the issue or behavior—and the "affective" component—feelings and emotions one associates with the behavior (Fabrigar et al., 2005; Rosenberg, 1960; Trafimow & Sheeran, 1998). The separability of attitudes into these components has been demonstrated for a variety of attitude objects (Abelson, Kinder, Peters, & Fiske, 1982; Breckler, 1984; Breckler & Wiggins, 1989; Crites, Fabrigar, & Petty, 1994; Stangor, Sullivan, & Ford, 1991; Trafimow & Sheeran, 1998). For example, from a cognitive component perspective, one may believe that the benefit of physical activity (e.g., weight loss, energy, body image) outweighs the costs that it entails (e.g., time, body soreness, boredom) and may therefore have an overall positive evaluation of activ-

ity behavior. By contrast, one may eat high-fat foods because they are associated with positive feelings of warmth, contentment, and comfort (affective component). Thus, to truly understand people's attitudes about a health behavior or a health issue, one must understand both what they think and how they feel about the issue.

Why is this important for understanding health issues? Most work on health decision making has focused on measuring and modifying the cognitive component of an attitude—factors such as perceived benefits of engaging in a behavior, beliefs about the relation of the behavior to health problems, and so forth. Many models of health decision making assume that attitudes are a function of the relative balance of perceived benefits to engaging in the behavior (or, more broadly, positive information one has about the behavior) and perceived costs or barriers to behavioral engagement. This construct is typically operationalized as the perceived value of the outcomes afforded by the behavior weighted by the perceived likelihood that it will occur. So, for example, a person might believe that it is equally likely that exercise will increase his or her cardiovascular fitness (a perceived benefit) and that it will take a lot of time (a perceived cost). Based on this operationalization of attitudes, if the person values the two outcomes equally, his or her overall attitude will be neutral, but if he or she values the increase in cardiovascular fitness more highly than the loss of time, his or her overall attitude will be positive. This expected utility construct forms the core of the attitude construct in theory of reasoned action/planned behavior (Ajzen, 1991; Fishbein, 1979) and the decisional balance construct in the transtheoretical model (Prochaska, DiClemente, & Norcross, 1992; for review and discussion, see Weinstein, 1993).

Although one might plausibly include affective components of attitudes as a special type of expected utility belief (e.g., "If I engage in this behavior, I expect that I will feel good"), models of attitudes and decision making that have addressed affect typically include it as a separate and distinct construct (e.g., Ajzen & Driver, 1991; Kiviniemi, Voss-Humke, & Seifert, 2007; Triandis, 1979). There is evidence that affectively based evaluations may also play a role in health behavioral decisions even after one accounts for the influence of cognitive components (e.g., Abelson et al., 1982; Kiviniemi et al., 2007; van den Berg, Manstead, van der Plight, & Wigboldus, 2005). The relation of affectively based attitudes to behavior has been demonstrated for alcohol and drug use (Simons & Carey, 1998), physical activity behavior (Kiviniemi et al., 2007), and dietary behavior (Aikman, Crites, & Fabrigar, 2006).

Given the evidence that both cognitive and affective components of attitudes can influence health behaviors, it is important to consider both components when trying to understand a person's health behavior patterns and to intervene to change their behaviors. To return to the example with which we started this section, a person who can well articulate the health advantages of a particular behavior but still does not engage in the behavior, the idea that people's attitudes can comprise both cognitive and affective components raises the possibility that the dissociation between people's beliefs and behavior occurs because of "ambivalence," a situation in which the components of a person's attitudes are not in alignment (Chaiken & Baldwin, 1981). For example, a person who may believe that having a colonoscopy would reduce his or her risk of colorectal cancer might also associate feelings of fear, embarrassment, and disgust with the procedure. In this case, the positive cognitive beliefs and the negative affective component would be pushing the person in opposite directions, creating ambivalence (for further discussion of the potential effects of cognitive–affective ambivalence on health behavior, see Kiviniemi & Bevins, 2007).

A second core feature concerns how strong attitudes are: "Attitude strength" refers to a variety of features of attitudes that relate to how stable (i.e., unlikely to change over time) an attitude is, how resistant to persuasion it is, and how impactful it is (i.e., how strong an influence it has over behavior, information processing, and so on; for further discussion and definition, see Krosnick & Petty, 1995). Two people might report that they hold equally favorable attitudes about a behavior (e.g., both might evaluate physical activity positively), but they might differ significantly in the strength of their attitudes. "Attitude strength" is an umbrella term for several features of attitudes that influ-

ence stability, resistance, and impact. One such feature follows from the idea of multiple attitude components discussed earlier—attitudes tend to be stronger when the components that make up the attitude are consistent (i.e., when cognitive and affective components of the attitude are equally positive or equally negative) or when different pieces of information/different emotions within a component are consistent (Chaiken & Baldwin, 1981; Chaiken & Yates, 1985; Thompson, Zanna, & Griffin, 1995).

Other strength features relate more to individuals' perceptions of their attitudes. For example, the degree to which one feels certain that one's attitude is correct (Abelson, 1988; Gross, Holtz, & Miller, 1995), one's feelings about the personal importance of an attitude (Krosnick, 1988), and how much knowledge one perceives having about the issue (Wood, Rhodes, & Biek, 1995) are associated with stronger attitudes.

A final definition of "attitude strength" deals with cognitive processing features of the attitude. Attitude "accessibility" refers to how quickly an attitude is brought to mind when the person is thinking about the issue (or, more technically, the strength of the association between a given attitude object and the attitude itself in memory; Fazio, 1989). Accessibility relates to the stability and impact of attitudes in a variety of ways. For example, accessible attitudes are more likely to guide behavior because accessible information is more likely to be available for use to guide a decision (Fazio, 1990). Because strong attitudes have been shown to be resistant to persuasion and to be better predictors of behavior, intervention strategies that target people's attitudes may be more effective if they not only change the valence of a person's attitude but also do so in a way that engenders a strong attitude. For example, direct experience with an attitude object has been shown to promote stronger, more durable attitudes (Regan & Fazio, 1977).

A final feature of attitudes that is worthy of note concerns attitude "specificity." People's attitudes about health issues can be thought of at a variety of levels. For example, if one were interested in the relation of attitudes to the behavior of jogging, one could examine people's attitudes about jogging, exercising more generally, health promotion behaviors at an even more general level, and the value of health at a yet more global level. Each of these levels of attitude has potential relevance to understanding whether or not a person jogs. In general, social psychological research has shown that researchers should assess attitudes at the same level of specificity as the behavior in which they are interested (Ajzen & Fishbein, 1977). Thus, if one wanted to understand jogging behavior, one should measure attitudes about jogging, but if the goal is to understand a variety of exercise behaviors, assessing attitudes about the general category of exercise behaviors would be more effective. One can also think about other types of specificity. Time and context are also important issues to consider: If one is interested in predicting a person's likelihood of reducing dietary fat consumption in the next 6 months, then attitude measures that ask specifically about the next 6 months are more effective predictors of behavior than those that ask about a different time span or no time span at all. Likewise, if a particular behavioral context is of interest (e.g., if one wants to predict likelihood of smoking in a bar setting), then assessing attitudes about the behavior in that particular setting is more effective.

How Do Attitudes Influence Health Behaviors?

Thus far, we have examined some of the features of people's attitudes about health behaviors. The role of attitudes about health behaviors receives a great deal of research attention because of a seemingly simple idea: One's attitudes about a behavior should influence whether one engages in the behavior. Research in the health domain shows that, overall, there is a relation between people's attitudes about an issue and their behaviors regarding the issue (for meta-analytic reviews, see Albarracin, Johnson, Fishbein, & Muellerleile, 2001; Godin & Kok, 1996; Hausenblas, Carron, & Mack, 1997; Sheeran, Abraham, & Orbell, 1999). As with many features of health and health behavior, the true relation between attitudes about health behaviors and engagement in the behavior is more complex: Although attitudes definitely can and do influence people's behavioral choices, there is not a one-to-one relation between one's attitudes and one's behavior, and additional factors are also necessary to understand the relation of at-

titudes and behaviors. Examining factors influencing the relation between attitudes and behavior, and exploring explanations for why attitudes at times do not predict behavior provide insight into the multitude of factors influencing people's behavioral choices and the processes by which psychosocial factors, such as attitudes, influence behavioral practices.

One complexity in the relation between attitudes and behavior is that attitudes are but one of several influences on people's behavioral practices. For example, the theory of reasoned action includes the idea of "social norms," one's perceptions of how other people view the behavior. For example, one might believe that one's friends and family members think that drinking is bad, and that those friends and family members would look unfavorably on the person drinking. Such a negative social norm would, all things being equal, lead the person to be less likely to engage in the behavior (Ajzen, 1991). For the most part, attitudes and other influences on behavior (e.g., social norms) are seen as independent, unconnected influences on behavior (and are theoretically unrelated to one another). Thus, if conflict exists between influences (e.g., one has a positive attitude but close others' thoughts and feelings about the behavior are predominantly negative), one might not see attitude–behavior correspondence if the other influences have a stronger role in predicting behavior.

Also, in most models that include attitudes as a construct (most notably, the theories of reasoned action and planned behavior; Ajzen, 1991; Fishbein, 1979), attitudes do not directly lead to behavior but rather influence behavioral intentions, the formation of a conscious decision/goal that one wishes to engage in the behavior. Although behavioral intentions are a strong, positive predictor of behaviors, the correspondence between the two is also not perfect (Webb & Sheeran, 2006). In fact, analysis of the relation between behavioral intentions and behavior has shown that a substantial portion of people are "inclined abstainers": They form an intention to engage in a behavior but do not actually translate that intention into behavioral action (Orbell & Sheeran, 1998). Here, too, there are a variety of possible reasons for the lack of correspondence. Of particular note, factors other than the individual's decision processes might lead to problems translating an intention into a behavior. For example, if one forms an intention to be more physically active but lives in a neighborhood without sidewalks, where activity outside is unsafe, or without access to exercise facilities, it is unlikely that the intention will translate into behavioral action. One means by which these environmental factors might influence behavior is by moderating the link between intentions and behaviors. Even if one forms an intention to perform a behavior, if the actual features of the environment do not allow for behavioral control, the intention is unlikely to lead to behavioral change (Ajzen & Fishbein, 2005).

Another key factor is that the decision-making and goal-setting processes that influence intention formation are not necessarily those that guide the process of acting on that intention. Translating an intention into a behavior requires a different set of planning processes, most notably, developing concrete action plans for enacting the behavior and considering how situational factors influence when and how the behavior can be enacted (Gollwitzer & Sheeran, 2006; Sheeran, Webb, & Gollwitzer, 2005). To the extent that one does not engage successfully in these implementation processes, the intention to engage in the behavior will not lead to behavior change.

A final note is important as we close out this section. All the work reviewed previously focuses on how and when attitudes influence behaviors. It is also the case that people's behaviors can influence their attitudes. This can happen through several mechanisms. First, people can use their behaviors as a source of information for inferring their attitudes (e.g., "I run regularly, so I must have a positive attitude about running"; Bem, 1967). Second, individuals are motivated to maintain consistency between their attitudes and their behaviors. When the two are inconsistent, individuals are motivated to maintain consistency by changing either their attitudes, their behavior, or both (Festinger, 1957). In some situations, this process acts to support patterns of unhealthy behavior. For example, because people are motivated to maintain a sense of themselves as healthy; when they engage in health risk behaviors such as smoking, they modify their beliefs about the behavior to support their self-perception of health (Gibbons, Eggleston, & Benthin, 1997). However, these processes have also been used by investigators to promote healthy behavior. For example, Stone, Aronson, Crain, and Winslow (1994) demonstrated that making people aware of the discrepancy between their beliefs and behavior—by inducing a sense of hypocrisy—can be an effective way to motivate people to modify their behavior.

Using This Knowledge to Affect Health Behaviors

So how does one address the person who has very positive beliefs about a behavior but does not engage in it? Are there situations where interventions to change attitudes, such as antidrug and proexercise messages, can influence behavioral practices? How does one incorporate knowledge of attitude structure and function, and of the complexity of attitude–behavior relations, into intervention design?

At the simplest level, there is a positive message for health professionals: Interventions that successfully change attitudes and behavioral intentions can have a positive impact on behavior (Webb & Sheeran, 2006). How might one most successfully change an attitude? We discuss this more fully in the next section on persuasion processes, but here we highlight one outcome from the literature on attitude structure. An implication of the attitude structure literature is that interventions to change one's attitudes need to take into account the structure of the attitude. One can try to change an attitude by altering either the cognitive component (e.g., arguing against current beliefs or trying to introduce new beliefs) or the affective component (e.g., trying to change the associated feelings).

Some work has shown that individuals differ in their receptivity to cognitive versus affective persuasion techniques; for example, individuals high in need for cognition are more receptive to cognitively based appeals (Haddock, Maio, Arnold, & Huskinson, 2008). Beyond individual differences, most research has shown that one should match one's persuasive technique to the type of attitude the person holds (Edwards, 1990; for an opposing viewpoint, see Millar & Tesser, 1986). If the person's attitude is primarily based on cognitive factors, a cognitively based message tends to be more effective, whereas a message designed to change affective components of attitudes is more effective if the attitude is affectively based.

The idea that attitudes directly influence behavioral intentions that in turn determine behavior has implications for intervention strategies. Given this multistep relation between attitudes and behavior, techniques to increase the likelihood that formed behavioral intentions will actually translate into behavior change are also important. One strategy here is to consider the differences in the processes involved in forming an intention to change a behavior versus those necessary actually to translate that intention into behavior change. Recent research has shown that interventions involving implementation intentions can target these processes and increase the likelihood of successful behavioral change. "Implementation intentions" involve having individuals consider *where* (i.e., in what situations) they will engage in a behavior and *how* (i.e., what concrete action steps they will take) they will do so (e.g., Armitage, 2007; for a review of this literature, see Gollwitzer & Sheeran, 2006). For example, if someone had formed an intention to lower the amount of fat in his or her diet, an effective implementation intention might take the form "When I am at a fast-food restaurant, I will select a salad and a baked chicken sandwich rather than a burger." Implementation intentions increase the likelihood that the intention will be brought to mind in the appropriate behavioral context because the context itself serves as a cue to remember the intention. Finally, given that intentions can be derailed by environmental circumstances that limit people's ability to engage in the behavior, the intention–behavior link can also be increased by community-level measures to change those environmental circumstances (Green & Kreuter, 1999; Sallis et al., 2003).

In summary, although attitudes about health issues are important and should influence behavioral practices, in reality, understanding attitudes and their relation to health behaviors involves both knowledge of the structure of one's attitudes and the complexity of the relation among attitudes, other influences, and behaviors. Even with this knowledge in hand, to utilize knowledge of attitudes to influence people's behavior effectively, health professionals must understand how to influence attitudes about health issues. We now turn to this topic—how one effectively communicates with people to change their attitudes about health-related issues.

Persuasion Processes

Although interventions to promote health and healthy behavior can take myriad forms, one feature that interventions often share is an attempt to persuade people to think, feel, or act in a particular manner. In some cases, the persuasive message is the primary feature of the intervention (e.g., an informational campaign to promote the benefits of eating fruits and vegetables); in other cases, the persuasive message is embedded within other facets of an intervention (e.g., a weight loss treatment program might include messages promoting the benefits of eating fruits and vegetables). However, in either case, investigators hope the message has the desired impact on how people think and feel about the issue at hand. In this section, we examine how principles of persuasion can and have been used to promote health and healthy behavior, including what persuasive messages are designed to do, and evaluate effectiveness of persuasive messages, different paths through which persuasion can operate, and persuasive strategies that have been employed effectively to promote healthy behavior.

What Should a Persuasive Message Do?

Although this may appear to be a rather simple question, specifying the purpose or goal of a persuasive message is critical because it guides both message development and evaluation. Persuasive messages are designed to create or reinforce a particular perspective on an issue and are therefore distinct from messages designed only to communicate information about an issue (e.g., communications regarding the risks associated with a surgical procedure). This is an important distinction because many health interventions involve messages designed to provide information in a manner that does not affect people's preferences systematically (for a discussion of this type of intervention, see Kaplan & Frosch, 2005). The effectiveness of a communication-focused message rests on how well people comprehend—and perhaps retain—the information provided.

Persuasive messages can target a range of outcomes. They can be deployed to create new beliefs about an issue such as an emerging health threat (e.g., severe acute respiratory syndrome [SARS]), or a newly developed behavior (e.g., taking the human papillovirus [HPV] vaccine), to change prevailing beliefs about an issue (e.g., normative beliefs about binge drinking), or to reinforce or render salient a prevailing belief about an issue (e.g., the importance of regular mammograms). A message is deemed effective to the extent that it elicits the desired outcome (e.g., a reduction in the perceived prevalence of binge drinking or an increase in the perceived importance of obtaining regular mammograms). However, in many cases, the observed changes in beliefs are considered intermediate outcomes and are thought to be of value only if they lead to changes in behavior. For example, a campaign might be designed to heighten perceptions of the importance of regular mammograms because that belief is in turn expected to lead to higher screening rates. However, as we discussed earlier, changes in beliefs do not always result in changes in behavior, which means that a persuasive message can be an effective but not sufficient method to promote behavior change.

Two Paths to Persuasion

How do persuasive appeals work? As McGuire (1985) noted, persuasion depends on the successful execution of a series of steps. In particular, before one can even begin to ascertain whether a message has elicited the desired response, the message recipient must receive and understand the message. However, assuming the successful execution of these initial steps, what processes regulate the effect a message has on people's beliefs?

To date, there are thought to be two primary paths through which a persuasive message can operate—a systematic or central route, and a heuristic or peripheral route (Chaiken, Liberman, & Eagly, 1989; Petty & Wegener, 1999). These routes primarily

reflect differences in the depth to which the information is processed. Systematic processing involves a careful analysis of the information provided in a message; thus, the persuasive impact of a message depends on the strength of the arguments provided. Beliefs that arise from systematic processing are thought to be stronger, more resistant to change, and more predictive of future behavior (Petty & Wegener, 1999). For this reason, most message-based interventions are designed to be processed systematically as investigators diligently work to develop strong, well-articulated reasons for a particular course of action. Yet the impact of even a strong message depends on two additional factors shown to regulate systematic processing: a person's ability and motivation to process the information. Investigators need to be sure to create conditions that not only support people's ability to reflect on the message but also ensure that they are motivated to do so. To the extent that someone is distracted and/or does not want to think about a potential health threat, systematic processing is likely to be constrained.

Although systematic processing involves careful analysis of the information provided, it would be a mistake to assume that this analysis is always unbiased. People's prior beliefs and goals have been shown to have a systematic effect on how they use, evaluate, and recall information (Kunda, 1990). For example, when faced with information indicating that one's behavior may be risky, people have been shown to evaluate the evidence in a biased manner (e.g., Liberman & Chaiken, 1992), to adopt more stringent criteria for evaluating the evidence (e.g., Ditto & Lopez, 1992; Ditto, Munro, Apanovitch, Scepansky, & Lockhart, 2003), and to have poorer memory for the information (Kiviniemi & Rothman, 2006).

When messages are processed heuristically, less attention is paid to the specific information provided. Typically, this occurs when people are unable or not motivated to process the message. At the extreme, people may be so distracted or depleted that a message has no meaningful impact. However, in other cases, people's response to the message depends less on the strength of the specific arguments provided and more on surface features of the message, such as its source (e.g., National Cancer Institute), or on its tone (e.g., happy). Although heuristic processing can lead to belief changes, these changes are not thought to be particularly stable. Investigators may not try to encourage heuristic processing, but it is important that they be mindful of the conditions under which it might occur.

Although understanding how a message is processed can be informative, it is important to note that processing models provide limited guidance as to content that should be included in the message. Systematic processing relies on the presence of strong arguments but offers no guidance as to what makes a particular argument strong. For instance, would it make a difference if a message about Lyme disease emphasized people's vulnerability to a health problem compared to the ease with which people can take precautions? Models of health behavior such as the theory of reasoned action (Ajzen & Driver, 1992), the theory of planned behavior (Ajzen & Fishbein, 1980), or social cognitive theory (Bandura, 1986) do offer predictions as to the type of information that should be emphasized and can therefore work synergistically with message processing models to guide the development of effective health messages. Efforts to integrate these two perspectives were the focus of a special issue of the *Journal of Communication* (Cappella & Rimer, 2006).

Persuasive Strategies

Health messages can utilize a broad range of communication strategies: They can be designed to reassure people or to scare people, to provide general information to the entire population, or information targeted to a specific group or person. Over the past 20 years, two strategies that have received considerable attention have been shown to be effective methods to motivate belief and behavior change: message tailoring and message framing.

"Message tailoring" is based on the premise that people pay more attention to and are more persuaded by information that speaks directly to their own needs and interests (for a recent review, see Hawkins, Kreuter, Resnicow, Fishbein, & Dijkstra, 2008). For example, a message designed to promote a healthy diet could emphasize fruits and vegetables that match a person's dietary prefer-

ences. Across a range of domains, research has primarily found tailored health messages to be more effective than generic messages that provide everyone with the same information (for reviews, see Hawkins et al., 2008; Skinner, Campbell, Rimer, Curry, & Prochaska, 1999).

Why are tailored messages effective? Because tailored messages are designed to be personally relevant, people should be motivated to process them systematically. In fact, several studies have shown that, compared to generic messages, tailored messages are perceived to be more interesting and engaging (e.g., Brug, Steenhuis, van Assema, & de Vries, 1996; Kreuter, Bull, Clark, & Oswald, 1999). To the extent that the message contains strong arguments, the elaboration process should lead people to form a stable set of beliefs that are in turn predictive of behavior (Petty, Barden, & Wheeler, 2002).

Research on "message framing" has worked to delineate when a message should emphasize the benefits of performing a behavior (a gain-framed message) and when it should emphasize the costs of failing to perform the behavior (a loss-framed message). Working from a framework initially derived from prospect theory (Tversky & Kahneman, 1981), Rothman and Salovey (1997; Rothman, Kelly, Hertel, & Salovey, 2003) developed a framework that specifies the factors that regulate the impact of gain- and loss-framed messages. In particular, they have demonstrated that when a behavior is perceived to pose some degree of risk (e.g., it might inform a person that he or she has a health problem), loss-framed messages are a more effective persuasive strategy, whereas when a behavior is perceived to afford a relatively certain, favorable outcome (e.g., it serves to maintain a person's current health), gain-framed messages are a more effective persuasive strategy (for reviews, see Rothman, Bartels, Wlaschin, & Salovey, 2006; Rothman, Stark, & Salovey, 2006; Rothman et al., 2008).

Although investigators have focused primarily on the match between message frame and how people construe the targeted behavior, several studies have also found that dispositional differences in people's sensitivity to favorable and unfavorable outcomes moderate their response to gain- and loss-framed messages (Cesario, Grant, & Higgins, 2004;

Lee & Aaker, 2004; Mann, Sherman, & Updegraff, 2004). The primary assumption underlying this work is that a message is more persuasive to the extent that it fits or is compatible with how the recipient thinks and reasons about his or her environment, a perspective that is consistent with the approach that underlies message tailoring. In fact, it may be that when features of the message fit a person's dispositional preferences, the message is more likely to be processed systematically.

Other People Matter

In many areas of human behavior, including health, our behaviors are not simply the product of our own individual thoughts and self-regulatory efforts; they are strongly influenced by other people. In the health domain, this impact of others influences both the behavioral choices people make and other aspects of their health status. We address three of these influences on health behaviors and health outcomes in this section: the role of social norms, social comparison information, and prejudice and discrimination.

Social Norms, Prototypes, and Behavior

Most adolescents begin smoking cigarettes in a group with other smoking peers (Friedman, Lichtenstein, & Biglan, 1985), and the extent to which teenagers think their peers view smoking favorably influences the decision to smoke (Chassin, Presson, Sherman, Corty, & Olshavsky, 1984). This influence of other people's perceptions of the behavior is not limited to peer pressure in adolescents. The extent to which women think that their family and friends approve of breast cancer screening is a predictor of their compliance with mammography recommendations (Allen, Sorensen, Stoddard, Peterson, & Colditz, 1999), and people with higher perceptions of the number of people who engage in a risk behavior are more likely to engage in the behavior themselves (for a review of this literature, see Blanton, Köblitz, & McCaul, 2008).

These research examples are illustrative of the power of social norms to influence behavior. "Social norms" are an individual's

beliefs about how other people in their social environment evaluate a behavior. Do the other people have positive or negative attitudes about the behavior? Would they approve or disapprove of someone who engaged in the behavior? Do they engage in the behavior themselves? Most theoretical perspectives on social norms distinguish between two classes of norms. Norms can be either "descriptive," providing individuals with information about what most people think about an issue or what most people do in a particular situation, or "injunctive," providing information on how people *should* think or act (Cialdini, Reno, & Kallgren, 1990; Miller & Prentice, 1996).

According to specifications of the theory of reasoned action, a theoretical perspective that includes social norms, norms are based on two pieces of information (Fishbein, 1979). First, what does the individual believe the social norms to be? Second, to what extent is the individual motivated to comply with those social norms? This dual construction illustrates an important point about social norms: They are a motivated influence on a person's behavior. Social norms have power because the individual values the perspective of the other people holding the normative belief, believes that those other people have insight into "correct" behavior in the situation, and/or is concerned about how those other people will evaluate him or her if the norm is violated (for further discussion of social norms as a motivated influence on behavior, see Blanton et al., 2008; Miller & Prentice, 1996).

Because social norms are a powerful influence on behavior, interventions that attempt to change social norms have been created. Some interventions try to change perceptions of the normality of a given behavioral choice by providing more accurate perceptions of the number of people who engage in a particular risk behavior (e.g., Hansen & Graham, 1991), whereas others address perceptions of others' attitudes about the behavior under consideration (e.g., Schroeder & Prentice, 1998; Suls & Green, 2003). It has been argued that interventions based on descriptive norms about behaviors can have unintended negative consequences by leading individuals whose behavior is healthier than the norm to shift to less healthy behavioral patterns (Schultz, Nolan, Cialdini,

Goldstein, & Griskevicius, 2007). Currently, evidence for the efficacy of these interventions is mixed, especially for those trying to address descriptive norms about other people's behaviors (for a review, see Blanton et al., 2008), and some evidence suggests that interventions targeting injunctive norms based on information about other people's attitudes may be more impactful than those addressing descriptive norms about behavior (Schultz et al., 2007).

A separate but related influence of others in the social setting involves one's image of the "type" of person who engages in a particular behavior or has a particular health problem. Most people can articulate a perception of the "typical" smoker, and most have an image in their heads of what "someone with AIDS" is like. These perceptions of the typical person who engages in a behavior, called "prototypes," have an influence on both engagement in health behaviors and perceptions of risk for health problems.

In general, the more favorable one's prototype of the type of person who engages in a behavior (i.e., the extent to which one sees that person as having positive, desirable attributes), the more likely one is to engage in the behavior (Gibbons, Gerrard, & Lane, 2003). As with social norms, prototype images have been found to influence adolescents' interest in risk behavior; adolescents with more favorable images of the type of teenager who engages in various risk behaviors are more likely to report interest in engaging in those risk behaviors themselves (Barton, Chassin, Presson, & Sherman, 1982; Chassin, Tetzloff, & Hershey, 1985), and the degree to which one has favorable images of adolescents who engage in various risk behaviors predicts one's adoption of those behaviors in the future (Gibbons & Gerrard, 1995; Gibbons, Gerrard, Blanton, & Russell, 1998). According to the prototype/willingness model, which directly incorporates prototype perception as an influence on behavior, prototypes may influence behavior by changing behavioral willingness. "Behavioral willingness," a construct that is independent of behavioral intentions, is based on an individual's willingness to engage in the behavior under certain circumstances (e.g., willingness to have unprotected sex if a condom is not available, even if in general one intends to use a condom during

sex) (see Gibbons & Gerrard, 1997; Gibbons et al., 2003).

Prototype images also impact perceptions of risk for various health problems. To the extent that a person's image of the "typical person" with a disorder is negative and dissimilar from his or her own self-image, the person will likely perceive him- or herself as being at low risk (Perloff, 1987). Moreover, there is some evidence that individuals who are objectively at high risk for a health problem may alter their perceptions of the "typical person" so as to minimize their own feelings of risk (van der Velde, van der Pligt, & Hooykaas, 1994). There is evidence that presenting a person with prototype images that are similar to him- or herself can increase feelings of risk (Misovich, Fisher, & Fisher, 1997).

Social Comparison and Health

One problem that laypeople often face when thinking about and interpreting information about their health is that the health information, more often than not, is ambiguous and difficult to interpret. For example, if your physician tells you that your cholesterol is 225, you have to then interpret what 225 means. Is that high? Low? Should you be concerned about it? Does it mean that you are going to have health problems? Similarly, being told that your risk of suffering from a particular health problem is 1 in 1,000 is difficult to interpret. Is that a high risk? A low risk?

One way in which individuals resolve this ambiguity is to rely on social comparison information. "Social comparison" involves comparing oneself to other people to gain information about one's own abilities, skills, traits, or standing in a particular domain (Festinger, 1954) In the health context, individuals use social comparison to interpret where they stand on behavioral risk factors for illnesses (e.g., "Do I exercise more or less than the average person?"), risk for health problems ("Is my risk higher or lower than the average person's?"), and coping with health problems ("Am I doing better or worse than others with the illness?"; Suls, 2003). This information is often very valuable and sought after by individuals in ambiguous medical situations; for example, individuals about to have major surgery express preferences for hospital roommates who have already gone through the surgery, so that they can use the roommate's experience as a source of information about their own likely outcomes (Kulik & Mahler, 1989), and having a roommate who has already gone through surgery is associated with lower anxiety and better outcomes following surgery (Kulik, Mahler, & Moore, 1996).

The use of social comparison information has major implications for understanding how individuals think about and conceptualize their risk, and for considering ways to communicate information to individuals more effectively. One example of how a social comparison perspective can shed light on how people think about health issue is the domain of risk perceptions. People can think about their risk for a health problem in two ways. First, individuals can think about their "absolute risk"—the chance that an event will happen to them in some period of time (e.g., "The chance that I'll suffer from heart disease is 15%"). Second, risk can be thought of in terms of "comparative risk"— how one's own risk compares to the risk associated with another person, often a typical or average person ("My risk of suffering from heart disease is higher than the average person's"). It turns out that comparative risk—risk information gained from comparing one's risk to that of others—can be more impactful than absolute risk information; for example, in an experimental study in which both absolute risk and comparative risk for a health problem were manipulated, participants were more motivated by their comparative risk than by their absolute risk for the health problem (Klein, 1997; but see Harris & Smith, 2005). Some evidence also shows that communicating risk in a comparative matter can be more impactful than absolute risk information for motivating behavior (Lipkus & Klein, 2006).

Social comparison information also has implications for how individuals respond to learning that they have a risk factor for a particular health problem. Here, individuals seem to use information about how many other people share the risk factor as a means of determining how concerned they should be. In general, if individuals believe that a risk factor is very prevalent, then they believe the problem to be less serious than if they believe the problem is comparatively rare (Ditto & Jemmott, 1989; Jemmott, Ditto, & Croyle, 1986). In a similar vein, individuals who engage in unhealthy behaviors perceive those behaviors to be more common (Suls, Wan, & Sanders, 1988).

Finally, social comparison information influences how individuals respond to and cope with having a chronic illness. Women with breast cancer report a much greater likelihood of comparing themselves to breast cancer patients who are worse off than they are (Taylor & Lobel, 1989; Wood, Taylor, & Lichtman, 1985), and making such downward comparisons is associated with better perceived outcomes (Suls, Marco, & Tobin, 1991). However, although downward social comparisons are useful for coping with chronic illness, research has also found that affiliating with others who have the disease and are coping better has substantial benefits: It provides information about how to cope successfully with the health problem and potential optimism for a positive outcome (Taylor & Lobel, 1989; Wood & VanderZee, 1997).

Prejudice, Discrimination, and Health

A third way in which beliefs and behavior of "other people" can affect an individual's health sheds light on a very different area of social psychological theory. It is well known that substantial racial and ethnic disparities exist for a variety of health-related outcomes (Levine et al., 2001; Wong, Shapiro, Boscardin, & Ettner, 2002). Numerous mechanisms help to explain these disparities; one with particular relevance to social psychology is that experiences with prejudice and discrimination have negative health effects on members of minority groups.

There are a variety of mechanisms through which experiences with prejudice and discrimination can influence health outcomes. First, such experiences and their psychological consequences can directly impact health. Repeated exposure to prejudice and discrimination is stressful (Clark, Anderson, Clark, & Williams, 1999) and can lead to chronically elevated cardiovascular response (Merritt, Bennett, Williams, Edwards, & Sollers, 2006). Because stress and the concomitant cardiovascular response is associated with cardiovascular problems (Smith & Ruiz, 2002), prejudice and discrimination can lead to a higher likelihood of cardiovascular disorders (Brondolo, Rieppi, Kelly, & Gerin, 2003; Steffen, McNeilly, Anderson, & Sherwood, 2003).

A second mechanism involves the relation between experiences of prejudice and discrimination, and health behaviors. In particular, several studies have shown a link between experiencing prejudice and discrimination and substance use, including alcohol use, smoking, and illicit drug use (Bennett, Wolin, Robinson, Fowler, & Edwards, 2005; Gibbons, Gerrard, Cleveland, Wills, & Brody, 2004). Racial/ethnic disparities exist in rates of other health-related behaviors, including diet (Lovejoy, Champagne, Smith, de Jonge, & Xie, 2001), exercise (Centers for Disease Control and Prevention, 2007), and preventive screening (Gilligan, Wang, Levin, Kantoff, & Avorn, 2004), although the link between rates of those behaviors and experiences with prejudice and discrimination is not known.

Finally, there is substantial evidence that prejudice and discrimination not only influence risk factors for illness but also contribute to racial and ethnic disparities in treatment for illnesses (for a comprehensive overview of data on health care disparities, see Agency for Healthcare Research and Quality, 2008). Members of racial and ethnic/minority groups are likely to be diagnosed at later stages of illness relative to majority group members (e.g., Jones et al., 2008) and to receive less aggressive treatment (Shavers & Brown, 2002).

Although this section has focused on examples based on race/ethnicity, there is also evidence that members of other social groups suffer negative health effects due to stereotyping, prejudice, and discrimination. For example, gender stereotypes about the "typical patient" influence how doctors diagnose and treat heart disease in men versus women; this leads to less likelihood of aggressive intervention treatment plans for female patients (Martin & Lemos, 2002). In another domain, the stress associated with identity concealment is associated with a variety of serious health problems for gay men (Cole, 2006; Cole, Kemeny, Taylor, & Visscher, 1996). Finally, biases based on socioeconomic status are found in both diagnosis and treatment of mental health issues (Garb, 1997).

Conclusions

We have been purposefully selective in this introduction to the relation between social psychology and health, choosing to introduce a small number of relevant areas of social psychological research in some detail rather than briefly mentioning every possible connection of social psychology to health. Other areas of social psychological research have strong connections to health behavior and are worthy of greater exploration. For example, social psychology has a long and rich research tradition in close relationships, a large body of work examines the impact of such relationships on both health behaviors and health outcomes (e.g., Heaney & Israel, 2002; House, Landis, & Umberson, 1988). In another domain, social psychological research on the self-concept and self-related motivations has implications for understanding behavioral choices (Leary, Tchividijian, & Kraxberger, 1994) and how people process health information (Ditto & Lopez, 1992; Kiviniemi & Rothman, 2006). The reader who is interested in learning more about these and other intersections of social psychology and health can find more broad-based introductions to the discipline in Salovey and Rothman (2003), Suls and Wallston (2003), and Rothman and Salovey (2007).

What value might the information presented here have for investigators and practitioners interested in promoting health and combating illness? First, understanding the roles of attitudes, social norms, and other individual perceptions on health behavior and health outcomes has value, as does appreciating both the ways in which the broader social context influences individual behavior and the complex factors that influence changes in health-related attitudes. For example, they can aid in understanding why individuals sometimes behave in ways that match health recommendations but often do not, and why they are at times not compliant with recommendations of health professionals. Second, each of these areas has implications for how health professionals might intervene to encourage individuals to make healthier behavioral choices, and to improve health outcomes in care and treatment settings. For example, understanding the effect of individual attitudes and social norms on behavior suggests ways in which health professionals might target interventions to encourage healthy behavioral practices. Moreover, each of the principles of persuasion described in the chapter can be applied in the health care setting.

Ultimately we believe that social psychology presents both a cautionary and an optimistic tale for professionals who design and deliver interventions. From a cautionary perspective, individuals' behaviors and outcomes are often more complicated than they first appear, in part because of the variety of ways in which individual perceptions and the social situation impact behavior. On the other hand, understanding these multiple and complex influences on health present myriad new opportunities for thinking of ways to intervene and change individuals' behaviors and improve health outcomes. A firm understanding of the role of social psychological principles in determining health behavior and health outcomes can help to advance the goal of increasing individual wellness and reducing disease morbidity and mortality.

Acknowledgment

Preparation of this chapter was funded by National Cancer Institute Grant No. K07CA106225 to Marc T. Kiviniemi.

Further Reading

Readers interested in learning more about the basic social psychological principles discussed in this chapter can find more in-depth discussions of these and other principles in the following:

Kunda, Z. (1999). *Social cognition: Making sense of people.* Cambridge, MA: MIT Press.
Ross, L., & Nisbett, R. E. (1991). *The person and the situation: Perspectives of social psychology.* New York: McGraw-Hill.

For more information about the application of social psychological principles to health issues, including additional information on the applications discussed here and additional examples, see the following:

Norman, P., Abraham, C., & Conner, M. (2000). *Understanding and changing health behaviour: From health beliefs to self-regulation.* Amsterdam: Harwood Academic.

Rothman, A. J., & Salovey, P. (2007). The reciprocal relation between principles and practice: Social psychology and health behavior. In A. W. Kruglanski & E. T. Higgins (Eds.), *Social psychology: Handbook of basic principles* (2nd ed., pp. 826–849). New York: Guilford Press.
Salovey, P., & Rothman, A. J. (Eds.). (2003). *Social psychology of health.* New York: Psychology Press.
Suls, J., & Wallston, K. A. (Eds.). (2003). *Social psychological foundations of health and illness.* Malden, MA: Blackwell.

References

Abelson, R. P. (1988). Conviction. *American Psychologist, 43,* 267–275.
Abelson, R. P., Kinder, D. R., Peters, M. D., & Fiske, S. T. (1982). Affective and semantic components in political person perception. *Journal of Personality and Social Psychology, 42,* 619–630.
Agency for Healthcare Research and Quality. (2008). 2007 *National Healthcare Disparities Report* (AHRQ Pub. No. 08-0041). Rockville, MD: U.S. Department of Health and Human Services.
Aikman, S. N., Crites, S. L., Jr., & Fabrigar, L. R. (2006). Beyond affect and cognition: Identification of the informational bases of food attitudes. *Journal of Applied Social Psychology, 36,* 340–382.
Ajzen, I. (1991). The theory of planned behavior. *Organizational Behavior and Human Decision Processes, 50,* 179–211.
Ajzen, I., & Driver, B. L. (1991). Prediction of leisure participation from behavioral, normative, and control beliefs: An application of the theory of planned behavior. *Leisure Sciences, 13,* 185–204.
Ajzen, I., & Driver, B. L. (1992). Application of the theory of planned behavior to leisure choice. *Journal of Leisure Research, 24,* 207–224.
Ajzen, I., & Fishbein, M. (1977). Attitude–behavior relations: A theoretical analysis and review of empirical research. *Psychological Bulletin, 84,* 888–918.
Ajzen, I., & Fishbein, M. (1980). *Understanding attitudes and predicting behavior.* Englewood Cliffs, NJ: Prentice-Hall.
Ajzen, I., & Fishbein, M. (2005). The influence of attitudes on behavior. In D. Albarracin, B. T. Johnson, & M. P. Zanna (Eds.), *The handbook of attitudes* (pp. 173–221). Mahwah, NJ: Erlbaum.
Albarracin, D., Johnson, B. T., Fishbein, M., & Muellerleile, P. A. (2001). Theories of rea-

soned action and planned behavior as models of condom use: A meta-analysis. *Psychological Bulletin, 127,* 142–161.

Allen, J., Sorensen, G., Stoddard, A., Peterson, K., & Colditz, G. (1999). The relationship between social network characteristics and breast cancer screening practices among employed women. *Annals of Behavioral Medicine, 21,* 193–200.

Andersen, B. L. (2002). Biobehavioral outcomes following psychological interventions for cancer patients. *Journal of Consulting and Clinical Psychology, 70,* 590–610.

Armitage, C. J. (2007). Effects of an implementation intention-based intervention on fruit consumption. *Psychology and Health, 22,* 917–928.

Bandura, A. (1986). *Social foundations of thought and action: A social cognitive theory.* Englewood Cliffs, NJ: Prentice-Hall.

Barton, J., Chassin, L., Presson, C. C., & Sherman, S. J. (1982). Social image factors as motivators of smoking initiation in early and middle adolescence. *Child Development, 53,* 1499–1511.

Bem, D. J. (1967). Self-perception: An alternative interpretation of cognitive dissonance phenomena. *Psychological Review, 74,* 183–200.

Bennett, G. G., Wolin, K. Y., Robinson, E. L., Fowler, S., & Edwards, C. L. (2005). Perceived racial/ethnic harassment and tobacco use among African American young adults. *American Journal of Public Health, 95,* 238–240.

Blanton, H., Köblitz, A., & McCaul, K. D. (2008). Misperceptions about norm misperceptions: Descriptive, injunctive, and affective "social norming" efforts to change health behaviors. *Social and Personality Psychology Compass, 2,* 1379–1399.

Breckler, S. J. (1984). Empirical validation of affect, behavior, and cognition as distinct components of attitude. *Journal of Personality and Social Psychology, 47,* 1191–1205.

Breckler, S. J., & Wiggins, E. C. (1989). Affect versus evaluation in the structure of attitudes. *Journal of Experimental Social Psychology, 25,* 253–271.

Brondolo, E., Rieppi, R., Kelly, K. P., & Gerin, W. (2003). Perceived racism and blood pressure: A review of the literature and conceptual and methodological critique. *Annals of Behavioral Medicine, 25,* 55–65.

Brug, J., Steenhuis, I., van Assema, P., & de Vries, H. (1996). The impact of a computer-tailored nutrition intervention. *Preventive Medicine, 25,* 236–242.

Cappella, J. N., & Rimer, B. K. (Eds.). (2006). The role of theory in developing effective health communications [Special issue]. *Journal of Health Communications, 56.*

Centers for Disease Control and Prevention. (2007). Prevalence of regular physical activity among adults—United States, 2001 and 2005. *Morbidity and Mortality Weekly Report, 56,* 1209–1212.

Cesario, J., Grant, H., & Higgins, E. T. (2004). Regulatory fit and persuasion: Transfer from "feeling right." *Journal of Personality and Social Psychology, 86,* 388–404.

Chaiken, S., & Baldwin, M. W. (1981). Affective–cognitive consistency and the effect of salient behavioral information on the self-perception of attitudes. *Journal of Personality and Social Psychology, 41,* 1–12.

Chaiken, S., Liberman, A., & Eagly, A. H. (1989). Heuristic and systematic information processing within and beyond the persuasion context. In J. S. Uleman & J. A. Bargh (Eds.), *Unintended thought* (pp. 212–252). New York: Guilford Press.

Chaiken, S., & Yates, S. (1985). Affective–cognitive consistency and thought-induced attitude polarization. *Journal of Personality and Social Psychology, 49,* 1470–1481.

Chassin, L., Presson, C. C., Sherman, S. J., Corty, E., & Olshavsky, R. W. (1984). Predicting the onset of cigarette smoking in adolescents: A longitudinal study. *Journal of Applied Social Psychology, 14,* 224–243.

Chassin, L., Tetzloff, C., & Hershey, M. (1985). Self-image and social-image factors in adolescent alcohol use. *Journal of Studies on Alcohol, 46,* 39–47.

Cialdini, R. B., Reno, R. R., & Kallgren, C. A. (1990). A focus theory of normative conduct: Recycling the concept of norms to reduce littering in public places. *Journal of Personality and Social Psychology, 58,* 1015–1026.

Clark, R., Anderson, N. B., Clark, V. R., & Williams, D. R. (1999). Racism as a stressor for African Americans: A biopsychosocial model. *American Psychologist, 54,* 805–816.

Cole, S. W. (2006). Social threat, personal identity, and physical health in closeted gay men. In A. M. Omoto & H. S. Kurtzman (Eds.), *Sexual orientation and mental health: Examining identity and development in lesbian, gay, and bisexual people* (pp. 245–267). Washington, DC: American Psychological Association.

Cole, S. W., Kemeny, M. E., Taylor, S. E., & Visscher, B. R. (1996). Elevated physical health risk among gay men who conceal their homosexual identity. *Health Psychology, 15,* 243–251.

Crites, S. L., Fabrigar, L. R., & Petty, R. E. (1994). Measuring the affective and cognitive properties of attitudes: Conceptual and methodological issues. *Personality and Social Psychology Bulletin, 20,* 619–634.

Ditto, P. H., & Jemmott, J. B. (1989). From rarity

to evaluative extremity: Effects of prevalence information on evaluations of positive and negative characteristics. *Journal of Personality and Social Psychology, 57,* 16–26.

Ditto, P. H., & Lopez, D. F. (1992). Motivated skepticism: Use of differential decision criteria for preferred and nonpreferred conclusions. *Journal of Personality and Social Psychology, 63,* 568–584.

Ditto, P. H., Munro, G. D., Apanovitch, A. M., Scepansky, J. A., & Lockhart, L. K. (2003). Spontaneous skepticism: The interplay of motivation and expectation in responses to favorable and unfavorable medical diagnoses. *Personality and Social Psychology Bulletin, 29,* 1120–1132.

Eagly, A. H., & Chaiken, S. (1993). *The psychology of attitudes.* New York: Harcourt Brace Jovanovich.

Eagly, A. H., Chaiken, S. (1998). Attitude structure and function. In D. T. Gilbert, S. T. Fiske, & G. Lindzey (Eds.), *The handbook of social psychology* (4th ed., Vol. 1, pp. 269–322). New York: McGraw-Hill.

Edwards, K. (1990). The interplay of affect and cognition in attitude formation and change. *Journal of Personality and Social Psychology, 59,* 202–216.

Engel, G. L. (1977). The need for a new medical model: A challenge for biomedicine. *Science, 196,* 129–136.

Fabrigar, L. R., MacDonald, T. K., & Wegener, D. T. (2005). The structure of attitudes. In D. Albarracin, B. T. Johnson, & M. P. Zanna (Eds.), *The handbook of attitudes* (pp. 79–125). Mahwah, NJ: Erlbaum.

Fazio, R. H. (1989). On the power and functionality of attitudes: The role of attitude accessibility. In A. R. Pratkanis, S. J. Breckler, & A. G. Greenwald (Eds.), *Attitude structure and function* (pp. 153–179). Hillsdale, NJ: Erlbaum.

Fazio, R. H. (1990). Multiple processes by which attitudes guide behavior: The MODE model as an integrative framework In M. P. Zanna (Ed.), *Advances in experimental social psychology* (Vol. 23, pp. 75–109). San Diego, CA: Academic Press.

Festinger, L. (1954). A theory of social comparison processes. *Human Relations, 7,* 117–140.

Festinger, L. (1957). *A theory of cognitive dissonance.* Oxford, UK: Row, Peterson.

Fishbein, M. (1979). A theory of reasoned action: Some applications and implications. *Nebraska Symposium on Motivation, 27,* 65–116.

Friedman, L. S., Lichtenstein, E., & Biglan, A. (1985). Smoking onset among teens: An empirical analysis of initial situations. *Addictive Behaviors, 10,* 1–13.

Garb, H. N. (1997). Race bias, social class bias, and gender bias in clinical judgment. *Clinical Psychology: Science and Practice, 4,* 99–120.

Gibbons, F. X., Eggleston, T. J., & Benthin, A. C. (1997). Cognitive reactions to smoking relapse: The reciprocal relation between dissonance and self-esteem. *Journal of Personality and Social Psychology, 72,* 184–195.

Gibbons, F. X., & Gerrard, M. (1995). Predicting young adults' health risk behavior. *Journal of Personality and Social Psychology, 69,* 505–517.

Gibbons, F. X., & Gerrard, M. (1997). Health images and their effects on health behavior. In B. P. Buunk & F. X. Gibbons (Eds.), *Health, coping, and well-being: Perspectives from social comparison theory* (pp. 63–94). Mahwah, NJ: Erlbaum.

Gibbons, F. X., Gerrard, M., Blanton, H., & Russell, D. W. (1998). Reasoned action and social reaction: Willingness and intention as independent predictors of health risk. *Journal of Personality and Social Psychology, 74,* 1164–1180.

Gibbons, F. X., Gerrard, M., Cleveland, M. J., Wills, T. A., & Brody, G. (2004). Perceived discrimination and substance use in African American parents and their children: A panel study. *Journal of Personality and Social Psychology, 86,* 517–529.

Gibbons, F. X., Gerrard, M., & Lane, D. J. (2003). A social reaction model of adolescent health risk. In J. Suls & K. A. Wallston (Eds.), *Social psychological foundations of health and illness* (pp. 107–136). Malden, MA: Blackwell.

Gilligan, T., Wang, P. S., Levin, R., Kantoff, P. W., & Avorn, J. (2004). Racial differences in screening for prostate cancer in the elderly. *Archives of Internal Medicine, 164,* 1858–1864.

Godin, G., & Kok, G. (1996). The theory of planned behavior: A review of its applications to health-related behaviors. *American Journal of Health Promotion, 11,* 87–98.

Gollwitzer, P. M., & Sheeran, P. (2006). Implementation intentions and goal achievement: A meta-analysis of effects and processes. *Advances in Experimental Social Psychology, 38,* 69–119.

Green, L. W., & Kreuter, M. W. (1999). *Health promotion planning: An educational and ecological approach.* Mountain View, CA: Mayfield.

Gross, S. R., Holtz, R., & Miller, N. (1995). Attitude certainty. In R. E. Petty & J. A. Krosnick (Eds.), *Attitude strength: Antecedents and consequences* (pp. 215–245). Hillsdale, NJ: Erlbaum.

Haddock, G., Maio, G. R., Arnold, K., & Huskinson, T. (2008). Should persuasion be affective or cognitive?: The moderating effects of need for affect and need for cognition. *Personality and Social Psychology Bulletin, 34*, 769–778.

Hansen, W. B., & Graham, J. W. (1991). Preventing alcohol, marijuana, and cigarette use among adolescents: Peer pressure resistance training versus establishing conservative norms. *Preventive Medicine, 20*, 414–430.

Harris, P. R., & Smith, V. (2005). When the risks are low: The impact of absolute and comparative information on disturbance and understanding in US and UK samples. *Psychology and Health, 20*, 319–330.

Hausenblas, H. A., Carron, A. V., & Mack, D. E. (1997). Application of the theories of reasoned action and planned behavior to exercise behavior: A meta-analysis. *Journal of Sport and Exercise Psychology, 19*, 36–51.

Hawkins, R. P., Kreuter, M., Resnicow, K., Fishbein, M., & Dijkstra, A. (2008). Understanding tailoring in communicating about health. *Health Education Research, 23*, 454–466.

Heaney, C. A., & Israel, B. A. (2002). Social networks and social support. In K. Glanz, B. K. Rimer, & F. M. Lewis (Eds.), *Health behavior and health education* (3rd ed., pp. 185–208). San Francisco: Jossey-Bass.

House, J. S., Landis, K. R., & Umberson, D. (1988). Social relationships and health. *Science, 241*, 540–545.

Huhman, M., Potter, L. D., Wong, F. L., Banspach, S. W., Duke, J. C., & Heitzler, C. D. (2005). Effects of a mass media campaign to increase physical activity among children: Year-1 results of the VERB campaign. *Pediatrics, 116*, e277–e284.

Janis, I. (1967). Effects of fear arousal on attitude change. In L. Berkowitz (Ed.), *Advances in experimental social psychology* (pp. 166–224). New York: Academic Press.

Jemmott, J. B., Ditto, P. H., & Croyle, R. T. (1986). Judging health status: Effects of perceived prevalence and personal relevance. *Journal of Personality and Social Psychology, 50*, 899–905.

Jones, B. A., Liu, W.-L., Araujo, A. B., Kasl, S. V., Silvera, S. N., Soler-Vila, H., et al. (2008). Explaining the race difference in prostate cancer stage at diagnosis. *Cancer Epidemiology Biomarkers and Prevention, 17*, 2825–2834.

Jones, E. E. (1985). Major developments in social psychology during the past five decades. In G. Lindzey & E. Aronson (Eds.), *Handbook of social psychology* (3rd ed., Vol. 1, pp. 47–108). New York: Random House.

Kaplan, R. M., & Frosch, D. L. (2005). Decision making in medicine and health care. *Annual Review of Clinical Psychology, 1*, 525–556.

Kelder, S. H., Maibach, E., Worden, J. K., Biglan, A., & Levitt, A. (2000). Planning and initiation of the ONDCP National Youth Anti-Drug Media Campaign. *Journal of Public Health Management and Practice, 6*, 14–26.

Kiviniemi, M. T., & Bevins, R. (2007). Affect–behavior associations in motivated behavioral choice: Potential transdisciplinary links. In P. R. Zelick (Ed.), *Issues in the psychology of motivation* (pp. 65–80). Hauppage, NY: Nova.

Kiviniemi, M. T., & Rothman, A. J. (2006). Selective memory biases in individuals' memory for health-related information and behavior recommendations. *Psychology and Health, 21*, 247–272.

Kiviniemi, M. T., Voss-Humke, A. M., & Seifert, A. L. (2007). How do I feel about the behavior?: The interplay of affective associations with behaviors and cognitive beliefs as influences on physical activity behavior. *Health Psychology, 26*, 152–158.

Klein, W. M. (1997). Objective standards are not enough: Affective, self-evaluative, and behavioral responses to social comparison information. *Journal of Personality and Social Psychology, 72*, 763–774.

Kreuter, M. W., Bull, F. C., Clark, E. M., & Oswald, D. L. (1999). Understanding how people process health information: A comparison of tailored and nontailored weight-loss materials. *Health Psychology, 18*, 487–494.

Krosnick, J. A. (1988). Attitude importance and attitude change. *Journal of Experimental Social Psychology, 24*, 240–255.

Krosnick, J. A., & Petty, R. E. (1995). Attitude strength: An overview. In R. E. Petty & J. A. Krosnick (Eds.), *Attitude strength: Antecedents and consequences* (pp. 1–24). Hillsdale, NJ: Erlbaum.

Kulik, J. A., & Mahler, H. I. (1989). Stress and affiliation in a hospital setting: Preoperative roommate preferences. *Personality and Social Psychology Bulletin, 15*, 183–193.

Kulik, J. A., Mahler, H. I. M., & Moore, P. J. (1996). Social comparison and affiliation under threat: Effects on recovery from major surgery. *Journal of Personality and Social Psychology, 71*, 967–979.

Kunda, Z. (1990). The case for motivated reasoning. *Psychological Bulletin, 108*, 480–498.

La Piere, R. T. (1934). Attitudes versus actions. *Social Forces, 13*, 230–237.

Leary, M. R., Tchividijian, L. R., & Kraxberger, B. E. (1994). Self-presentation can be hazardous to your health: Impression management and health risk. *Health Psychology, 13*, 461–470.

Lee, A. Y., & Aaker, J. L. (2004). Bringing the frame into focus: The influence of regulatory fit on processing fluency and persuasion. *Journal of Personality and Social Psychology, 86*, 205–218.

Leventhal, H. (1970). Findings and theory in the study of fear communications. In L. Berkowitz (Ed.), *Advances in experimental social psychology* (Vol. 5, pp. 119–186). New York: Academic Press.

Levine, R. S., Foster, J. E., Fullilove, R. E., Fullilove, M. T., Briggs, N. C., Hull, P. C., et al. (2001). Black–white inequalities in mortality and life expectancy, 1933–1999: Implications for healthy people 2010. *Public Health Reports, 116,* 474–483.

Liberman, A., & Chaiken, S. (1992). Defensive processing of personally relevant health messages. *Personality and Social Psychology Bulletin, 18,* 669–679.

Lipkus, I. M., & Klein, W. M. P. (2006). Effects of communicating social comparison information on risk perceptions for colorectal cancer. *Journal of Health Communication, 11,* 391–407.

Lovejoy, J. C., Champagne, C. M., Smith, S. R., de Jonge, L., & Xie, H. (2001). Ethnic differences in dietary intakes, physical activity, and energy expenditure in middle-aged, premenopausal women: The Healthy Transitions Study. *American Journal of Clinical Nutrition, 74,* 90–95.

Mann, T., Sherman, D., & Updegraff, J. (2004). Dispositional motivations and message framing: A test of the congruency hypothesis in college students. *Health Psychology, 23,* 330–334.

Martin, R., & Lemos, K. (2002). From heart attacks to melanoma: Do common sense models of somatization influence symptom interpretation for female victims? *Health Psychology, 21,* 25–32.

McGuire, W. J. (1985). Attitudes and attitude change. In G. Lindzey & E. Aronson (Eds.), *Handbook of social psychology* (3rd ed., Vol. 2, pp. 233–346). New York: Random House.

Merritt, M. M., Bennett, G. G., Jr., Williams, R. B., Edwards, C. L., & Sollers, J. J., III. (2006). Perceived racism and cardiovascular reactivity and recovery to personally relevant stress. *Health Psychology, 25,* 364–369.

Millar, M. G., & Tesser, A. (1986). Effects of affective and cognitive focus on the attitude–behavior relation. *Journal of Personality and Social Psychology, 51,* 270–276.

Miller, D. T., & Prentice, D. A. (1996). The construction of social norms and standards. In E. T. Higgins & A. W. Kruglanski (Eds.), *Social psychology: Handbook of basic principles* (pp. 799–829). New York: Guilford Press.

Misovich, S. J., Fisher, J. D., & Fisher, W. A. (1997). Social comparison processes and AIDS risk and AIDS preventive behavior. In B. P. Buunk & F. X. Gibbons (Eds.), *Health, coping, and well-being: Perspectives from social comparison theory* (pp. 95–123). Mahwah, NJ: Erlbaum.

Orbell, S., & Sheeran, P. (1998). "Inclined abstainers": A problem for predicting health-related behaviour. *British Journal of Social Psychology, 37,* 151–165.

Perloff, L. S. (1987). Social comparison and illusions of invulnerability to negative life events. In C. R. Snyder & C. E. Ford (Eds.), *Coping with negative life events: Clinical and social psychological perspectives* (pp. 217–242). New York: Plenum Press.

Petty, R. E., Barden, J., & Wheeler, S. C. (2002). The elaboration likelihood model of persuasion: Health promotions that yield sustained behavioral change. In R. J. DiClemente, R. A. Crosby, & M. C. Kegler (Eds.), *Emerging theories in health promotion practice and research* (pp. 71–99). San Francisco: Jossey-Bass.

Petty, R. E., & Wegener, D. T. (1999). The elaboration likelihood model: Current status and controversies. In S. Chaiken & Y. Trope (Eds.), *Dual-process theories in social psychology* (pp. 37–72). New York: Guilford Press.

Pratkanis, A. R., Breckler, S. J., & Greenwald, A. G. (1989). *Attitude structure and function.* Hillsdale, NJ: Erlbaum.

Prochaska, J. O., DiClemente, C. C., & Norcross, J. C. (1992). In search of how people change: Applications to addictive behaviors. *American Psychologist, 47,* 1102–1114.

Regan, D. T., & Fazio, R. (1977). On the consistency between attitudes and behavior: Look to the method of attitude formation. *Journal of Experimental Social Psychology, 13,* 28–45.

Rosenberg, M. J. (1960). A structural theory of attitude dynamics. *Public Opinion Quarterly, 24,* 319–340.

Ross, L., & Nisbett, R. E. (1991). *The person and the situation: Perspectives of social psychology.* New York: McGraw-Hill.

Rothman, A. J., Bartels, R. D., Wlaschin, J., & Salovey, P. (2006). The strategic use of gain- and loss-framed messages to promote healthy behavior: How theory can inform practice. *Journal of Communication, 56,* S202–S220.

Rothman, A. J., Kelly, K. M., Hertel, A. W., & Salovey, P. (2003). Message frames and illness representations: Implications for interventions to promote and sustain healthy behavior. In L. D. Cameron & H. Leventhal (Eds.), *The self-regulation of health and illness behaviour* (pp. 278–296). New York: Routledge.

Rothman, A. J., & Salovey, P. (1997). Shaping perceptions to motivate healthy behavior: The role of message framing. *Psychological Bulletin, 121,* 3–19.

Rothman, A. J., & Salovey, P. (2007). The reciprocal relation between principles and practice: Social psychology and health behavior. In A.

W. Kruglanski & E. T. Higgins (Eds.), *Social psychology: Handbook of basic principles* (2nd ed., pp. 826–849). New York: Guilford Press.

Rothman, A. J., Stark, E., & Salovey, P. (2006). Using message framing to promote healthy behavior: A guide to best practices. In J. Trafton (Ed.), *Best practices in the behavioral management of chronic diseases* (Vol. 3, pp. 31–48). Los Altos, CA: Institute for Disease Management.

Rothman, A. J., Wlaschin, J. T., Bartels, R. D., Latimer, A., & Salovey, P. (2008). How persons and situations regulate message framing effects: The study of health behavior. In A. J. Elliot (Ed.), *Handbook of approach and avoidance motivation* (pp. 475–486). New York: Psychology Press.

Sallis, J. F., McKenzie, T. L., Conway, T. L., Elder, J. P., Prochaska, J. J., Brown, M., et al. (2003). Environmental interventions for eating and physical activity: A randomized controlled trial in middle schools. *American Journal of Preventive Medicine, 24,* 209–217.

Salovey, P., & Rothman, A. J. (Eds.). (2003). *Social psychology of health.* New York: Psychology Press.

Schroeder, C. M., & Prentice, D. A. (1998). Exposing pluralistic ignorance to reduce alcohol use among college students. *Journal of Applied Social Psychology, 28,* 2150–2180.

Schultz, P. W., Nolan, J. M., Cialdini, R. B., Goldstein, N. J., & Griskevicius, V. (2007). The constructive, destructive, and reconstructive power of social norms. *Psychological Science, 18,* 429–434.

Shavers, V. L., & Brown, M. L. (2002). Racial and ethnic disparities in the receipt of cancer treatment. *Journal of the National Cancer Institute, 94,* 334–357.

Sheeran, P., Abraham, C., & Orbell, S. (1999). Psychosocial correlates of heterosexual condom use: A meta-analysis. *Psychological Bulletin, 125,* 90–132.

Sheeran, P., Webb, T. L., & Gollwitzer, P. M. (2005). The interplay between goal intentions and implementation intentions. *Personality and Social Psychology Bulletin, 31,* 87–98.

Simons, J., & Carey, K. B. (1998). A structural analysis of attitudes toward alcohol and marijuana use. *Personality and Social Psychology Bulletin, 24,* 727–735.

Skinner, C. S., Campbell, M. K., Rimer, B. K., Curry, S., & Prochaska, J. O. (1999). How effective is tailored print communication? *Annals of Behavioral Medicine, 21,* 290–298.

Smith, T. W., & Ruiz, J. M. (2002). Psychosocial influences on the development and course of coronary heart disease: Current status and implications for research and practice. *Journal of Consulting and Clinical Psychology, 70,* 548–568.

Stangor, C., Sullivan, L. A., & Ford, T. E. (1991). Affective and cognitive determinants of prejudice. *Social Cognition, 9,* 359–380.

Steffen, P. R., McNeilly, M., Anderson, N., & Sherwood, A. (2003). Effects of perceived racism and anger inhibition on ambulatory blood pressure in African Americans. *Psychosomatic Medicine, 65,* 746–750.

Stone, J., Aronson, E., Crain, A. L., & Winslow, M. P. (1994). Inducing hypocrisy as a means of encouraging young adults to use condoms. *Personality and Social Psychology Bulletin, 20,* 116–128.

Suls, J. (2003). Contributions of social comparison to physical illness and well-being. In J. Suls & K. A. Wallston (Eds.), *Social psychological foundations of health and illness* (pp. 226–255). Malden, MA: Blackwell.

Suls, J., & Green, P. (2003). Pluralistic ignorance and college student perceptions of gender-specific alcohol norms. *Health Psychology, 22,* 479–486.

Suls, J., Marco, C. A., & Tobin, S. (1991). The role of temporal comparison, social comparison, and direct appraisal in the elderly's self-evaluations of health. *Journal of Applied Social Psychology, 21,* 1125–1144.

Suls, J., & Rothman, A. (2004). Evolution of the biopsychosocial model: Prospects and challenges for health psychology. *Health Psychology, 23,* 119–125.

Suls, J., & Wallston, K. A. (Eds.). (2003). *Social psychological foundations of health and illness.* Malden, MA: Blackwell.

Suls, J., Wan, C. K., & Sanders, G. S. (1988). False consensus and false uniqueness in estimating the prevalence of health-protective behaviors. *Journal of Applied Social Psychology, 18,* 66–79.

Taylor, S. E., & Lobel, M. (1989). Social comparison activity under threat: Downward evaluation and upward contacts. *Psychological Review, 96,* 569–575.

Thompson, M. M., Zanna, M. P., & Griffin, D. W. (1995). Let's not be indifferent about (attitudinal) ambivalence. In R. E. Petty & J. A. Krosnick (Eds.), *Attitude strength: Antecedents and consequences* (pp. 361–386). Hillsdale, NJ: Erlbaum.

Trafimow, D., & Sheeran, P. (1998). Some tests of the distinction between cognitive and affective beliefs. *Journal of Experimental Social Psychology, 34,* 378–397.

Triandis, H. C. (1979). Values, attitudes, and interpersonal behavior. In M. M. Page (Ed.), *Nebraska Symposium on Motivation* (Vol. 27, pp. 195–259). Lincoln: University of Nebraska Press.

Tversky, A., & Kahneman, D. (1981). The framing of decisions and the psychology of choice. *Science, 211,* 453–458.

van den Berg, H., Manstead, A. S. R., van der Pligt, J., & Wigboldus, D. L. H. J. (2005). The role of affect in attitudes toward organ donation and donor-relevant decisions. *Psychology and Health, 20,* 789–802.

van der Velde, F. W., van der Pligt, J., & Hooykaas, C. (1994). Perceiving AIDS-related risk: Accuracy as a function of differences in actual risk. *Health Psychology, 13,* 25–33.

Webb, T. L., & Sheeran, P. (2006). Does changing behavioral intentions engender behavior change?: A meta-analysis of the experimental evidence. *Psychological Bulletin, 132,* 249–268.

Weinstein, N. D. (1993). Testing four competing theories of health-protective behavior. *Health Psychology, 12,* 324–333.

Wong, M. D., Shapiro, M. F., Boscardin, W. J., & Ettner, S. L. (2002). Contribution of major diseases to disparities in mortality. *New England Journal of Medicine, 347,* 1585–1592.

Wood, J. V., Taylor, S. E., & Lichtman, R. R. (1985). Social comparison in adjustment to breast cancer. *Journal of Personality and Social Psychology, 49,* 1169–1183.

Wood, J. V., & VanderZee, K. (1997). Social comparisons among cancer patients: Under what conditions are comparisons upward and downward? In B. P. Buunk & F. X. Gibbons (Eds.), *Health, coping, and well-being: Perspectives from social comparison theory* (pp. 299–328). Mahwah, NJ: Erlbaum.

Wood, W., Rhodes, N., & Biek, M. (1995). Working knowledge and attitude strength: An information-processing analysis. In R. E. Petty & J. A. Krosnick (Eds.), *Attitude strength: Antecedents and consequences* (pp. 283–313). Hillsdale, NJ: Erlbaum.

CHAPTER 6

Clinical Psychology and Health Psychology

Toward an Integrated Perspective on Health

Perry M. Nicassio
Melanie A. Greenberg
Sarosh J. Motivala

Historical Foundations

Clinical psychology has evolved into a major professional field over the last century to have a significant impact on mental health services delivery. Since its inception, clinical psychology has undergone many transformations, addressed numerous obstacles from other disciplines, and worked through various crises of identity. While the scientific study of psychology as an academic discipline already had an established history, the field of clinical psychology developed gradually because of a growing need to assess and quantify human traits, abilities, and cognitive processes for a variety of populations, including children with mental deficiencies and academic limitations, institutionalized psychiatric patients, and veterans of World War I who returned with debilitating posttraumatic symptoms, mood disturbances, and myriad adjustment problems associated with their reentry into civilian life (Benjamin, 2005). As clinical psychologists addressed these demands, they began to establish their identity as professionals by fulfilling an important role in the development and implementation of mental health services.

Over the next several decades, clinical psychology expanded as an independent professional field as it distinguished itself from psychiatry. A key feature of this growth was the contribution of psychologists in psychotherapy, patient management, and consultation. Opportunities for formal clinical psychology training, however, were limited in the first half of the 20th century, and the demand for mental health treatment far exceeded the supply of clinicians who could serve the public. Recognizing this need, the federal government supported the expansion of clinical psychology by directing the Veterans Administration and U.S. Public Health Service to facilitate the growth of mental health professionals. Federal funding became available to support the development of university-based clinical psychology doctoral education and training programs. The emergence of PhD programs legitimized clinical psychology as both an academic discipline and a profession, preparing students to conduct research and render service. Since the 1970s, independent professional schools of clinical psychology have provided additional opportunities for clinical training at the doctoral level to meet the demand for clinicians to serve the public. Currently, more than 200 accredited university-based and professional school clinical psychology doctoral programs in the United States and Canada provide training under the auspices of the American Psychological Association. Several thousand students graduate from these programs on a yearly basis, with the goal of obtaining a professional license to practice within their respective states. As a result of these developments, the capacity to address the mental health needs of the public has increased dramatically over the past 50 years, as has the awareness of the lay public regarding the value and importance of the field of clinical psychology to human welfare.

Clinical psychologists currently function in a range of settings, including academic departments of psychology, medical centers, industry, government, and private practice. The influence of clinical psychology has broadened as greater numbers of doctoral-level trained professionals have occupied roles in these settings, along with the recognition that their skills as diagnosticians, therapists, and problem solvers are relevant to many other fields and populations. In this chapter, we describe the relevance and contributions of clinical psychology to the burgeoning field of health psychology, highlighting key areas that constitute a foundation for understanding the interdependence of these fields in research and practice.

Scientist-Practitioner Training

As clinical psychology grew in importance as a profession, the American Psychological Association recognized the need to establish an appropriate training model and educational curriculum for academic programs. The Boulder Conference, held at the University of Colorado campus in 1949, addressed the basic elements of training in clinical psychology and promoted the view that both scientific and clinical training are essential factors in the preparation of psychologists who enter clinical practice (Raimy, 1950). This conference led to the establishment of the scientist-practitioner model as the preeminent framework for the education and training of clinical psychologists. Although professional psychologists and academics have offered different interpretations of this model, Belar (2000) has made the point that the integra-

tion of science and practice throughout curricula and applied training sites is the critical feature of scientist-practitioner training. An important element of this model is the synergistic relationship between science and practice, such that research findings inform all aspects of clinical decision making, and that patient interactions yield valuable insights and testable hypotheses for researchers.

Emerging later were doctoral programs in independent professional schools that promoted alternative practitioner models, de-emphasizing this integrated framework by offering the Doctor of Psychology (PsyD) to prepare students for clinical roles but not as researchers. A major reason for the development of the PsyD was to increase the number of clinically trained professionals because academic clinical psychology programs were not preparing a sufficient number of psychologists to function in service delivery roles. While meeting this need, the awarding of the PsyD has raised concerns among academic and scientist-practitioner clinicians that such training would lead clinical psychology away from its empirical roots by emphasizing clinical training at the expense of research and jeopardize clinical care. A key issue has been whether the PsyD would prepare clinicians to integrate research findings into their diagnostic and treatment decisions. Although ongoing debate persists between academics and professional psychologists about this model of training and the professional qualifications of PsyD clinicians, the American Psychological Association has formally recognized the PsyD as an accredited degree in clinical psychology for over two decades. Several thousand psychologists with the PsyD currently function in clinical roles throughout the United States.

Definition of Clinical Psychology and Its Relation to Health Psychology and Clinical Health Psychology

Clinical psychology is evolving at a rapid rate in response to changing demographic trends in the United States, new scientific developments, and the increased relevance of the field to other disciplines (Belar, Nelson, & Wasik, 2003). Clearly, the scope of clinical psychology has transcended its earlier roles in assessment and psychotherapy to have far-reaching significance as a health-related discipline. The American Psychological Association's Commission for the Recognition of Specialties and Proficiencies (2004) defined "clinical psychology" as a general practice and health service provider specialty in professional psychology, and noted that clinical psychologists provide a vast range of services, including assessment, diagnosis, prediction, prevention, and treatment of psychopathology and behaviors to improve personal effectiveness and satisfaction.

This characterization of clinical psychology illustrates the breadth of the field and its role in promoting quality of life and positive psychosocial functioning. The American Psychological Association's recognition of clinical psychology as a health-related discipline also represents a departure from its historical emphasis on psychopathology diagnostics and treatment, reinforcing its independence from psychiatry and its potential alliance with medicine. The implications of this transformation in emphasis are striking. As health service providers, clinical psychologists face the challenge and responsibility of understanding the interface between psychology and health, developing assessment and therapeutic skills that address this interface, and rendering clinical services that focus both on mental health and physical health outcomes. The role of health services provider places special importance on the identity and professional activities of clinical psychologists in the future. Many clinical psychologists will continue to see their role as restricted to mental health services delivery, while others will assume a broader professional identity that encompasses interdisciplinary perspectives. Importantly, clinical psychologists will continue to have opportunities to influence the health and welfare of diverse populations and enhance health care delivery in the future. Clinical psychology's leaders can further this agenda by establishing, monitoring, and reevaluating criteria for education and training that are commensurate with this expanded role, and by promoting the relevance of clinical psychology to areas such as medicine, public health, rehabilitation, and allied health.

From an interdisciplinary perspective, the expanded definition of clinical psychology raises questions about its relationship with health psychology. Over the last 30 years, the field of health psychology has emerged as a new field of study and has experienced an expansion that has paralleled the growth and development of clinical psychology. The definition of the field of health psychology offered by Matarazzo (1982) in the field's nascent years sheds light on its relationship with clinical psychology. Specifically, he referred to "health psychology" as the aggregate of the specific educational, scientific, and professional contributions of the discipline of psychology to (1) the promotion and maintenance of health; (2) the prevention and treatment of illness; (3) the identification of etiological and diagnostic correlates of health, illness, and related dysfunction; and (4) the analysis and improvement of the health care system and health policy formation. Division 38 (Health Psychology) of the American Psychological Association adopted the central elements of this definition in its mission statement and objectives.

A key distinction between the fields is that health psychology is inclusive of all areas of psychology, thus espousing a broader perspective on the contribution of psychological factors affecting health and illness. Importantly, Matarazzo's (1982) definition incorporates the professional contributions of psychology to the four areas mentioned earlier, highlighting the relevance of clinical services and patient care. The field of clinical health psychology emerged soon after formal recognition of health psychology, further substantiating the importance of the role of clinicians in areas such as chronic illness management, health promotion and diseases prevention, chronic pain, stress management, and the treatment of psychophysiological disorders (e.g., insomnia, tension headache, hypertension).

As clinicians became increasingly involved in health care settings, the American Psychological Association made it a priority to address the educational and training requirements for professionals providing service as clinical health psychologists. In 1983, the National Working Conference on Education and Training in Health Psychology, sponsored by the Division of Health Psychology, made three recommendations regarding the field that continue to shape professional activities and training today (Belar & Gesser, 1995; Stone, 1983). The first recommendation was an endorsement of the scientist-practitioner model of clinical training. The second recommendation was that clinical health psychologists should have core education and training in professional psychology, as well as additional training in areas such as the biological bases of health and disease, psychological and social factors in health and disease, health assessment and intervention, and interdisciplinary collaboration. The final recommendation was that clinical health psychologists should have supervised training in a health care setting by professional health psychology mentors at predoctoral and postdoctoral levels. These criteria set the stage for the development and implementation of curricula and training guidelines for PhD programs that would specifically train clinical health psychologists.

The emergence of clinical health psychology is an explicit confirmation of the relevance of clinical psychology to health care. The guidelines set forth by the National Training Conference also distinguish clinical health psychology from its parent field of clinical psychology. The requirement that clinical health psychologists must have core education and training in professional psychology, in addition to specialty knowledge and skills in health, reflects the unique demands and responsibilities of these clinicians compared to their counterparts who exclusively render "mental health" services. It also raises questions about the role of clinical psychologists who are not clinical health psychologists. An important question concerns the appropriateness and clinical advisability of rendering mental health services without taking into account the health circumstances of patients or the potential causal association between psychosocial factors and health outcomes. For example, can clinicians be effective in managing depression in patients with chronic pain without understanding how to conceptualize the influence of pain on mood? While professional psychologists may not agree on this issue, a health psychology perspective would promote the view that clinical effectiveness is likely to be compromised when such issues are not correctly addressed, and the psychological functioning of the patient is not framed in a broader, integrative context. The advent of health psychology has caused these issues to be relevant for all clinicians, not just those who have received specific training to do so (see Table 6.1). To a significant degree, the

TABLE 6.1. Comparison between Clinical Psychology and Clinical Health Psychology

Clinical psychology	Clinical health psychology
Theoretical foundations	
Social learning theory	Systems theory/eclectic
Psychodynamic theory	Social learning theory
Attachment theory	Community/public health
Treatment foci	
Psychological distress	Prevention of disease
Psychiatric disorders	Management of comorbidity
Enhance adaptive role functioning	Reduction of pain, stress
Reduction of risk/self-harm	Management of chronic illness
Populations	
Psychiatric outpatients	Chronically medically ill
Psychiatric inpatients	Patients at health risk
Families/couples	Chronic pain patients
Children/adolescents	Communities at health risk
Contemporary treatment approaches	
Psychotherapy	Cognitive-behavioral therapy
Group therapy	Meditation/mindfulness
Cognitive-behavioral therapy	Exercise
Stress management	Applied psychophysiology
Exposure therapy	Community behavioral strategies
Written expressive therapy	Written expressive therapy

separate existence of clinical psychology and clinical health psychology reflects an artificial distinction between mental and physical health that will experience continued erosion given the accumulation of future scientific evidence that the welfare of patients cannot be dichotomized in such a manner.

Perhaps the future will embrace a unitary model of training in which all clinicians have the knowledge and skills to render health care services to patients with health problems and to understand the increased health risk of patients with psychological disorders, maladaptive coping, or inadequate social supports. Short of such a significant paradigmatic change, all clinical psychologists may in the future be required to receive additional education and training in health, while clinical health psychologists will continue to be the experts. Such a change, it seems, would be in the interests of the profession and the public.

General Applicability of the Biopsychosocial Model

Health psychology since its inception has embraced the biopsychosocial model (Engel, 1980) as a way of understanding the association between psychosocial factors and health, and of managing patients in clinical settings. It is a foundational element of the field of health psychology. The biopsychosocial model is a conceptual framework that stresses the importance of considering the contribution of psychological, social, and cultural factors in conjunction with biological influences when analyzing the determinants of disease, symptoms, and treatments. Although it does not promote a particular theory, it fosters the view that the expression of health or illness depends on the way that various systems are organized within the individual (e.g., cellular, nervous), and between the individual and the broader social (e.g., family, cultural) environment (Nicassio & Smith, 1995). An important corollary is that human problems may have multiple etiologies, and their manifestations can vary markedly between individuals, depending on the systems factors (e.g., cultural, biological, psychological) involved.

In addition to these elements, the biopsychosocial model promotes the importance of interdisciplinary collaboration and problem solving with regard to human welfare. This perspective is necessary given the potential relevance of biological, social, psychological, and societal factors in explaining mental and physical health outcomes. Expertise from medicine, anthropology, and public policy may be required to address the prevention and treatment of complex human problems and disorders, and to develop creative approaches in the future. By espousing an integrated view of mental and physical health, the biopsychosocial model also leads to novel research questions that continue to have a far-reaching impact. For example, this framework has contributed to the examination of divergent questions such as the efficacy of behavioral treatment approaches for patients with chronic arthritis pain (e.g., Dixon, Keefe, Scipio, Perri, & Abernethy, 2007), analyses of the relationship between poverty and poor health outcomes (e.g., Kaler, 2008), and studies of the effects of depression on the immune system (Irwin & Miller, 2007). The implications of such findings have both theoretical and clinical significance, and simultaneously affect our interpretation of the complexity of human problems and the associations among related disciplines in studying them. Without question, the biopsychosocial model has been a major factor in the development and success of health psychology as a research and clinical discipline.

Because the biopsychosocial model does not make a distinction between mental and physical health problems, or between the types of systems factors that may contribute to either dimension of functioning, the argument can be made that it is as relevant to clinical psychology as it is to health psychology. Clinical psychology, however, has not openly promulgated this framework. Ironically, many clinical psychologists became clinical health psychologists to embrace this "new" model, without realizing its relevance to mental health and the tradition of clinical psychology. The adoption of the biopsychosocial model could unify clinical psychology and clinical health psychology under the same conceptual umbrella (see Table 6.2). In essence, the union of clinical psychology and clinical health psychology could emerge as a new professional discipline that promotes an integrated framework for understanding

TABLE 6.2. Elements of the Biopsychosocial Model Applicable to Both Clinical and Clinical Health Psychology

- Adoption of systems perspective for evaluation and treatment
- Synergistic, integrated relationship between mental and physical health
- Multiple factors affect mental and physical health outcomes
- Focus on individual differences in adjustment and patterns of causation
- Promotion of positive psychosocial functioning and quality of life
- Prevention of adverse mental and physical health outcomes
- Interdisciplinary collaboration
- Importance of ethnicity and culture in human welfare
- Importance of biological underpinnings of disease processes
- Adoption of empirically supported treatments

human functioning that is ambitious in its objectives, holistic in its approach, and comprehensive in scope. A unified framework would also clarify many issues related to education and training, and provide a new direction for the entire field of clinical psychology. Importantly, the biopsychosocial model would provide a more appropriate and necessary foundation for clinical psychologists to function as health service providers. This change is in keeping with the development and expansion of the field into new areas of inquiry. The following sections of this chapter further illustrate the relevance of examining the association between clinical psychology and health through an integrated conceptual framework.

Comorbidity between Psychological and Physical Dimensions of Health: The Case of Depression

The biopsychosocial model implies that physiological and psychological factors coexist, and systems can overlap and affect each other. Thus, disorders that are conceptualized as "psychological" may have consistent physiological correlates. For example, depressive disorders are associated with altered autonomic and endocrine function, and increased inflammatory processes. Similarly, disorders that are conceptualized as "physiological" can also have consistent psy-

chological correlates. For example, hypertension is associated with stress (e.g., Wirtz, Ehlert, Bartschi, Redwine, & von Kanel, 2009), and chronic pain is associated with depression (e.g., Angst, Verra, Lehmann, Aeschlimann, & Angst, 2008). For psychiatric disorders, the fourth edition of the *Diagnostic and Statistical Manual of Mental Disorders* (DSM-IV; American Psychiatric Association, 1994) formally acknowledges the relationship between psychological and physical dimensions of functioning through the diagnosis of "Psychological Factors Affecting Medical Condition," to be used in cases in which stress or depression, for example, may be causing social impairment in patients with chronic illness. Furthermore, the biopsychosocial model emphasizes the identification of psychological and physiological mediators and moderators of functioning. Health psychology research has been incredibly varied in its approach to analyzing such relationships. We use research on the relationship between depression and cardiovascular disease to illustrate the relevance of this approach to studying comorbidity.

Almost 1 in 3 deaths in the United States is due to cardiovascular disease (CVD). The American Heart Association estimates that over 80 million Americans have at least one form of CVD, including high blood pressure, stroke, heart failure, or coronary heart disease (including angina and myocardial infarction). Traditional risk factors include smoking status, serum cholesterol, and high blood pressure, which may play a causative role in CVD (Schneiderman, Antoni, Saab, & Ironson, 2001). In addition, there are a number of predisposing factors, such as obesity, sedentary lifestyle, and family history of CVD, that impact these causative factors. There is considerable evidence that psychopathology, expressed via chronic depressive symptoms and hostility, is associated with CVD. A recent meta-analysis demonstrated that in patients with coronary heart disease, clinically significant depressive symptoms are associated with a twofold increase in mortality (Barth, Schumacher, & Herrmann-Lingen, 2004).

Researchers have addressed the question of whether depression influences disease risk. It seems clear that depression can impact disease risk through multiple pathways, including smoking risk, obesity, and sedentary behavior (Whooley et al., 2008). Indeed, a core symptom of depression is behavioral inactivity. Thirty minutes of aerobic exercise three times per week leads to improvement in depressive symptoms that rival pharmacotherapy (Babyak et al., 2000).

Through the perspective of the biopsychosocial model, depression emerges as a multiaxial disorder, with core symptoms that include not only disturbances in affect but also prominent dysregulation of physiological parameters. Core symptoms of depression include poor energy, fatigue, behavioral inactivity, and poor sleep. Major depression is associated with increased low-grade inflammation, cortisol dysfunction, and heightened sympathetic nervous system activity.

Atherosclerotic plaque development requires active involvement of the immune system, which primes and directs immune cells to the plaque. Immune cells communicate via a complex panoply of "cytokines," signaling molecules that stimulate or inhibit inflammation, as well as coordinate the body's response to infectious challenge (Libby, 2002). Proinflammatory cytokines such as interleukin-6 (IL-6) stimulate a cascade of effects, including production of acute phase proteins (including C-reactive protein, or CRP) by the liver. Inflammatory cytokines stimulate inflammation and host defense against infection by modulating vascular permeability (associated with swelling in damaged areas), recruiting immune cells to the sites of damage or infection, and activating immune cells to clear damaged cells or attack pathogens. Unfortunately, chronic elevations of these inflammatory cytokines in circulation reflect a poorly working system. Higher levels of these cytokines, such as IL-6, in healthy adults confer a higher risk of development of CVD (Ridker, Rifai, Stampfer, & Hennekens, 2000).

Depressed patients with CVD have higher IL-6 and CRP than nondepressed patients with CVD (Lespérance, Frasure-Smith, Theroux, & Irwin, 2004). Furthermore, even depressed patients without CVD have higher levels of IL-6 (Motivala, Sarfatti, Olmos, & Irwin, 2005). A number of factors may drive inflammatory processes in depression, including poor sleep, increased sympathetic nervous system activity, and hypercortisolemia. Poor sleep, common in as many as 90% of depressed patients, also likely plays

a role in explaining the association between major depression and CVD. In patients with major depression, sleep-onset time is positively correlated with IL-6 and is a better predictor of elevated IL-6 than depressive status (Motivala et al., 2005). If sleep loss is related to patients' increased low-grade inflammatory processes, then one would expect experimental sleep deprivation studies to reveal increases in inflammation. Irwin, Wang, Campomayor, Collado-Hidalgo, and Cole (2006) found that just one night of partial sleep deprivation could produce increased gene expression of inflammatory markers. These findings are corroborated in other sleep-disordered populations as well. Insomnia patients without clinically significant depressive symptoms also have elevated levels of IL-6 (Burgos et al., 2005; Vgontzas et al., 2002).

Although sleep difficulties may promote elevations in inflammatory indicators, these same cytokines appear to exert effects on the central nervous system as well. In animal and human studies, administration of inflammatory cytokines such as IL-6, interleukin-1 (IL-1), and tumor necrosis factor-alpha (TNFa) affect sleep (for reviews on these topics, see Motivala & Irwin, 2007; Opp, 2005). These effects may be part of a broader system of interaction where cells of the immune system communicate with the central nervous system (CNS) via cytokine–autonomic mechanisms (Tracey, 2002). Peripheral inflammatory cytokines can trigger a pattern of CNS-mediated behaviors that include sleep and appetite changes, behavioral inactivity, and social withdrawal. These behaviors taken together are called "sickness behaviors" (Dantzer, O'Connor, Freund, Johnson, & Kelley, 2008). In response to infection, these behaviors are highly adaptive; however, dysregulation of this cytokine–CNS system can lead to chronic behavioral changes mimicking depressive symptoms, including fatigue, poor sleep, and depressed affect (Raison et al., 2009). This dysregulation could explain why levels of inflammatory markers are elevated in depressed patients. In patients with cancer and hepatitis C who undergo treatment via infusion of inflammatory cytokines, a consistent pattern of sickness behaviors is elicited (Musselman et al., 2001). Like depressed patients, chronically stressed adults also show progressive increases in levels of inflammatory cytokines (Glaser & Kiecolt-Glaser, 2005), and a recent meta-analysis indicates that short-term psychological stress can also up-regulate levels of inflammatory cytokines (Steptoe, Hamer, & Chida, 2007). Taken together, these findings highlight how psychological processes such as stress and poor sleep impact peripheral cytokines, which in turn affect behavioral outcomes, including depressive symptoms.

Depression also may be associated with a shift in autonomic balance toward sympathetic overactivity and impaired vagal control (Carney, Freedland, & Veith, 2005). High sympathetic activity drives a positive feedback loop promoting high blood pressure, insulin resistance, hyperinsulinemia, and low-grade inflammation. Why depressed patients develop elevated sympathetic nervous system (SNS) activity is unclear. But the allostatic model (McEwen, 1998) suggests that these physiological pathways are activated in host responses to environmental challenges (i.e., stressors). Frequent and intense responses to environmental demands in highly stress-responsive individuals eventually overtax these systems, promoting increased SNS activity at rest. Gradual progressive increases in SNS activity are a normal part of aging, possibly as a method to regulate thermogenesis (Seals & Esler 2000); however, it seems that this increase accelerates in vulnerable populations, such as those with major depression or chronic insomnia (see Figure 6.1).

The links between depression and CVD clearly involve behavioral and physiological pathways. A broader conception of depression via the biopsychosocial approach will expand the possibilities in terms of conceptualization, progression of the disorder, and antecedents, as well as opening up novel treatment possibilities. Aerobic exercise may be an effective strategy for treating depressive symptoms. Although the mechanisms are unclear (Blumenthal et al., 1999), there is some evidence that autonomic function improves with exercise and is measured by increased heart rate variability (Blumenthal et al., 2005). Increased physical activity and fitness and improved autonomic function would also confer benefits for CVD as well. Novel pharmacological approaches may also be effective. Patients with CVD and depres-

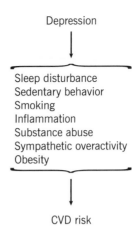

FIGURE 6.1. Potential mediational pathways between depression and cardiovascular disease risk.

sion have elevated markers of inflammation, but not if they are taking statin medications (Lespérance et al., 2004). Statin medications may be effective in CVD because of their effects not only on cholesterol but also inflammatory markers (Koh, 2000). There is also some evidence that statin use is associated with fewer depressive symptoms (Yang, Jick, & Jick, 2003; Young-Xu, Chan, Liao, Ravid, & Blatt, 2003). These findings suggest a possible pathway in which statins reduce inflammation, which could in turn reduce depressive symptoms. The studies described here highlight the connection between psychological and physiological systems, and suggest that compartmentalizing mental health separately from physical health is at best overly simplified, and at worst is misleading in regard to assessment, conceptualization, and treatment.

The Interface of Clinical and Health Psychology in Assessment and Screening

The relationship between depression and health outcomes illustrates the need to detect mood disturbance and psychological distress in patients seen in health care settings. Thus, an important area of interface between clinical and health psychology concerns assessment and screening of patients. Within the clinical context, screening is important to determine whether patients would be best served by a health psychology intervention designed primarily to improve health status and reduce pain, disability, and disease-related symptoms, or by a clinical psychology intervention designed to improve mental and social functioning, and reduce negative thoughts and mood or inappropriate behaviors. In practice, many health psychology interventions improve mood and cognitions as well, but these outcomes are often secondary to the physical health and functional outcomes. Within a research context, health psychology researchers frequently need to screen potential participants for serious mental disorders that may confound mood and functional status outcomes. Furthermore, they may want to characterize the mental health of a population or assess mental disorders as a possible covariate or change in mental health diagnoses as a clinical outcome. These issues are discussed in more detail below.

Abundant evidence demonstrates a high degree of comorbidity between chronic medical conditions and psychiatric disorders (e.g., Berardi et al., 1999; Wells et al., 1988). Often, the mental disorder is secondary to a chronic disease or syndrome. For example, facing the possibility of dying or enduring negative treatment side effects, physical disfigurement, or financial burden may lead to increased anxiety and depression that, for a subset of patients, meet criteria for diagnosis of a mental disorder. In many instances, these illness-related stressors may cause significant emotional symptoms that do not reach the threshold of a mental disorder. Other types of mental disorders, such as bipolar disorder or schizophrenia, have a stronger genetic component and are less likely to be secondary to a physical health condition, although their existence may complicate disease course or threaten patient compliance with health regimens. In other cases, the mental disorder may be primary. Patients with untreated depression may attempt to regulate their negative moods by engaging in behaviors (e.g., smoking or drug use) that increase vulnerability for physical diseases such as lung cancer or hepatitis. Finally, certain types of life events, such as childhood abuse or severe trauma, may increase vulnerability for a variety of diseases, psychiatric disorders, and negative health outcomes, ranging from posttraumatic stress disorder (PTSD),

depression, and substance abuse to chronic pain syndromes and heart disease (Taylor, Repetti, & Seeman, 1997).

Because of this comorbidity, health psychologists in both clinical and research settings should acquire knowledge about diagnostic systems, screening tools, and treatments to address mental health problems and diagnoses. Within the context of an integrated health care system, individuals may be referred by their physicians to the behavioral medicine service for specialized health psychology interventions, such as pain management, smoking cessation, stress management, or health promotion treatments, that complement traditional medical care. The intake coordinator typically conducts an assessment to determine whether the patient is appropriate for a health psychology/behavioral medicine intervention. Patients who have serious untreated mental disorders, such as major depression, bipolar disorder, PTSD, substance abuse/dependence, or a psychotic disorder, may be referred to behavioral medicine for stress management when they would be treated more appropriately by psychiatry for medication management, or by the psychology service for cognitive-behavioral or other clinical interventions. Individuals with substance abuse or dependence disorders likewise require specialized intervention to address these issues before they are considered suitable for behavioral medicine intervention.

Because certain types of acute mental disorders and personality disorders carry high risk for immediate negative consequences, such as suicide attempts, drug overdose, or behavior that is dangerous to self or others, treatment of these conditions is often considered a higher priority than health psychology interventions that address conditions, such as smoking or lack of exercise, whose risks are more long term. Basic stress management and coping techniques may be helpful but not sufficient to treat serious mood or thought disorders. Additionally, the existence of a serious comorbid mental disorder may compromise a patients' ability to understand and participate constructively in a health psychology intervention and may negatively affect motivation and compliance. On the other hand, it may be possible to conduct mental and behavioral health interventions simultaneously, such as smoking cessation, pain management, or exercise groups for individuals in treatment for substance abuse issues. In these cases, the health interventions may actually enhance the clinical intervention by providing alternative ways to handle stress or avoid triggers.

Within primary care, rates of depression are substantial. One study of nearly 2,000 primary care patients found that 13.5% had major depression and 22.6% had any type of depressive disorder (Coyne, Fechner-Bates, & Schwenk, 1994). Research also reports high prevalence (19.5%) in primary care of the four most common anxiety disorders (generalized anxiety disorder, panic disorder, social anxiety disorder, and PTSD) (Kroenke, Spitzer, Williams, Monahan, & Löwe, 2007). Anxiety and depressive disorders have been linked to a variety of negative physical health outcomes, including more somatic symptoms, functional impairment, and increased medical utilization and health care cost (Katon et al., 1990; Kroenke et al., 2007; Wells et al., 1988). Whereas detection and treatment of depression in primary care have improved in recent years, detection and management of anxiety disorders are less than optimal. A recent study found that more than 40% of primary care patients with an anxiety disorder were not receiving any concurrent mental health treatment (Kroenke et al., 2007).

Primary care practitioners treat the majority of patients with major depression, with prescription of antidepressants being the most common approach. However, despite this prevalence, the most recent American Preventive Services Task Force clinical guidelines (Pignone, Gaynes, Mulrow, Orleans, & Lohr, 2002) do not advocate routine screening for depression in primary care. Screening may not directly improve clinical outcomes unless resources are available and procedures are in place for accurately diagnosing, treating or referring, and following up patients so identified. Because depression can substantially elevate the risk for heart disease and mortality (Ferketich, Schwartzbaum, Frid, & Moeschberger, 2000), routine screening for depression is becoming a standard of care in cardiology practice and has been recommended in the latest American Heart Association clinical guidelines (Lichtman et al., 2008). However, barriers to treatment of depression exist at the level of patient, health provider, and health care system that make it difficult for depressed patients to receive effective treatment (Nicassio, 2008).

In addition, patients commonly present with anxiety in medical settings and create challenges in clinical management. For example, panic attack symptoms may mimic heart attack symptoms, leading to unnecessary emergency room or cardiologist visits, and the need for psychiatric and medical screening for differential diagnosis. At other times, anxious patients may somatize their distress and lack awareness of the nature of their psychological state and how it is affecting them. Such patients are typically very difficult to manage because they do not have medical conditions and also refuse to accept that psychological factors could be causing their symptoms. Early identification of anxious patients who present in this manner is critical to effective long-term management and the prevention of disability and excessive seeking of health care.

In a research context, a health psychologist wanting to study a particular disease group to determine predictors of health outcomes, or to assess effects of an intervention will consider it appropriate to screen for, and exclude, participants with serious mental disorders. A patient with psychosis or bipolar disorder and a comorbid disease diagnosis is generally considered to belong to a different population than other patients with the same disease because these disorders require long-term maintenance on powerful medications and are associated with more severe impairment in cognitive, affective, and behavioral functioning. Even less severe comorbid mental health conditions, such as unipolar depression, anxiety, or substance abuse disorders, can seriously impair functional status and confound the effects of health intervention on functional outcomes. The issue is complicated because depression and anxiety are often assessed as predictors, criterion variables, or clinical outcomes in studies of medical populations. Excluding all patients with a lifetime history of major depression may lead to low base rates of depressed mood, which makes it more difficult to show effects of intervention on this outcome or to reduce within-group variability and attenuate correlations between depressed mood and disease-related variables.

A middle ground taken by many researchers studying medical populations is to exclude patients with current, active, untreated mental disorders and those with thought disorder but include individuals whose mental disorders are in remission or successfully controlled by medication.

A related issue is the use of psychotropic drugs. A substantial proportion of medical patients take antidepressants, antianxiety drugs, or sedative–hypnotic drugs to treat subclinical or clinical symptoms of comorbid mental disorders (Pincus et al., 1998). Therefore, health researchers should assess use and change in psychotropic medication as a potential confound. Participants with unstable use should be excluded or held for a month or two, until use is stable.

Since the risk for chronic diseases increases with age, health psychologists may often research or treat elderly populations at higher risk for dementia and Alzheimer's disease. Individuals with these conditions may also need to be excluded from health psychology research studies not specifically designed to address comorbidity, due to the same confounding of health status described earlier. Furthermore, these conditions interfere with patients' reporting accuracy on self-report measures of clinical status. Within a clinical context, dementia presents unique disease management challenges and requires specialized assessments to determine neuropsychological status and functional ability. Often social workers need to become involved as well to help determine the optimal level of care and living arrangements needed for this patient, and to support families in finding appropriate resources.

This section addressed the *why* of clinical screening and assessment for mental health disorders by health psychologists. In the next section we discuss *how* to screen for these disorders.

Clinical Assessment and Screening Instruments

The "gold standard" in screening instruments for mental disorders is standardized diagnostic interviews based on DSM-IV (American Psychiatric Association, 1994). In addition to screening for exclusionary conditions, these interviews may characterize the diagnostic status of a particular sample or assess psychiatric diagnosis as a potential covariate or change in clinical status associated with intervention. These measures have the strengths and weaknesses of the DSM diagnostic system. They are based on expert consensus, extensive validity data, and a descriptive system that characterizes symptoms but does not infer underlying causality. On the other hand, it has been suggested that psychopathology may be more dimensional than categorical in nature, and that substantial differences may exist between individuals within a particular diagnostic category. Furthermore, these measures may become outdated as new diagnostic systems and methodologies are developed.

A widely used, validated, and comprehensive diagnostic interview measure that is suitable for research use is the Structured Clinical Interview for DSM-IV Axis I Disorders (SCID-I; First, Spitzer, Gibbon, & Williams, 2002), which comprises 10 modules based on DSM-IV-TR Axis I diagnostic categories. Separate versions of the SCID are available for clinical and research use and for patients and nonpatients, and a version is available for assessing Axis II (personality) disorders (SCID-II; First, Gibbon, Spitzer, Williams, & Benjamin, 1997). The different modules stand alone, allowing researchers to customize the measure for their needs. Its developers designed the SCID to be administered by mental health professionals familiar with clinical diagnostic criteria. In some cases, research assistants without such specialized mental health qualifications may appropriately administer the SCID following more extensive training by a clinically trained professional. Use of these measures typically requires collaboration with a clinical psychologist or psychiatrist. For research purposes, interrater reliability should be established and, ideally, raters should be blind to study hypotheses.

Like its counterpart, the National Institute of Mental Health Diagnostic Interview Schedule, Version IV (DIS-IV; Robins, Cottler, Bucholz, & Compton, 1995) is a fully structured interview, designed to assess for presence or absence of DSM-IV psychiatric disorders. The DIS-IV mimics the format of a clinical interview, and questions determine whether specific symptoms are present that cannot be attributed to a medical condition or substance use. The major difference between the DIS-IV and SCID is that the DIS-IV was designed to be administered by a trained nonclinician. In a clinical context, DIS-IV diagnoses should be supplemented by professional clinical judgment, or the DIS-IV can be used in a medical setting to screen for referral to a mental health professional for further evaluation.

One issue with the aforementioned diagnostic interviews is that the DSM diagnostic system was developed within a North American cultural context and validated on U.S. samples, limiting its cross-cultural applicability. A more recent measure, the Composite International Diagnostic Interview (CIDI; Kessler & Ustun, 2004), based on the 10th edition of the World Health Organization's *International Classification of Diseases* (ICD-10; 1993), as well as the DSM-IV, is therefore more suitable for use with individuals from diverse cultural backgrounds and nationalities.

Interview measures are generally considered the "gold standard"; however, they are more expensive and time-consuming to administer than self-report measures. For situations in which time and resources are limited, such as a primary care setting, it may be sufficient to administer validated self-report questionnaires to screen for psychological distress or negative moods of sufficient magnitude to necessitate medical intervention or referral to a clinical psychologist or clinical health psychologist. Widely used mood or distress questionnaires typically have cutoffs for clinically significant symptom levels that have been validated against objective interview measures. While not sufficient to establish clinical diagnoses, these questionnaires are also useful in research to characterize a sample or assess change in symptoms over time in relation to data from normative samples and standardized criteria for clinically significant symptom elevations.

Some validated self-reported distress questionnaires that are widely used for screening in medical clinical and research settings include the General Health Questionnaire (GHQ; Goldberg, 1978), the Hospital Anxiety and Depression Scale (HADS; Zigmond & Snaith, 1983), the Center for Epidemiologic Studies Depression Scale (CES-D; Radloff, 1977), the Beck Depression Inventory–II (BDI-II; Beck, Steer, & Brown, 1996), and the Beck Anxiety Inventory (BAI; Beck &

Steer, 1990). One difference among these questionnaires concerns validation samples, which consisted of medical outpatients for the first two measures, community residents for the third, and psychiatric outpatients for the last two. Additionally, whereas some questionnaires have a single cutoff for clinically significant distress (CES-D), others have cutoffs for mild, moderate, and severe symptomatology (BDI-II). Somatic symptoms of depression, such as fatigue or sleep disturbance, overlap with sequelae of chronic pain; therefore, higher cutoffs for clinically significant symptoms have been recommended for chronic pain and other medical samples (e.g., Geisser, Roth, & Robinson, 1997).

In settings such as primary care, where time is limited, or in research settings, where assessment of clinical symptoms is not the primary focus, a brief screening instrument may suffice. One example is the Beck Depression Inventory—Fast Screen (BDI-FS; Beck, Steer, & Brown, 2000), a seven-item inventory for medical patients, specifically designed to assesses the cognitive and affective criteria for depression specified in DSM-IV, but omitting somatic criteria that may be confounded with medical problems. The measure has adequate-to-good sensitivity and specificity in diagnosing depression using a cutoff of 4. The BDI-FS can be used with adolescents, adults, and geriatric patients, and has recently been validated for use with multiple sclerosis patients, a disease for which depression prevalence is very high.

Another validated instrument that can be used to screen for depression and assess its severity is the nine-item Patient Health Questionnaire (PHQ-9; Kroenke, Spitzer, & Williams, 2001), which is based on DSM-IV diagnostic criteria and has been validated in primary care and gynecology practice. An alternative, very brief depression screener, the PHQ-2 (Kroenke, Spitzer, & Williams, 2003), comprises the first two items of the PHQ-9, which assess for depressed mood and anhedonia. Although sufficiently sensitive to the presence of depression, briefer measures tend to have poor specificity and high rates of false positives. These instruments may still be appropriate if the goal is to identify patients for referral to a clinician for further diagnosis and evaluation, but they are not appropriate as diagnostic tools. Until recently, the variety of anxiety disorders present in primary care made screening a formidable challenge. However, a new screening scale, the Generalized Anxiety Disorder–7 (GAD-7; Spitzer, Kroenke, Williams, & Löwe, 2006) and its two core items (GAD-2; Kroenke et al., 2007) have demonstrated appropriate psychometric criteria for detection of the four most prevalent anxiety disorders (Kroenke et al., 2007).

Clinical Interventions

The overlap of clinical psychology and health psychology is also apparent in the sphere of intervention. While based on a systems perspective, most health psychology interventions are derived from behavioral or cognitive-behavioral theories of behavior change that have their origins in early animal studies of learning and were initially used in clinical treatment of human fears, phobias, or depressive disorders. The concept of self-efficacy (Bandura, 1977), frequently used in health psychology interventions as a pathway to symptom control or behavior change, had its origins in Bandura's early studies of snake phobics. Acceptance and commitment therapy (Hayes, Strosahl, & Wilson, 2003), now widely used with pain patients, developed out of a behavioral theory that focused on the acquisition of reinforcing properties of thought and language, and on a therapy initially used to treat patients with substance abuse.

Health psychology interventions are not entirely based on behavioral or cognitive-behavioral clinical theories, however. Mindfulness meditation interventions (Kabat-Zinn, 1982), which are now frequently integrated into cognitive-behavioral treatments, were based on principles of calming the mind, derived from ancient Indian and Buddhist philosophies. Expressive writing interventions (e.g., Pennebaker & Beall, 1986; Smyth, Stone, Hurewitz, & Kaell, 1999) that have shown efficacy in enhancing health status in rheumatoid arthritis, cancer, and hypertension are based on Breuer and Freud's (1895/1957) early theories related to hysteria, emotional repression, and the talking cure, as well as cognitive processing concepts derived from cognitive and psychodynamic theories of trauma. Health psychology theorists have also added unique theoretical elements, such as the stages of change model (Prochaska & DiClemente, 1983), which suggests that interventions need to be tailored to the patient's level of readiness for behavior change. Biofeedback interventions based on psychophysiological theories suggest that patients can learn to change their physiological behaviors (e.g., muscle tension, blood pressure) to improve mood and reduce stress-related symptoms.

While health and clinical psychology interventions are often based on similar theories of cognition and behavior change, they often differ in intervention targets. Although cognitive-behavioral treatments for both anxiety (e.g., Borkovec & Costello, 1993) and chronic pain (e.g., Turk, Meichenbaum, & Genest, 1987) target catastrophic thoughts and expectations, and encourage exposure to feared situations, the nature of the fears and the triggering situations differ. For example, a patient with social anxiety might fear public humiliation in social settings, whereas the pain patient's fears generally focus on the never-ending nature, anhedonic quality, intensity, disability, and subjective suffering associated with pain. At times, the distinction can become somewhat blurred. Although the specific feared symptoms differ, both patients with chronic pain and those with panic disorder fear bodily symptoms and avoid situations where such symptoms might be exacerbated, leading to disability and impaired quality of life.

Because both chronic illness and clinical depression interfere with social and occupational functioning, there are, of necessity, many similarities between treatment foci and targets for these disorders. For example, behavioral treatments for depression teach patients to identify and schedule pleasant events, even if they do not feel like doing them. Similarly, a focus in behavioral treatment of chronic illness is to function and to carry out one's regular daily activities despite the symptoms and catastrophic cognitions, while structuring breaks or reducing extraneous commitments. In both types of therapies, reinforcement, reassurance, and encouragement from the therapist initially motivate patients' behavior changes, which, once initiated, are reinforced by their natural environmental consequences.

In summary, clinical psychology and health psychology share important similarities in underlying theories, as well as research and practice applications. Knowledge of diagnostic criteria, screening instruments, theories, and interventions of clinical psychology can help health psychologists to develop more effective interventions and research designs, and to facilitate more seamless integration of behavioral medicine within the overall health care system. The adoption of the biopsychosocial model as a unifying paradigm for both clinical and health psychology has the potential to strengthen the influence of both disciplines within medicine and to promote better health outcomes in diverse patient groups. It is important for researchers and clinicians to recognize the complementarity and synergy of these disciplines to frame meaningful scientific questions, and to develop creative and innovative approaches to treatment and management.

Evidence-Based Treatments and Practices

As empirical disciplines, clinical psychology and health psychology have historically embraced the importance of integrating scientifically validated diagnostic and treatment approaches into clinical practice settings. The contribution of science to practice has grown as empirical knowledge from clinical trials has highlighted the efficacy of specific therapeutic approaches. The promotion of science in clinical care reflects not only the need to provide to patients quality service that meets objective standards but also a growing demand for accountability in our health care system. The public health and policy implications of this view are profound inasmuch as professional organizations may foster the establishment of standards of care that delineate the importance of adopting certain treatment approaches for specific disorders or health conditions (Institute of Medicine, 2001; Sackett, Straus, Richardson, Rosenberg, & Haynes, 2000).

Both clinical psychologists and health psychologists face the challenge of providing scientifically supported treatments to their patients. In this regard, Kazdin (2008) has noted a distinction between "evidence-based treatment" (EBT) and "evidence-based practice" (EBP). Whereas EBT involves the application of interventions that have demonstrated efficacy in randomized controlled

trials, EBP is a broader term, referring to the type of clinical practice that integrates effective interventions, professional expertise, and patient needs and values into decision making about individual patient care. The latter term recognizes the complexity of clinical practice by acknowledging the importance of professional competence and individual differences in patients (e.g., culture, age, gender) in case formulation and management (Collins, Leffingwell, & Belar, 2007; Sackett et al., 2000). Importantly, EBP also addresses concerns raised by professional psychologists that effective clinical care involves managing a process rather than simply implementing an EBT in a rote, linear fashion for a particular problem. EBP is compatible with the spirit of the biopsychosocial model, in that it emphasizes the importance of recognizing individual differences in patients in delivering effective treatments. For example, while there is an established literature supporting the efficacy of cognitive-behavioral therapy for chronic arthritis pain (e.g., Dixon et al., 2007), considerable professional expertise is required to tailor such treatment to patients from different socioeconomic backgrounds and with divergent psychiatric histories. Since empirical guidelines and clinical algorithms often are unavailable to help clinicians address such issues systematically, psychologists must rely on their professional competence and experience in making sound clinical decisions. While the role of professional expertise will always be a critical element in clinical practice, the time has arrived for research to focus greater attention on the process of individualizing care using an EBP approach. A closer collaboration between clinical scientists and professional psychologists would contribute to the development of this agenda.

Conclusions

Clinical psychology and health psychology should face the challenge of disseminating EBTs to clinical sites and to patient populations in need of help. From a public health perspective, it is desirable to render effective treatments to as many patients as possible who may potentially benefit from them. While health psychology has made substantial progress in this area by emphasizing health promotion and integrating effective behavioral treatments into medical settings and a variety of specialty clinics (e.g., pain, cancer, diabetes), there is an equal, if not more, compelling need for clinical psychology to develop better mechanisms for delivering EBTs to patients with psychiatric disorders. Disorders such as depression, anxiety, and substance abuse are very common in the general population, and are particularly prevalent in populations that face barriers in accessing care or are underserved for cultural or socioeconomic reasons. An important question facing clinical psychology is whether, as a discipline, it will promote a public health framework that allows such broader questions to be addressed more meaningfully and eventually answered.

To a significant degree, health psychology has advocated the importance of public health approaches through its association with allied health and medicine, and by emphasizing interdisciplinary models and research methodologies. However, as a more insular discipline, clinical psychology has focused primarily on the delivery of services to individual patients. Notwithstanding the benefits that have resulted from this approach, clinical psychology has historically has found itself several steps removed from the public health arena. Importantly, the time has come for change. Clinical psychology's evolution as a health care discipline and a closer working alliance with health psychology may lead to a more thorough appreciation of the importance of this goal and the mechanisms needed to achieve it. This evolution could lead to greater visibility for the profession and enhanced clinical care for a broader range of patient populations.

Further Reading

Belar, C. D., & Gesser, M. D. (1995). Roles of the clinical health psychologists in the management of chronic illness. In P. M. Nicassio & T. W. Smith (Eds.), *Managing chronic illness: A biopsychosocial approach* (pp. 33–57). Washington, DC: American Psychological Association.

Belar, C. D., Nelson, P. D., & Wasik, B. H. (2003). Rethinking education in psychology and psychology in education: The inaugural education leadership conference. *American Psychologist, 58*, 678–684.

Benjamin, L. T. (2005). A history of clinical psychology as a profession in America (and a glimpse at its future). *Annual Review of Clinical Psychology, 1*, 1–30.

Dixon, K. E., Keefe, F. J., Scipio, C. D., Perri, L. M., & Abernethy, A. P. (2007). Psychological interventions for arthritis pain management in adults: A meta-analysis. *Health Psychology, 26*, 241–250.

Ferketich, A. K., Schwartzbaum, J. A., Frid, D. J., & Moeschberger, M. L. (2000). Depression as an antecedent to heart disease among women and men in the NHANES I Study. *Archives of Internal Medicine, 160*, 1261–1268.

Kazdin, A. E. (2008). Evidence-based treatment and practice: New opportunities to bridge clinical research and practice, enhance the knowledge base, and improve patient care. *American Psychologist, 63*, 146–159.

Nicassio, P. M. (2008). The problem of detecting and managing depression in the rheumatology clinic. *Arthritis and Rheumatism, 59*, 155–158.

Nicassio, P. M., & Smith, T. W. (1995). *Managing chronic illness: A biopsychosocial approach*. Washington, DC: American Psychological Association.

References

American Psychiatric Association. (1994). *Diagnostic and statistical manual of mental disorders* (4th ed.). Washington, DC: Author.

Angst, F., Verra, M. L., Lehmann, S., Aeschlimann, A., & Angst, J. (2008). Refined insights into the pain–depression association in chronic pain patients. *Clinical Journal of Pain, 24*, 808–816.

Babyak, M., Blumenthal, J. A., Herman, S., Khatri, P., Doraiswamy, M., Moore, K., et al. (2000). Exercise treatment for major depression: Maintenance of therapeutic benefit at 10 months. *Psychosomatic Medicine, 62*, 633–638.

Bandura, A. (1977). Self-efficacy: Toward a unifying theory of behavioral change. *Psychological Review, 84*, 191–215.

Barth, J., Schumacher, M., & Herrmann-Lingen, C. (2004). Depression as a risk factor for mortality in patients with coronary heart disease: A meta-analysis. *Psychosomatic Medicine, 66*, 802–813.

Beck, A. T., & Steer, R. A. (1990). *Manual for the Beck Anxiety Inventory*. San Antonio, TX: Psychological Corporation.

Beck, A. T., Steer, R. A., & Brown, G. K. (1996). *Manual for the Beck Depression Inventory-II*. San Antonio, TX: Psychological Corporation.

Beck, A. T., Steer, R. A., & Brown, G. K. (2000).

BDI: Fast Screen for medical patients. San Antonio, TX: Psychological Corporation.

Belar, C. D. (2000). Scientist-practitioner does not equal science + practice: Boulder is bolder. *American Psychologist, 55,* 249–250.

Belar, C. D., & Gesser, M. D. (1995). Roles of the clinical health psychologists in the management of chronic illness. In P. M. Nicassio & T. W. Smith (Eds.), *Managing chronic illness: A biopsychosocial approach* (pp. 33–57). Washington, DC: American Psychological Association.

Belar, C. D., Nelson, P. D., & Wasik, B. H. (2003). Rethinking education in psychology and psychology in education: The inaugural education leadership conference. *American Psychologist, 58,* 678–684.

Benjamin, L. T. (2005). A history of clinical psychology as a profession in America (and a glimpse at its future). *Annual Review of Clinical Psychology, 1,* 1–30.

Berardi, D., Cerroni, G. B., Leggieri, G., Rucci, P., Ustun, B., & Ferrari, G. (1999). Mental, physical and functional status in primary care attenders. *International Journal of Psychiatry in Medicine, 29,* 133–148.

Blumenthal, J. A., Babyak, M. A., Moore, K. A., Craighead, W. E., Herman, S., Khatri, P., et al. (1999). Effects of exercise training on older patients with major depression. *Archives of Internal Medicine, 159,* 2349–2356.

Blumenthal, J. A., Sherwood, A., Babyak, M. A., Watkins, L. L., Waugh, R., Georgiades, A., et al. (2005). Effects of exercise and stress management training on markers of cardiovascular risk in patients with ischemic heart disease: A randomized controlled trial. *Journal of the American Medical Association, 293,* 1626–1634.

Borkovec, T. D., & Costello, E. (1993). Efficacy of applied relaxation and cognitive-behavioral therapy in the treatment of generalized anxiety disorder. *Journal of Consulting and Clinical Psychology, 61,* 611–619.

Breuer, J., & Freud, S. (1957). *Studies on hysteria.* New York: Basic Books. (Original work published 1895)

Burgos, I., Richter, L., Klein, T., Fiebich, B., Feige, B., Lieb, K., et al. (2005). Increased nocturnal interleukin-6 excretion in patients with primary insomnia: A pilot study. *Brain, Behavior, and Immunity, 20,* 246–253.

Carney, R. M., Freedland, K. E., & Veith, R. C. (2005). Depression, the autonomic nervous system, and coronary heart disease. *Psychosomatic Medicine, 67*(Suppl. 1), S29–S33.

Collins, F. L., Leffingwell, T. R., & Belar, C.D. (2007). Teaching evidence-based practice: Implications for psychology. *Journal of Clinical Psychology, 63,* 657–670.

Commission for Recognition of Specialties and Proficiencies. (2004). *Archival description of clinical psychology.* Retrieved April 5, 2010, from *www.apa.org/crsppp/clipsych.html.*

Coyne, J. C., Fechner-Bates, S., & Schwenk, T. L. (1994). Prevalence, nature, and comorbidity of depressive disorders in primary care. *General Hospital Psychiatry, 16,* 267–276.

Dantzer, R., O'Connor, J. C., Freund, G. G., Johnson, R. W., & Kelley, K. W. (2008). From inflammation to sickness and depression: When the immune system subjugates the brain. *National Review of Neuroscience, 9,* 46–56.

Dixon, K. E., Keefe, F. J., Scipio, C. D., Perri, L. M., & Abernethy, A. P. (2007). Psychological interventions for arthritis pain management in adults: A meta-analysis. *Health Psychology, 26,* 241–250.

Engel, G. L. (1980). The clinical application of the biopsychosocial model. *American Journal of Psychiatry, 137,* 535–544.

Ferketich, A. K., Schwartzbaum, J. A., Frid, D. J., & Moeschberger, M. L. (2000). Depression as an antecedent to heart disease among women and men in the NHANES I Study. *Archives of Internal Medicine, 160,* 1261–1268.

First, M. B., Gibbon, M., Spitzer, R. L., Williams, J. B. W., & Benjamin, L. S. (1997). *Structured Clinical Interview for DSM-IV Axis II Personality Disorders (SCID-II).* Washington, DC: American Psychiatric Press.

First, M. B., Spitzer, R. L., Gibbon, M., & Williams, J. B. W. (2002). *Structured Clinical Interview for DSM-IV-TR Axis I Disorders, Research Version, Patient Edition (SCID-I/P).* New York: Biometrics Research, New York State Psychiatric Institute.

Geisser, M. E., Roth, R. S., & Robinson, M. E. (1997). Assessing depression among persons with chronic pain using the Center for Epidemiologic Studies—Depression Scale and the Beck Depression Inventory: A comparative analysis. *Clinical Journal of Pain, 13,* 163–170.

Glaser, R., & Kiecolt-Glaser, J. K. (2005). Stress-induced immune dysfunction: Implications for health. *National Review of Immunology, 5,* 243–251.

Goldberg, D. P. (1978). *Manual of the General Health Questionnaire.* Slough, UK: National Foundation for Educational Research.

Hayes, S. C., Strosahl, K. D., & Wilson, K. G. (2003). *Acceptance and commitment therapy: An experiential approach to behavior change.* New York: Guilford Press.

Institute of Medicine. (2001). *Crossing the quality chasm: A new health system for the 21st century.* Washington, DC: National Academy Press.

Irwin, M. R., & Miller, A. H. (2007). Depressive disorders and immunity: 20 years of discovery. *Brain, Behavior, and Immunity, 21,* 374–383.

Irwin, M. R., Wang, M., Campomayor, C. O., Collado-Hidalgo, A., & Cole, S. (2006). Sleep deprivation and activation of morning levels of cellular and genomic markers of inflammation. *Archives of Internal Medicine, 166,* 1756–1762.

Kabat-Zinn, J. (1982). An outpatient program in behavioral medicine for chronic pain patients based on the practice of mindfulness mediation: Theoretical considerations and preliminary results. *General Hospital Psychiatry, 4,* 33–47.

Kaler, S. G. (2008). Diseases of poverty with high mortality in infants and children: Malaria, measles, lower respiratory infections, and diarrheal illnesses. *Annals of the New York Academy of Science, 1136,* 28–31.

Katon, W., Von Korff, M., Lin, E., Lipscomb, P., Russo, J., Wagner, E., et al. (1990). Distressed high utilizers of medical care: DSM-III-R diagnoses and treatment needs. *General Hospital Psychiatry, 12,* 355–362.

Kazdin, A. E. (2008). Evidence-based treatment and practice: New opportunities to bridge clinical research and practice, enhance the knowledge base, and improve patient care. *American Psychologist, 63,* 146–159.

Kessler, R. C., & Ustun, T. B. (2004). The World Mental Health (WMH) Survey Initiative Version of the World Health Organization (WHO) Composite International Diagnostic Interview (CIDI). *International Journal of Methods in Psychiatric Research, 13,* 93–121.

Koh, K. K. (2000). Effects of statins on vascular wall: Vasomotor function, inflammation, and plaque stability. *Cardiovascular Research, 47,* 648–657.

Kroenke, K., Spitzer, R. L., & Williams, J. B. W. (2001). The PHQ-9: Validity of a brief depression severity measure. *Journal of General Internal Medicine, 16,* 606–613.

Kroenke, K., Spitzer, R. L., & Williams, J. B. W. (2003). The Patient Health Questionnaire-2: Validity of a two-item depression screener. *Medical Care, 41,* 1284–1292.

Kroenke, K., Spitzer, R. L., Williams, J. B. W., Monahan, P. O., & Löwe, B. (2007). Anxiety disorders in primary care: Prevalence, impairment, comorbidity, and detection. *Annals of Internal Medicine, 146,* 317–325.

Lespérance, F., Frasure-Smith, N., Theroux, P., & Irwin, M. (2004). The association between major depression and levels of soluble intercellular adhesion molecule 1, interleukin-6, and C-reactive protein in patients with recent acute coronary syndromes. *American Journal of Psychiatry, 61,* 271–277.

Libby, P. (2002). Inflammation in atherosclerosis. *Nature, 420,* 868–874.

Lichtman, J. H., Bigger, J. T., Jr., Blumenthal, J. A., Frasure-Smith, N., Kaufman, P. G., Lespérance, F., et al. (2008). Depression and coronary heart disease: Recommendations for screening, referral, and treatment: A science advisory from the American Heart Association Prevention Committee of the Council on Cardiovascular Nursing, Council on Clinical Cardiology, Council on Epidemiology and Prevention, and Interdisciplinary Council on Quality of Care and Outcomes Research: Endorsed by the American Psychiatric Association. *Circulation, 118,* 1768–1775.

Matarazzo, M. D. (1982). Behavioral health's challenge to academic, scientific, and professional psychology. *American Psychologist, 37,* 1–14.

McEwen, B. S. (1998). Stress, adaptation, and disease: Allostasis and allostatic load. *Annals of the New York Academy of Sciences, 840,* 33–44.

Motivala, S. J., & Irwin, M. R. (2007). Sleep and immunity: Cytokine pathways linking sleep and health outcomes. *Current Directions in Psychological Science, 16,* 21–25.

Motivala, S. J., Sarfatti, A., Olmos, L., & Irwin, M. R. (2005). Inflammatory markers and sleep disturbance in major depression. *Psychosomatic Medicine, 67,* 187–194.

Musselman, D. L., Miller, A. H., Porter, M. R., Manatunga, A., Gao, F., Penna, S., et al. (2001). Higher than normal plasma interleukin-6 concentrations in cancer patients with depression: Preliminary findings. *American Journal of Psychiatry, 158,* 1252–1257.

Nicassio, P. M. (2008). The problem of detecting and managing depression in the rheumatology clinic. *Arthritis and Rheumatism, 59,* 155–158.

Nicassio, P. M., & Smith, T. W. (1995). *Managing chronic illness: A biopsychosocial approach.* Washington, DC: American Psychological Association.

Opp, M. R. (2005). Cytokines and sleep. *Sleep Medicine Review, 9,* 355–364.

Pennebaker, J. W., & Beall, S. K. (1986). Confronting a traumatic event: Toward an understanding of inhibition and disease. *Journal of Abnormal Psychology, 95,* 274–281.

Pignone, M., Gaynes, B., Mulrow, C., Orleans, T., & Lohr, K. (2002). Screening for depression in adults: A systematic review for the U.S. Preventive Services Task Force. *Annals of Internal Medicine, 136,* 765–776.

Pincus, H. A., Tanielian, T. L., Marcus, S. C., Olfson, M., Zarin, D. A., Thompson, J., et al. (1998). Prescribing trends in psychotropic medications: Primary care, psychiatry, and other medical specialties. *Journal of the American Medical Association, 279,* 526–531.

Prochaska, J. O., & DiClemente, C. C. (1983).

Stages and processes of self-change of smoking: Toward an integrative model of change. *Journal of Consulting and Clinical Psychology, 51,* 390–395.

Radloff, L. S. (1977). The CES-D scale: A self-report depression scale for research in the general population. *Applied Psychological Measurement, 1,* 385–401.

Raimy, V. C. (1950). *Training in clinical psychology.* Englewood Cliffs, NJ: Prentice-Hall.

Raison, C. L., Borisov, A. S., Majer, M., Drake, D. F., Pagnoni, G., Woolwine, B. J., et al. (2009). Activation of central nervous system inflammatory pathways by interferon-alpha: Relationship to monoamines and depression. *Biological Psychiatry, 65*(4), 296–303.

Ridker, P. M., Rifai, N., Stampfer, M. J., & Hennekens, C. H. (2000). Plasma concentration of interleukin-6 and the risk of future myocardial infarction among apparently healthy men. *Circulation, 101,* 1767–1772.

Robins, L. N., Cottler, L., Bucholz, K., & Compton, W. (1995). *The Diagnostic Interview Schedule, Version IV.* St. Louis, MO: Washington University.

Sackett, D. L., Straus, S. E., Richardson, W. S., Rosenberg, W., & Haynes, R. B. (2000). *Evidence-based medicine: How to practice and teach EMB* (2nd ed.). Edinburgh, UK: Churchill Livingstone.

Schneiderman, N., Antoni, M. H., Saab, P. G., & Ironson, G. (2001). Health psychology: Psychosocial and biobehavioral aspects of chronic disease management. *Annual Review of Psychology, 52,* 555–580.

Seals, D. R., & Esler, M. D. (2000). Human ageing and the sympathoadrenal system. *Journal of Physiology, 528*(3), 407–417.

Smyth, J. M., Stone, A. A., Hurewitz, A., & Kaell, A. (1999). Effects of writing about stressful experiences on symptom reduction in patients with asthma or rheumatoid arthritis: a randomized trial. *Journal of the American Medical Association, 281,* 1304–1309.

Spitzer, R. L., Kroenke, K., Williams, J. B. W., & Löwe, B. (2006). A brief measure for assessing generalized anxiety disorder: The GAD-7. *Archives of Internal Medicine, 166,* 1092–1097.

Steptoe, A., Hamer, M., & Chida, Y. (2007). The effects of acute psychological stress on circulating inflammatory factors in humans: A review and meta-analysis. *Brain, Behavior, and Immunity, 21,* 901–912.

Stone, G. C. (1983). Proceedings of the National Working Conference on Education and Training in Health Psychology. *Health Psychology,* 2(Suppl. 1), 1–153.

Taylor, S. E., Repetti, R. L., & Seeman, T. (1997). Health psychology: What is an unhealthy environment and how does it get under the skin? *Annual Review of Psychology, 48,* 411–447.

Tracey, K. J. (2002). The inflammatory reflex. *Nature, 420,* 853–859.

Turk, D. C., Meichenbaum, D., & Genest, M. (1987). *Pain and behavioral medicine: A cognitive-behavioral perspective.* New York: Guilford Press.

Vgontzas, A. N., Zoumakis, M., Papanicolaou, D. A., Bixler, E. O., Prolo, P., Lin, H. M., et al. (2002). Chronic insomnia is associated with a shift of interleukin-6 and tumor necrosis factor secretion from nighttime to daytime. *Metabolism, 51,* 887–992.

Wells, K. B., Stewart, A., Hays, R. D., Burnam, M. A., Rogers, W., Daniels, M., et al. (1988). The functioning and well-being of depressed patients: Results from the Medical Outcomes Study. *Journal of the American Medical Association, 262,* 914–919.

Whooley, M. A., de Jonge, P., Vittinghoff, E., Otte, C., Moos, R., Carney, R. M., et al. (2008). Depressive symptoms, health behaviors, and risk of cardiovascular events in patients with coronary heart disease. *Journal of the American Medical Association, 300,* 2379–2388.

Wirtz, P. H., Ehlert, U., Bartschi, C., Redwine, L. S., & von Kanel, R. (2009). Changes in plasma lipids with psychosocial stress are related to hypertension status and the norepinephrine stress response. *Metabolism, 58,* 30–37.

World Health Organization. (1993). *The ICD-10 classification of mental and behavioral disorders: Diagnostic criteria for research.* Geneva: Author.

Yang, C. C., Jick, S. S., & Jick, H. (2003). Lipid-lowering drugs and the risk of depression and suicidal behavior. *Archives of Internal Medicine, 163,* 1926–1932.

Young-Xu, Y., Chan, K. A., Liao, J. K., Ravid, S., & Blatt, C. M. (2003). Long-term statin use and psychological well-being. *Journal of the American College of Cardiology, 4,* 690–697.

Zigmond, A. S., & Snaith, R. P. (1983). The Hospital Anxiety and Depression Scale. *Acta Psychiatrica Scandinavica, 67,* 361–370.

CHAPTER 7

Contributions of Personality to Health Psychology

Howard S. Friedman
Margaret L. Kern

At a most basic and important level, a key goal of health psychology is to improve health, well-being, and longevity. Reaching this goal means understanding not only the correlates and predictors of health but also the causal processes. Too often, health research uncovers a variable connected to good health but has no way of knowing whether an intervention involving this new variable will lead to better health. For example, the traditional Mediterranean diet, full of nutrient-rich vegetables, fruits, and olive oil, is associated with good health, but should individuals tilt their behavior toward olive and tomato consumption, vitamin and nutrient pills, or sailing in the sunshine-filled Mediterranean? Or might none of these be effective in causing improvements in health? Conversely, unhappy, distressed loners are at high risk for poor health, but should we find them marriage partners, conscript them to church, and feed them antidepressant pills to lower their risk of cancer and heart disease? Or might none of these be effective in reducing disease risk?

In health psychology, the problem of appropriate interventions over the long term is especially complex for two reasons. First, it is often impossible to conduct optimal randomized clinical trials; that is, we cannot randomly assign some adolescents to spend the next 20 years becoming smokers, marathon runners, well-educated professionals, good spouses, sound sleepers, or religious worshippers. Second, there is tremendous individual variation as early individual temperamental predispositions encounter diverse social environments and differing sociobehavioral patterns develop (Friedman, 2007; Hampson & Friedman, 2008). This extensive individual variation then interacts with subsequent threats to health as people grow and age. Understanding the likelihood of disease for the unique individual often turns out to be as important as knowing the general causes of disease.

Modern understanding of personality provides a sophisticated entry into these complex matters. Personality encapsulates a blend of biological, familial, social, and cultural fundamentals. Furthermore, personality not only has a certain temporal stability but it also gradually matures and changes. Thus, "personality"—the individual's biopsychosocial patterns of behavior—is a construct that connects well with biopsychosocial approaches to health, and it is especially well suited to understanding the complex causal pathways to better health and longevity. In fact, modern notions of personality, which include ideas of situation selection and evocative effects, are well matched to the most sophisticated models of healthy development and health promotion (Aldwin, Spiro, & Park, 2006; Bolger & Zuckerman, 1995; Hampson & Friedman, 2008; Roberts, Walton, & Viechtbauer, 2006; Scarr & McCartney, 1983; Suls & Rothman, 2004).

Contemporary personality psychology looks quite different from the personality psychology of half a century ago—it is more nuanced, scientific, and multifaceted. Early personality approaches to health were based primarily on psychoanalytic concepts, which proved impossible to test. For example, neoanalytic psychosomatic theorists proposed vague notions of inner psychological conflicts causing physical symptoms. Ulcers, asthma, heart disease, migraines, and other complex or puzzling conditions were blamed on the inner conflicts of disturbed patients (Alexander, 1950; Dunbar, 1955). Although loosely grounded in the psychophysiological models of Claude Bernard (1880) and the "fight-or-flight" discoveries of Walter Cannon (1932), such approaches were rich in theory and insight but lacking in reliable measurement and empirical validation.

As a counterpoint, empiricists focused attention on quantifying and operationalizing personality variables. For example, medical students at Johns Hopkins University were classified as either slow and solid, rapid and facile, or irregular and uneven. Years later, members of the last category were more likely to develop a serious medical disorder (Betz & Thomas, 1979). Taking empiricism to the extreme, researchers of the Type A behavior pattern purposely disregarded construct validity and psychological theory in an attempt to make the phenomenon of coronary proneness more objective (Chesney & Rosenman, 1985). Type A behavior was seen as a medical syndrome (collection of symptoms) stripped of all conceptual grounding. The actual result, however, was not objectivity but thousands of often meandering and unfocused studies that produced more confusion than clarity—a sad lesson that is still important for current research in this field. Individual differences need not only to be

defined and assessed rigorously but also to be framed in a deep conceptual understanding of biopsychosocial patterns.

Humanistic perspectives on personality, and "interactionist perspectives" (seeing behavior as a joint function of person and environment), attempted to repatriate the whole person and social context, even while biological perspectives expanded the reach of the models through new understandings of genetics and temperament. Today, many researchers focus on understanding individual life paths within a complex socioenvironmental framework. This fresh perspective includes aspects of previous approaches, but these are now interwoven in a dynamic, mutually influential fashion that more closely mirrors reality viewed from an interdisciplinary lifespan perspective (Baltes, Lindenberger, & Staudinger, 2006; Conley, 1985; Kuh & Ben-Shlomo, 1997; McCrae et al., 2000; Smith & MacKenzie, 2006). We call this a "lifespan epidemiological personality approach."

In this chapter, we contend that personality, as part of a lifespan developmental model, is an important contributor to our understanding of biopsychosocial processes, health, and disease. Drawing examples from our research and that of others, we illustrate both the direct and indirect pathways between personality and disease. We argue that personality is one of the major constructs that links mental and physical health, and that by using time-dependent techniques grounded in lifespan developmental theories, we can better address the complex health trajectories that people travel during their lives.

Disease-Prone Personalities and Self-Healing Personalities

To provide a comprehensive approach that relies on a full nomological net (Campbell & Fiske, 1959; Cronbach & Meehl, 1955), Friedman and Booth-Kewley (1987) reviewed and meta-analyzed the associations between emotional aspects of personality and chronic diseases (including heart disease) thought to be especially influenced by psychosomatic factors. Two key conclusions emerged. First, the surprisingly similar pattern of associations that appeared between predictors and multiple disease outcomes contradicted then-prevailing notions of a "coronary-prone personality," a distinct "ulcer-prone personality," and so on. Friedman and Booth-Kewley referred to this broader pattern as pointing to a "disease-prone personality," suggesting that negative traits such as hostility, anxiety, depression, and aggressiveness are markers of increased risk for disease in general.

A second consequence of these analyses was greater appreciation of the importance of employing multiple predictors in the same study. The best studies now employ multiple predictors and several disease and well-being outcomes (Friedman, 2007; Friedman, Kern, & Reynolds, 2010; Smith & Gallo, 2001). In particular, often there is now a primary focus on the five-factor model of personality (the traits of conscientiousness, neuroticism, extraversion, agreeableness, and openness), an advance that we take up later in this chapter.

Another benefit of this broader approach has been a less exclusive focus on negativity and disease-proneness and a more active consideration of the potential health-promoting effects of often salutary traits, such as optimism, extraversion, hardiness, and conscientiousness. Complementing the disease-prone personality, Friedman (1991) suggested the notion of a "self-healing personality," a cluster of characteristics that promotes health and well-being. Although characterized by traits such as hardiness (control, commitment, and challenge; Maddi & Kobasa, 1984) and sociability, the crux of the construct is the match between the person and the environment that will best maintain biopsychosocial balance, thus promoting health and well-being. For example, a driven and competent business executive who may be quite happy and successful with his or her fast-paced lifestyle may become ill and depressed if forced to slow down and take a break. This notion fits well with the lifespan epidemiological personality approach because it simultaneously considers the individual's resources, the socioenvironmental challenges, and the trajectories of change over time.

Moreover, it is now becoming clear that multiple outcomes should be considered. It was decades ago that the World Health Organization (1948) defined health as a multidimensional construct, consisting of physical, mental, social, cognitive, and functional components, but only recently has attention extended beyond the physical health dimension. Length of life is also important because many studies of psychosocial predictors and well-being outcomes rely on measures that share method and definitional variance (i.e., both predictors and outcomes are self-reported measures of the individual's feelings, self-perceived symptoms, complaints, and perceptions of health and well-being). In contrast, longevity offers a valid, reliable health outcome that temporally follows other variables. One good way to combine subjective and objective aspects of health is to use the concept of quality-adjusted life years, which incorporates years of life and the health quality of each year (Diehr & Patrick, 2003; Kaplan, 1994, 2003) and takes into account multiple predictors, multiple pathways, and multiple well-being outcomes (Bogg, Voss, Wood, & Roberts, 2008; Friedman et al., 2010; Gruenewald, Mroczek, Ryff, & Singer, 2008; Hampson, Goldberg, Vogt, & Dubanoski, 2007; Korotkov & Hannah, 2004; Steel, Schmidt, & Shultz, 2008).

Ironically, research on subjective well-being has often stumbled into the same biases in measurement and narrow constructs that plagued the field of personality and health in studies of Type A behavior and negative affect. Claims of the far-reaching health benefits of happiness and optimism permeate the scientific and lay literatures despite mixed evidence (Howell, Kern, & Lyubomirsky, 2007; Lyubomirsky, King, & Diener, 2005; Pressman & Cohen, 2005). It is true that in some cases of challenged individuals, dispositional optimism can speed recovery (e.g., after surgery). But it is also true that optimism can be detrimental if it leads to riskier activities, skipping needed medical treatment, or ignoring health warnings. Furthermore, although it is true that a sense of well-being is associated with health correlates such as better immune function and lower mortality risk, the causal relations are murky. For example, it is not at all clear whether psychoneuroimmunological effects are a key factor in explaining links between personality and health, or whether becoming happier causes better health (Friedman, 2008; Held, 2004; Kemeny, 2007; Segerstrom, 2000, 2005; Segerstrom & Miller, 2004).

A meta-analytic review of subjective well-being as predictor of objective health outcomes included study design, how health outcomes and well-being were operationalized and measured, and various sample characteristics (Howell et al., 2007). Here, again, the relations between health and individual differences in subjective well-being were complex, with bidirectional relationships and psychosocial factors interacting with health and well-being predictors and outcomes. Simple models are insufficient (Friedman, 2007; Suls & Bunde, 2005).

Pathways Linking Personality and Health

Personality and health are linked at multiple levels, including the health-related behaviors in which individuals engage, physiological reactions to stress, situation selection, interactions with other people, and biological aspects of the person (Friedman, 2008; Hampson & Friedman, 2008; Roberts, Walton, & Bogg, 2005; Smith, 2006; Smith & MacKenzie, 2006). In general, health psychology has moved beyond the traditional biomedical or mechanical model of disease, and it is important that work in personality and health do so as well.

The Health Behavioral Model

The health behavioral model postulates that personality causes disease through its effects on habitual unhealthy behavior. The focus here is generally on harmful or risky behaviors such as poor diet, smoking, alcohol abuse, unsafe recreation, unprotected sex, dangerous driving, and lack of physical activity. Increasing evidence suggests personality affects the behaviors in which people engage, which in turn are linked to health, well-being, and mortality risk (e.g., Caspi et al., 1997; Hampson et al., 2007; Markey, Markey, & Tinsley, 2003; U.S. Department of Health and Human Services, 2000).

Research addresses this model in several ways. First, personality predictors of more or less healthy and risky behaviors are assessed. For example, higher levels of extraversion and conscientiousness predict engagement in more physical activity (Rhodes & Smith, 2006). It is important not to stop at this point and assume that health has been assessed. *Predictors* of health—exercise, cholesterol, drinking—are not the same as health. In the second step, health behaviors are tested as mediators; that is, once a link is established between a personality predictor and a health outcome, one or more behaviors are added to the regression model to see whether the personality–health association diminishes. For example, studies have linked conscientiousness to lower mortality risk; the effect is somewhat attenuated when alcohol use and smoking are added to the model, suggesting some behavioral pathways (Bogg & Roberts, 2004; Friedman et al., 1995; Hampson et al., 2007). Third, the relations among the personality trait, the health behavior, and the health outcome are evaluated across long periods of time. Fourth, behavioral modification intervention programs are applied to multiple subgroups (e.g., children, young adults, middle-aged adults, and older adults) to examine age-relevant intervention effects. Finally, it is important to evaluate whether interventions affect the whole sequence—the individual, the behavior, and health. Treating the overeating behavior of a neurotic, obese individual should not be considered effective if he or she later turns to smoking instead.

The Psychophysiological Stress and Coping Model

The internal stress and coping model focuses on how negative traits may trigger and maintain maladaptive chronic stress responses, and how positive traits may either buffer activation from stress or quickly restore balance to the physiological system (Fredrickson, 2001; Pressman & Cohen, 2005). From a life course perspective, change occurs throughout life as both internal and external losses and challenges occur (Aldwin et al., 2006; Baltes et al., 2006; Rook, Charles, & Heckhausen, 2007; Schultz & Heckhausen, 1996). People vary in both how they perceive stressors and how successfully they cope with challenges. For example, when two coworkers lose their jobs, one may view the layoff as an opportunity to start a new career direction or pursue further education, whereas the other may view it as a failure and succumb to a life as an unemployed alcoholic. A certain degree of stress motivates change and growth, but chronically high stress levels become maladaptive, disrupting physiological processes and increasing susceptibility to illness and disease (Graham, Christian, & Kiecolt-Glaser, 2006; Kemeny, 2007; McEwen, 2006).

Studies addressing this model typically measure personality in concert with physiological markers, such as blood pressure, immune and endocrine function, or cardiovascular reactivity. There may also be reports of chronic stress or acute stressful life events (e.g., Miller, Cohen, Rabin, Skoner, & Doyle, 1999; Puttonen et al., 2008). For example, personality, blood pressure, neuroendocrine, and immune function parameters were assessed in healthy adults under quarantine conditions (Miller et al., 1999). Participants scoring low on agreeableness and extraversion demonstrated increased sympathetic nervous system activity and, for extraversion, higher natural killer cell cytotoxicity, suggesting that personality is associated with basal physiological levels. An assumption of this model is that cross-sectional and short-term associations between personality and physiological function extend to disease outcomes later in life; however, studies have yet to test the entire causal model across long time periods. In one of the few exceptions, links between blood pressure and personality were examined cross-sectionally and longitudinally across a 10-year period (Leclerc, Rahn, & Linden, 2006). Hostility predicted higher systolic blood pressure at baseline and higher diastolic blood pressure 10 years later, but no other consistencies between cross-sectional and longitudinal personality–health relationships were evident. Importantly, there is good evidence that immune disruptions are sometimes a *cause* of psychological distress (rather than vice versa). For example, proinflammatory cytokines may be a partial cause of depression. As Kemeny (2007) put it, "A relationship between a psychological factor and a change in the immune system may be due to the simple impact of the mind on the immune system, the effects of the immune system on the mind, both, or neither" (p. 111).

Underlying Biological (Third-Variable) Models

Third-variable models propose that relations between personality and health stem from an underlying "propensity" (i.e., a genetic or temperamental factor) toward both

patterns of responding and health or disease. Personality differences in health and well-being may begin before birth and be influenced by genetic–environmental interactions throughout life (Hampson & Friedman, 2008). For example, prenatal stress predicts infant activity, sleep, and attention at 3 months (Jones, 2008; Wadhwa, 2005). These models are important because they suggest that changing personality will not necessarily have any effect on the likelihood of the associated disease. Personality–health relations are thus sometimes termed "spurious" associations—the correlations are real, but the causality is specious.

Because multiple genetic and biological (prenatal and neonatal) variables may unfold and interact with the early environment to influence personality and health outcomes, this model adds a complex temperamental pathway. Research using laboratory animals, behavioral genetics, and psychoimmunology is increasingly informative of such biological processes (Friedman, 2008). Animal research has been often ignored in personality psychology, but cross-species research suggests that extraversion, neuroticism, agreeableness, dominance, and curiosity (a facet of openness) have correlates across multiple animal species, (Gosling & John, 1999; Mehta & Gosling, 2008). Animal research overcomes several of the limitations of personality and health research: such research does not rely on self-report measures; the short-lived nature of many animals allow consideration of lifespan patterns within a short period of time; and traits can be selected for through trait-specific breeding programs (Cavigelli, 2005). Importantly, individual animals can be assigned to different socio-environmental conditions, and ongoing physiological measures can be obtained.

In humans, twin studies can be informative about pre-natal genetic factors, early experiences that shape subsequent trajectories, and differential genetic effects at different ages across the lifespan. Using a behavior genetic covariance analysis, a study of twins found the familiar five-factor structure in both the phenotype and genotype, suggesting both a strong biological and environmental structure to the five factors (McCrae, Jang, Livesley, Riemann, & Angleitner, 2001). Using data from the Swedish Adoption/Twin Study of Aging study, both genetic and environmental influences on personality appear to be relatively stable, although environmental effects show increasing variability with age (Pedersen & Reynolds, 1998).

Developments in neuroscience also offer possibilities in studying brain patterns, reactions across different situations, individual characteristics, and health outcomes. For example, using structured magnetic resonance imaging (MRI) scans, higher scores on harm avoidance and other anxiety-prone traits showed a specific relation to the right hippocampus for both males and females (Yamasue et al., 2008). Individual differences in extraversion and neuroticism demonstrate differential activation patterns, which in turn relate to positive or negative attributions, judgments, and memories (Canli, 2004). Such studies may help to untangle cognitive-level mechanisms linking personality and health outcomes.

Disease-Caused Personality Changes

Although personality is often considered a predictor and underlying cause of health outcomes, bidirectional relations can occur. For example, a friendly, easygoing person can slowly become harsh and critical as Alzheimer's disease slowly (and without the person or observer knowing) attacks brain tissue. Later, it may appear that personality (or personality change) caused the disease, when in reality the disease caused the shift in the long-term behavioral patterns of the person. Even outside of pathological cases, evidence suggests that age and time make a difference; for example, people often become more conscientious and less neurotic as they grow older and establish more stable lifestyles (e.g., increasing work responsibilities, stable marriages) (Roberts, Wood, & Caspi, 2008). Both changes and continuity in the internal and external environment impact personality–health linkages.

The Importance of Time

Medical care is organized to take care of acute diseases and acute manifestations of chronic illnesses. The traditional biomedical approach to disease generally works well with such matters: When symptoms appear, one seeks medical care, goes through diagnostic tests, and is prescribed a drug or surgery to address the problem. But many health problem of the 21st century involve chronic conditions that the biomedical models and the accompanying public policies are poorly designed to handle. There is far less than optimal allocation of resources for the long-term prevention of disease and promotion of health (Kaplan, 2007).

Medical research studies typically focus on treating acute manifestations of disease, or sometimes on "secondary prevention"—actions taken once a disease begins to develop. Interventions involving drugs to reduce hypertension or to combat osteoporosis are taking a longer-term perspective but still follow a one-factor approach in a web that demands multifactor, multioutcome designs. It is relatively rare for a study to focus on "primary prevention"—actions designed to prevent illness from developing in the first place. Such studies are costly, unwieldy, and even if feasible, would take a long time. Complex causal linkages tend to be underexplored or even totally overlooked. We know relatively little about effective long-term societal approaches to promote health, healthy aging, and longevity. Here is where personality becomes important, since by nature it considers the individual across time.

Tropisms and Cumulative Continuity

"Tropisms" are forces that pull phototropic plants toward a source of light, and pull some individuals toward healthier environments (Friedman, 2000). Personality development begins early in life as temperament encounters environmental pressures and socialization factors. Studies of personality across decades indicate that temperament-related factors in childhood are good predictors of personality traits later on, and that personality traits become more stable with age (Allemand, Zimprich, & Hertzog, 2007; Allemand, Zimprich, & Martin, 2008; Caspi & Silva, 1995; McCrae et al., 2000; Roberts, Helson, & Klohnen, 2002). But they also show that as people move nonrandomly in and out of contexts and environments, aspects of their personalities are altered by these experiences (Srivastava, John, Gosling, & Potter, 2003; Twenge, 2000, 2001). There is a cumulative continuity (Caspi & Bem, 1990; Caspi et al., 1997), in which change occurs but often follows a consistent and predictable pattern. Thus, if we understand the underlying components and can accurately assess the life path trajectory, we can predict a variety of meaningful health outcomes. An important but often overlooked point is that part of what maintains this continuity is people's frequent selection of their own stressful or unstressful environments (Bandura, 1999; Buss, 1987; Caspi, Roberts, & Shiner, 2005; Scarr & McCartney, 1983), in which they essentially choose or are pulled toward (perhaps unconsciously) the very experiences that will mold and shape them. Extraverted individuals are both subjectively and objectively more likely to do more and to engage in activities that are potentially highly enjoyable and rewarding, whereas neurotic individuals may do less and engage in mundane activities (Bolger & Zuckerman, 1995; Magnus, Diener, Fujita, & Payot, 1993; Roberts, Caspi, & Moffitt, 2003).

Similar issues apply to research involving environmental stressors and their contributions to physical manifestations of disease. These models of stress, coping, and adaptation have typically viewed stressors as random events to which the individual must respond, but many life events may not be random and might instead be evoked by or selected according to characteristics of the individual (Bolger & Zuckerman, 1995; Buss, 1987; Ickes, Snyder, & Garcia, 1997; Magnus et al., 1993; Van Heck, 1997). For example, some people are more likely to select marriages that will end in divorce (Johnson, McGue, Krueger, & Bouchard, 2004; Larson & Holman, 1994; Tucker, Friedman, Wingard, & Schwartz, 1996).

During the past 18 years, we have worked extensively to expand the Terman Life-Cycle Study, an archival study that began in 1922 and has followed over 1,500 individuals prospectively throughout their lives. Participants completed assessments every 5–10 years, offering a picture of many psychosocial aspects of their lives. In this sample, children who experienced parental divorce were both more likely to have their own marriages end in divorce and to face premature mortality than were children who came from stable homes (Schwartz et al., 1995; Tucker et al., 1997). Early life experiences may begin a trajectory of ill-being (or sometimes recovery) that can only be captured in a long-term developmental perspective (Baltes, Saudinger, & Lindenberger, 1999; McCrae et al., 2000; Roberts & Pomerantz, 2004; Rutter, Kim-Cohen, & Maughan, 2006; Sroufe, Carlson, Levy, & Egeland, 1999).

What Time-Sensitive Trajectory Analyses Can Reveal

As new statistical methods have developed, lifespan models that address both individual- and group-level factors across time can now be evaluated more directly. Multilevel modeling techniques can create estimates of an overall average trajectory for a sample (e.g., increasing, remaining steady, decreasing over time), individual variation around this trajectory, and reasons for this variation (Singer & Willett, 2003). Structural equation modeling techniques allow complex relationships across time to be estimated, while they address the problematic issues in classical regression techniques of unreliability in measurement, indirect pathways, correlated error, and mild to moderate violation of regression assumptions (Little, Bovaird, & Slegers, 2006). Other cross-time techniques include cross-lagged panel designs (which allow estimation of lagged and simultaneous effects by two or more variables; Hertzog & Nesselroade, 2003), measurement burst designs (macro- and micro-level linkages are studied by nesting intensive periods of measurement within long-term longitudinal studies; Nesselroade, 1991), joint growth–survival analyses (which combine growth and survival techniques; McArdle, Small, Backman, & Fratiglioni, 2005), and dynamic growth models (which consider the dynamic interplay of two or more variables over time). For example, using data from the Veterans Affairs Normative Aging Study, Mroczek and Spiro (2007) found that change in neuroticism over a 12-year period was important to longevity outcomes; individuals who are high in neuroticism at baseline and become more neurotic with age face a significantly higher mortality risk than do individuals at lower levels or without a late-life increase in neuroticism.

The Five-Factor Approach to Personality

The five-factor model of personality (FFM, or the Big Five) provides a conceptual framework for investigating the relations among personality, health, and longevity (Carver &

Miller, 2006; Duberstein, Seidlitz, Lyness, & Conwell, 1999; Smith, 2006). Although some uncertainty about the best labels and structure remains, the factors—conscientiousness, agreeableness, extraversion, openness to experience, and neuroticism—have been linked to important life outcomes (Goldberg, 1993; Ozer & Benet-Martinez, 2006; Roberts, Kuncel, Shiner, Caspi, & Goldberg, 2007).

Conscientiousness and Health: Associations and Causal Mechanisms

Conscientiousness includes traits such as organization, thoroughness, perseverance, competence, order, dutifulness, achievement striving, self-discipline, and deliberation. Though often ignored by earlier studies involving Type A behavior, hostility, and health, conscientiousness has clearly been linked to positive health outcomes. In addition to being valued employees and successful in general, conscientious individuals are more likely to have good social relationships, marital stability, more community involvement, and better health and longevity (Barrick & Mount, 1991; Bogg & Roberts, 2004; Gelissen & de Graaf, 2006; Kern & Friedman, 2008; Kern, Friedman, Martin, Reynolds, & Luong, 2009; Ozer & Benet-Martinez, 2006; Roberts et al., 2007; Schmidt & Hunter, 1992).

In our work with the Terman Life-Cycle Study, both child and adult conscientiousness are associated with benefits across multiple domains. Conscientiousness predicted less alcohol abuse, less smoking, more successful careers, stable marriages, and physical and mental health in old age (Friedman et al., 1995, 2010; Kern et al., 2009; Tucker et al., 1996). Most notably, our early studies found that childhood conscientiousness, as rated by parents and teachers in 1922, predicted lower mortality risk across seven decades (Friedman et al., 1993, 1995). Adult conscientiousness was also protective, even when childhood conscientiousness was controlled (Martin & Friedman, 2000; Martin, Friedman, & Schwartz, 2007). Using diverse samples and study designs, others followed up on these intriguing results, all finding support for this protective effect (e.g., Christensen et al., 2002; Deary, Batty, Pattie, & Gale, 2008; Terracciano, Locken-

hoff, Zonderman, Ferrucci, & Costa, 2008; Weiss & Costa, 2005; Whiteman, 2006; Wilson, Mendes de Leon, Bienias, Evans, & Bennett, 2004). Meta-analysis confirms that across 20 samples and over 8,900 participants, conscientiousness is indeed protective against mortality risk (Kern & Friedman, 2008).

Simple explanations for this protective effect remain elusive, and the web of causal mechanisms exemplifies the complexity of the personality–health puzzle. Conscientious individual are more likely to engage in health-protective behaviors and to avoid risky behaviors, clearly supporting the behavioral model (Bogg & Roberts, 2004). Yet health behaviors alone do not explain this relationship (Friedman et al., 1995; Hampson et al., 2007; Martin et al., 2007; Weiss & Costa, 2005; Wilson et al., 2004). Successful careers, academic success, and good social relationships all offer protection from mortality risk, suggesting multiple social pathways. Studies with animals, twins, and biological markers show links between conscientiousness-related traits and more stable biological function, suggesting biological pathways (Figueredo et al., 2005; O'Cleirigh, Ironson, Weiss, & Costa, 2007; Williams, Kuhn, et al., 2004). Serotonin is linked to conscientiousness, impulsiveness, and genetic variations of cortisol responses (Carver & Miller, 2006; Evans & Rothbart, 2007; Kusumi et al., 2002; Manuck et al., 1998; Wand et al., 2002).

Agreeableness, Extraversion, and Health: Interpersonal Traits

Agreeableness involves characteristics such as cooperativeness, consideration, empathy, kindness, and generosity. Limited evidence suggests that higher agreeableness may be health protective, although research has linked it more to subjective health status than to objective health outcomes (e.g., Korotkov & Hannah, 2004). In the Midlife Development in the United States Survey (MIDUS), a nationally representative sample of the U.S. population, agreeableness related to higher levels of perceived health (Goodwin & Engstrom, 2002). In some studies, high agreeableness has been weakly related to lower mortality risk (Weiss & Costa, 2005), but others have found no such relationship

(Martin & Friedman, 2000; Wilson et al., 2004). Links among agreeableness, health behaviors, and subsequent health outcomes are stronger for women than for men (Chapman, Duberstein, & Lyness, 2007; Costa, Terracciano, & McCrae, 2001; Jerram & Coleman, 1999). To the extent that agreeableness is a sign or cause of good social relations, social integration, and lack of isolation and depression, it should be a marker of or influence on health. But to the extent that it interacts with life challenges leading to less optimal life pathways, it could have less positive or even negative effects.

Extraversion includes traits such as sociability, assertiveness, dominance, and energy/activity. Like agreeableness, extraversion has been inconsistently linked to health—there are both positive and negative health outcomes. For example, in one study, moderate levels of extraversion predicted better self-assessed health, whereas very high levels, especially in combination with neuroticism, predicted worse health outcomes (Williams, O'Brien, & Colder, 2004). Evidence suggests that extraverted individuals are more likely to engage in risky health behaviors, such as smoking, drinking, and risky driving, but other studies suggest protective effects, such as staying physically active. Not surprisingly, this trait has been inconsistently linked to mortality risk (Cloninger, 2005; Wilson et al., 2004, 2005).

Conflicting findings involving agreeableness, extraversion, and health illustrate and confirm the importance of considering multiple causal life pathways. Extraversion has both strong biological and interpersonal components, and its implications are susceptible to situational influences. For example, the extraverted individual who likes adventure and often goes to parties may also smoke, abuse alcohol, and engage in risky hobbies in certain cultures, creating a behavioral risk to health. At the same time, social individuals may have more friends and health-supportive social contacts. Likewise, a highly agreeable person may develop a strong social network offering protective effects, but he or she may also be taken advantage of, leading to ill-being. Extraversion and agreeableness quite possibly work in combination with other traits and social factors, such that when considered alone, personality–health links wash out.

Openness, Intelligence, and Health

Openness to experience includes characteristics such as being imaginative, creative, tolerant, and intelligent. It is the least distinct trait within the FFM. Although the overall openness factor has shown few consistent health outcomes, the intellect facet does predict health. Across several well-controlled studies, intelligence predicts lower rates of morbidity and mortality (Batty et al., 2009; Deary et al., 2008; Deary, Whiteman, Starr, Whalley, & Fox, 2004; Hemmingsson, Essen, Melin, Allebeck, & Lundberg, 2007; O'Toole, 1990; Whalley & Deary, 2001).

Intelligence is often correlated with other protective psychosocial factors. Intelligent individuals are often better educated, come from a moderate to high socioeconomic level, have the ability to understand medical advice, engage in more health-protective and fewer risky health behaviors, and are better equipped to draw on social resources as needed (Batty, Deary, & Gottfredson, 2007; Batty, Deary, Schoon, & Gale, 2007; Beier & Ackerman, 2003; Hart et al., 2004; Taylor et al., 2003). In turn, each of these factors relates to better health and longevity. Aside from intelligence, openness has not been clearly linked to mortality risk (Roberts et al., 2007). In the Terman sample, all participants had an IQ of 135 or greater, but despite this high level of intelligence, participants varied dramatically across most biopsychosocial variables, including health behaviors, social activities, work status, and health and longevity outcomes (Friedman, 2000; Friedman & Markey, 2003; Schwartz et al., 1995; Tucker et al., 1996). Attempts to make individuals smarter will not necessarily produce health benefits, unless the relevant mediating mechanisms are identified and changed.

Neuroticism and Health

Among the most difficult issues to untangle are the relations between neuroticism and health. Neuroticism includes proneness to anxiety and depression, emotional instability, and a tendency to experience the world as distressful. There is no doubt that anxiety, depression, and hostility are linked to illness, but controversies about validity and causality abound.

For many of the reasons described earlier, it is not at all clear whether "treating" neuroticism promotes better health. One basic issue involves subjective versus objective health outcomes. Neuroticism clearly relates to lower levels of perceived health and subjective well-being (Costa & McCrae, 1987; DeNeve & Cooper, 1998; Smith & Gallo, 2001; Watson & Pennebaker, 1989), leading some researchers to declare that it is simply a noninformative marker of psychopathology (Guarino, Roger, & Olason, 2007; Ormel, Rosmalen, & Farmer, 2004). Objective evidence is mixed, with some studies reporting more physical symptoms and increased mortality risk (Charles, Gatz, Kato, & Pedersen, 2008; Friedman & Booth-Kewley, 1987; Neupert, Mroczek, & Spiro, 2008; Suls & Bunde, 2005; Terracciano et al., 2008), others reporting no relation; and still others suggesting a protective effect (Korten et al., 1999; Taga, Friedman, & Martin, 2009; Weiss & Costa, 2005). In the Western Electric Study, neuroticism was unrelated to mortality risk, after researchers controlled for cynicism, blood pressure, cholesterol, smoking, and alcohol use (Almada et al., 1991). A population-based study in Australia found no effect of neuroticism on mortality risk for females and a protective effect for males, when other demographic and psychosocial variables were controlled for (Korten et al., 1999). In a group of frail older adults, neuroticism was protective (Weiss & Costa, 2005).

Furthermore, there are multiple causal linkages between neuroticism and health. Neuroticism is associated with cardiovascular disease (Suls & Bunde, 2005) and with eating disturbances/obesity, lack of exercise, and various measures of stress, but in the Enhancing Recovery in Coronary Heart Disease (ENRICHD; 2003) study, it was surprising to the investigators that treating depression in patients who previously had a heart attack did not impact the likelihood of subsequent heart attacks. Notably, disease can predict subsequent increased anxiety and anger, and proinflammatory cytokines may be a partial cause of depression (Kemeny, 2007; Räikkönen, Matthews, & Kuller, 2002).

There is also evidence of a biological third variable here. There may be common genetic vulnerability to depression and to coronary artery disease (Bondy, 2007; McCaffrey et al., 2006). To the extent that such a relation holds, the ordinary risk factor intervention ("treat depression") will fail. To the extent that both depression and coronary heart disease develop from genetically based vulnerability in the serotonin and dopamine systems, or in prenatal experiences, interventions to affect hostility or depression will not have expected effects on disease risk (see also Barker, Osmond, Forsén, Kajantie, & Eriksson, 2005).

In the Terman sample, we examined neuroticism (measured in 1940 when the participants were in their 30s) as a predictor of older adults' health (measured in 1986, when participants were in their 70s) and mortality risk through 2007 (Friedman et al., 2010). As expected, high levels of neuroticism predicted lower subjective well-being and, to a lesser extent, physical health. For mortality, however, a different picture emerged. For males, neuroticism was somewhat protective. In particular, neuroticism was protective for widowed men, again suggesting that neuroticism may in certain cases become protective (Taga et al., 2009). In stressful times, neurotic individuals, despite reporting more health distress, may be the most resilient, with their tendency to worry possibly leading to better self-care, regular doctor visits, or better health behaviors. Neuroticism predicts increased susceptibility to pain, which may influence reports and experiences of poor health (Charles et al., 2008), but other pathways may include negative self-stereotypes, an altered stress response, and changed interactions with others (Moor, Zimprich, Schmitt, & Kliegel, 2006; Neupert et al., 2008; Terracciano et al., 2008).

Nonlinear Relationships, Moderating Effects, and Trait Interactions

The picture of the relations between personality and health is further complicated by nonlinear relationships and trait interactions (Aldwin, Spiro, Levenson, & Cupertino, 2001; Cloninger, 2005; MacKinnon, & Luecken, 2008; Smith & MacKenzie, 2006; Suls & Bunde, 2005; Vollrath & Torgersen, 2008). For example, in a 20-year follow-up study of a nationally representative sample, there was a nonlinear relationship between psychological distress (neuroticism) and mortality risk for men, such that moderate amounts of distress were protective, whereas high levels substantially increased risk (Ferraro & Nuriddin, 2006). In a student sample, there was a nonlinear relation between extraversion and symptom reporting, such that more symptoms were reported, both retrospectively and concurrently, only for individuals high on extraversion compared to those at moderate or low levels (Williams, O'Brien, & Colder, 2004). In the Medicare Demonstration Study, when conscientiousness was trichotomized, there was a significant predictive effect of mortality for high conscientiousness but not moderate or low levels of conscientiousness (Weiss & Costa, 2005). In the Terman sample, conscientiousness moderated an association between career success and longevity, such that conscientiousness made little difference for successful individuals but attenuated the negative effect of an unsuccessful career (Kern et al., 2009).

Although the FFM suggests intriguing relations between personality and health, lower-order trait-level analyses, using more narrowly defined traits (e.g., "self-control," "energy/activity," "anxious distress"), may be more predictive (Adams & Mowen, 2005; Brown, Cober, Kane, Levy, & Shalhoop, 2006; Crant, 2000; Erdogan & Bauer, 2005; Greven, Chamorro-Premuzic, Arteche, & Furnham, 2008; O'Connor & Paunonen, 2007; Seibert, Crant, & Kraimer, 1999; Watson & Hubbard, 1996; Zweig & Webster, 2004). Studies that address these more nuanced relationships within and between traits are in their infancy but provide an area ripe for future research.

Implications for Interventions and Interventional Research

A key goal of health psychology is to find ways to improve people's health and well-being across the lifespan. If we are to intervene effectively in some way to change lives, we must understand the causal paths: What influences health outcomes, how, for whom, and when (MacKinnon & Luecken, 2008)? Longitudinal studies have clearly shown that personality is a key factor, answering the "what" question, yet the mix of findings and mechanisms underscores the challenges ahead.

In traditional approaches to health promotion, insufficient consideration is given to the trajectories individuals are following—where they come from (in a biopsychosocial sense);

the contemporary biopsychosocial context (with its challenges and stress buffers); and future paths, goals, and aspirations. When personality is measured as part of a study or assessment, it is a snapshot of the person within his or her unique personal trajectory. Personality research suggests that one size does not fit all: An intervention may be quite effective but only for certain people, at certain times, under certain conditions. As we begin to understand the causal mechanisms, including the contexts in which a particular relationship holds, meaningful and enduring change becomes a greater possibility. Adding even a few questions to major health studies can be costly, but core aspects of personality can be simply and powerfully measured and should be incorporated into investigations and interventions. A side benefit is that as we better understand relations of health and personality, we better understand the nature of personality itself.

Conclusions

Health psychology has clearly established that long-term biopsychosocial processes are important to understanding and predicting health, well-being, and longevity. Such processes are a crucial complement to the traditional biomedical focus on treating acute disease and managing chronic illness, but there must be a new emphasis on preventing disease and promoting health throughout the lifespan. Interventions for this purpose have often been hard to imagine and difficult to study and implement due to the psychosocial complexity of human behavior and development. Modern understanding of personality provides a valuable tool with which to approach these multifaceted health issues.

Personality encapsulates a blend of the crucial elements. Personality has a biological base, revealed in studies of genetics, temperament, and psychophysiology. Personality is shaped by early intimate and family experiences, by socialization processes, and by later social relations. Personality emerges in a culture, which shapes behaviors, situations, and trajectories. Furthermore, personality has a certain temporal stability, yet it matures and changes. Thus, many of the fundamentals of the needed causal models and interventions are illuminated by a deeper understanding of personality and health.

The individual travels certain life courses or trajectories that have implications for health promotion. All in all, personality approaches suggest that there are multiple causal pathways between earlier psychosocial behavior patterns and later health and longevity, but they can gradually be teased apart. The same recommendations are not appropriate for each individual, but sensible and effective interventions will likely be available in the foreseeable future.

Acknowledgments

Preparation of this chapter was supported in part by National Institute on Aging Grant No. AG027001. Opinions expressed are those of the authors and not necessarily those of the National Institute on Aging.

Further Reading

Caspi, A., Roberts, B. W., & Shiner, R. L. (2005). Personality development: Stability and change. *Annual Review of Psychology, 56,* 453–484.

Friedman, H. S. (2007). Personality, disease, and self-healing. In H. S. Friedman & R. C. Silver (Eds.), *Foundations of health psychology* (pp. 172–199). New York: Oxford University Press.

Friedman, H. S. (2008). The multiple linkages of personality and disease. *Brain, Behavior, and Immunity, 22,* 668–675.

Hampson, S. E., & Friedman, H. S. (2008). Personality and health: A lifespan perspective. In O. P. John, R. W. Robins, & L. A. Pervin (Eds.), *The handbook of personality: Theory and research* (3rd ed., pp. 770–794). New York: Guilford Press.

Roberts, B. W., Kuncel, N. R., Shiner, R., Caspi, A., & Goldberg, L. R. (2007). The power of personality: The comparative validity of personality traits, socioeconomic status, and cognitive ability for predicting important life outcomes. *Perspectives on Psychological Science, 2,* 313–345.

Smith, T. W., & MacKenzie, J. (2006). Personality and risk of physical illness. *Annual Review of Clinical Psychology, 2,* 435–467.

Suls, J., & Bunde, J. (2005). Anger, anxiety, and depression as risk factors for cardiovascular disease: The problems and implications of overlapping affective dispositions. *Psychological Bulletin, 131,* 260–300.

References

Adams, T. B., & Mowen, J. C. (2005). Identifying the personality characteristics of healthy eaters and exercisers: A hierarchical model approach. *Health Marketing Quarterly, 23,* 21–42.

Aldwin, C. M., Spiro, A., Levenson, M. R., & Cupertino, A. P. (2001). Longitudinal findings from the Normative Aging Study: III. Personality, individual health trajectories, and mortality. *Psychology and Aging, 16,* 450–465.

Aldwin, C. M., Spiro, A., & Park, C. L. (2006). Health, behavior, and optimal aging: A life span developmental perspective. In J. E. Birren & K. W. Schaire (Eds.), *Handbook of the psychology of aging* (6th ed., pp. 85–104). Amsterdam: Elsevier.

Alexander, F. (1950). *Psychosomatic medicine: Its principles and applications.* New York: Norton.

Allemand, M., Zimprich, D., & Hertzog, C. (2007). Cross-sectional age differences and longitudinal age changes of personality in middle adulthood and old age. *Journal of Personality, 75,* 323–358.

Allemand, M., Zimprich, D., & Martin, M. (2008). Long-term correlated change in personality traits in old age. *Psychology and Aging, 23,* 545–557.

Almada, S. J., Zonderman, A. B., Shekelle, R. B., Dyer, A. R., Daviglus, M. L., Costa, P. T., Jr., et al. (1991). Neuroticism and cynicism and risk of death in middle-aged men: The Western Electric Study. *Psychosomatic Medicine, 53,* 165–175.

Baltes, P. B., Lindenberger, U., & Staudinger, U. M. (2006). Life span theory in developmental psychology. In R. M. Lerner & W. Damon (Eds.), *Handbook of child psychology: Vol. 1. Theoretical models of human development* (6th ed., pp. 569–664). Hoboken, NJ: Wiley.

Baltes, P. B., Staudinger, U. M., & Lindenberger, U. (1999). Lifespan psychology: Theory and application to intellectual functioning. *Annual Review of Psychology, 50,* 471–507.

Bandura, A. (1999). Social cognitive theory of personality. In L. A. Pervin & O. P. John (Eds.), *Handbook of personality: Theory and research* (2nd ed., pp. 154–196). New York: Guilford Press.

Barker, D. J. P., Osmond, C., Forsén, T. J., Kajantie, E., & Eriksson, J. G. (2005). Trajectories of growth among children who have coronary events as adults. *New England Journal of Medicine, 353,* 1802–1809.

Barrick, M. R., & Mount, M. K. (1991). The Big Five personality dimensions and job performance: A meta-analysis. *Personality Psychology, 44,* 1–26.

Batty, G. D., Deary, I. J., & Gottfredson, L. S. (2007). Premorbid (early life) IQ and later mortality risk: Systematic review. *Annals of Epidemiology, 17,* 278–288.

Batty, G. D., Deary, I. J., Schoon, I., & Gale, C.

R. (2007). Childhood mental ability in relation to food intake and physical activity in adulthood: The 1970 British Cohort Study. *Pediatrics, 119,* E38–E45.

Batty, G. D., Wennerstad, K. M., Smith, G. D., Gunnell, D., Deary, I. J., Tynelius, P., et al. (2009). IQ in early adulthood and mortality by middle age: Cohort study of 1 million Swedish men. *Epidemiology, 20,* 100–109.

Beier, M. E., & Ackerman, P. L. (2003). Determinants of health knowledge: An investigation of age, gender, abilities, personality, and interests. *Journal of Personality and Social Psychology, 84,* 439–448.

Bernard, C. (1880). *Leçons de pathologie expérimentale: Et leçons sur les propriétésde la moelle épinière* [Lessons of experimental pathology: And lessons on the properties of the spinal cord]. Paris: Librarie J.-B. Baillière.

Betz, B., & Thomas, C. (1979). Individual temperament as a predictor of health or premature disease. *John Hopkins Medical Journal, 44,* 81–89.

Bogg, T., & Roberts, B. W. (2004). Conscientiousness and health-related behaviors: A meta-analysis of the leading behavioral contributors to mortality. *Psychological Bulletin, 130,* 887–919.

Bogg, T., Voss, M. W., Wood, D., & Roberts, B. W. (2008). A hierarchical investigation of personality and behavior: Examining neo-socioanalytic models of health-related outcomes. *Journal of Research in Personality, 42,* 183–207

Bolger, N., & Zuckerman, A. (1995). A framework for studying personality in the stress process. *Journal of Personality and Social Psychology, 69,* 890–902.

Bondy, B. (2007). Common genetic factors for depression and cardiovascular disease. *Dialogues in Clinical Neuroscience, 9,* 19–28.

Brown, D. J., Cober, R. T., Kane, K., Levy, P. E., & Shalhoop, J. (2006). Proactive personality and the successful job search: A field investigation with college graduates. *Journal of Applied Psychology, 91,* 717–726.

Buss, D. M. (1987). Selection, evocation, and manipulation. *Journal of Personality and Social Psychology, 53,* 1214–1221.

Campbell, D. T., & Fiske, D. W. (1959). Convergent and discriminant validation by the multitrait–multimethod matrix. *Psychological Bulletin, 56,* 81–105.

Canli, T. (2004). Functional brain mapping of extraversion and neuroticism: Learning from individual differences in emotion processing. [Special issue]. *Journal of Personality, 72,* 1105–1132.

Cannon, W. B. (1932). *Wisdom of the body.* New York: Norton.

Carver, C. S., & Miller, C. J. (2006). Relations of serotonin function to personality: Current views and a key methodological issue. *Psychiatry Research, 144,* 1–15.

Caspi, A., Begg, D., Dickson, N., Harrington, H., Langley, J., Moffitt, T. E., et al. (1997). Personality differences predict health-risk behaviors in young adulthood: Evidence from a longitudinal study. *Journal of Personality and Social Psychology, 73,* 1052–1063.

Caspi, A., & Bem, D. J. (1990). Personality continuity and change across the life course. In L. Pervin (Ed.), *Handbook of personality: Theory and research* (pp. 549–575). New York: Guilford Press.

Caspi, A., Roberts, B. W., & Shiner, R. L. (2005). Personality development: Stability and change. *Annual Review of Psychology, 56,* 453–484.

Caspi, A., & Silva, P. A. (1995). Temperamental qualities at age 3 predict personality traits in young adulthood: Longitudinal evidence from a birth cohort. *Child Development, 66,* 486–498.

Cavigelli, S. A. (2005). Animal personality and health. *Behaviour, 142,* 1223–1244.

Chapman, B., Duberstein, P., & Lyness, J. M. (2007). Personality traits, education, and health-related quality of life among older adult primary care patients. *Journals of Gerontology B: Psychological Sciences and Social Sciences, 62,* P343–P352.

Charles, S. T., Gatz, M., Kato, K., & Pedersen, N. L. (2008). Physical health 25 years later: The predictive ability of neuroticism. *Health Psychology, 27,* 369–378.

Chesney, M. A., & Rosenman, R. H. (Eds.). (1985). *Anger and hostility in cardiovascular and behavioral disorders.* Washington, DC: Hemisphere.

Christensen, A. J., Ehlers, S. L., Wiebe, J. S., Moran, P. J., Raichle, K., Ferneyhough, K., et al. (2002). Patient personality and mortality: A 4-year prospective examination of chronic renal insufficiency. *Health Psychology, 21,* 315–320.

Cloninger, C. R. (2005). How does personality influence mortality in the elderly? *Psychosomatic Medicine, 67,* 839–840.

Conley, J. J. (1985). Longitudinal stability of personality traits: A multitrait–multimethod–multioccasion analysis. *Journal of Personality and Social Psychology, 49,* 1266–1282.

Costa, P. T., & McCrae, R. R. (1987). Neuroticism, somatic complaints, and disease: Is the bark worse than the bite? [Special issue]. *Journal of Personality, 55,* 299–316.

Costa, P. T., Terracciano, A., & McCrae, R. R. (2001). Gender differences in personality traits across cultures: Robust and surprising findings. *Journal of Personality and Social Psychology, 81,* 322–331.

Crant, J. M. (2000). Proactive behavior in organizations. *Journal of Management, 26,* 435–462.

Cronbach, L. J., & Meehl, P. E. (1955). Construct validity in psychological tests. *Psychological Bulletin, 52*, 281–302.

Deary, I., Batty, G. D., Pattie, A., & Gale, C. R. (2008). More intelligent, more dependable children live longer: A 55-year longitudinal study of a representative sample of the Scottish nation. *Psychological Science, 19*, 874–880.

Deary, I. J., Whiteman, M. C., Starr, J. M., Whalley, L. J., & Fox, H. C. (2004). The impact of childhood intelligence on later life: Following up the Scottish Mental Surveys of 1932 and 1947. *Journal of Personality and Social Psychology, 86*, 130–147.

DeNeve, K. M., & Cooper, H. (1998). The happy personality: A meta-analysis of 137 personality traits and subjective well-being. *Psychological Bulletin, 124*, 197–229.

Diehr, P., & Patrick, D. L. (2003). Trajectories of health for older adults over time: Accounting fully for death. *Annuals of Internal Medicine, 139*, 416–420.

Duberstein, P. R., Seidlitz, L., Lyness, J. M., & Conwell, Y. (1999). Dimensional measures and the five-factor model: Clinical implications and research directions. In E. Rosowsky, R. C. Abrams, & R. A. Zweig (Eds.), *Personality disorders in older adults: Emerging issues in diagnosis and treatment* (pp. 95–117). Mahwah, NJ: Erlbaum.

Dunbar, F. (1955). *Mind and body: Psychosomatic medicine* (2nd ed.). New York: Crown.

ENRICHD Investigators. (2003). Effects of treating depression and low perceived social support on clinical events after myocardial infarction: The Enhancing Recovery in Coronary Heart Disease Patients (ENRICHD) randomized trial. *Journal of the American Medical Association, 289*, 3106–3116.

Erdogan, B., & Bauer, T. N. (2005). Enhancing career benefits of employee proactive personality: The role of fit with jobs and organizations. *Personnel Psychology, 58*, 859–891.

Evans, D. E., & Rothbart, M. K. (2007). Developing a model for adult temperament. *Journal of Research in Personality, 41*, 868–888.

Ferraro, K. F., & Nuriddin, T. A. (2006). Psychological distress and mortality: Are women more vulnerable? *Journal of Health and Social Behavior, 47*, 227–241.

Figueredo, A. J., Vásquez, G., Brumbach, B. H., Sefcek, J. A., Kirsner, B. R., & Jacobs, W. J. (2005). The K-factor: Individual differences in life history strategy. *Personality and Individual Differences, 39*, 1349–1360.

Fredrickson, B. L. (2001). The role of positive emotions in positive psychology: The broaden-and-build theory of positive emotions. *American Psychologist, 56*, 218–226.

Friedman, H. S. (1991). *The self-healing personality*. New York: Holt.

Friedman, H. S. (2000). Long-term relations of personality, health: Dynamisms, mechanisms, and tropisms. *Journal of Personality, 68*, 1089–1107.

Friedman, H. S. (2007). Personality, disease, and self-healing. In H. S. Friedman & R. C. Silver (Eds.), *Foundations of health psychology* (pp. 172–199). New York: Oxford University Press.

Friedman, H. S. (2008). The multiple linkages of personality and disease. *Brain, Behavior, and Immunity, 22*, 668–675.

Friedman, H. S., & Booth-Kewley, S. (1987). The "disease-prone personality": A meta-analytic view of the construct. *American Psychologist, 42*, 539–555.

Friedman, H. S., Kern, M. L., & Reynolds, C. A. (2010). Personality and health, subjective well-being, and longevity as adults age. *Journal of Personality, 78*, 179–215.

Friedman, H. S., & Markey, C. N. (2003). Paths to longevity in the highly intelligent Terman cohort. In C. E. Finch, J.-M. Robine, & Y. Christen (Eds.), *Brain and longevity* (pp. 165–175). New York: Springer.

Friedman, H. S., Tucker, J. S., Schwartz, J. E., Martin, L. R., Tomlinson-Keasey, C., Wingard, D., et al. (1995). Childhood conscientiousness and longevity: Health behaviors and cause of death. *Journal of Personality and Social Psychology, 68*, 696–703.

Friedman, H. S., Tucker, J. S., Tomlinson-Keasey, C., Schwartz, J. E., Wingard, D. L., & Criqui, M. H. (1993). Does childhood personality predict longevity? *Journal of Personality and Social Psychology, 65*, 176–185.

Gelissen, J., & de Graaf, P. M. (2006). Personality, social background, and occupational career success. *Social Science Research, 35*, 702–726.

Goldberg, L. R. (1993). The structure of phenotypic personality traits. *American Psychologist, 48*, 26–34.

Goodwin, R., & Engstrom, G. (2002). Personality and the perception of health in the general population. *Psychological Medicine, 32*, 325–332.

Gosling, S. D., & John, O. P. (1999). Personality dimensions in nonhuman animals: A cross-species review. *Current Directions in Psychological Science, 8*, 69–75.

Graham, J. E., Christian, L. M., & Kiecolt-Glaser, J. K. (2006). Stress, age, and immune function: Toward a lifespan approach. *Journal of Behavioral Medicine, 29*, 389–400.

Greven, C., Chamorro-Premuzic, T., Arteche, A., & Furnham, A. (2008). A hierarchical integration of dispositional determinants of general health in students: The Big Five, trait emotional intelligence and humour styles. *Personality and Individual Differences, 44*, 1562–1573.

Gruenewald, T. L., Mroczek, D. K., Ryff, C. D., & Singer, B. H. (2008). Diverse pathways to positive and negative affect in adulthood and later life: An integrative approach using recursive partitioning. *Developmental Psychology, 44,* 330–343.

Guarino, L., Roger, D., & Olason, D. T. (2007). Reconstructing N: A new approach to measuring emotional sensitivity. *Current Psychology, 26,* 37–45.

Hampson, S. E., & Friedman, H. S. (2008). Personality and health: A lifespan perspective. In O. P. John, R. W. Robins, & L. A. Pervin (Eds.), *The handbook of personality: Theory and research* (3rd ed., pp. 770–794). New York: Guilford Press.

Hampson, S. E., Goldberg, L. R., Vogt, T. M., & Dubanoski, J. P. (2007). Mechanisms by which childhood personality traits influence adult health status: Educational attainment and healthy behaviors. *Health Psychology, 26,* 121–125.

Hart, C. L., Taylor, M. D., Smith, G. D., Whalley, L. J., Hole, D. J., Wilson, V., et al. (2004). Childhood IQ and cardiovascular disease in adulthood: Prospective observational study linking the Scottish Mental Survey 1932 and the midspan studies. *Social Science and Medicine, 59,* 2131–2138.

Held, B. B. (2004). The negative side of positive psychology. *Journal of Humanistic Psychology, 44,* 9–46.

Hemmingsson, T., Essen, J. V., Melin, B., Allebeck, P., & Lundberg, I. (2007). The association between cognitive ability measured at ages 18–20 and coronary heart disease in middle age among men: A prospective study using the Swedish 1969 conscription cohort. *Social Science and Medicine, 65,* 1410–1419.

Hertzog, C., & Nesselroade, J. R. (2003). Assessing psychological change in adulthood: An overview of methodological issues. *Psychology and Aging, 18,* 639–657.

Howell, R., Kern, M. L., & Lyubomirsky, S. (2007). Health benefits: Meta-analytically determining the impact of well-being on objective health outcomes. *Health Psychology Review, 1,* 83–136.

Ickes, W., Snyder, M., & Garcia, S. (1997). Personality influences on the choice of situations. In R. Hogan, J. Johnson, & S. Briggs (Eds.), *Handbook of personality psychology* (pp. 165–195). San Diego, CA: Academic Press.

Jerram, K. L., & Coleman, P. G. (1999). The Big Five personality traits and reporting of health problems and health behaviour in old age. *British Journal of Health Psychology, 4,* 181–192.

Johnson, W., McGue, M., Krueger, R. J., & Bouchard, T. J., Jr. (2004). Marriage and personality: A genetic analysis. *Journal of Personality and Social Psychology, 86,* 285–294.

Jones, S. M. (2008). Maternal cortisol as a mediator of prenatal stress and infant regulation development. *Dissertation Abstracts International B: Sciences and Engineering, 69,* 681.

Kaplan, R. M. (1994). The Ziggy theorem: Toward an outcomes-focused health psychology. *Health Psychology, 13,* 451–460.

Kaplan, R. M. (2003). The significance of quality of life in health care. *Quality of Life Research, 12,* 3–16.

Kaplan, R. M. (2007). Uncertainty, variability, and resource allocation in the health care decision process. In H. S. Friedman & R. C. Silver (Eds.), *Foundations of health psychology* (pp. 358–383). New York: Oxford University Press.

Kemeny, M. E. (2007). Psychoneuroimmunology. In H. S. Friedman & R. C. Silver (Eds.), *Foundations of health psychology* (pp. 92–116). New York: Oxford University Press.

Kern, M. L., & Friedman, H. S. (2008). Do conscientious individuals live longer?: A quantitative review. *Health Psychology, 27,* 505–512.

Kern, M. L., Friedman, H. S., Martin, L. R., Reynolds, C. A., & Luong, G. (2009). Conscientiousness, career success, and longevity: A lifespan analysis. *Annals of Behavioral Medicine, 37,* 154–163.

Korotkov, D., & Hannah, T. E. (2004). The five-factor model of personality: Strengths and limitations in predicting health status, sick-role and illness behaviour. *Personality and Individual Differences, 36,* 187–199.

Korten, A. E., Jorm, A. F., Jiao, Z., Letenneur, L., Jacomb, P. A., Henderson, A. S., et al. (1999). Health, cognitive, and psychosocial factors as predictors of mortality in an elderly community sample. *Journal of Epidemiology and Community Health, 53,* 83–88.

Kuh, D., & Ben-Shlomo, Y. (Eds.). (1997). *A life course approach to chronic disease epidemiology.* New York: Oxford University Press.

Kusumi, I., Suzuki, K., Sasaki, Y., Kameda, K., Sasaki, T., & Koyama, T. (2002). Serotonin $5\text{-}HT_{2A}$ receptor gene polymorphism, $5\text{-}HT_{2A}$ receptor function and personality traits in healthy subjects: A negative study. *Journal of Affective Disorders, 68,* 235–241.

Larson, J. H., & Holman, T. B. (1994). Premarital predictors of marital quality and stability. *Family Relations: Interdisciplinary Journal of Applied Family Studies, 43,* 228–237.

Leclerc, J., Rahn, M., & Linden, W. (2006). Does personality predict blood pressure over a 10-year period? *Personality and Individual Differences, 40,* 1313–1321.

Little, T. D., Bovaird, J. A., & Slegers, D. W. (2006). Methods for the analysis of change. In D. K. Mroczek & T. D. Little (Eds.), *Handbook of personality development* (pp. 181–211). Mahwah, NJ: Erlbaum.

Lyubomirsky, S., King, L., & Diener, E. (2005). The benefits of frequent positive affect: Does happiness lead to success? *Psychological Bulletin, 131,* 803–855.

MacKinnon, D. P., & Luecken, L. J. (2008). How and for whom?: Mediation and moderation in health psychology. *Health Psychology, 27,* S99–S100.

Maddi, S. R., & Kobasa, S. C. (1984). *The hardy executive: Health under stress.* Chicago: Dow Jones-Irwin.

Magnus, K., Diener, E., Fujita, F., & Payot, W. (1993). Extraversion and neuroticism as predictors of objective life events: A longitudinal analysis. *Journal of Personality and Social Psychology, 65,* 1046–1053.

Manuck, S. B., Flory, J. D., McCaffery, J. M., Matthews, K. A., Mann, J. J., & Muldoon, M. F. (1998). Aggression, impulsivity, and central nervous system serotonergic responsivity in a nonpatient sample. *Neuropsychopharmacology, 19,* 287–299.

Markey, C. N., Markey, P. M., & Tinsley, B. J. (2003). Personality, puberty, and preadolescent girls' risky behaviors: Examining the predictive value of the five-factor model of personality. *Journal of Research in Personality, 37,* 405–419.

Martin, L. R., & Friedman, H. S. (2000). Comparing personality scales across time: An illustrative study of validity and consistency in life-span archival data. *Journal of Personality, 68,* 85–110.

Martin, L. R., Friedman, H. S., & Schwartz, J. E. (2007). Personality and mortality risk across the lifespan: The importance of conscientiousness as a biopsychosocial attribute. *Health Psychology, 26,* 428–436.

McArdle, J. J., Small, B. J., Backman, L., & Fratiglioni, L. (2005). Longitudinal models of growth and survival applied to early detection of Alzheimer's disease. *Journal of Geriatric Psychiatry and Neurology, 18,* 234–241.

McCaffrey, J. M., Frasure-Smith, N., Dubé, M. P., Théroux, P., Rouleau, G. A., Duan, Q., et al. (2006). Common genetic vulnerability to depressive symptoms and coronary artery disease: A review and development of candidate genes related to inflammation and serotonin. *Psychosomatic Medicine, 68,* 187–200.

McCrae, R. R., Costa, P. T., Jr., Ostendorf, F., Angleitner, A., Hrebickova, M., Avia, M. D., et al. (2000). Nature over nurture: Temperament, personality, and lifespan development. *Journal of Personality and Social Psychology, 78,* 173–186.

McCrae, R. R., Jang, K. L., Livesley, W. J., Riemann, R., & Angleitner, A. (2001). Sources of structure: Genetic, environmental, and artifactual influences on the covariation of personality traits. *Journal of Personality, 69,* 511–535.

McEwen, B. S. (2006). Protective and damaging effects of stress mediators: Central role of the brain. *Dialogues in Clinical Neuroscience, 8,* 283–293.

Mehta, P. H., & Gosling, S. D. (2008). Bridging human and animal research: A comparative approach to studies of personality and health. *Brain, Behavior, and Immunity, 22,* 651–661.

Miller, G. E., Cohen, S., Rabin, B. S., Skoner, D. P., & Doyle, W. J. (1999). Personality and tonic cardiovascular, neuroendocrine, and immune parameters. *Brain, Behavior, and Immunity, 13,* 109–123.

Moor, C., Zimprich, D., Schmitt, M., & Kliegel, M. (2006). Personality, aging self-perceptions, and subjective health: A mediation model. *International Journal of Aging and Human Development, 63,* 241–257.

Mroczek, D. K., & Spiro, A., III. (2007). Personality change influences mortality in older men. *Psychological Science, 18,* 371–376.

Nesselroade, J. R. (1991). The warp and woof of the developmental fabric. In R. Downs, L. Liben, & D. Palarmo (Eds.), *Visions of development, the environment, and aesthetics: The legacy of Joachim F. Wohlwill* (pp. 213–240). Hillsdale, NJ: Erlbaum.

Neupert, S. D., Mroczek, D. K., & Spiro, A., III. (2008). Neuroticism moderates the daily relation between stressors and memory failures. *Psychology and Aging, 23,* 287–296.

O'Cleirigh, C., Ironson, G., Weiss, A., & Costa, P. T. (2007). Conscientiousness predicts disease progression (CD4 number and viral load) in people living with HIV. *Health Psychology, 26,* 473–480.

O'Connor, M. C., & Paunonen, S. V. (2007). Big Five personality predictors of post-secondary academic performance. *Personality and Individual Differences, 43,* 971–990.

Ormel, J., Rosmalen, J., & Farmer, A. (2004). Neuroticism: A non-informative marker of vulnerability to psychopathology. *Social Psychiatry and Psychiatric Epidemiology, 39,* 906–912.

O'Toole, B. I. (1990). Intelligence and behaviour and motor vehicle accident mortality. *Accident Analysis and Prevention, 22,* 211–221.

Ozer, D. J., & Benet-Martinez, V. (2006). Personality and the prediction of consequential outcomes. *Annual Review of Psychology, 57,* 401–421.

Pedersen, N. L., & Reynolds, C. A. (1998). Stability and change in adult personality: Genetic and environmental components. *European Journal of Personality, 12,* 365–386.

Pressman, S. D., & Cohen, S. (2005). Does positive affect influence health? *Psychological Bulletin, 131,* 925–971.

Puttonen, S., Elovainio, M., Kivimäki, M., Koskinen, T., Pulkki-Råback, L., Viikari, J. S.

A., et al. (2008). Temperament, health-related behaviors, and autonomic cardiac regulation: The cardiovascular risk in young Finns study. *Biological Psychology, 78,* 204–210.

Räikkönen, K., Matthews, K. A., & Kuller, L. H. (2002). The relationship between psychological risk attributes and the metabolic syndrome in healthy women: Antecedent or consequences? *Metabolism, 51,* 1573–1577.

Rhodes, R. E., & Smith, N. E. I. (2006). Personality correlates of physical activity: A review and meta-analysis. *British Journal of Sports Medicine, 40,* 958–965.

Roberts, B. W., Caspi, A., & Moffitt, T. (2003). Work experiences and personality development in young adulthood. *Journal of Personality and Social Psychology, 84,* 582–593.

Roberts, B. W., Helson, R., & Klohnen, E. C. (2002). Personality development and growth in women across 30 years: Three perspectives. *Journal of Personality, 70,* 79–102.

Roberts, B. W., Kuncel, N. R., Shiner, R., Caspi, A., & Goldberg, L. R. (2007). The power of personality: The comparative validity of personality traits, socioeconomic status, and cognitive ability for predicting important life outcomes. *Perspectives on Psychological Science, 2,* 313–345.

Roberts, B. W., & Pomerantz, E. M. (2004). On traits, situations, and their integration: A developmental perspective. *Personality and Social Psychology Review, 8,* 402–416.

Roberts, B. W., Walton, K. E., & Bogg, T. (2005). Conscientiousness and health across the life course. *Review of General Psychology, 9,* 156–168.

Roberts, B. W., Walton, K. E., & Viechtbauer, W. (2006). Patterns of mean-level change in personality traits across the lifespan: A meta-analysis of longitudinal studies. *Psychological Bulletin, 132,* 1–25.

Roberts, B. W., Wood, D., & Caspi, A. (2008). The development of personality traits in adulthood. In O. P. John, R. W. Robins, & L. A. Pervin (Eds.), *The handbook of personality: Theory and research* (3rd ed., pp. 375–398). New York: Guilford Press.

Rook, K. S., Charles, S. T., & Heckhausen, J. (2007). Aging and health. In H. S. Friedman & R. C. Silver (Eds.), *Foundations of health psychology* (pp. 234–262). New York: Oxford University Press.

Rutter, M., Kim-Cohen, J., & Maughan, B. (2006). Continuities and discontinuities in psychopathology from childhood to adult life. *Journal of Child Psychology and Psychiatry, 47,* 276–295.

Scarr, S., & McCartney, K. (1983). How people make their own environments: A theory of genotype → environment effects. *Child Development, 54,* 424–435.

Schmidt, F. L., & Hunter, J. E. (1992). Development of a causal model of processes determining job performance. *Current Directions in Psychological Science, 1,* 89–92.

Schultz, R., & Heckhausen, J. (1996). A life span model of successful aging. *American Psychologist, 51,* 702–714.

Schwartz, J. E., Friedman, H. S., Tucker, J. S., Tomlinson-Keasey, C., Wingard, D. L., & Criqui, M. H. (1995). Sociodemographic and psychosocial factors in childhood as predictors of adult mortality. *American Journal of Public Health, 85,* 1237–1245.

Segerstrom, S. C. (2000). Personality and the immune system: Models, methods, and mechanisms. *Annals of Behavioral Medicine, 22,* 180–190.

Segerstrom, S. C. (2005). Optimism and immunity: Do positive thoughts always lead to positive effects? *Brain, Behavior, and Immunity, 19,* 195–200.

Segerstrom, S. C., & Miller, G. E. (2004). Psychological stress and the human immune system: A meta-analytic study of 30 years of inquiry. *Psychological Bulletin, 104,* 601–630.

Seibert, S. E., Crant, J. M., & Kraimer, M. L. (1999). Proactive personality and career success. *Journal of Applied Psychology, 84,* 416–427.

Singer, J. D., & Willett, J. B. (2003). *Applied longitudinal data analysis: Modeling change and event occurrence.* Oxford, UK: Oxford University Press.

Smith, T. W. (2006). Personality as risk and resilience in physical health. *Current Directions in Psychological Science, 15,* 227–231.

Smith, T. W., & Gallo, L. C. (2001). Personality traits as risk factors for physical illness. In A. Baum, T. Revenson, & J. Singer (Eds.), *Handbook of health psychology* (pp. 139–172). Hillsdale, NJ: Erlbaum.

Smith, T. W., & MacKenzie, J. (2006). Personality and risk of physical illness. *Annual Review of Clinical Psychology, 2,* 435–467.

Srivastava, S., John, O. P., Gosling, S. D., & Potter, J. (2003). Development of personality in early and middle adulthood: Set like plaster or persistent change? *Journal of Personality and Social Psychology, 84,* 1041–1053.

Sroufe, L. A., Carlson, E. A., Levy, A. K., & Egeland, B. (1999). Implications of attachment theory for developmental psychopathology. *Development and Psychopathology, 11,* 1–13.

Steel, P., Schmidt, J., & Shultz, J. (2008). Refining the relationship between personality and subjective well-being. *Psychological Bulletin, 134,* 138–161.

Suls, J., & Bunde, J. (2005). Anger, anxiety, and depression as risk factors for cardiovascular disease: The problems and implications of overlapping affective dispositions. *Psychological Bulletin, 131,* 260–300.

Suls, J., & Rothman, A. (2004). Evolution of the biopsychosocial model: Prospects and challenges for health psychology. *Health Psychology, 23,* 119–125.

Taga, K. A., Friedman, H. S., & Martin, L. R. (2009). Early personality traits as predictors of mortality risk following conjugal bereavement. *Journal of Personality, 77,* 669–690.

Taylor, M. D., Hart, C. L., Davey Smith, G., Starr, J. M., Hole, D. J., Whalley, L. J., et al. (2003). Childhood mental ability and smoking cessation in adulthood: Prospective observational study linking the Scottish Mental Survey 1932 and the Midspan studies. *Journal of Epidemiology and Community Health, 57,* 464–465.

Terracciano, A., Lockenhoff, C. E., Zonderman, A. B., Ferrucci, L., & Costa, P. T. (2008). Personality predictors of longevity: Activity, emotional stability, and conscientiousness. *Psychosomatic Medicine, 70,* 621–627.

Tucker, J. S., Friedman, H. S., Schwartz, J. E., Criqui, M. H., Tomlinson-Keasey, C., Wingard, D. L., et al. (1997). Parental divorce: Effects on individual behavior and longevity. *Journal of Personality and Social Psychology, 73,* 381–391.

Tucker, J. S., Friedman, H. S., Wingard, D. L., & Schwartz, J. E. (1996). Marital history at midlife as a predictor of longevity: Alternative explanations to the protective effect of marriage. *Health Psychology, 15,* 94–101.

Twenge, J. M. (2000). The age of anxiety?: Birth cohort change in anxiety and neuroticism, 1952–1993. *Journal of Personality and Social Psychology, 79,* 1007–1021.

Twenge, J. M. (2001). Birth cohort changes in extraversion: A cross-temporal meta-analysis, 1966–1993. *Personality and Individual Differences, 30,* 735–748.

U.S. Department of Health and Human Services. (2000). *Healthy People 2010: Understanding and improving health* (2nd ed.). Washington, DC: U.S. Government Printing Office.

Van Heck, G. (1997). Personality and physical health: Toward an ecological approach to health-related personality research. *European Journal of Personality, 11,* 415–443.

Vollrath, M. E., & Torgersen, S. (2008). Personality types and risky health behaviors in Norwegian students. *Scandinavian Journal of Psychology, 49,* 287–292.

Wadhwa, P. D. (2005). Psychoneuroendocrine processes in human pregnancy influence fetal development and health. *Psychoneuroendocrinology, 30,* 724–743.

Wand, G. S., McCaul, M., Yang, X., Reynolds, J., Gotjen, D., Lee, S., et al. (2002). The mu-opinid receptor gene polymorphism (A118G) alters HPA axis activation induced by opioid receptor blockade. *Neuropsychopharmacology, 26,* 106–114.

Watson, D., & Hubbard, B. (1996). Adaptational style and dispositional structure: Coping in the context of the five-factor model. *Journal of Personality, 64,* 737, 774.

Watson, D., & Pennebaker, J. W. (1989). Health complaints, stress, and distress: Exploring the central role of negative affectivity. *Psychological Review, 96,* 234–254.

Weiss, A., & Costa, P. T. (2005). Domain and facet personality predictors of all-cause mortality among Medicare patients aged 65 to 100. *Psychosomatic Medicine, 67,* 724–733.

Whalley, L. J., & Deary, I. J. (2001). Longitudinal cohort study of childhood IQ and survival up to age 76. *British Medical Journal, 322,* 819–822.

Whiteman, M. C. (2006). Personality, cardiovascular disease and public health. In M. E. Vollrath (Ed.), *Handbook of personality and health* (pp. 13–34). Hoboken, NJ: Wiley.

Williams, P. G., O'Brien, C. D., & Colder, C. R. (2004). The effects of neuroticism and extraversion on self-assessed health and health-relevant cognition. *Personality and Individual Differences, 37,* 83–94.

Williams, R. B., Kuhn, C. M., Helms, M. J., Siegler, I. C., Barefoot, J. C., Ashley-Kocy, A., et al. (2004). *Central nervous system (CNS) serotonin function and NEO-PI personality profiles.* Presented at the 62nd Annual Meeting of the American Psychosomatic Society, Orlando, FL.

Wilson, R. S., Krueger, K. R., Gu, L., Bienias, J. L., Mendes de Leon, C. F., & Evans, D. A. (2005). Neuroticism, extraversion, and mortality in a defined population of older persons. *Psychosomatic Medicine, 67,* 841–845.

Wilson, R. S., Mendes de Leon, C. F., Bienias, J. L., Evans, D. A., & Bennett, D. A. (2004). Personality and mortality in old age. *Journals of Gerontology B: Psychological Sciences and Social Sciences, 59,* P110–P116.

World Health Organization. (1948). Preamble to the constitution of the World Health Organization as adopted by the International Health Conference. *Official Records of the World Health Organization, 2,* 100.

Yamasue, H., Abe, O., Suga, M., Yamada, H., Inoue, H., Tochigi, M., et al. (2008). Gender-common and -specific neuroanatomical basis of human anxiety-related personality traits. *Cerebral Cortex, 18,* 46–52.

Zweig, D., & Webster, J. (2004). What are we measuring?: An examination of the relationships between the Big-Five personality traits, goal orientation, and performance intentions. *Personality and Individual Differences, 36,* 1693–1708.

CHAPTER 8

Anger, Anger Expression, and Health

Padmini Iyer
Maya Rom Korin
Laura Higginbotham
Karina W. Davidson

Although all emotions play a pivotal role in physical and mental health, anger holds a special place in past research, clinical care delivery, and the future of health psychology. All other emotions are to some extent diagnosed, investigated, and treated by other professions. Anger, on the other hand, is the "orphan" emotion whose definition, measurement, development, and interaction with health are all intimately entwined in the development of the field of health psychology (DiGiuseppe & Tafrate, 2007). Authoritative reviews of this history already exist (Siegman, 1994), so we focus on the evidence base developed by health psychology about the interplay of anger, angry expression or behavior, and health. We briefly review the multidimensional definitions of anger and related constructs, then provide information on the major theories from psychology and related fields on anger. Major findings on the ways that anger and its expression predict health are then reviewed, as well as possible biological and behavioral mechanisms that might be implicated in the association of anger and health. Finally, intervention studies that have attempted to modify anger and anger behavior are reviewed. Due to the paucity of research solely on anger, our focus is on anger and anger expression, even though some of the findings are about highly correlated constructs, such as hostility and aggression. We conclude with ways that health psychologists can continue to advance our knowledge and understanding of anger, anger expression, and health.

The Multidimensional Nature of Anger

Anger may be defined as "an emotional state that consists of feelings that vary in intensity from mild irritation or annoyance to intense fury and rage" (Spielberger, Jacobs, Russell, & Crane, 1983, p. 160), most often in response to perceived mistreatment, provocation, or exploitation (Kassinove & Sukhodolsky, 1995; Nesse, 1990). Moreover, anger can be perceived as both an emotional response and an enduring personality trait (Spielberger et al., 1985). Although older definitions of anger were simplistic, newer definitions treat it as a complex set of physiological, cognitive, and emotional variables

(Eckhardt, Norlander, & Deffenbacher, 2004; Kassinove & Sukhodolsky, 1995). The one commonality among the many conceptualizations, however disparate they may be, is that anger is a basic emotion that sometimes leads to aggressive or anger expression and is subjectively aversive (Luutonen, 2007; Mayne & Ambrose, 1999). There has been considerable debate about the definitions of anger and hostility (Barefoot, 1992; Houston, 1994; Martin, Watson, & Wan, 2000; Miller, Smith, Turner, Guijarro, & Hallet, 1996; Siegman, 1994), and although the discussion continues, we adopt the conceptualization of Martin and colleagues (2000) and others (Barefoot, Dodge, Peterson, Dahlstrom, & Williams, 1989), who describe anger/hostility as having three dimensions: an affective dimension that includes feelings of anger, irritation, rage, and disgust; a cognitive dimension that includes cynical attitudes and suspiciousness; and finally, a behavioral dimension that includes verbal and physical aggression. The first and last dimensions are the focus of this chapter.

Various scales (e.g., Anger Inventory, Reaction Inventory, Anger Response Scale, Framingham Anger Scale, Anger Self-Report Scale, and Multidimensional Anger Inventory) have been created to measure the different dimensions of anger (Biaggio, 1980; Biaggio, Supplee, & Curtis, 1981; Catchlove, Cohen, Braha, & Demers-Desrosiers, 1985; Siegel, 1985; Spielberger et al., 1985; Spielberger, Reheiser, & Sydeman, 1995). Common measures of anger include the Spielberger Trait Anger Scale, a 20-item self-report measure; and the Minnesota Multiphasic Personality Inventory (MMPI) Anger subscale and various other subscales. The Cook–Medley Scale has most commonly measured hostility. Other assessment tools, such as the Buss–Durkee Hostility Inventory and the Cook–Medley Hostility Scale, although they assess hostility, are sometime used to assess specific dimensions of anger (Biaggio, 1980; Biaggio et al., 1981; Gidron & Davidson, 1996). A major issue, then, is the number of basic anger and anger expression dimensions. From an empirical perspective, factor analyses of the various measures of anger have generally resulted in a two-factor structure (Bendig, 1962; Buss & Durkee, 1957; Edmunds & Kendrick, 1980; Musante, MacDougall, Dembroski,

& Costa, 1989; Zelin, Adler, & Myerson, 1972). These two factors are typically labeled the "experience" and "expression" of anger/hostility. When three factors are found, the third is typically a "cognitive" or "attitudinal" facet of anger/hostility (Musante et al., 1989). Stoney and Engebretson (1994) considered the multidimensionality of anger from a theoretical perspective. They reviewed biological, social learning, social cognitive, and drive theories as they relate to the development, maintenance, and control of anger behavior, and concluded that there may be dimensions of anger expression that are typically not assessed, such as communicative anger expression. They urged researchers to consider these additional anger behavior dimensions and suggested that the motivation for anger expression is a particularly important consideration.

The Multidimensional Nature of Angry Expression/Behavior

There are a number of conceptualizations and measures of the behavioral dimension of anger/hostility. For example, Friedman and Rosenman (1959) first described extremes of competitiveness–achievement striving, aggressiveness–hostility, and speed–impatience as a manifestation of the Type A behavioral pattern, which is thought to put persons at considerable risk for stress and disease. This conceptualization resulted in a standardized interview (Dembroski, MacDougall, Shields, Petitto, & Lushene, 1978) to assess anger expression. Buss and Durkee (1957) conceptualized aggressiveness as including assault, indirect aggression, irritability, and verbal aggression, and they developed a self-report measure for assessing these behavioral tendencies. This measure was then substantially revised by (Buss & Perry, 1992) to assess four dimensions, of which the first two are behavioral (physical aggression, verbal aggression, anger, and hostility). Spielberger and colleagues (1985) constructed a self-report measure of anger expression based on a unidimensional classification system (Gentry, Chesney, Gary, Hall, & Harburg, 1982; Harburg, Gleiberman, Russell, & Cooper, 1991; Julius, Harburg, Schork, & DiFranceisco, 1992) but found that self-reported anger-in and anger-out items comprised two separate and independent factors rather than a single dimension. The Anger-In/Anger-Out subscale, developed by Harburg and colleagues (1973), asks respondents to imagine a number of difficult interpersonal situations and indicate their likely response (Martin & Watson, 1997). This conceptualization of anger-in (how often angry feelings are experienced but not expressed) and anger-out (how often angry feelings are expressed in verbally or physically aggressive behavior) has remained the predominant view of anger expression (Spielberger et al., 1995). But the Anger-In/Anger-Out subscale has been criticized for its limitations, particularly due to its dichotomous nature (Martin &Watson, 1997). Siegel (1985) has additionally offered a self-report measure of anger experience and behavior, the Multidimensional Anger Inventory, which contains five subscales: Anger-In, Anger-Out, Anger Talk, Anger Frequency, and Hostility. Therefore, some scales have been developed not only to measure anger but also to analyze style of anger expression. While many measures of anger experience, hostility, and anger expression exist, no "gold standard" measure exists for assessing anger and its dimensions.

Conceptualizations and Theories of Anger

In terms of theories and research, anger has received far less attention than other negative emotions, which may stem in part from the lack of agreement about the definition and dimensionality of the anger construct. While theories on anger and its cognitive and behavioral correlates, hostility and anger expression, have been topics of discussion since ancient times, there is an obvious lack of unity among them. Scholars in the ancient and medieval periods tended to regard anger as an extremely negative emotion, to the degree that a fit of anger signified uncontrollability and madness (Kemp & Strongman, 1995). The general trend of animosity toward and condemnation of anger was the *zeitgeist* of those eras. More recently, however, attitudes toward the experience and expression of anger have changed considerably, with a shift of focus to its functionality as well. This has also brought forth developments and alternative thinking toward treatment of anger and associated negative emotions.

Emotions are generally seen as functionally appropriate responses that motivate persons to be receptive to changing environments and stressors (Kubzansky, Kawachi, Weiss, & Sparrow, 1998). As with other basic emotions, such as fear, disgust, sorrow and happiness, anger is said to be biological in nature and has an inherent adaptive value (Luutonen, 2007; Thomas, 2007). Contemporary researchers such as Plutchik (1980) and Ekman (1972) expanded on Darwin's idea of emotions as having adaptive value for survival. In conjunction with this idea, anger may be positive or negative, depending on the individual who experiences it, or the individual or group upon whom it is inflicted (Harmon-Jones & Harmon-Jones, 2006). Besides aiding in the organization and regulation of psychological processes such as self-defense and mastery, anger monitors and organizes interpersonal behaviors to help with goal-directed actions (Harmon-Jones & Harmon-Jones, 2006). Hence, anger's function in a hostile situation is to overcome obstacles and achieve a goal—most often one that has positive value to the individual (Harmon-Jones & Harmon-Jones, 2006; Robins & Novaco, 1999).

To date, theories of anger have varied, with each seeking to expound a particular aspect. For example, appraisal theorists assert that a person's anger experience is related to his or her subjective appraisal of the situation (Lazarus, 1991). Other theorists claim that anger is not always a result of an external stimulus; it may be caused by internal physical discomfort or unpleasantness (Berkowitz & Harmon-Jones, 2004). They found that anger-related muscular movements can also lead to anger-related feelings, memories, cognitions, and autonomic responses. There is a lack of consistency among these theories, with each encompassing a different perspective of the construct.

Some researchers suggest that anger theory and research are lagging due to the lack of diagnostic categories within the *Diagnostic and Statistical Manual of Mental Disorders* (4th ed. [DSM-IV]; American Psychiatric Association, 1994) for this negative emotion (Eckhardt & Deffenbacher, 1995). DSM-IV does not recognize anger as the core feature of any clinical diagnosis (Brondolo, DiGiuseppe, & Tafrate, 1997; Eckhardt & Deffenbacher, 1995; Novaco, 1985;

Thomas, Smucker, & Droppleman, 1998). Thus, in an attempt to broaden the scope of diagnostic criteria used by clinicians, researchers have proposed a working model of anger to provide some conceptual clarity of the construct. These criteria are designed to provide a framework under which clinicians can assess and treat clients who seek help for anger-related problems (DiGiuseppe & Tafrate, 2007).

Eckhardt and Deffenbacher (1995) have proposed that three anger disorders should be added to DSM-IV: adjustment disorder with angry mood, situational anger disorder, and generalized anger disorder. Adjustment disorder with angry mood is characterized by an angry affect; people with situational anger disorder experience intense anger reactions related to certain situations; and generalized anger disorder is characterized by persistent and pervasive anger (Eckhardt & Deffenbacher, 1995; Thomas et al., 1998). The proposed criteria are in the preliminary stages, and further research is needed to provide additional clarification on the nuances of the anger construct.

Anger theorists have considered more beneficial aspects of anger expression that are important. From both theoretical and empirical viewpoints, anger expression may be considered to result from one of two motivations: destructive or constructive. Traditional anger-in and anger-out measures typically have been created with destructive motivations in mind (Deffenbacher, Oetting, Lynch, & Morris, 1996; Harburg et al., 1973; Spielberger et al., 1985), although some anger behaviors may be motivated by the impulse to resolve or improve the anger-provoking situation (Averill, 1982; Stoney & Engebretson, 1994; Thomas, 1989, 1997), even though constructively motivated anger expression appears to characterize many persons (Averill, 1982; Tangney, Hill-Barlow, et al., 1996; Tangney, Wagner, Hill-Barlow, Marschall, & Gramzow, 1996; Thomas, 1989, 1997). This type of anger expression has received less empirical attention, particularly in the study of physical health. While constructive anger expression was hypothesized to be protective of health, a standardized measure of this aspect of anger expression was not available. Davidson, MacGregor, Stuhr, Dixon, and MacLean (2000) created an observer-based measure, which is coded from

the Extended Structured Interview (ESI; Hall, Davidson, MacGregor, & MacLean, 1998), entitled the Constructive Anger Behavior—Verbal Style (CAB-V) scale. Persons who have high scores tend to discuss anger in an assertive, calm manner, with the motivation to resolve or improve the situation.

Anger's Unknown Prevalence and Course

Due to the continuing absence of common nomenclature and assessment strategies for anger, as well as the absence of accepted diagnostic categories and/or clinical cutoffs with existing measures, evidence for anger prevalence, course, and gender and cultural features is not presented. These basic descriptive studies are desperately needed to understand the extent to which anger and its dysfunctional extremes are prevalent in populations, and therefore possibly affect mental and physical health.

Evidence Base for Anger and Illness

To date there have been few systematic meta-analyses of anger as it relates to illness in general; yet accumulated data link anger to various conditions. In this section we outline the current evidence base linking anger or anger expression to health effects.

There have been a number of studies investigating the links between anger and cardiovascular disease. Friedman and Rosenman (1959), as we mentioned earlier, were the first to identify the Type A behavior pattern (TABP), and they launched a major epidemiological study to test the TABP–coronary heart disease (CHD) link. Results from this study showed that people with Type A personalities were twice as likely to show clinical manifestations of CHD, although further studies of this anger expression complex reported null findings (Siegman, 1994).

A large systematic meta-analysis (Chida & Steptoe, 2009) found that anger and hostility are significantly associated with both increased CHD events in healthy populations and poor prognosis in patients with existing CHD. Harmful effects of anger were said to be greater in men than in women. Another meta-analysis (Suls & Bunde, 2005), which separated the anger construct into cynical hostility, anger expression, and trait anger, found the strongest evidence for cynical hostility and anger expression in its relation to CHD risk.

For over 20 years there has been evidence of the relationship between anger and headaches, particularly migraines. People with headaches, as one study found, tend to suppress their anger more (anger-in), even after researchers control for depression and anxiety (Nicholson, Gramling, Ong, & Buenaver, 2003; Venable, Carlson, & Wilson, 2001). Low anger control has been an important predictor of tension headaches as well; patients with migraines and tension headaches also show higher levels of angry temperament and reaction (Perozzo et al., 2005). The biological mechanisms for these associations have not been fully explored, but there is some evidence to suggest that anger manifests itself in acute general vasomotor reflexes that increase cerebral blood flow (Sugahara, 2004).

Specific anger expression styles have been linked with chronic pain intensity. Anger-out has been shown in several studies to be associated with increased pain sensitivity, possibly through mediation of endogenous opioid dysfunction (Bruehl, Burns, Chung, & Quartana, 2008; Bruehl, Chung, & Burns, 2006; Burns & Bruehl, 2005). On the other hand, anger inhibition, or anger-in, has been associated with increased pain severity, through augmenting perception of pain (Burns et al., 2008; Quartana & Burns, 2007). Thus, not only the presence but also the expression of anger can have detrimental effects for how pain is perceived and tolerated.

Anger is also linked with other mental conditions, such as anxiety and depression (Fava, Anderson, & Rosenbaum, 1990; Newman, Gray, & Fuqua, 1999). Research has shown that persons who experience high levels of anger also experience symptoms of anxiety (Deffenbacher, Demm, & Brandon, 1986; Fava et al., 1990; Zwemer & Deffenbacher, 1984). Deffenbacher and colleagues (1986) found that anxiety was as predictive of anger as other general measures. Studies have also indicated that depressed participants report higher levels of anger than do nondepressed participants (Riley & Treiber, 1989; Robbins & Tanck, 1997). Fava and Rosenbaum (1998) found that depressed patients were 70% more likely than non-depressed patients to experience what they called "anger attacks." Tedlow and colleagues (1999) have further demonstrated that patients with depression who experience these "anger attacks" have significantly higher rates of dependent, avoidant, narcissistic, borderline, and antisocial personality disorders than those who do not experience these attacks. In addition, support of the relation between anger and depression has been shown at the pharmacological level. Persons treated with tricyclic antidepressants reported a reduction in their feelings of anger (Fava et al., 1990; Fava & Rosenbaum, 1998).

The relationship between anger and other illnesses, such as diabetes, irritable bowel syndrome and various skin conditions, has not been as conclusive (Golden et al., 2006; Keltikangas-Jarvinen, Räikkönen, Hautanen, & Adlercreutz, 1996; Yi, Yi, Vitaliano, & Weinger, 2008). Further research is needed to understand possible biological mechanisms and temporality of the associations found. Given that many studies have shown that anger and anger expression predict illness, it is important to ascertain the mechanisms through which this association occurs. The next two sections review biological and behavioral mechanisms or pathways by which anger and anger expression might confer risk for mental and physical illness.

Possible Biological Mechanisms for the Association of Anger, Anger Expression, and Health

Mechanistic research exploring the link between anger and illness has primarily focused on the effect of anger and anger expression on cardiovascular disease. Like other emotions, anger is processed by the brain's limbic system, particularly the amygdala. Limbic projections to the hypothalamus lead to activation of the hypothalamic–pituitary–adrenal (HPA) axis and the sympathetic nervous system (Roppers & Samuels, 2009).

In response to anger, the hypothalamus releases corticotropin-releasing factor (CRF). CRF acts on the anterior pituitary to trigger release of adrenocorticotropic hormone (ACTH) into the bloodstream. ACTH then elicits cortisol secretion from the adrenal cortex. The body normally maintains cortisol within a fine range due to extensive negative feedback. Research suggests, however, that anger causes overstimulation of the HPA axis, resulting in increased levels of circulating cortisol (al'Absi & Bongard, 2006; Everson-Rose & Lewis, 2005; Kubzansky & Kawachi, 2000). Supporting this, several studies found greater cortisol concentrations in hostile participants compared to nonhostile controls (Izawa, Hirata, Kodama, & Nomura, 2007; Pope & Smith, 1991). Hypercortisolemia is in turn associated with insulin resistance, central obesity, hyperlipidemia, hypertension, and leukocytosis (Fitzgerald, 2009).

Hypothalamic detection of negative emotions such as anger or stress also leads to activation of the sympathetic nervous system. Sympathetic fibers release norepinephrine that results in increased heart rate and cardiac contractile force. They also stimulate peripheral secretion of norepinephrine and epinephrine at the adrenal medulla. Norepinephrine and epinephrine bind receptors in endothelial smooth muscle, which triggers vasoconstriction and increased resistance in the vessels ("total peripheral resistance") (Fitzgerald, 2007). The combination of increased contractile force and total peripheral resistance leads to greater cardiac output and increased blood pressure. Some studies demonstrate an acute rise in blood pressure in participants responding to an anger stimulus (Sargent, Flora, & Williams, 1999; Shapiro, Goldstein, & Jamner, 1995; Vella & Friedman, 2009), though this result is not consistently replicated. If anger does promote acute blood pressure increase, then individuals with chronic anger or angry temperament may be at risk for hypertension. Hypertension and elevated heart rate generate greater shear force against the endothelial wall, causing potential damage that is thought to be the initial step in atherosclerotic plaque development (Fisher, Chien, Barakat, & Nerem, 2001). In addition to cardiac and endothelial actions, norepinephrine and epinephrine also stimulate platelet aggregation (Fitzgerald, 2007), which encourages development of thrombosis and may explain anger's association with acute coronary syndrome (ACS).

Increased sympathetic activity may also promote arrhythmia. Normal heart rate varies as the sympathetic and parasympathetic divisions respond to internal and external environmental cues. One study revealed decreased heart rate variability (HRV) in female participants unable to relieve anger, but this result is not well supported (Horsten et al., 1999). Reduced HRV predicts arrhythmia, sudden cardiac death after heart attack (myocardial infarction), and all-cause mortality (Carpeggiani et al., 2004; Singh, Mironov, Armstrong, Ross, & Langer, 1996; Vaishnav et al., 1994). The Framingham Offspring Study demonstrated that hostile patients are also at increased risk for atrial fibrillation (Eaker, Sullivan, Kelly-Hayes, D'Agostino, & Benjamin, 2004).

Inflammation is another potential mechanism linking anger to cardiovascular disease. C-reactive protein (CRP), tumor necrosis factor–alpha (TNF-alpha), and interleukin–6 (IL-6) exist at greater levels in healthy men and women with high anger indices than in healthy low-anger individuals (Suarez, 2003, 2004; Suarez, Lewis, & Kuhn, 2002). Further research is required to determine how anger might lead to increases in these proinflammatory markers.

Pathophysiological research has also explored the role of anger in migraine, irritable bowel syndrome, and pain. In a recent article, Sugahara (2004) discussed the brain blood perfusion hypothesis as an explanation for the commonalities seen in anger and migraine. In the proposed model, sympathetic hyperactivity caused by anger leads to cerebral vasoconstriction. The resulting reduced cerebral blood flow triggers reflex hyperperfusion and the development of migraine.

Recent work explored the role of CRF in the altered gut environment of irritable bowel syndrome. CRF injected into the hypothalamus of mice causes increased colonic motility, defecation, and release of mucus and watery stool (Tache, Martinez, Wang, & Million, 2004). As we mentioned earlier, anger causes increased CRF release from the hypothalamus. This seems like a plausible mechanism linking anger and irritable bowel syndrome.

Finally, several theories exist for the role of anger in pain. The most popular mechanistic theory focuses on "endogenous opioid dysfunction," a decrease in opioids leading to anger and decreased analgesic effect (Bruehl et al., 2006). Imaging studies show that anger and exogenous opioid administration both activate the anterior cingulate cortex, a region known to contain many opioid receptors.

Possible Behavioral Mechanisms for the Association of Anger, Anger Expression, and Health

Anger and anger expression have also been associated with increased psychosocial vulnerability (e.g., increased interpersonal conflict, lack of social support, more stressful life events, and depression) and an unhealthy lifestyle (e.g., smoking, excess fat intake). These behavioral variables are in turn often linked to poor physical health (Miller et al., 1996). As studies have shown (Knox, 2002), hostility and anger can account for a great deal of detrimental health behaviors that mediate long-term health outcomes. For example, smokers with high levels of hostility may use cigarettes to cope with anger-provoking situations. Studies (e.g., al'Absi, Carr, & Bongard, 2007; Kahler et al., 2009) have demonstrated a high level of trait anger associated with risk for relapse among smokers interested in cessation. High trait anger has been linked with greater increases in withdrawal symptoms and craving during the first 24 hours of abstinence, as well as an increased risk for early relapse. Anger and hostility have also been related to smoking initiation in adolescents, as well as more frequent smoking (Hampson, Andrews, & Barckley, 2007; Weiss et al., 2005).

As with smoking, people often use alcohol, drugs, and food as coping mechanisms for anger-provoking situations. Hostility has been shown to impact drinking patterns negatively, with more hostility related to relatively high intake per drinking occasion. Additionally, among adolescents, hostility has predicted intentions to use alcohol over time (Hampson, Andrews, Barckley, & Severson, 2006), as well as marijuana (Nichols, Mahadeo, Bryant, & Botvin, 2008). On the other hand, anger can be a result of alcohol consumption (Giancola, Saucier, & Gussler-Burkhardt, 2003; Parrott, Zeichner, & Stephens, 2003), and alcohol-induced anger is also associated with trait anger (Parrott & Giancola, 2004). Poor eating habits and physical inactivity have both been linked to

hostility and anger (Anton & Miller, 2005) (Carmody, Brunner, & St. Jeor, 1999), with those having high hostility scores more likely to report eating disinhibition, hunger, and dietary helplessness.

Poor sleep habits can have a deleterious effect on health and have been shown to be affected by anger and hostility. Large-scale studies in both Finland and Korea (Grano, Vahtera, Virtanen, Keltikangas-Jarvinen, & Kivimaki, 2008; Shin et al., 2005) have revealed that hostility is an independent risk factor for sleep disturbances, and that transient hostility may also predispose individuals to shorter sleep duration. Additionally, negative affect and anger rumination (the cognitive dimension for anger) were found to mediate the relationship between forgiveness and sleep quality; maintaining feelings of anger and hostility was related to poorer sleep quality (Stoia-Caraballo et al., 2008).

Other behavioral mechanisms that may be implicated in the association between anger and poor health outcome are more social in nature. For example, Fitzgerald, Haythornthwaite, Suchday, and Ewart (2003) showed that low levels of job control and social support, and high levels of job dissatisfaction were independently associated with increased work-related anger, and that anger experienced at work may be an early marker of job stress, which has been prospectively related to cardiovascular disease. Another study found that aggressive behavior in childhood was related to ongoing temporary employment status in adulthood among individuals in low socioeconomic positions, suggesting that hostility and aggressiveness are related to labor market prospects among certain individuals (Virtanen et al., 2005). And job insecurity in turn has been linked to increased cardiovascular disease (Lee, Colditz, Berkman, & Kawachi, 2004).

Poor social support and social isolation have been associated with worse health outcomes (Rozanski, Blumenthal, & Kaplan, 1999). People who have high trait anger and are hostile have been shown to have poor social skills, a greater degree of interpersonal conflict, and less social support, which can in turn be detrimental to physical health (Smith, 1992; Smith & Pope, 1990). In summary, anger and hostility can impact health through a range of pathways.

Anger and Anger Expression Interventions

The past two decades have witnessed an accumulation of research on treatment outcome studies focusing on anger/hostility and its many manifestations (Beck & Fernandez, 1998; Fields et al., 1998; Mayne & Ambrose, 1999). However, research in this area is still lacking compared to that of anxiety and depression treatment (DiGiuseppe, 1999; Fields et al., 1998). Tafrate (1995) conducted a meta-analysis of treatment outcome studies focusing on anger. Only 17 studies found in the literature met inclusion criteria (e.g., adults seeking treatment for their anger problems, attendance at two sessions, and comparison with another experimental condition). The studies were grouped into the following psychotherapy treatment strategies: cognitive therapies (e.g., self-instructional training), relaxation-based therapies (e.g., systematic desensitization; exposing patients to increasingly aggravating situations, while they practice relaxing), skills-training therapies (e.g., assertiveness training), and multicomponent treatments (e.g., stress inoculation and cognitive-behavioral therapy) (Tafrate, 1995). The results of Tafrate's meta-analysis revealed that systematic desensitization was most effective in treating anger, followed by multicomponent and self-instruction therapies. Cognitive therapy was also found to be effective.

Beck and Fernandez (1998) conducted a meta-analysis solely on the cognitive-behavioral treatments of anger. Their sample consisted of 50 studies, including dissertations and nonpublished manuscripts of predominantly clinical samples (inmates, abusive parents/spouses, etc.). The results of the meta-analysis revealed that cognitive-behavioral treatment was effective, but the strength of this treatment was weaker than that found by Tafrate (1995).

In a more recent meta-analysis, DiGiuseppe and Tafrate (2003) examined the efficacy of 92 psychosocial treatments of anger that incorporated 1,841 participants. The investigators found that participants who received treatment showed a reduction in anger and an increase in positive behaviors compared with untreated participants. Anger interventions produced reductions in anger and aggressive behaviors, and increases in positive behaviors. However, whereas some specific treatments seemed helpful, others did not. These findings suggest that, under certain conditions, some treatments for anger could potentially produce iatrogenic effects (Olatunji & Lohr, 2004).

For those interested in conducting anger intervention studies or treating angry clients, there are now research reviews as well as books that are helpful to practitioners (Deffenbacher, 1994; DiGiuseppe & Tafrate, 2003, 2007), although much work remains to be done in this area.

Conclusions

The evidence testing the association among anger, anger expression, and illness and their possible mechanisms has proliferated in recent years. But identifying observationally what predicts disease development does not necessarily reveal what caused the disease. Because many of the studies reviewed here used nonstandardized measures of anger or one of its related components, combining these studies into larger systematic reviews is not possible. These limitations notwithstanding, anger and anger expression demonstrate some observational association with disease across populations and designs, sufficient biological plausibility, and initial interventional data indicating they are modifiable. This initial evidence suggests that research on anger and anger expression warrants vigorous further investigation. We hope this overview might prompt our readers to be among the new generation of investigators to test how anger and anger expression might influence health.

Further Reading

al'Absi, M., & Bongard, S. (2006). Neuroendocrine and behavioral mechanisms mediating the relationship between anger expression and cardiovascular risk: Assessment considerations and improvements. *Journal of Behavioral Medicine, 29*(6), 573–591.

DiGiuseppe, R., & Tafrate, R. C. (2003). Anger treatment for adults: A meta-analytic review. *Clinical Psychology: Science and Practice, 10*, 70–84.

Kassinove, H., & Sukhodolsky, D. G. (1995). Anger disorders: Basic science and practice issues [Review]. *Issues in Comprehensive Pediatric Nursing, 18*(3), 173–205.

Martin, R., Watson, D., & Wan, C. K. (2000). A three-factor model of trait anger: Dimensions of affect, behavior, and cognition. *Journal of Personality, 68*(5), 869–897.

Suls, J., & Bunde, J. (2005). Anger, anxiety, and depression as risk factors for cardiovascular disease: The problems and implications of overlapping affective dispositions. *Psychological Bulletin, 131*(2), 260–300.

References

al'Absi, M., & Bongard, S. (2006). Neuroendocrine and behavioral mechanisms mediating the relationship between anger expression and cardiovascular risk: Assessment considerations and improvements. *Journal of Behavioral Medicine, 29*(6), 573–591.

al'Absi, M., Carr, S. B., & Bongard, S. (2007). Anger and psychobiological changes during smoking abstinence and in response to acute stress: Prediction of smoking relapse. *International Journal of Psychophysiology, 66*(2), 109–115.

American Psychiatric Association. (1994). *Diagnostic and statistical manual of mental disorders* (4th ed.). Washington, DC: Author.

Anton, S. D., & Miller, P. M. (2005). Do negative emotions predict alcohol consumption, saturated fat intake, and physical activity in older adults? *Behavior Modification, 29*(4), 677–688.

Averill, J. R. (1982). *Anger and aggression: An essay on emotion.* New York: Springer-Verlag.

Barefoot, J., Dodge, K., Peterson, B., Dahlstrom, W., & Williams, R., Jr. (1989). The Cook–Medley Hostility Scale: Item content and ability to predict survival. *Psychosomatic Medicine, 51*(1), 46–57.

Barefoot, J. C. (1992). Developments in the measurement of hostility. In H. S. Friedman (Ed.), *Hostility, coping, and health* (pp. 13–31). Washington, DC: American Psychological Association.

Beck, R., & Fernandez, E. (1998). Cognitive-behavioral therapy in the treatment of anger: A meta-analysis. *Cognitive Therapy and Research, 22*(1), 63–74.

Bendig, A. W. (1962). Factor analytic scales of covert and overt hostility. *Journal of Consulting Psychology, 26,* 200.

Berkowitz, L., & Harmon-Jones, E. (2004). More thoughts about anger determinants. *Emotion, 4,* 151–155.

Biaggio, M. K. (1980). Assessment of anger arousal. *Journal of Personality Assessment, 44,* 289–298.

Biaggio, M. K., Supplee, K., & Curtis, N. (1981).

Reliability and validity of four anger scales. *Journal of Personality Assessment, 45,* 639–648.

Brondolo, E., DiGiuseppe, R., & Tafrate, R. C. (1997). Exposure-based treatment for anger problems: Focus on the feeling. *Cognitive and Behavioral Practice, 4*(1), 75–98.

Bruehl, S., Burns, J. W., Chung, O. Y., & Quartana, P. (2008). Anger management style and emotional reactivity to noxious stimuli among chronic pain patients and healthy controls: The role of endogenous opioids. *Health Psychology, 27*(2), 204–214.

Bruehl, S., Chung, O. Y., & Burns, J. W. (2006). Anger expression and pain: An overview of findings and possible mechanisms. *Journal of Behavioral Medicine, 29*(6), 593–606.

Burns, J. W., & Bruehl, S. (2005). Anger management style, opioid analgesic use, and chronic pain severity: A test of the opioid-deficit hypothesis. *Journal of Behavioral Medicine, 28*(6), 555–563.

Burns, J. W., Holly, A., Quartana, P., Wolff, B., Gray, E., & Bruehl, S. (2008). Trait anger management style moderates effects of actual ("state") anger regulation on symptom-specific reactivity and recovery among chronic low back pain patients. *Psychosomatic Medicine, 70*(8), 898–905.

Buss, A., & Durkee, A. (1957). An inventory for assessing different kinds of hostility. *Journal of Consulting Psychology, 21,* 343–349.

Buss, A. H., & Perry, M. (1992). The Aggression Questionnaire. *Journal of Personality and Social Psychology, 63,* 452–459.

Carmody, T. P., Brunner, R. L., & St. Jeor, S. T. (1999). Hostility, dieting, and nutrition attitudes in overweight and weight-cycling men and women. *International Journal of Eating Disorders, 26*(1), 37–42.

Carpeggiani, C., L'Abbate, A., Landi, P., Michelassi, C., Raciti, M., Macerata, A., et al. (2004). Early assessment of heart rate variability is predictive of in-hospital death and major complications after acute myocardial infarction. *International Journal of Cardiology, 96*(3), 361–368.

Catchlove, R. F., Cohen, K. R., Braha, R. E., & Demers-Desrosiers, L. A. (1985). Incidence and implications of alexithymia in chronic pain patients. *Journal of Nervous and Mental Disease, 173*(4), 246–248.

Chida, Y., & Steptoe, A. (2009). The association of anger and hostility with future coronary heart disease: A meta-analytic review of prospective evidence. *Journal of the American College of Cardiology, 53*(11), 936–946.

Davidson, K., MacGregor, M. W., Stuhr, J., Dixon, K., & MacLean, D. (2000). Constructive anger verbal behavior predicts blood pressure in a population-based sample. *Health Psychology, 19*(1), 55–64.

Deffenbacher, J. L. (1994). Anger reduction: Issues, assessment, and intervention strategies. In A. W. Siegman & T. W. Smith (Eds.), *Anger, hostility, and the heart* (pp. 239–269). Hillsdale, NJ: Erlbaum.

Deffenbacher, J. L., Demm, P. M., & Brandon, A. D. (1986). High general anger: Correlates and treatment. *Behaviour Research and Therapy, 24*(4), 481–489.

Deffenbacher, J. L., Oetting, E. R., Lynch, R. S., & Morris, C. D. (1996). The expression of anger and its consequences. *Behaviour Research and Therapy, 34*(7), 575–590.

Dembroski, T. M., MacDougall, J. M., Shields, J. L., Petitto, J., & Lushene, R. (1978). Components of the type A coronary-prone behavior pattern and cardiovascular responses to psychomotor performance challenge. *Journal of Behavioral Medicine, 1*, 159–176.

DiGiuseppe, R. (1999). End piece: Reflections on the treatment of anger. *Journal of Clinical Psychology, 55*(3), 365–379.

DiGiuseppe, R., & Tafrate, R. C. (2003). Anger treatment for adults: A meta-analytic review. *Clinical Psychology: Science and Practice, 10*, 70–84.

DiGiuseppe, R., & Tafrate, R. C. (2007). *Understanding anger disorders.* New York: Oxford University Press.

Eaker, E. D., Sullivan, L. M., Kelly-Hayes, M., D'Agostino, R. B., & Benjamin, E. J. (2004). Anger and hostility predict the development of atrial fibrillation in men in the Framingham Offspring Study. *Circulation, 109*(10), 1267–1271.

Eckhardt, C., & Deffenbacher, J. (1995). Diagnosis of anger disorders. In H. Kassinove (Ed.), *Anger disorders: Definition, diagnosis, and treatment.* Washington, DC: Taylor & Francis.

Eckhardt, C., Norlander, B., & Deffenbacher, J. (2004). The assessment of anger and hostility: A critical review. *Aggression and Violent Behavior, 9*(1), 17–43.

Edmunds, G., & Kendrick, D. C. (1980). *The measurement of human aggressiveness.* Chichester, UK: Horwood.

Ekman, P. (1972). Universals and cultural differences in facial expression of emotion. In J. R. Cole (Ed.), *Nebraska Symposium on Motivation* (Vol. 19, pp. 207–283). Lincoln: University of Nebraska Press.

Everson-Rose, S. A., & Lewis, T. T. (2005). Psychosocial factors and cardiovascular diseases. *Annual Review Public Health, 26*, 469–500.

Fava, M., Anderson, K., & Rosenbaum, J. F. (1990). "Anger attacks": Possible variants of panic and major depressive disorders. *American Journal of Psychiatry, 147*(7), 867–871.

Fava, M., & Rosenbaum, J. (1998). Anger attacks in depression. *Depression and Anxiety, 8*(Suppl. 1), 59–63.

Fields, B., Reesman, K., Robinson, C., Sims, A., Edwards, K., McCall, B., et al. (1998). Anger of African-American women in the South. *Issues in Mental Health Nursing, 19*, 353–373.

Fisher, A. B., Chien, S., Barakat, A. I., & Nerem, R. M. (2001). Endothelial cellular response to altered shear stress. *American Journal of Physiology: Lung Cellular and Molecular Physiology, 281*(3), L529–L533.

Fitzgerald, P. A. (2007). Adrenal medulla and paraganglia. In D. G. Gardner & D. Shoback (Eds.), *Greenspan's basic and clinical endocrinology* (8th ed.). New York: McGraw-Hill.

Fitzgerald, P. A. (2009). Endocrine disorders. In S. J. McPhee & M. Papadakis (Eds.), *Current medical diagnosis and treatment* (pp. 965–1050). New York: McGraw-Hill.

Fitzgerald, S. T., Haythornthwaite, J. A., Suchday, S., & Ewart, C. K. (2003). Anger in young black and white workers: Effects of job control, dissatisfaction, and support. *Journal of Behavioral Medicine, 26*(4), 283–296.

Friedman, M., & Rosenman, R. H. (1959). Association of specific overt behavior pattern with blood and cardiovascular findings. *Journal of the American Medical Association, 169*, 1286–1296.

Gentry, W. D., Chesney, A. P., Gary H. E., Jr., Hall, R. P., & Harburg, E. (1982). Habitual anger-coping styles: I. Effect on mean blood pressure and risk for essential hypertension. *Psychosomatic Medicine, 44*, 195–202.

Giancola, P. R., Saucier, D. A., & Gussler-Burkhardt, N. L. (2003). The effects of affective, behavioral, and cognitive components of trait anger on the alcohol-aggression relation. *Alcoholism: Clinical and Experimental Research, 27*(12), 1944–1954.

Gidron, Y., & Davidson, K. (1996). Development and preliminary testing of a brief intervention for modifying CHD-predictive hostility components. *Journal of Behavioral Medicine, 19*(3), 203–220.

Golden, S. H., Williams, J. E., Ford, D. E., Yeh, H.-C., Sanford, C. P., Nieto, F. J., et al. (2006). Anger temperament is modestly associated with the risk of Type 2 diabetes mellitus: The atherosclerosis risk in communities study. *Psychoneuroendocrinology, 31*(3), 325–332.

Grano, N., Vahtera, J., Virtanen, M., Keltikangas-Jarvinen, L., & Kivimaki, M. (2008). Association of hostility with sleep duration and sleep disturbances in an employee population. *International Journal of Behavioral Medicine, 15*(2), 73–80.

Hall, P., Davidson, K., MacGregor, M., & MacLean, D. (1998). *Expanded structured in-*

terview administration training manual. Halifax: Heart Health of Nova Scotia.

Hampson, S. E., Andrews, J. A., & Barckley, M. (2007). Predictors of the development of elementary-school children's intentions to smoke cigarettes: Hostility, prototypes, and subjective norms. *Nicotine and Tobacco Research*, 9(7), 751–760.

Hampson, S. E., Andrews, J. A., Barckley, M., & Severson, H. H. (2006). Personality predictors of the development of elementary school children's intentions to drink alcohol: The mediating effects of attitudes and subjective norms. *Psychology of Addictive Behaviors*, 20(3), 288–297.

Harburg, E., Erfurt, J. C., Hauenstein, L. S., Chape, C., Schull, W. J., & Schork, M. A. (1973). Socio-ecological stress, suppressed hostility, skin color, and black–white male blood pressure: Detroit. *Psychosomatic Medicine*, 35(4), 276–296.

Harburg, E., Gleiberman, L., Russell, M., & Cooper, M. (1991). Anger-coping styles and blood pressure in black and white males: Buffalo, New York. *Psychosomatic Medicine*, 53(2), 153–164.

Harmon-Jones, E., & Harmon-Jones, C. (2006). Anger: Causes and components. In T. A. Cavell & K. T. Malcolm (Eds.), *Anger, aggression and interventions for interpersonal violence* (pp. 99–117). Mahwah, NJ: Erlbaum.

Horsten, M., Ericson, M., Perski, A., Wamala, S. P., Schenck-Gustafsson, K., & Orth-Gomer, K. (1999). Psychosocial factors and heart rate variability in healthy women. *Psychosomatic Medicine*, 61(1), 49–57.

Houston, B. K. (1994). Anger, hostility, and psychophysiological reactivity. In A. W. Siegman & T. W. Smith (Eds.), *Anger, hostility, and the heart* (pp. 97–115). Hillsdale, NJ: Erlbaum.

Izawa, S., Hirata, U., Kodama, M., & Nomura, S. (2007). [Effect of hostility on salivary cortisol levels in university students]. *Shinrigaku Kenkyu*, 78(3), 277–283.

Julius, M., Harburg, E., Schork, M. A., & DiFrancesco, W. (1992). *Role of suppressed anger in cause-specific deaths for married pairs (Tecumseh 1971–1988)*. Paper presented at the annual meeting of the Second International Congress of Behavioral Medicine, Hamburg, Germany.

Kahler, C. W., Spillane, N. S., Leventhal, A. M., Strong, D. R., Brown, R. A., & Monti, P. M. (2009). Hostility and smoking cessation treatment outcome in heavy social drinkers. *Psychology of Addictive Behaviors*, 23(1), 67–76.

Kassinove, H., & Sukhodolsky, D. G. (1995). Anger disorders: Basic science and practice issues [Review]. *Issues in Comprehensive Pediatric Nursing*, 18(3), 173–205.

Keltikangas-Jarvinen, L., Räikkönen, K., Hautanen, A., & Adlercreutz, H. (1996). Vital exhaustion, anger expression, and pituitary and adrenocortical hormones: Implications for the insulin resistance syndrome. *Arteriosclerosis, Thrombosis and Vascular Biology*, 16(2), 275–280.

Kemp, S., & Strongman, K. T. (1995). Anger theory and management: A historical analysis. *American Journal of Psychology*, 108(3), 397–417.

Knox, S. S. (2002). Psychosocial factors in cardiovascular disease: Implications for therapeutic outcomes. *Expert Review of Pharmacoeconomics and Outcomes Research*, 2(2), 147–159.

Kubzansky, L. D., & Kawachi, I. (2000). Going to the heart of the matter: Do negative emotions cause coronary heart disease? *Journal of Psychosomatic Research*, 48(4–5), 323–337.

Kubzansky, L. D., Kawachi, I., Weiss, S. T., & Sparrow, D. (1998). Anxiety and coronary heart disease: A synthesis of epidemiological, psychological, and experimental evidence. *Annals of Behavioral Medicine*, 20(2), 47–58.

Lazarus, R. S. (1991). *Emotion and adaptation*. Oxford, UK: Oxford University Press.

Lee, S., Colditz, G. A., Berkman, L. F., & Kawachi, I. (2004). Prospective study of job insecurity and coronary heart disease in U.S. women. *Annals of Epidemiology*, 14(1), 24–30.

Luutonen, S. (2007). Anger and depression—theoretical and clinical considerations [Review]. *Nordic Journal of Psychiatry*, 61(4), 246–251.

Martin, R., & Watson, D. (1997). Style of anger expression and its relation to daily experience. *Personality and Social Psychology Bulletin*, 23(3), 285–294.

Martin, R., Watson, D., & Wan, C. K. (2000). A three-factor model of trait anger: Dimensions of affect, behavior, and cognition. *Journal of Personality*, 68(5), 869–897.

Mayne, T. J., & Ambrose, T. K. (1999). Research review on anger in psychotherapy [Review]. *Journal of Clinical Psychology*, 55(3), 353–363.

Miller, T. Q., Smith, T. W., Turner, C. W., Guijarro, M. L., & Hallet, A. J. (1996). A meta-analytic review of research on hostility and physical health. *Psychological Bulletin*, 119(2), 322–348.

Musante, L., MacDougall, J., Dembroski, T., & Costa, P. T. (1989). Potential for hostility and dimensions of anger. *Health Psychology*, 8(3), 343–354.

Nesse, R. (1990). Evolutionary explanations of emotions. *Human Nature*, 1(3), 261–289.

Newman, J. L., Gray, E. A., & Fuqua, D. R. 1999). Sex differences in the relationship of anger and depression: An empirical study. *Journal of Counseling and Development*, 84, 157–162.

Nichols, T. R., Mahadeo, M., Bryant, K., & Botvin, G. J. (2008). Examining anger as a predictor of drug use among multiethnic middle school students. *Journal of School Health, 78*(9), 480–486.

Nicholson, R. A., Gramling, S. E., Ong, J. C., & Buenaver, L. (2003). Differences in anger expression between individuals with and without headache after controlling for depression and anxiety. *Headache, 43*(6), 651–663.

Novaco, R. W. (1985). Anger and its therapeutic regulation. In M. A. Chesman & R. M. Roseman (Eds.), *Anger and hostility in cardiovascular and behavioural disorders* (pp. 203–226). New York: Hemisphere.

Olatunji, B. O., & Lohr, J. M. (2004). Nonspecific factors and the efficacy of psychosocial treatments for anger. *Scientific Review of Mental Health Practice, 3*, 3–18.

Parrott, D. J., & Giancola, P. R. (2004). A further examination of the relation between trait anger and alcohol-related aggression: The role of anger control. *Alcoholism: Clinical and Experimental Research, 28*(6), 855–864.

Parrott, D. J., Zeichner, A., & Stephens, D. (2003). Effects of alcohol, personality, and provocation on the expression of anger in men: A facial coding analysis. *Alcoholism: Clinical and Experimental Research, 27*(6), 937–945.

Perozzo, P., Savi, L., Castelli, L., Valfre, W., Lo Giudice, R., Gentile, S., et al. (2005). Anger and emotional distress in patients with migraine and tension-type headache. *Journal of Headache and Pain, 6*(5), 392–399.

Plutchik, R. (1980). A general psychoevolutionary theory of emotion. In R. Plutchik & H. Kellerman (Eds.), *Emotion: Theory, research, and experience: Vol. 1. Theories of emotion* (pp. 3–33). New York: Academic Press.

Pope, M. K., & Smith, T. W. (1991). Cortisol excretion in high and low cynically hostile men. *Psychosomatic Medicine, 53*(4), 386–392.

Quartana, P. J., & Burns, J. W. (2007). Painful consequences of anger suppression. *Emotion, 7*(2), 400–414.

Riley, W. T., & Treiber, F. A. (1989). The validity of multidimensional self-report anger and hostility measures. *Journal of Clinical Psychology, 45*(3), 397–404.

Robbins, P. R., & Tanck, R. H. (1997). Anger and depressed effect: Interindividual and intraindividual perspectives. *Journal of Psychology, 131*(5), 489–500.

Robins, S., & Novaco, R. W. (1999). Systems conceptualization and treatment of anger. *Journal of Clinical Psychology, 55*(3), 325–337.

Roppers, A., & Samuels, M. (2009). The limbic lobes and the neurology of emotion. In *Adams and Victor's principles of neurology* (9th ed.). New York: McGraw-Hill Professional.

Rozanski, A., Blumenthal, J. A., & Kaplan, J.

(1999). Impact of psychological factors on the pathogenesis of cardiovascular disease and implications for therapy. *Circulation, 99*(16), 2192–2217.

Sargent, C. A., Flora, S. R., & Williams, S. L. (1999). Vocal expression of anger and cardiovascular reactivity within dyadic interactions. *Psychological Reports, 84*(3, Pt. 1), 809–816.

Shapiro, D., Goldstein, I. B., & Jamner, L. D. (1995). Effects of anger/hostility, defensiveness, gender, and family history of hypertension on cardiovascular reactivity. *Psychophysiology, 32*(5), 425–435.

Shin, C., Kim, J., Yi, H., Lee, H., Lee, J., & Shin, K. (2005). Relationship between trait-anger and sleep disturbances in middle-aged men and women. *Journal of Psychosomatic Research, 58*(2), 183–189.

Siegel, J. M. (1985). The measurement of anger as a multidimensional construct. In M. A. Chesney & R. H. Rosenman (Eds.), *Anger and hostility in cardiovascular and behavioral disorders* (pp. 59–62). Washington, DC: Hemisphere.

Siegman, A. W. (1994). From Type A to hostility to anger: Reflections on the history of coronary-prone behavior. In A. W. Siegman & T. W. Smith (Eds.), *Anger, hostility, and the heart* (pp. 1–21). Hillsdale, NJ: Erlbaum.

Singh, N., Mironov, D., Armstrong, P. W., Ross, A. M., & Langer, A. (1996). Heart rate variability assessment early after acute myocardial infarction: Pathophysiological and prognostic correlates. *Circulation, 93*(7), 1388–1395.

Smith, T. W. (1992). Hostility and health: Current status of a psychosomatic hypothesis. *Health Psychology, 11*(3), 139–150.

Smith, T. W., & Pope, M. K. (1990). Cynical hostility as a health risk: Current status and future directions. *Journal of Social Behavior and Personality, 5*(1), 77–88.

Spielberger, C. D., Jacobs, G., Russell, S., & Crane, R. (1983). Assessment of anger: The State–Trait Anger Scale. In J. N. Butcher & C. D. Spielberger (Eds.), *Advances in personality assessment* (Vol. 2, pp. 159–187). Hillsdale, NJ: Erlbaum.

Spielberger, C. D., Johnson, E. H., Russell, S. F., Crane, R. J., Jacobs, G. A., & Worden, T. J. (1985). The experience and expression of anger: Construction and validation of an anger expression scale. In M. A. Chesney & R. H. Rosenman (Eds.), *Anger and hostility in cardiovascular and behavioral disorders* (pp. 5–30). New York: Hemisphere.

Spielberger, C. D., Reheiser, E. C., & Sydeman, S. J. (1995). Measuring the experience, expression, and control of anger. In H. Kassinove (Ed.), *Anger disorders: Definitions, diagnosis, and treatment* (pp. 49–67). Washington, DC: Taylor & Francis.

Stoia-Caraballo, R., Rye, M. S., Pan, W., Brown Kirschman, K. J., Lutz-Zois, C., & Lyons, A. M. (2008). Negative affect and anger rumination as mediators between forgiveness and sleep quality. *Journal of Behavioral Medicine, 31*(6), 478–488.

Stoney, C. M., & Engebretson, T. O. (1994). Anger and hostility: Potential mediators of the gender difference in coronary heart disease. In A. W. Siegman & T. W. Smith (Eds.), *Anger, hostility, and the heart* (pp. 215–237). Hillsdale, NJ: Erlbaum.

Suarez, E. C. (2003). Plasma interleukin-6 is associated with psychological coronary risk factors: Moderation by use of multivitamin supplements. *Brain, Behavior, and Immunity, 17*(4), 296–303.

Suarez, E. C. (2004). C-reactive protein is associated with psychological risk factors of cardiovascular disease in apparently healthy adults. *Psychosomatic Medicine, 66*(5), 684–691.

Suarez, E. C., Lewis, J. G., & Kuhn, C. (2002). The relation of aggression, hostility, and anger to lipopolysaccharide-stimulated tumor necrosis factor (TNF)-alpha by blood monocytes from normal men. *Brain, Behavior, and Immunity, 16*(6), 675–684.

Sugahara, H. (2004). Brain blood perfusion hypothesis for migraine, anger, and epileptic attacks. *Medical Hypotheses, 62*(5), 766–769.

Suls, J., & Bunde, J. (2005). Anger, anxiety, and depression as risk factors for cardiovascular disease: The problems and implications of overlapping affective dispositions. *Psychological Bulletin, 131*(2), 260–300.

Tache, Y., Martinez, V., Wang, L., & Million, M. (2004). CRF1 receptor signaling pathways are involved in stress-related alterations of colonic function and viscerosensitivity: Implications for irritable bowel syndrome. *British Journal of Pharmacology, 141*(8), 1321–1330.

Tafrate, R. C. (1995). Evaluation of treatment of strategies for adult anger disorders. In H. Kassinove (Ed.), *Anger disorders: Definition, diagnosis, and treatment* (pp. 109–129). Washington, DC: Taylor & Francis.

Tangney, J. P., Hill-Barlow, D., Wagner, P. E., Marschall, D. E., Borenstein, J. K., Sanftner, J., et al. (1996). Assessing individual differences in constructive versus destructive responses to anger across the lifespan. *Journal of Personality and Social Psychology, 70*(4), 780–796.

Tangney, J. P., Wagner, P. E., Hill-Barlow, D., Marschall, D. E., & Gramzow, R. (1996). Relation of shame and guilt to constructive versus destructive responses to anger across the lifespan. *Journal of Personality and Social Psychology, 70*(4), 797–809.

Tedlow, J., Leslie, V., Keefe, B. R., Alpert, J., Nierenberg, A. A., Rosenbaum, J. F., et al. (1999). Axis I and Axis II disorder comorbidity in unipolar depression with anger attacks. *Journal of Affective Disorders, 52*(1–3), 217–223.

Thomas, S. (2007). Trait anger, anger expression, and themes of anger incidents in contemporary undergraduate students. In E. I. Clausen (Ed.), *Psychology of anger* (pp. 23–69). New York: Nova Science.

Thomas, S., Smucker, C., & Droppleman, P. (1998). It hurts most around the heart: A phenomenological exploration of women's anger. *Journal of Advanced Nursing, 28*(2), 311–322.

Thomas, S. P. (1989). Gender differences in anger expression: Health implications. *Research in Nursing and Health, 12*(6), 389–398.

Thomas, S. P. (1997). Angry? Let's talk about it! *Applied Nursing Research, 10*(2), 80–85.

Vaishnav, S., Stevenson, R., Marchant, B., Lagi, K., Ranjadayalan, K., & Timmis, A. D. (1994). Relation between heart rate variability early after acute myocardial infarction and long-term mortality. *American Journal of Cardiology, 73*(9), 653–657.

Vella, E. J., & Friedman, B. H. (2009). Hostility and anger in: Cardiovascular reactivity and recovery to mental arithmetic stress. *International Journal of Psychophysiology, 72*(3), 253–259.

Venable, V. L., Carlson, C. R., & Wilson, J. (2001). The role of anger and depression in recurrent headache. *Headache, 41*(1), 21–30.

Virtanen, M., Kivimaki, M., Elovainio, M., Vahtera, J., Kokko, K., & Pulkkinen, L. (2005). Mental health and hostility as predictors of temporary employment: Evidence from two prospective studies. *Social Science and Medicine, 61*(10), 2084–2095.

Weiss, J. W., Mouttapa, M., Chou, C.-P., Nezami, E., Johnson, C., Palmer, P. H., et al. (2005). Hostility, depressive symptoms, and smoking in early adolescence. *Journal of Adolescence, 28*(1), 49–62.

Yi, J. P., Yi, J. C., Vitaliano, P. P., & Weinger, K. (2008). How does anger coping style affect glycemic control in diabetes patients? *International Journal of Behavioral Medicine, 15*(3), 167–172.

Zelin, M. L., Adler, G., & Myerson, P. G. (1972). Anger Self-Report: An objective questionnaire for the measurement of aggression. *Journal of Consulting and Clinical Psychology, 39*(2), 340.

Zwemer, W. A., & Deffenbacher, J. L. (1984). Irrational beliefs, anger and anxiety. *Journal of Counseling Psychology, 31*(3), 391–393.

CHAPTER 9

Developmental Influences in Understanding Child and Adolescent Health Behaviors

Dawn K. Wilson
Sara M. St. George
Nicole Zarrett

Children's health behaviors are influenced by a multitude of biological, cognitive, social, and environmental factors. Approaching the study of health behaviors from a developmental perspective increases our understanding of the changing influence of biological, cognitive, social, and environmental processes on the health behaviors of children and adolescents (Bronfenbrenner 2005; Bronfenbrenner & Morris, 2006; Wilson & Lawman, 2009). This chapter provides a framework for understanding determinants of health behaviors, including both health-promoting (e.g., physical activity, healthy diet) and health-compromising (e.g., smoking prevention, drug prevention) behaviors, at different developmental periods during childhood and adolescence. The goal of understanding determinants of youths' health behaviors within a developmental framework is to provide direction for improving implementation of effective interventions by targeting relevant factors that influence youths' health behaviors as they mature. This may be especially important for identifying how biological, cognitive, social, and environmental factors may serve to inform

intervention development and to increase understanding of barriers that are specific to studying health behaviors in youths.

Theoretical Framework

The theoretical framework outlined in this chapter integrates reciprocal determinism theories and developmental systems (Bandura, 1997; Bronfenbrenner, 2005; Bronfenbrenner & Morris, 2006; Schwartz, 1982). Bandura's social cognitive theory (SCT) assumes that individual cognitive factors, environmental events, and behavior are interacting and reciprocal determinants of each other (Bandura, 1991, 1997). SCT theory provides not only a broad perspective for explaining behavior but also more specific direction on how various cognitive, social, and environmental factors interact to influence health behaviors. For example, the reciprocal interaction of cognitive factors, such as self-efficacy, and social factors, such as instrumental and emotional support from parents and peers, have been important predictors of positive health trajectories across the lifespan (Bandura, 2002). SCT is commonly used as the guiding framework for behavior change interventions (Bandura, 2002).

Although the theoretical approach has been shown to be effective at some points in the lifespan, a major limitation is that this theory does not account for differences in these processes (determinants) by developmental age or differences in the needs, resources, and challenges of youths as they mature. To more clearly integrate age-appropriate influences on health behaviors, we propose the integration of SCT with a biological and developmental perspective (Bronfenbrenner, 2005; Bronfenbrenner & Morris, 2006; Schwartz, 1982). Factors influential at one point in development may not function as predominant influences at other points in development. Addressing youths' health and health behaviors from this integrated perspective is particularly important for identifying the multiple factors that need consideration to make sure that intervention strategies are developmentally appropriate, and that help guide parents and other important socializers to foster children's development and maintenance of healthy lifestyles as they mature. Given the increasing prevalence rate of obesity and Type 2 diabetes in youths (Ogden, Carroll, Curtin, Lamb, & Flegal, 2010), it is essential to gain a better perspective on social and environmental conditions that may contribute to increased risk among youths at critical points in their development.

Understanding youths' health behaviors requires an examination of development that results from the interaction of biological, psychological, and social factors over time. Scientists have begun to apply systems-based theories/models as a more effective/comprehensive means for understanding health behaviors (Baranowski, Cullen, Nicklas, Thompson, & Baranowski, 2003; Wilson, 2008; Wilson & Lawman, 2009; Zarrett, 2007; Zarrett & Eccles, 2009). Although a number of different ecological models exist, all share the core belief that behavior is influenced by the synergistic relation between individuals and their multiple levels of environmental subsystems over time (Bronfenbrenner, 2005; Bronfenbrenner & Morris, 2006; Sallis et al., 2006). The bioecological model outlined by Bronfenbrenner and Morris (2006) provides a framework for understanding health and health behaviors

as shaped by environmental subsystems that include the integration of intrapersonal factors, microsystemic factors (families and institutions), mesosystemic factors (interactions between family and institutions), exosystemic factors (communities, policies), and macrosystemic effects (all systems, micro-, meso-, and exo-, are related to a culture or subculture). Bronfenbrenner and Morris noted that the direct person–context interactions that occurred at the "microsystem" level are of particular importance. Although distal ecologies, such as the parents' workplace, or a federal policy, influence the type and quality of interactions that occur within the microsystem, development is directly influenced by the moment-to-moment pattern of exchange between the individual and his or her surroundings. Furthermore, within the bioecological model, each part of the system (e.g., the individual, the family, the peer group, the neighborhood) is considered to be only one important part of a complex multilevel system. Therefore, if we are to understand how to influence youths to engage in healthy behaviors, we must consider all of the parts of the developmental system and how they interact with one another to promote positive attitudes and behavior (Mahoney, Vandell, Simpkins, & Zarrett, 2009; Zarrett & Eccles, 2009). The bioecological model, and systems theory more generally, provides a strong macroparadigm for understanding development as the complex relation between youths and their environments over time. Thus, the theoretical approach proposed in this chapter integrates biological, cognitive, social, and environmental influences in understanding of health behaviors at different ages and developmental stages.

The biopsychosocial model (Schwartz, 1982) has been a particularly effective application of systems theory for approaching issues regarding health and health behaviors across the lifespan. This model places a strong emphasis on the biological factors that influence healthy choices and behaviors, while considering the integrated nature of these biological factors with psychological and social factors. Specifically, this model proposes that these three factors—biological, psychological, and social—interact in understanding individuals' overall health behaviors through a dynamic reciprocal process. Biological factors such as genetics (Allison, Heshka, Neale, Lakken, & Heymsfield, 1994), as well as metabolism and taste-related factors (Logue, 1991), have been shown to influence health behaviors such as weight and eating preferences. Taste preferences, metabolism, body type, and addictive traits are then nurtured, maintained, or altered given the cultural influence of the family, the availability of food and activities in the home, and the beliefs and values about health and healthy behaviors of parents and other key socializers (e.g., peers, teachers).

Developmental theories have been in existence since the inception of the field of psychology; however, successful integration of developmental theories in understanding the formation and development of long-term health-related lifestyle preferences in youths has not been forthcoming. Much progress in understanding the appropriate theoretical approaches to influencing health behaviors depend on fully understanding and integrating critical elements of developmental theory into systematic and scientifically designed studies. Previous investigators have proposed that a future orientation be given to prevention and the promotion of positive lifestyle development from very early on in a child's lifetime (Maddux, Roberts, Sledden, & Wright, 1986). Other investigators have also argued that, from a developmental perspective, prevention and treatment approaches must target specific issues during each critical period of a child's developmental lifespan (Maddux et al., 1986). For example, during preschool and elementary stages of life, children are much more dependent on their parents (Flavell, 1999) for their basic daily needs, including food availability and consumption patterns. As youths mature into adolescence, they gain autonomy (Inhelder & Piaget, 1964) and begin to make more independent decisions regarding their choice of leisure activities, food consumption patterns, and risky health behaviors (e.g., substance use), and they are more greatly influenced by the social environment external to the family context, including peers and institutionalized social norms (e.g., school breakfast and/or lunch programs). Thus, a major objective of this chapter is to integrate biopsychosocial and developmental processes in understanding how to intervene effectively during critical developmental stages in childhood and adolescence to promote health and healthy behaviors.

Developmental Stages and Influences

Biological, psychosocial, and environmental determinants of health/health behaviors vary in their influence as children mature from infancy through adolescence. The specific stages that we have organized as critical include toddler and preschool years, early elementary school years, late elementary school years, middle school years, and high school years. The integration of key biological, cognitive, social, and environmental factors during each of these critical periods is outlined in this section, and specific studies are reviewed as examples and summarized in Table 9.1.

Infancy to Toddlerhood

Even as early as the infancy and toddlerhood years, children are able to recognize their parents' simple health beliefs and respond to simple behavioral and environmental cues (Flavell, 1999). Parenting styles that encourage attachment are believed to play a part in establishing positive parent–child interactions early on in a child's life (Flavell, 1999). For example, in previous research, an authoritative parenting style and parent warmth were found to predict higher rates of participation in positive activities and lower participation in unconstructive activities (Bohnert, Martin, & Garber, 2007; Fletcher, Elder, & Mekos, 2000; Huebner & Mancini, 2003; Larson, Richards, Sims, & Dworkin, 2001; Mahoney & Stattin, 2000; Mahoney, Stattin, & Lord, 2004; Persson, Kerr, & Stattin, 2007). Researchers believe that these more general parenting behaviors impact youths indirectly, by promoting their socioemotional adjustment, although these mediation models have not been tested. Biological factors, in terms of taste preferences and genetic-related risk factors, continue to interact with environmental influences to influence child health behaviors. During these early years, the home environment may be particularly important in terms of food availability and of early preferences for foods that may be introduced to children. Introducing vegetables and fruits at this critical period is important for future taste preferences (Birch, McPhee, Shoba, Pirok, & Steinberg, 1987).

The study by Spurrier, Magarey, Golley, Curnow, and Sawyer (2008) provides an ex-

TABLE 9.1. Determinants of Health Behaviors (Diet, Physical Activity, Smoking) across Developmental Stages of Children and Adolescents

Developmental stage	Author	Sample	Study design	Determinants of behavior	Primary outcomes	Findings
Preschool	Spurrier et al. (2008)	Homes of preschool children in South Australia (N = 280, mean age = 4.8 ± .21 years)	Cross-sectional survey and direct observation	• *Social:* Parental behaviors associated with food (e.g., eating in front of TV, rewarding good behavior with food) and physical activity (e.g., role modeling) • *Environmental:* Nutritional home environment (e.g., quantity of fruit and vegetables, fat content of dairy products, presence of sweetened drinks) and physical characteristics of the home (e.g., size of backyard).	• Parent report of children's dietary patterns • Parent report of children's outdoor playtime	• Higher fruit and vegetable scores were associated with parental factors such as the use of less food rewards/incentives ($p < .05$) and not allowing the child to eat in front of the TV ($p < .01$). • Higher outdoor play scores were associated with factors such as mothers' walking ($p < .01$), mothers' involvement in organized sports ($p < .05$), size of backyard ($p < .01$), and items of outdoor play equipment ($p < .01$).
Early elementary	Weir et al. (2006)	Total N = 307 (n = 204 inner-city youth, mean age = 7.4 ± 1.9, 76% Hispanic, 11% African American; N = 103 suburban youth, mean age = 6.9 ± 1.6, 50% European American, 17% African American)	Cross-sectional survey completed by parents	• *Demographic variables:* Age, gender, parents' education, race • *Social/environmental:* Parents' perceptions of neighborhood safety (anxiety about gangs, crime, aggression by other children, traffic, and neighborhood safety in general) • *Environmental:* Inner-city versus suburban surroundings	Parent report of youth physical activity	• Inner-city children engaged in less physical activity than did suburban children ($p < .001$). • A greater percentage of the inner city versus suburban parents worried about their child being threatened by gangs, felt that there was no safe area to play in their neighborhood, believed it was dangerous to let a child play outside, believed that neighborhood crime made it unsafe to play outdoors, and felt personally unsafe in their own neighborhood ($p < .0001$ for each comparison). • In the inner-city group, parental anxiety about neighborhood safety was negatively associated with children's physical activity levels ($r = -.18, p < .05$).
	Fisher et al. (2002)	Non-Hispanic white families with 5-year-old girls (N = 191)	Cross-sectional	• *Social:* Parents' fruit and vegetable intake, parents' use of pressure to eat in child feeding	Parent report of child fruit, vegetable, micronutrient,	• Girls' fruit and vegetable intake was positively related to their parents' reported fruit and vegetable intake ($r = .23, p < .05$).

	Study	Sample	Design	Variables	Outcome measure	Findings
					and fat intake	• Girls who received more pressure to eat tended to have lower fruit and vegetable ($r = -.18$, $p < .05$) and micronutrient intakes ($r = -.12$, $p < .05$).
Late elementary	Côté et al. (2004)	French-speaking public school students from Quebec ($N = 373$, 191 girls and 182 boys)	Repeated measures: Beginning of fifth grade; beginning of sixth grade (Time 1); end of sixth grade (Time 2); middle of first year of secondary school (Time 3)	*Cognitive:* Intention over time, perceived self-efficacy *Social:* Perceived smoking behavior of friends, perceived smoking behavior of a brother, parental supervision, socioeconomic status	Self-reported abstinence from cigarettes	• 76.14% of the sample remained abstinent from cigarettes • Perceived behavior of friends ($p = .0001$), intention interaction with time ($p = .0037$), perceived behavior of a brother ($p = .0314$), perceived self-efficacy ($p = .0206$), socioeconomic index ($p = .0002$), and parental supervision ($p = .0113$), all independently and significantly predicted maintenance of abstinence from cigarettes.
Middle school	Springer et al. (2006)	Girls in Texas ($N = 718$, 71.8% European American, 11.6% Hispanic, 16.6% other)	Cross-sectional baseline data from an osteoporosis prevention intervention study	*Social:* Type of social support (social participation, social encouragement for physical activity), sources of social support (family, friends)	Self-reported daily minutes of physical activity and sedentary behavior	• Social encouragement from friends was the only variable positively related to vigorous physical activity ($r = .11$, $p = .005$). • Social participation in physical activity by friends (partial correlation coefficient [r] = .10, $p = .009$) and friend ($r = .12$) and family encouragement ($r = .11$) ($p < .01$, respectively) were positively related to moderate-to-vigorous physical activity. • Social participation in physical activity by family had the strongest negative correlation with total minutes of TV viewing and computer video playing ($r = -0.08$, $p < .05$).

(cont.)

TABLE 9.1. (*cont.*)

Developmental stage	Author	Sample	Study design	Determinants of behavior	Primary outcomes	Findings
Middle school–high school	Dornelas et al. (2005)	Youth who had smoked at least 100 cigarettes in their lifetime and were current smokers ($N = 181$, European American = 138, African American = 24, Hispanic = 19)	Cross-sectional	• *Demographic variables*: Ethnicity, age, gender, tobacco use history • *Social*: Social factors associated with smoking (i.e., smokes with smoking friends, smokes with family, perception of support for quitting smoking) • *Social/cognitive*: Situational factors associated with smoking (i.e., stress, hunger, boredom, after meals) • *Environmental*: Places that were likely sites for smoking (i.e., school, inside the home)	Youth smoking based on self-report	• 96% of the African American adolescents lived with another smoker compared to 68% of Hispanic and 60% of European Americans ($p = .004$). • African American teenagers were more likely to smoke with family members (50%) than Hispanics (5%) or European Americans (25%) ($p = .003$). • 50% of African American teenagers versus 5% of Hispanics and 12% of European American teenagers reported smoking to fit in ($p < .0001$). • Higher rates of role modeling by members of the household, more prevalent beliefs that smoking is a way to achieve belonging, acceptance of smoking by family, and lack of perceived support for quitting by friends influence cigarette smoking more for African American than for European American or Hispanic youths.
High school	Neumark-Sztainer et al. (2005)	Students participating in TACOS (Trying Alternative Cafeteria Options in Schools) school-based intervention	Cross-sectional	• *Environmental*: School food-related polices (regarding open vs. closed campus at lunch time, regarding hours of operation of vending machines), food environment (number of vending machines serving snacks or soft drinks, types of food served in vending machines)	Self-report of students' lunch patterns (regular school lunch, à la carte lunch, bring lunch, fast food, convenience	• Boys ate meals from the main lunch line more frequently than girls ($p < .001$) and brought lunch from home less frequently than girls ($p < .001$). • 68.4% of schools had closed campus lunchtime policies, and only 15.8% of schools had policies regarding the types of foods that could be sold in vending machines.

138

Study	Sample	Design	Variables	Results
	trial (N = 1,088, 47% male, 53% female; 84.3% European American, 4.6% Asian, 2.5% Hispanic, 2.4% African American, 6.2% American Indian/other)		store). Vending machine practices (snacks, soft drinks)	• Students who attended schools with open campus lunchtime policies were significantly more likely to eat lunch at a fast food restaurant than students at schools with closed campus lunchtime policies (0.7 days/week vs. 0.2 days/week, $p < .001$). • At schools with food-related policies, students reported purchasing significantly more snack food than students from schools without food-related policies ($p < .001$).
Smith et al. (2007)	Students from three high schools (N = 785, 53% female, 80% European American, 14% African American, 6% other ethnic groups)	Cross-sectional	• *Demographic variables:* Grade in school, ethnicity, sex • *Cognitive:* Attitudes toward remaining tobacco-free, perceived risks of tobacco use, subjective norms, perceived behavioral control to avoid smoking, perceived difficulty to quit smoking • *Social:* Peer tobacco use, presence of a male guardian, perceived prevalence of smoking among age group	Intentions to try smoking, smoking status based on self-report	• 21.2% reported smoking in the past 30 days. • Students with no intentions to smoke in the next 6 months had significantly more favorable attitudes toward remaining tobacco free (M = 4.17) and perceived greater risk of tobacco use (M = 4.50) than those with intentions to smoke (M = 3.69, 4.12) and those who already smoke (M = 3.57, 4.16). • The likelihood of having intentions to try to smoke in the next 6 months significantly decreased with more positive attitudes toward staying tobacco-free (odds ratio [OR] 0.56, 95% confidence interval [CI] 0.34, 0.92; $p < .05$) and increased levels of perceived difficulty to quit (OR 0.67, 95% CI 0.52, 0.85; $p < .001$), and significantly increased with more peer smoking (OR 1.42, 95% CI 1.04, 1.95).

ample of the importance of both social and environmental factors in determining diet and physical activity patterns in preschool children (Table 9.1). Specifically, this study illustrates critical factors related to social and environmental contexts. Health behaviors at this developmental stage revolve around children's interactions with parents and their experience of home surroundings. For example, parental behaviors, such as mothers' frequently taking walks with children, were associated with physical activity scores in youths (Spurrier et al., 2008). Similarly, aspects of the physical home environment (e.g., number of items of outdoor play equipment, amount of fruit available) were related both to more positive diet and to physical activity scores in youth (Spurrier et al., 2008). At this developmental stage, parents are key facilitators of positive health behaviors in terms of creating a positive context (both socially and physically) that supports their child's engagement in healthy eating and physical activity practices.

Preschool Years

As children move into the preschool years they develop short-term memory and concrete cognitive abilities, such as being able to understand simple notions of self-oriented beliefs (Flavell, 1999). In addition, children of preschool age begin to understand the concepts of simple positive and negative reinforcers of behavior (Flavell, 1999). This also implies that children at this developmental stage can begin to be influenced by parental modeling and behavioral consequences. For example, parents regularly act as role models, with active engagement in their own set of healthy physical activities. In fact, research suggests both a concurrent relation between parents' and youths' activity levels (e.g., Babkes & Weiss, 1999) as well as a longitudinal influence of parents' own activity involvement on their children's subsequent participation in the activity through adolescence (Huebner & Mancini, 2003; Simpkins, Fredricks, Davis-Kean, & Eccles, 2006). Moreover, during this stage of their children's development, parents are able to begin encouraging them to pursue healthy behaviors by exposing them to these behaviors in various ways. Such support can include parental participation in activi-

ties (coactivity), which gives parents the opportunity actively to coach and teach their children skills, and to provide performance feedback, including direct positive and negative reinforcements for participating (Eccles, Wigfield, & Schiefele, 1998; Fredricks & Eccles, 2005). This is the time when early lifestyle patterns begin to be established. In particular, the home and neighborhood environments begin to establish the availability of physical activity opportunities, as well as patterns of sedentary behaviors. The availability of playgrounds, play spaces, and opportunities for viewing television and movies all begin to impact the establishment of healthy behaviors during this developmental period in the lifespan.

Several studies of children at this critical age (Fisher, Mitchell, Smiciklas-Wright, & Birch, 2002; Weir, Etelson, & Brand, 2006) have demonstrated that an integration of both social and environmental factors related to parents continues to impact the health behaviors of youths in the early elementary school years (Table 9.1). For example, Weir and colleagues (2006) studied the influence of parent perceptions of neighborhood safety on children's physical activity levels. Greater parent perceptions of neighborhood crime were negatively correlated with reported levels of children's physical activity. Fisher and colleagues (2002) examined the social impact of parent modeling and parenting style around child intake of fruit and vegetable consumption. Parents who ate more fruits and vegetables had daughters who ate more fruits and vegetables. Together, these studies capture the fact that both environmental factors, such as perceptions of neighborhood safety, and parental factors, such as role modeling, influence health behaviors in elementary school–age youths.

Early Elementary School Years

Children in their early elementary school years begin to understand the concept of time and time-based images of reality (Flavell, 1999). Most children in this age group develop concrete operational thinking, and the ability to reason begins. In addition, they begin to understand external causes of behavior (Erikson, 1968). This suggests that children of this age begin to develop health beliefs and understand the concept of health behaviors, such as the importance of diet and physical activity. This is the developmental point at which a shift in social interactions involves schools, afterschool youth programs, and availability of leisure time activities with peers and family members. This is a time when social interaction begins to be a part of children's lives and has some impact on play experiences at recess. The availability of playgrounds and play spaces is important to youths at this age. During this development stage the availability of computers, television, and electronic devices, such as handheld games, sets the stage for children's expectations as they move into the late elementary and middle school years. Parental role modeling continues to be very instrumental at this age, although peer influences begin to have some impact on children's health behaviors.

Late Elementary School Years

By the late elementary school years, children begin to formulate their own health attitudes, beliefs, goals, and intentions with respect to health behaviors (Flavell, 1999). Beliefs about self-efficacy, perceived personal control, perceived vulnerability to health problems, and behavioral goal setting are concepts that many late elementary school-age children now comprehend. This is also a developmental stage in which some children undergo pubertal changes that can impact emotions, and social interactions that can ultimately impact health behaviors (Brooks-Gunn, 1993). Although parents continue to play a major role in establishing lifestyle patterns around healthy behaviors, peers begin to have a more significant role in late elementary school-age children's lives (Brooks-Gunn, 1993). Environmental factors related to cultural, family, and institutional factors all become increasingly important in shaping the eating and activity patterns of youths in the late elementary school years.

Additionally, youths begin to be at greater risk for developing other health-related risks, such as substance use during the later elementary school years, when peers begin to have more influence on youths' behaviors. Côté, Godin, and Gagné (2004) examined both social and cognitive factors as they relate to abstinence from cigarettes in a cohort of elementary school children (Table 9.1).

This study illustrates that unlike earlier developmental stages in which social factors affecting health behaviors mainly revolve around parents and the home, smoking behaviors of children in the process of transitioning into middle school are affected by other social networks, namely, peers. Côté and colleagues found that participants were more likely to abstain from smoking if they perceived fewer friends smoking in their surroundings. In addition, this study also illustrates the importance of the children's own cognitions in impacting behavior. Children were more likely to remain abstinent if they had higher perceived self-efficacy to do so (Côté et al., 2004).

Middle School Years

During the middle school years, children and adolescents develop formal operational thoughts and now have the ability to consider multiple, interacting determinants of behavior (Inhelder & Piaget, 1964). This includes knowledge of real, as well as abstract, phenomena and an understanding about the complex interactions of personal, social, cultural, and environmental influences on health behaviors, which may expand approaches that can be used to increase positive health behaviors at this age. In this developmental stage, social interactions with peers become increasingly important. Parental supervision is an important part of this developmental stage as well. In particular, the home environment becomes a key setting in providing opportunities for transportation to physical activity opportunities or for having physical activity equipment and healthy foods available for consumption on a regular basis. Youths at this developmental stage continue to experience pubertal changes and also become more aware of safety-related issues in their neighborhood and community environment (Fauth, Roth, & Brooks-Gunn, 2007; Weir, Etelson, & Brand, 2006).

Springer, Kelder, and Hoelscher (2006) examined the importance of understanding social determinants of health behaviors at the middle school age, when children's interactions with peers become more important (Table 9.1). In this study, encouragement from friends was the only variable associated positively with vigorous physical activity in youths. Still, the home context (including social and environmental factors) continues to play a role in providing opportunities that either support or inhibit a particular health behavior. For example, child sedentary behavior (i.e., minutes watching television and playing computer/video games) had the strongest negative association with family participation in physical activity (Springer et al., 2006). In terms of adolescents' smoking, Dornelas and colleagues (2005) showed how an integration of social, cognitive, and environmental factors contributes to ethnic differences in this behavior. For example, African American adolescents (compared to European American and Hispanic youth) were more likely to live with another smoker, smoke with family members, and to smoke because they believed it would help them fit in. In addition, African American adolescents felt the least support from others for quitting smoking (Dornelas et al., 2005). As evidenced by this study, the health behaviors of adolescents in middle school are impacted by myriad interacting determinants.

High School Years

As adolescents move into the high school years, they demonstrate formal operational thinking and are able to apply these sophisticated cognitive processes to a broader array of personal, social, and physical domains (Gerrard, Gibbons, Benthin, & Hessling, 1996). Self-regulatory cognitions, including self-efficacy, future orientation, social comparison orientation, and perceived behavior of peers, are concepts that are comprehended at this developmental stage (Gerrard et al., 1996). Puberty may also continue for some youths as they move into the high school years. For others, puberty may be completed and no longer a part of their developmental life stage. Social interactions with peers become a major aspect of this developmental stage, while parents continue to have some influences in the home environment. Community opportunities for engaging in physical activity and health-related opportunities become more essential from an environmental perspective; however, there may also be fewer community programs that target this age group (Fauth et al., 2007; Simpkins, Ripke, Huston, & Eccles, 2005). Access to neighborhood resources, such as parks, community centers, playing fields,

and positive adult mentors that implement and oversee the activity are significantly associated with increases in youths' participation (Duncan & Brooks-Gunn, 2000; Mahoney, Cairns, & Farmer, 2003; Pedersen & Seidman, 2005; Quinn, 1999; Rural School and Community Trust, 2005). During early and middle adolescence, not only do almost all youths attend school, but many of them receive additional support from community youth organizations. By late adolescence, when community and school may be most needed, these supports diverge or disappear altogether, with fewer community programs and recreational leagues targeting high schoolers, and fewer school-based opportunities to engage in physical activity such as sports teams become more competitive/selective (Eccles & Gootman, 2002; Zarrett & Eccles, 2006). Despite these challenges during late adolescence, early participation (during middle childhood and adolescence), when youths build their activity-specific skills set and increase internal motivation, predicts sustained participation in healthy physical activities (Busseri, Rose-Krasnor, Willoughby, & Chalmers, 2006; Jordan & Nettles, 2000; Mahoney et al., 2003) even when activities become competitive in high school (Quiroz, 2000; Simpkins, Ripke, Huston, & Eccles, 2005).

Several studies (e.g., Neumark-Sztainer, French, Hannan, Story, & Fulkerson, 2005; Smith, Bean, Mitchell, Speizer, & Fries, 2007) provide examples of how determinants of health behaviors expand and become more complex as youths get older (see Table 9.1). For instance, Smith and colleagues (2007) showed how cognitive factors, such as attitudes toward remaining tobacco-free, perceived risks of tobacco use, subjective norms, perceived behavioral control to avoid smoking, and perceived difficulty to quit smoking, impact older youths' smoking behavior. These cognitions are affected by the social climate and the physical environment. For example, from an environmental perspective, Neumark-Sztainer and colleagues (2005) examined the relationship between school food-related policies and students' lunchtime patterns, and found that at schools with food-related policies, students reported purchasing significantly more snack food than students from schools without food-related policies.

Conclusions

In summary, due to changing cognitive, biological, social, and environmental variables across the critical developmental stages, there are distinct opportunities for influencing children's and adolescents' health behaviors. For example, although parents have a major role in their children's behavioral choices at younger ages (infancy through late elementary years), peer influence becoming increasingly important from middle to high schools years. Biological influences begin at birth, but wide variations in biological changes, such as those experienced during puberty, vary across individual youths. The community, school, and home environments are all key in a child's life, but as a child moves through the developmental stages, more profound environmental influences may come into play, such as community opportunities for physical activity and the availability of equipment, and tangible parental support to engage in physical activity. Food availability in the home continues to be important throughout the entire development spectrum; however, as youths mature, food options in other contexts in which they are embedded (e.g., school, friends' homes) become increasingly more influential. Smoking behavior is influenced by peers and family members during middle and high school years.

This chapter has provided a developmental framework for understanding youths' health choices and behaviors from infancy through the high school years. Biological, cognitive, social, and environmental factors play a key role in whether youths are more likely to eat healthy food, be physically active, and not initiate smoking behavior. The studies reviewed in this chapter provide a basis for understanding developmental issues of correlates of health behaviors in youths. In general, early participation in positive health behaviors (during middle childhood and adolescence) have been shown to predict sustained health behaviors over time (Busseri et al., 2006; Jordan & Nettles, 2000; Mahoney et al., 2003). Previous investigators have shown that intrapersonal factors such as motivation (values and ability beliefs) often develop as a result of external motivating factors (Pearce & Larson, 2006). Thus, the influence of other people (e.g., encouraging parents, participating friends and teachers) is a common external source that may be instrumental in influencing youths to engage in healthy behavioral choices (Loder & Hirsch, 2003). Thus, the social influences of parents, friends, and significant others are important in understanding developmental approaches to promoting positive health in early childhood. Further research is needed to compare more extensively different developmentally relevant approaches to promoting positive health behaviors across childhood and adolescence. More research is needed that focuses on longitudinal designs to understand better youths' differing needs at various ages. To advance the work in this area, it will also be important for researchers and scientists to develop critical studies that test competing theories. For example, environmental supports for physical activity are not well understood across developmental stages. While parental and home environmental variables may be more important influences on these behaviors in younger children, it is not clear to what extent cognitive beliefs (health beliefs, self-efficacy, etc.) versus social interaction approaches (social norms, etc.) are more effective for improving health behaviors in youths in the middle to high school years of development.

The most fundamental notion that needs to be incorporated into future research is a clear and well-implemented theoretical approach to designing interventions. Longitudinal studies should be coupled with intervention models, and both should include predicted mediational influences. Theory is essential to understanding mediational influences that may be critical during the various developmental stages outlined in this chapter (Baranowski et al., 2003; Wilson, 2008). For example, previous research has demonstrated that interventions are more likely to have the desired impact on an outcome if the mediating variables are strongly related to the behaviors of interest, and if effective procedures are used in the intervention to manipulate these variables in desired directions (Baranowski et al., 1997). Mediators or mediating variables, such as biological, psychological, and social/environmental influences, can also be analyzed to test how some of these variables are integrated into cause–effect sequences that affect behavior as youths mature.

In summary, research that has addressed the health behaviors of youths within a developmental framework has in general been scarce. This chapter was developed to highlight how a developmental approach that integrates the impact of biological, cognitive, social, and environmental influences can contribute to our understanding of the critical components needed to promote healthy youth behaviors. Given the increasing prevalence of obesity and chronic disease in children and adolescents, the perspective presented in this chapter should be very useful to researchers, scientists, and scholars, and to a wide range of health professionals interested in promoting positive health behaviors in youths.

Acknowledgment

Preparation of this chapter was supported in part by Grant No. R01 HD 045693 from the National Institute of Child Health and Human Development to Dawn K. Wilson.

Further Reading

Gordon-Larsen, P., Nelson, M. C., & Popkin, B. M. (2004). Longitudinal physical activity and sedentary behavior trends: Adolescence to adulthood. *American Journal of Preventive Medicine, 27*(4), 277–283.

Janz, K. F., Dawson, J. D., & Mahoney, L. T. (2000). Tracking physical fitness and physical activity from childhood to adolescence: The Muscatine Study. *Medicine and Science in Sports and Exercise, 32*(7), 1250–1257.

Malina, R. M. (2001). Physical activity and fitness: Pathways from childhood to adulthood. *American Journal of Human Biology, 13*(2), 162–172.

Nelson, M. C., Neumark-Stzainer, D., Hannan, P. J., Sirard, J. R., & Story, M. (2006). Longitudinal and secular trends in physical activity and sedentary behavior during adolescence. *Pediatrics, 118*(6), 1627–1634.

Neumark-Sztainer, D., Story, M., Hannan, P. J., Tharp, T., & Rex. J. (2003). Factors associated with changes in physical activity: A cohort study of inactive adolescent girls. *Archives of Pediatric and Adolescent Medicine, 157*, 803–810.

Sallis, J. F., Prochaska, J. J., & Taylor, W. C. (2000). A review of correlates of physical activity of children and adolescents. *Medicine and Science in Sports and Exercise, 32*(5), 963–975.

Simpkins, S. D., Fredricks, J., Davis-Kean, P., & Eccles, J. S. (2006). Healthy minds, healthy habits: The influence of activity involvement in middle childhood. In A. C. Huston & M. N. Ripke (Eds.), *Developmental contexts in middle childhood* (pp. 283–302). New York: Cambridge University Press.

Taylor, R. W., Grant, A. M., Goulding, A., & Williams, S. M. (2005). Early adiposity rebound: Review of papers linking this to subsequent obesity in children and adults. *Current Opinions in Clinical Nutrition and Metabolic Care, 8*(6), 607–661.

Wilson, D. K., Zarrett, N., & Kitzman-Ulrich, H. (in press). Physical activity and health: Current research trends and critical issues. In H. Friedman (Ed.), *Oxford handbook of health psychology*. New York: Oxford University Press.

References

Allison, D. B., Heshka, S., Neale, M. C., Lakken, D. T., & Heymsfield, S. B. (1994). A genetic analysis of relative weight among 4,020 twin pairs, with an emphasis on sex effects. *Health Psychology, 13*, 362–365.

Babkes, M. L., & Weiss, M. R. (1999). Parent influence on cognitive and affective responses in children's competitive soccer participation. *Pediatric Exercise Science, 11*, 44–62.

Bandura, A. (1991). Self-regulation of motivation through anticipatory and self-reactive mechanisms. In R. Dienstbier (Ed.), *Nebraska Symposium on Motivation: Perspectives on motivation* (pp. 69–164). Lincoln: University of Nebraska Press.

Bandura, A. (1997). Self-efficacy: The exercise of control. New York: Freeman.

Bandura, A. (2002). Health promotion by social cognitive means. *Health Education and Behavior, 31*, 143–164.

Baranowski, T., Cullen, K. W., Nicklas, T., Thompson, D., & Baranowski, J. (2003). Are current health behavioral change models helpful in guiding prevention of weight gain efforts? *Obesity Research, 11*, 23S–43S.

Birch, L. L., McPhee, L., Shoba, B. C., Pirok, E., & Steinberg, L. (1987). What kind of exposure reduces children's food neophobia?: Looking vs. tasting. *Appetite, 9*, 171–178.

Bohnert, A. M., Martin, N. C., & Garber, J. (2007). Predicting adolescents' organized activity involvement: The role of maternal depression history, family relationship quality, and adolescent cognitions. *Journal of Research on Adolescence, 17*(1), 221–244.

Bronfenbrenner, U. (2005). *Making human beings human: Bioecological perspectives on human development*. Thousand Oaks, CA: Sage.

Bronfenbrenner, U., & Morris, P. (2006). The bioecological model of human development. In W. Daman & R. M. Lerner (Editors-in-Chief) and R. M. Lerner (Vol. Ed.), *Handbook of child psychology: Vol. 1. Theoretical models of human development* (pp. 793–828). Hoboken, NJ: Wiley.

Brooks-Gunn, J. (1993). Why do adolescents have difficulty adhering to health regimes. In N. A. Krasnegor, L. Epstein, S. Bennett Johnson, & S. J. Yaffe (Eds.), *Developmental aspects of health compliance behavior* (pp. 125–152). Hillsdale, NJ: Erlbaum.

Busseri, M. A., Rose-Krasnor, L., Willoughby, T., & Chalmers, H. (2006). A longitudinal examination of breadth and intensity of youth activity involvement and successful development. *Developmental Psychology, 42,* 1313–1326.

Côté, F., Godin, G., & Gagné, C. (2004). Identification of factors promoting abstinence from smoking in a cohort of elementary schoolchildren. *Preventive Medicine, 39,* 695–703.

Dornelas, E., Patten, C., Fischer, E., Decker, P. A., Offord, K., Barbagallo, J., et al. (2005). Ethnic variation in socioenvironmental factors that influence adolescent smoking. *Journal of Adolescent Health, 36,* 170–177.

Duncan, G. J., & Brooks-Gunn, J. (2000). Family poverty, welfare reform, and child development. *Child Development, 71*(1), 188–196.

Eccles, J. S., & Gootman, J. A. (Eds.). (2002). *Community programs to promote youth development.* Washington, DC: National Academy Press.

Eccles, J. S., Wigfield, A., & Schiefele, U. (1998). Motivation to succeed. In W. Damon (Series Ed.), & N. Eisenberg (Vol. Ed.), *Handbook of child psychology: Vol. 3. Social, emotional and personality development* (5th ed., pp. 1017–1094). New York: Wiley.

Erikson, E. H. (1968). *Identity: Youth and crisis.* New York: Norton.

Fauth, R. C., Roth, J. L., & Brooks-Gunn, J. (2007). Does the neighborhood context alter the link between youth's after-school activities and developmental outcomes?: A multilevel analysis. *Developmental Psychology, 43,* 760–777.

Fisher, J. O., Mitchell, D. C., Smiciklas-Wright, H., & Birch, L. L. (2002). Parental influences on young girls' fruit and vegetable, micronutrient, and fat intakes. *Journal of the American Dietetic Association, 102,* 58–64.

Flavell, J. H. (1999). Cognitive development: Children's knowledge about mind. *Annual Review of Psychology, 50,* 21–45.

Fletcher, A. C., Elder, G. H., Jr., & Mekos, D. (2000). Parental influences on adolescent involvement in community activities. *Journal of Research on Adolescence, 10*(1), 29–48.

Fredricks, J. A., & Eccles, J. S. (2005). Family socialization, gender, and sport motivation and involvement. *Journal of Sport and Exercise Psychology, 27,* 3–31.

Gerrard, M., Gibbons, F. X., Benthin, A. C., & Hessling, R. M. (1996). A longitudinal study of the reciprocal nature of risk behaviors and cognitions in adolescents: What you do shapes what you think, and vice versa. *Health Psychology, 15,* 344–354.

Huebner, A. J., & Mancini, J. A. (2003). Shaping structured out-of-school time use among youth: The effects of self, family, and friend systems. *Journal of Youth and Adolescence, 32*(6), 453–463.

Inhelder, B., & Piaget, J. (1964) *The early growth of logic in the child* (E. A. Lunzer & D. Papert, Trans.). London: Routledge & Kegan Paul.

Jordan, W. J., & Nettles, S. M. (2000). How students invest their time outside of school: Effects on school-related outcomes. *Social Psychology of Education, 3,* 217–243.

Larson, R. W., Richards, M. H., Sims, B., & Dworkin, J. (2001). How urban African American young adolescents spend their time: Time budgets for locations, activities, and companionship. *American Journal of Community Psychology, 29,* 565–597.

Loder, T. L., & Hirsch, B. J. (2003). Inner-city youth development organizations: The salience of peer ties among early adolescent girls. *Applied Developmental Science, 7*(1), 2–12.

Logue, A. W. (1991). *The psychology of eating and drinking: An introduction* (2nd ed.). New York: Freeman.

Maddux, J. E., Roberts, M. C., Sledden, E. A., & Wright, L. (1986). Developmental issues in child health psychology. *American Psychologist, 41,* 25–34.

Mahoney, J. L., Cairns, B. D., & Farmer, T. W. (2003). Promoting interpersonal competence and educational success through extracurricular activity participation. *Journal of Educational Psychology, 95,* 409–418.

Mahoney, J. L., & Stattin, H. (2000). Leisure activities and adolescent antisocial behavior: The role of structure and social context. *Journal of Adolescence, 23,* 113–127.

Mahoney, J. L., Stattin, H., & Lord, H. (2004). Unstructured youth recreation centre participation and antisocial behaviour development: Selection influences and the moderation role of antisocial peers. *International Journal of Behavioral Development, 28,* 553–560.

Mahoney, J. L., Vandell, D., Simpkins, S., & Zarrett, N. (2009). Adolescents' out-of-school activities. In R. M. Lerner & L. Steinberg (Eds.), *Handbook of adolescent psychology* (3rd ed.). New York: Wiley.

Neumark-Sztainer, D., French, S. A., Hannan, P. J., Story, M., & Fulkerson, J. A. (2005).

School lunch and snacking patterns among high school students: Associations with school food environment and policies. *International Journal of Behavioral Nutrition and Physical Activity, 2*, 14–20.

Ogden, C. L., Carroll, M. D., Curtin, L. R., Lamb, M. M., & Flegal, K. M. (2010). Prevalence of high body mass index in U.S. children and adolescents. *Journal of the American Medical Association, 303*, 242–249.

Pearce, N. J., & Larson, R. W. (2006). How teens become engaged in youth development programs: The process of motivational change in a civic activism organization. *Applied Developmental Science, 10*, 121–131.

Pedersen, S., & Seidman, E. (2005). Contexts and correlates of out-of-school activity participation among low-income urban adolescents. In J. L. Mahoney, R. W. Larson, & J. S. Eccles (Eds.), *Organized activities as contexts of development: Extracurricular activities, after-school and community programs* (pp. 85–110). Mahwah, NJ: Erlbaum.

Persson, A., Kerr, M., & Stattin, H. (2007). Staying in or moving away from structured activities: Explanations involving parents and peers. *Developmental Psychology, 43*, 197–207.

Quinn, J. (1999). Where needs meet opportunity: Youth development programs for early teens. In R. Behrman (Ed.), *The future of children: When school is out* (pp. 96–116). Washington, DC: David and Lucile Packard Foundation.

Quiroz, P. (2000). A comparison of the organizational and cultural contexts of extracurricular participation and sponsorship in two high schools. *Educational Studies, 31*, 249–275.

Rural School and Community Trust. (2005). Retrieved January 7, 2008, from *www.ruraledu.org/site/c.bejmizocirh/b.2820295*.

Sallis, J. F., Cervero, R. B., Ascher, W., Henderson, K. A., Kraft, M. K., & Kerr, J. (2006). An ecological approach to creating active living communities. *Annual Review of Public Health, 27*, 297–322.

Schwartz, G. E. (1982). Testing the biopsychosocial model: The ultimate challenge facing behavioral medicine? *Journal of Consulting and Clinical Psychology, 50*, 1040–1053.

Simpkins, S. D., Fredricks, J., Davis-Kean, P., & Eccles, J. S. (2006). Healthy minds, healthy habits: The influence of activity involvement in middle childhood. In A. Huston & M. N. Ripke (Eds.), *Developmental contexts in middle childhood: Bridges to adolescence and adulthood* (pp. 283–302). New York: Cambridge University Press.

Simpkins, S. D., Ripke, M., Huston, A. C., & Eccles, J. S. (2005). Predicting participation and outcomes in out-of-school activities: Similarities and differences across social ecologies. In G. G. Noam (Series Ed.), H. B. Weiss, P. M. D. Little, & S. M. Bouffard (Vol. Eds.), *New directions for youth development: No. 105. Participation in youth programs: Enrollment, attendance, and engagement* (pp. 51–70). New York: Wiley.

Smith, B. N., Bean, M. K., Mitchell, K. S., Speizer, I. S., & Fries, E. A. (2007). Psychosocial factors associated with non-smoking adolescents' intentions to smoke. *Health Education Research, 22*, 238–247.

Springer, A. E., Kelder, S. H., & Hoelscher, D. M. (2006). Social support, physical activity and sedentary behavior among 6th-grade girls: a cross-sectional study. *International Journal of Behavioral Nutrition and Physical Activity, 3*, 8. Retrieved from *www.ijbnpa.org/content/pdf/1479-5868-3-8.pdf*.

Spurrier, N. J., Magarey, A. A., Golley, R., Curnow, F., & Sawyer, M. G. (2008). Relationships between the home environment and physical activity and dietary patterns of preschool children: A cross-sectional study. *International Journal of Behavioral Nutrition and Physical Activity, 5*, 31–42.

Weir, L. A., Etelson, D., & Brand, D. A. (2006). Parents' perceptions of neighborhood safety and children's physical activity. *Preventive Medicine, 43*, 212–217.

Wilson, D. K. (2008). Theoretical advances in diet and physical activity interventions. *Health Psychology, 27*(1, Suppl.), S1–S2.

Wilson, D. K., & Lawman, H. G. (2009). Health promotion in children and adolescent: An integration of the biopsychosocial model and ecological approaches to behavior change. In M. C. Roberts & R. G. Steele (Eds.), *Handbook of pediatric psychology* (4th ed., pp. 603–617). New York: Guilford Press.

Zarrett, N. (2007). The dynamic relation between out-of-school activities and adolescent development (Doctoral dissertation, University of Michigan, 2006). *Dissertation Abstracts International, 67*(10), 6100B.

Zarrett, N., & Eccles, J. S. (2006). The passage to adulthood: Challenges of late adolescence. In S. Piha & G. Hall (Eds.), *New directions for youth development: Preparing youth for the crossing: From adolescence to early adulthood* (Issue 111, pp. 13–28). Hoboken, NJ: Wiley.

Zarrett, N., & Eccles, J. S. (2009). The role of the family and community in extracurricular activity [Peer-reviewed chapter]. *AERA Monographs Series: Promising practices for family and community involvement during high school* (Vol. 4, pp. 27–51). Charlotte, NC: Information Age.

CHAPTER 10

Adult Development, Aging, and Gerontology

Ilene C. Siegler
Karen Hooker
Hayden B. Bosworth
Merrill F. Elias
Avron Spiro

Advancing age is often the strongest risk factor for morbidity and mortality. It is impossible, in a short chapter, to cover all of the relevant literature. Fortunately, there are specialized volumes such as the *Handbook of Health Psychology and Aging* (Aldwin, Park, & Spiro, 2007) and the *Encyclopedia of Health and Aging* (Markides, 2007) that may interest the readers of this chapter and provide detailed reviews of relevant literature.

Maturing longitudinal studies in the psychology of aging are now publishing data that have been collected for over 50 years (Seattle Longitudinal Study: Schaie, 2005; Baltimore Longitudinal Study of Aging: Terracciano, Lockenhoff, Zonderman, Ferrucci, & Costa, 2008; Normative Aging Study: Mroczek & Spiro, 2007). In addition, findings from a second generation of psychologically based longitudinal studies (e.g., Maine–Syracuse Longitudinal Study: Elias, Robbins, et al., 2004; Berlin Aging Study: Baltes & Mayer, 1999; Gerstof, Ram, Rocke, Lindenberger, & Smith, 2008; Victoria Longitudinal Study: MacDonald, Hultsch, & Dixon, 2008) have incorporated health and cognitive measures into their de-

signs, resulting in an increased understanding of stability and change in basic psychological processes and their implications for health and survival. Long-term prospective epidemiological studies that generally focus on understanding a specific disease outcome have also grown older and have incorporated psychosocial variables into their designs (e.g., Framingham Heart Study: Elias et al., 2000, 2005; Elias, Sullivan, et al., 2005; Terry, 2007; Wulsin et al., 2005) adding to a developing literature on the epidemiology of aging (Fried, 2000; Rush Memory and Aging Study: Buchman, Boyle, Wilson, Tang, & Bennett, 2007; Wilson, Beck, Bienias, & Bennett, 2007; The Nun Study: Snowden, 2001; Tyas et al., 2007; Whitehall II Study: Singh-Manoux et al., 2007).

There are a few "truisms" about aging that should be kept in mind:

1. The 35 years between ages 65 and 100 are quite variable. Rates of nursing home residence range from 3% at ages 65–69 up to 15% for those ages 85–89 and approximately 48% for persons age 100.
2. An individual's age is also an index of the birth cohort, reflecting a particular

period in historical time with potentially important age × time of measurement interactions.

3. Numbers of chronic conditions and sensory problems increase with advancing age.

4. Independent of disease status, the older the organism, the longer it will take to recover from a particular stressor (Siegler, Bosworth, & Elias, 2003).

In a recent review in a textbook for geriatric psychiatrists, we suggested the following key points that summarize what we know about normal aging:

1. Individual decline in cognitive performance before age 60 is generally not normal aging. By the mid-70s, average decrement is observed for all abilities, and by the 80s this decrement is widespread except for verbal ability.

2. Empirical data from centenarian studies suggest that dementia is not inevitable.

3. Cognitive abilities that depend on perceptual speed and contextual memory tend to decline with age, even for healthy adults, while abilities that rely on semantic knowledge and highly overlearned patterns decline less or may even improve.

4. Continuity of personality and social preferences is expected across the adult lifespan; thus, changes have potential diagnostic significance.

5. Health effects of Alzheimer's disease (AD) on patients and their caregivers vary in diverse populations (Siegler et al., 2009).

This concern with normal aging is important for health psychologists to keep in mind to separate effects of the particular disease process under study from the impact of advanced age.

In developmental health psychology, there has been interest in the role of psychosocial factors in the prediction of survival (see Siegler, Elias, & Bosworth, in press). Here we extend our review to focus on the prediction of cognitive decline and dementia and on studies that describe the functioning of long-term survivors; to highlight some of the methodological contributions of studies of developmental change; and to work toward developing a health psychology of

an aging population. The study of psychology of aging has always had two traditions. Experimental aging research with cross-sectional studies of age differences has been the starting point. These are important and give a snapshot of the prevalence of diseases and competencies at one point in time. To understand aging as a process, longitudinal or prospective studies are required. We adopt the lifespan approach as detailed by Spiro (2007), in which age is descriptive not causal, longitudinal data are fundamental to understand aging, and complex methods we employ have the ability to model change that focuses on variation, as well as average trends. In addition, the socioeconomic scale (SES) gradient in health is ubiquitous and interacts with age, such that lower SES individuals have worse health than their higher SES age peers (Adler & Stewart, 2007).

Personality and Health

It is impossible to study the full lifespan in a single study. However, one can take advantage of existing data and add new measures. This strategy has been successfully for Friedman and his colleagues in the Terman studies (see Friedman & Kern, Chapter 7, this volume). Our work on the University of North Carolina Alumni Heart Study (UNCAHS, Siegler, Peterson, Barefoot, Harvin, et. al., 1992; Siegler, Peterson, Barefoot, & Williams, 1992; Siegler, Costa, et al., 2003) provides data on the cohort of the baby boomers—born after World War II—who are now in their early 60s. The UNCAHS was designed to test the hypotheses that hostility is a predictor of coronary heart disease (CHD), and that health habits are a potential mechanism of that relationship. Developmental trends provide important information about predictors. If trends are stable, one can expect that they have similar effects at different points in the lifespan. It they change over time, the interpretation is more complex. Comparisons of longitudinal versus cross-sectional data provide inferences about the role of cultural change and secular trends (see Schaie, 2005). Developmental trends of hostility are shown in Figure 10.1. Note that this is unaffected by selection factors when comparing the 2,000 persons with data at all four measurement points and the

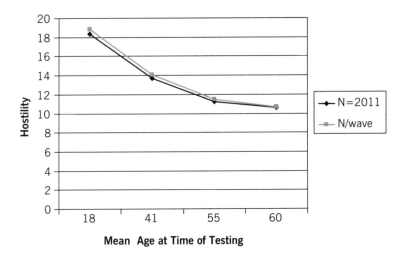

FIGURE 10.1. Longitudinal change in hostility from age 18 to 60. Data from Siegler (2007).

group present at each measurement. Ongoing analyses of these data suggests that this normative pattern describes approximately 75% of the sample, that an additional 23% decline more slowly, while 3% show an increase from ages 18 to 60. These patterns are related to the accumulation of disease by age 60 (Siegler, 2007; Siegler et al., in press) and, we expect, will predict longer-term outcomes within the next 5–10 years. These results also suggest that studies of older adults that have a broader population base (about 25% of the U.S. population has attended college) would have higher mean levels at comparable ages. We do not know whether the rates of change would be the same. However, Mroczek and Spiro (2007) in the Normative Aging Study found patterns of change in neuroticism related to 12-year survival, such that patterns including initial levels and rates of change were both important, with personality measured at a mean age of 63, suggesting that we should expect similar outcomes in the UNCAHS. These findings also highlight the potential clinical importance of high hostility in later life because it is non-normative.

Personality, or personality change, as a risk factor for dementia may suggest some new avenues for targeted intervention with individuals before the disease is evident (Crowe, Andel, Pedersen, Fratiglioni, & Gatz, 2006; Siegler, Dawson, & Welsh, 1994). Because individuals with dementia cannot report on their status, research using informant reports is necessary. Balsis, Carpenter, and Storandt (2005) reported on informant ratings on the Blessed Dementia Scale for nondemented individuals who entered a longitudinal study. In the next 4 years they observed individuals who remained normal, developed dementia, or died without a clinical diagnosis but were found to have dementia on autopsy. They found that personality change on any of eight dimensions occurred in twice as many individuals who developed dementia as in those who did not. Major changes were increases in rigidity, apathy, egocentricity, and impaired emotional control. In a cross-sectional study, Duchek, Balota, Storandt, and Larsen (2007) administered the NEO Five-Factor Inventory (FFI; Costa & McCrae, 1992) to four groups—healthy middle-aged and older persons, and those with very mild dementia at the time of the clinic visit. The same personality instrument was also filled out by a family member about the patient's current state. All five factors were significantly different on the informant ratings, such that increased neuroticism and decreased extraversion, openness, and agreeableness were seen in a comparison of normal controls and persons with mild dementia, while decreases in conscientiousness were associated with dementia onset and severity. In logistical regression models comparing normal controls to persons with very mild dementia, increases in neuroticism and decreases in conscientiousness added explained variance to cognitive factors and suggested that personality enhances the ability to detect very mild or early dementia. These important cross-sectional findings suggest that it will be useful to follow cohorts with personality measures to assess the onset of dementia and/or cognitive decline. Wilson, Beck, Bienias, and Bennett (2007) gave the NEO FFI to 997 members of the Religious Orders Study and followed them for the development of AD and mild cognitive impairment (MCI) over a 12-year period in which 176 persons developed AD and 728 did not. At baseline, there were significant differences in age, depression, and cognitive indicators, as well as all five personality factors: increased neuroticism and extraversion, and decreased openness, agreeableness, and conscientiousness were found in a comparison of those who developed AD and those who did not. Proportional hazard regression models adjusted for age, sex, and education found that higher conscientiousness was a protective factor. These findings suggest that examination of personality earlier in the life cycle will help us to understand the development of cognitive impairments and dementing disorders.

Hooker (1999, 2002) and Hooker and McAdams (2003) have taken a social psychological process approach and combined it with emphases in personality theory (e.g., McAdams, 1995) on structure, resulting in the "six-foci" model of personality, which holds promise for understanding the myriad ways in which personality relates to health and may be particularly useful for health psychologists. A basic premise of aging research is that heterogeneity increases between individuals over time (e.g., Maddox, 1987), so that a population of older individuals comprises people with large inter-individual differences in cognitive abilities, health, personality, and emotional functioning. Identifying personality structures and processes that drive these individual differences can provide insight into linkages between personality and important health and life outcomes (e.g., Roberts, Kuncel, Shiner, Caspi, & Goldberg, 2007).

Incorporation of this more process-oriented approach is an important addition to the overwhelming evidence that already confirms the "Big Five" trait models of personality (e.g., Goldberg, 1993; McCrae

& Costa, 2003). The five "megatraits" derived through factor analyses that have been found to be universal across all periods of the lifespan and across cultures (McCrae & Terracciano, 2005) are neuroticism, extraversion, openness to experience, agreeableness, and conscientiousness. However, critics of this approach (Block, 1995) argued for a definition of personality that emphasizes its dynamic nature and speaks to the importance of the organization that personality lends to behavior. As well, earlier works of pioneers in the field of adult development, such as Neugarten (1968, 1979), highlighted a life course perspective in which social roles and sequencing of life events are integrated into personality frameworks.

Today, the field is putting less emphasis on whether personality changes and is moving toward an understanding of change as an individual-difference variable in and of itself (Mroczek, Spiro, & Griffin, 2006). Numerous longitudinal studies have shown that individuals tend to retain their relative ranking on traits over a period spanning several years, even decades. This type of rank-order stability, captured in correlation coefficients, does not speak to mean-level changes, which can take place within individuals over short- or long-term time frames. Measurement strategies, such as "burst" measurements over periods of days embedded within widely spaced measurements more typical of longitudinal studies (over months or years), allow researchers to disentangle short-term variability from long-term change (e.g., Nesselroade & Boker, 1994; Nesselroade & Featherman, 1991; Sliwinski & Mogle, 2008).

The six-foci model (Hooker, 2002; Hooker & McAdams, 2003) pairs structures with processes in a levels-of-analysis framework. McAdams (1995) helped organize thinking about the personality change versus stability issue by describing three very different levels on which personality operates structurally: traits, personal action constructs (or goals), and life stories (see McAdams, 1995; McAdams & Pals, 2006).

Traits are relatively stable, and are paired with state processes that change and even bring about trait change (cf. Fleeson, 2001). In general, it has been shown that neuroticism, the part of extraversion related to social vitality, and openness to experience tend to decrease slightly with age (McCrae & Costa, 2003; Mroczek & Spiro, 2003), whereas agreeableness, the part of extraversion related to social dominance, and conscientiousness tend to increase over the adult lifespan (Roberts, Walton, & Viechtbauer, 2006). Even among centenarians (e.g., Adkins, Martin, & Poon, 1996), traits are malleable.

"Personal action constructs" are goal structures that change in relation to normative developmental tasks and life events. Self-regulatory processes (e.g., self-efficacy, outcome expectancy) in domains where goals exist provide the willpower to motivate behavior. For example, if one has a goal of being physically fit, the self-efficacy for sticking to an exercise regimen helps one put in the necessary time on the treadmill or bike, or in the pool to become fit and to stay fit. Self-evaluation, regulation of emotion, and goal setting are among the most established and potent of these self-regulatory processes (Staudinger & Kunzmann, 2005).

Life stories are generated via narrative processes that—while showing continuity—constantly evolve to fit the sociohistorical moment and be responsive to what the social "audience" affords (Adams, Smith, Pasupathi, & Vitolo, 2002). For example, in telling one's life story to one's grandchildren, different events, characters, and emotions are recounted than if one is telling one's life story to a group of new friends at the senior center.

Researchers should consider the role that other foci of personality, such as goals, beliefs, and narrative processes related to identity and life story, play in health outcomes. For example, a sense of coherence and mastery has been linked with lower rates of all-cause mortality, even after adjusting for disease (Surtees, Wainwright, Luben, Khaw, & Day, 2006). Hooker and Kaus (1992) found that older adults who had self-related health goals were more likely to report engaging in health behaviors. Adults appear to maintain and regain levels of subjective well-being and adjust to life tasks more effectively with age (Staudinger & Kunzmann, 2005). Heckhausen's (2001) research has drawn attention to the ways in which middle-aged adults use compensatory strategies and adaptive behaviors to limit losses. Similarly, despite the increasing likelihood in old age of having experiences that are encountered rather than elicited, most older adults still maintain their sense of control and personal agency (Staudinger & Kunzmann, 2005), perhaps by winnowing areas in which control "matters" to those that are most important to them (Hooker, 1999).

A model of lifespan development used to explain successful aging has emphasized a trio of developmental processes: selection, optimization, and compensation, giving this model the moniker SOC (Baltes & Baltes, 1990; Baltes & Carstensen, 1999). These three universal adaptive processes allow older adults to manage, self-regulate, and be proactive about maintenance of competence against a backdrop of age-related losses (Baltes, 1997). As we age, we become more selective about areas or domains in which to invest our time and resources; thus, we can regulate loss by optimizing behavior in those selected domains, and when losses do occur, we can compensate to some extent—though our ability to do so does become more compromised in the "fourth age," when losses clearly outnumber gains. Baltes and Carstensen (1999), for example, found that many older adults select goals related to maintenance of family relationships, optimize these goals by investing more time in family as opposed to other relationships, and compensate for loss of friendships due to relocation or deaths by maximizing the salience of family ties (Bolkan, Mierdiercks, & Hooker, 2008).

Studying Change: Developmental Methods of Use in Health Psychology

Spiro (2007) presents a more detailed account of these issues that are abstracted here. We focus on two that are of particular interest—how to index time in developmental studies and recommended methods for longitudinal health research.

How to Index Time

Depending on the variable in question, data can be collected over intervals of seconds (e.g., heart rate variability), hours or days (e.g., blood pressure, mood), or months and years (e.g., for personality traits). Age seems most appropriate for use in developmental studies, but other options include time since an event (e.g., randomization in a clinical trial, first heart attack), or time until an event (e.g., death, or until first stroke). In repeated measures studies, time can be defined relative to the sample as a whole (e.g., mean age = age 50) or to the individual (e.g., age 50 for one person and age 40 for another). However, centering time relative to the person rather than to the sample can result in incorrect estimates, as can use of occasion as the time axis (Mehta & West, 2000; Sliwinski & Mogle, 2008). In survival analysis, use of time on study rather than age can likewise result in mistaken inferences (Lamarca, Alonso, Gomez, & Munoz, 1998; Thiebaut & Benichou, 2004). By using age in survival analysis, the hazard function is the age-specific incidence of the outcome. In observational studies, in which participants are enrolled based on the time of their assessment, and may or may not have the outcome in question, age would be the preferred choice. In clinical studies, in which enrolled participants are screened and do not have (or have not yet experienced) the outcome, then time since enrollment is reasonable. Under certain conditions, results based on time versus age as the temporal axis will agree, but the results can diverge even when age is used as a stratification variable (Thiebaut & Benichou, 2004).

Recommended Methods for Longitudinal Studies

Foremost among these are growth curve (i.e., multilevel, random effects, or hierarchical) models (Singer & Willett, 2003) that models take into consideration the hierarchical structure of data, such as the nesting of multiple testing occasions within persons or the nesting of persons within geographic areas (e.g., neighborhoods) or social structures (e.g., marital dyads). Applied to longitudinal data, such models can be used to assess whether there are individual differences in change in personality traits (Mroczek & Spiro, 2003), in measures of affect (Griffin, Mroczek & Spiro, 2006), or in changes in couples for each member of the pair separately (Yorgason, Almeida, Neupert, Hoffman, & Spiro, 2006).

Growth curves can also be used in situations where the temporal process under investigation has multiple phases or components. For example, Llabre, Spitzer, Saab,

and Schneiderman (2001) used piecewise growth curves to model two phases of a stress response, reactivity and recovery, simultaneously in a laboratory challenge task. Multiple measures of blood pressure were taken over a 10-minute span, before and after a cold pressor test. The investigators were able to model the two phases of the process simultaneously, and to consider both predictors and consequences of the two phases. In this example, the two phases were contiguous rather than discrete, but in other applications (e.g., interrupted time series designs) or studies with multiple assessments both before and after an intervention, piecewise growth curves could also be useful.

A second recent development in growth curves involves multivariate applications, or examining correlated change (between individuals) or coupled change (within individuals) in outcomes (Sliwinski & Mogle, 2008). For example, Sliwinski, Hofer, and Hall (2003) examined correlations of change in multiple cognitive abilities over time in an aging sample, some of whom had preclinical dementia. Using age as the time axis, correlations among changes in the cognitive dimensions were moderate in the overall sample; however, when the sample was stratified into cases and noncases, the correlations among ability declines were stronger in the cases. When time until disease onset was used as the time axis for the cases, the extent of decline was much greater than that in the age-based model, but the correlations among changes in abilities were lower than those in the overall sample, although higher than those among the noncases. Other approaches to examining change between or within individuals include the use of structural equation modeling (SEM). The final set of methods, known as latent class or growth mixture models, has as its objective the identification of subgroups within the population studied. A common element among these methods is the recognition that the sample under study may be heterogeneous, comprised of subgroups with different patterns or correlates of change. Alternative approaches have been proposed by Muthén (2001) and Nagin (1999), but in both cases, the intent is to identify latent classes that have different patterns of change. In a related approach, Aldwin, Spiro, Levenson, and Cupertino (2001) used growth curves to identify individual trajectories of self-reported health, then cluster analysis to identify groups of persons with similar health trajectories.

Cognition and Health

Two different areas of current research suggest how cognition is important in terms of the use of cognitive decline as an indicator of function and the extent to which it may lead to dementia, and in understanding nongenetic risk factors and the role of cognitive decline in the ability of older persons to contribute to their own care.

There are many nongenetic risk factors for the dementias, including age, myocardial infarction, midlife hypertension, hypertension, low blood pressure, atherosclerosis, atrial fibrillation, diabetes mellitus, obesity, smoking, low alcohol consumption, low physical activity at midlife, lack of fish in the diet, low rate of decline in body mass index (BMI), low level of social and mental activities, less education, low intake of antioxidants, raised markers of inflammation, raised plasma total homocysteine, low plasma concentrations of folate and vitamin B_{12}, low testosterone in men, hormone replacement therapy in women after age 65, head injury in men, depression, and poor perceived health (Smith, 2008).

Many of these variables are also risk factors for modest cognitive deficit and longitudinal decline in cognitive functioning (Elias, Robbins, et al., 2004; Waldstein & Elias, 2001). Mild cognitive deficit is of concern because it has a negative impact on quality of life in our competitive society. Possibly of greater concern, it is a risk factor for dementia (e.g., Elias et al., 2000). In the Framingham Heart Study, decrements in cognitive performance in stroke-free and nondemented individuals predicted dementia 22 years before it was diagnosed (Elias et al., 2000).

There are still many unanswered questions regarding the prediction of dementia from earlier, predementia cognitive deficits. Among these are the following:

1. Why do some individuals progress from poor cognitive performance to dementia while others do not?
2. What pattern of cognitive deficit prior to dementia predicts the various types of dementia?

Therefore, investigations of cognitive and cardiovascular factors leading to conversion to dementia from milder forms of cognitive impairment are extremely important, as is characterization of the pattern of these milder, predementia deficits (Gamaldo et al., 2006; Grober et al., 2008).

For example, the Baltimore Longitudinal Study investigators reported that clinical stroke is a risk factor for conversion from mild cognitive impairment to dementia, but only in persons diagnosed with mild cognitive impairment prior to stroke (Gamaldo et al., 2006). Deficits in episodic memory occur early in the course of the progression from mild cognitive impairment to AD, executive functions decline later, and decrements in verbal intelligence occur near the time of diagnosis (Grober et al., 2008).

The pattern of cognitive deficits that predict vascular dementia and mixed forms (e.g., AD and vascular dementia) has received less attention. Studies of vascular and mixed forms of dementia are important because neuropathology studies based on autopsy data indicate that changes in the brain associated with AD are different than those associated with vascular dementia Among other changes in the brain, AD is characterized by atrophy of the cerebral cortex of the brain; decrease in brain substance and enlargement of the folds of the brain (gyri); and microscopic changes, such as neurofibrillary tangles resulting in the death of brain cells (e.g., Salmon & Hodges, 2001; Stevens & Fox, 2001). In contrast, vascular dementia is characterized by ischemic changes in the arterial vessels, that is, blockage, obstruction, or constriction leading to a decrease in cerebral blood flow, and hence oxygenation of brain tissue (e.g., Salmon & Hodges, 2001; Stevens & Fox, 2001). There is evidence suggesting that changes in the brain seen on autopsy may occur years before the dementia manifests and are responsible for the differences in pattern of cognitive deficits preceding dementia (Hodges & Graham, 2001). Mild deficits in "episodic memory" (i.e., memory for events) appear to predominate in the preclinical state prior to the diagnosis of AD. In vascular dementia, decline in memory is seen prior to the diagnosis of dementia, but memory loss is not predominant and is accompanied by deficits in other cognitive skills, such as visual–spatial ability, attention, and executive function (e.g.,

Salmon & Hodges, 2001). Thus, it is important not to miss an early diagnosis of dementia (and early intervention) because memory impairment is not prominent in cognitive loss, and it is most important to characterize the pattern of cognitive decline prior to dementia because it indicates the specific type of dementia involved and the most effective treatment strategy (Knopman et al., 2001). It is also important to note that not all individuals who have risk factors for cardiovascular disease, or who show memory loss and other deficits, progress to dementia, and that there is a far from perfect correlation between changes in brain structure and cognition (Hodges & Graham, 2001; Knopman et al., 2001).

Whereas much attention has focused on the important issue of patterns of cognitive deficit preceding dementia, more research is needed on the course of cognitive decline following the diagnosis of dementia, so as to recognize skills that are lost and those that remain as dementia progresses. This information is valuable in the treatment of dementia, so that therapists may work effectively with remaining skills and abilities. In this context, it is important that we continue to identify risk factors for lowered cognitive performance and mild cognitive impairment. Because of a vast literature in this area we can highlight several risk factors as examples of ongoing studies.

We focus on studies of hypertension and homocysteine as active areas of research because they illustrate the role health psychology can play in improving work in the psychology of aging that is dealing with the prediction and prevention of dementia.

Arterial hypertension is a risk factor for dementia (Birns & Kalra, 2008; Waldstein, 1995; Waldstein & Katzel, 2001). But a lifespan approach to prevention of dementia is important by virtue of three major findings: (1) Higher levels of systolic and diastolic blood pressure (BP) in middle age, or earlier, are related to lowered cognitive performance in old age (Elias, Wolf, D'Agostino, Cobb, & White, 1993; Launer, Masaki, Petrovitch, Foley, & Havlik, 1995); (2) for fluid-type abilities, the rate of hypertension-related decline over time is similar for younger and older persons (P. K. Elias, Elias, Robbins, & Budge, 2004); and (3) functional and structural changes in the brain begin early

in adulthood, even for essential and uncomplicated forms of hypertension (Jennings et al., 2008). Clinical trials that feature lowering of BP will be necessary to establish further the likelihood of a causal link between BP and cognition. A recent review (Birns & Kalra, 2008) indicates that only eight randomized clinical trials of antihypertensive medications with a placebo arm have been completed, and the results are inconclusive. Current antihypertensive medications (e.g., some types of calcium channel–blocking agents and angiotensin-converting enzyme inhibitors or blockers) do have the potential for restoration of cognitive functioning either via prevention of undesirable hypertension-related changes in the vasculature or by their direct effects on neurons (see Elias & Dore, 2008; Staessen & Birkenhäger, 2004). Controlled clinical trials of antihypertensive medications are very important because of the observation of U- and L-shaped relations between BP and cognition (Birns & Kalra, 2008; Waldstein, Giggey, Thayer, & Zonderman, 2005). Creative work by the Pittsburgh Group (Jennings et al., 2008) offers new methods to evaluate efficacy of drug treatment in relation to functional and structural changes in the brain, including changes in regional cerebral blood flow response to specific cognitive tasks (see editorial by Elias & Dore, 2008).

Many risk factors for lowered cognitive performance, other than hypertension, have received attention in recent years; homocysteine in particular. Homocysteine is an amino acid produced during 1-carbon metabolism. In the 1990s several studies indicated higher levels of fasting total homocysteine (tHcy) in patients with cognitive deficits or dementia (Smith, 2008). Early in 2008, there were 77 cross-sectional studies and 33 prospective studies indicating relations between higher levels of tHcy (or lower folate, B_6 and B_{12} status) and lowered cognitive performance and dementia. Aside from homocysteineuria, high tHcy levels have not been defined clinically, but many studies use the median of the distribution as a cutoff point or relate tHcy concentrations to performance. A number of mechanisms have been proposed as mediators of this association between homocysteine and cognition. The most direct hypothesis is that higher blood levels of tHcy have an adverse influence on cognition because they are neurotoxic. However, inverse associations between tHcy and cognition are seen at less than toxic levels (Elias et al., 2005, 2006), and there is evidence that higher tHcy levels serve as markers for cardiovascular disease and for folic acid, vitamin B_{12}, and vitamin B_6 deficiencies (see Smith, 2008). Ongoing clinical trails are examining the possibility that tHcy lowering by B vitamins improves cognitive performance in persons who exhibit decline in cognitive ability. Until these trials are completed, it is not certain that B vitamins are an effective treatment for cognitive deficit associated with high tHcy levels.

We have touched briefly on only a few risk factors. Many other risk factors are associated with decline in cognitive performance in older and elderly persons: diabetes mellitus, obesity, central adiposity, metabolic syndrome, atrial fibrillation and heart arrhythmias, chronic kidney disease, and inflammatory markers. A discussion of these and other cardiovascular risk factors for lowered cognitive performance can be found in Siegler and colleagues (in press) and in Waldstein and Elias (2001).

Everyday Cognition in Older Adults

Within the past couple of decades, there has been increased interest in everyday cognition, or how older adults address complex cognitive tasks in their everyday lives. This interest has been driven by both methodological and theoretical concerns. Methodologically, researchers who study everyday cognition emphasize external validity as opposed to laboratory-based researchers, who emphasize internal validity (Puckett, Reese, & Pollina, 1993). Theoretically, researchers have argued that traditional laboratory-based tests of cognition do not adequately capture older adults' cognitive functioning in everyday life due to the contextual richness of the environment and the frequency with which everyday tasks are faced (Denney & Pearce, 1989; Puckett et al., 1993). Despite this increased focus on everyday cognition, applying basic research to "real-world" settings remains one of the biggest challenges identified by cognitive aging researchers (Bosworth & Hertzog, 2009; Hershey, Boyd, Coutant, & Turner, 1999). The

addition of cognitive measures to national surveys holds great promise as well (e.g., McArdle, Fisher, & Kadlec, 2007).

Cognitive decline among older adults may be particularly problematic because of the disproportionate amount of health care consumed by older adults and the increased demands required for organizing and maintaining their complex medical regimens (Bosworth & Schaie, 1995; Park & Kidder, 1996; Salthouse, 1991). An example of the importance of examining the impact of cognitive function among older adults on health/disease is the context of medication adherence. Prior research has shown that only 50–60% of patients are adherent in taking prescribed medications over a 1-year period (Bosworth, 2006; Haynes et al., 2005; Sabate, 2003), even medications that are essential for the treatment of chronic diseases (Avorn et al., 1998). Medication nonadherence costs an estimated $100 billion annually in the United States, and medications errors and adverse drug reactions account for 10% of hospital administrations (Vermeire, Hearnshaw, Van Royen, & Denekens, 2001).

Cognitive factors are related to all of the components, or "stages," of medication adherence, including comprehension, formulating plans, and actually taking medication. For example, nonadherence may be due to patients' poor understanding of instructions about their medications (Ad Hoc Committee on Health Literacy for the Council on Scientific Affairs, American Medical Association, 1999; Hoffman & Proulx, 2003). Several recent studies have demonstrated that patients frequently have difficulty reading and understanding medication labels (Davis, Wolf, Bass, Middlebrooks, et al., 2006; Davis, Wolf, Bass, Thompson, et al., 2006; Wolf, Davis, Tilson, Bass, & Parker, 2006). Although patients should receive medication counseling from their health care providers, including physician and pharmacists, numerous studies have shown that discussions about drugs are often limited (Sleath, Rubin, Campbell, Gwyther, & Clark, 2001; Tarn et al., 2006), and because patients frequently do not remember those conversations (Post & Roter, 1988; Stewart & Liolitsa, 1999), many rely on drug labels for information. Unfortunately, older adults are more likely than younger adults to misunderstand instructions on prescription drug labels, leading to an increased number of mistakes (Morrell, Park, & Poon, 1989). One way to organize components of cognition required for medication adherence is through the construct of medication management capacity (MMC). This important aspect of adherence is defined as "the cognitive and functional ability to self-administer a medication regimen as it has been prescribed" (Maddigan, Farris, Keating, Wiens, & Johnson, 2003, p. 333). Measures of MMC typically assess functional skills, such as correctly identifying medications, opening containers, selecting the proper dose, and taking the medication at the proper time (MacLaughlin et al., 2005). Low MMC predicts greater emergency department utilization, functional decline, and subsequent residence in assisted-living facilities (Edelberg, Shallenberger, Hausdorff, & Wei, 2000). Developing methods to help older adults and their families deal with declines in everyday cognition should be an excellent venue for future research in developmental health psychology.

Gerontological Contributions

"Gerontology" is the study of aging across disciplines. Access to information about the aging of the population is no longer a secret known only to gerontologists. A trip to the website of the U.S. Census Bureau (*www.census.gov*) provides a wealth of detailed, up-to-date information. Of particular interest here are new projections for life expectancy from 1999 to 2100. Life expectancy is when half of a birth cohort will die. It varies by gender and race. If we just look at the figures for the total U.S. population, the current ages are 74.0 for men and 79.7 for women. Future projections of the most optimistic scenario project life expectances of 92.3 for men and 95.2 for women by 2100. As summarized by Hollmann, Mulder, and Kallan (2000), "Demographic projections for populations 50 to 100 years in the future are highly subject to behavioral decisions by individuals, policy decisions by governments at home and abroad and possible unexpected developments in health and morbidity" (p. 22). Projections such as these make understanding the behavioral decisions of individuals who determine their own health

in later life and predictors of morbidity and mortality critical, and highlight the role that health psychology has to play for the future of the nation.

For example, Gerstof and colleagues (2008) reported on data from the Berlin Aging Study (BASE) to evaluate whether changes in life satisfaction in later life are due to age or distance from death. They applied multilevel modeling to 12-year longitudinal data from 414 individuals who died, tested terminal decline versus drop in rates of change, then looked at potential covariates of the process. There were 516 participants with a mean age of 84.92 in the BASE (range, 70–103). Mortality was assessed 15 years after baseline in 2005, when only 83 persons (16%) were still alive. Results indicated that life satisfaction changes are due to distance from death rather than age, are more likely to be described as a decline (linear) model than as a drop (curvilinear) model, and that the number of medical comorbidities is a significant covariate, whereas cognitive indicators are not. Buchman and colleagues (2007), who used a composite measure of frailty to predict 3-year incident AD in the Rush Memory and Aging Study, found that both baseline frailty and increases in frailty predicted incident AD and cognitive decline, suggesting that frailty occurs before the diagnosis of incident AD.

Papers presented at a conference celebrating the 20th anniversary of the Georgia Centenarian Study indicate that research into the genetic bases of AD and longevity have both developed and may be converging. While life expectancy at birth is approaching 80 years at present, about half of those who reach the age of 92 will become centenarians. Estimates of health in centenarians suggest that in the population, one-third are in exceptional health, one-third have significant impairments, and one-third are moribund. Whether the distribution of these health status figures will remain the same or change is a topic of intense discussion. The study of "extreme aging"—a new term for the oldest-old—or centenarian studies (Poon & Perls, 2007) requires multidisciplinary perspectives and international collaboration. Although centenarians and supercentenarians (older than 110 years old) are increasing in number, they are still rare. Terry (2007) compared elderly children of centenarian parents and elderly children of parents with average life expectancy. The results indicated that centenarian offspring have reduced odds of heart disease, hypertension, and diabetes but similar rates of cancer, stroke, dementia, osteoporosis, glaucoma, macular degeneration, depression, Parkinson's disease, thyroid disease, and chronic obstructive pulmonary disease. Such studies may provide important clues about genetic, as well as environmental, phenotypes of exceptional longevity.

Conclusions

Individuals are expanding the time period of middle age. Baby boomers are a demographic cohort that is pushing the limits. Personality and social factors lead to risk behaviors that can change the picture of late life in good or poor health focusing on the decades from the 40s to the 60s (Lachman, 2004). Individuals tend not to consider themselves as old or aging until health declines set in, and this is often closer to age 85+ for those at the upper end of the SES gradient; thus, the term "successful aging" has lost any meaning beyond not feeling or seeming old at all. This is not just an individual problem. The entire world population is aging. Individuals, as well as societies, must prepare for longer lives and seek ways to reduce age-related disabilities (National Institute on Aging, 2007), and to care for those who survive them, as centenarian studies show. Older adults of the future will be more diverse than those of today.

Psychology of aging that uses a lifespan approach and appropriate multivariate methods for the study of change has produced important data showing how personality, cognition, and other psychosocial indicators change over time; health psychology has produced important data showing how these constructs are related to health, specific disease outcomes, and survival. Putting them together is the task for a developmental health psychology of aging.

Acknowledgments

Preparation of this chapter was supported by National Institutes of Health Grant No. R01 HL55356 from the National Heart, Lung and Blood Institute (NHLBI) with cofunding by the National Institute on Aging, Grant No. P01 HL36587 from the NHLBI, grants from the Marchionne Foundation, Grant No. IRG-08-89565 from the Alzheimer's Association, and the Duke Behavioral Medicine Research Center (to Ilene C. Siegler); the Oregon State University Center for Healthy Aging Research (to Karen Hooker); NHLBI Grant No. R01 HL070713, VA Health Services Research and Development Grant No. 20-034, an Established Investigator Award from the American Heart Association, and a VA Career Scientist Award (to Hayden B. Bosworth); Grant Nos. 1RO1-HL67358 and 1R01-HL081290 from the NHLBI (to Merrill F. Elias); and a VA Merit Award and Grant No. AG018346 from the National Institute on Aging (to Avron Spiro). We wish to acknowledge the editorial work by Ms. Danielle Briggeman at the University of Maine.

Further Reading

Aldwin, C. M., Park, C. L., & Spiro, A. (Eds.). (2007). *Handbook of health psychology and aging.* New York: Guilford Press.

Baum, A., Revenson, T. A., & Singer, J. E. (Eds.). (in press). *Handbook of health psychology* (2nd ed.). New York: Psychology Press.

Blazer, D. B., & Steffens, D. C. (Eds.). (2009). *Textbook of geriatric psychiatry.* Washington, DC: American Psychiatric Press.

Schaie, K. W. (2005). *Developmental influences on adult intelligence: The Seattle Longitudinal Study.* New York: Oxford University Press.

Waldstein, S. R., & Elias, M. F. (Eds.). (2001). *Neuropsychology of cardiovascular disease.* Mahwah, NJ: Erlbaum.

References

Ad Hoc Committee on Health Literacy for the Council on Scientific Affairs, American Medical Association. (1999). Health literacy: Report of the council on scientific affairs. *Journal of the American Medical Association, 281,* 552–557.

Adams, C., Smith, M. C., Pasupathi, M., & Vitolo, L. (2002). Social context effects on story recall in older and younger women: Does the listener make a difference? *Journals of Gerontology B: Psychological Sciences and Social Sciences, 57,* 28–40.

Adkins, G., Martin, P., & Poon, L. W. (1996). Personality traits and states as predictors of subjective well-being in centenarians, octogenarians, and sexagenarians. *Psychology and Aging, 11,* 408–416.

Adler, N. (Dir.) & Stewart, S. (Network Admin.). (2007). Reaching for a healthier life: Facts on socioeconomic status and health in the U.S.: Report from the John D. and Catherine T. Mac Arthur Foundation Research Network on Socioeconomic Status and Health. Available at *www.macfound.org*.

Aldwin, C. M., Park, C. L., & Spiro, A. (Eds.). (2007). *Handbook of health psychology and aging*. New York: Guilford Press.

Aldwin, C. M., Spiro, A., III, Levenson, M. R., & Cupertino, A. P. (2001). Longitudinal findings from the Normative Aging Study: III. Personality, health trajectories, and mortality. *Psychology and Aging, 16(3), 450–465*.

Avorn, J., Monette, J., Lacour, A., Bohn, R. L., Monane, M., Mogun, H., et al. (1998). Persistence of use of lipid-lowering medications: A cross-national study. *Journal of the American Medical Association, 279, 1458–1462*.

Balsis, S., Carpenter, B. D., & Storandt, M. (2005). Personality change precedes diagnosis of dementia of the Alzheimer type. *Journals of Gerontology B: Psychological Sciences and Social Sciences, 60, P98–P101*.

Baltes, M. M., & Carstensen, L. L. (1999). Social psychological theories and their applications to aging: From individual to collective. In V. Bengtson & K.W. Schaie (Eds.), *Handbook of theories of aging* (pp. 209–226). New York: Springer.

Baltes, P. B. (1997). On the incomplete architecture of human ontogeny: Selection, optimization, and compensation as foundation of developmental theory. *American Psychologist, 52, 366–380*.

Baltes, P. B., & Baltes, M. M. (1990). Psychological perspectives on successful aging: The model of selective optimization with compensation. In *Successful aging: Perspectives from the behavioral sciences* (pp. 1–34). New York: Cambridge University Press.

Baltes, P. B., & Mayer, K. U. (Eds.). (1999). *The Berlin Aging Study: From 70 to 100*. New York: Cambridge University Press.

Birns, J., & Kalra, L. (2008). Cognitive function and hypertension. *Journal of Human Hypertension, 23(2), 86–96*.

Block, J. (1995). A contrarian view of the five-factor approach to personality description. *Psychological Bulletin, 117, 187–215*.

Bolkan, C. R., Mierdiercks, P., & Hooker, K. (2008). Stability and change in the six-foci model of personality: Personality development in midlife and beyond. In M. C. Smith & T. G. Reio, Jr. (Eds.), *Handbook of research on adult development and learning* (pp. 220–240). Mahwah, NJ: Erlbaum.

Bosworth, H. (2006). Medication adherence. In H. B. Bosworth & M. Weinberger (Eds.), *Patient treatment adherence: Concepts, interventions, and measurement* (pp. 147–194). Mahwah, NJ: Erlbaum.

Bosworth, H. B., & Hertzog, C. (Eds.). (2009). *Aging and cognition: Research methodologies and empirical advances*. Washington, DC: American Psychological Association.

Bosworth, H. B., & Schaie, K. W. (1995). Medication knowledge and health status in the Seattle Longitudinal Study. *Gerontologist, 35,* 24.

Buchman, A. S., Boyle, P. A., Wilson, R. S., Tang, Y., & Bennett, D. A. (2007). Frailty is associated with incident Alzheimer's disease and cognitive decline in the elderly. *Psychosomatic Medicine, 69, 483–489*.

Costa, P. T., & McCrae, R. R. (1992). *NEO PI-R professional manual: Revised NEO Personality Inventory (NEO PI-R) and NEO Five Factor Inventory (FFI)*. Odessa, Fl: Psychological Assessment Resources.

Crowe, M., Andel, R., Pedersen, N. L., Fratiglioni, L., & Gatz, M. (2006). Personality and risk of cognitive impairment 25 years later. *Psychology and Aging, 21, 573–580*.

Davis, T., Wolf, M. S., Bass, P. F., Middlebrooks, M., Kennen, E., Baker, D. W., et al. (2006). Low literacy impairs comprehension of prescription drug warning labels. *Journal of General Internal Medicine, 21, 847–851*.

Davis, T., Wolf, M. S., Bass, P. F., Thompson, J. A., Tilson, H. H., Neuberger, M., et al. (2006). Literacy and misunderstanding prescription drug labels. *Annals of Internal Medicine, 145, 887–894*.

Denney, J. A., & Pearce, K. A. (1989). A developmental study of practical problem solving in adults. *Psychology and Aging, 4, 438–442.*

Duchek, J. M., Balota, D. A., Storandt, M., & Larsen, R. (2007). The power of personality in discriminating between healthy aging and early stage Alzheimer's disease. *Journals of Gerontology B: Psychological Sciences and Social Sciences, 62(6), 353–361*.

Edelberg, H. K., Shallenberger, E., Hausdorff, J. M., & Wei, J. Y. (2000). One-year follow-up of medication management capacity in highly functioning older adults. *Journals of Gerontology A: Biological Sciences and Medical Sciences, 55, M550–M553*.

Elias, M. F., Beiser, A., Wolf, P. A., Au, R., White, R. F., & D'Agostino, R. B. (2000). The preclinical phase of Alzheimer disease: A 22-year prospective study of the Framingham cohort. *Archives of Neurology, 57, 808–813*.

Elias, M. F., & Dore, G. A. (2008). Brain indices predict blood pressure control: Aging brains and new predictions. *Hypertension, 52, 1–2*.

Elias, M. F., Robbins, M. A., Budge, M. M., Elias, P. K., Brennan, S. L., Johnston, C., et al. (2006). Homocysteine, folate, and vitamins B_6 and B_{12} blood levels in relation to cognitive performance: The Maine–Syracuse Study. *Psychosomatic Medicine, 68,* 547–554.

Elias, M. F., Robbins, M. A., Budge, M. M., Elias, P. K., Hermann, B. A., & Dore, G. A. (2004). Studies of aging, hypertension and cognitive functioning: With contributions from the Maine–Syracuse study. In P. T. Costa & I. C. Siegler (Eds.), *Advances in cell aging in gerontology: Vol. 15. Recent advances in psychology and aging.* Amsterdam: Elsevier.

Elias, M. F., Sullivan, L. M., D'Agostino, R. B., Elias, P. K., Jacques, P. F., Selhub, J., et al. (2005). Homocysteine and cognitive performance in the Framingham Offspring Study: Age is important. *American Journal of Epidemiology, 162,* 644–653.

Elias, M. F., Wolf, P. A., D'Agostino, R. B., Cobb, J., & White, L. R. (1993). Untreated blood pressure level is inversely related to cognitive functioning: The Framingham Study. *American Journal of Epidemiology, 138,* 353–364.

Elias, P. K., Elias, M. F., Robbins, M. A., & Budge, M. M. (2004). Blood pressure-related cognitive decline: Does age make a difference? *Hypertension, 44,* 631–636.

Fleeson, W. (2001). Toward a structure- and process-integrated view of personality: Traits as density distribution of states. *Journal of Personality and Social Psychology, 80*(6), 1011–1027.

Fried, L. P. (2000). Epidemiology of aging. *Epidemiologic Reviews, 22,* 95–106.

Gamaldo, A., Mogherkar, A., Kilada, S., Resnick, S. M., Zonderman, A. B., & O'Brien, R. (2006). Effect of a clinical stroke on the risk of dementia in a prospective cohort. *Neurology, 67,* 1363–1369.

Gerstof, D., Ram, N., Rocke, C., Lindenberger, U., & Smith, J. (2008). Decline in life satisfaction in old age: Longitudinal evidence for the links to distance to death. *Psychology and Aging, 23,* 154–168.

Goldberg, L. (1993). The structure of phenotypic personality traits. *American Psychologist, 48,* 26–34.

Griffin, P. W., Mrozek, D. K., & Spiro, A., III. (2006). Variability in affective change among aging men: Findings from the VA Normative Aging Study. *Journal of Research in Personality, 40,* 942–965.

Grober, E., Hall, C. B., Lipton, R. B., Zonderman, A. B., Resnick, S. M., & Kawas, C. (2008). Memory impairment, executive dysfunction, and intellectual decline in preclinical AD. *Journal of International Neuropsychological Society, 14,* 266–278.

Haynes, R. B., Yao, X., Degani, A., Kripalani, S., Garg, A., & McDonald, H. P. (2005). Interventions to enhance medication adherence. *Cochrane Database of Systematic Reviews,* Issue 4 (Article No. CD000011), DOI: 10.1002/14651858.CD000011.pub3.

Heckhausen, J. (2001). Adaptation and resilience in midlife. In M. E. Lachman (Ed.), *Handbook of midlife development* (pp. 345–394). New York: Wiley.

Hershey, D. A., Boyd, M. L., Coutant, K. M., & Turner, K. (1999). Cognitive aging psychology: Significant advances, challenges, and training issues. *Educational Gerontology, 25,* 349–364.

Hodges, J. R., & Graham, N. L. (2001). Vascular dementias. In J. R. Hodges (Ed.), *Early onset dementia: A multidisciplinary approach* (pp. 47–65). Oxford, UK: Oxford University Press.

Hoffman, J., & Proulx, S. M. (2003). Medication errors caused by confusion of drug names. *Drug Safety, 26,* 445–454.

Hollmann, F. W., Mulder, T. J., & Kallan, J. E. (2000). *Methodology and assumptions for the population projections of the United States: 1999 to 2100* (U.S. Census Bureau, Population Division Working Paper No. 38). Retrieved October 28, 2008, from *www.census.gov.*

Hooker, K. (1999). Possible selves in adulthood: Incorporating teleonomic relevance into studies of the self. In T. M. Hess & F. Blanchard-Fields (Eds.), *Social cognition and aging* (pp. 97–122). New York: Academic Press.

Hooker, K. (2002). New directions for research in personality and aging: A comprehensive model for linking levels, structures and processes. *Journal of Research in Personality, 35,* 318–334.

Hooker, K., & Kaus, C. R. (1992). Possible selves and health behaviors in later life. *Journal of Aging and Health, 4,* 390–411.

Hooker, K., & McAdams, D. P. (2003). Personality reconsidered: A new agenda for aging research. *Journals of Gerontology B: Psychological Sciences and Social Sciences, 58,* 296–304.

Jennings, J. R., Muldoon, M. F., Whyte, E. M., Scanion, J., Price, J., & Melizer, C. C. (2008). Brain imaging findings predict blood pressure response to pharmacological treatment. *Hypertension, 52,* 1113–1119.

Knopman, D. S., DeKosky, S. T., Cummings, J. L., Chui, H., Corey-Bloom, J., & Relkin, N. (2001). Practice parameter: Diagnosis of dementia (an evidence-based review): Report of the quality standards subcommittee of the American Academy of Neurology. *Neurology, 56,* 1143–1153.

Lachman, M. (2004). Development in midlife. *Annual Review of Psychology, 55,* 305–331.

Lamarca, R., Alonso, J., Gomez, G., & Munoz,

A. (1998). Left-truncated data with age as time scale: An alternative for survival analysis in the elderly population. *Journals of Gerontology B: Psychological Sciences and Social Sciences, 53*(5), M337–M343.

Launer, L. J., Masaki, K., Petrovitch, H., Foley, D., & Havlik, R. J. (1995). The association between mid-life blood pressure and late-life functioning. *Journal of the American Medical Association, 274,* 1846–1851.

Llabre, M. M., Spitzer, S. B., Saab, P. G., & Schneiderman, N. (2001). Piecewise latent growth curve modeling of systolic blood pressure reactivity and recovery from the cold pressor test. *Psychophysiology, 38*(6), 951–960.

MacDonald, S. W. S., Hultsch, D. F., & Dixon, R. A. (2008). Predicting impending death: Inconsistency in speed is an a selective and early marker. *Psychology and Aging, 23,* 595–607.

Maddox, G. (1987). Aging differently. *Gerontologist, 27,* 557–64.

MacLaughlin, E. J., Raehl, C. L., Treadway, A. K., Sterling, T. L., Zoller, D. P., & Bond, C. A. (2005). Assessing medication adherence in the elderly: Which tools to use in clinical practice? *Drugs and Aging, 22,* 231–255.

Maddigan, S. L., Farris, K. B., Keating, N., Wiens, C. A., & Johnson, J. A. (2003). Predictors of older adults' capacity for medication management in a self-medication program: A retrospective chart review. *Journal of Aging and Health, 15,* 332–352.

Markides, K. S. (2007). *Encyclopedia of health and aging.* Thousand Oaks, CA: Sage.

McAdams, D. P. (1995). What do we know when we know a person? *Journal of Personality, 63,* 365–396.

McAdams, D. P., & Pals, J. (2006). A new Big Five: Fundamental principles for an integrative science of personality. *American Psychologist, 61*(3), 204–217.

McArdle, J. J., Fisher, G. G., & Kadlec, K. M. (2007). Latent variable analyses of age trends on cognition in the Health and Retirement Study 1992–2004. *Psychology and Aging, 22,* 525–545.

McCrae, R. R., & Costa, P. T. (2003). *Personality in adulthood: A five-factor theory perspective* (2nd ed.). New York: Guilford Press.

McCrae, R. R., & Terracciano, A. (2005). Universal features of personality traits from the observer's perspective: Data from 50 cultures. *Journal of Personality and Social Psychology, 88*(3), 547–561.

Mehta, P. D., & West, S. G. (2000). Putting the individual back into individual growth curves. *Psychological Methods, 5*(1), 23–43.

Morrell, R. W., Park, D. C., & Poon, L. W. (1989). Quality of instructions on prescription drug labels: Effects on memory and compre-

hension in young and old adults. *Gerontologist, 29,* 345–354.

Mroczek, D. K., & Spiro, A., III (2003). Modeling intraindividual change in personality traits: Findings from the Normative Aging Study. *Journals of Gerontology B: Psychological Sciences and Social Sciences, 58,* P153–P165.

Mroczek, D. K., & Spiro, A. (2007). Personality change influences mortality in older men. *Psychological Science, 18,* 371–376.

Mroczek, D. K., Spiro, A., & Griffin, P. (2006). Personality and aging. In J. E. Birren & K. W. Schaie (Eds.), *Handbook of the psychology of aging* (6th ed., pp. 69–84). San Diego, CA: Elsevier.

Muthén, B. (2001). Second-generation structural equation modeling with a combination of categorical and continuous latent variables: New opportunities for latent class/latent growth modeling. In L. M. Collins & A. Sayer (Eds.), *New methods for the analysis of change* (pp. 291–322). Washington, DC: American Psychological Association.

Nagin, D. S. (1999). Analyzing developmental trajectories: A semi-parametric, group-based approach. *Psychological Methods, 4,* 139–177.

National Institute on Aging. (2007). *Why population aging matters.* Bethesda, MD: Author.

Nesselroade, J. R., & Boker, S. M. (1994). Assessing constancy and change. In T. F. Heatherton & J. L. Weinberger (Eds.), *Can personality change?* (pp. 121–147). Washington, DC: American Psychological Association.

Nesselroade, J. R., & Featherman, D. L. (1991). Intraindividual variability in older adults depression scores: Some implications for developmental theory and longitudinal research. In D. Magnusson, R. L. Bergman, G. Rudinger, & B. Torestad (Eds.), *Problems and methods in longitudinal research: Stability and change* (pp. 47–66). Cambridge, UK: Cambridge University Press.

Neugarten, B. L. (1968). Adult personality. In *Middle age and aging* (pp. 137–147). Chicago: University of Chicago Press.

Neugarten, B. L. (1979). Time, age, and the life cycle. *American Journal of Psychiatry, 136*(7), 887–894.

Park, D., & Kidder, D. P. (1996). Prospective memory and medication adherence. In G. E. M. Brandimonte & M. A. McDaniel (Eds.), *Prospective memory theory and application* (pp. 369–390). Hillsdale, NJ: Erlbaum.

Poon, L. W., & Perls, T. T. (Eds.). (2007). *Annual review of gerontology and geriatrics: Biosocial approaches to longevity.* New York: Springer.

Post, K., & Roter, D. (1988). Predictors of recall of medication regimens and recommendations for lifestyle change in elderly patients. *Gerontologist, 27,* 510–515.

Puckett, J. M., Reese, H. W., & Pollina, L. K. (1993). An integration of life-span research in everyday cognition: Four issues. In J. M. Puckett & H. W. Reese (Eds.), *Mechanisms of everyday cognition* (pp. 3–19). Hillsdale, NJ: Erlbaum.

Roberts, B. W., Kuncel, N. R., Shiner, R., Caspi, A., & Goldberg, L. R. (2007). The power of personality: The comparative validity of personality traits, socioeconomic status, and cognitive ability for predicting important life outcomes. *Perspectives on Psychological Science, 2,* 313–345.

Roberts, B. W., Walton, K., & Viechtbauer, W. (2006). Patterns of mean-level change in personality traits across the life course: A meta-analysis of longitudinal studies. *Psychological Bulletin, 132,* 1–25.

Sabate, E. (2003). *Adherence to long-term therapies: Evidence for action.* Geneva: World Health Organization.

Salmon, D. P., & Hodges, J. R. (2001). Neuropsychological assessment of early onset dementia. In J. R. Hodges (Ed.), *Early onset dementia: A multidisciplinary approach* (pp. 47–65). Oxford, UK: Oxford University Press.

Salthouse, T. (1991). *Theoretical perspectives in cognitive aging.* Hillsdale, NJ: Erlbaum.

Schaie, K. W. (2005). *Developmental influences on adult intelligence: The Seattle Longitudinal Study.* New York: Oxford University Press.

Siegler, I. C. (2007). *Psychology of aging and the public health: 2007 Developmental Health Award Lecture.* Divisions 20 and 38, American Psychological Association, San Francisco, CA.

Siegler, I. C., Bosworth, H. B., & Elias, M. F. (2003). Adult development and aging. In A. M. Nezu, C. M. Nezu, & P. A. Geller (Eds.), *Handbook of psychology: Vol. 9. Health psychology* (pp. 487–510). New York: Wiley.

Siegler, I. C., Costa, P. T., Brummett, B. H., Helms, M. J., Barefoot, J. C., Williams, R. B., et al. (2003). Patterns of change in hostility from college to midlife in the UNC Alumni Heart Study predict high-risk status. *Psychosomatic Medicine, 65,* 738–745.

Siegler, I. C., Dawson, D. V., & Welsh, K. A. (1994). Caregiver ratings of personality change in Alzheimer's disease patients: A replication. *Psychology and Aging, 9,* 464–466.

Siegler, I. C., Elias, M. F., & Bosworth, H. B. (in press). Health and aging. In A. Baum, T. Revenson, & J. E. Singer (Eds.), *Handbook of health psychology* (2nd ed.). New York: Psychology Press.

Siegler, I. C., Peterson, B. L., Barefoot, J. C., Harvin, S. H., Dahlstrom, W. G., Kaplan, B. H., et al. (1992). Using college alumni populations in epidemiologic research: The UNC Alumni Heart Study. *Journal of Clinical Epidemiology, 45*(11), 1243–1250.

Siegler, I. C., Peterson, B. L., Barefoot, J. C., & Williams, R. B. (1992). Hostility during late adolescence predicts coronary risk factors at midlife. *American Journal of Epidemiology, 136*(2), 146–154.

Siegler, I. C., Poon, L. W., Madden, D. J., Dilworth-Anderson, P., Schaie, K. W., Willis, S. E., et al. (2009). Psychological aspects of normal aging. In D. G. Blazer & D. C. Steffens (Eds.), *Textbook of geriatric psychiatry* (pp. 137–155). Washington, DC: American Psychiatric Association Press.

Singer, J. D., & Willett, J. B. (2003). *Applied longitudinal data analysis: Modeling change and event occurrence.* New York: Oxford University Press.

Singh-Manoux, A., Gueguen, A., Martikainen, P., Ferrie, J., Marmot, M., & Shipley, M. (2007). Self-rated health and mortality: Short and long-term associations in the Whitehall II Study. *Psychosomatic Medicine, 69,* 138–143.

Sleath, B., Rubin, R. H., Campbell, W., Gwyther, L., & Clark, T. (2001). Physician–patient communication about over-the-counter medications. *Social Science and Medicine, 53,* 357–369.

Sliwinski, M. J., Hofer, S. M., & Hall, C. (2003). Correlated and coupled cognitive change in older adults with and without preclinical dementia. *Psychology and Aging, 18,* 672–683.

Sliwinski, M., & Mogle, J. (2008). Time-based and process-based approaches to analysis of longitudinal data. In S. M. Hofer & D. F. Alwin (Eds.), *Handbook of cognitive aging: Interdisciplinary perspectives* (pp. 477–491). Thousand Oaks, CA: Sage.

Smith, A. D. (2008). The worldwide challenge of the dementias: A role for B vitamins and homocysteine? *Food and Nutrition Bulletin, 29,* S143–S172.

Snowden, D. A. (2001). *Aging with grace.* New York: Bantam Books.

Spiro, A. (2007). The relevance of a lifespan developmental approach to health. In C. M. Aldwin, C. L. Park, & A. Spiro (Eds.), *Handbook of health psychology and aging* (pp. 75–93). New York: Guilford Press.

Staessen, J. A., & Birkenhäger, W. H. (2004). Cognitive impairment and blood pressure: Quo usque tandem abutere patientia nostra? *Hypertension, 44,* 612–613.

Staudinger, U., & Kunzmann, U. (2005). Positive adult personality development: Adjustment and/or growth? *European Psychologist, 10*(4), 320–329.

Stevens, J. M., & Fox, N. C. (2001). Structural imaging. In J. R. Hodges (Ed.), *Early onset dementia: A multidisciplinary approach* (pp. 47–65). Oxford, UK: Oxford University Press.

Stewart, R., & Liolitsa, D. (1999). Type 2 diabetes mellitus, cognitive impairment and dementia. *Diabetes Medicine, 16*, 93–112.

Surtees, P., Wainwright, N., Luben, R., Khaw, K., & Day, N. (2006). Mastery, sense of coherence, and mortality: Evidence of independent associations from the EPIC-Norfolk prospective cohort study. *Health Psychology, 25*(1), 102–110.

Tarn, D., Heritage, J., Paterniti, D. A., Hays, R. D., Kravitz, R. L., & Wenger, N. S. (2006). Physician communication when prescribing new medications. *Archives of Internal Medicine, 166*, 1855–1862.

Terracciano, A., Lockenhoff, C. E., Zonderman, A. B., Ferrucci, L., & Costa, P. T. (2008). Personality predictors of longevity: Activity, emotional stability and conscientiousness. *Psychosomatic Medicine, 70*, 621–627.

Terry, D. F. (2007). Centenarian offspring: A model for successful aging. In L. W. Poon & T. T. Perls (Eds.), *Annual review of gerontology and geriatrics* (Vol. 27, pp. 79–87). New York: Springer.

Thiebaut, A. C., & Benichou, J. (2004). Choice of time-scale in Cox's model analysis of epidemiologic cohort data: A simulation study. *Statistics in Medicine, 23*(24), 3803–3820.

Tyas, S. L., Salazar, J. C., Snowdon, D. A., Desrosiers, M. F., Riley, K. P., Mendiondo, M. S., et al. (2007). Transitions to mild cognitive impairments, dementia and death: Findings from the Nun Study. *American Journal of Epidemiology, 165*, 1231–1238.

Vermeire, E., Hearnshaw, H., Van Royen, P., & Denekens, J. (2001). Patient adherence to treatment: Three decades of research: A comprehensive review. *Journal of Clinical Pharmacy and Therapeutics, 26*, 331–342.

Waldstein, S. R. (1995). Hypertension and neuropsychological function: A lifespan perspective. *Experimental Aging Research, 21*, 321–352.

Waldstein, S. R., & Elias, M. F. (Eds.). (2001). *Neuropsychology of cardiovascular disease.* Mahwah, NJ: Erlbaum.

Waldstein, S. R., Giggey, P. P., Thayer, J. F., & Zonderman, A. B. (2005). Nonlinear relations of blood pressure to cognitive function: The Baltimore Longitudinal Study of Aging. *Hypertension, 45*, 374–379.

Waldstein, S. R., & Katzel, L. I. (2001). Hypertension and cognitive function. In S. R. Waldstein & M. F. Elias (Eds.), *Neuropsychology of cardiovascular disease* (pp. 15–36). Mahwah, NJ: Erlbaum.

Wilson, R. S., Beck, T. L., Bienias, J. L., & Bennett, D. A. (2007). Terminal cognitive decline: Accelerated loss of cognition in the last years of life. *Psychosomatic Medicine, 69*, 131–137.

Wilson, R. S., Schneider, J. A., Arnold, S. E., Bienias, J. L., & Bennett, D. A. (2007). Conscientiousness and the incidence of Alzheimer's disease and mild cognitive impairment. *Archives of General Psychiatry, 64*, 1204–1212.

Wolf, M., Davis, T. C., Tilson, H. H., Bass, P. F., & Parker, R. M. (2006). Misunderstanding of prescription drug warning labels among patients with low literacy. *American Journal of Health-System Pharmacy, 63*, 1048–1055.

Wulsin, L. R., Evans, J. C., Vasan, R. S., Murabito, J. M., Kelley-Hayes, M., & Benjamin, E. J. (2005). Depressive symptoms, coronary heart disease and overall mortality in the Framingham Heart Study. *Psychosomatic Medicine, 67*, 697–702.

Yorgason, J. B., Almeida, D., Neupert, S., Hoffman, L., & Spiro, A., III (2006). A dyadic examination of daily health symptoms and emotional well-being in later life couples. *Family Relations, 55*, 613–624.

CHAPTER 11

Animal Models in Health Psychology Research

Daniel A. Nation
Neil Schneiderman
Philip M. McCabe

An important challenge for health psychology researchers is to integrate basic biobehavioral findings with applied fields of research and clinical treatment, that is, "translational research." Understanding the fundamental processes by which biobehavioral factors can influence human disease is important for not only delineation of pathophysiological processes but also the prevention, diagnosis, and treatment of disease. Animal models of human disease have played a major role in our understanding of the relationship between behavior and disease. The best animal models allow the investigation of the etiology, pathogenesis, symptomatology, and responsiveness to preventive measures and therapeutic strategies. Moreover, these models provide researchers with greater control over experimental variables (e.g., environmental, genetic, dietary) than that in many human studies, and allow for more invasive investigation of physiological mechanisms.

The current chapter examines some of the most important animal models, and research strategies within these models, used in health psychology/behavioral medicine. These models have provided useful information regarding the role of behavior in cardiovascular disorders, diabetes/obesity, immunological disorders, cancer, and gastrointestinal disorders. Finally, the chapter describes in detail a recently developed animal model in health psychology, the Watanabe heritable hyperlipidemic rabbit, and how this model has helped us to understand the relationship among social environment, behavior, and the progression of atherosclerosis.

Historical Perspectives on the Use of Animal Models in Health Psychology

The use of animals as models to study the structure and function of the human body in health and disease may have begun with the second-century Roman physician Galen, who used animals to study anatomy when dissection of humans was forbidden (Bendick, 2002). Today, as in Galen's time, animal models are utilized to explore hypotheses that cannot be tested in humans. These highly controlled experiments are capable of transforming our understanding of human disease from theory and passive observation to knowledge of pathophysiology and therapeutic efficacy. In medical science, animal models often involve the translation of theoretical or cell and tissue culture findings to living animals, but they can also be used to pursue mechanistic explanations for clinical observations. The results of animal studies investigating the efficacy of treatments or the pathophysiology of disease can then be translated into human research.

The major discovery of 20th-century medicine that would lead to the creation of the field of health psychology resulted from a series of animal experiments by the Hungarian physician and scientist Hans Selye. Early in his career, Selye, who is often regarded as the "Einstein of medicine," noted the apparent homogeneity of symptoms presented by patients across a broad range of pathological conditions (Cooper & Dewe, 2004). This puzzling clinical observation was fueled by frustrating results from a number of Selye's ongoing experiments in animals. In his studies of endocrine function, Selye was injecting organ extracts into rats. He discovered that regardless of the particular solution injected into the rats, postmortem examination of the internal organs tended to reveal the same general pattern of pathology. This included adrenal hypertrophy, thymic atrophy, and gastric and duodenal ulceration. The similarity of response regardless of the stimulus was consistent with his clinical observation that sick patients tended to present with similar symptoms regardless of the cause. His findings suggested that the body may react in the same fashion to any event that disrupts homeostasis. This was the birth of the notion that the body responds to environmental stimuli with a stereotyped stress response, which Selye termed the "general adaptive response." Thus, the revelation that an endogenously produced response to environmental stimuli can result in organic pathology was largely based on animal studies that would have been impossible to perform in human beings.

The term "stress," which Selye would later lament and attempt to replace with "strain," was broken into the "stressor," or stimulus, and the "distress," or response. It quickly became clear that not all stressors elicited the same distress, and the disconnect between stressors used in animal research (e.g., immobilization, electric shock) and those occurring in human ecology (e.g., be-

reavement, divorce) became apparent. More recent research into the biology of the stress response and its effects on disease has expanded the definition of "stress" to include many different kinds of psychological factors, while focusing on social factors that are more relevant to human circumstances. This has led to advances in our understanding of how social dominance or hostility, social defeat or subordination, social deprivation or isolation, and other social contexts may impact biological functioning in health and disease. Other researchers in health psychology have used animal models to reach beyond the stressor construct to study the importance of positive psychosocial factors in disease, such as affiliative social behavior and stable social environment. Thus, as the relative importance of different psychosocial constructs has evolved within the field of health psychology, so have animal models used to investigate the biological mechanisms responsible for the effects of psychosocial factors on disease.

Animal Models in Behavioral Medicine

Diabetes and Cardiovascular Disease

As with Selye's early work, many areas of animal research in contemporary health psychology were initially driven by clinical observations that suggested an association between psychological factors and disease. An early example of this approach can be found in the diabetes literature. Clinical observations at least as early as the mid-19th century noted that stress may precipitate the onset of diabetes through increases in blood glucose levels (Helz & Templeton, 1990). Partially fueled by these reports, eminent physiologist Walter Cannon (1928) demonstrated that restraint stress can induce increases in glucose production in cats. With the subsequent development of numerous animal models of both Type 1 and Type 2 diabetes (e.g., BB [biobreeding] Wistar rat, streptozotocin-treated rat) the effect of stress on diabetes pathophysiology could be directly studied experimentally (Surwit & Schneider, 1993). Studies utilizing these models were able to demonstrate that stress can precipitate the onset of diabetes in animals vulnerable to the disease. These findings have been attributed to increases in circulating catecholamine concentrations and direct adrenergic stimulation of pancreatic and liver cells through sympathetic innervation of these organs. Behavioral interventions designed to prevent the onset of Type 2 diabetes in at-risk individuals now include stress reduction, in an effort to reduce activation of the sympathetic nervous system (SNS) in vulnerable individuals.

Another example of animal research verifying clinical observation comes from the cardiovascular disease literature. One of the more successful lines of research in behavioral medicine began with an observation by two cardiologists, Friedman and Rosenman (1959), that a particular personality type was associated with increased prevalence and severity of cardiovascular disease (CVD). The term "Type A personality" came to represent a constellation of characterological features consistent with predisposition toward increased hostility, anger, and time-pressured anxiety (for a review, see Rozanski, Blumenthal, & Kaplan, 1999). In addition to a large number of human studies investigating the association between these personality factors and CVD, this observation was partially responsible for the initiation of an elegant series of behavioral studies in the cholesterol-fed cynomolgus monkey model of atherosclerosis. In these primate studies, Kaplan, Manuck, and colleagues were not only able to demonstrate a causal link between social hostility and coronary artery atherosclerosis but also to provide a mechanistic explanation for these observations based on increased SNS activation (Kaplan, Manuck, Clarkson, Lusso, & Taub, 1982; for a review, see Kaplan & Manuck 1999).

In this model, monkeys fed a "Western diet," with approximately 40% of calories from fat, develop extensive atherosclerosis in the coronary arteries that is remarkably similar to what occurs in humans (Kaplan & Manuck, 1999). In the wild these animals live in groups with a clear hierarchy of dominance–subordination relationships. Adolescent males form smaller bands that live on the outskirts of these groups as they await their opportunity to move in and compete for membership in an established group. These encounters with novel young males represent a disruptive social event within the hierarchy of the group. Thus, by manipulating the composition of the social group,

investigators were able to implement an ecologically valid psychosocial stressor defined by the degree of stability in the social environment (Kaplan & Manuck, 1997). This was accomplished by housing the animals in one of two social conditions. Creation of the unstable social group entailed the periodic reorganization of group members, necessitating the continual reestablishment of dominance–subordination relationships. The stable social group comprised the same individuals, with the dominance–subordination hierarchy left intact throughout the study. Results from the initial study indicated that within the unstable social group, dominant male monkeys displayed increased coronary artery atherosclerosis relative to subordinate males. Importantly, the effect of social environment on atherosclerosis was determined to be independent of lipid profile, suggesting that factors unrelated to cholesterol metabolism were responsible for these observations. A subsequent study in monkeys fed a low-fat diet confirmed that an unstable social environment potentiates the development of atherosclerotic lesions in socially dominant males, even in the absence of dietary risk factors (Kaplan et al., 1983).

Further investigation of the mechanisms responsible for this experimental observation revealed that excessive SNS activation in response to psychosocial stress is associated with increased atherosclerosis, and that blockade of SNS activity abrogates the effects of an unstable social environment on disease (Kaplan & Manuck, 1994). These findings came from studies demonstrating that animals with more elevated cardiac responsivity to threat of capture showed cardiac hypertrophy and increased coronary artery lesion area (Manuck, Kaplan, & Clarkson, 1983). Furthermore, administration of the nonspecific beta-adrenoceptor antagonist, propranolol, protected dominant male monkeys from developing increased atherosclerosis (Kaplan, Manuck, Adams, Weingand, & Clarkson, 1987). An interpretation of these findings that is consistent with human studies of hostility in CVD holds that under unstable social conditions, socially dominant males are under increased pressure to continually maintain their hierarchical position. The strain of constant hostile confrontations with novel males competing for status translates into excessive and prolonged SNS activation (Kaplan & Manuck, 1994). Chronic SNS overactivation is thought to exacerbate atherosclerotic lesion development through a variety of mechanisms, including increased hemodynamic strain, oxidative stress, inflammation, and endothelial dysfunction (Black, 2006; Nation et al., 2008; Strawn et al., 1991).

Additional studies using the cholesterol-fed cynomolgus monkey have significantly advanced our understanding of how psychosocial factors can lead to increased atherosclerosis in females. Investigation of female monkeys kept on an atherogenic diet revealed that subordination is associated with hypercortisolism, ovarian dysfunction, and increased coronary artery atherosclerosis (Clarkson, Adams, Kaplan, Shively, & Koritnik, 1989). Unlike the effect of social dominance in male monkeys, which occurred only under unstable social circumstances, the impact of social subordination on atherosclerosis in female monkeys occurred regardless of the stability of the housing condition (Shively & Clarkson, 1994). Increases in coronary artery atherosclerosis observed in subordinate female monkeys were similar to those of dominant males. Subordinate females also show an increase in the number of anovulatory cycles, luteal-phase deficiencies, and adrenal weight (Kaplan et al., 1996). These findings are consistent with the triad of hypercortisolism, ovarian dysfunction, and CVD observed in humans. The fact that experimentally induced subordination stress was able to produce this syndrome in the laboratory further suggests that psychosocial stress may lead to ovarian dysfunction and, subsequently, to increased atherosclerosis. Further studies demonstrated that ovariectomy (Adams, Kaplan, Koritnik, & Clarkson, 1985), pregnancy (Adams, Kuplan, Koritnik, & Clarkson, 1987), or oral contraceptive (Kaplan et al., 1995) negated the differences between dominant and subordinate females, further supporting the hypothesis that psychosocial stress impacts atherosclerotic disease through its effects on estrogen.

Social isolation, or social deprivation, was also found to impact the progression of atherosclerosis in female cholesterol-fed cynomolgus monkeys (Shively, Clarkson, & Kaplan, 1989). The extent of atherosclerosis in socially deprived females was greater than that of dominant females, but less than that found in subordinates. Findings from a later study suggested that social deprivation was affecting disease progression through increased SNS activation, as indexed by elevated resting heart rate (Watson, Shively, Kaplan, & Line, 1998).

Taken together the results of studies in the cholesterol-fed cynomolgus monkey model of atherosclerosis have not only provided powerful evidence for the role of social stability, social status, and social deprivation in the progression of atherosclerosis, but they have also revealed specific mechanisms responsible for mediating the effects of these psychosocial factors on disease.

Immunological Disorders and Cancer

Along with the significant advances in cardiovascular behavioral medicine during the previous century, rapid development in our understanding of the connection between the central nervous system (CNS) and the immune system has highlighted the importance of psychological factors in diseases related to immune functioning (for a review, see Moynihan & Ader, 1996). Prior to the 1950s there was the long-held assumption that the immune system was a relatively autonomous physiological entity not under direct control of the CNS. Early research provided anatomical evidence to the contrary by demonstrating neural innervation of key immune organs, such as the lymph nodes and the spleen (for a review, see Nance & Sanders, 2007). These findings were followed by groundbreaking animal studies that indicated important aspects of immune functioning, including immunosuppression, could be behaviorally conditioned using a classic Pavlovian paradigm (Ader & Cohen, 1993).

In one such study, two groups of lupus-prone (MRL-lpr/lpr) mice were given injections of the immunosuppressant cyclophosphamide (Ader & Cohen, 1982). Injections were paired with consumption of saccharin-flavored water in one group, while no such pairing was provided to the other group. When the medication was discontinued, the animals with no pairing between injections and saccharin died rapidly, whether or not they drank the flavored water. However, those that received the pairing of saccharin with the injections and continued to drink the flavored water lived nearly as long as those continuing to receive the drug. This and other similar studies demonstrated that stimuli could be conditioned to produce alterations in immune function significant enough to prolong survival, suggesting that the CNS is capable of exerting profound modulation of immune function. These seminal discoveries led to the creation of the field of "psychoneuroimmunology," dedicated to describing the relationships between behavior, brain, and immune function.

To date, animal paradigms of social defeat (Engler, Engler, Bailey, & Sheridan, 2005), isolation (Chida, Sudo, & Kubo, 2005), depression (Bartolomucci, 2007), and other psychosocial factors have been used to examine how behavioral contexts can alter the progression of many diseases through changes in immunological function. It has been hypothesized that psychosocial stress may convey increased susceptibility to infectious disease through suppression of immune function. Support for this hypothesis has come from early studies involving multiple models of bacterial and viral infection, where restraint, foot shock, fear conditioning , and social crowding have been used to investigate the effects of stress on immune functioning (for a review, see Sheridan, Dobbs, Brown, & Zwilling, 1994). Findings have demonstrated that various stress induction paradigms are associated with decreased antibody titers (Edwards & Dean, 1977), proinflammatory cytokine (e.g., interferon-gamma [IFN-gamma], tumor necrosis factor–alpha [TNF-a], interleukin-2 [IL-2]) production (Jessop & Bayer, 1989), immune cell proliferation (Stefanski & Engler, 1999), and T cell and natural killer (NK) cell cytotoxicity (Ben-Eliyahu, Shakhar, Page, Stefanski, & Shakhar, 2000). These stress-induced alterations in immune function have been associated with increased bacterial growth, viral replication, symptoms of infection, and mortality (for a review, see Sheridan et al., 1994).

The immunosuppressive effects of psychological stress are thought be mediated by some combination of glucocorticoid (GCC) activity controlled by the hypothalamic–pituitary–adrenal (HPA) axis (Webster, Tonelli, & Sternberg, 2002), and catecholamine activity controlled by the sympathetic–adrenal medullary axis (Sanders & Straub, 2002). Support for this hypothesis comes from studies in which the immunosuppressive effects of psychosocial stress are reversed by adrenalectomy (Bonneau, Sheridan, Feng, & Glaser, 1993), hypophysectomy (Keller et al., 1988), sympathectomy (Cao, Filipov, & Lawrence, 2002), or administration of exogenous GCCs or adrenergic receptor antagonists (Dobbs, Vasquez, Glaser, & Sheridan, 1993). The immunosuppressive effects of pharmacological doses of GCCs or their synthetic analogues are well established. These effects are thought to occur through GCC receptor mediated suppression of the immunomodulatory transcription factor, nuclear factor kappa-B (NF-kappa-B), which is largely responsible for inflammatory and cell-mediated immune responses to infection (Webster et al., 2002). The ability of psychosocial stress to induce immunosuppression through endogenous GCC release is one of the most consistent mechanistic observations in animal studies in health psychology.

Results from studies of infectious disease are easily generalized to investigation of the effects of psychosocial stress on tumor development and metastasis. The finding that psychological stress inhibits NK cell function is one of the most consistently observed immunological results of stress (Bartolomucci, 2007). The effect of stress on NK cell function is particularly important in cancer, as these cells are the first line of defense against tumor growth and metastasis (Vivier, Tomasello, Baratin, Walzer, & Ugolini, 2008). Multiple models of tumor induction have demonstrated suppression of NK cell function, and increased tumor development and metastasis associated with different stress paradigms, particularly those involving social confrontation and subordination (Stefanski, 2001). While contrary reports also exist, these are likely due to a host of methodological differences across studies. For example, studies involving social confrontation may find immunosuppression on the part of both dominant and subordinate animals at an early time point, when both animals are acclimating to the new social environment. Subsequent interactions then stabilize the hierarchy, and the immunological profile of the dominant mouse may normalize, while the subordinate mouse continues to endure the stress of being dominated. There are also many different types of cancers, as well as methods of cancer induction, and measurement of disease in different animals under different stress paradigms. Research suggests that lung metastasis in rat mammary tumors are strictly modulated by NK cell activity, which is particularly susceptible to the immunosuppressive effects of stress. Repeated use of this paradigm has shown that the psychosocial stress of social defeat, produced by repeated exposure to dominant conspecifics, can lead to diminished NK cell function and increased tumor growth and metastasis to the lungs (Stefanski, 2001).

Hepatology and Special Immunology

Other behavioral paradigms have demonstrated that factors related to social environment can impact progression and metastasis in liver cancer. For example, social isolation stress has also been shown to increase the incidence of hepatocellular carcinoma in mice that are genetically susceptible to tumor development through overexpression of transforming growth factor–alpha (TGF-alpha) (Hilakivi-Clarke & Dickson, 1995). Another study utilizing the social isolation paradigm in mice given colonic injections of carcinoma cells found that this stressor increased metastasis to the liver (Wu et al., 2000). The mechanism proposed to be responsible for these effects involves decreased hepatic blood flow and suppression of immune functioning in stressed mice (Chida, Sudo, & Kubo, 2006).

There is also powerful evidence that psychosocial factors may impact the progression of diseases that attack the immune system itself. While results from human research have long suggested that psychosocial factors may play a role in the course of the human immunodeficiency virus (HIV), little has been done with animal research (Glaser, Rabin, Chesney, Cohen, & Natelson, 1999). Recent utilization of the simian model of HIV, referred to as SIV, has allowed for well-controlled studies of the impact of complex social interactions on histopathological measures of disease and mortality in infected animals. Studies using *in vitro* models indicate that norepinephrine (NE) is capable of increasing viral replication in isolated T lymphocytes through impairment of the Type 1 interferon responses known to inhibit HIV replication (Cole, Korin, Fahey, & Zack, 1998). This is consistent with clinical studies demonstrating that increased SNS activity is associated with poor prognosis in humans with HIV (Cole et al., 2001), suggesting that stress-induced SNS activity could accelerate key aspects of disease progression.

Recently, the SIV model was used to test the hypothesis that an unstable and stressful social environment can lead to chronic changes in SNS structure and function that accelerate disease processes (Sloan et al., 2007). In this study, male rhesus macaques were placed into either unstable or stable social conditions for 100 minutes per day for 39 weeks. The stable condition entailed a meeting of the same three animals throughout the study. In the unstable condition, between two and four animals met each day, with the number and identity of the animals differing each day. The unstable environment necessitates the continual reestablishment of dominance and subordination relationships, creating an environment characterized by chronic stress and SNS activation. Animals were inoculated with SIV, and after months of exposure to differential social housing lymph nodes were biopsied. Results indicated that animals housed in an unstable social environment had enhanced sympathetic innervation of the primary lymph nodes, with a greater number of varicosities (branching synaptic terminals), particularly in the paracortex. Animals in the unstable social environment also displayed greater density of viral replication within the lymph nodes, which are major sites for viral replication. Further investigation into gene expression within the lymph nodes of socially stressed animals showed that some Type 1 interferons known to inhibit HIV replication *in vitro* were suppressed relative to animals housed in a stable social environment. Finally, quantification of circulating CD4+ T lymphocyte levels revealed that animals in the unstable social condition also had fewer CD4+ cells, indicating accelerated disease progression. This cutting edge research is capable of powerfully demonstrating how the body can generate specific adaptive responses to different social environments that lead to alterations in immune functioning directly related to disease progression. It is in part the ability to perform invasive examination of body compartments (i.e., lymph nodes) that allowed researchers to uncover the otherwise mysterious effects of psychosocial stress on HIV progression.

While the hypotheses described thus far primarily concern diseases impacted by stress through suppression of various aspects of immune functioning, many diseases that involve hyperactivation of specific immune functions are also negatively impacted by psychosocial stress. These apparently contradictory findings are nonetheless quite consistent. Studies using animal models of a host of autoimmune diseases, including systemic lupus erythematosus (Chida et al., 2005), arthritis (Cutolo & Straub, 2006), insulin-dependent diabetes (Surwit & Schneider, 1993), and two models of multiple sclerosis (Gold & Heesen, 2006), have revealed that psychosocial stress can exacerbate these diseases. For example, chronic social isolation significantly reduced serum levels of antiinflammatory cytokines (IL-4 and IL-10), increased proinflammatory cytokine (IFN-gamma) levels, enhanced autoimmune nephritis, and reduced survival rate in lupus-prone MRL/lpr mice (Chida et al., 2005). Early in the study, socially isolated animals exhibited increased corticosterone levels relative to group-housed controls, likely due to the stress of isolation, but soon showed a corticosterone "burnout" effect, with no further increases after 9 weeks. Conversely, the group-housed animals showed a steady increase in corticosterone concentrations throughout the study, eventually exhibiting higher levels than animals in the isolation condition. This steady rise in circulating corticosterone is consistent with previous findings from a number of autoimmune diseases. As the disease progresses, part of the animal's adaptive response is to suppress the excessive inflammation associated with a T helper cell type 1 (Th1) cytokine response by producing more corticosterone. The inability to produce an effective HPA-axis response to proinflammatory cytokine activation has been found in a number of diseases associated with excessive inflammation, including fibromyalgia and chronic fatigue syndrome (Gur & Oktayoglu, 2008). Other studies have shown that chronic stress can produce a blunted HPA axis response to stress similar to the "burnout" effect observed in these isolated MRL/lpr mice (Miller et al., 2008). These findings suggest that while GCC responses to stress may increase susceptibility to infectious disease in exposed individuals, stress can lead to HPA axis dysfunction and

an inability to control excessive inflammation in those predisposed to inflammatory conditions.

Another possible explanation for the negative effects of stress on diseases characterized by excessive inflammation is the so-called "glucocorticoid resistance" hypothesis (Stark et al., 2001). According to this theory, even in the presence of sufficient HPA axis activity, prolonged exposure to stressful conditions may lead to the development of GCC resistance within immune cells and tissues responsible for the inflammatory response. In one study, chronic social defeat in male mice led to GCC resistance, measured as resistance to corticosterone-induced splenocyte antiproliferative responses (Engler et al., 2005). This decreased GCC sensitivity in splenocytes was associated with increased GCC sensitivity in bone marrow cells, suggesting that psychosocial stress causes a redistribution of GCC insensitive cells to the spleen. In addition to reduced function of the HPA axis and redistribution of GCC insensitive cells, it is also possible that down-regulation of GCC receptor activity itself could be responsible for the stress-induced exacerbation of autoimmune diseases. Another study revealed that while chronic social defeat led to GCC resistance in splenocytes, GCC resistance was not detected in peritoneal macrophages (Avistur, Stark, Dhabhar, Padgett, & Sheridan, 2002). This further indicates that GCC resistance is site-specific and may not generalize to all tissues and immune cell types. Additional animal studies are needed to elucidate the specific mechanisms governing the relationship between GCC sensitivity and inflammatory disease.

Psychological stress is also thought to exacerbate liver diseases (e.g., cirrhosis and hepatitis C) and cardiovascular disease through alterations in blood flow and increased inflammation within specific tissue compartments (for a review, see Chida et al., 2006). Basic animal research has shown that while stressors can cause suppression of systemic proinflammatory cytokine responses, local release of these inflammatory mediators within specific tissues actually increases during stress. This phenomenon has been extensively investigated in the liver, where sympathetic nerve terminals that directly innervate the tissue have been found to release NE in response to restraint stress (Kitamura et al., 1997). Studies conducted both *in vitro* (Dong Jung et al., 2000), using cultured hepatocytes, and *in vivo* during restraint have shown that stress-induced SNS activity within the liver causes increased IL-6 production by hepatocytes (Kitamura et al., 1997). The finding that behavioral contexts can increase inflammation locally within a particular tissue, while differentially impacting other tissues, has far reaching implications for the study of inflammatory diseases in behavioral medicine. These results underscore the necessity of analyzing tissue-specific changes in response to behavioral manipulations. Early theories regarding SNS function focused on the stereotyped nature of SNS responses, but more recent empirical findings have demonstrated that both sympathetic and parasympathetic branches are capable of differential responses within specific tissue compartments. Studying such changes within tissues typically requires animal research because of the invasiveness of tissue collection procedures.

The diverse effects of psychosocial stress detailed in the preceding review of animal models research indicates that the impact of stress on disease must be examined within the context of the adaptive response produced by the particular disease under investigation. This implies that psychological stress involves disruption in homeostasis, which is not a static set point but a dynamic equilibrium that is always responding to internal and external conditions. Accumulated evidence from human studies suggests that psychosocial factors directly impact many other important diseases that have yet to receive attention from health psychologists utilizing animal models. These include Grave's disease, fibromyalgia, Parkinson's disease, and cerebrovascular disease, to name only a few. Some of these diseases have simply been ignored within health psychology, while others lack appropriate animal models. As more animal models are developed and greater numbers of researchers utilize them, novel biological mechanisms capable of transducing the effects of psychosocial stress are likely to be uncovered.

Increasing the Breadth of Investigation

While most animal studies examining psychosocial factors in disease focus on nega-

tive risk factors, such as social stress and social deprivation, other studies suggest that there may be important physiological pathways mediating the beneficial effects of positive psychosocial factors. A series of sophisticated animal and cell culture studies have demonstrated that acetylcholine release from parasympathetic nerve terminals plays an important role in the regulation of local inflammatory responses within specific tissue compartments (for a review, see Tracey, 2007). Furthermore, stimulation of the vagus nerve, the primary efferent parasympathetic pathway, has been shown to decrease inflammatory responses to vascular injury (Borovikova et al., 2000). These findings suggest that increased vagal nerve activity could have health benefits, particularly for those with diseases involving excessive inflammation. This hypothesis is consistent with numerous human studies suggesting that increased heart rate variability, an index of vagal nerve activity, is associated with decreased mortality and improved health (Thayer & Lane, 2007). Interventions frequently utilized by health psychologists, such as biofeedback, conditioned relaxation, controlled breathing, yoga, and meditation, are thought to involve targeted increases in vagal nerve activity (Kattab, Kharrab, Ortak, Richardt, & Bonnemeier, 2007; Nolan et al., 2005). While the potential health benefits provided by such interventions cannot be addressed directly by animal studies, these studies can take advantage of more invasive measures and methods of inducing nerve activity. This work could increase our understanding of the efficacy and physiology behind these treatments. As health psychologists attempt to disseminate information regarding biobehavioral interventions and to promote their increased acceptance and utilization by the general medical community, well-controlled animal studies may provide powerful evidence for the biological basis of these treatments and their impact on disease.

The necessity of animal research in any biomedical field lies in its ability both to provide a high degree of experimental control and to allow the invasive examination of biological functioning and disease. These strengths are particularly useful in new fields, such as health psychology, where a basic understanding of the relationship between proposed risk factors and a particular disease is often lacking. In this context, animal research can clarify the extent to which psychosocial factors, such as anxiety, distress, depression, social isolation, hopelessness, or hostility, impact different kinds of diseases. These models may also inform behavioral interventions by testing whether modification of specific psychosocial factors impacts disease. Furthermore, investigation of physiological pathways linking behavioral contexts to disease outcomes may suggest particular pharmacological interventions.

Along with the strengths of experimental control and the ability to utilize invasive procedures, animal research also has a number of weaknesses. The most obvious of these is the tacit assumption that animals are useful analogues of homeostatic and pathophysiological processes in human beings. Many basic biological functions, aspects of disease, treatment responses, and behavioral factors are species-specific. The extent to which any particular animal model of human disease is characterized by these species-specific properties determines its usefulness in medical research. This variable is especially important in health psychology, where behavioral factors are just as important as pathophysiology, and where so few animal species have a behavioral repertoire remotely approaching that of human beings. However, if an animal model bears similarity to certain aspects of human disease and human behavior, it often involves problems similar to those encountered in human studies. For example, experiments using primate models of chronic diseases, such as CVD, necessitate years of data collection. During the same period of time, multiple rodent experiments can be conducted, potentially answering the same questions using a simpler model. Other examples of such studies include those examining the effects of early rearing environment on disease susceptibility in adulthood, mortality in chronic diseases, or disease processes associated with aging.

An additional complication of primate models is that animals more similar to human beings make ethical considerations more problematic. This issue is particularly salient in health psychology because of the importance of fundamentally aversive (i.e., stressful) stimuli in theories relating behavior to disease. Nonetheless, given the significance of psychosocial factors in disease and the difficulties involved in the scientific study of such phenomena, it is clear that animal research is a necessity for the advancement of health psychology.

Another important consideration in choosing animal species for studies of psychosocial factors in disease is the availability of appropriate models. Early studies examining the impact of psychological stress on hypertension involved the use of rats because of the availability of numerous models, including spontaneously hypertensive (SHR), borderline hypertensive (BHR), and Dahl salt-sensitive rats. Research in BHR and Dahl salt-sensitive rats demonstrated that restraint and other stressors could precipitate the onset of hypertension in genetically predisposed animals (for a review, see Zimmerman & Frolich, 1990). While use of animals selectively bred for the development of specific diseases provided crucial information regarding the role of psychological factors in human diseases during the early years of behavioral medicine research, the usefulness of these animals is limited by a lack of clarity regarding the genetic underpinnings of their disease susceptibility. Under these circumstances, disease vulnerability is conveyed by an unknown or multifaceted genetic mechanism that greatly reduces the ability of experimenters to propose and test specific mechanistic hypotheses regarding the effects of psychological factors on disease. In some cases, investigation of the genetics of selectively bred animals has revealed "naturally" occurring mutations in a single gene to convey disease vulnerability; however, these single-gene mutations are not the rule with inbred strains. The increased availability of transgenic and gene knockout mice, coupled with the extensive information available regarding murine genetics, makes mouse models particularly powerful tools in animal research. These models allow investigators to approach the disease from a mechanistically informed perspective on both pathophysiology and stress physiology, and to manipulate the genetic underpinnings of each. Increased use of these animals in health psychology should provide not only important facts regarding the role of psychosocial factors in a greater variety of diseases but also critical information about the underlying physiological pathways responsible for such observations.

Social Environment and the Progression of Atherosclerosis in the Watanabe Heritable Hyperlipidemic Rabbit

An example of the utility of animal models in behavioral medicine research is work from our laboratory examining the influence of social and emotional factors on the progression of atherosclerosis in the Watanabe heritable hyperlipidemic rabbit (WHHL). The WHHL is an inbred strain that exhibits profound hypercholesterolemia, severely elevated plasma low-density lipoprotein (LDL) levels, and hypertriglyceridemia from birth due to a single gene mutation leading to aberrant LDL receptors (Buja, Clubb, Bilheimer, & Willerson, 1990; Buja, Kita, Goldstein, Watanabe, & Brown, 1983; Kondo & Watanabe, 1975). These animals have a genotype and phenotype that is similar to human familial hypercholesterolemia, which afflicts approximately 0.2% of the population (Buja et al., 1990). WHHLs spontaneously develop atherosclerotic lesions in the aortic arch as early as 2 months of age, and by 6 months of age, 100% of these animals have severe atherosclerosis throughout the aorta (Buja et al., 1983). At about 8–10 months of age, disease progresses through the coronary arteries, and beginning at approximately 1 year of age, WHHLs begin to die from CHD (Buja et al., 1983, 1990). Therefore, this is an animal model of disease with strong genetic determinants.

Although genetic factors greatly influence a number of human diseases (e.g., human familial hypercholesterolemia), it has been demonstrated that the expression of disease can vary as a result of environmental factors (Kaplan et al., 1982; Manuck, Kaplan, & Matthews, 1986). With this in mind, we decided to examine the role of social environment, and associated behavior, in disease progression using the WHHL as an experimental model. An advantage of the WHHL model is that since atherosclerosis develops and progresses spontaneously, one can assess factors that both attenuate disease progression and accelerate the development of disease. An additional advantage of the WHHL over some of the other animal models is that atherosclerosis develops rapidly during the first 6 months of life, and this compressed time frame can facilitate mechanistic studies of the relationship of behavior and disease.

In our initial study (McCabe et al., 2002), 3-month-old male WHHLs were assigned to one of three social/behavioral groups: an unstable group, in which unfamiliar rabbits were paired for 4 hours daily, with the pairing switched each week; a stable group, in which littermates were paired daily for the entire study; and an individually caged group, in which animals never had any social contact with other rabbits. These social conditions were maintained for 4 months, with the study terminated when the animals were 7 months of age. Over the course of the study, the stable group exhibited significantly more affiliative social behavior (e.g., nuzzling, cuddling, grooming cagemates) and less agonistic behavior than the unstable group. Importantly, the stable group developed significantly less aortic atherosclerosis than the other two groups (see Figure 11.1). Although the unstable and individually caged groups had comparable aortic lesion areas, the severity of the disease progressed faster in the unstable group, as indexed by a larger area of calcification and increased fibrous cap thickness in complex lesions. In addition to showing increased agonistic behavior, the unstable group also had increased corticosterone levels and testicular hypertrophy compared to the individually caged group, and greater adrenal weight/body weight than either of the other groups, suggesting relative adrenal hypertrophy in the unstable group. Many of the lesions in the individually caged group consisted pri-

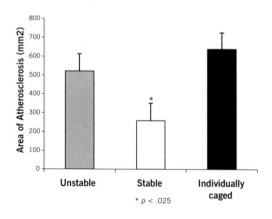

FIGURE 11.1. Total area of aortic atherosclerosis in WHHLs at 7 months of age as a function of social environment. Data from McCabe et al. (2002).

marily of foams cells and fatty streaks. Over the course of the study, the individually caged group was behaviorally relatively sedentary, spending over two-thirds of the time in inactivity. Not surprisingly, these animals gained more weight and were hyperinsulinemic compared to the other groups.

The major finding of this study was that a stable social environment, characterized by increased affiliative behavior and relatively less agonistic behavior, can slow the progression of atherosclerosis relative to unstable social conditions or individual caging. This suggests that the behavioral profile exhibited in the stable environment may protect by slowing the progression of disease, even in animals genetically predisposed to disease. The findings are interesting in light of human studies that have shown that social isolation and a lack of social support predict mortality from CVD (Berkman & Orth-Gomer, 1996; Syme, 1996). For the unstable group, it is proposed that the severe progression of disease is related to chronic emotional stress, as is suggested by increased agonistic behavior, elevated glucocorticoids, and adrenal and testicular hypertrophy. This notion is consistent with human and animal studies suggesting that chronic sympathetic and HPA activation during emotional stress plays an important role in atherosclerotic disease (Manuck, Marsland, Kaplan, & Williams, 1995; Williams, 1996). Finally, individually caged WHHLs exhibited a great deal of aortic atherosclerosis; however, the severity of the lesions was less than that observed in the unstable group. Because the individually housed animals did not show overt behavioral signs of distress or glucocorticoid activation, it is proposed that disease progressed in this group primarily due to insulin metabolic factors (i.e., behavioral inactivity, dyslipidemia, increased body weight, hyperinsulinemia). Regardless of the specific mechanisms underlying these group differences, the results of this first study emphasize the importance of behavioral factors in atherogenesis, even in a model of disease with strong genetic determinants.

Social Environment, Oxytocin, and Atherosclerosis

Given our finding that a stable social environment and associated affiliative behavior slows the progression of atherosclerosis in

WHHLs, we began to look for physiological mechanisms that might account for this effect. There is a large literature that suggests the neuropeptide oxytocin (OT) is involved in the mediation of complex social behaviors in a variety of species. For example, in rodents, central OT has been associated with affiliative behavior, pair-bonding, sexual behavior, and social recognition (Carter, 1998; Insel & Young, 2000). It has also been demonstrated that OT is released in the brain in response to stress (Englemann, Ebner, Landgraf, Holsboer, & Wotjak, 1999). Others have suggested that OT may exert potent antistress effects (Unväs-Möberg, 1998; Unväs-Möberg, Ahlenius, Hillegaart, & Alster, 1994). Brain administration of OT has been shown to attenuate autonomic (Morris, Callahan, Li, & Lucion, 1995), stressful behavioral (Windle, Shanks, Lightman, & Ingram, 1997) and neuroendocrine responses (Neumann, Wigger, Torner, Holsboer, & Landgraf, 2000; Windle et al., 2004). Based on this literature, we hypothesized that the central regulatory influence of OT on affiliative social behaviors, and on the HPA and sympathetic axes, may be an important mechanism underlying the protective effects of a stable social environment in the WHHL model.

In order to explore the notion that OT may be related to social behavior and the progression of disease in the WHHL model, we used chronic microdialysis (Paredes et al., 2006) to measure the release of OT from the paraventricular nucleus (PVN) of the hypothalamus, a major source of brain OT, from male WHHLs in the three social conditions in our initial study (i.e., unstable, stable, individually caged). WHHLs were chronically implanted with a guide cannula terminating in the PVN. Following recovery from surgery, a microdialysis probe was inserted through the guide cannula into the PVN and the region was perfused with artificial cerebrospinal fluid and dialysate samples, and venous blood samples were taken. Following the baseline measures, animals were placed in either an unstable, stable, or individually caged social condition for 1 hour, and their behavior was videotaped and scored throughout the pairing. After the behavioral manipulation, the animals were separated, and the microdialysis procedure and blood draw were repeated. Following this first day, the WHHLs were placed in the same social condition daily for 3 weeks, then the microdialysis procedure was repeated at the end of the study (when the animals were 4.5 months old).

Significant changes in PVN OT were not observed in any of the social groups on the first day of social experience (i.e., Day 1). Following 3 weeks of daily social exposure, however, PVN OT was significantly elevated in the unstable group following social pairing, whereas the other social groups did not exhibit a hypothalamic PVN response. Animals in the unstable group also exhibited increased plasma catecholamines, greater agonistic behavior, and less affiliative behavior in response to their social pairing at the end of the study. These data suggest that social environment modulates PVN OT responses; however, PVN OT was preferentially influenced in the relatively "high stress" unstable group rather than in the stable or individually caged groups. Since the PVN OT response was not present on the first day of social experience, the data suggests that the PVN OT response develops over time and is related to emotionally stressful experience, perhaps as a mechanism to attenuate the effects of stress. An important aspect of this study is that we were able to replicate the finding of our first study (McCabe et al., 2002) that a stable social environment slows the progression of atherosclerosis relative to the other social environments. Interestingly, this study found the effect at 4.5 months of age, after only 3 weeks of social manipulation. There was a 70% attenuation of disease in the stable group, demonstrating the power of social experience early in the disease process.

During this study we also measured plasma OT as a function of social environment. Although not statistically significant, there was a strong trend indicating elevated plasma OT levels in the stable group relative to the other groups. Thus, the data suggest that peripheral OT, produced in hypothalamic magnocellular neurons and released via the posterior pituitary, can be dissociated from central OT pools, which are produced primarily from dendrites and perikarya of magnocellular neurons (Ludwig & Pittman, 2003; Pow & Morris, 1989) in response to stressful experiences (Engelmann et al., 1999). Dendritically released peptides generally have autoregulatory actions on mag-

nocellular neurons or autocrine–paracrine actions nearby. We were particularly interested in the plasma OT elevations in stable animals because it has been suggested that OT may also function as a cardiovascular hormone (Gutkowska, Jankowski, Mukaddam-Daher, & McCann, 2000). OT receptors have been found on cardiac cells (Jankowski et al., 1998), in the vasculature (including the aorta) (Jankowski et al., 2000), and on human vascular endothelial cells (Thibonnier et al., 1999).

Another interesting observation pertaining to peripheral OT is that this hormone appears to have important anti-inflammatory actions. It has been demonstrated that OT ameliorates oxidative colonic inflammation through a neutrophil-dependent mechanism (Iseri et al., 2005) and inflammation associated with tissue injury (carrageenan injection model) in rats (Petersson, Wiberg, Lundeberg, & Uvnäs-Möberg, 2001). Finally, it was reported that OT, and other secretory peptides, scavenge free peroxyl radicals, prevent the oxidation of LDL, and inhibit lipid peroxidation in membranes, suggesting that OT may also function as a natural antioxidant (Moosman & Behl, 2002). Taken together, the presence of OT receptors in cardiovascular tissue and its putative effects on mechanisms underlying atherosclerosis (i.e., inflammation and oxidative stress) led us to hypothesize that peripheral OT, perhaps preferentially released during stable social conditions, may work directly on vascular OT receptors to attenuate vascular inflammation and oxidative stress, thereby slowing the progression of atherosclerosis.

Modulation of Oxidative Stress and Inflammation by Social Environment and OT

As mentioned earlier, increased vascular oxidative stress and inflammation are known to be critical early events in the progression of atherosclerosis (Griendling, Sorescu, & Ushio-Fukai, 2000; Ross, 1999). The primary vascular oxidative stress pathway is through nicotinamide adenine dinucleotide phosphate (NADPH) oxidase, found in endothelial cells, smooth muscle cells, and macrophages within the vessel (Warnholtz et al., 1999). Early inflammatory events in atherogenesis involve monocyte interaction with the endothelial cell layer, migration into the subendothelial space, and differentiation into macrophages (Ross, 1999). Once present in the vessel wall, the macrophages release a variety of chemokines and cytokines that propagate the atherogenic process.

In a recent study we examined the effect of social environment on markers of oxidative stress and inflammation in WHHLs (Nation et al., 2008). Three-month-old male WHHLs were assigned to one of the three social groups used in our previous studies (i.e., unstable, stable, individually caged), and the social manipulations continued until the animals were 5 months old. Over the course of the 2-month study, the stable group engaged in more affiliative social behavior than did the unstable group. The unstable group showed more agonistic behavior compared to the stable group and higher C-reactive protein (CRP, a circulating marker of inflammation) levels than did the individually caged group. The individually caged animals were behaviorally sedentary, had higher 24-hour urinary catecholamine levels than the other groups, and exhibited higher NADPH oxidase activity in the aortic arch relative to the stable group. The results from this study suggest that social environment creates distinct behavioral contexts that can affect markers of inflammation and oxidative stress early in the development of atherosclerosis. These pathophysiological markers may help to explain some of the behaviorally related differences in the extent of atherosclerosis observed in prior studies; however, this study did not address the potential role of OT in the progression of disease.

Recently, we conducted a study (Szeto et al., 2008) using *in vitro* cultured human vascular cells and macrophages designed to test whether OT modulates oxidative stress and inflammatory response in these cells, thereby providing a mechanism that may slow the progression of atherosclerosis. Although it is possible to culture WHHL vascular cells, it is difficult to obtain antibodies and reagents that work well in rabbits. The goals of this study were to identify the presence of OT receptors in cultured human vascular cells, including monocytes and macrophages, and examine the influence of OT on vascular oxidative stress and inflammation in these cultured cells, as measured by NADPH oxidase activity and IL-6 secretion, respectively.

The results from this study demonstrated the presence of OT receptor protein and its transcribed messenger ribonucleic acid (mRNA) in monocytes and macrophages (THP-1 leukemia cell line). Incubation of cells at physiological levels of OT (i.e., picomolar range) significantly decreased basal activity and stimulated NADPH-dependent superoxide activity in vascular cells, monocytes, and macrophages by 25–50%. OT also attenuated IL-6, a potent proinflammatory cytokine, secretion from stimulated THP-1 macrophages and endothelial cells by 50 and 30%, respectively. These findings suggest that OT attenuates vascular oxidative stress and inflammation, two important pathophysiological processes in atherosclerosis. The fact that OT receptors are found in monocytes and macrophages, and that OT decreases both superoxide production and release of a proinflammatory cytokine from these cells, suggests a potentially larger role for OT in the attenuation of diseases other than atherosclerosis and heart disease.

In order to support this notion that OT may have broad anti-inflammatory actions in the body that could attenuate a variety of disease processes, Larry Brooks in our laboratory recently examined the influence of OT on cultured rat adipocytes. Adipose tissue is a major source of circulating proinflammatory cytokines (Gimeno & Klaman, 2005), and obesity has been linked to many disorders and diseases. We verified the presence of OT receptor on cultured adipocytes, using immunoblotting to measure this protein. Following incubation with physiological concentrations of OT, the adipocytes were stimulated with either lipopolysaccharide (LPS), an endotoxin that stimulates IL-6 secretion, or epinephrine, which also stimulates IL-6 secretion from these cells. It was found that OT attenuated the LPS and epinephrine-stimulated release of IL-6 from the adipocytes by approximately 25%. By decreasing the release of proinflammatory cytokines from fat cells, OT may be an important component of an organism's ability to suppress inflammation throughout the body.

We recently tested these *in vitro* observations in an *in vivo* model of atherosclerosis (Nation et al., in press). The apolipoprotein E knockout (apoE$^{-/-}$) mouse model of atherosclerosis spontaneously develops the disease due to defective clearance of cholesterol and triglyceride, exhibiting early lesion development within the aorta by 3 months of age (Meir & Leitersdorf, 2004). ApoE$^{-/-}$ mice were chronically infused with either OT or vehicle solutions from 12 to 24 weeks of age through subcutaneously implanted osmotic minipumps (Alzet model 2006, DURECT Corporation). Analysis of postmortem aortic samples indicated that animals treated with OT for 12 weeks exhibited significantly less lesion area within the thoracic aorta than vehicle controls. Additionally, adipose tissue extracted from OT-treated animals at necropsy and incubated in culture media produced significantly less IL-6 than samples taken from vehicle-treated animals. Importantly, OT and vehicle control animals did not differ on measures of lipids, insulin, blood pressure, heart rate, or physical activity. These findings indicated that increases in peripheral OT may slow the progression of atherosclerosis in animals prone to develop the disease and suggested that OT was not exerting these effects through lipid clearance, insulin-metabolic, hemodynamic, or behavioral pathways. These results also confirmed and extended cell and tissue culture findings demonstrating that OT has anti-inflammatory effects on adipose tissue inflammation *in vivo*.

The Effect of Behavioral Interventions on Insulin Metabolic Variables and Atherosclerosis in WHHLs

In our initial study (McCabe et al., 2002,) individually caged WHHLs developed significant aortic atherosclerosis and exhibited hyperinsulinemia, increased body weight, elevated heart rate, and sedentary behavior relative to the other social groups. We hypothesized that insulin metabolic variables may play an important role in the progression of disease in this social condition. Interestingly, Zhang and colleagues (1991, 1994) reported that WHHLs are hyperinsulinemic and insulin resistant relative to healthy Japanese rabbit controls. In these studies, the individually housed adult rabbits were over 10 months old and food-restricted (i.e., 80 g/day). In contrast, in our study, young WHHLs were examined during a period of early disease progression (i.e., between 3 and 7 months old) and were given unlimited access to food. Therefore, we conducted a study

(Gonzales et al., 2005) to examine whether the young individually caged WHHLs in our studies were insulin resistant, as assessed by an intravenous glucose tolerance test, relative to young New Zealand White (NZW) rabbits (a strain without dyslipidemia). In addition, we assessed whether dietary or aerobic exercise interventions over the course of the 4-month study could alter insulin sensitivity and the progression of atherosclerosis in these individually caged WHHLs.

The results of this study demonstrated that WHHLs, as early as 3 months of age, are insulin resistant compared to NZWs. In addition, the WHHLs exhibited elevated systolic blood pressure, urinary catecholamines, and plasma leptin relative to the NZWs at this early time point when disease is beginning (Buja et al., 1983). In terms of the interventions, whereas the dietary restriction (25% less food) was effective in controlling insulin resistance, WHHLs in the exercise group (60 minutes/day on a motorized treadmill, without dietary restriction) and the no-treatment control group exhibited significant increases in insulin resistance. Interestingly, neither intervention significantly influenced the progression of atherosclerosis. Therefore, although dietary restriction can reduce cardiovascular risk factors, such as insulin resistance, it is not effective in slowing the development of disease in these genetically dyslipidemic rabbits. Similarly, aerobic exercise did not effectively prevent disease or insulin resistance in this model.

Summary

This series of studies emphasizes the importance of social environment in the progression of cardiovascular disease. Although the WHHL is genetically predisposed to the development of profound dyslipidemia and atherosclerosis, we have shown that social conditions, and resulting behavior, alter the course of disease. Whereas several investigators have utilized animal models to demonstrate that social environment and/ or emotional behavior can accelerate the progression of atherosclerosis, we have been able to show that prosocial behavior, as seen in a stable social environment, can slow the progression of disease in this genetically deterministic model. The power of social behavior is illustrated further when one considers that other behavioral interventions, such as dietary restriction and exercise, did not influence the course of disease in these animals. A variety of potential physiological mechanisms could account for the influence of a stable social environment and affiliative social behavior on disease progression. Our research suggests that one important mechanism is that social environment may lead to the preferential release of OT, which then acts on vascular and adipocyte OT receptors to attenuate vascular inflammation and oxidative stress, thereby slowing the development of atherosclerosis. Future research will test this hypothesis through chronic infusion of OT in WHHLs.

Conclusions

Claude Bernard (1865/1961) contended that the maintenance of life depends on an organism's keeping its internal environment constant despite changes in the external environment. Subsequently, Walter Cannon (1928) used the term "homeostasis" to describe how organisms maintain such stability. He also showed that homeostasis can be threatened by psychosocial, as well as physical, challenges. As previously mentioned, Hans Selye (1956) used the term "stress" to describe the effects of agents that seriously threaten homeostasis. Selye, of course, recognized that responses to stress are designed to be adaptive, but he also determined that severe, prolonged stress responses can result in tissue damage. With the development of animal models, investigators have been able to demonstrate that stress can precipitate the onset of diabetes in animals vulnerable to the disease (Surwit & Schneider, 1993), that the interaction of diet and stress can produce atherosclerosis in primates, and that behavioral contexts can alter the progression of many animal models of disease by producing changes in catecholamines (Sloan et al., 2007), or by inducing immunosuppression through endogenous release of GCCs (Webster et al., 2002).

Although several landmark animal behavior studies have shown that stress can exacerbate disease processes (Kaplan et al., 1982), a number of studies have suggested that psychosocial (McCabe et al., 2002) or pharmacological (Kaplan et al., 1987) interventions

can attenuate such processes. Furthermore, some studies examining the relationship between behavior and pathophysiological processes have now begun to elucidate the ways by which psychosocial and pharmacological interventions may be achieving such goals (Nation et al., 2008).

Further Reading

Chida, Y., Sudo, N., & Kubo, C. (2006). Does stress exacerbate liver diseases? *Journal of Gastroenterology and Hepatology, 20,* 202–208.

Kaplan, J. R., Adams, M. R., Clarkson, T. B., Manuck, S. B., Shively, C. A., & Williams, J. K. (1996). Psychosocial factors, sex differences, and atherosclerosis: Lessons from animal models. *Psychosomatic Medicine, 58*(6), 598–611.

Moynihan, J. A., & Ader, R. (1996). Psychoneuroimmunology: Animal models of disease. *Psychosomatic Medicine, 58,* 546–558.

Pavlov, V. A., & Tracey, K. J. (2005). The cholinergic anti-inflammatory pathway. *Brain, Behavior, and Immunity, 19*(6), 493–499.

Rozanski, A., Blumenthal, J. A., & Kaplan, J. (1999). Impact of psychological factors on the pathogenesis of cardiovascular disease and implications for therapy. *Circulation, 99*(16), 2192–217.

References

Adams, M. R., Kaplan, J. R., Koritnik, D. R., & Clarkson, T. B. (1985). Ovariectomy, social status, and atherosclerosis in cynomolgus monkeys. *Arteriosclerosis, 5,* 192–200.

Adams, M. R., Kaplan, J. R., Koritnik, D. R., & Clarkson, T. B. (1987). Pregnancy-associated inhibition of coronary artery atherosclerosis in monkeys: Evidence of a relationship with endogenous estrogen. *Arteriosclerosis, 7,* 378–384.

Ader, R., & Cohen, N. (1982). Behaviorally conditioned immunosuppression and murine systemic lupus erythematosus. *Science, 215,* 1534–1536.

Ader, R., & Cohen, N. (1993). Psychoneuroimmunology: Conditioning and stress. *Annual Reviews in Psychology, 44,* 53–85.

Avistur, R., Stark, J. L., Dhabhar, F. S., Padgett, D. A., & Sheridan, J. F. (2002). Social disruption-induced glucocorticoid resistance: Kinetics and site specificity. *Journal of Neuroimmunology, 124,* 54–61.

Bartolomucci, A. (2007). Social stress, immune

function and disease in rodents. *Frontiers in Neuroendocrinology, 28,* 28–49.

Bendick, J. (2002). *Galen and the gateway to medicine.* Ft. Collins, CO: Ignatius Press.

Ben-Eliyahu, S., Shakhar, G., Page, G. G., Stefanski, V., & Shakhar, K. (2000). Suppression of NK cell activity and of resistance to metastasis by stress: A role for adrenal catecholamines and beta-adrenoceptors. *NeuroImmunoModulation, 8,* 154–164.

Berkman, L. F., & Orth-Gomer, K. (1996). Prevention of cardiovascular morbidity and mortality: Role of social relations. In K. Orth-Gomer & N. Schneiderman (Eds.), *Behavioral medicine approaches to cardiovascular disease prevention* (pp. 51–67). Mahwah, NJ: Erlbaum.

Bernard, C. (1961). *An introduction to the study of experimental medicine* (H. C. Greene, Trans.). New York: Collier. (Original work published 1865)

Black, P. H. (2006). The inflammatory consequences of psychologic stress: Relationship to insulin resistance, obesity, atherosclerosis and diabetes mellitus, Type 2. *Medical Hypotheses, 67,* 869–871.

Bonneau, R. H., Sheridan, J. F., Feng, N., & Glaser, R. (1993) Stress-induced modulation of the primary cellular immune response to herpes simplex virus infection is mediated by both adrenal-dependent and independent mechanisms. *Journal of Neuroimmunology, 42*(2), 167–176.

Borovikova, L. V., Ivanova, S., Zhang, M., Yang, H., Botchkina, G. I., Watkins, L. R., et al. (2000). Vagus nerve stimulation attenuates the systemic inflammatory response to endotoxin. *Nature, 405,* 458–462.

Buja, L. M., Clubb, F. J., Bilheimer, D. W., & Willerson, J. T. (1990). Pathobiology of human familial hypercholesterolaemia and a related animal model, the WHHL. *European Heart Journal, 11*(Suppl. E), 41–52.

Buja, L. M., Kita, T., Goldstein, J. L., Watanabe, Y., & Brown, M. S. (1983). Cellular pathology of progressive atherosclerosis in the WHHL rabbit. *Arteriosclerosis, 3,* 87–101.

Cannon, W. B. (1928). The mechanism of emotional disturbance of bodily functions. *New England Journal of Medicine, 198,* 165–172.

Cao, L., Filipov, N. M., & Lawrence, D. A. (2002). Sympathetic nervous system plays a major role in acute cold/restraint stress inhibition of host resistance to *Listeria* monocytogenes. *Journal of Neuroimmunology, 125*(1–2), 94–102.

Carter, C. S. (1998). Neuroendocrine perspectives on social attachment and love. *Psychoneuroendocrinology, 23,* 779–818.

Chida, Y., Sudo, N., & Kubo, C. (2005). Social isolation stress exacerbates autoimmune disease in MRL/lpr mice. *Journal of Neuroimmunology, 158,* 138–144.

Chida, Y., Sudo, N., & Kubo, C. (2006). Does stress exacerbate liver diseases? *Journal of Gastroenterology and Hepatology, 20,* 202–208.

Clarkson, T. B., Adams, M. R., Kaplan, J. R., Shively, C. A., & Koritnik, D. R. (1989). From menarche to menopause: Coronary artery atherosclerosis and protection in cynomolgus monkeys. *American Journal of Obstetrics and Gynecology, 160,* 1280–1285.

Cole, S. W., Korin, Y. D., Fahey, J. L., & Zack, J. A. (1998). Norepinephrine accelerates HIV replication via protein kinase A-dependent effects on cytokine production. *Journal of Immunology, 161*(2), 610–616.

Cole, S. W., Naliboff, B. D., Kemeny, M. E., Griswold, M. P., Fahey, J. L., & Zack, J. A. (2001). Impaired response to HAART in HIV-infected individuals with high autonomic nervous system activity. *Proceedings of the National Academy of Sciences USA, 98*(22), 12695–12700.

Cooper, C. L., & Dewe, P. (2004). *Stress: A brief history.* Hoboken, NJ: Wiley.

Cutolo, M., & Straub, R. H. (2006). Stress as a risk factor in the pathogenesis of rheumatoid arthritis. *NeuroImmunoModulation, 13*(5–6), 277–282.

Dobbs, C. M., Vasquez, M., Glaser, R., & Sheridan, J. F. (1993). Mechanisms of stress-induced modulation of viral pathogenesis and immunity. *Journal of Neuroimmunology, 48,* 151–160.

Dong Jung, B., Kimura, K., Kitamura, H., Makondo, K., Okita, K., Kawasaki, M., et al. (2000). Norepinephrine stimulates interleukin-6 mRNA expression in primary cultured rat hepatocytes. *Journal of Biochemistry, 127,* 205–209.

Edwards, E. A., & Dean, L. M. (1977). Effects of crowding of mice on humoral antibody formation and protection to lethal antigenic challenge. *Psychosomatic Medicine, 39,* 19–24.

Engelmann, M., Ebner, K., Landgraf, R., Holsboer, F., & Wotjak, C. T. (1999). Emotional stress triggers intrahypothalamic but not peripheral release of oxytocin in male rats. *Journal of Neuroendocrinology, 11,* 867–872.

Engler, H., Engler, A., Bailey, M. T., & Sheridan, J. F. (2005). Tissue-specific alterations in the glucocorticoid sensitivity of immune cells following repeated social defeat in mice. *Journal of Neuroimmunology, 163,* 110–119.

Friedman, M., & Rosenman, R. H. (1959). Association of specific overt behavior pattern with blood and cardiovascular findings: Blood cholesterol level, blood clotting time, incidence of arcus senilis, and clinical coronary artery disease. *Journal of the American Medical Association, 169,* 1286–1296.

Gimeno, R. E., & Klaman, L. D. (2005). Adipose tissue as an active endocrine organ: Recent advances. *Current Opinion in Pharmacology, 5*(2), 122–128.

Glaser, R., Rabin, B., Chesney, M., Cohen, S., & Natelson, B. (1999). Stress-induced immunomodulation: Implications for infectious diseases? *Journal of the American Medical Association, 281*(24), 2268–2270.

Gold, S. M., & Heesen, C. (2006). Stress and disease progression in multiple sclerosis and its animal models. *NeuroImmunoModulation, 13*(5–6), 318–326.

Gonzales, J. A., Szeto, A., Mendez, A. J., Zaias, J., Paredes, J., Caperton, C. V., et al. (2005). Effect of behavioral interventions on insulin sensitivity and atherosclerosis in the Watanabe heritable hyperlipidemic rabbit. *Psychosomatic Medicine, 67,* 172–178.

Griendling, K. K., Sorescu, D., & Ushio-Fukai, M. (2000). NAD(P)H oxidase: Role in cardiovascular biology and disease. *Circulation Research, 86,* 494–501.

Gur, A., & Oktayoglu, P. (2008). Central nervous system abnormalities in fibromyalgia and chronic fatigue syndrome: New concepts in treatment. *Current Pharmaceutical Design, 14*(13), 1274–1294.

Gutkowska, J., Jankowski, M., Mukaddam-Daher, S., & McCann, S. M. (2000). Oxytocin is a cardiovascular hormone. *Brazilian Journal of Medical and Biological Research, 33,* 625–633.

Helz, J. W., & Templeton, B. (1990). Evidence of the role of psychosocial factors in diabetes mellitus: A review. *American Journal of Psychiatry, 147*(10), 1275–1282.

Hilakivi-Clarke, L., & Dickson, R. B. (1995). Stress influence on development of hepatocellular tumors in transgenic mice overexpressing TGF-α. *Acta Oncologia, 34,* 907–912.

Insel, R. R., & Young, L. J. (2000). Neuropeptides and the evolution of social behavior. *Current Opinion in Neurobiology, 10*(6), 784–789.

Iseri, S. O., Sener, G., Saglam, B., Gedik, N., Ercan, F., & Yegen, B. Ç. (2005). Oxytocin ameliorates oxidative colonic inflammation by a neutrophil-dependent mechanism. *Peptides, 26,* 483–491.

Jankowski, M., Hajjar, F., Kawas, S. A., Mukaddam-Daher, S., Hoffman, G., McCann, S. M., et al. (1998). Rat heart: A site of oxytocin production and action. *Proceedings of the National Academy of Sciences USA, 95,* 14558–14563.

Jankowski, M., Wang, D., Hajjar, F., Mukaddam-Daher, S., McCann, S. M., & Gutkowska, J. (2000). Oxytocin and its receptors are synthesized in the rat vasculature. *Proceedings of the National Academy of Sciences USA, 97,* 6207–6211.

Jessop, J. J., & Bayer, B. M. (1989). Time-dependent effects of isolation on lymphocyte and adrenocortical activity. *Journal of Neuroimmunology, 23,* 143–147.

Kaplan, J. R., Adams, M. R., Anthony, M. S., Morgan, T. M., Manuck, S. B., & Clarkson, T. B. (1995). Dominant social status and contraceptive hormone treatment inhibit atherogenesis in premenopausal monkeys. *Atherosclerosis, Thrombosis, and Vascular Biology, 15,* 2094–2100.

Kaplan, J. R., Adams, M. R., Clarkson, T. B., Manuck, S. B., Shively, C. A., & Williams, J. K. (1996). Psychosocial factors, sex differences, and atherosclerosis: Lessons from animal models. *Psychosomatic Medicine, 58*(6), 598–611.

Kaplan, J. R., & Manuck, S. B. (1994). Anti-atherogenic effects of ß-adrenergic blocking agents: Theoretical, experimental, and epidemiologic considerations. *American Heart Journal, 128*(6), 1316–1328.

Kaplan, J. R., & Manuck, S. B. (1997). Using ethological principles to study psychosocial influences on coronary atherosclerosis in monkeys. *Acta Physiologica Scandinavica Supplementum, 640,* 96–99.

Kaplan, J. R., & Manuck, S. B. (1999). Status, stress, and atherosclerosis: The role of environment and individual behavior. *Annals of the New York Academy of Sciences, 896,* 145–161.

Kaplan, J. R., Manuck, S. B., Adams, M. R., Weingand, K. W., & Clarkson, T. B. (1987). Inhibition of coronary atherosclerosis by propranolol in behaviorally predisposed monkeys fed an atherogenic diet. *Circulation, 76,* 1364–1372.

Kaplan, J. R., Manuck, S. B., Clarkson, T. B., Lusso, F. M., & Taub, D. M. (1982). Social status, environment, and atherosclerosis in cynomolgus monkeys. *Atherosclerosis, 2,* 359–368.

Kaplan, J. R., Manuck, S. B., Clarkson, T. B., Lusso, F. M., Taub, D. M., & Miller, E. W. (1983). Social stress and atherosclerosis in normocholesterolemic monkeys. *Science, 220,* 733–735.

Kattab, K., Kharrab, A. A., Ortak, J., Richardt, G., & Bonnemeier, H. (2007). Iyengar yoga increases cardiac parasympathetic nervous modulation among healthy yoga practitioners. *Evidence-Based Complementary and Alternative Medicine, 4*(4), 511–517.

Keller, S. E., Schleifer, S. J., Liotta, A. S., Bond, R. N., Farhoody, N., & Stein, M. (1988). Stress-induced alterations of immunity in hypophysectomized rats. *Proceedings of the National Academy of Sciences USA, 85*(23), 297–301.

Kitamura, H., Konno, A., Morimatsu, M., Jung, B. D., Kimura, K., & Saito, M. (1997). Immobilization stress increases hepatic IL-6 expression in mice. *Biochemical and Biophysical Research Communications, 238,* 707–711.

Kondo, T., & Watanabe, Y. (1975). A heritable hyperlipidemic rabbit. *Experimental Animals, 24,* 89–94.

Ludwig, M., & Pittman, Q. J. (2003). Talking back: Dendritic neurotransmitter release. *Trends in Neurosciences, 26,* 255–261.

Manuck, S. B., Kaplan, J. R., & Clarkson, T. B. (1983). Behaviorally induced heart rate reactivity and atherosclerosis in cynomolgus monkeys. *Psychosomatic Medicine, 45*(2), 95–108.

Manuck, S. B., Kaplan, J. R., & Matthews, K. A. (1986). Behavioral antecedents of coronary heart disease and atherosclerosis. *Arteriosclerosis, 6,* 2–14.

Manuck, S. B., Marsland, A. L., Kaplan, J. R., & Williams, J. K. (1995). The pathogenicity of behavior and its neuroendocrine mediation: An example from coronary artery disease. *Psychosomatic Medicine, 57,* 275–283.

McCabe, P. M., Gonzales, J., Zaias, J., Szeto, A., Kumar, M., Herron, A., et al. (2002). Social environment influences the progression of atherosclerosis in the Watanabe heritable hyperlipidemic rabbit. *Circulation, 105,* 354–359.

Meir, K. S., & Leitersdorf, E. (2004). Atherosclerosis in the apolipoprotein E-deficient mouse: A decade of progress. *Arteriosclerosis, Thrombosis, and Vascular Biology, 24,* 1006–1014.

Miller, G. E., Chen, E., Sze, J., Marin, T., Arevalo, J. M., Doll, R., et al. (2008). A functional genomic fingerprint of chronic stress in humans: Blunted glucocorticoid and increased NF-kappaB signaling. *Biological Psychiatry, 64,* 66–72.

Moosman, B., & Behl, C. (2002). Secretory peptide hormones are biochemical antioxidants: Structure–activity relationship. *Molecular Pharmacology, 61,* 260–268.

Morris, M., Callahan, M. F., Li, P., & Lucion, A. B. (1995). Central oxytocin mediates stress-induced tachycardia. *Journal of Neuroendocrinology, 7,* 455–459.

Moynihan, J. A., & Ader, R. (1996). Psychoneuroimmunology: Animal models of disease. *Psychosomatic Medicine, 58,* 546–558.

Nance, D. M., & Sanders, V. M. (2007). Autonomic innervation and regulation of the immune system (1987–2007). *Brain, Behavior, and Immunity, 21*(6), 736–745.

Nation, D. A., Gonzales, J. A., Mendez, A. J., Zaias, J., Szeto, A., Paredes, J., et al. (2008). The effect of social environment on markers of vascular oxidant stress and inflammation in the Watanabe heritable hyperlipidemic rabbit. *Psychosomatic Medicine, 70*(3), 269–275.

Nation, D. A., Szeto, A., Mendez, A. J., Brooks, L. G., Zaias, J., Herderick, E. E., et al. (in press). Oxytocin inhibits atherosclerosis and adipose tissue inflammation in apoE–/– mice. *Psychosomatic Medicine.*

Neumann, I. D., Wigger, A., Torner, L., Holsboer, F., & Landgraf, R. (2000). Brain oxytocin inhibits basal and stress-induced activity of the hypothalamo–pituitary–adrenal axis in male and female rats: Partial action within the paraventricular nucleus. *Journal of Neuroendocrinology, 12,* 235–243.

Nolan, R. P., Kamath, M. V., Flores, J. S., Stanley, J., Pang, C., Picton, P., et al. (2005). Heart rate variability biofeedback as a behavioral neurocardiac intervention to enhance vagal heart rate control. *American Heart Journal, 149*(6), 1137.

Paredes, J., Szeto, A., Levine, J. E., Zaias, J., Gonzales, J. A., Mendez, A. J., et al. (2006). Social experience influences hypothalamic oxytocin in the WHHL rabbit. *Psychoneuroendocrinology, 31,* 1062–1075.

Petersson, M., Wiberg, U., Lundeberg, T., & Uvnäs-Möberg, K. (2001). Oxytocin decreases carrageenan induced inflammation in rats. *Peptides, 22,* 1479–1484.

Pow, D. V., & Morris, J. F. (1989). Dendrites of hypothalamic magnocellular neurons release neurohypophysial peptides by exocytosis. *Neuroscience, 32,* 435–439.

Ross, R. (1999). Atherosclerosis—an inflammatory disease. *New England Journal of Medicine, 340,* 115–126.

Rozanski, A., Blumenthal, J. A., & Kaplan, J. (1999). Impact of psychological factors on the pathogenesis of cardiovascular disease and implications for therapy. *Circulation, 99*(16), 2192–2217.

Sanders, V. M., & Straub, R. H. (2002). Norepinephrine, the beta-adrenergic receptor, and immunity. *Brain, Behavior, and Immunity, 16*(4), 290–332.

Selye, H. (1956). *The stress of life.* New York: McGraw-Hill.

Sheridan, J. F., Dobbs, C., Brown, D., & Zwilling, B. (1994). Psychoneuroimmunology: Stress effects on pathogenesis and immunity during infection. *Clinical Microbiology Reviews, 7*(2), 200–212.

Shively, C. A., & Clarkson, T. B. (1994). Social status and coronary artery atherosclerosis in female monkeys. *Arteriosclerosis and Thrombosis, 14*(5), 721–726.

Shively, C. A., Clarkson, T. B., & Kaplan, J. R. (1989). Social deprivation and coronary artery atherosclerosis in female cynomolgus monkeys. *Atherosclerosis, 77*(1), 69–76.

Sloan, E. K., Capitanio, J. P., Tarara, R. P., Mendoza, S. P., Mason, W. A., & Cole, S. W. (2007). Social stress enhances sympathetic innervations of primate lymph nodes: Mechanisms and implications for viral pathogenesis. *Journal of Neuroscience, 27*(33), 8857–8865.

Stark, J. L., Avitsur, R., Padgett, D. A., Campbell, K. A., Beck, F. M., & Sheridan, J. F. (2001). Social stress induces glucocorticoid resistance in macrophages. *American Journal of Physiology: Regulatory, Integrative and Comparative Physiology, 280*(6), R1799–R1805.

Stefanski, V. (2001). Social stress in laboratory rats: Behavior, immune function, and tumor metastasis. *Physiology and Behavior, 73*(3), 385–391.

Stefanski, V., & Engler, H. (1999). Social stress, dominance and blood cellular immunity. *Journal of Neuroimmunology, 94*, 144–152.

Strawn, W. B., Bondjers, G., Kaplan, J. R., Manuck, S. B., Schwenke, D. C., Hansson, G. K., et al. (1991). Endothelial dysfunction in response to psychosocial stress in monkeys. *Circulation Research, 68*(5), 1270–1279.

Surwit, R. S., & Schneider, M. S. (1993). Role of stress in the etiology and treatment of diabetes mellitus. *Psychosomatic Medicine, 55*(4), 380–393.

Syme, S. L. (1996). Social class and cardiovascular disease. In K. Orth-Gomer & N. Schneiderman (Eds.), *Behavioral medicine approaches to cardiovascular disease prevention* (pp. 43–50). Mahwah, NJ: Erlbaum.

Szeto, A., Nation, D. A., Mendez, A. J., Dominguez-Bendala, J., Brooks, L. G., Schneiderman, N., et al. (2008). Oxytocin attenuates NADPH-dependenvt superoxide activity and IL-6 secretion in macrophages and vascular cells. *American Journal of Physiology: Endocrinology and Metabolism, 295*(6), E1495–E1501.

Thayer, J. F., & Lane, R. D. (2007). The role of vagal function in the risk for cardiovascular disease and mortality. *Biological Psychology, 74*(2), 224–242.

Thibonnier, M., Conarty, D. M., Preston, J. A., Plesnicher, C. L., Dweik, R. A., & Erzurum, S. C. (1999). Human vascular endothelial cells express oxytocin receptors. *Endocrinology, 140*, 1301–1309.

Tracey, K. J. (2007). Physiology and immunology of the cholinergic anti-inflammatory pathway. *Journal of Clinical Investigation, 117*(2), 289–296.

Uvnäs-Möberg, K. (1998). Oxytocin may mediate the benefits of positive social interaction and emotions. *Psychoneuroendocrinology, 23*, 819–835.

Uvnäs-Möberg, K., Ahlenius, S., Hillegaart, V., & Alster, P. (1994). High doses of oxytocin cause sedation and low doses cause an anxiolytic-like effect in male rats. *Pharmacology Biochemistry and Behavior, 23*, 819–835.

Vivier, E., Tomasello, E., Baratin, M., Walzer, T., & Ugolini, S. (2008). Functions of natural killer cells. *Nature Immunology, 9*(5), 503–510.

Warnholtz, A., Nickenig, G., Schulz, E., Macharzina, R., Bräsen, J. H., Skatchkov, M., et al. (1999). Increased NADH-oxidase–mediated superoxide production in the early stages of atherosclerosis: Evidence for involvement of the renin–angiotensin system. *Circulation, 99*, 2027–2033.

Watson, S. L., Shively, C. A., Kaplan, J. R., & Line, S. W. (1998). Effects of chronic social separation on cardiovascular disease risk factors in female cynomolgus monkeys. *Atherosclerosis, 137*(2), 259–266.

Webster, J. I., Tonelli, L., & Sternberg, E. M. (2002). Neuroendocrine regulation of immunity. *Annual Review of Immunology, 20*, 125–163.

Williams, R. B. (1996). Coronary-prone behaviors, hostility, and cardiovascular health: Implications for behavioral and pharmacological interventions. In K. Orth-Gomer & N. Schneiderman (Eds.), *Behavioral medicine approaches to cardiovascular disease prevention* (pp. 161). Mahwah, NJ: Erlbaum.

Windle, R. J., Kershaw, Y. M., Shanks, N., Wood, S. A., Lightman, S. L., & Ingram, C. D. (2004). Oxytocin attenuates stress-induced c-*fos* mRNA expression in specific forebrain regions associated with modulation of hypothalamo–pituitary–adrenal activity. *Journal of Neuroscience, 24*, 2974–2982.

Windle, R. J., Shanks, N., Lightman, S. L., & Ingram, C. D. (1997). Central oxytocin administration reduces stress-induced corticosterone release and anxiety behavior in rats. *Endocrinology, 138*, 2829–2834.

Wu, W., Yamaura, T., Murakami, K., Murata, J., Matsumoto, K., Watanabe, H., et al. (2000). Social isolation stress enhanced liver metastasis of murine colon 26-L5 carcinoma cells by suppressing immune responses in mice. *Life Science, 66*, 1827–1838.

Zhang, B., Saku, K., Hirata, K., Liu, R., Tateishi, K., Shiomi, M., et al. (1994). Quantitative characterization of insulin–glucose response in Watanabe heritable hyperlipidemic and cholesterol-fed rabbits and the effect of cilazapril. *Metabolism, 43*, 360–366.

Zhang, B., Saku, K., Hirata, K., Liu, R., Tateishi, K., Yamamoto, K., et al. (1991). Insulin resistance observed in WHHL rabbits. *Atherosclerosis, 91*, 277–278.

Zimmerman, R. S., & Frolich, E. D. (1990). Stress and hypertension. *Journal of Hypertension Supplement, 8*(4), S103–S107.

CHAPTER 12

All Roads Lead to Psychoneuroimmunology

Christopher L. Coe

[handwritten annotation: Lymphocyte - is one of the sub types of white blood cell in vertebrates Immune System]

The field of "psychoneuroimmunology" (PNI) has come of age. Once focused primarily on the topic of stress and negative life events, and investigating a relatively delimited set of infectious diseases and malignancies, it now figures more prominently in many aspects of health psychology and behavioral medicine research. The range of clinical illnesses to which PNI findings apply has also been considerably broadened by the realization that inflammatory processes can aggravate many conditions, including the blood vessel pathology that underlies cardiovascular disease. In addition, the increasing sophistication of studies investigating immune mechanisms that account for the effects seen in PNI research has attracted the interest and enthusiasm of a wider group of new researchers, including neuroscientists and immunologists.

A Brief History

It is of historical note that initially there was considerable debate and controversy over what term to choose as the official name for this field. Some wanted this corpus of knowledge to be designated by the moniker "neuroimmunomodulation" (NIM), in order to emphasize the central role of the brain in effecting the alterations in immunity (Spector, 1995). At the time there was also concern about the willingness of immunologists to accept a field that endorsed the view that psychological factors could influence not only health but also the functioning of lymphocytes and their competence. I personally recall a comment in the mid-1980s from the Chair of my university's Department of Medicine, after he found out that I conducted research in the still nascent area of PNI. He remarked, "Oh, you work in that field of *voodoo medicine*." It would take a while before the main premises of PNI became more readily accepted.

Even today, many remain skeptical about the clinical and applied relevance of the observation that immune responses can be negatively or positively influenced by emotional state and lifestyle. Are these effects really large enough to cause an autoimmune disorder to become manifest or seriously compromise host defense against an infectious bacterial or viral pathogen? Does this mean that immune responses can be shaped or activated in a specific way by behavioral interventions to be of actual value in patient care? A high priority for the field is more demonstrations that psychological processes and lifestyle changes can be meaningfully incorporated into treatments to improve clinical outcomes for patient populations with immune-related disorders. It is heartening that a growing number of published studies now document that exercise regimens, the practice of meditation, and cognitive-behavioral therapies do act in a positive way on immune responses and appear to be of practical benefit for improving health (Antoni et al., 2006; Antoni, Schneiderman, & Penedo, 2007; Irwin, Pike, Cole, & Oxman, 2003).

The early days of PNI in the late 1970s and 1980s were especially exciting because each year brought new discoveries that validated the central tenet that psychological processes can influence the immune system (Ader, 2003; Kemeny & Schedlowlski, 2007). Many studies in both humans and animals showed that the mediating pathways were ones familiar to us from an even earlier period of research on the endocrine and autonomic nervous system (Figure 12.1). When individuals are aroused or challenged, the increased secretion of hormones, including the potent glucocorticoids from the adrenal gland, provide a direct means to influence the number of leukocytes, their location, and responsiveness (Munck, Guyre, & Holbrook, 1984). It has also been known for a long time that cortisol can affect the ability of cells to proliferate and will suppress the capacity of leukocytes to phagocytose and kill bacteria, or to produce antibody.

Indeed, these immunosuppressive actions were the cornerstone of the stress response described in pioneering observations by Hans Selye (1936). His concept of a general adaptation syndrome was based on the prominent triadic reaction in the body following physical or psychological challenge: (1) activation of the endocrine system; (2) changes in gastrointestinal activity; and (3) immune alterations, including a thymolymphatic involution. If one were to adhere strictly to this view of the stress response, by definition, an organism should be considered to be in a stressed state only if there are also immune changes. At that time, these effects were detected primarily by gross changes, such as the smaller size and reduced weight of the lymphoid tissue or the disappearance of certain cells from circulation, including the sudden absence of eosinophils from the bloodstream. By the 1980s, however, many other techniques had become available to track immune function (see Table 12.1). It was possible to measure lymphocyte responses and antibody levels with increasing sophistication. Soon many papers reported that the antibody responses of animals to bacterial and viral pathogens, and the capacity of cells to proliferate, were reduced by stressful conditions (Coe & Laudenslager, 2007).

While the effects of corticosteroids on immunity were well characterized, and cortisol remained the prototypical hormone modulator of immune responses, it became clear that many other endocrine secretions had immune-modulating effects, including prolactin, thyroid, gonadal, growth, and opioid hormones (Grossman, 1985; Heijnen, Kavelaars, & Ballieux, 1991; Kelley, Arkins, Minshall, Liu, & Dantzer, 1996; Kelley, Weigent, & Kooijman, 2007). In addition, investigators found that norepinephrine (NE) and epinephrine could induce equally important effects on immunity once the autonomic nervous system became activated (Madden et al., 1997). This additional influence really should not have been surprising. Nearly 100 years ago, Walter Cannon and others had described changes in circulating leukocyte numbers in rats after they had been exposed to the frightening presence of a cat, and similar cellular alterations were seen in aroused humans (Cannon, 1929; Mora, Amtmann, & Hoffman, 1926). In these instances, the cellular redistribution appeared to be linked to activation of the sympathetic nervous system (SNS), the classic "fight or flight" reaction (Madden et al., 1997).

The full significance of those seminal observations was to become evident later, following the demonstration that most lymphoid tissue, including the thymus and spleen, is innervated by the SNS, and in many cases by parasympathetic nerves as well (Bullock & Moore, 1981; Felten et al., 1987). In addition, many leukocytes bear noradrenergic receptors on their cell surface, which enables NE to change the functional state of these cells (Sanders & Kavelaars, 2007). Exposure to neurotransmitters released from nerve endings, as well as to neuromodulators such as substance P, has a

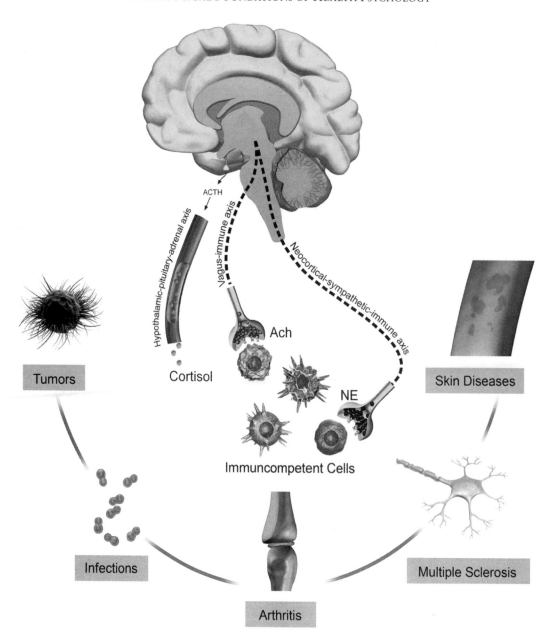

FIGURE 12.1. PNI studies investigate the influence of psychological and neural factors on immunity and several major categories of immune-related illness. Downstream effects of neuroendocrine and autonomic activity on immune responses, along with reciprocal immune-to-brain feedback via cytokines and the vagus nerve, are believed to account for most of the observed influences on immunity and disease. From Kemeny and Schedlowski (2007). Copyright 2007 by the Psychoneuroimmunology Research Society. Reprinted with permission from Elsevier.

TABLE 12.1. Representative Measures and Assays Commonly Used to Assess Immunity in PNI Research

Quantitative determinations

Complete blood counts (number of white blood cells, lymphocytes, neutrophils, etc.)

Cell subset enumeration (percentages of T and B cells, activated monocytes, etc.)

Salivary antibody levels (secretory immunoglobulin A, total or specific)

Serum cytokine levels (single cytokine, such as interleukin-6, or multicytokine array)

In vitro functional assays

Lymphocyte proliferation (stimulation with mitogens such as phytohemagglutinin or lipopolysaccharide)

Cell-killing assays (natural killer cell lysis of cancer cells)

Phagocytosis of bacteria (engulfment by neutrophils)

Tumoricidal activity (chemotaxis and killing of tumor cells by macrophages)

In vivo measures

Antibody responses to immunization (e.g., influenza or tetanus vaccine)

Delayed type hypersensitivity (cutaneous reaction to recall antigen)

Herpes virus reactivation (e.g., antibody titers to Epstein–Barr virus or Herpes simplex virus)

---

large influence on inflammatory reactions, as cells course to a site of injury or to inflamed and infected tissue (Straub, Dhabhar, Bijlsma, & Cutolo, 2005). Many of the more rapid immune changes that occur after an arousing stimulus are either induced or influenced by the SNS. For example, an appreciation of noradrenergic action helps one to understand the quick changes in the number and type of leukocytes seen in psychological studies of persons who become aroused by delivering a speech to a disapproving audience (Buske-Kirschbaum, Kern, Ebrecht, & Hellhammer, 2007). This cell "margination," or trafficking of leukocytes between tissue and blood, is driven to a large degree by the SNS and endocrine system, as cells detach from the blood vessel wall and are stimulated to translocate from one compartment to another, or are pushed along by the increased rate of blood flow.

Even more surprising than the diverse autonomic and endocrine influences on immunity was the discovery that lymphoid cells themselves can synthesize hormones. While this novel source of hormone is not very prominent in the nonchallenged host, once the immune system begins to respond to a pathogen, or after lymphoid cells are directly infected by a virus, we now know that leukocytes can be induced to secrete a number of different hormones with immune-modulating actions (Blalock, 1984; Blalock & Smith, 2007). It is believed that this hormone release helps to foster changes in cell-to-cell interactions, acting on the cells in an autocrine- and paracrine-like manner, and may also assist in some signaling feedback to the endocrine system.

The latter findings helped to set the stage for other discoveries that would garner considerably more attention for the field of PNI. While most of the research had been focused on the downstream effects on immunity, there was already an appreciation that immune processes could in turn affect the nervous system. It was known that psychological factors and lifestyle influenced symptom expression and disease progression in some autoimmune conditions, such as multiple sclerosis, in which the pathology results from errant immune responses directed toward neural tissue (Grant et al., 1989; Meagher, Johnson, Good, & Welsh, 2007). In addition, other research had implicated a dysregulation of immune responses as either a causal factor or a consequence of certain types of psychopathology, including depression (Herbert & Cohen, 1992). A disturbance in immunity was also suspected to be of special significance in schizophrenia because of repeated observations that many of these individuals' lymphocytes exhibited an abnormal morphology of the nucleus, as well as elevated antibody in their cerebrospinal fluid against herpes viruses or neural proteins (Fessel, Hirata-Hibi, & Shapiro, 1965; Yolken & Torrey, 1997). Much greater credence for this belief about the importance of immune system-to-brain communication would be obtained when it became possible to measure cytokine levels routinely. These proteins secreted by white blood cells normally serve as growth promoters, chemoattractants for other cells, and regulators of immune responses, but they also have many functions that go beyond the immune system.

When cytokine concentrations in the blood reach a high enough level, they act as one of the primary conduits of information about the state of the immune system to the central nervous system (CNS). Many laboratories have worked in parallel to figure out how this cytokine feedback to the brain occurs (Dantzer, O'Connor, Freund, Johnson, & Kelley, 2008; Watkins & Maier, 2000;). Cytokines from systemic circulation can diffuse through the more porous regions of the blood–brain barrier (BBB). There is also some receptor-mediated active transport of certain cytokines into the brain (Banks, Kastin, & Gutierrez, 1994). Furthermore, it has also been shown that endothelial cells comprising the capillary walls of BBB produce their own cytokines, which are then released as second messengers into the CNS on the abluminal side of the BBB (Reyes, Fabry, & Coe, 1999). But one especially permissive and quick route for immune system-to-brain communication turned out to be via transmission of information up the vagus nerve (Goehler et al., 1999; Maier, Gleher, Fleshner, & Watkins, 1998). Although this major cranial nerve was traditionally thought to have mostly effector functions, enabling parasympathetic regulation of the lung, heart, and gut, it also has a unique sensory role as it branches throughout the upper body cavity, with receptors for proinflammatory cytokines such as interleukin-1 (IL-1). In this way, the vagus nerve provides a ready means for feedback of information about infections and inflammation to the brainstem. Once it makes connections there,

all of the major monoamine neurotransmitter pathways that emanate from the medulla and midbrain become accessible to the immune system (Wieczorek & Dunn, 2006). These discoveries helped to provide an anatomical and biochemical road map to explain the phenomena of "sickness behavior," an important area of PNI research that continues to be a subject of active study today (Kelley et al., 2003; see Figure 12.2).

The Broader Implications of Sickness Behavior

We can look back to early Greek medicine and the writings of the Roman physician Galen to trace some of the formative ideas that first laid the foundation for the belief that there are links between behavior and immunity that account for illness. If one thinks about the four cardinal signs of injury and infection—*calor, dolor, rubor,* and *tumor*—each involves aspects of cytokine biology. Similarly, the feelings of malaise and fatigue associated with disease are also common responses when cytokine levels are high. Here, it is of interest to reflect upon the fact that the subjective feelings and symptoms associated with cytokines and illness probably contributed to both the ancient schema of body humors in Western medicine and to the Eastern views about energy and yin–yang balance in Asian thought. In contemporary science we now have the tools and knowledge to determine the physiological mediators. The sickness reaction—seen in both the ill patient and an animal infected with a bacterial pathogen—appears to be an organized set of behavioral and physiological changes orchestrated in large part by cytokines (Hart, 1988).

It includes both beneficial and maladaptive components. Among the most prominent features are fever, fatigue, and anorexia. In addition, the sick animal or debilitated human host often experiences a loss of libido, withdraws from social interactions with others, and finds it difficult to learn, to retain memories, or to be happy. This state of sickness can be re-created in animals without a virus or bacterial infection. It can be induced by simply injecting a cytokine, such as IL-1-beta or tumor necrosis factor–alpha (TNF-alpha). Similar sickness reactions are also evinced when patients receive certain

---

Cytokine-Induced Sickness Behavior

- malaise
- loss of appetite
- social withdrawal
- loss of libido
- fever
- fatigue
- inability to learn
- depression

FIGURE 12.2. One of the more important discoveries in PNI research is that cytokines play a major role in the phenomena of sickness behavior. These effects account for many of the symptoms experienced by chronically ill patients, as well as the malaise experienced during infection and after many immune-modulating clinical treatments.

immune-modulating therapies. It occurs in cancer patients given interleukin-2 (IL-2) to boost their immune responses, as well as hepatitis patients administered interferon-alpha (IFN-alpha) for its antiviral properties (Capuron, Ravaud, Miller, & Dantzer, 2004). In both cases, the feelings of malaise and fatigue can become a major concern and deleterious side effect of treatment.

From a behavioral point of view, this reaction is more distinctive than just a generalized stress response to an aversive stimulus. From the physiological vantage point, it is also more than a shift in energy balance from an anabolic to a catabolic state. Insightful researchers quickly realized that this cytokine-induced condition includes psychological features reminiscent of certain symptoms of psychopathology. To the observer, an animal injected with IL-1-beta appears to be not only somnolescent but also depressed (Dantzer et al., 2008). Beyond their hunched posture, these animals lose interest in previously positive stimuli. For example, cytokine-treated rats no longer appear to experience the hedonic reward and pleasure normally felt when consuming a sweetened drink. Several different cytokines, when secreted at high levels into systemic circulation or following direct administration into the brains of rats and mice, can quickly induce this type of depressive reaction.

Based on these observations, the field of PNI could lay claim to an example of a neuroimmune effect that was clearly relevant to clinical practice. The anxiousness and depression frequently seen in many chronically ill patients seem to be natural sequelae, a consequence of the physiological activation associated with host defense. Ongoing studies continue to refine this interpretation and are discerning how the depressive state induced by cytokines is similar or different from an affective disorder of purely psychogenic origin. Most of the somatic manifestations can be replicated by the administration of cytokines to people, but not all of the cognitive features of depressive disorders are induced.

These findings remain a stellar example of the value of basic science, enabling PNI researchers to respond in the affirmative when queried about whether their field can really provide useful information for the practicing clinician engaged in patient care.

As an adjunctive medication, when patients are treated with biological response modifiers that stimulate cytokine release, or if they receive cytokines such as IFN directly as the therapeutic modality, it is advisable to consider the preemptive use of an antidepressant, such as paroxetine, to prevent the induction of dysphoria as an unwanted side effect (Musselman et al., 2001).

It's More Than Just a Simple Immune Suppression

Even today, it is not uncommon to see textbooks describe the primary effect of stress on immunity as simply suppressive, and that general conclusion is the end of the story. The inhibition of immune responses is then given as the reason for increased susceptibility to disease in stressed individuals. Certainly, a stress-induced reduction in some aspects of immunity does help to explain a greater susceptibility to upper respiratory infections or the capacity of latent viruses, such as *Herpes simplex* virus (HSV), to reactivate after having lain dormant for a long time (Cohen, Tyrrel, & Smith, 1991; Glaser et al., 1999). But there has long been other evidence indicating that such a unidimensional view is too simplistic. When an individual is challenged by stressful situations, some immune responses actually seem to be turned on rather than off (see Figure 12.3).

Looking back on these findings collectively, it becomes evident that the activated responses are most often components of innate immunity (Black, 2002; Johnson et al., 2005). These more ancestral aspects of the immune system go back in evolutionary time before fish. They serve as the first line of defense, including the complement proteins, heat shock proteins, and the phagocytic neutrophils, a "first responder" cell in response to bacterial infection. Research in both animals and humans has shown, for example, that the production of antibacterial products by neutrophils is increased, not decreased, during times of stress. During the week of final exams in the school semester, the release of superoxide molecules by neutrophils is markedly elevated in students (Kang, Coe, McCarthy, & Ershler, 1997). This enhancement can still be detected for several weeks afterwards if the students' cells are cultured with phorbol myristate acetate

(PMA) *in vitro* (Figure 12.3). It is as if the psychological demands of test-taking evoke the same basic cellular response that would have been induced by a wound or following the detection of endotoxin, a biochemical signal warning of a bacterial invasion. In the stressed state, there seems to be a greater reliance on these ancestral, formative building blocks of the immune system, which occurs concurrently with the suppression of many lymphocyte responses, more recently evolved components of adaptive immunity.

This more complex reaction induced by stressors should have been anticipated from the early descriptions of how stress affects cellular margination. Even in the general trafficking of cells, we can see a similar duality in the way leukocytes move in and out of tissue during infection or following a psychological challenge (Dhabhar, Miller, McEwen, & Spencer, 1995). As the number of lymphocytes decreases in the bloodstream, there is usually a commensurate surge in the number of neutrophils. In fact, the outpouring of neutrophils may be so great that it results in an overall elevation in the total white cell count, despite a much lower percentage of lymphocytes in the blood.

Even among the different types of lymphocytes, fluctuations in the number and location of the various cell subsets are not identical. For example, if one closely tracks the temporal kinetics of one specific lymphocyte,

the natural killer (NK) cell, its numbers first rise dramatically for 30–60 minutes, before showing a more sustained drop in peripheral blood. This biphasic aspect of the change in NK cell numbers has sometimes led to confusion in the literature. Today, investigators commonly use whole blood assays rather than isolating the lymphocytes first, in order to determine the functional ability of NK cells to kill virally transformed cells or cancer cell targets. Using this type of assay method, the number of cells in the specimen will then influence the *in vitro* lytic results. An aroused individual may initially appear to show an acute rise in cytolytic activity, which is really due to there being more NK cells in the assay. In contrast, signs of a more protracted suppression emerge over several hours and days as a consequence of both a sustained decrease in NK cell numbers and a lower lytic capacity per cell (Aronson et al., 1997). One should expect to see comparable idiosyncratic variation in the profiles of other lymphocyte subsets across time. During the long-term response to natural disasters and trauma, some lymphocytes may remain elevated, while others tend to be lower than the level found in the undisturbed individual (e.g., the number of B lymphocytes may be increased, whereas T cells with the cluster of differentiation #4 [CD4+] are frequently found to be below normal levels) (Ironson et al., 1997).

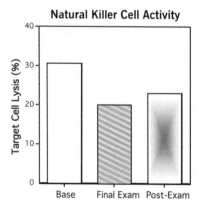 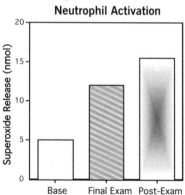

FIGURE 12.3. Although it is commonly stated that stress and psychological disturbance result in a general suppression of immunity, some immune responses are actually activated. In this study of high school students assessed before, during, and after final exams, natural killer cell activity was decreased, but the release of superoxides by neutrophils was increased during the test period and for 2 weeks afterwards. Modified from Kang et al. (1997).

Returning to our larger take-home message, this differential pattern of response seen for specific cell populations requires one to qualify simply, overarching statements about there being a single, monolithic immune system. However, the finer-grained analysis does help to provide deeper insights into the diverse effects that psychological processes have on so many different immune-related diseases. If stressful and negative events were simply suppressive, one might even hypothesize that stress could sometimes be beneficial when the pathological disorders are due to an immune overreaction. Some degree of immune inhibition might then potentially help individuals with rheumatoid arthritis given that their tissue pathology involves inappropriate immune responses directed against joint proteins. Similarly, a suppression of inflammatory responses in Crohn's disease might ameliorate symptoms caused by the presence of activated cells along an inflamed large intestine. In contrast, it is the more complex reactions, with some arms of immunity turned on and others suppressed, that help us to understand the broad impact of psychological factors on many different types of disease.

In the case of allergies and asthma, for example, a stress-induced increase in the release of proinflammatory cytokines could be problematic. We specifically investigated this question in 20 asthmatic students by obtaining mononuclear cells from their upper airways at two different points in the school semester, during the stressful demands of final exam week and during a non-test-period (Liu et al., 2002). On each occasion, they inhaled an allergen (dust mite, cat dander, or ragweed), and we collected blood and sputum specimens from the airways over the next 24 hours. During exam week, their cells were predisposed to produce higher levels of IL-5, a cytokine with chemotactic actions. Larger cytokine reactions to the allergens in the stressed students were associated with a greater influx of activated lymphocytes and eosinophils into their airways.

The various types of T lymphocytes are also each differentially affected by psychological factors in terms of how their numbers change, the relative predominance of certain subsets, and the tilting of the overall balance of the immune reaction in one direction or another (i.e., whether biased toward generat-ing primarily a cellular or humoral immune response). Today, we can easily count and distinguish lymphocyte subsets by marking their unique cell surface proteins with fluorescent monoclonal antibodies (MOABs), then determining the percentages of each cell type on a flow cytometer. Utilizing this methodology, we know that the T cells expressing CD4 proteins, often described as the helper/inducer subset, are affected differently by psychological factors than are the CD8+ cells, which include the T suppressor and cytotoxic T subsets. In general, it seems that CD4+ T cells are somewhat more sensitive to psychological stimuli, at least acutely. During arousing and stressful events, therefore, one can frequently find a decrease in the ratio of CD4+ to CD8+ lymphocytes. Such an inversion in the T cell ratio could be of particular concern for an HIV+ individual who already has a lower number of CD4+ lymphocytes (Cole, Kemeny, Fahey, Zack, & Naliboff, 2003).

Even this fairly detailed level of analysis can be refined further as one reflects on what might be learned from additional marking and subdivision of the T cell subsets. For example, there is now considerable interest in a particular type of CD4+ lymphocyte, the regulatory T cell (T reg) because of its pivotal role in guiding the type of immune response that will be generated. The T reg also prevents overreactions by the immune system. To discern this particular T cell subset, one must employ three MOABs simultaneously and use multicolor flow cytometry to mark both cell surface and intracellular nuclear proteins (i.e., the T reg is a CD4+CD25+FOXP3+ cell) (Roncador et al., 2005). It is an exciting time for the PNI researchers who can master these new techniques. For those of us who began our PNI studies a few decades ago with bioassays and petri dishes, or used light microscopes to count cells, these are truly major methodological advances.

The steps forward and recent achievements are occurring not just because of the new instruments and assays. The realization that the normal process of aging may also be associated with a proinflammatory bias has considerably broadened the potential reach of PNI (Bruunsgaard, Pedersen, & Pedersen, 2001). Many investigators are now determining how inflammation and age-related alterations in cellular immune responses contribute to the vascular pathology underlying hypertension and heart disease, as well as the neural changes associated with dementia and Alzheimer's disease. Monocytes and macrophages, an important group of mononuclear leukocytes, appear to be implicated specifically in these effects on the vasculature. Monocytes play a critical role in immune surveillance and are responsive to any indicators of infection or tissue damage, including irregularities in the arterial wall. Once activated and transformed into macrophages, they can assist in sculpting and remodeling tissue, and can stimulate the growth of new blood vessels (i.e., angiogenesis). It now appears that these cellular processes related to the activation or regulation of immunity have a lot in common with the pathways leading to cardiovascular disease, as well as to the disturbed glucoregulation that goes along with the metabolic syndrome and diabetes. The fact that many cytokines are also produced by nonlymphoid cells, including adipocytes, fibroblasts, and endothelial cells, further emphasizes the importance of this back-and-forth talk across our physiological systems. These findings offer new ways of thinking about the relationship between immunity and health. Elevated levels of some cytokines, such as IL-6, also help to explain why these associations are often compounded by obesity. The body's adipocytes, especially in the abdominal region, are a major producer of the IL-6 found in systemic circulation.

Think Global, Act Locally

Having discussed a number of ways of thinking about PNI in broad brushstrokes, it is necessary to add another caveat. While the immune system can mount a bodywide general reaction, such as in the case of septic shock, the more typical response is a localized one. Immune responses are energetically demanding, and also have the potential to damage healthy tissue when allowed to proceed unchecked (Straub, Cutolo, Buttgereit, & Pongratz, 2010). It is usually safer and more efficient to minimize the scope of the response if possible. Why involve millions of lymphocytes in the spleen if the pathogen can be contained and managed within

a local lymph node? Why sustain a long-term antibody response over several weeks if it is possible to rely on phagocytic cells to engulf more quickly and kill a bacterial pathogen? Thus, when interested in determining the influence of psychological factors on an immune process or a particular disease, ideally it makes the most sense to focus on a specific region of the body. Cold and influenza viruses infect the upper respiratory tract. In contrast, HSV type 2 is usually found in the genital region. If interested in the immune control of these particular viruses, why study mucosal immunity in a different, unrelated part of the body? When using animal models, it is optimal to harvest tissue in the local region and to assess cytotoxic lymphocytes (CTLs) or other cellular responses where the virus would normally be confronted, rather than just to test undifferentiated and noncommitted lymphocytes from the bloodstream.

When thinking about immune defense in this way, it is also worth pausing for a moment to reflect that the optimal situation is not to have to mount an immune response at all. Our first and best line of defense against infectious agents is really a physical barrier, our skin. Only when broken by a wound or trauma would a substantive immune response normally be required. An especially innovative series of studies utilized the response to skin injury as a means to gauge the influence of psychological state on a person's biological vitality and restorative vigor (Christian, Graham, Padgett, Glaser, & Kiecolt-Glaser, 2006). For example, when challenged by the responsibilities and emotional demands of caring for an incapacitated spouse with a chronic illness, the healing of wounds was found to be significantly slower (Kiecolt-Glaser, Marucha, Malarkey, Mercado, & Glaser, 1995). Similarly, psychological factors were shown to delay the healing of other tissue, including the gums, after small biopsy incisions were made in the mouths of dental students (Marucha & Engeland, 2007). Detailed analyses of the physiological reactions at the site of the incisions revealed how the immediate cellular response when the barrier is first broken affects the likelihood of an opportunistic bacterial invasion, then the rate of tissue repair.

While a traumatic break in the skin surface creates a moment of higher risk, at all times we are most vulnerable to bacterial and viral pathogens at the exposed surfaces of the mouth and eyes, and within the respiratory and reproductive tracts. These orifices permit infectious agents easier access, and the specific type of immunity dedicated to this essential defense at mucosal surfaces is related to but distinct from systemic immunity. One particularly exposed surface is the gastrointestinal tract. In fact, while not visibly apparent to us, it is the largest surface area to protect (i.e., approximately 400 square meters versus the mere 2 square meters of skin for most people). Mucosal immune responses are vital to the containment of bacterial pathogens within the gut because it would be far more serious if these bacteria were able to translocate through the intestinal wall into systemic circulation. To appreciate the full significance of this aspect of immunity related to the digestive tract, one has only to reflect on the sheer number of bacteria that comprise the resident microbiota of the gut. Estimates of the bacteria residing within and on us are thought to be over 10^{14}, exceeding the number of cells that comprise our own body (10^{13})!

Fortunately, over the course of evolution, many bacterial species have developed a symbiotic relationship with their hosts and actually serve beneficial functions, aiding in digestion and competing in a helpful way with the disease-causing, pathogenic bacteria. Two bacterial species thought to serve this type of supportive role within the gut are *Lactobacillus* and *Bifidobacterium*. For a number of years, our laboratory has investigated how the concentrations of these two strains are affected by both psychological disturbance and change with age in the very young and the old (Bailey & Coe, 1999; Bailey, Lubach, & Coe, 2004). Specifically, in studies with infant monkeys, we found that when the beneficial lactobacilli are reduced by stressful conditions, there is an increased likelihood of infection with enteric pathogens, including both *Shigella* and *Campylobacter*. The latter can cause diarrheal symptoms and, if unchecked by antibiotic medications, can even result in death from dehydration. In nonindustrialized countries with limited access to clean water, good sanitation, and health care, these types of infections remain a major killer of human infants worldwide. More studies taking a PNI approach are needed to investigate how psychosocial factors, familial living conditions, and nutrition influence the developmental health of children and the likelihood of bacterial and parasitic infestations. This translational application is one way to apply these findings meaningfully in a real-world setting.

The Miner's Canary for PNI Research: Herpes Viruses

The significance of localized immune responses and containment is also of importance when considering the control of herpes, a latent virus infection that has been very popular in PNI research. These viruses are of special interest because psychological and lifestyle factors appear to influence the latency phase after the initial infection, and between the periodic episodes of viral shedding, when the virus should normally remain quiescent in tissue for an extended time. Pioneering studies by Ronald Glaser and Janice Kiecolt-Glaser demonstrated that a number of different stressful life events can result in a partial reactivation of at least one type of herpes virus, Epstein–Barr virus (EBV), the cause of mononucleosis (Glaser & Kiecolt-Glaser, 2005). During the latent phase, each herpes virus usually hones and returns to a different type of tissue. *Herpes zoster*, the cause of chicken pox and shingles, is typically found in the spinal cord; HSV type 1, the viral vector for cold sores, most commonly is found in facial nerves when inactive. It is now known that a localized immune surveillance for early viral proteins by CD8+ T lymphocytes is required to prevent many herpes viruses from recrudescing. If this cellular containment fails, then there may be complete reactivation, viral shedding, and clinical symptoms, typically in the region of the body proximal to where the virus had been residing. For PNI studies, this weakening of immune control over herpes viruses provides a unique biomarker and a sensitive outcome measure to track the immune status of an individual. As the virus recrudesces, B lymphocytes with an affinity and memory for the particular virus are provoked to produce antibody. Thus, one can gauge the viral reactivation relatively easily by a rise in antibody levels directed toward specific viral proteins.

Building upon the prior papers showing that antibody against EBV is higher in a stressed person, we investigated whether a similar association between psychological factors and antibody levels would be evident for HSV. Given the proximity of HSV type 1 to the oral cavity when activated, we quantified the levels of HSV-specific antibody secreted into saliva, which is predominantly of the secretory immunoglobulin A class (sIgA). This survey of salivary HSV–specific sIgA concentrations in 155 adolescents indicated that the ones from disturbed and problematic rearing backgrounds had the highest antibody levels (Shirtcliff, Coe, & Pollak, 2009). Higher HSV–sIgA concentrations were found in both adolescents with a history of maltreatment as children and teenagers who had been adopted from institutions when young but living in better family situations now (Figure 12.4).

The occurrence of elevated antibody against several different herpes viruses can thus be one way to obtain a general measure of an individual's immune status. In these particular examples, it also served as a sensitive biological barometer of the strong influence of interpersonal relationships on our health and physiology. Similar assessment methods provided an immune index of the impact of abusive marital relationships on the emotional well-being and physical health of adult women (Garcia-Linares, Sanchez-Lorente, Coe, & Martinez, 2004). Higher levels of sIgA against HSV type 1 were also found in the saliva of these women experiencing psychological and physical abuse from their domestic partners compared to antibody levels for married women in better, supportive relationships. Moreover, when the specimens from the abused women were specifically tested *in vitro* to determine if they could neutralize HSV with a Vero cell bioassay, their saliva showed less antiviral bioactivity. These results suggested a further influence of the women's difficult personal situation and emotional distress on the salivary cystatins and mucins that can inhibit virus attachment and growth.

Who's Hosting the Response?

As evidenced by our review, an association between psychological factors, lifestyle, and immunity can be found at any point in the lifespan, but these relationships are likely to be of special significance for health at two particular times, during childhood and old age (Figure 12.5). There are number of reasons for this belief. Both are periods when the immune system is undergoing intrinsic change, and the regulatory set points that facilitate immune competence in the adult are either not yet established or are in flux. Especially in the very young infant, many immune processes are still maturing. For example, the capacity of the antigen-presenting cells to detect a foreign pathogen and to recruit lymphocytes to join in mounting an integrated immune response is not yet well developed. Even later in childhood, the immune response to an infection may still be a first-time, primary one, without the benefits garnered from prior exposures to the pathogen for generating the more robust secondary or memory response. Subsequently, in the senescent host, there will be a progressive decline in immune competence. Thus, perturbations in both the very young and the old may result in larger and more persistent effects after periods of stress.

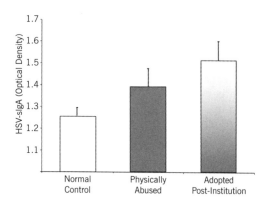

FIGURE 12.4. Many different stressful life events have been shown to affect the immune containment of herpes viruses. Higher antibody levels against HSV type 1 were found in the saliva of adolescents in maltreating families, as well as teenagers living in supportive families, but after adoption from institutional settings as young children, which is suggestive of poorer control over viral activation. From Shirtcliff et al. (2009). Copyright 2009 by the National Academy of Sciences. Adapted by permission.

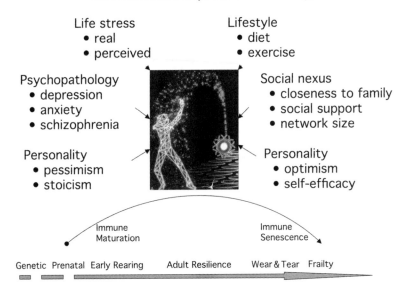

Life stress
- real
- perceived

Lifestyle
- diet
- exercise

Psychopathology
- depression
- anxiety
- schizophrenia

Social nexus
- closeness to family
- social support
- network size

Personality
- pessimism
- stoicism

Personality
- optimism
- self-efficacy

Immune
Maturation

Immune
Senescence

Genetic Prenatal Early Rearing   Adult Resilience   Wear & Tear Frailty

FIGURE 12.5. Many different psychological factors and lifestyle variables have been shown to affect the trajectory of immune development and the subsequent decline of immunity at the end of the lifespan. From Coe and Laudenslager (2007). Copyright 2007 by the Psychoneuroimmunology Research Society. Reprinted with permission from Elsevier.

Not coincidentally, at both of these times there is a greater susceptibility to infectious disease. As the rigor of immunity wanes in old age, the reduced resistance to infectious pathogens is accompanied by a general decline in immune surveillance, which accounts for the greater likelihood that mutagenic cells will become cancerous conditions. An age-related dysregulation of immunity in some older adult individuals also contributes to the increased incidence of autoimmune conditions. Collectively, this decline in antiviral and antitumor immunity has been described as a process of "immune senescence" (i.e., the going to sleep of the immune system) (Pawelec et al., 2002). When this warranty on immunity begins to run out varies markedly across individuals and is not set by chronological age only. It demarcates a point in the lifespan when it is especially important to learn more about how psychological and lifestyle variables affect our immune biology. For example, it is already known that the protective benefits of immunizations are frequently reduced in older adults. As many as one-third of older individuals may not really benefit from annual influenza vaccinations by mounting a sufficiently protective antibody response.

Thus, it is a time when behavioral interventions such as exercise and meditation may be especially helpful for enhancing vaccine efficacy and promoting health.

We actually know considerably more about how early life events can stimulate or impair the development of immune competence at the beginning of the lifespan, at least in animal models. In addition to the substantial literature on how maternal care, antigen stimulation, and rearing conditions affect immune responses in young animals, considerable evidence documents how the path toward health or illness can be strongly influenced by prenatal events affecting the gravid female during pregnancy (Coe & Lubach, 2008). Here the story for PNI and behavioral medicine researchers becomes especially interesting because one can discern an influence of maternal factors and pregnancy conditions projecting onto the next generation. Studies in farm animals, laboratory rats and mice, as well as nonhuman primates have all demonstrated that experimental perturbations of fetal development can result in offspring that mount different immune responses to the environment and to infections during infancy. This type of research on infant development from a PNI perspective is also proving to have direct clinical relevance in the applied pediatric topic area of allergies and asthma. In addition to the known effects of allergen exposure and smoking, stressful social and familial conditions during prenatal and early postnatal periods can influence whether a baby has a physiological bias toward atopic disorders (Chen & Miller, 2007). Neonates who are predisposed to allergy and asthma already may at birth have elevated levels of immunoglobulin E (IgE; a class of antibody associated with allergies). Cells from their cord blood are more likely to produce higher levels of IL-12, a specific cytokine response indicative of a bias toward atopy (i.e., a stronger T helper cell type 2 [Th2] cytokine profile). Combining a developmental perspective with the psychobiological models from PNI can thus inform us about etiological factors that account for a number of different illnesses in childhood.

One further corollary of the argument that we should take a number of host factors into consideration when weighing the ramifications of PNI for clinical medicine is that the significance of psychological influences on immunity is probably most germane to the immune-compromised and sick individual. In this case, behavioral and lifestyle factors that impair or promote immunity take on a special meaning because they can aggravate symptoms and impede or speed recovery. The same conclusion applies to individuals who may have a high genetic risk for particular illness, such as an autoimmune condition. Stressful events or a certain type of lifestyle may precipitate onset at an earlier age. There have already been many retrospective studies documenting how major life events can be associated with the emergence of illnesses such as rheumatoid arthritis and multiple sclerosis (Grant et al., 1989). With animal models, it has also been possible to show how these linkages among psychological state, pathophysiology, and disease expression emerge prospectively. One dramatic example was reported by Robert Ader and Nicholas Cohen (1982) during the early, formative years of PNI. They took advantage of established behavioral conditioning techniques to suppress immune responses transiently and were able to delay the age of disease onset in a strain of mice prone to lupus. Many other investigators have also shown

that the animal's age at weaning from the mother, as well as its social housing conditions, can affect the time when symptoms first appear, as well as the severity and pace of a disease's course.

This line of thinking goes along with the long-standing view that the field of PNI is of particular relevance for understanding the progression of cancer and may ultimately offer important insights into how best to care for patients postdiagnosis. Several landmark studies have already provided strong evidence to back up the claim that social support and psychotherapy can reduce morbidity and extend the lifespan for certain types of cancer (Spiegel, 1992). We need more research on this subject to know which interventions are most effective, and to determine for which types of cancer an immune modulation achievable through behavioral means will be most meaningful. Especially exciting and informative are recent studies demonstrating that psychological factors can even affect immune responses within the immediate tissue surrounding the malignancy itself (Lutgendorf et al., 2002, 2005). Showing that both the invasion of the tumor by immune cells and angiogenesis are malleable processes helps to explain how behavioral factors can affect neoplastic growth. It also opens the possibility that behavioral interventions may one day assist in modifying the physiology that supports the blood supply essential to sustain the rapid growth of an enlarging tumor. These clinical studies are building upon a large number of prior PNI experiments with animal models that have documented an influence of psychological factors on the immune surveillance for mutagenic cells and, specifically, the role of NK cells in containing the spread of metastases (Ben-Eliyahu, 2003; Ben-Eliyahu et al., 1991).

Delineating the Salience of Psychological Factors

The prior sections might make it seem that the most exciting PNI research in the future will take place at the cellular level using the latest state-of-the-art assay techniques. But equally important work remains to be done at the conceptual level of analysis with regard to refining our thoughts on the psychological and lifestyle variables of most significance.

We need to learn more about which psychological variables are truly salient, and able to exert the largest and most sustained effects on immune responses. The preponderance of prior research has also focused on negative factors, especially related to stressful conditions. As a consequence, many more studies are required to characterize the positive factors that have the most salubrious influences on immunity and health (Prather, Marsland, Muldoon, & Manuck, 2007).

Even at this point we do not have a systematic, comprehensive way to catalogue major life events that can influence immune responses. Perhaps as important, we need a coherent taxonomic framework for classifying these types of events in terms of their intensity or biological impact. The list of negative events that can undermine immune competence is already fairly long: It includes the loss of a loved one, marital discord, unemployment, natural disasters, and interpersonal trauma. But it is not yet known whether each situation affects our immune biology in a similar way. Do the different sources of cognitive and emotional distress all act through the same neuroendocrine and autonomic pathways to alter our immune responses? The answer is, probably not. There are also other critical lacunae in PNI that need filling. While a substantial literature describes how our immune responses change transiently following acute challenges, such as after delivering a speech or taking school exams, we know far less about the immune effects of more enduring attributes such as personality traits. There is some evidence already to indicate that many personality traits that affect other aspects of our physiological reactivity, such as emotional expressiveness, sociality, exuberance, and neuroticism, are also associated with immune responses. It is just as likely that some distinct aspects of our cognitive and temperamental makeup are uniquely salient for the maintenance and promotion of immune competence.

Especially when discussing the influence of psychological processes that are really remote from the immune system, that act indirectly via the brain to impinge on this dispersed cellular physiology, we have to ask what allows a particular psychological factor to have penetrance, to intrude and reorient, and sometimes to even reorganize immune responses. The essential role of the immune system in protecting us against infectious disease is what first led immunologists to believe that its functioning had to be largely autonomous of psychological state and even the nervous system. For a psychological factor to reach across this boundary line and to impinge upon cellular immune processes in more than a transient way, requires that it reach a high level of salience. The same logic also works in reverse. Only when the immune system is activated, and cytokine levels are high, can we clearly discern its influence on the brain and psychological state. In this review, I have described how this type of immune system-to-brain feedback can become emergent in the sick individual and contribute to some of the symptomatology seen in an affective disorder such as depression. It remains to be determined whether the immune abnormalities found in some individuals with schizophrenia also act on the nervous system in this way, or whether their immune dysregulation is really a consequence of the downstream effects of their psychopathology and altered neurochemistry.

Conclusions

The field of PNI has certainly come a long way. Initially, the idea that immune responses could be significantly impacted by psychological factors was greeted with considerable skepticism by immunologists and by many clinicians. As detailed in this chapter, over the last three decades, research ranging from the conditioning of immunity to the numerous demonstrations that many cellular processes are compromised in a stressed host helped to convince even the most skeptical that immune responses are far more malleable than once thought (Ader, 2003; Kemeny & Schedlowski, 2007). Cautious and reserved opinions about the veracity of the PNI perspective have also become less jaundiced and have given way as mounting evidence indicates that the traditional boundaries between the immune, nervous, and endocrine systems are not so clearly delineated. Indeed, the National Institutes of Health today considers the field of PNI to be a stellar exemplar of interdisciplinary research. The fact that many soluble factors secreted by immune cells are also released by other tissues now provides a common biochemical medium to account for the extensive crosstalk between these physiological systems. The 19th-century division of the body into major biological systems (i.e., nervous, endocrine, and immune) was invaluable for learning about the functioning of each, but to understand the biology of health and disease, especially from the perspectives of health psychology, it is essential to put the body systems back together.

Not surprisingly, much of the early research focused on downstream effects of psychological processes on immunity. More work still needs to be done to understand the neuroendocrine processes that mediate the effects of thoughts, feelings, and behaviors on immunity, and to describe the extent and duration of the many immune alterations that occur following various types of events. Certainly one of the more important contributions of PNI was the demonstration of equally potent immune system-to-brain effects. The significance becomes immediately evident as a means to explain the sickness behavior of animals administered cytokines or the symptoms of the ill patient. As highlighted in this review, it is a wonderful example of translational relevance, from bench to bedside, offering a cogent explanation for the malaise and depression often associated with chronic disease. These findings, in turn, will help us to refine better interventions as we learn more about how sleep, diet, exercise, and even social support and positive emotions influence cytokine biology and cellular functioning.

Many of these research findings also have social policy and public health implications that go beyond the scope of this review. If one can show that the well-being of an expectant mother has an effect on the future health and immune competence of her child, then there is a compelling need for the provision of better prenatal care. From a PNI perspective, what does the U.S. government No Child Left Behind policy really mean? We already know that early rearing conditions can influence the developmental trajectory toward health or deflect it in another direction, toward vulnerability and illness. The PNI research showing psychological effects on the biology of aging has an equally clear societal message. Here one is more inclined to invoke the 13th-century proverb "Prevention is worth a pound of cure." We know that bereavement, the stress of relocation, and the demands of being a caregiver can weaken immune responses, undermine the control of herpes viruses, and slow wound healing, but we know far less about how best to maintain or restore immunity.

Metaphorically speaking, the field of PNI can be described as having successfully navigated a remarkable path to productive middle age. The initial developmental tasks required for PNI to prove its worth have been accomplished, and PNI is now an accepted and established discipline. The next important stage will be to show how this knowledge about the body's intricate physiology can best be applied to restore the strength of the infirm, to lessen the suffering of the impaired and, of course, to sustain the vitality and vigor of the healthy.

Further Reading

Ader, R. (2007). *Psychoneuroimmunology* (4th ed.). San Diego, CA: Academic Press.

Daruna, J. H. (2004). *Introduction to psychoneuroimmunology*. San Diego, CA: Elsevier.

Fleshner, M., & Laudenslager, M. L. (2004). Psychoneuroimmunology: Then and now. *Behavioral and Cognitive Neuroscience Reviews* 3(2), 114–130.

Kiecolt-Glaser, J. K., McGuire, L., Robles, T. F., & Glaser R. (2002). Emotions, morbidity, and mortality: New perspectives from psychoneuroimmunology. *Annal Review of Psychology, 53*(1), 83–107.

Kiecolt-Glaser, J. K., McGuire, L., Robles, T. F., & Glaser, R. (2002). Psychoneuroimmunology: Psychological influences on immune function and health. *Journal of Consulting and Clinical Psychology, 70*, 537–547.

Kop, W. (2003). The integration of cardiovascular behavioral medicine and psychoneuroimmunology: New developments based on converging research fields. *Brain, Behavior, and Immunity, 17*(4), 233–237.

Miller, A. H. (2009). Mechanisms of cytokine-induced behavioral changes: Psychoneuroimmunology at the translational interface. *Brain, Behavior, and Immunity, 23*(2), 149–158.

Miller, G. E., Cohen, S., Pressman, S., Barkin, A., Rabin, B. S., & Treanor, J. J. (2004). Psychological stress and antibody response to influenza vaccination: When is the critical period for stress, and how does it get inside the body? *Psychosomatic Medicine, 66*(2), 215–223.

Vedhara, K., & Irwin, M. R. (2005). *Human psychoneuroimmunology.* London: Oxford University Press.

Watkins, L. R., & Maier, S. F. (2000). The pain of being sick: Implications of immune to-brain communication for understanding pain. *Annal Review of Psychology, 51,* 29–57.

References

Ader, R. (2003). Conditioned immunomodulation: Research needs and directions. *Brain, Behavior, and Immunity, 17*(Suppl. 1), 51–57.

Ader, R., & Cohen, N. (1982). Behaviorally conditioned immunosuppression and murine systemic lupus erythematosus. *Science, 215,* 1534–1536.

Antoni, M. H., Lutgendorf, S. K., Cole, S., Dhabhar, F. S., Sephton, S. E., McDonald, P. G., et al. (2006). The influence of bio-behavioural factors on tumour biology: Pathways and mechanisms, *Nature Reviews Cancer, 6,* 240–248.

Antoni, M. H., Schneiderman, N., & Penedo, F. (2007). Behavioral interventions: Immunologic mediators and disease outcomes. In R. Ader (Ed.), *Psychoneuroimmunology* (pp. 675–703). San Diego, CA: Academic Press.

Aronson, G., Wynings, C., Schneiderman, N., Baum, A., Rodriguez, M., Greenwood, B., et al. (1997). Posttraumatic stress symptoms, intrusive thoughts, loss, and immune function after Hurricane Andrew. *Psychosomatic Medicine, 59,* 128–141.

Bailey, M. T., & Coe, C. L. (1999). Maternal separation disrupts indigenous microflora of infant monkeys. *Developmental Psychobiology, 35*(2), 146–155.

Bailey, M. T., Lubach, G. R., & Coe, C. L. (2004). Prenatal conditions alter the bacterial colonization of the gut in the infant monkey. *Journal of Pediatric Clinical Gastroenterology and Nutrition, 38,* 414–421.

Banks, W. A., Kastin, A. J., & Gutierrez, E. G. (1994). Penetration of interleukin-6 across the murine blood–brain barrier. *Neuroscience Letters, 179,* 53–56.

Ben-Eliyahu, S. (2003). The promotion of tumor metastasis by surgery and stress: Immunological basis and implications for psychoneuroimmunology. *Brain, Behavior, and Immunity, 17,* 27–36.

Ben-Eliyahu, S., Yirmiya, R., Liebeskind, J. C., Taylor, A. N., & Gale, R. P. (1991). Stress increases metastatic spread of a mammary tumor in rats: Evidence of mediation by the immune system. *Brain, Behavior, and Immunity, 5*(2), 193–205.

Black, P. H. (2002). Stress and the inflammatory response: A review of neurogenic inflammation. *Brain, Behavior, and Immunity, 16*(6), 622–653.

Blalock, J. E. (1984). Immune system as a sensory organ. *Journal of Immunology, 132,* 1067–1070.

Blalock, J. K., & Smith, E. M. (2007). Conceptual development of the immune system as a sixth sense. *Brain, Behavior, and Immunity, 21,* 23–33.

Bruunsgaard, H., Pedersen, M., & Pedersen, B. K. (2001). Aging and proinflammatory cytokines. *Current Opinion in Hematology, 8,* 131–136.

Bullock, K., & Moore, R. Y. (1981). Thymus gland innervation by brain stem and spinal cord in mouse and rat. *American Journal of Anatomy, 162,* 157–166.

Buske-Kirschbaum, A., Kern, S. M., Ebrecht, M., & Hellhammer, D. H. (2007). Altered distribution of leukocyte subsets and cytokine production in response to acute psychosocial stress in patients with psoriasis vulgaris. *Brain, Behavior, and Immunity, 21,* 92–99.

Cannon, W. B. (1929). *Bodily changes in pain, hunger, fear and rage* (2nd ed.). New York: Appleton.

Capuron, L., Ravaud, A., Miller, A. H., & Dantzer, R. (2004). Baseline mood and psychosocial characteristics of patients developing depressive symptoms during interleukin-2 and/or interferon-alpha cancer therapy. *Brain, Behavior, and Immunity, 18,* 205–213.

Chen, E., & Miller, G. E. (2007). Stress and inflammation in exacerbations of asthma. *Brain, Behavior, and Immunity, 221*(8), 993–999.

Christian, L. M., Graham, J. E., Padgett, D. A., Glaser, R., & Kiecolt-Glaser, J. K. (2006). Stress and wound healing. *NeuroImmunoModulation, 13,* 337–346.

Coe, C. L., & Laudenslager, M. L. (2007). Psychosocial influences on immunity, including effects on immune maturation and senescence. *Brain, Behavior, and Immunity, 221*(8), 1000–1008.

Coe, C. L., & Lubach, G. R. (2008). Fetal programming: Prenatal origins of health and illness. *Current Directions in Psychological Science, 17*(1), 36–41.

Cohen, S., Tyrrel, D. A. G., & Smith, A. P. (1991). Psychological stress and susceptibility to the common cold. *New England Journal of Medicine, 325,* 606–612.

Cole, S. W., Kemeny, M. E., Fahey, J. L., Zack, J. A., & Naliboff, B. D. (2003). Psychological risk factors for HIV pathogenesis: Mediation by the autonomic nervous system. *Biological Psychiatry, 54,* 1444–1456.

Dantzer, R., O'Connor, J. C., Freund, G. G., Johnson, R. W., & Kelley, K. W. (2008). From inflammation to sickness and depression: When the immune system subjugates the brain. *Nature Reviews Neuroscience, 9,* 46–56.

Dhabhar, F. S., Miller, A. H., McEwen, B. S., & Spencer, R. L. (1995). Effects of stress on immune cell distribution: Dynamics and hormonal mechanisms. *Journal of Immunology, 154,* 5511–5527.

Felten, D. L., Felten, S. Y., Bellinger, D. L., Carlson, S. L., Ackerman, K. D., Madden, K. S., et al. (1987). Noradrenergic sympathetic neural interactions with the immune system: Structure and function. *Immunological Reviews, 100,* 225–260.

Fessel, W. J., Hirata-Hibi, M., & Shapiro, I. M. (1965). Genetic and stress factors affecting the abnormal lymphocyte in schizophrenia. *Journal of Psychiatric Research, 3,* 275–283.

Garcia-Linares, M. I., Sanchez-Lorente, S., Coe, C. L., & Martinez, M. (2004). Intimate partner violence impairs immune control over *Herpes simplex* virus type 1 in physically and psychologically abused women. *Psychosomatic Medicine, 66,* 965–972.

Glaser, R., Friedman, S. B., Smyth, J., Ader, R., Bijur, P., Brunell, P., et al. (1999). The differential impact of training stress and final examination stress on herpesvirus latency at the United States Military Academy at West Point. *Brain, Behavior, and Immunity, 13,* 240–251.

Glaser, R., & Kiecolt-Glaser, J. K. (2005). Stress-induced immune dysfunction: Implications for health. *Nature Reviews Immunology, 5,* 243–251.

Goehler, L. E., Gaykema, R. P. A., Nguyen, K. T., Lee, J. E., Tilders, F. J. H., Maier, S. F., et al. (1999). Interleukin-1 in immune cells of the abdominal vagus nerve: A link between the immune and nervous systems? *Journal of Neuroscience, 19*(7), 2799–2806.

Grant, I., Brown, G. W., Harris, T., McDonald, W. I., Patterson, T., & Trimble, M. R. (1989). Severely threatening events and marked life difficulties preceding onset or exacerbation of multiple sclerosis. *Journal of Neurology, Neurosurgery and Psychiatry, 52,* 8–13.

Grossman, C. J. (1985). Interactions between the gonadal steroids and the immune system. *Science, 227,* 257–261.

Hart, B. L. (1988). Biological basis of the behavior of sick animals. *Neuroscience and Biobehavioral Reviews, 12,* 123–137.

Heijnen, C. J., Kavelaars, A., & Ballieux, R. E. (1991). Beta-endorphin: Cytokine and neuropeptide. *Immunological Reviews, 119,* 41–63.

Herbert, T. B., & Cohen, S. (1992). Depression and immunity: A meta-analytic review. *Psychological Bulletin, 113,* 472–486.

Ironson, G., Wynings, C., Schneiderman, N., Baum, A., Rodriguez, M., Greenwood, D., et al. (1997). Posttraumatic stress symptoms, intrusive thoughts, loss, and immune function after Hurricane Andrew. *Psychosomatic Medicine, 50,* 128–141.

Irwin, M. R., Pike, J. L., Cole, J. C., & Oxman, M. N. (2003). Effects of a behavioral intervention, *tai chi chih,* on varicella–zoster virus specific immunity and health functioning in older adults. *Psychosomatic Medicine, 65,* 824–830.

Johnson, J. D., Campisi, J., Sharkey, C. M., Kennedy, S. L., Nickerson, M., & Fleshner, M. (2005). Adrenergic receptors mediate stress-induced elevations in extracellular Hsp72. *Journal of Applied Physiology, 99,* 1789–1795.

Kang, D.-H., Coe, C. L., McCarthy, D. O., & Ershler, W. B. (1997). Immune responses to final exams in healthy and asthmatic adolescents. *Nursing Research, 46,* 12–19.

Kelley, K. W., Arkins, S., Minshall, C., Liu, Q., & Dantzer, R. (1996). Growth hormone, growth factors and hematopoiesis. *Hormone Research, 45,* 38–45.

Kelley, K. W., Bluthé, R.-M., Dantzer, R., Zhou, J.-H., Shen, W.-H., Johnson, R. W., et al. (2003). Cytokine-induced sickness behavior. *Brain, Behavior, and Immunity, 17*(Suppl. 1), 112–118.

Kelley, K. W., Weigent, D. A., & Kooijman, R. (2007). Protein hormones and immunity. *Brain, Behavior, and Immunity, 21,* 384–392.

Kemeny, M. E., & Schedlowski, M. (2007). Understanding the interaction between psychosocial stress and immune-related diseases: A stepwise progression. *Brain, Behavior, and Immunity, 21*(8), 1009–1018.

Kiecolt-Glaser, J. K., Marucha, P. T., Malarkey, W. B., Mercado, A. M., & Glaser, R. (1995). Slowing of wound healing by psychological stress. *Lancet, 346,* 1194–1196.

Liu, L. Y., Coe, C. L., Swenson, C. A., Kelley, E. A., Kita, H., & Busse, W. W. (2002). School examinations enhance airway inflammation to antigen challenge. *American Journal of Respiratory and Critical Care Medicine, 265,* 1062–1067.

Lutgendorf, S., Johnsen, E., Cooper, B., Anderson, B., Sorsoky, J. I., Buller, R. E., et al. (2002). Vascular endothelial growth factor and social support in patients with ovarian carcinoma. *Cancer, 95,* 808–815.

Lutgendorf, S. K., Sood, A. K., Anderson, B., McGinn, S., Maiseri, H., Dao, M., et al. (2005). Social support, psychological distress, and natural killer cell activity in ovarian cancer. *Journal of Clinical Oncology, 23,* 7106–7113.

Madden, K. S., Bellinger, D. L., Felten, S. Y., Snyder, E., Maida, M. E., & Felten, D. (1997). Alterations in sympathetic innervation of thymus and spleen in aged mice. *Mechanisms of Ageing and Development, 94*(1–3), 165–175.

Maier, S. F., Glehler, L. E., Fleshner, M., & Watkins, L. R. (1998). The role of the vagus nerve in cytokine-to-brain communication. *Annals of the New York Academy of Sciences, 840*, 289–301.

Marucha, P. T., & Engeland, C. G. (2007). Stress, neuroendocrine hormones, and wound healing: Human models. In R. Ader (Ed.), *Psychoneuroimmunology* (pp. 825–835). San Diego, CA: Academic Press.

Meagher, M. W., Johnson, R., Good, E., & Welsh, C. J. (2007). Social stress alters the severity of a virally initiated model of multiple sclerosis. In R. Ader (Ed.), *Psychoneuroimmunology* (pp. 1107–1124). San Diego, CA: Academic Press.

Mora, J. M., Amtmann, L. E., & Hoffman, S. J. (1926). Effect of mental and emotional states on the leukocyte count. *Journal of the American Medical Association, 86*, 945–946.

Munck, A., Guyre, P. M., & Holbrook, N. J. (1984). Physiological functions of glucocorticoids in stress and their relation to pharmacological actions. *Endocrinology Reviews, 5*, 25–44.

Musselman, D. L., Lawson, D. H., Gumnick, J. F., Manatunga, S., Penna, R. S., Goodkin, K., et al. (2001). Paroxetine for the prevention of depression induced by high-dose interferon alpha. *New England Journal of Medicine, 344*, 961–966.

Pawelec, G., Barnett, Y., Forsey, R., Frasca, D., Globerson, A., McLeod, J., et al. (2002). T cells and aging. *Frontiers in Bioscience, 7*, 1056–2183.

Prather, A. A., Marsland, A. L., Muldoon, M. F., & Manuck, S. B. (2007). Positive affective style covaries with stimulated IL-6 and IL-10 production in a middle-aged community sample. *Brain, Behavior, and Immunity, 21*, 1033–1037.

Reyes, T. M., Fabry, Z., & Coe, C. L. (1999). Brain endothelial cell production of a neuroprotective cytokine, interleukin-6, in response to noxious stimuli. *Brain Research, 851*, 215–220.

Roncador, G., Garcia, G. F., Garcia, J. F., Maestre, L., Lucas, E., Menarguez, J., et al. (2005). T-cell leukemia and lymphoma (TCL and T lymphoma) FOXP3, a selective marker for a subset of adult T-cell leukaemia/lymphoma. *Leukemia, 19*, 2247–2253.

Sanders, V. M., & Kavelaars, A. (2007). Adrenergic regulation of immunity. In R. Ader (Ed.), *Psychoneuroimmunology* (pp. 63–84). San Diego, CA: Academic Press.

Selye, H. (1936). A syndrome produced by diverse nocuous agents. *Nature, 138*, 32.

Shirtcliff, E. A., Coe, C. L., & Pollak, S. D. (2009). Early childhood stress is associated with elevated antibody levels to *Herpes simplex* virus type 1. *Proceedings of the National Academy of Sciences USA, 106*(8), 2963–2967.

Spector, N. H. (1995). Three leaders in neuroimmunomodulation research: A tribute to Branislva D. Jankovic, Linus Pauling, and Vladmir Dilman. *NeuroImmunoModulation, 2*(4), 182–183.

Spiegel, D. (1992). Effects of psychosocial support on women with metastatic breast cancer. *Journal of Psychosocial Oncology, 10*, 113–120.

Straub, R. H., Cutolo, M., Buttgereit, F., & Pongratz, H. G. (2010). Energy regulation and neuroendocrine-immune control in chronic inflammatory diseases. *Journal of Internal Medicine, 267*(6), 543–560.

Straub, R. H., Dhabhar, F. S., Bijlsma, J. W., & Cutolo, M. (2005). How psychological stress via hormones and nerve fibers may exacerbate rheumatoid arthritis. *Arthritis and Rheumatism, 52*, 16–26.

Watkins, L. R., & Maier, S. F. (2000). The pain of being sick: Implications of immune-to-brain communication for understanding pain. *Annal Review of Psychology, 51*, 29–57.

Wieczorek, M., & Dunn, A. J. (2006). Effect of subdiaphragmatic vagotomy on the noradrenergic and HPA axis activation induced by intraperitoneal interleukin-1 administration in rats. *Brain Research, 1101*(1), 73–84.

Yolken, R. H., & Torrey, E. (1997). Viruses as etiologic agents of schizophrenia. *Advances in Biological Psychiatry, 18*, 1–12.

PART III

CONTRIBUTIONS OF OTHER SCIENCES TO HEALTH PSYCHOLOGY

CHAPTER 13

Behavioral Epidemiology

Robert M. Kaplan

The popular media often state, "Doctors know that a high-fat diet and lack of exercise may cause heart disease." Yet how did doctors come to know this? Clinical experience in medicine rarely allows a doctor to follow the same people throughout their lifespan. Although the weight of the evidence supports the use of cholesterol lowering to prevent deaths from heart disease (Barter et al., 2007; Kastelein et al., 2008; See et al., 2008), some authors have challenged the belief that heart disease can be prevented with current medications (Criqui & Golomb, 2004, 2008; Golomb, McGraw, Evans, & Dimsdale, 2007; Golomb, Stattin, & Mednick, 2000). "Epidemiologists" are scientists devoted to the study of health determinants, the distribution of disease in communities, and the validity of disease risk factors. This science provides much of the foundation for preventive medicine and preventive health care. Few heath care providers are actually involved in epidemiological research, but many pay close attention to the findings of epidemiological studies. This chapter provides an introductory overview of this important science. I hope this will provide some foundation for the interpretation of epidemiological findings.

What Is Epidemiology?

"Epidemiology" is the study of the determinants and distribution of disease (Ferenczi & Muirhead, 2006). Epidemiologists (scientists who study epidemiology) measure disease, then attempt to relate the development of diseases to characteristics of people and the environments in which they live. The word "epidemiology" is derived from Greek. The Greek word *epi* translates to "among," while the Greek word *demos* means "people." *Logos* indicates a scholarly discipline. The stem *-ology* means "the study of." Epidemiology, then, is the study of what happens among people. For as long as there has been recorded history, people have been interested in what causes disease. It has been obvious, for example, that diseases are not equally distributed within populations of people. Some people are at greater risk for certain problems than others.

Traditionally, epidemiologists primarily have been interested in infectious diseases. For example, people who live in close contact are most likely to get similar illnesses or to be "infected" by one another. Ancient doctors also recognized that people who became ill from certain diseases, and subsequently recovered, seldom got the same disease again. Thus, the notions of communicability of diseases and of immunity were known many years before specific microorganisms and antibodies were understood. Epidemiological history was made by Sir John Snow, who studied cholera in London in the mid-19th century (Timmreck, 1994). Cholera is a horrible disease that causes severe diarrhea and eventually kills its victims through dehydration. Snow systematically studied those who developed cholera and compared them to people who did not get the disease. His detective-like investigation demonstrated that those who obtained their drinking water from a particular source were more likely to develop cholera. Thus, he was able to link a specific environmental factor to the development of the disease (Snow, Frost, & Richardson, 1936). This occurred many years before the specific organism that causes cholera was identified.

It is common to think of epidemics as major changes in infectious disease rates. For example, we are experiencing a serious epidemic of acquired immune deficiency syndrome (AIDS). Yet there are other, less dramatic epidemics. For instance, we are also experiencing a major epidemic of coronary heart disease (CHD) in the United States.

In 1900, heart disease accounted for about 6.2% of all deaths, while infectious diseases, such as influenza and tuberculosis, accounted for nearly 25% of all deaths. By the year 2000, cardiovascular (heart and circulatory system) diseases had caused more than 34% of all deaths, while the effect of influenza and tuberculosis had been reduced to less than 4%. The days when infectious diseases were the major killers in the industrialized world appear to be over. AIDS, although rapidly increasing in incidence in some parts of the world, still accounts for a very small percentage of all deaths. Today, the major challenge is from chronic illnesses. The leading causes of death include heart disease, cancer, stroke, chronic obstructive pulmonary disease (COPD), and diabetes. Each of these may be associated with a long period of disability. In addition, personal habits and health behaviors may be associated with both the development and the maintenance of these conditions (Kaplan, Sallis, & Patterson, 1993). Figure 13.1 shows the number of deaths in the United States in 2005 by cause of death. Each of the top six causes of death is associated with behavior. Smoking is a major risk factor of heart disease, cancer, stroke, and COPD. Poor diet and obesity are associated with heart disease, cancer,

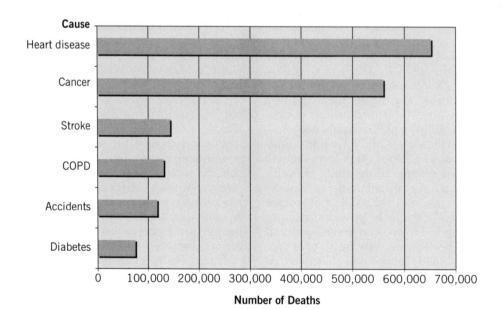

FIGURE 13.1. Leading causes of death in the United States: 2005. Data from National Center for Health Statistics (2008). COPD, chronic obstructive pulmonary disease.

stroke, COPD, and diabetes. Alcohol misuse is a leading risk factor for unintentional injuries.

Big numbers are sometimes difficult to interpret. So, to place these into context, I present a graph of the major causes of death and also homicides in 2009 (see Figure 13.2). Homicides are included because we all fear being murdered and many people acknowledge that they practice particular behaviors to avoid being a murder victim. Yet murder is a relatively less common cause of death, with about 14,000 cases reported in 2007. In fact, deaths from suicide in 2007 (about 32,000 cases) were more common than murders.

I am not suggesting that murder and suicide are unimportant. We often change our behaviors to avoid these dramatic problems because the linkage between our activities and these outcomes is obvious. However, there are similar linkages between behaviors and each of the other major causes of death. In some cases, altering behavior may have substantial effects upon causes of death in the United States and throughout the world. For example, we might have a major impact upon world health by changing cigarette smoking behavior (Lopez & the Disease Control Priorities Project, 2006).

In the following sections, I explore some of the relationships between health behaviors and health outcomes.

Behavioral Epidemiology

We use the term "behavioral epidemiology" to describe the study of individual behaviors and habits in relation to health outcomes. Wise observers have been aware of the relationship between lifestyle and health for many centuries. This is evidenced by the following statement from Hippocrates in approximately 400 B.C.:

> Whoever wishes to investigate medicine properly, should proceed thus: . . . and the mode in which the inhabitants live, and what are their pursuits, whether they are fond of drinking and eating to excess, and given to indolence, and are fond of exercise and labor, and not given to excess eating and drinking.

"Behavioral epidemiology," a term that has been used in the literature since the late 1970s, has not yet been clearly defined. In the context of behavioral medicine research, behavioral epidemiology can be considered

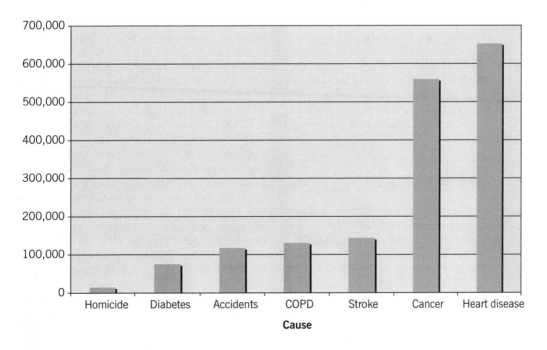

FIGURE 13.2. Causes of death including homicide.

a subset of research that studies the distribution and etiology of health-related behaviors in populations, as contrasted with research on clinical cases. Furthermore, behavioral epidemiology concerns itself with research that has the explicit purpose of understanding and influencing healthful behavior patterns, as part of populationwide initiatives to prevent disease and promote health (Kaplan, Criqui, & North Atlantic Treaty Organization Scientific Affairs Division, 1985).

Despite long-standing suspicion about the detrimental influence of unhealthy habits, most systematic studies have been reported only within the last 25 years. These studies suggest significant associations between lifestyle variables and cancer, CHD, and other major causes of death. It has been less than 50 years since the Surgeon General released the first report on smoking and health (United States Surgeon General's Advisory Committee on Smoking and Health, 1964), summarizing evidence on the detrimental effects of cigarette smoking. During the last 45 years, the evidence that cigarette smoking is harmful has mushroomed. There are now several thousand published studies documenting the health consequences of cigarette use (Owing, 2005).

In recognition of these relationships, the Institutes of Medicine of the National Academy of Sciences (Institute of Medicine [U.S.] Committee on Health and Behavior: Research Practice and Policy, 2001) implicated the role of individual behavior in the cause and maintenance of many disease states. I explore some of these linkages in more detail. First, however, it is important to review the methodologies used to establish them.

Epidemiological Methodology

Epidemiologists and social scientists use very similar research methodologies. The methodologies used by epidemiologists can be divided into two broad categories: descriptive and inferential. "Descriptive epidemiology" refers to the description of health outcomes and their determinants in terms of person, place, and time. "Inferential epidemiology" uses statistical methods to estimate characteristics of a population on the basis of a sample.

Person variables include age of members of the population, their sex, and other characteristics, and their racial or ethnic origin, marital status, and socioeconomic status. Person variables are sometimes referred to as "host variables," because some diseases may develop more in those with particular biological or social characteristics. Breast cancer, for example, occurs more commonly in women with a family history of similar problems (Welsh et al., 2009).

Place variables are also important in descriptive epidemiology. We know that certain problems are more common in some regions of the country than in others. For example, in studies of Lyme disease, which is a musculoskeletal problem associated with a bite by a specific deer tick, the original epidemiological studies identified a preponderance of cases in Lyme, Connecticut. It was noted that people on one side of a river were much more likely than those on the other side to develop the problem. Thus, place was associated with greater likelihood of exposure. We know that place is associated with a variety of different problems. For instance, people who live in the Sunbelt have much higher chances of developing skin cancer than those who live in areas with less sun exposure. Multiple sclerosis becomes more common with greater distance from the equator.

Time is also an important consideration in descriptive epidemiology. Rapid changes in the rate of death are also very important from an epidemiological standpoint. For example, the rapid increase in the number of persons infected with and succumbing to AIDS is a matter of major concern. AIDS is still not a major cause of death in the United States. Yet the rate of increase in the 1980s suggested that this condition was becoming a very serious public health problem. Epidemiologists often want to know about the duration between exposure to an infectious agent and the eventual outcome. The duration between exposure to the human immunodeficiency virus (HIV) and development of clinical AIDS may be several years. For other diseases the duration may be even longer. Cigarette smoking may take 20–30 years to cause COPD, and overexposure to saturated fat in the diet could take several decades to have an impact on any health outcome. To understand these linkages, very long-term studies are required.

Epidemiological Measures

A variety of epidemiological measures are commonly used in behavioral research. Epidemiological studies typically focus on outcomes expressed as "morbidity" (illness) and "mortality" (death). Morbidity and mortality are usually reported as rates divided into two major types: incidence and prevalence. "Incidence" refers to the rate at which new cases are occurring and is defined as the number of new cases within a specific population within a defined time interval. Typically, the *incidence* rate is expressed per 1,000 in the population. Conceptually it is:

$$\text{Incidence rate per 1,000} = \frac{\text{New cases per unit of time}}{\text{Persons exposed or at risk per unit of time}} \times 1,000$$

Prevalence rates describe the number of diagnosed cases at a particular point in time:

$$\text{Prevalence rate per 1,000} = \frac{\text{Cases at specific time point}}{\text{Persons exposed or at risk at specific time point}} \times 1,000$$

The prevalence rate is equal to the incidence rate times the duration of the disease. For example, if the average duration of dementia is 5 years and its incidence is 3 per 1,000 per year, the prevalence would be 15 per 1,000. Figure 13.3 shows the incidence of obesity or overweight between 1960 and 2004, based on the National Health and Nutrition Examination Survey (NHANES). As the figure shows, overweight had a lower prevalence in 1960 in comparison to more recent times. However, being overweight very rapidly increases rate of incidence, suggesting the seriousness of the epidemic. Conversely, heart disease has decreasing incidence (see Figure 13.4) but very high prevalence.

Virtually all research designs common to clinical and experimental research are used in behavioral epidemiology. In this section I provide a brief overview of observational and experimental studies. Observational studies do not attempt to manipulate variables in a systematic fashion. Instead, inferences are made on the basis of an ongoing series of observations. Some of the most common observational studies include the cohort study, the panel study, and the case–control study.

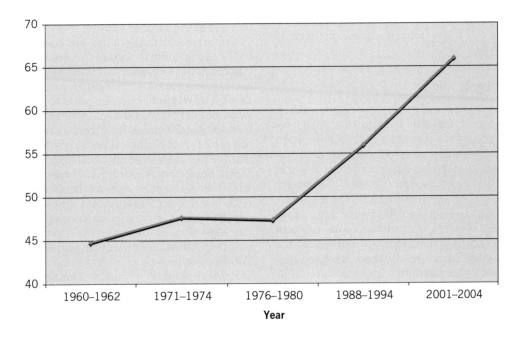

FIGURE 13.3. Percent overweight or obese by year in NHANES.

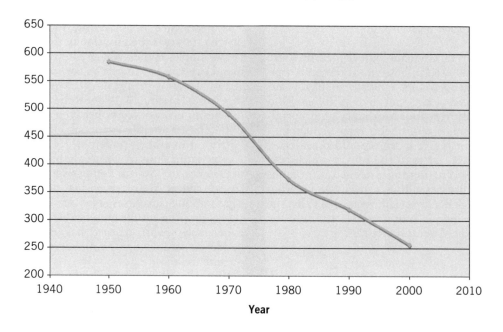

FIGURE 13.4. Heart disease deaths by year.

Cohort Studies

In cohort studies, groups of people who share some common characteristics are followed over the course of time. These studies, which are often prospective, resample the same population of individuals on repeated occasions. However, the exact participants in the study may not be the same on repeated observations.

Panel Studies

Panel studies are similar to cohort studies. However, panel studies have the stricter requirement that the same individuals in the original sample are followed at each repeated assessment. An example of a panel study is Coronary Artery Risk Development in Young Adults (CARDIA). This investigation was designed to determine how heart disease develops over the course of time. In 1986, a group of 5,115 black and white men and women ages 18–30 years were selected in four cities: Birmingham, Alabama; Chicago, Illinois; Minneapolis, Minnesota; and Oakland, California. The subjects completed baseline assessments and were followed in 1987–1988 (Year 2), 1990–1991 (Year 5), 1992–1993 (Year 7), 1995–1996 (Year 10), 2000–2001 (Year 15), and 2005–2006 (Year

20). Measures include traditional biological factors, such as blood pressure, cholesterol, and other lipids. In addition, the dataset includes behavioral variables, such as substance use (tobacco and alcohol), dietary and exercise patterns, and personality measures (Janicki-Deverts, Cohen, Matthews, & Cullen, 2008; Ohira et al., 2008).

Cohort and panel studies are considered to be longitudinal designs. Longitudinal studies make inferences about changes over the course of time. The most respected epidemiological studies use the prospective longitudinal panel study design. A variety of epidemiological studies have considered both behavioral and biological predispositions toward CHD. For example, the Framingham Heart Study began with 5,127 participants who had no visible signs of heart disease. Each participant was given a physical examination and a detailed interview, including lifestyle and demographic characteristics, then followed every other year (Kaplan, 2004).

Epidemiologists typically evaluate risk factors in terms of ratios. For example, if 30% of all smokers and 24% of all nonsmokers in a population-based study died from a fatal heart attack, then 0.30/0.24 = 1.25. Thus, smoking increased the risk of a fatal heart attack 25% over the risk attributable to all other risk factors combined. The relative risk, in this example, is a measure of the importance of smoking as a cause for fatal heart attack.

Cross-sectional studies differ from longitudinal studies in that they examine different groups of individuals at the same point in time. To make inferences about drug use in college, for example, the cross-sectional method would require sampling of each current class. Then, freshmen could be compared with sophomores, juniors, and seniors. These individuals would not be members of the same class or birth cohort.

Case–Control Studies

This methodology compares a group of people with a diagnosed disease (cases) with one or more groups that have not been given the same diagnosis. Case–control studies are typically retrospective because they make inferences about events that have caused currently diagnosed cases. Longitudinal studies are often prospective and have the advantage of documenting antecedents of new cases.

In observational studies, variables that are uncontrolled throughout the experimental design are often adjusted for using statistical methods. However, these statistical adjustments are often incomplete and known to introduce some errors.

Experimental Studies

In contrast to observational studies in which important variables are not controlled, experimental studies typically involve the systematic manipulation of variables. Illnesses have natural histories, and in most instances their course fluctuates considerably without treatment. One of the difficulties in determining the effects of an intervention is that the intervention may occur at a crisis time. For example, patients with an illness might seek care on days when they are most sick. If the illness is likely to get better on its own (as in the case of most common illnesses), any treatment will appear to have "worked." A control group can help sort out the effect of treatment from other factors. In this way, a group receiving the intervention under study is compared with the control group that does not receive treatment to determine whether there are differences attributable to the intervention.

It is widely accepted among medical and biobehavioral scientists that a control or comparison group is required to establish causal inference. In some cases, investigators are willing to accept "quasi-experimental" data in which an ad hoc control is used, or a stable baseline of observations exists prior to an intervention. However, several authors have argued that an experiment characterized by a single observation, an intervention, and a second observation is virtually impossible to interpret from a causal perspective (Yusuf, Collins, & Peto, 1984).

Bias occurs when the design of a study does not ensure an impartial assessment of the treatment. For experiments using control groups, random assignment to treatment and control conditions is very desirable. Simply stated, randomized clinical trials remove several sources of bias. The value of randomized clinical trials has been emphasized by Sacks, Chalmers, and Smith (1982), who reviewed six therapies for which approximately equal numbers of randomized clinical trials and nonrandomized trials were reported in the literature. They found that 79% of the studies in which patients were not randomly assigned to groups reported that the therapy was better than the control regimen. In contrast, the same therapies were found to be effective in only 20% of the studies in which patients had been randomly assigned to the treatment or control condition. In a related review, Chalmers, Celano, Sacks, and Smith (1983) analyzed 145 scientific reports divided into three categories: those in which the randomization process was blinded, those in which the randomization was unblinded, and those in which assignment to treatment or control was by a nonrandom process. "Blinding" refers to the process of keeping investigators ignorant of the treatment assignments. Review of these studies suggested a systematic relationship between the rigor of the experimental design and the probability of finding a treatment benefit. There was a significant treatment benefit in 58% of the studies in which subjects were not randomly assigned. The same benefit was observed in 24% of the unblinded randomized studies and in approximately 9% of the blinded randomized studies. These reviews have convinced many leaders in medicine to discount results that have not been observed in a randomized clinical trial (Sackett, Straus, Richardson, Rosenberg, & Haynes, 2000).

For example, most protocols for evaluating the quality of research in evidence-based medicine reviews give significantly more weight to randomized clinical trials than to studies using other methodologies (Petitti et al., 2009; Sawaya, Guirguis-Blake, LeFevre, Harris, & Petitti, 2007)

In summary, there are many sources of bias in studies that do not use control groups, and the end result is frequently an overestimation of the effects of the therapy under study. These biases are reduced in experimental studies, but the rigor of the experimental design is systematically related to the chances of not finding a treatment benefit. Valid scientific inferences must be built upon a solid experimental foundation.

Major Epidemiological Studies

Much of what we know about behavioral risk factors comes from a limited number of major epidemiological investigations. Several major studies have been conducted in the United States, Canada, Europe, and Australia. To provide a flavor of these studies, I review three of the major investigations: the Framingham Heart Study, the Alameda County Population Study, and the China Stroke Prevention Trial. These studies are mentioned repeatedly throughout the rest of the book because they provide some of the basic justifications for behavioral interventions.

Framingham Heart Study

The Framingham Heart Study is the oldest and perhaps best-known population study in the United States. In 1948, a group of medical researchers entered an average New England town of Framingham, Massachusetts (population about 68,000), to begin one of the largest and most important epidemiological studies in the history of medicine. The purpose of the Framingham Heart Study was to determine the causes of stroke and heart failure. Before this study, most investigations of heart disease had been retrospective. Retrospective studies start with a group of people who have already developed heart trouble, then look into their pasts to determine what they have in common. In contrast, the researchers in the Framingham study started with healthy people and attempted to predict which ones would eventually die of heart and circulatory problems. This approach is called "prospective" and is considered to produce superior and more convincing scientific data than the retrospective method. The study began by identifying every other man and woman in Framingham between the ages of 30 and 60 who had no signs of heart disease. In the beginning, there were 5,127 participants. Each time a new subject was enrolled, he or she was given a thorough physical exam and a detailed interview about lifestyle. The subjects were remeasured every 2 years.

Within a few decades, the picture of the "heart disease–prone" individual began to emerge because many of the Framingham subjects had suffered heart attacks or strokes. Some of the predictors of heart disease were identified as being beyond the subject's control, such as age (older people are more prone); sex (males are more prone); and certain diseases, such as diabetes, and race (blacks are more prone). However, a major finding of the study was that some of the best predictors of heart disease and early death are direct consequences of our own behavior. These predictors of heart disease include smoking, obesity, high cholesterol levels (perhaps associated with a high animal fat diet), physical inactivity, and possibly excessive tension and stress.

The Framingham Heart Study has been very important in establishing that some risk factors for heart disease are "mutable," or subject to change. Thus, much of the current practice of preventive medicine was launched. Risk factors were identified, and important recommendations for behavior change were offered. The Framingham Heart Study has continued to follow the original group of participants. After nearly 60 years, the study continues to contribute scientific insights (Kannel, 2000b). In addition, the study has been expanded to include the offspring of the original participants and, more recently, their grandchildren. Literally hundreds of scientific papers have been based on observations from this important New England community. However, the general risk factors identified in the original Framingham study continue to be confirmed in newer studies (D'Agostino et al., 2008).

Alameda County Study

The Alameda County Study originally identified 8,300 adults who lived in 4,735 households. Eighty-six percent of the eligible adults completed questionnaires, and these 6,928 individuals have been followed by the investigators for more than 40 years. The study began in 1965, and by the mid-1970s, a variety of interesting findings began to emerge. For example, a series of important analyses (Berkman & Kawachi, 2000; Maty, Lynch, Raghunathan, & Kaplan, 2008; Turrell, Lynch, Leite, Raghunathan, & Kaplan, 2007; Yen & Kaplan, 1999) demonstrated that health habits are a major predictor of survival for the residents of this urban California community. The specific predictors of surviving (not dying early) included not smoking cigarettes, using alcohol in moderation, being average weight, engaging in moderate leisure time physical activity, and obtaining 7–9 hours of sleep each night. In some of the analyses, the investigators simply counted the number of good health habits in which the participants engaged. They found systematic relationships between the number of these activities and both morbidity (illness) and mortality (early death). For example, those who engaged in none of these practices were 3.11 times more likely to die of heart disease than those who engaged in five of the activities.

The Alameda County Study also broke new ground by demonstrating the relationship between social support and health outcomes (Yen & Kaplan, 1999). Those who were more "socially connected," as measured by number of social contacts, had significantly greater chances of survival than those who were less connected (Maty et al., 2008; Turrell et al., 2007).

China Stroke Prevention Trial

People in the urban areas of China have a high rate of death from stroke. In the 1990s, stroke was the leading cause of death in several urban areas of China. Methods for reducing stroke, primarily the control of blood pressure, are well understood, but it was not known whether these methods for controlling stroke could be disseminated at a community level. To explore these issues, a community-based intervention trial was designed and implemented in major urban areas of Beijing, Shanghai, and Changsha. In 1991, two well-matched communities were chosen within each of the three major urban areas. In each urban area, one community was chosen as the intervention site and the other as the control site. Each intervention or control site had approximately 50,000 residents.

The intervention communities received health education and health promotion services to help participants avoid cigarettes and control blood pressure, while these treatments were not given in the control communities. Residents in each intervention community received counseling on how to control high blood pressure, and those with definite high blood pressure (systolic blood pressure [SBP] > 160) got special attention and advice on the use of antihypertensive drugs. During the second phase, patients with diabetes and smokers were targeted. Those with diabetes were invited to trimonthly sessions on control or maintenance of blood sugar through diet and physical activity. Smokers attended quarterly meetings on tobacco control, use of nicotine gum, and cigarette substitutes. Every 2 or 3 months, intervention community members received flyers and booklets on stroke prevention. Public bulletins, also issued quarterly, emphasized weight control, smoking cessation, and refraining from alcoholic beverages.

The long-term effects of the interventions were measured by considering the number of fatal and nonfatal stroke cases in each community. Using 10 years of follow-up, there were 2,273 first-ever stroke cases in the intervention communities and 3,015 in the control communities. Through 10 years of intervention, incidence rates of all types of stroke decreased by 11.4% in the intervention compared with control communities. This community-based study offers very good evidence that comprehensive, community-based interventions have the potential to reduce the burden of stroke in large populations. Overall, the results are quite impressive: They demonstrate that counseling methods can be used on a large scale to reduce the threat of stroke. Suffice it to say, however, that epidemiological studies include both observation and, in some cases, manipulation of experimental variables (Wang et al., 2007).

Person, Place, and Time in Epidemiological Studies

Epidemiologists are interested in the influence of person, place, and time upon health outcomes. Most epidemiological studies involve all three components. In the next few sections I consider studies that focus primarily on person, time, and place.

Person

Characteristics of individuals can affect health outcomes. Clearly, genetic endowment is a major contributor to the health status we achieve or the health problems we suffer. In addition, personality characteristics may also be associated with disease development and recovery from illness. One example comes from a study of restenosis following coronary angioplasty. Stenosis is narrowing and "coronary stenosis" refers to the narrowing of the major arteries in the heart that predispose people to heart disease. "Coronary angioplasty" is a procedure to expand the artery to reduce the stenosis. However, the arteries often narrow again within a year of the procedure, referred to as "restenosis." Studies have shown that personality characteristics can predict restenosis. For example, some people exhibit "overcommitment," which is defined as excessive striving in combination with an unusually strong desire to be approved of and respected. One study demonstrated that among people who had coronary angioplasty, overcommitted persons were at least 2.5 times more likely to have restenosis than those who were not overcommitted (Joksimovic et al., 1999). Person influences go beyond our genetic predispositions. This and many other studies show how personalities and personal choices can predispose people to serious illnesses, and how lifestyles can affect the recovery process.

Place

Numerous examples show the relationship between place of residence and susceptibility to illness. One example of the importance of place concerns the relationship between sunlight exposure and the development of cancer. One group of researchers believes that exposure to sunlight may be helpful in preventing certain cancers. For example, they have demonstrated that skin cancers are more common in regions of the world where people are exposed to more ultraviolet light from the sun. However, sunlight is also an important source of vitamin D, and some cancers may be related to deficiencies in this important vitamin. For example, vitamin D may play an important role in reducing the risk of colon and breast cancer (Garland, Gorham, Baggerly, & Garland, 2008; Garland, Gorham, et al., 2007; Garland, Grant, Mohr, Gorham, & Garland, 2007). One hypotheses is that the high levels of air pollutants causing haze block ultraviolet light and may result in vitamin D deficiencies (Garland, Garland, & Gorham, 1999). A study evaluated the relationships between sulfur dioxide and other components of air pollution that blocked sunlight in 20 Canadian cities. There were significant relationships between the presence of this type of air pollution and the development of colon cancer in both men and women, as well as significant relationships between the pollutants and breast cancer in women. Mortality rates for cancer not believed to be associated with vitamin D were not associated with these levels of aerosols (Garland et al., 1999).

Prevalence of many diseases differs by location. For example, deaths rates from heart disease are much more common in the Deep South than in other parts of the United States. Rates tend to be the lowest in the band that runs from Arizona and New Mexico up to Idaho and Montana (see Figure 13.5).

In conclusion, place may be very important because people in some areas have greater toxic exposures to contaminants in the air, difficult weather, water systems, or other environmental factors. The studies described earlier suggest that air pollution may block sunlight. This can ultimately result in increased risk of cancers of the breast and colon (Garland et al., 2008; Garland, Gorham, et al., 2007; Mohr, Garland, Gorham, & Garland, 2008).

Time

Many illnesses develop slowly. Thus, the epidemiologist must consider time in addition to person and place variables. The epidemiology of heart disease is a good example. Heart disease may develop slowly over the course

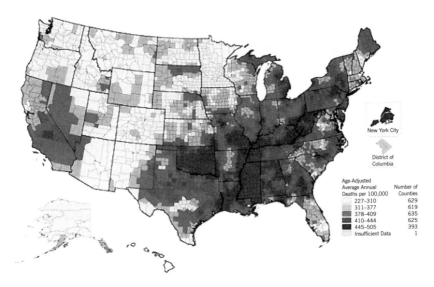

FIGURE 13.5. Heart disease deaths in the United States: 2000–2005. From Centers for Disease Control and Prevention (2009).

of 40 or 50 years, and behavioral variables have been shown to be a major contributing cause. Before we consider the time issue, it is necessary to give an overview of heart disease epidemiology.

It has been estimated that nearly 60 million Americans have CHD, and an additional 4.4 million have cerebrovascular disease (problems with blood flow to the brain). Furthermore, about 50 million people have high blood pressure (American Heart Association, 2008). In the United States, there are about 3,000 heart attacks every day. In the 1 minute the reader spends reading this paragraph, about two people will have had heart attacks. *Prospective* epidemiological studies have identified a variety of major risk factors for CHD and stroke. It is difficult to do anything about some of these risk factors. For example, men die of heart disease more often than do women, particularly in the younger age categories. Blacks are more likely than whites to have high blood pressure and eventually die of heart disease (American Heart Association, 2008). Family history is also an important predictor of death due to heart disease. Those with family histories of heart attack or stroke are more likely to develop these problems themselves.

Although it is difficult to do something about many risk factors, epidemiological studies have demonstrated that most of the risk factors for heart disease are under our

personal control, including cigarette smoking, cholesterol, obesity, and high blood pressure (D'Agostino et al., 2008). Some studies have tried to compare the population attributable risk relevant to four risk factors for heart disease. Among these, high blood pressure is the most important risk factor, followed by cigarette smoking. High blood pressure may be the cause of 30% of all cardiovascular deaths. It has been estimated that one-half of those suffering a first heart attack and two-thirds of those suffering a stroke have high blood pressure (Kannel, 2000a, 2000b; Kannel & Wolf, 2008). Several studies have now demonstrated that we can reduce the burden of suffering by controlling high blood pressure. Treatments for high blood pressure depend on behavior change. Some treatments involve changing long-standing habits, such as reducing dietary salt, increasing daily exercise, and reducing weight. Other treatments involve the use of medications. Although substantial evidence suggests that blood pressure can be reduced with medications, compliance with these treatments is often disturbingly low. In other words, patients simply do not take their medications on a regular basis. Behavioral interventions may be very important in helping people find ways to comply with these difficult medical regimens (Catz, Kelly, Bogart, Benotsch, & McAuliffe, 2000).

In addition to elevated blood pressure, high blood cholesterol is also a major risk factor for death due to heart disease. It is widely believed that "luxury" diets with high percentages of calories from animal fats increase the probability of death from heart disease. Several epidemiological studies have identified high levels of cholesterol in blood serum as a risk factor for death, and it is assumed that high dietary fat contributes to these high blood cholesterol levels (D'Agostino et al., 2008). Thus, consuming a high-fat diet may be a risk factor for CHD.

Perhaps the most important controllable risk factor for heart disease is cigarette smoking. Although smoking is on the decline, more than 20 percent of all adults still smoke cigarettes. As many as 17 percent of all heart disease deaths may be attributed to cigarette smoking. This translates into about 78,000 deaths per year (American Heart Association, 2008). Others have estimated that smoking causes many more deaths. For example, the American Heart Association estimates that about 1 in 5 deaths from cardiovascular disease can be attributed to smoking. The World Health Organization estimated that there were about 3 million smoking related deaths in 1990. It estimates that by the year 2020, the number will reach 10 million (Peto, Chen, & Boreham, 1999). It is important to consider the number of smoking-related CHD deaths in relation to deaths from other causes. For example, consider deaths due to murder. There are approximately 14,000 murders per year in the United States, and we have come to think of murder as very common. Thus, we spend considerable resources on more police and stricter laws, and we deal with murderers very harshly. Yet we have been relatively lenient with those who promote and sell cigarettes. Considering only heart disease (just one of the many diseases caused by cigarette smoking), there may be four to eight people who die from cigarette use compared to each person who is murdered.

The risk factors for heart disease were almost all identified and confirmed in the major epidemiological studies. The studies evaluated people's habits while they were healthy. Then the participants were followed over the course of time, and the researchers observed differences in adverse health outcomes among those with the various risk factors. Time is important in these epidemiological studies

because we have witnessed genuine epidemics of heart disease in this century. At the turn of the 20th century, heart disease was relatively uncommon. However, there were rapid increases in the numbers of people who die from heart disease over the first half of that century. Since about 1968, the number of people who die of heart disease has been declining. Many believe that these reductions are associated with the identification of heart disease risk factors. The declines coincide with greater awareness of some of the behavioral factors that cause these ailments. For example, tobacco use systematically declined at about the same time that heart disease diminished.

Conclusions

This chapter provides an overview of the science of epidemiology, the basic science that offers the foundation for preventive medicine. It uses methods of social sciences alongside techniques of the biological sciences. In recent years, epidemiologists have discovered that many risk factors for the major causes of death are behavioral. Heart disease may be associated with high dietary fat consumption, physical inactivity, and cigarette smoking. Cancer may be caused by smoking cigarettes and by eating a high-fat and low-fiber diet. Epidemiologists have also shown that women are less at risk for some of the major causes of death and have a longer life expectancy in the Western World. However, they may be at higher risk for some other disabling diseases, such as rheumatoid arthritis. Despite advances in modern medicine, there are substantial differences between white and nonwhite populations in the chances of suffering from most of the major diseases.

Further Reading

Berkman, L. F., & Kawachi, I. (2000). *Social epidemiology.* New York: Oxford University Press.

D'Agostino, R. B., Vasan, R. S., Pencina, M. J., Wolf, P. A., Cobain, M., Massaro, J. M., et al. (2008). General cardiovascular risk profile for use in primary care: The Framingham Heart Study. *Circulation, 117*(6), 743–753.

Gilpin, E. A., Choi, W. S., Berry, C., & Pierce, J. P. (1999). How many adolescents start smoking each day in the United States? *Journal of Adolescent Health, 25*(4), 248–255.

Glasgow, R. E., Fisher, E. B., Anderson, B. J., LaGreca, A., Marrero, D., Johnson, S. B., et al. (1999). Behavioral science in diabetes: Contributions and opportunities. *Diabetes Care, 22*(5), 832–843.

Kannel, W. B., & Wolf, P. A. (2008). Framingham Study insights on the hazards of elevated blood pressure. *Journal of the American Medical Association, 300*(21), 2545–2547.

Kaplan, G. A. (1998). Socioeconomic considerations in the health of urban areas. *Journal of Urban Health, 75*(2), 228–235.

Kaplan, G. A., & Lynch, J. W. (1999). Socioeconomic considerations in the primordial prevention of cardiovascular disease. *Preventive Medicine, 29*(6, Pt. 2), S30–S35.

Kaplan, R. M. (2000). Two pathways to prevention. *American Psychologist, 55*(4), 382–396.

Sawaya, G. F., Guirguis-Blake, J., LeFevre, M., Harris, R., & Petitti, D. (2007). Update on the methods of the U.S. Preventive Services Task Force: Estimating certainty and magnitude of net benefit. *Annals of Internal Medicine, 147*(12), 871–875.

References

American Heart Association. (2008). *2008 heart and stroke statistical update.* Dallas: Author.

Barter, P., Gotto, A. M., LaRosa, J. C., Maroni, J., Szarek, M., Grundy, S. M., et al. (2007). HDL cholesterol, very low levels of LDL cholesterol, and cardiovascular events. *New England Journal of Medicine, 357*(13), 1301–1310.

Berkman, L. F., & Kawachi, I. (2000). *Social epidemiology.* New York: Oxford University Press.

Catz, S. L., Kelly, J. A., Bogart, L. M., Benotsch, E. G., & McAuliffe, T. L. (2000). Patterns, correlates, and barriers to medication adherence among persons prescribed new treatments for HIV disease. *Health Psychology, 19*(2), 124–133.

Centers for Disease Control and Prevention. (2009). *Preventing heart disease and stroke.* Atlanta, GA: Author. Available at *www.cdc.gov/chronicdisease/resources/publication.*

Chalmers, T. C., Celano, P., Sacks, H. S., & Smith, H., Jr. (1983). Bias in treatment assignment in controlled clinical trials. *New England Journal of Medicine, 309*(22), 1358–1361.

Criqui, M. H., & Golomb, B. A. (2004). Low and lowered cholesterol and total mortality. *Journal of the American College of Cardiology, 44*(5), 1009–1010.

Criqui, M. H., & Golomb, B. A. (2008). Lipid lowering: What and when to monitor. *Lancet, 372,* 516–517.

D'Agostino, R. B., Vasan, R. S., Pencina, M. J., Wolf, P. A., Cobain, M., Massaro, J. M., et al. (2008). General cardiovascular risk profile for use in primary care: The Framingham Heart Study. *Circulation, 117*(6), 743–753.

Ferenczi, E., & Muirhead, N. (2006). *Statistics and epidemiology.* London: Hodder Arnold.

Garland, C. F., Garland, F. C., & Gorham, E. D. (1999). Calcium and vitamin D: Their potential roles in colon and breast cancer prevention. *Annals of the New York Academy of Sciences, 889*(Suppl. 1), 107–119.

Garland, C. F., Gorham, E. D., Baggerly, C. A., & Garland, F. C. (2008). Re: Prospective study of vitamin D and cancer mortality in the United States. *Journal of the National Cancer Institute, 100*(11), 826–827.

Garland, C. F., Gorham, E. D., Mohr, S. B., Grant, W. B., Giovannucci, E. L., Lipkin, M., et al. (2007). Vitamin D and prevention of breast cancer: Pooled analysis. *Journal of Steroid Biochemistry and Molecular Biology, 103*(3–5), 708–711.

Garland, C. F., Grant, W. B., Mohr, S. B., Gorham, E. D., & Garland, F. C. (2007). What is the dose–response relationship between vitamin D and cancer risk? *Nutrition Reviews, 65*(8, Pt. 2), S91–S95.

Golomb, B. A., McGraw, J. J., Evans, M. A., & Dimsdale, J. E. (2007). Physician response to patient reports of adverse drug effects: Implications for patient-targeted adverse effect surveillance. *Drug Safety, 30*(8), 669–675.

Golomb, B. A., Stattin, H., & Mednick, S. (2000). Low cholesterol and violent crime. *Journal of Psychiatric Research, 34*(4–5), 301–309.

Hippocrates. (ca. 400 B.C.). *On airs, waters, and places* (F. Adams, Trans.). Available at *www.literaturemaster.com/literature/ancient/3179.*

Institute of Medicine (U.S.) Committee on Health and Behavior: Research Practice and Policy. (2001). *Health and behavior: The interplay of biological, behavioral, and societal influences.* Washington, DC: National Academy Press.

Janicki-Deverts, D., Cohen, S., Matthews, K. A., & Cullen, M. R. (2008). History of unemployment predicts future elevations in C-reactive protein among male participants in the Coronary Artery Risk Development in Young Adults (CARDIA) Study. *Annals of Behavioral Medicine, 36*(2), 176–185.

Joksimovic, L., Siegrist, J., Meyer-Hammer, M., Peter, R., Franke, B., Klimek, W. J., et al. (1999). Overcommitment predicts restenosis after coronary angioplasty in cardiac patients. *International Journal of Behavioral Medicine, 6*(4), 356–369.

Kannel, W. B. (2000a). Elevated systolic blood pressure as a cardiovascular risk factor. *American Journal of Cardiology, 85*(2), 251–255.

Kannel, W. B. (2000b). Fifty years of Framingham Study contributions to understanding hypertension. *Journal of Human Hypertension, 14*(2), 83–90.

Kannel, W. B., & Wolf, P. A. (2008). Framingham Study insights on the hazards of elevated blood pressure. *Journal of the American Medical Association, 300*(21), 2545–2547.

Kaplan, R. M. (2004). Framingham Heart Study. In N. B. Anderson (Ed.), *Encyclopedia of health and behavior* (Vol. 1, pp. 343–344). Thousand Oaks: Sage.

Kaplan, R. M., Criqui, M. H., & the North Atlantic Treaty Organization Scientific Affairs Division. (1985). *Behavioral epidemiology and disease prevention.* New York: Plenum Press.

Kaplan, R. M., Sallis, J. F., & Patterson, T. L. (1993). *Health and human behavior.* New York: McGraw-Hill.

Kastelein, J. J., van der Steeg, W. A., Holme, I., Gaffney, M., Cater, N. B., Barter, P., et al. (2008). Lipids, apolipoproteins, and their ratios in relation to cardiovascular events with statin treatment. *Circulation, 117*(23), 3002–3009.

Lopez, A. D., & the Disease Control Priorities Project. (2006). *Global burden of disease and risk factors.* New York: Oxford University Press; Washington, DC: World Bank.

Maty, S. C., Lynch, J. W., Raghunathan, T. E., & Kaplan, G. A. (2008). Childhood socioeconomic position, gender, adult body mass index, and incidence of type 2 diabetes mellitus over 34 years in the Alameda County Study. *American Journal of Public Health, 98*(8), 1486–1494.

Mohr, S. B., Garland, C. F., Gorham, E. D., & Garland, F. C. (2008). The association between ultraviolet B irradiance, vitamin D status and incidence rates of type 1 diabetes in 51 regions worldwide. *Diabetologia, 51*(8), 1391–1398.

National Center for Health Statistics. (2008). Leading causes of death. Available at *www.cdc.gov/nchs/fastats.lcod.htm.*

Ohira, T., Hozawa, A., Iribarren, C., Daviglus, M. L., Matthews, K. A., Gross, M. D., et al. (2008). Longitudinal association of serum carotenoids and tocopherols with hostility: The CARDIA Study. *American Journal of Epidemiology, 167*(1), 42–50.

Owing, J. H. (2005). *Trends in smoking and health research.* New York: Nova Biomedical Books.

Petitti, D. B., Teutsch, S. M., Barton, M. B., Sawaya, G. F., Ockene, J. K., & DeWitt, T. (2009). Update on the methods of the U.S. Preventive Services Task Force: Insufficient evidence. *Annals of Internal Medicine, 150*(3), 199–205.

Peto, R., Chen, Z. M., & Boreham, J. (1999). Tobacco—the growing epidemic [news]. *Nature Medicine, 5*(1), 15–17.

Sackett, D. L., Straus, S. E., Richardson, W. S., Rosenberg, W., & Haynes, R. B. (2000). *Evidence-based medicine* (2nd ed.). Edinburgh, UK: Churchill Livingston.

Sacks, H., Chalmers, T. C., & Smith, H., Jr. (1982). Randomized versus historical controls for clinical trials. *American Journal of Medicine, 72*(2), 233–240.

Sawaya, G. F., Guirguis-Blake, J., LeFevre, M., Harris, R., & Petitti, D. (2007). Update on the methods of the U.S. Preventive Services Task Force: Estimating certainty and magnitude of net benefit. *Annals of Internal Medicine, 147*(12), 871–875.

See, R., Lindsey, J. B., Patel, M. J., Ayers, C. R., Khera, A., McGuire, D. K., et al. (2008). Application of the screening for Heart Attack Prevention and Education Task Force recommendations to an urban population: Observations from the Dallas Heart Study. *Archives of Internal Medicine, 168*(10), 1055–1062.

Snow, J., Frost, W. H., & Richardson, B. W. (1936). *Snow on cholera.* New York: The Commonwealth Fund; London: Humphrey Milford, Oxford University Press.

Timmreck, T. C. (1994). *An introduction to epidemiology.* Boston: Jones & Bartlett.

Turrell, G., Lynch, J. W., Leite, C., Raghunathan, T., & Kaplan, G. A. (2007). Socioeconomic disadvantage in childhood and across the life course and all-cause mortality and physical function in adulthood: Evidence from the Alameda County Study. *Journal of Epidemiology and Community Health, 61*(8), 723–730.

U.S. Surgeon General's Advisory Committee on Smoking and Health. (1964). *Smoking and health: Report of the Advisory Committee to the Surgeon General of the Public Health Service.* Princeton, NJ: Van Nostrand.

Wang, W. Z., Jiang, B., Wu, S. P., Hong, Z., Yang, Q. D., Sander, J. W., et al. (2007). Change in stroke incidence from a population-based intervention trial in three urban communities in China. *Neuroepidemiology, 28*(3), 155–161.

Welsh, M. L., Buist, D. S., Aiello Bowles, E. J., Anderson, M. L., Elmore, J. G., & Li, C. I. (2009). Population-based estimates of the relation between breast cancer risk, tumor subtype, and family history. *Breast Cancer Research and Treatment, 14*(3), 549–558.

Yen, I. H., & Kaplan, G. A. (1999). Neighborhood social environment and risk of death: Multilevel evidence from the Alameda County Study. *American Journal of Epidemiology, 149*(10), 898–907.

Yusuf, S., Collins, R., & Peto, R. (1984). Why do we need some large, simple randomized trials? *Statistics in Medicine, 3*(4), 409–422.

CHAPTER 14

Depression and Illness

Madeline Li
Gary Rodin

Medical illnesses and depressive disorders commonly coexist in the general population, and their comorbidity occurs more frequently than would be expected on the basis of their coincidental association. Depressive disorders may occur with increased frequency in chronic medical conditions because of multiple nonspecific risk factors, and perhaps because of specific depressogenic factors in particular medical conditions. Alternatively, the relationship between depressive disorders and medical illness could be mediated through shared biological mechanisms (Capuron et al., 2008).

The World Health Organization projects that by the year 2020, depression will be the second leading cause of disability, after cardiovascular disease. Medical illness is associated with the exacerbation of depressive disorders, increased treatment resistance, and higher rates of depressive relapse (Iosifescu, 2007). Depressive disorders, in turn, may worsen quality of life, reduce treatment compliance, and increase morbidity and mortality in many medical illnesses. Depression is also associated with higher rates of health care utilization, with medical costs up to 50% higher than those

attributed to medical illness alone, unrelated to the costs of specialty mental health care (Unutzer et al., 2009).

Depression remains underdiagnosed and undertreated in medical settings, despite the availability of pharmacological and psychological interventions with demonstrated efficacy. Barriers to the identification of depressive symptoms in the medically ill include stigma associated with psychological distress, difficulty distinguishing normative from pathological distress and physical symptoms of depression from those of medical illness, lack of training or comfort of medical caregivers with emotional inquiry, and mistaken beliefs about the untreatability of depression that has a realistic or understandable basis.

This chapter reviews the clinical features and diagnostic issues, epidemiology, psychobiology, and approaches to treatment of depressive disorders in medical illness. Clinically relevant unanswered questions are emphasized, with suggestions for future research directions. Throughout the text, the term "depression" refers to the spectrum of depressive disorders, including major depressive disorder, dysthymic disorder, and subthreshold or minor depressive disorders. The chapter focuses on the common mechanisms by which depression may emerge in a range of medical conditions.

The Continuum of Depression

Currently, the *Diagnostic and Statistical Manual of Mental Disorders*, fourth edition, text revision (DSM-IV-TR; American Psychiatric Association, 2000) specifies six categories of depressive disorders, including (1) major depressive disorder (MDD), (2) dysthymic disorder (DD), (3) mood disorder due to a (specified) general medical condition (GMC), (4) substance-induced mood disorder, (5) adjustment disorder with depressed mood, and (6) depressive disorder not otherwise specified (NOS), which includes subthreshold depressive disorders that do not meet full criteria for the other specified depressive disorders. However, although such diagnostic systems categorize discrete syndromes, depressive symptoms occur on a fluid continuum. At the milder end of this continuum are symptoms that may be regarded as nonpathological sadness and grief. In the middle, lie adjustment disorders and subthreshold depressions, which are the most prevalent depressive disorders among medically ill patients. At the more severe end of the continuum are depressive symptoms that may clearly meet diagnostic criteria for MDD, particularly severe MDD. These categories have heuristic and communicative value, but the boundaries between them are somewhat arbitrary and often difficult to establish.

Normative Responses to Medical Illness

Serious illness is frequently associated with changes in physical appearance, distressing physical symptoms, impairment of psychosocial and occupational functioning, alterations in the life trajectory of those affected, increased uncertainty about the future, and the threat of mortality. These consequences most often evoke at least transient feelings of grief and sadness that can be regarded as normative and nonpathological. The question of what should or should not be considered a psychiatric disorder is complex and involves equal risks of pathologizing normal

sadness and of neglecting clinically significant and treatable depressive symptoms.

Adjustment Disorder with Depressed Mood

The category of adjustment disorder lies in a transitional zone on the continuum of distress between normative responses and psychopathology. It is conceptualized in the DSM-IV-TR as emotional and/or behavioral symptoms "in excess of what would be expected" from exposure to a given stressor. The lack of operational criteria for this diagnosis, and the difficulty in establishing the boundary between normative and "excessive" responses to the multiple and chronic stressors of medical illness, raise questions about its validity in this context. However, the diagnosis of adjustment disorder may be of clinical value when used to capture prodromal or transient states of distress that are amenable to preventive or early interventions.

Subthreshold Depression

The rubric of subthreshold depression includes minor depressive disorder, which refers to the presence of two to four depressive symptoms for more than 2 weeks, and DD, which is characterized by less severe depressive symptoms that have been continuously present for at least 2 years. The latter may be found in association with medical illness because of the multiple, repetitive, and persistent stressors and disability that may occur. These are the most common depressive syndromes in medical populations. They do not usually progress to MDD but deserve clinical attention because they can substantially impair quality of life and the capacity to comply with medical treatment.

Diagnostic Complexity of MDD in Medical Illness

A categorical diagnosis of MDD is based on the presence of five or more symptoms, which must include a depressed mood or anhedonia for at least 2 weeks, most of the day, nearly every day that represents a significant change from previous functioning. Neurovegetative criteria include impairment in sleep, altered appetite with weight change, loss of energy, and psychomotor retardation or agitation. Psychological criteria include feelings of worthlessness, hopelessness, or excessive guilt; cognitive impairment; and recurrent suicidal ideation.

The heterogeneity of MDD is captured in the clinical subtypes, including atypical depression (increased appetite and hypersomnia), melancholia (diurnal variation in mood and early morning awakening), psychotic or catatonic depression (mood-congruent delusions or hallucinations, or extreme psychomotor disturbance), and anxious depression (prominent anxiety symptoms). These subtypes of MDD have been shown in the general population to have different treatment responsiveness, but relatively little attention has been paid to such differences in the context of medical illness. Furthermore, the diagnosis of MDD in the medically ill is complicated by the overlap of symptoms of MDD with those of medical illness. Diagnostic uncertainty related to this overlap may arise from the following:

1. The difficulty distinguishing depressive anhedonia from illness-related functional impairment. However, the index of suspicion for depression should be heightened when limitations in activity appear to be disproportionate to the expected functional capacity.

2. The overlap of symptoms of depression with those directly related to the medical illness. Many medical illnesses, such as cancer or AIDS, are associated with neurovegetative symptoms, such as fatigue, anorexia, weight loss, insomnia, psychomotor retardation, and cognitive impairment. In neurological conditions, such as stroke, "emotionalism," or pathological crying, can be mistaken for depression. It may also be difficult to distinguish the cognitive and motor slowing of depression from that associated with hypoactive delirium, common in the terminally ill, or from the apathy associated with the dementias. Parkinson's disease, in particular, is characterized by akinesia and masked facies, which can easily be mistaken for MDD.

3. The atypical presentation with somatic symptoms of MDD in medical populations. In such cases, somatic symptoms due to depression may be difficult to distinguish from symptoms of the medical illness itself. Furthermore, behavioral manifestations of depression, such as treatment noncompliance or refusal, may also be unrecognized as depressive in origin.

4. The difficulty distinguishing depressive suicidality from nonpathological thoughts of death, a desire for hastened death, or demoralization. The core features of demoralization, which overlaps with but is distinct from depression, are subjective feelings of incompetence, a negative view of self in relation to the future; feelings of panic and threat; and existential despair. Demoralization has a prevalence of up to 30% in some medical populations and may deserve clinical attention, although it is not recognized within DSM-IV classification.

5. The overlap of the categories of MDD, mood disorder due to a GMC, and substance-induced mood disorder in the context of medical illness. The diagnoses of mood disorder due to a GMC and substance-induced mood disorder both imply that the etiology of the depression is a direct physiological consequence of the specified GMC or substance. However, no specific pathophysiology, medical illness, or substance has been shown to have a linear causal relationship to depression. Instead, the bulk of recent evidence suggests that depression has a multifactorial etiology with biological, psychological, and social contributors.

Epidemiology of Depression in Illness

The lifetime prevalence of depression in the general population of adults in the United States is 17% (Kessler et al., 2003). Prevalence in medical populations is higher, but there is large variability in the reported prevalence rates, presumably due to diagnostic, methodological, clinical, and social factors. Simon, Goldberg, Von Korff, and Ustun (2002) demonstrated a 15-fold variation in the prevalence of current MDD, in the context of medical illness, in a study of depression in 25,000 primary care patients across 14 countries. In that regard, rates of depression in cancer have varied from 8 to 57%, depending on the cancer type, hospitalization status, diagnostic strategy, measurement tool, diagnostic thresholds, and stage of cancer (Massie, 2004).

The timing of the assessment of depression in the medically ill is an important variable because the presence and severity of symptoms may fluctuate over time. This complicates comparisons, since most studies have assessed rates of depression in medical illness cross-sectionally and at variable time points in the illness. Furthermore, some prevalence estimates are based on depression rating scales, for which there are no established cutoff points or thresholds for a categorical determination of MDD, DD, or subthreshold depression. Rates of MDD, which are based on such measures, vary considerably depending on the cutoff points employed.

The prevalence of MDD in medical illness increases with the severity of the illness. Accordingly, the prevalence of MDD progressively increases from 2 to 4% in community samples, 5 to 10% in primary care settings, and 6 to 14% in medical inpatient wards (Burvill, 1995). Minor depressive disorders are likely even more common, and are reported in up to 16% of medical outpatients and 64% of medical inpatients (Beck & Koenig, 1996; Burvill, 1995). Table 14.1 lists prevalence rates of MDD in specific medical illnesses, including cancer, diabetes, cardiovascular disease, HIV/AIDS, stroke, epilepsy, multiple sclerosis, Alzheimer's disease, and Parkinson's disease.

Psychobiology of Depression in Illness

A plethora of factors increase the risk of depression in medical illness, including younger age, personal or family history of depression, less social support, greater attachment anxiety, poorer communication with medical caregivers, greater illness intrusiveness and disability, maladaptive coping strategies, greater pain and treatment intensity, more advanced disease, and proximity to death (Lo, Li, & Rodin, 2008). Indeed, depression can be understood as the final common pathway of the interaction of disease-related, psychological, and social factors.

Depression in the context of medical illness is a prime example of the biopsychosocial model of psychiatric formulation. Mechanisms of comorbidity between depression and medical illness include both pathophysiological and psychosocial factors. The former include medications, systemic inflammation, neurological disorders, and genetic vulnerability. Psychosocial factors include demographic characteristics, personality traits, and relational factors, all of which may contribute to the stigma and personal meaning associated with illness. A model for the interaction of these multiple risk and protective factors in the emergence of depression is depicted in Figure 14.1.

Medications

A broad range of prescription medications have been linked etiologically to depression. No medications have been shown to cause the typical MDD syndrome, although evidence links corticosteroids, interferon-alpha, interleukin-2, gonadotrophin-releasing hormone agonists, and mefloquine to depression (Patten & Barbui, 2004). Cytokines, such as the interferons and interleukin-2, are immunomodulatory agents that result in "sickness behaviors," behavioral changes that overlap with depressive symptoms, in-

TABLE 14.1. Prevalence of Major Depressive Disorder in Select Medical Illnesses

Medical illness	Prevalence (%)	Reference
Cancer	8–57	Massie (2004)
Diabetes	9–26	Musselman et al. (2003)
Cardiovascular disease	17–27	Rudisch & Nemeroff (2003)
HIV/AIDS	5–20	Cruess et al. (2003)
Stroke	14–19	Robinson (2003)
Epilepsy	20–55	Kanner (2003)
Multiple sclerosis	40–60	Wallin et al. (2006)
Alzheimer's disease	30–50	Lee & Lyketos (2003)
Parkinson's disease	4–75	McDonald et al. (2003)

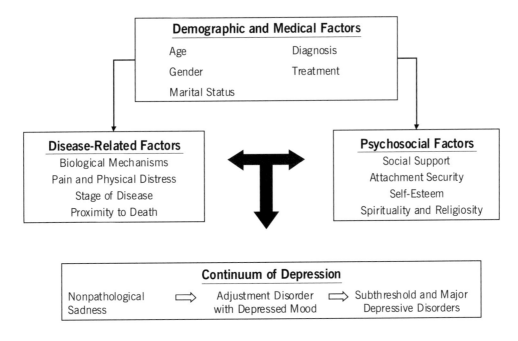

FIGURE 14.1. Model of pathways to depressive disorders in medical illness.

cluding anhedonia, fatigue, cognitive disturbance, anxiety, irritability, psychomotor slowing, anorexia, sleep alterations, and hyperalgesia (Dantzer, O'Connor, Freund, Johnson, & Kelley, 2008). These "sickness behaviors" occur in up to 45% of hepatitis patients treated with interferon, appear soon after cytokine administration, and disappear shortly after termination of treatment. The demonstration that prophylactic treatment with the antidepressant paroxetine prevents the development of the depressive symptoms supports the "cytokine hypothesis of depression," which postulates that depression may be linked to immune-activated systemic inflammation and elaboration of proinflammatory cytokines (Raison, Capuron, & Miller, 2006).

Immune-Activated Systemic Inflammation

Classically, the pathophysiology of depression has been described in terms of alterations in monoamine neurotransmitters such as serotonin, norepinephrine, and dopamine. Hypersecretion of the neuropeptide hormone corticotropin-releasing hormone (CRH) and subsequent activation of the hypothalamic–pituitary–adrenal (HPA) axis

and sympathetic nervous system are also well known biological substrates in the link between psychosocial stress and depression. The association between systemic immune activation and cytokines as mediators of depression is a new and rapidly expanding area of research, in which several pathophysiological mechanisms for cytokine-induced depression have been proposed, specifically involving alterations of monoamine metabolism and HPA axis function (Dantzer et al., 2008; Raison et al., 2006).

The evidence for immune-activated systemic inflammation in MDD in nonmedical populations has been inconsistent (Raison et al., 2006). However, this pathophysiological mechanism may have greater plausibility in the context of depression in medical illness. It has been evoked in such cases to explain the bidirectional relationship between depression and medical illnesses associated with inflammation. Although most often studied as a contributor to depression in the context of cancer, there is now a growing appreciation that inflammatory processes are central to a number of common illnesses, including diabetes, cardiovascular disease (CVD), and infectious diseases, such as HIV/AIDS.

Cancer

Psychological distress in cancer arises from both physical and psychosocial disease-related factors that impact every domain of daily life. Depression in patients with more advanced disease may be related not only to the psychological consequences of this state but also to tumor cell burden and tissue destruction that contribute to the release of proinflammatory cytokines. In this regard, a few studies have demonstrated increases in plasma interleukin-6 and neuroendocrine alterations in cancer patients with depression (Miller, Ancoli-Israel, Bower, Capuron, & Irwin, 2008).

Diabetes

Depression is an independent risk factor for the development of Type 2 diabetes mellitus, possibly mediated through its association with increased serum glucocorticoids, catecholamines, growth hormones, insulin resistance, and cytokine secretion (Musselman, Betan, Larsen, & Phillips, 2003). Depression is also associated with poor glycemic control, either through decreased treatment compliance or metabolic abnormalities increasing insulin resistance, and with increased mortality. Conversely, diabetes may also contribute to the development of depression, possibly through the common metabolic abnormalities and the associated psychosocial adversities, including diet restrictions, daily insulin injections, and living with the risks of complications such as blindness, renal failure, neuropathy, and vascular disease.

Cardiovascular Disease

The strongest evidence for a specific mechanism to account for bidirectional comorbidity may be in the relationship between depression and CVD (Parissis et al., 2007). Depression is both an independent cardiac risk factor and is also common in patients with CVD (including coronary artery disease, unstable angina, acute myocardial infarction, congestive heart failure, and coronary artery bypass graft surgery). This association is of great clinical concern, in view of the correlations that have been found between depression and post–myocardial

infarction mortality. Although some studies have challenged this finding, a recent meta-analysis confirms the association between depression and cardiac mortality. Its authors suggest that improvements in treatment and decreases in overall cardiac fatalities account for the lack of association in later studies (van Melle et al., 2004).

There are at least five hypothesized mechanisms to account for a specific comorbidity for depression and CVD:

1. Systemic inflammation involving cytokines, C-reactive protein, and tryptophan degradation pathways that promote atherothrombosis.
2. HPA and sympathoadrenal dysregulation, resulting in increased plasma catecholamines.
3. Decreased heart rate variability, which may result from excess catecholamines altering parasympathetic and sympathetic nervous system control.
4. Excessive platelet aggregation, which is associated with thrombosis, atherosclerosis, and acute coronary syndromes, and that may result from abnormal platelet serotonin ($5\text{-}HT_2$) receptors.
5. Poor health behaviors, including smoking, alcohol consumption, and lack of exercise and compliance with treatment (Huffman, Smith, Quinn, & Fricchione, 2006).

In addition, there has been speculation about the role of other depression-related affective states that may be comorbid with CVD, including anxiety, anger/hostility, and a mixed negative emotional syndrome (Huffman et al., 2006). These affective states may also adversely affect engagement in heart-healthy lifestyle changes and treatment compliance.

HIV/AIDS

Depression, one of the most common psychiatric disorders in people with HIV, is associated with poor compliance with antiretroviral treatment, deterioration in psychosocial functioning, more rapid progression to AIDS, and higher mortality (Cruess et al., 2003). It has also been suggested that depression-related increases in cortisol and cytokine secretion might affect HIV entry and replication, thereby increasing the risk of infection (Leserman, 2003). Alternatively, depression and HIV infection may share a common association with dysregulation of the HPA axis and the sympathetic nervous system, which may account for their comorbidity. Numerous psychosocial stressors unique to HIV/AIDS infection may contribute to the development of depression in these patients, including stigma, poor social support, antiretroviral-induced body image changes, and increased frequency of bereavement in social support networks.

Multiple Medical Comorbidities

HPA axis dysfunction and cytokine elevations have been implicated in several other chronic conditions in association with depression. These include hypertension, ulcers, chronic obstructive pulmonary disease (COPD), arthritis, obesity, chronic pain, and osteoporosis (Iosifescu, 2007). The lifetime prevalence of depression increases from 9 to 13% in patients when the medical comorbidity increases from one to more than one associated condition, and this multiple comorbidity defines a population with increased functional disability. In addition to disease-specific psychosocial stressors, systemic inflammation may represent a common denominator that mediates the relationship of these diverse conditions to depression.

Neurological Disorders

High rates of depression are seen in both cortical and subcortical neurological disorders, including cerebrovascular disease (Robinson, 2003), epilepsy (Kanner, 2003), dementia (Lee & Lyketsos, 2003), Parkinson's disease (McDonald, Richard, & DeLong, 2003), and multiple sclerosis (Wallin, Wilken, Turner, Williams, & Kane, 2006). Each of these disorders is associated with significant psychosocial stress related to living with a progressive and incurable disease that may directly affect cognitive functioning, psychological coping strategies, or the capacity to engage in psychological treatments. Neurological compromise significantly impairs activities of daily living and increases caregiver burden, which may increase the risk of depression. In addition to

these psychosocial stressors, depression in neurological disorders may also be related to neurochemical and structural changes affecting brain function.

The pathogenesis of depression in neurological disorders may be related to neuroanatomical pathways involved in depression. The limbic–cortical–striatal–pallidal–thalamic tract is thought to be involved in emotional regulation and is associated with tract volume loss in patients with depression. Damage to structures involved in this tract, including the frontal cortex, hippocampus, thalamus, amygdala, and basal ganglia, can be identified in neurological disorders (Sheline, 2003) and may be related to central inflammation, recapitulating the peripheral immune-mediated inflammatory mechanisms implicated in depression.

Associations of depression with brain lesion localization have been reported for epilepsy, poststroke depression, and multiple sclerosis (Benedetti, Bernasconi, & Pontiggia, 2006). Postseizure depression has been correlated with temporal lobe epilepsy and abnormalities in 5HT receptor binding outside of the epileptogenic zone. Left-sided anterior lesions were postulated to be implicated in poststroke depression, but a large recent meta-analysis did not confirm this association (Carson et al., 2000). Neuroimaging studies have defined microangiopathic insults resulting in hyperintensities of white and deep gray matter in the basal ganglia and frontal lobes as correlates of "vascular depression." Depression was also found to be associated with lesions in the left inferior medial frontal region and atrophy in left anterior temporal regions in patients with multiple sclerosis.

Degenerative changes may underlie the pathogenesis of depression in conditions such as dementia, Parkinson's disease, and Huntington's disease (Benedetti et al., 2006). Depression in Alzheimer's dementia has been associated with noradrenergic neuronal loss in the locus coeruleus and serotonergic cell loss in the dorsal raphe nucleus. Subcortical white matter infarcts have been associated with depression in both vascular and Alzheimer's dementia. The overlapping symptoms of psychomotor retardation, apathy, and neurovegetative disturbance in depression and Parkinson's disease may reflect a common pathophysiology involving dopamine depletion in the basal ganglia–thalmus–frontal cortex circuit, although monoaminergic deficits resulting from extensive cell loss in the locus coeruleus and raphe nuclei have also been implicated.

Stroke, Alzheimer's disease, and multiple sclerosis all can be considered to be neuroinflammatory disorders, in which immune-mediated central inflammation may contribute to the development of depression. The same platelet reactivity and adrenocortical hyperreactivity implicated in the bidirectional risk of depression and CVD, may also explain the association between depression and stroke. The role of neuroinflammation in the pathology of Alzheimer's disease is now well recognized (Leonard, 2007). In multiple sclerosis, an inflammatory demyelinating disease, increased expression of the cytokine interferon-gamma is related to depression severity, with decreased levels associated with psychotherapy or pharmacotherapy (Mohr, Goodkin, Islar, Hauser, & Genain, 2001). Thus far, however, the prevalence of depression in neurological disease has not been shown to be greater than in any other medical conditions when comparisons control for the severity of disease and the extent of disability.

Genetic Vulnerability

Genetic vulnerability is clearly a risk factor in depression. Family studies indicate that the risk of developing depression is three to four times higher in relatives of patients with MDD, and twin studies estimate that 30–40% of the variance in liability to develop MDD is attributable to genetic factors (Levinson, 2006). In the context of specific medical illnesses, susceptibility to depression has been linked to apolipoprotein E (*ApoE4*) alleles in Alzheimer's disease (Kim, Shin, & Yoon, 2002) and the low-activity serotonin transporter polymorphism (*5-HTTLPR*) allele in Parkinson's disease (Mossner et al., 2001), although these results have yet to be consistently replicated. Common genetic vulnerabilities accounting for the frequent comorbidity of depression and CVD have also been suggested, with almost 20% of the genetic influence on depression and CVD being commonly shared (Scherrer et al., 2003).

Psychosocial Risk Factors

Depression in medical populations has been associated with demographic, psychological, and social factors. In that regard, it has been found consistently that age is inversely related to the severity of depressive symptoms (Cleland, Lee, & Hall, 2007). The explanation for this finding is not known, but speculations have included the greater disruption of life trajectory caused by medical illness in younger individuals, the diminishing tendency to experience or communicate distress with advanced age, the potentially greater stigma associated with emotional distress in older patients, or a biologically determined reduction in affective intensity with advanced age. An association of depression has been found with gender in many studies of depression in the general population. This finding has been attributed to factors such as education, socioeconomic status, and adverse life events that occur disproportionately in women, although biological factors have also been postulated. However, many studies of depression in medical populations have not found a gender difference in the prevalence of depression (Rodin, Walsh, et al., 2007). It may be that the overriding common stressors related to the medical illness obliterate differences due to gender.

Individual differences related to social and psychological factors have also been shown to affect the risk of depression. Factors such as self-esteem and spirituality (Rodin, Walsh, et al., 2007) and the capacity to express affect (Classen et al., 2008) have been shown to correlate with the severity of depressive symptoms. Social support has also been shown in a variety of studies to buffer the stresses of more severe illness and physical symptoms, and to protect against the emergence of more severe depressive symptoms. More recent evidence suggests that expectations of support and the capacity for flexible use of social support, captured in the construct of attachment security, may protect against the emergence of depressive symptoms in medically ill patients (Rodin, Walsh, et al., 2007). Those with less attachment security may be more likely to become depressed and may be in double jeopardy, since they may also have less ability to attract and to experience social support. There is also a literature that has linked specific coping strategies to depression (Lynch, Kroencke, & Denney, 2001), although it has been difficult in some studies to distinguish between what is a cause and what is an effect of depression.

Diagnostic Considerations

Various strategies have been proposed for diagnosing depression in the context of medical illness, none of which has demonstrated consistent validity. Four main approaches have been described (Trask, 2004):

1. The inclusive approach, which accepts all of the DSM-IV diagnostic criteria for MDD, regardless of whether they are attributed to depression or to physical illness. This approach maximizes sensitivity at the expense of specificity, and may be appropriate in clinical situations in which resources are available to assess a larger proportion of screened patients. The DSM-IV utilizes the etiological approach, counting symptoms only if they clearly are not due to the physical illness. However, this distinction relies heavily on inference by a clinician who may not be able to determine whether a physical or psychological symptom is normal or excessive in the context of a particular illness.

2. The exclusive approach, which removes symptoms if they do not occur more frequently in depressed than in nondepressed patients with illness. This primarily excludes the somatic symptoms of fatigue and of appetite and weight changes, thereby reducing the number of diagnostic criteria. It maximizes specificity but identifies only the most severe cases of depression. This may be preferable in specific research applications, in which the wish is to minimize false-positive diagnoses.

3. The substitutive approach, which replaces physical symptoms (e.g., fatigue, weight loss, impaired concentration) with symptoms that are more affective and cognitive in origin (e.g., indecisiveness, irritability, social withdrawal). However, there is no established standard by which somatic or affective–cognitive symptoms should be selected.

Depression and anxiety commonly occur together as manifestations of psychological distress in medical illness. A detailed discussion of anxiety disorders in medical illness is beyond the scope of this chapter, although there are several recent reviews on this topic (Roy-Byrne et al., 2008). However, many of the risk factors, possibly the psychobiology, and even the treatment of anxiety overlap with depression. Most psychological distress screening tools capture both anxiety and depressive symptoms, emphasizing the importance of recognizing anxiety in the diagnosis of depression. In fact, many depression rating scales include anxiety symptoms, which contributes to their low specificity and poor positive predictive value (PPV) when used as screening tools for depression.

Measurement and Screening for Depression in Medical Populations

There is no "gold standard" for the diagnosis of depression, particularly in the context of medical illness, although clinical interviews are considered to be most valid. They include unstructured inclusive or substitutive interviews, or more structured diagnostic instruments, such as the Schedule for Affective Disorders and Schizophrenia (SADS), the Structured Clinical Interview for DSM Disorders (SCID), Research Diagnostic Criteria (RDC), the Diagnostic Interview Schedule (DIS), the Mini-International Neuropsychiatric Interview, the Present State Examination (PSE), or the Primary Care Evaluation of Mental Disorders (PRIME-MD) (Rush, First, & Blacker, 2008).

Numerous psychometric measures have been developed to assess depression, with variable reliability and validity depending upon the applications. The cutoff scores utilized with such measures determine their sensitivity and specificity. Higher cutoffs are more likely to yield true prevalence rates of depression and may be preferable for research studies and the determination of resource allocation, while lower thresholds may be preferable in treatment settings where there is a high priority on not missing cases and on identifying subthreshold disorders.

The use of depression rating scales ensures that relevant symptoms are assessed comprehensively and in a standardized fashion, and provides consistency of assessment across time and across examiners. Such tools can be used for multiple clinical purposes, including measurement of depression severity or symptom change with time, as diagnostic aids, or as screening tools to identify patients in need of further assessment. Most tools demonstrate good reliability and validity for measuring and monitoring symptom severity in populations with diagnosed mood disorders. However, they cannot be used independently to establish a diagnosis of depression. Therefore, a two-stage approach is required; a first-stage screen to identify individuals likely to have depression, followed by a second-stage clinical diagnostic interview.

Missed diagnoses of depression in the medically ill result in a lost opportunity to improve quality of life and treatment compliance, and to decrease the length of hospital stays and suicide risk. Yet numerous barriers limit the identification of depression in medical populations. Most medical visits last less than 15 minutes, and the majority of that time is devoted to medical symptoms. Such time constraints may limit disclosure or elaboration of psychological symptoms. In addition, some clinicians lack experience and comfort with responding to the emotions that may be elicited by inquiry about patients' psychological state. Some patients may be reluctant to disclose depressive symptoms for fear of stigma, or their own lack of knowledge about the importance and availability of treatment for depression. For these reasons, there has been a move to introduce standardized depression screening into medical clinics as part of the routine general health assessment. A screening program can facilitate psychosocial resource planning and referral of patients for psychosocial and psychiatric treatment. Requirements of a screening tool are that it be accurate and rapid, easy to administer and score, and acceptable to patients.

Depression Rating Scales

The Center for Epidemiologic Studies Depression Scale (CES-D; Radloff, 1977) was developed to measure depressive symptoms in community populations. It does not include items that assess changes in appetite or sleep, anhedonia, guilt, psychomotor changes, or suicidal thoughts. In fact, only four of 20 items on the CES-D measure somatic symptoms. The CES-D has been used exten-

sively in medical populations and has good reliability, although there is a lack of consensus regarding the optimal cutoff score. The low PPV of the CES-D to detect depression in some studies suggests that it might better be considered a measure of general distress than of depression.

The Hospital Anxiety and Depression Scale (HADS; Zigmond & Snaith, 1983) was specifically designed for use in primary care or hospital settings and excludes somatic symptoms of depression. It has separate 7-item subscales for anxiety and depression, and has been used extensively in medical populations. The HADS has good concurrent and discriminant validity, and is sensitive to changes in severity. However, it has not been well validated as a screening instrument; some studies report acceptable accuracy, whereas others report unacceptably low sensitivity, specificity, and PPV (Rush et al., 2008). There is also a lack of consensus about whether the total HADS score or the Depressive subscale score should be used for screening. These conflicting data suggest that the HADS may be of limited value as a screening tool in medical populations.

The Beck Depression Inventory–II (BDI-II; Beck, Steer, & Brown, 1996) is a newer version of the BDI, which was originally developed to measure depression severity in psychiatric patients. Its modifications were intended to reflect DSM-IV criteria better than the BDI and, accordingly, it contains a preponderance of somatic items, with 13 out of 21 items contributing to a Somatic subscale score. There have been concerns about its validity in medical populations and its acceptability to patients, due to its forced-choice format and complex response alternatives. However, it has been used in numerous studies of depression in medical illness, and it has been found to be accurate as a screening tool in these populations.

The PHQ-9 is the 9-item Depression module of the Patient Health Questionnaire, a self-report version of the PRIME-MD, a diagnostic instrument to assess mental disorders in primary care settings (Spitzer, Kroenke, & Williams, 1999). The PHQ-9 scores each of the nine DSM-IV diagnostic criteria for a major depressive episode from 0 (*Not at all*) to 3 (*Nearly every day*). It also has demonstrated sensitivity to changes in severity, with scores of 5, 10, 15, and 20 representing *Mild*, *Moderate*, *Moderately Severe*, and *Severe* depression, respectively. The PHQ-9 is therefore the only tool that can be used as both a screening and a diagnostic tool, and a cutoff score of 10 has been recommended for screening purposes.

Ultrabrief Screening Scales

Ultrabrief screening tools, involving fewer than five questions, are a simple method for detecting depression in medical illness, based on their ability to exclude possible cases of depression. Such tools include the single-item Distress Thermometer, a 10-point visual analogue distress scale advocated by the National Comprehensive Cancer Network, single-item questions (e.g., "Are you depressed?" or "Do you often feel sad or depressed?"), the 4-item Geriatric Depression Scale, and the 2-item PHQ-2 (reviewed in Mitchell, 2007). Recent pooled analyses of such tools in cancer (Mitchell, 2007) and primary care (Mitchell & Coyne, 2007) populations reveal overall PPVs of 34% and 38%, respectively. Such tools can therefore be considered a first-stage screen but are best suited to situations where there are sufficient resources for second-stage assessment to establish diagnoses in those who screen positive.

The amount of time required for patients to complete the measure is one of several practical considerations in choosing a screening tool. Clinician time to administer, to score, and to interpret the measure, training requirements for evaluators, and copyright costs are others. Most significantly, recent critical reviews of depression screening suggest that patient outcomes are only improved by such screening when accompanied by effective treatment and follow-up (Palmer & Coyne, 2003). Instituting depression screening programs is a costly process that is unlikely to be beneficial unless sufficient resources are available to ensure parity, accessibility, delivery, and monitoring of treatment.

Treatment of Depression in Medically Ill Persons

Clinical treatment of depression in the context of medical illness is largely extrapolated from what is known about pharmacotherapy and psychotherapy in nonmedical populations. Pharmacotherapy and psychotherapy are equally effective in treating mild to moderate depression in primary care populations (Cipriani, Geddes, Furukawa, & Barbui, 2007; Schulberg, Raue, & Rollman, 2002). People with more severe depression may respond better to a combination of both modalities. The preponderance of evidence suggests that these treatment modalities are effective in depressed medically ill patients (Rodin, Lloyd, et al., 2007; Vamos, 2006), although some have suggested that depression in medical illness is associated with more treatment resistance, slower response rates, and higher relapse rates (Iosifescu, 2007). However, the relative absence of psychiatric comorbidity in medical populations suggests that the potential for treatment responsiveness may actually be greater than that in psychiatric populations.

Determination of the effectiveness of depression treatments in medically ill patients is important in weighing the costs and potential adverse effects of such treatment. The evidence base in this area is limited by a paucity of methodologically sound studies. Studies have often been difficult to compare because of variability in case identification, treatment, outcomes measures, follow-up, and missing data due to high dropout rates, likely related to the illness. The limited number of treatment studies for depression in the medically ill is likely a reflection of undertreatment in this population. Depression treatment is rarely included in general medical practice guidelines, and it is estimated that 60% of primary care patients with depression do not receive adequate treatment (Kessler et al., 2003).

Pharmacological Treatment

The effectiveness of antidepressant treatment has been demonstrated for many medical disorders (Krishnan, 2005). A recent Cochrane Review of randomized controlled trials comparing antidepressants to placebo for depression in medical illness provided evidence that all classes of antidepressants improve depressive symptoms in patients with a wide range of medical disorders (odds ratio of 2.33, 95% confidence interval 1.80–3.00, $p < 0.00001$). No one antidepressant was found to be more effective than another

(Rayner et al., 2010). Several recent systematic reviews of the treatment of depression in cancer suggest that, overall, antidepressants may be effective, but the evidence is limited at present (Rodin, Lloyd, et al., 2007). The weak evidence base is not equivalent to evidence of ineffectiveness, but it calls for more robust research in the treatment of depression in illness to inform the development of effective practice guidelines.

There are at least eight pharmacological classes of antidepressants, not one of which has been shown to be most effective for treating depression in illness, and all of which have differing risks and benefits in specific medical disorders.

Tricyclic/Heterocyclic Antidepressants and Monoamine Oxidase Inhibitors

These older classes of antidepressants have demonstrated effectiveness for depression in multiple medical conditions, as well as for neuropathic pain syndromes and the treatment of insomnia, which frequently accompanies medical conditions. However, they are discontinued in one-third of medical patients because of adverse effects. They have significant central and peripheral anticholinergic and antihistaminic side effects, and are strong antagonists at alpha-adrenergic receptors. These properties limit their use in cardiac disease due to hypotension and the potential for arrhythmias, in diabetes due to their anticholinergic and cardiac adverse effects, and in dementias due to their association with delirium and risk of hip fracture due to sedation and orthostatic hypotension. Finally, both tricyclic/heterocyclic antidepressants and monoamine oxidase inhibitors can be lethal in overdose. For these reasons, their role in the treatment of depression in illness has largely been replaced by newer antidepressant classes that have wider therapeutic windows, and are better tolerated and easier to administer.

Selective Serotonin Reuptake Inhibitors

The selective serotonin reuptake inhibitors (SSRIs) are generally regarded as first-line treatment for MDD in illness, along with psychological treatments, due to their relative safety and tolerability. SSRIs may also have additional benefits beyond treating depression in specific medical disorders. They may possess analgesic properties that alleviate the symptoms of diabetic neuropathy and of chronic pain syndromes. Fluoxetine has been shown to improve glycemic control in diabetes, and motor function and cognitive performance in stroke patients. Fluoxetine may ameliorate severe refractory orthostatic hypotension, and recent studies point to potential protective effects of SSRIs in the biology of cardiovascular disease (Paraskevaidis, Parissis, Fountoulaki, Filippatos, & Kremastinos, 2006). Paroxetine and sertraline effectively reduce hot flashes related to tamoxifen use in women with breast cancer, and in men requiring hormone therapy for prostate cancer.

Despite their benefits, caution must be exercised with SSRIs in medical illness, particularly in the presence of hepatic disease, due to their significant potential for drug interactions and altered pharmacokinetics. For example, paroxetine is a strong inhibitor of cytochrome P450-2D6, which has been found to decrease levels of the active metabolite of tamoxifen. Sertraline and citalopram appear to present the lowest risk of drug interactions. In addition, adverse effects of SSRIs may be problematic in some conditions, such as worsening the motor symptoms of Parkinson's disease. Short-term adverse effects of SSRIs include nausea and gastrointestinal disturbance, anxiety, headache, sedation, and tremor. Long-term potential side effects include sexual dysfunction, weight gain, the syndrome of inappropriate antidiuretic hormone secretion, and platelet dysfunction leading to bleeding.

Novel Antidepressants

The remaining pharmacological classes of antidepressants are newer agents that have become available in the last 15 years. These include the serotonin–norepinephrine reuptake inhibitors (SNRIs) (venlafaxine, duloxetine), norepinephrine–dopamine modulators (bupropion), norepinephrine reuptake inhibitors (reboxetine), reversible inhibitors of monoamine oxidase A (moclobemide), and noradrenergic and specific serotonergic antidepressants (mirtazapine). These agents are increasingly being used as alternatives to SSRIs in medical populations, although the empirical evidence for their safety and efficacy in these patients remains limited. Dual-action agents such as the SNRIs may be more effective than SSRIs for remission of depression.

The main adverse effects of these medications are hypertension with high doses of venlafaxine, and possible elevation of serum transaminases and bilirubin with duloxetine, limiting its use in patients with hepatic insufficiency or significant renal impairment. Bupropion has a favorable side effect profile in medical illness, in that it is not sedating, has little cardiotoxicity, and is not associated with sexual dysfunction. It may have particular application in medical populations with prominent fatigue and in the treatment of the neurovegetative symptoms of cytokine-induced depression. At higher doses, bupropion is associated with seizure risk and is therefore best avoided in patients with brain tumors or a history of seizures. Mirtazapine has a unique mechanism of action, in that it increases norepinephrine and serotonin levels through blockade of inhibitory alpha-2 adrenergic receptors. Unlike the SSRIs, it does not cause gastrointestinal disturbance, insomnia, anxiety, or sexual dysfunction, and it is associated with minimal drug interactions. Rather, it is associated with sedation, increased appetite and antiemetic effects, for which it has been proposed for multiple symptom palliation in advanced cancer.

Augmenting Agents

Psychostimulants such as methylphenidate or modafinil are often used in advanced illness and in palliative care settings due to their rapid onset of action and limited side effects. They are used either as single agents or in combination with other antidepressant medication. Methylphenidate can elevate mood rapidly, increase appetite, diminish fatigue, improve attention and concentration, and decrease sedation from opiates.

New directions in the pharmacotherapy of depression in patients with medical illness include targeting novel mechanisms of action, with a focus on more specific illness-related pathophysiology (Holmes, Heilig, Rupniak, Steckler, & Griebel, 2003). Potential targets include neurobiological treatments (e.g., CRH antagonists and cyclooxygenase [COX] inhibitors), as well as immunological treatments (e.g., cytokine antagonists, immunosuppressants, prostaglandin inhibitors, nitric oxide synthase inhibitors, and substance P inhibitors). Preliminary evidence exists for the antidepressant action of a corticotropin-releasing factor–1 (CRF_1) receptor antagonist (Nielsen, 2006). More recently, tumor necrosis factor–alpha (TNF-α) receptor inhibitors have demonstrated effectiveness on subthreshold depressive symptoms in psoriasis (Tyring et al., 2006).

Neurological Treatments

Electroconvulsive therapy (ECT) may be indicated in the medically ill with cases of severe or treatment-resistant depression, and in those with medical illnesses that contraindicate the use of antidepressants (e.g., severe renal, cardiac, or hepatic disease). ECT has been effective in the treatment of depression in Parkinson's disease, stroke, cancer, epilepsy, multiple sclerosis, endocrine disorders, and renal failure (Weiner & Coffey, 1993). Newer modalities of treatment for depression include repetitive transcranial magnetic stimulation (rTMS), and vagus nerve stimulation (Fitzgerald & Daskalakis, 2008). They have demonstrated impressive response rates in patients with neurological disorders, but this effect is short-lived. Given their limited side effects, absence of drug interactions, and safety in medical populations, these modalities are important directions for research on the treatment of depression in the medically ill.

Psychosocial Treatment

Psychological therapies have several advantages over pharmacological therapies in medical illness. They are free of physical side effects and drug–drug interactions. Also, they can be used not only to treat depressive symptoms but also to modify health behaviors that may adversely affect disease outcomes. Their use may be limited in patients with significant pain, fatigue, cognitive impairment, or more severe illness, or when there is a lack of motivation on the part of the patient.

Psychotherapy in medical populations may be distinguished by the collaborative relationships between the therapist and the patient's medical caregivers (Vamos, 2006), and by the frequent shifts in the patient's physical well-being and capacity to participate in and attend psychotherapeutic sessions. A recent Cochrane Review of psychotherapy for depression among incurable cancer patients concluded that psychotherapy is effective in decreasing depressive symptoms, but no studies were identified that focused on psychotherapy for the syndrome of MDD in advanced cancer (Akechi, Okuyama, Onishi, Morita, & Furukawa, 2008). The relationship with the primary medical health care provider and disease-specific support groups may also protect the patient from depression by maintaining morale, diminishing stigma, and promoting self-efficacy and a sense of mastery. Referral for a specific psychotherapeutic intervention should take into account the severity of depressive symptoms; the availability of social supports; the patient's motivation for psychological assistance; and his or her capacity for adaptation, introspection, and emotional expression.

Many psychosocial interventions have been studied in medical populations, including psychoeducational interventions, problem-solving therapy, cognitive-behavioral therapy (CBT), interpersonal therapy (IPT), and supportive–expressive therapy, on an individual or group basis. There has been some limited evidence that psychological interventions either reduce or prevent the emergence of depressive symptoms in patients with cancer (Jacobson, Rosenfeld, Pessin, & Breitbart, 2008), cardiovascular disease (Rivelli & Jiang, 2007), diabetes (Musselman et al., 2003), HIV/AIDS (Olatunji, Mimiaga, O'Cleirigh, & Safren, 2006), and multiple sclerosis (Wallin et al., 2006). Evidence for the effectiveness of psychological therapies in stroke and other neurological disorders is lacking. A randomized trial of CBT for poststroke depression found no evidence for benefit of the intervention (Lincoln & Flannaghan, 2003).

In cancer research there is considerable debate over the effectiveness and acceptability of psychosocial interventions for distress. Some researchers (Coyne, Lepore, & Palmer, 2006) argue that the evidence is not compelling enough to warrant an investment in psychosocial interventions. Others (Andrykowski & Manne, 2006) argue that the preponderance of evidence supports the benefit of psychosocial interventions. Resolution of this debate will have important implications for psychosocial intervention research in other medical conditions, where the number of studies is currently very limited.

Treatment Outcomes

Overall, the weight of evidence suggests that depression in the medically ill is responsive to psychological and/or pharmacological treatment. Although the negative impact of depression on illness is unequivocal and the bidirectional relationship between depression and medical illness is strong, evidence that treatment of depression improves medical outcomes is more equivocal. This question has been most extensively investigated in CVD and cancer, in several studies that have explored the relationship between treatment of depression and survival.

In CVD, randomized trials of pharmacological treatment for depression, such as the Sertraline Antidepressant Heart Attack Randomized Trial (SADHART; Glassman et al., 2002) and Myocardial Infarction and Depression-Intervention Trial (MIND-IT; van den Brink et al., 2002) studies, failed to demonstrate a statistically significant reduction in risk for cardiac events. Similarly, no beneficial effects on cardiac outcomes were found in studies of psychotherapeutic interventions, such as the Montreal Heart Attack Readjustment Trial (M-HEART; Frasure-Smith, 1995) and Enhancing Recovery in Coronary Heart Disease (ENRICHD; Berkman et al., 2003) trial, and, conversely, female patients demonstrated worse cardiac outcomes. It has been suggested that these studies in fact lacked power to detect significant differences given the modest effectiveness of treatment and the fact that certain antidepressant treatments (tricyclics, psychotherapy) may have pleiotropic effects that worsen cardiac outcomes (Rivelli & Jiang, 2007).

In cancer, supportive–expressive group therapy in women with metastatic breast cancer was found to prevent the emergence of depression (Kissane et al., 2007). It may be that the effectiveness of currently available treatments for depression in medical illness is too limited to overcome the physiological disease burden of advanced illness. Ultimately, the question of whether treatment of depression in medical illness has a significant impact on disease outcomes awaits the development of more effective treatments, possibly targeting common disease and depression-related pathophysiology.

Conclusions

Accumulated evidence has shown that depression is common in medical populations and is associated with impaired quality of life, reduced medical treatment compliance, and increased health care utilization. Although many factors can obscure the diagnosis of depression, failure to identify it most often results from a simple lack of inquiry. Screening measures may increase detection rates but are unlikely to improve outcomes, unless accompanied by the infusion of resources for treatment and follow-up.

The relationship between medical illness and depression appears to be reciprocal, with depression as both a common consequence of medical illness and a factor that influences the course of medical illness. The question of whether specific mechanisms link depression and a variety of medical conditions is an intriguing subject of much fruitful research that may help to illuminate the pathogenesis of depression. Further studies are warranted in medical populations, with attention to dimensional measures and subthreshold depression, the longitudinal course of depression, and the use of study designs that concurrently measure psychosocial and biological variables.

The overwhelming weight of evidence suggests that depression in the medically ill is directly related to the severity of the illness and arises as a result of a final common pathway of multiple risk and protective factors. Early and preventive measures may be valuable in high-risk groups to interrupt this cascade effect. Both psychological and pharmacological treatments have been shown to be effective in the treatment of major depression in medical populations. However, current evidence suggests that what is likely to be most effective is a multimodal approach that includes pain and symptom relief, information, assistance with active coping strategies, and empathetic understanding.

Further Reading

Benton, T., Staab, J., & Evans, D. L. (2007). Medical co-morbidity in depressive disorders. *Annals of Clinical Psychiatry, 19*(4), 289–303.

Krishnan, K. R. (2005). Treatment of depression in the medically ill. *Journal of Clinical Psychopharmacology, 25*(4, Suppl. 1), S14–S18.

Rodin, G., Lo, C., Mikulincer, M., Donner, A., Gagliese, L., & Zimmermann, C. (2009). Pathways to distress: The multiple determinants of depression, hopelessness, and the desire for hastened death in metastatic cancer patients. *Social Science and Medicine, 68*, 562–569.

Steptoe, A. (Ed.). (2007). *Depression and physical illness*. Cambridge, UK: Cambridge University Press.

Trask, P. C. (2004). Assessment of depression in cancer patients. *Journal of the National Cancer Institute Monographs, 32*, 80–92.

References

Akechi, T., Okuyama, T., Onishi, J., Morita, T., & Furukawa, T. A. (2008). Psychotherapy for depression among incurable cancer patients. *Cochrane Database of Systematic Reviews*, Issue 2 (Article No. CD005537), DOI: 10.1002/14651858/CD005537.

American Psychiatric Association. (2000). *Diagnostic and statistical manual of mental disorders* (4th ed., text rev.). Washington, DC: Author.

Andrykowski, M. A., & Manne, S. L. (2006). Are psychological interventions effective and accepted by cancer patients? I. Standards and levels of evidence. *Annals of Behavioral Medicine, 32*(2), 93–97.

Beck, A. T., Steer, R. A., & Brown, G. K. (1996). *Manual for the Beck Depression Inventory–II*. San Antonio, TX: Psychological Corporation.

Beck, D. A., & Koenig, H. G. (1996). Minor depression: A review of the literature. *International Journal of Psychiatry in Medicine, 26*(2), 177–209.

Benedetti, F., Bernasconi, A., & Pontiggia, A. (2006). Depression and neurological disorders. *Current Opinion in Psychiatry, 19*(1), 14–18.

Berkman, L. F., Blumenthal, J., Burg, M., Carney, R. M., Catellier, D., Cowan, M. J., et al. (2003). Effects of treating depression and low perceived social support on clinical events after myocardial infarction: The Enhancing Recovery in Coronary Heart Disease Patients (ENRICHD) randomized trial. *Journal of the American Medical Association, 289*(23), 3106–3116.

Burvill, P. W. (1995). Recent progress in the epidemiology of major depression. *Epidemiologic Reviews, 17*(1), 21–31.

Capuron, L., Su, S., Miller, A. H., Bremner, J. D., Goldberg, J., Vogt, G. J., et al. (2008). Depressive symptoms and metabolic syndrome: Is inflammation the underlying link? *Biological Psychiatry, 64*(10), 896–900.

Carson, A. J., MacHale, S., Allen, K., Lawrie, S. M., Dennis, M., House, A., et al. (2000). Depression after stroke and lesion location: A systematic review. *Lancet, 356*, 122–126.

Cipriani, A., Geddes, J. R., Furukawa, T. A., & Barbui, C. (2007). Metareview on short-term effectiveness and safety of antidepressants for depression: An evidence-based approach to inform clinical practice. *Canadian Journal of Psychiatry, 52*(9), 553–562.

Classen, C. C., Kraemer, H. C., Blasey, C., Giese-Davis, J., Koopman, C., Palesh, O. G., et al. (2008). Supportive–expressive group therapy for primary breast cancer patients: A randomized prospective multicenter trial. *Psycho-Oncology, 17*(5), 438–447.

Cleland, J. A., Lee, A. J., & Hall, S. (2007). Associations of depression and anxiety with gender, age, health-related quality of life and symptoms in primary care COPD patients. *Family Practice, 24*(3), 217–223.

Coyne, J. C., Lepore, S. J., & Palmer, S. C. (2006). Efficacy of psychosocial interventions in cancer care: Evidence is weaker than it first looks. *Annals of Behavioral Medicine, 32*(2), 104–110.

Cruess, D. G., Petitto, J. M., Leserman, J., Douglas, S. D., Gettes, D. R., Ten Have, T. R., et al. (2003). Depression and HIV infection: Impact on immune function and disease progression. *CNS Spectrums, 8*(1), 52–58.

Dantzer, R., O'Connor, J. C., Freund, G. G., Johnson, R. W., & Kelley, K. W. (2008). From inflammation to sickness and depression: When the immune system subjugates the brain. *Nature Reviews Neuroscience, 9*(1), 46–56.

Fitzgerald, P. B., & Daskalakis, Z. J. (2008). The use of repetitive transcranial magnetic stimulation and vagal nerve stimulation in the treatment of depression. *Current Opinion in Psychiatry, 21*(1), 25–29.

Frasure-Smith, N. (1995). The Montreal Heart Attack Readjustment Trial. *Journal of Cardiopulmonary Rehabilitation, 15*(2), 103–106.

Glassman, A. H., O'Connor, C. M., Califf, R. M., Swedberg, K., Schwartz, P., Bigger, J. T., Jr., et al. (2002). Sertraline treatment of major depression in patients with acute MI or unstable angina. *Journal of the American Medical Association, 288*(6), 701–709.

Holmes, A., Heilig, M., Rupniak, N. M., Steck-ler, T., & Griebel, G. (2003). Neuropeptide systems as novel therapeutic targets for depression and anxiety disorders. *Trends in Pharmacological Sciences, 24*(11), 580–588.

Huffman, J. C., Smith, F. A., Quinn, D. K., & Fricchione, G. L. (2006). Post-MI psychiatric syndromes: Six unanswered questions. *Harvard Review of Psychiatry, 14*(6), 305–318.

Iosifescu, D. V. (2007). Treating depression in the medically ill. *Psychiatric Clinics of North America, 30*(1), 77–90.

Jacobson, C. M., Rosenfeld, B., Pessin, H., & Breitbart, W. (2008). Depression and IL-6 blood plasma concentrations in advanced cancer patients. *Psychosomatics, 49*(1), 64–66.

Kanner, A. M. (2003). Depression in epilepsy: Prevalence, clinical semiology, pathogenic mechanisms, and treatment. *Biological Psychiatry, 54*(3), 388–398.

Kessler, R. C., Berglund, P., Demler, O., Jin, R., Koretz, D., Merikangas, K. R., et al. (2003). The epidemiology of major depressive disorder: Results from the National Comorbidity Survey Replication (NCS-R). *Journal of the American Medical Association, 289*(23), 3095–3105.

Kim, J. M., Shin, I. S., & Yoon, J. S. (2002). Apolipoprotein E among Korean Alzheimer's disease patients in community-dwelling and hospitalized elderly samples. *Dementia and Geriatric Cognitive Disorders, 13*(3), 119–124.

Kissane, D. W., Grabsch, B., Clarke, D. M., Smith, G. C., Love, A. W., Bloch, S., et al. (2007). Supportive–expressive group therapy for women with metastatic breast cancer: Survival and psychosocial outcome from a randomized controlled trial. *Psycho-Oncology, 16*(4), 277–286.

Krishnan, K. R. (2005). Treatment of depression in the medically ill. *Journal of Clinical Psychopharmacology, 25*(4, Suppl. 1), S14–S18.

Lee, H. B., & Lyketsos, C. G. (2003). Depression in Alzheimer's disease: Heterogeneity and related issues. *Biological Psychiatry, 54*(3), 353–362.

Leonard, B. E. (2007). Inflammation, depression and dementia: Are they connected? *Neurochemical Research, 32*(10), 1749–1756.

Leserman, J. (2003). The effects of stressful life events, coping, and cortisol on HIV infection. *CNS Spectrums, 8*(1), 25–30.

Levinson, D. F. (2006). The genetics of depression: A review. *Biological Psychiatry, 60*(2), 84–92.

Lincoln, N. B., & Flannaghan, T. (2003). Cognitive behavioral psychotherapy for depression following stroke: A randomized controlled trial. *Stroke, 34*(1), 111–115.

Lo, C., Li, M., & Rodin, G. (2008). The assessment and treatment of distress in cancer patients: Overview and future directions. *Minerva Psichiatrica, 49,* 129–143.

Lynch, S. G., Kroencke, D. C., & Denney, D. R. (2001). The relationship between disability and depression in multiple sclerosis: The role of uncertainty, coping, and hope. *Multiple Sclerosis, 7*(6), 411–416.

Massie, M. J. (2004). Prevalence of depression in patients with cancer. *Journal of the National Cancer Institute Monographs, 32,* 57–71.

McDonald, W. M., Richard, I. H., & DeLong, M. R. (2003). Prevalence, etiology, and treatment of depression in Parkinson's disease. *Biological Psychiatry, 54*(3), 363–375.

Miller, A. H., Ancoli-Israel, S., Bower, J. E., Capuron, L., & Irwin, M. R. (2008). Neuroendocrine–immune mechanisms of behavioral comorbidities in patients with cancer. *Journal of Clinical Oncology, 26*(6), 971–982.

Mitchell, A. J. (2007). Pooled results from 38 analyses of the accuracy of distress thermometer and other ultra-short methods of detecting cancer-related mood disorders. *Journal of Clinical Oncology, 25*(29), 4670–4681.

Mitchell, A. J., & Coyne, J. C. (2007). Do ultra-short screening instruments accurately detect depression in primary care?: A pooled analysis and meta-analysis of 22 studies. *British Journal of General Practice, 57*(535), 144–151.

Mohr, D. C., Goodkin, D. E., Islar, J., Hauser, S. L., & Genain, C. P. (2001). Treatment of depression is associated with suppression of nonspecific and antigen-specific T(H)1 responses in multiple sclerosis. *Archives of Neurology, 58*(7), 1081–1086.

Mossner, R., Henneberg, A., Schmitt, A., Syagailo, Y. V., Grassle, M., Hennig, T., et al. (2001). Allelic variation of serotonin transporter expression is associated with depression in Parkinson's disease. *Molecular Psychiatry, 6*(3), 350–352.

Musselman, D. L., Betan, E., Larsen, H., & Phillips, L. S. (2003). Relationship of depression to diabetes types 1 and 2: Epidemiology, biology, and treatment. *Biological Psychiatry, 54*(3), 317–329.

Nielsen, D. M. (2006). Corticotropin-releasing factor type-1 receptor antagonists: The next class of antidepressants? *Life Sciences, 78*(9), 909–919.

Olatunji, B. O., Mimiaga, M. J., O'Cleirigh, C., & Safren, S. A. (2006). Review of treatment studies of depression in HIV. *Topics in HIV Medicine, 14*(3), 112–124.

Palmer, S. C., & Coyne, J. C. (2003). Screening for depression in medical care: Pitfalls, alternatives, and revised priorities. *Journal of Psychosomatic Research, 54*(4), 279–287.

Paraskevaidis, I., Parissis, J. T., Fountoulaki, K.,

Filippatos, G., & Kremastinos, D. (2006). Selective serotonin re-uptake inhibitors for the treatment of depression in coronary artery disease and chronic heart failure: Evidence for pleiotropic effects. *Cardiovascular and Hematological Agents in Medicinal Chemistry, 4*(4), 361–367.

Parissis, J. T., Fountoulaki, K., Filippatos, G., Adamopoulos, S., Paraskevaidis, I., & Kremastinos, D. (2007). Depression in coronary artery disease: Novel pathophysiologic mechanisms and therapeutic implications. *International Journal of Cardiology, 116*(2), 153–160.

Patten, S. B., & Barbui, C. (2004). Drug-induced depression: A systematic review to inform clinical practice. *Psychotherapy and Psychosomatics, 73*(4), 207–215.

Radloff, L. (1977). The CES-D Scale: A self-report depression scale for research in the general population. *Applied Psychological Measurement, 1,* 385–401.

Raison, C. L., Capuron, L., & Miller, A. H. (2006). Cytokines sing the blues: Inflammation and the pathogenesis of depression. *Trends in Immunology, 27*(1), 24–31.

Rayner, L., Price, A., Evans, A., Valsraj, K., Higginson, I. J., & Hotopf, M. (2010). Antidepressants for depression in physically ill people. *Cochrane Database of Systematic Reviews,* Issue 3.

Rivelli, S., & Jiang, W. (2007). Depression and ischemic heart disease: What have we learned from clinical trials? *Current Opinion in Cardiology, 22*(4), 286–291.

Robinson, R. G. (2003). Poststroke depression: Prevalence, diagnosis, treatment, and disease progression. *Biological Psychiatry, 54*(3), 376–387.

Rodin, G., Lloyd, N., Katz, M., Green, E., Mackay, J. A., & Wong, R. K. (2007). The treatment of depression in cancer patients: A systematic review. *Supportive Care in Cancer, 15*(2), 123–136.

Rodin, G., Walsh, A., Zimmermann, C., Gagliese, L., Jones, J., Shepherd, F. A., et al. (2007). The contribution of attachment security and social support to depressive symptoms in patients with metastatic cancer. *Psycho-Oncology, 16*(12), 1080–1091.

Roy-Byrne, P. P., Davidson, K. W., Kessler, R. C., Asmundson, G. J., Goodwin, R. D., Kubzansky, L., et al. (2008). Anxiety disorders and comorbid medical illness. *General Hospital Psychiatry, 30*(3), 208–225.

Rudisch, B., & Nemeroff, C. B. (2003). Epidemiology of comorbid coronary artery disease and depression. *Biological Psychiatry, 54*(3), 227–240.

Rush, A., First, M., & Blacker, D. (2008). *Handbook of psychiatric measures* (2nd ed.). Washington, DC: American Psychiatric Association.

Scherrer, J. F., Xian, H., Bucholz, K. K., Eisen, S. A., Lyons, M. J., Goldberg, J., et al. (2003). A twin study of depression symptoms, hypertension, and heart disease in middle-aged men. *Psychosomatic Medicine, 65*(4), 548–557.

Schulberg, H. C., Raue, P. J., & Rollman, B. L. (2002). The effectiveness of psychotherapy in treating depressive disorders in primary care practice: Clinical and cost perspectives. *General Hospital Psychiatry, 24*(4), 203–212.

Sheline, Y. I. (2003). Neuroimaging studies of mood disorder effects on the brain. *Biological Psychiatry, 54*(3), 338–352.

Simon, G. E., Goldberg, D. P., Von Korff, M., & Ustun, T. B. (2002). Understanding cross-national differences in depression prevalence. *Psychological Medicine, 32*(4), 585–594.

Spitzer, R. L., Kroenke, K., & Williams, J. B. (1999). Validation and utility of a self-report version of PRIME-MD: The PHQ Primary Care Study. *Journal of the American Medical Association, 282*(18), 1737–1744.

Trask, P. C. (2004). Assessment of depression in cancer patients. *Journal of the National Cancer Institute Monographs, 32*, 80–92.

Tyring, S., Gottlieb, A., Papp, K., Gordon, K., Leonardi, C., Wang, A., et al. (2006). Etanercept and clinical outcomes, fatigue, and depression in psoriasis: Double-blind placebo-controlled randomised phase III trial. *Lancet, 367*, 29–35.

Unutzer, J., Schoenbaum, M., Katon, W. J., Fan, M. Y., Pincus, H. A., Hogan, D., et al. (2009). Healthcare costs associated with depression in medically ill fee-for-service Medicare participants. *Journal of the American Geriatrics Society, 57*(3), 506–510.

Vamos, M. (2006). Psychotherapy in the medically ill: A commentary. *Australian and New Zealand Journal of Psychiatry, 40*(4), 295–309.

van den Brink, R. H., van Melle, J. P., Honig, A., Schene, A. H., Crijns, H. J., Lambert, F. P., et al. (2002). Treatment of depression after myocardial infarction and the effects on cardiac prognosis and quality of life: Rationale and outline of the Myocardial INfarction and Depression-Intervention Trial (MIND-IT). *American Heart Journal, 144*(2), 219–225.

van Melle, J. P., de Jonge, P., Spijkerman, T. A., Tijssen, J. G., Ormel, J., van Veldhuisen, D. J., et al. (2004). Prognostic association of depression following myocardial infarction with mortality and cardiovascular events: A meta-analysis. *Psychosomatic Medicine, 66*(6), 814–822.

Wallin, M. T., Wilken, J. A., Turner, A. P., Williams, R. M., & Kane, R. (2006). Depression and multiple sclerosis: Review of a lethal combination. *Journal of Rehabilitation Research and Development, 43*(1), 45–62.

Weiner, R., & Coffey, C. (1993). *Psychiatric care of the medical patient.* New York: Oxford University Press.

Zigmond, A. S., & Snaith, R. P. (1983). The Hospital Anxiety and Depression Scale. *Acta Psychiatrica Scandinavica, 67*(6), 361–370.

CHAPTER 15

Self-Direction toward Health
Overriding the Default American Lifestyle

John Mirowsky
Catherine E. Ross

The default American lifestyle is unhealthy. It is not a default in the old sense of a failure to perform a task or fulfill an obligation. It is a default in the newer sense of an option, assigned automatically by an operating system, that remains in effect unless canceled or overridden by the operator. The automatic routines of 21st-century affluent society are set by the economic system and physical infrastructure. They developed from two related, centuries-old trends: the progressive increase in per capita productivity and wealth, and the progressive substitution of mechanical energy and work for human labor. These have nearly eliminated the threats to health and survival common in 1900, increasing life expectancy but leaving as residue the diseases of affluence.

Abundance has its risks. The industrial production of food products provides an excess of cheap calories always ready at hand. The food is engineered as much or more for production, transportation, marketing, and convenience as for nutrition. Gas engines, electric motors, and electronic communication make travel, work, play, and commerce increasingly sedentary. The locales of daily activity are separated by distances and ob-

stacles that are forbidding and dangerous to anyone not in a motorized vehicle. So people eat lots of packaged and prepared foods, drive from place to place, and sit while working, playing, and socializing. Their physiological systems, evolved for physical effort in contexts of scarcity, drift further and further from balance. Their muscles become atrophied, their joints inflamed and calcified, their bones brittle and misaligned, their hearts weak, and their arteries clogged. They take medicines to control blood pressure, cholesterol, and glucose; to regulate bowel movements, urination, stomach acidity and reflux; and to stifle anxiety, depression and pain. This is the unhealthy lifestyle that remains in effect unless canceled or overridden by the operator.

Given the legacy of caloric glut and deficient physical activity, health depends on one's ability to override the standard mode of life. Doing so requires insight, knowledge, critical analysis, long-range strategic thinking, and willful self-design. Three things in particular develop that ability: education, creative work, and a sense of controlling one's own life. These are becoming, or perhaps have become, the preeminent factors distinguishing individual and group levels of health.

Ironically, the diseases of affluence disproportionately afflict the least affluent individuals and groups. This has little to do with material deprivation. For the most part, the problem is not that food, transportation, goods, and treatments need to get cheaper and more abundant. The problem is that many individuals cannot see the dangers of the ordinary way of life or lack the ability to redesign their lives. Health depends on power: the power of knowledge, the power of critical thinking, and the power to design and direct one's own life toward better ends.

This chapter introduces a sociological view of health disparities, particularly as they relate to the psychology of self-direction and biological accumulation. Sociology and psychology have a long history of overlapping research on mental and physical health. Scientists in each field read and apply findings from the other. Sociology distinctively addresses questions about social strata and statuses. "Strata" are the layers, levels, and divisions of society composed of people with similar social and economic status. "Status" is simply a position or standing relative to that of others. The core sociological fact about health is that lower status and poorer health go together, and this is becoming more and more the case. Sociologists try to understand why and how these health disparities exist and grow. Psychology provides the elemental facts about human behavior. Economics and demographics reveal the large-scale human context that sets the default lifestyle. Considering the behavior in context reveals the statuses and traits of individuals who successfully override the default.

The rest of this chapter has four sections. The first gives a brief history of how health problems and their social distributions have gotten to be what they are today. The others summarize observations and ideas relating health to formal education, creative work, and the sense of controlling one's own life, the main tributaries of self-direction. The education section introduces the concept of "accumulators," which are economic, social, behavioral or biological reservoirs of advantage and disadvantage. Self-direction toward health requires understanding and guiding those accumulations.

A Brief History of the Default Lifestyle

Programs for public, occupational, and environmental heath protect all individuals in modern nations, particularly those of lower status who otherwise would be most at risk. Economic and industrial trends toward greater wealth and productivity provide a general level of material prosperity that in 1900 was enjoyed only by the well-to-do. The average per capita income in the United States, adjusted for inflation, was eight times greater in 2000 than in 1900 (Fisk, 2003). Ironically, the widely beneficial programs and trends create a growing association between social status and health mediated by behaviors with an irreducible element of personal choice and self-determination (Mirowsky & Ross, 2003; Stroebe, 2000). Individuals increasingly face health problems that have solutions requiring personal knowledge, choice, effort, and effectiveness. This does not imply that wayward self-destructiveness is the primary cause of modern health problems. Rather, it implies that too many individuals lack the tools needed to gain effective control of their own lives and overcome the default lifestyle. Given these tools, they would seek health as willingly and effectively as others do.

During the 20th century, the advanced industrial nations made enormous progress in public health programs that benefit all citizens, especially workers and the poor (Cutler & Miller, 2005; McKinlay & McKinlay, 1977; Stroebe, 2000). Everyone benefits from public supplies of monitored and treated water; testing and regulation of private wells, public sanitary sewers, and sewage treatment; regulation of septic systems; removal of trash and garbage to sanitary landfills or incinerators; rat, mosquito, fire, and flood control; safety standards for buildings; environmental and occupational health and safety standards and programs; transportation safety standards and agencies; regulation of food purity and vitamin content; evaluation and regulation of product safety and of dangerous medical interventions; programs that mandate or promote vaccination against childhood infectious diseases; and agencies that scan ceaselessly for and combat as early as possible outbreaks of epidemics.

Health scientists know the value and effectiveness of the public health systems. At the beginning of the previous century, in the early 1900s, life expectancy at birth was 47 years (Bogue, 1985; Hobbs & Stoops, 2002). Infectious diseases were the major causes of death, including pneumonia and influenza, tuberculosis, diarrhea, and enteritis (intestinal infections), nephritis (kidney infections), and diphtheria and measles (Haines, 2006; McKeown, 1979; McKinlay & McKinlay, 1977; Stroebe, 2000). Many also died from whooping cough, smallpox, typhus, typhoid fever, rheumatic fever, syphilis, and mumps. Deaths in infancy and childhood were common. One infant in seven died within a year of birth (Hobbs & Stoops, 2002; Olshansky & Ault, 1987). Individuals who survived to adulthood had less than an even chance of living to age 65. Dangerous and grueling jobs contributed to the risks (Fisk, 2003; Wyatt & Hecker, 2006). Farming and farm labor were the most common occupations, accounting for about 35% of all jobs, with other labor and mining accounting for another 12%. Common jobs often had horrendous risks. Coal miners, for example, working in dark, cramped, wet, and cold tunnels, faced immediate risks from explosions, asphyxiating gases, cave-ins, and crushing or mangling machinery, with longer term risks from breathing coal dust and other mineral particles. Workers' compensation for injuries was essentially nonexistent.

By the end of the 20th century the median life expectancy at birth had increased to age 76.9 (Haines, 2006; Hobbs & Stoops, 2002; Stroebe, 2000). Deaths of children and working-age adults were unusual. Over 99% of newborns are expected to survive into adulthood. More than half of those that do will live into their 80s, if adulthood mortality rates stay as low as in the year 2000. Almost all deaths that year occurred among older adults, with a median age at death of 78 years. The leading causes of death were heart disease, cancer, stroke, accidents, diabetes, liver disease, suicide, kidney disease, high blood pressure, septicemia, and pneumonia and influenza. In 1900, pneumonia and influenza were chiefly deaths among children and adults weakened by poverty and poor nutrition. By 2000, they were increasingly deaths among very old individuals who had been healthy throughout life and had avoided all the other causes of death but eventually became frail and susceptible.

Two important things characterize the other, current leading causes of death. Most of them are chronic diseases that develop over several decades. All are heavily influenced by lifestyle, particularly sedentary work and leisure; diets of packaged and prepared food products with too much fat, sugar, and protein; tobacco smoking and drug or alcohol abuse; driving many miles a day (often in fast or dense traffic, or engaged in distracting activities); chronic psychophysiological stress; and uncritical reliance on dangerous prescriptions and procedures to alleviate the growing consequences.

Accidents also remain on the list from 1900 but were in 2000 more often associated with motor vehicles, home, and recreation than with paid work (Haines, 2006). Occupational conditions improved greatly by the end of the 20th century (Fisk, 2003; Toscano, 1997; Toscano & Windau, 1994; Wyatt & Hecker, 2006). Workplaces now are remarkably safe. For almost all occupations, workers face far greater short-run risks to life and health at home and on the way to and from home. Few jobs require the grueling labor in aversive conditions that was once common. The most common occupations now involve clerical, managerial, or analytic desk work. Most jobs are safe.

The new problem is that few jobs require or even allow the development of aerobic capacity, muscle strength, bone density, and joint flexibility (Brownson & Boehmer, 2004; Brownson, Boehmer, & Luke, 2005; Lakdawalla & Philipson, 2009; Philipson, 2001). Even factory and construction workers increasingly use machines to do what once required human labor. The riskiest jobs are outdoors and use powerful machinery, such as lumbering and commercial fishing, which have the long-term counterbalancing benefit of requiring physical activity (Toscano, 1997; Toscano & Windau, 1994). The next most risky jobs, which are far more common, involve use of motor vehicles or handling money while in contact with the public. They lack long-term physical benefits. In many jobs, the combination of physical restriction and psychological tension encourage bad dietary habits. Workers drink sugary, caffeinated beverages to stay alert and eat high-fat snacks to regulate stress. Far more workplaces have vending machines or coffee and doughnut pools than exercise facilities and programs.

The same economic and technological forces that have taken the physical activity out of work have taken it out of transportation and communication. Suburbanization is the clearest large-scale indicator (Brownson et al., 2005; Duany, Plater-Zyberk, & Speck, 2000; Ewing, Schmid, Killingsworth, Zlot, & Raudenbush, 2003; Hobbs & Stoops, 2002). In 1900, only 28.4% of Americans lived in metropolitan areas, and only 25% of those lived in the suburbs. By 2000, 80.3% lived in metropolitan areas, with 62.3% of those in the suburbs. Urban scale has increased enormously, whereas urban density has decreased. From 1950, when the statistics were first collected, to 2000, the population density of metropolitan areas decreased by 25%, from 407 persons per square mile to a little over 300. Some of this reflected the dramatic decline of density in the urban core, from 7,515 persons per square mile to 2,716. Most of it, though, reflected the move to suburbs. The number of Americans living in metropolitan urban cores declined slightly between 1950 and 2000, whereas the number living in the suburbs increased by 105 million.

The decline in metropolitan density may seem a good thing, giving everyone more space and air. Unfortunately, much of the space is taken up by roads and parking places, and the air is filled with exhaust. The increasing geographic scale means that time in transit takes up more and more of the day, with people chiefly sitting in motor vehicles rather than walking or bicycling (National Household Travel Survey, 2001a, 2001b; Transportation Research Board, 2005). Americans drive an average of 13,600 miles per person a year, and the average vehicle is driven about 15,000 miles a year. The number of miles driven is increasing steadily in all categories, not just in commuting (about 19% of all miles driven) and at work (about 8% of miles). Americans spend more and more of their time motoring around getting to and from work, running errands, shopping, socializing, and doing their jobs.

With little time for leisure, Americans increasingly rely on take-out, restaurant, and packaged food products for meals. Food and diet trends are another major contribution to the unhealthy default lifestyle (Cook & Daponte, 2008; Cutler, Glaeser, & Shapiro, 2003; Pollan, 2006; Rashad, Grossman, & Chou, 2006; Schlosser, 2002). Historically, nearly all American households prepared most of the food eaten, and many produced it, too. Purchased food was usually grown locally, often bought directly from the producers. Over the 20th century, food has been industrialized, from production to distribution, preparation, and serving. The amount of agricultural product per acre has increased. The cost per unit of output has decreased. Storage and shipping have gotten less expensive. Traceable food items now travel an average of 1,500 miles from producer to consumer. Much food, however, is no longer traceable. Agricultural products are increasingly commodity raw materials, fractionated into components sold to the manufacturers of food products (Pollan, 2006). As a familiar example, high-fructose corn syrup is a fraction made from commodity corn. It is sold and shipped in bulk to manufacturers that assemble products ranging from cookies to heat-and-serve meat loaf. Many food components are used to make animal feed, with the animal parts in turn becoming components of mass production. Vitamins and minerals from a variety of sources are also acquired in bulk and used to make food products.

The industrialization of food has solved the dietary problems of 1900. Workers then could burn over 4,000 calories a day in heavy labor. They needed plentiful, inexpensive food. The brawn for that labor was most readily built and maintained with animal protein, containing all the amino acids required for human protein that cannot be made by the human body itself. For the hard laborers of 1900, the triglyceride fat layered on or marbled through meat was converted to glucose burned in physical exertions. So were the sugars and complex carbohydrates from vegetables and fruits. Because food was local and seasonal, even a person fed enough calories could suffer from deficiency diseases such as rickets or pellagra. Adding vitamins and minerals to food products effectively eliminated those deficiencies.

The dietary problem of the 21st century is excess, not deficiency. It occurs when the proteins, fats, and carbohydrates eaten exceed amounts needed to maintain lean body mass and fuel activity and cellular processes (Campbell & Campbell, 2005; Koplan & Dietz, 1999; Rosenbaum, Leibel, & Hirsch, 1997). Excess triglycerides and other fats go into subcutaneous storage. Excess sugars and complex carbohydrates become blood glucose, which eventually is made into more triglycerides for subcutaneous storage. Amino acids from excess protein combine with some of the excess fat to make circulating low-density lipoprotein (the bad cholesterol). They also promote cancer growth by providing needed materials. Digesting the excess protein creates acids that must be neutralized with calcium drawn from bones and then excreted. These dietary excesses contribute to disabling and life-threatening chronic conditions that include obesity, atherosclerosis, hypertension, diabetes, and osteoporosis.

Education and Learned Effectiveness

Being "healthy" means feeling sound, well, vigorous, and physically able to do the things most people ordinarily can do. The word can refer to a dimension that is graded from very unhealthy to ideally healthy, to an individual's current place on that dimension, or to the apex of that dimension, the ideal state of health. Population surveys use five types of health measures: individual reports of subjective health, feelings of vitality and well-being, physical impairments, diagnoses of serious chronic disease, and expected longevity. Health, by all of these definitions and measures, increases with the level of education.

Education forms a unique dimension of social status, with qualities that make it especially important to health (Mirowsky & Ross, 2003, 2005a, 2005b; Ross & Wu, 1995, 1996). Educational attainment marks social status at the beginning of adulthood, functioning as the main bridge between the status of one generation and that of the next, and also as the main avenue of upward mobility. It precedes and substantially influences the other achieved social statuses, including occupation and occupational status, earnings, personal and household income and wealth, and freedom from economic hard-

ship. Education creates desirable outcomes because it trains individuals to acquire, evaluate, and use information. It teaches individuals to tap the power of knowledge. As a result, education influences health in ways that are varied, present at all stages of adult life, cumulative, self-amplifying, and uniformly positive. Education develops the learned effectiveness that enables self-direction toward any and all values sought, including health (Mirowsky & Ross, 2003).

Schooling builds the real skills, abilities, and resources called "human capital" on several levels. On the most general level, education teaches people to learn. It develops the ability to write, communicate, solve problems, analyze data, develop ideas, and implement plans. It develops broadly useful analytic skills, such as mathematics and logic, and, on a more basic level, observing, experimenting, summarizing, synthesizing, interpreting, classifying, and so on. In school, one encounters and solves problems that are progressively more difficult, complex, and subtle. The more years of schooling, the greater one's cognitive development, characterized by flexible, rational, complex strategies of thinking. Higher education teaches people to think logically and rationally, to see many sides of an issue, and to analyze problems and solve them. In addition, the occupational skills one learns in school have generic value.

Education also develops broadly effective habits and attitudes such as dependability, judgment, motivation, effort, trust, and confidence, as well as skills and abilities. In particular, the process of learning creates confidence in the ability to solve problems. Education instills the habit of meeting problems with attention, thought, action, and perseverance. Thus, education increases effort that, along with ability, is a fundamental component of problem solving. Apart from the value of the skills and abilities learned in school, the process of learning builds the confidence, motivation, and self-assurance needed to *attempt* to solve problems. Because it develops competence on many levels, education gives people the ability and motivation to shape and control their lives.

In the United States, socioeconomic differences in health are large and growing. Education is increasingly the fundamental element of socioeconomic status linked to health. Today, education is more important than income and wealth, more important than occupational category and rank in connecting better health with higher social status. Education's beneficial effects are pervasive, cumulative, and self-amplifying, growing across the life course (Mirowsky & Ross, 2003, 2005a, 2005b; Ross & Wu, 1995, 1996). Of particular importance to social policy, education moderates or eliminates the harm to health of disadvantaged origins (Mirowsky & Ross, 2005a). Education develops the capacity to find out what needs to be done and how to do it, and the habits and skills of self-direction, which together prove effective when seeking health. They make individuals better at identifying and avoiding risky situations or habits, at more quickly exiting the risky situations or correcting risky ways, and better able to manage health problems that occur, to minimize the damage, and to return to health as fully and quickly as possible.

For decades American health scientists have acted as if social status has no great bearing on health (Mirowsky & Ross, 2003). Researchers knew that life expectancy was increasing; that programs in public, occupational, and environmental health were widespread and effective; and that medical technology was expanding in scope and availability. Not until the last quarter of the 20th century did American researchers begin to look for evidence that socioeconomic differences in health were disappearing. The results were a surprise and a wake-up call. Although mortality rates were going down, the differences in mortality rates across social strata were growing (Elo & Preston, 1996; Lauderdale, 2001; Pappas, Queen, Hadden, & Fisher, 1993).

At first American researchers suspected that the absence of a U.S. national medical care system might explain the growing disparities. American scientists who turned to the British literature were disabused of that idea. In Great Britain, the Black Report (named after the study's leader) was commissioned to examine the success of the National Health Service in its core mission of reducing social inequality in health and survival. The report and its offspring showed the same growing disparities as in the United States (Bartley, Blane, & Davey Smith,

1998), as did studies in Canada and Sweden, too. Clearly, providing basic medical care to all citizens did not avert the trend (Kunst & Mackenbach, 1994; Ross & Mirowsky, 2000).

Some researchers thought that perhaps the standard publicly funded care was falling behind powerful new interventions available chiefly outside the national health care systems. The British Whitehall Study of civil servants cast doubt on that explanation. It found substantial gradients in heart disease morbidity and mortality across civil service grades, despite seemingly quite adequate pay and benefits even at the lowest levels (Marmot & Mustard, 1994). In the United States, physicians at Vanderbilt School of Medicine made similar observations. Pincus and his colleagues, who were conducting clinical studies of treatments for rheumatoid arthritis and other debilitating and deadly autoimmune diseases (Pincus, 1986; Pincus, Esther, DeWalt, & Callahan, 1998), noticed large differences in functional decline and survival across patients' education levels, despite the fact that all of them were treated by teams of doctors following the same research protocols, specifying the best known forms of care. Education was a far better predictor of outcome than a host of clinical and laboratory assessments. Turning to the literature, they found similar patterns for heart disease survival. Indeed, the differences in survival across levels of education far outstripped those between patients treated with beta-blockers and those given placebos (Pincus et al., 1998). Pincus believes firmly in the value of medical intervention and the desirability of a national health care system. Even so, he argues that some powerful extramedical force must account for the substantial differences in outcome across levels of education in clinical studies that provide a uniformly high standard of care (Pincus, 1996).

The differences in health and survival across levels of education are remarkably large. One way to gauge their size is to compare them to the differences across age groups. For example, each additional year of education decreases the expected mortality rate to roughly the same degree as being 1–2 years younger (Hadden & Rockswold, 2008; Rogers, Hummer, & Nam, 2000). A year spent in school takes 1–2 years off mortality risk. Subjective health and physical function show even larger benefits. Estimates vary depending on the survey but show that a year of education improves one's subjective health and physical functioning by an amount equivalent to being 2–6 years younger (Mirowsky & Ross, 2005a). In terms of subjective health, physical function, and survival, formal education apparently pays back the time spent and more.

The association of education with health is not just a coincidence due to childhood advantages. Individuals from socially advantaged backgrounds do get more schooling because of better childhood health and other benefits. They are healthier than others in adulthood largely *because of* more schooling and its consequences, such as better jobs and incomes (Blackwell, Hayward, & Crimmins, 2001; Hayward & Gorman, 2004). Individuals with poorly educated parents generally get less schooling than others, but they also get the biggest health benefits from more schooling (Mirowsky & Ross, 2005a). As a result, statewide increases in compulsory education reduce adulthood mortality by even larger amounts than do individual voluntary increases (Lleras-Muney, 2005). This is not because compulsion is good for personal development. Rather, mandated increases pertain largely to children from the most disadvantaged backgrounds, who otherwise would not get more schooling. They also apply to an entire disadvantaged population, perhaps thereby multiplying benefits. Adults from educationally disadvantaged backgrounds show the strongest association between their health and personal educational attainment (Mirowsky & Ross, 2005a). Individuals with poorly educated parents depend on personal education to counteract the health effects of childhood disadvantage.

The age equivalents given earlier actually understate the health benefits of education because they average across adults of all ages. The health benefits of education actually grow across adulthood as people age. Many things in life produce effects that fade over time as individuals adjust to their circumstances, as times change, and as new experiences intervene. Education's effects work the opposite way, growing with time. They do so because education transforms the person, putting his or her life on a different track. To fully understand education's

positive impact on health, one must envision that benefit unfolding across the lifetime. Education's health-related effects are present throughout adulthood. Even if they are small in any single year, they accumulate and compound over a lifetime, producing ever larger health differences between persons with different levels of education.

The health-related consequences of education accumulate on many levels, from socioeconomic (employment, job quality, earnings, income, and wealth) and behavioral (habits such as smoking or exercising, beliefs such as perceived control over one's own life, personal relationships) levels to physiological (blood pressure, cholesterol levels, aerobic capacity), anatomical (body fat, joint deterioration, arterial fatty plaque) and perhaps even intracellular (insulin resistence, free radical damage) levels. Many consequences of educational attainment influence each other, creating self-amplifying feedback, or interact with each other to produce cascading results (Mirowsky & Ross, 2003).

A growth curve model of rising physical impairment illustrates how the large socioeconomic differences among older Americans develop over the life course. Figure 15.1 shows a vector graph of the growth curve model (Mirowsky & Kim, 2007; Mirowsky & Ross, 2005b;). The vectors are arrows representing the predicted origin and change in level of impairment over the 6-year period of the study, from 1995 to 2001. Researchers measured impairment by asking individuals how much trouble they had climbing stairs, kneeling, or stooping; lifting or carrying objects under 10 pounds, such as a bag of groceries; preparing meals or cleaning; doing other household work; shopping or getting around town; seeing, even with glasses; and hearing. No difficulty was coded 0, Some difficulty was coded 1, and A great deal of difficulty was coded 2. The impairment score is the average level of difficulty with the seven functions. The analysis divided the sample into three groups: less than high school degree (382 persons), high school degree but no college degree at the bachelors level or higher (1,533), and college degree or higher (660). The growth curve model predicts the level of impairment at the beginning and the change in it over the follow-up as a polynomial function of age at the beginning. The age effects can be any

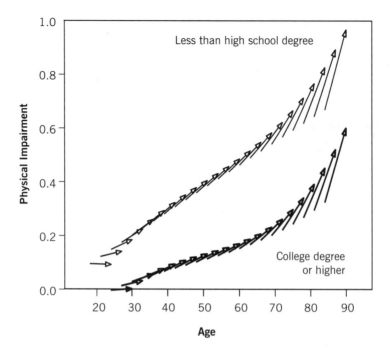

FIGURE 15.1. Origin and change in physical impairment predicted for Americans with a college degree or higher ($N = 663$) compared to those with less than a high school degree ($N = 383$), based on a growth curve model of self-reports in 1995, 1998, and 2001.

combination of linear, quadratic, and cubic functions with significant coefficients. The predictions fit the observations quite well. (The probability is .721 that the observed deviations from the model's predictions occurred purely by chance.) To simplify, Figure 15.1 only shows the vector arrow for every third one-year age group. It also shows only the arrows for those with a college degree or higher compared to those with less than a high school degree.

The impairment vectors in Figure 15.1 illustrate several important observations about education and health. First, persons with college degrees have lower levels of impairment in every age group. The differences are quite large. The persons with less than a high school degree report impairment levels roughly equal to those of college-educated persons who are 20–30 years older. (The high school graduates, not shown, report impairment levels similar to those reported by college graduates who are 15–20 years older.) Second, impairment increases faster over the follow-up for those with less than a high school degree than for those with col-

lege degrees. At all ages, the arrow above has a steeper upward slope than the arrow below. (The same is true for high school graduates compared to college graduates.) This is most pronounced among the young and middle-aged groups. Each group shows an essentially constant rate of increase in impairment from the mid-20s up to the mid-60s, with college-educated groups on a flatter slope. This difference in the growth rate progressively enlarges the differences in impairment. Third, beyond age 65, the age-specific slopes become more similar but are added to very different base levels of impairment. The differences in impairment still grow, but by progressively smaller amounts. Vectors of self-rated health show similar patterns (Mirowsky & Ross, 2008).

Taken together, the observations suggest that the large socioeconomic differences in impairment among older Americans accumulated earlier in life. By definition, a "cumulative advantage" is a benefit acquired by successive addition (O'Rand, 1996). Education's cumulative health advantage rests on three underlying phenomena: permeation, accumulation, and amplification. Education affects virtually all aspects of life. A range of things influenced by education in turn affect health, including habits, interpersonal relationships, family responsibilities, occupational exposures and opportunities, economic sufficiency and security, neighborhood qualities, autonomous and creative activities, and a sense of controlling one's own life. Education's effects add up over time. Many of education's consequences influence or regulate each others' effects in ways that enlarge differences (Mirowsky & Ross, 2003).

Accumulation is especially important in explaining how the default American lifestyle undermines health, and how to override the default. "Accumulation" refers to gathering many smaller effects into a larger one. Some accumulations benefit health, and others harm it. Education tends to speed or advance the beneficial accumulations and slow or delay the detrimental ones. Accumulation occurs when consequences, once present, tend to stay present. The health-related consequences of education accumulate on many levels, from socioeconomic down to cellular levels (Mirowsky & Ross, 2003).

Socioeconomic Accumulation

On the socioeconomic level, individuals generally stay in the same line of work, accumulating experience and seniority and gaining access to the more desirable and lucrative positions (Mirowsky & Ross, 2003). The norms and rules in an organization, occupation, or profession generally lay out a sequence of stages and discourage both skipping ahead or going backward in line. As a consequence, the extrinsic and intrinsic work rewards that influence health tend to accumulate. Some almost take on a life of their own, becoming accumulations of accumulations. For example, pay generally increases the longer someone works, with each raise a multiple of the previous amount, which means the raises generally get larger as pay increases. As income goes up, larger amounts are used to acquire wealth in the form of durable goods, real estate, savings, and investments, which themselves accumulate over time. Some of that wealth generates interest or capital gains, increasing the rate of accumulation.

Behavioral Accumulation

Accumulation happens on the behavioral level, too (Mirowsky & Ross, 1998). Humans naturally form "habits," which are recurrent and often unconscious patterns of behavior acquired through frequent repetition, established dispositions of the mind or character, and customary manners or practices. Habits relevant to health include physical and social activities, diet, smoking, drinking, and so on. Education influences many habits and activities by increasing one's sense of control over one's own life, which is itself a learned and stable worldview summing a lifetime of experience. The sense of control influences a person's habitual approach to risks and problems. The more control one feels he or she has, the more effort one makes to detect and avoid risks, and the more actively and practically he or she responds to problems that arise. This tends to make individuals more effective. In addition, a higher sense of control generally reduces the psychophysiological distress associated with crises by reducing the sense of helplessness and hopelessness. The stability of activities, health-related behaviors, and sense of control create persistent effects throughout long portions of life.

Humans also form sustaining personal relationships that can be viewed as habits of association and interaction. Relationships tend to be stable over time. Education generally improves the quality of relationships, making them seem to participants more fair, equal, respectful, and sustaining (Ross & Wu, 1995). Partly because of this, education makes marital relationships more enduring, increasing the prevalence of marriage and reducing the risk of exposure to the stress of divorce. Marriage, marital quality, and social support all contribute to health. To the extent that education's health-promoting interpersonal consequences persist, they contribute to accumulating health benefits.

Biological Accumulation

The socioeconomic and behavioral accumulations necessarily influence health through biological states, many of which accumulate, too. Health scientists know of many biological accumulators that affect health, and probably will discover many more. The accumulation of body fat may be the most obvious and best known one because of its place in popular culture. It serves as a good example of biological accumulators in general. The buildup of body fat happens slowly over a period of years. Once gained, the fat persists. There is no quick and easy way to get rid of it. On the other hand, not accumulating the fat takes much less intensive effort. An extra cookie's worth of calories a day adds up to 5 pounds of fat a year, or 50 pounds in 10 years. It takes only 20 extra minutes a day of gardening, bicycling, or brisk walking to burn those calories. A person who habitually parks an extra 5 minutes away, and takes stairs instead of elevators and escalators, easily burns an extra 5 pounds of fat a year instead of accumulating it. Lifestyle differences may look small on any given day, but they add up greatly over the years.

Desirable and Undesirable Accumulators

The human body has many less obvious biological accumulators that influence health. Many of the desirable ones contribute to aerobic capacity, including lung capacity, the number of mitochondria and nuclei in muscle cells, and the number of small arteries supplying muscles. Some undesirable biological accumulations get defined as diseases or medical conditions when they progress beyond a clearly dangerous point. They include high resting blood pressure, buildup of fatty plaque in arteries, a low ratio of high-density to low-density lipoprotein in the blood, cellular resistence to insulin and the resulting increase in blood glucose, declining bone density, deposits of uric acid crystals in the soft tissues of joints, softening and fraying of cartilage, and the calcification of ligaments. Some undesirable accumulations eventually provoke damaging and deadly crises, such as embolism, fibrillation, heart failure, infarction, hemorrhage, stroke, or respiratory arrest.

Stress, Allostatic Load, and Neuroendocrine Accumulators

Most of the better understood biological accumulators influenced by education reflect elements of health lifestyle, such as smoking, diet, and exercise (Mirowsky & Ross, 1998). However, differences in the levels of stress over the lifetime probably also influence biological accumulators directly, apart from health lifestyle (Taylor, Repetti, & Seeman, 1997). As used here, the word "stress" refers to the neuroendocrine reaction, called the "stress response," to threatening events or conditions, called "stressors."

Much current biobehavioral research examines "allostatic load," which is the impact of intense, recurring, or chronic stress on neuroendocrine accumulators that influence health (McEwen, 1998; Seeman, Singer, Rowe, Horwitz, & McEwen, 1997; Taylor et al., 1997). "Allostasis" refers to the fluctuation in physiological systems to meet demands from external events or exposures. "Allostatic load" refers to persistent and potentially harmful changes in the regulatory system itself, in response to its own history of activity. The harmful changes include hair-trigger activation, failure to relax in a normal amount of time, failure to adapt to a stressor with experience, or abnormal suppression of response. Over time, these affect the states of other accumulators, such as resting blood pressure, body fat, insulin resistance, and so on. Education reduces allostatic load by giving individuals the skills, resources, standing, and confidence to master their own lives and cope with life's challenges effectively and efficiently.

Prevention and Correction

The health benefits of education flow primarily from the "ounce of prevention" taken daily. Healthy accumulations forestall damaging and deadly crises, and also improve recovery from the injuries and crises that do happen. However, education also increases the likelihood of sensible and effective responses among those who experience a health crisis (Pincus, 1996; Pincus et al., 1998). For example, among middle-aged cigarette smokers who have a heart attack, the probability of quitting goes up dramatically with the level of education (Wray, Herzog, Willis, & Wallace, 1998). Only about 33% of smokers with less than a high school degree quit after a heart attack, compared to over 80% of those with 4 years or more of college. Higher education improves the odds of a healthy response at every step. Education reduces the likelihood of ever smoking.

Among those who smoke, education increases the likelihood of quitting before a health crisis occurs. Among smokers who have a health crisis, such as a heart attack, higher education increases the odds of quitting in response to the crisis.

Dangerous and damaging medical events (e.g., a heart attack) often result from the decline of desirable accumulations (e.g., aerobic capacity) and the development of undesirable ones (e.g., the buildup of fatty plaques in arteries). Undesirable accumulations typically can be reversed, even after a crisis, but generally only over a period of time as a result of concerted and multifaceted effort. Education helps individuals to avoid and to correct undesirable accumulations before they precipitate a crisis and, failing that, to heed the implications of a crisis and take the difficult but necessary corrective action.

Creative Work

"Work" is physical or mental effort or activity directed toward production or accomplishment. The relationship of work to human health goes deeper than physical exposures, economic benefits, and place in the pecking order. Humans express themselves through work. Apparently, productive self-expression acts as an elemental motivation in humans, and its suppression, frustration, or neglect undermines human health (Mirowsky & Ross, 2007a; Ross & Wright, 1998). Creative work is productive activity that individuals find interesting, challenging, complex, nonroutine, and enjoyable (Mirowsky & Ross, 2007a). As used here, the term "creative work" refers to the qualities of main daily activities (paid or not) as experienced by the individual. It does not refer directly to employment in arts and entertainment or in occupations and industries categorized as creative. It does not require that others ascribe novelty or unique value to the product or service, or that they ascribe insight or intuition to its production. In creative work, individuals solve problems, figure things out, learn new things, and do different things in different ways, using their skills in the design and production of something.

Ideas about the psychological attributes of healthy work go back to the 19th-century writings of Marx and Engels (1884/1964). They contrasted the oppressiveness of industrial working conditions with an ideal of expressive work. They wrote of jobs that were physically exhausting and mentally debasing, of humans used as replaceable and disposable parts in an inhuman productive apparatus, and of life sold off by the hour, until there was little of value left. In particular, they wrote about wage slavery, about turning over one's own body and mind to be used as the instrument of someone else's will. They contrasted this oppressed work with an ideal typified in the craft work of earlier eras. Craftsmen owned the tools, materials, and workshop; designed and made the products; and sold them and got the profit. Each product was the physical embodiment of the person's skill and a potential source of pride. By nature, human beings create things. Marx and Engels thought that humans inherently enjoy the things they create and the process of creating them. Somehow the joy of creation had been lost in the 19th-century industrial machine. It made food, clothing, shelter, transportation, and wealth but crushed something at the core of human nature: productive self-expression.

Contrasting wage labor with an idealized craftsmanship illustrates the issue well but can obscure the real options in modern society. Paid employment can provide access to tools, equipment, and materials that provide the means of productive self-expression. The same may be said of a place in a bureaucratic hierarchy, which puts the labor of some under the direction of others. In organizations, the work of other people becomes a medium of production and, thus, of self-expression. A hierarchy provides more control over that medium to some than to others, partly at the expense of those others. Even so, most employed individuals gain more than they lose, just as composers, conductors, and musicians all gain an opportunity for creative work despite their hierarchical relationships (Mirowsky & Ross, 2007a). Moreover, beyond the tools of production, paid jobs provide a theater for self-expression: a locus of performance with an audience capable of appreciation.

In data from the end of the 20th century, creative work has an association with health that equals or exceeds those of education and household income in size (Mirowsky &

Ross, 2007a). To put it in perspective, the 40th and 60th percentiles of a normal distribution are about half a standard deviation apart. A half standard deviation difference in work creativity has an association with current health equivalent to that of being 6.7 years younger, or of having 2 more years of education or 15 times higher household income. A half standard deviation increase in work creativity has an association with change in health over a 6-year follow-up equivalent to that of being 8.7 years younger or of having 2.8 more years of education at baseline, or to that of a 3.5-fold increase in household income over the period. While these comparisons should not be taken too literally, they reveal that access to creative work may be among the major social factors in health.

It might seem that the jobs available give less room for varied, enjoyable, interesting, and challenging activity to the poorly educated than they might find outside of employment through unpaid activities. Results do not support this idea (Mirowsky & Ross, 2007a). Even among the poorly educated, the gain in creative work associated with employment equals the gain expected from 4 additional years of education. Paid employment gives people at all levels of education more of a chance for creative self-expression. The paid work of the poorly educated is less creative than that of the well educated, but the gain in creativity from paid work compared to unpaid activities is as great.

Over the 20th century, the focus of research on work and health progressed from occupational hazards to work strains to work control. To some extent this shift in focus reflects the success of occupational health and safety efforts and the shift to postindustrial economies. To some extent it represents a progression of discovery about the factors relevant to human health. Scientists originally thought any link between work and health must result from physical exposures. Toward the end of the 20th century, studies shifted focus from physical exposures to psychological strains and work control. Karasek and Theorell (1990) found that work-related health problems are the product of high demands and "low decision latitude" (their term for low autonomy and creativity). Health correlates more strongly with

job latitude than with job demands because latitude regulates the psychological impact of demands, shifting the effect from detrimental toward neutral or even beneficial. Periods or circumstances of high demand but low latitude increase the likelihood of accidents and injuries, and also make it difficult to maintain a healthy lifestyle. However, the correlation of low control with poor health outcomes remains substantial in the absence of injury and when the standard lifestyle factors are held constant (Karasek & Theorell, 1990). Apparently the health impact of low job control goes beyond the risk of injury or the short-run difficulty of maintaining a healthy lifestyle.

The Whitehall Studies by Marmot and Mustard (1994) find a similar pattern for British civil servants. The studies find a substantial gradient in morbidity and mortality related to employment grade or rank after adjustment for standard lifestyle risk factors, despite the relatively clean, safe work conditions and good employment benefits enjoyed by all. Civil service grades link job categories to pay ranges, but adjustment for earnings and income, as well as for education and status of origin, accounts for only part of the health association. Apparently something else indexed by service grade or rank creates much of the association with morbidity and mortality. Mediator analyses indicate that low work control predicts high levels of fibrinogen in the blood. Fibrinogen is a protein that stimulates clotting, and high levels raise the risk of coronary heart disease and stroke. The greater work control associated with higher civil service grade may provide at least part of the advantage with regard to morbidity and mortality.

Why does creative work benefit health, while routine, boring, monotonous, unchallenging work impairs health? One theory distinguishes between chronic, unresolved threats that ultimately impair health, and intermittent manageable challenges that ultimately improve health (Epel, McEwen, & Ickovics, 1998). Successfully resolved challenges instigate the same fight-or-flight response in the alarm and resistance stages but differ in a third recovery or rebuilding phase. Following successfully resolved challenges, anabolic hormones are released that increase muscle growth, relaxation, and energy; promote healing; and lead to quicker cortisol habituation (Epel et al., 1998). Perhaps the problem solving and learning of creative work provide a stream of successfully resolved challenges that trigger healthful anabolic responses.

Research on the biological mechanisms linking creative work to health may need to go beyond the fight-or-flight stress response and look for health benefits of a well developed and well trained cerebral cortex. The biological links between creative work and health may include paths that are distinctively human. In the human brain, the prefrontal cortex apparently controls planning, the holding and sorting of information while performing a task, the regulation of current behavior with respect to future consequences, the evaluation of conflicting information or values, the prediction of outcomes, and similar executive functions (Miller & Cohen, 2001). It also may be a center of self-awareness, including self-concept, social comparison, and self-relevant feedback (Morin, 2004). It is heavily connected to the limbic system, which includes the amygdala and hippocampus, and controls aggression, fear, and pleasure. The connection may be a mechanism of the pleasure obtained from solving problems. A well-exercised prefrontal cortex may give individuals a greater ability to regulate behavior toward long-range goals, such as health. It also may give them a greater ability to transform the expression of hypothalamic–pituitary–adrenal axis activation from stressful and destructive to invigorating and constructive. Physical fitness of the prefrontal cortex may require and also promote creative work.

The Sense of Personal Control

Formal education and creative work help individuals to become active and effective agents in their own lives. A sense of personal control is a learned, generalized expectation that outcomes are contingent on one's own choices and actions (Mirowsky & Ross, 2003, 2007b). Controlling one's own life means exercising authority and influence over it by directing and regulating it oneself. People who feel in control of their own lives seek information by which to guide their lives and improve their outcomes. As a result, people who feel in control of their own lives tend to adopt a lifestyle that produces health (Mirowsky & Ross, 1998).

People vary in the sense of control they feel over their own lives (Mirowsky & Ross, 1998, 2003, 2007b). Perceptions range by degree from fatalism and a deep sense of helplessness to agency and a firm sense of mastery. Individuals with a sense of control see themselves as active and consequential agents in their own lives. They feel responsible for their own successes and failures. They feel they can do just about anything they set their minds to, and they view personal misfortunes as results of mistakes that can be corrected. On the other end of the continuum, some individuals believe that situations and outcomes are determined by forces external to themselves, such as powerful others, luck, fate, or chance. They feel that any good things that happen are mostly luck: fortunate outcomes that they desire but do not design. They see their personal problems as results of bad breaks or the callous selfishness of others, and feel little ability to regulate or avoid bad things in the future. A number of social and behavioral sciences recognize the importance of a sense of personal control. The concept appears in a number of related forms with various names, including internal locus of control, mastery, instrumentalism, self-efficacy, agency, personal autonomy, self-direction and, at the other end of the continuum, fatalism, helplessness, perceived helplessness, and perceived powerlessness. A low or negative sense of control may represent human awareness that corresponds to "learned helplessness," a behavioral state of suppressed attention and action (Hiroto, 1974).

A sense of control, as do education and creative work, encourages the development of habits, skills, resources, and abilities that enable individuals to achieve a better life. To the extent that people want health, these three tributaries of self-direction provide the intellectual and motivational means toward that end, through a lifestyle that promotes health. Educated, creative, self-designing persons merge otherwise unrelated habits and ways into a healthy lifestyle that consequently behaves as a coherent trait. The three tributaries of self-direction make individuals more effective users of information. Purposeful individuals coalesce a healthy lifestyle from otherwise incoherent or diametric practices. Usually, individuals tend to do whatever others like them do, particularly if it distinguishes the people with whom they identify from the ones with whom they do not. Some of these things make health better, and others make it worse. For example, men exercise more frequently than do women; women restrict body weight more closely. Likewise, young adults smoke more than do older adults, but they also exercise more. Individuals putting together a healthy lifestyle must adopt the healthy habits of men and women, young and old. In doing so they create positive correlations among traits that otherwise would be uncorrelated or even negatively correlated.

Conclusions

Health is not just a lucky but unintended consequence of the prosperity that results from education, creative work, and a sense of control. Rather, the three tributaries of self-direction help individuals to recognize the health risks of the default American lifestyle, to evaluate claims about health risks and benefits, to coalesce health-producing behaviors into a coherent lifestyle, and to overcome the temptations and obstacles built into the usual way of life. More than ever, health depends on knowledge, critical thinking, self-design, and self-direction.

Further Reading

Brownson, R. C., Boehmer, T. K., & Luke, D. A. (2005). Declining rates of physical activity in the United States: What are the contributors? *Annual Review of Public Health, 26,* 421–443.

Duany, A., Plater-Zyberk, E., & Speck, J. (2000). *Suburban nation: The rise of sprawl and the decline of the American Dream.* New York: North Point Press.

Ewing, R., Schmid, T., Killingsworth, R., Zlot, A., & Raudenbush, S. (2003). Relationship between urban sprawl and physical activity, obesity, and morbidity. *American Journal of Health Promotion, 18,* 47–57.

Mirowsky, J., & Ross, C. E. (2003). *Education,*

social status, and health. New York: Aldine de Gruyter/Transaction.

Pollan, M. (2006). *The omnivore's dilemma: A natural history of four meals.* New York: Penguin.

Schlosser, E. (2002). *Fast food nation.* New York: HarperCollins.

References

Bartley, M., Blane, D., & Davey Smith, G. (2000). Beyond the Black Report. *Sociology of Health and Illness, 20,* 563–577.

Blackwell, D. L., Hayward, M. D., & Crimmins, E. M. (2001). Does childhood health affect chronic morbidity in later life? *Social Science and Medicine, 52,* 1261–1284.

Bogue, D. J. (1985). *The population of the United States: Historical trends and future projections.* New York: Free Press.

Brownson, R. C., & Boehmer, T. K. (2004). Patterns and trends in physical activity, occupation, transportation, land use, and sedentary behaviors. Retrieved September 30, 2008, from *trb.org/downloads/sr282papers/ sr282brownson.pdf.*

Brownson, R. C., Boehmer, T. K., & Luke, D. A. (2005). Declining rates of physical activity in the United States: What are the contributors? *Annual Review of Public Health, 26,* 421–443.

Campbell, T. C., & Campbell, T. M. (2005). *The China Study: The most comprehensive study of nutrition ever conducted and the startling implications for diet, weight loss and long-term health.* Dallas, TX: BenBella Books.

Cook, A., & Daponte, B. O. (2008). A demographic analysis of the rise in the prevalence of the US population overweight and/or obese. *Population Research and Policy Review, 27,* 403–426.

Cutler, D., & Miller, G. (2005). The role of public health improvements in health advances: The twentieth century United States. *Demography, 42,* 1–22.

Cutler, D. M., Glaeser, E. L., & Shapiro, J. M. (2003). Why have Americans become more obese? *Journal of Economic Perspectives, 17,* 93–118.

Duany, A., Plater-Zyberk, E., & Speck, J. (2000). *Suburban nation: The rise of sprawl and the decline of the American Dream.* New York: North Point Press.

Elo, I. T., & Preston, S. H. (1996). Educational differentials in mortality: United States, 1979– 85. *Social Science and Medicine, 42,* 47–57.

Epel, E. S., McEwen, B. S., & Ickovics, J. R. (1998). Embodying psychological thriving:

Physical thriving in response to stress. *Journal of Social Issues, 54*, 301–322.

Ewing, R., Schmid, T., Killingsworth, R., Zlot, A., & Raudenbush, S. (2003). Relationship between urban sprawl and physical activity, obesity, and morbidity. *American Journal of Health Promotion, 18*, 47–57.

Fisk, D. M. (2003). American labor in the 20th century. Retrieved September 30, 2008, from *www.bls.gov/opub/cwc/print/cm20030124ar02pl.htm.*

Hadden, W. C., & Rockswold, P. D. (2008). Increasing differential mortality by educational attainment in adults in the United States. *International Journal of Health Services, 36*, 47–61.

Haines, M. R. (2006). Death rate, by cause: 1900–1998. In S. B. Carter, S. S. Gartner, M. R. Haines, A. L. Olmstead, R. Sutch, & G. Wright (Eds.), *Historical statistics of the United States* [millennial edition online, Table Ab929-951). Retrieved September 30, 2008, from *hsus.cambridge.org/hsusweb/hsusentry-servlet.*

Hayward, M. D., & Gorman, B. K. (2004). The long arm of childhood: The influence of early-life social conditions on men's mortality. *Demography, 41*, 87–107.

Hiroto, D. S. (1974). Locus of control and learned helplessness. *Journal of Experimental Psychology, 102*, 187–193.

Hobbs, F., & Stoops, N. (2002). *Demographic trends in the 20th century: Census 2000 special report CENSR-4.* Washington, DC: U.S. Government Printing Office.

Karasek, R. A., & Theorell, T. (1990). *Healthy work, stress, productivity, and the reconstruction of working life.* New York: Basic Books.

Koplan, J. P., & Dietz, W. H. (1999). Caloric imbalance and public health policy. *Journal of the American Medical Association, 282*, 1579–1581.

Kunst, A. E., & Mackenbach, J. P. (1994). The size of mortality differences associated with educational level in nine industrialized countries. *American Journal of Public Health, 84*, 932–937.

Lakdawalla, D., & Philipson, T. (2009). The growth of obesity and technological change: A theoretical and empirical examination. *Economics and Human Biology, 7*, 283–293.

Lauderdale, D. S. (2001). Education and survival: Birth cohort, period, and age effects. *Demography, 38*, 551–561.

Lleras-Muney, A. (2005). The relationship between education and adult mortality in the United States. *Review of Economic Studies, 72*, 189–221.

Marmot, M. G., & Mustard, J. F. (1994). Coro-

nary heart disease from a population perspective. In R. G. Evans, M. L. Barer, & T. R. Marmor (Eds.), *Why are some people healthy and others not?* (pp. 189–214). New York: Aldine de Gruyter.

Marx, K., & Engels, F. (1964). Economic and philosophical manuscripts. In *Karl Marx: Early writings* (pp. 221–247) (T. R. Bottomore, Ed., Trans.). New York: McGraw-Hill. (Original work published 1884)

McKinlay, J. B., & McKinlay, S. M. (1977). The questionable contribution of medical measures to the decline of mortality on the United States in the twentieth century. *Milbank Memorial Fund Quarterly, 55*, 405–428.

McEwen, B. S. (1998). Stress, adaptation, and disease: Allostasis and allostatic load. *Annals of the New York Academy of Sciences, 840*, 33–44.

McKeown, T. (1979). The direction of medical research. *Lancet, 2*, 1281–1284.

Miller, E. K., & Cohen, J. D. (2001). An integrative theory of prefrontal cortex function. *Annual Review of Neuroscience, 24*, 167–202.

Mirowsky, J., & Kim, J. (2007). Graphing age trajectories: Vector graphs, synthetic and virtual cohort projections, and cross-sectional profiles of depression. *Sociological Methods and Research, 37*, 497–541.

Mirowsky, J., & Ross, C. E. (1998). Education, personal control, lifestyle and health: A human capital hypotheses. *Research on Aging, 20*, 415–449.

Mirowsky, J., & Ross, C. E. (2003). *Education, social status, and health.* New York: Aldine de Gruyter/Transaction.

Mirowsky, J., & Ross, C. E. (2005a). Education, learned effectiveness and health. *London Review of Education, 3*, 205–220.

Mirowsky, J., & Ross, C. E. (2005b). Education, cumulative advantage and health. *Aging International, 30*, 27–62.

Mirowsky, J., & Ross, C. E. (2007a). Creative work and health. *Journal of Health and Social Behavior, 48*, 385–403.

Mirowsky, J., & Ross, C. E. (2007b). Life course trajectories of perceived control and their relationship to education. *American Journal of Sociology, 112*, 1339–1382.

Mirowsky, J., & Ross, C. E. (2008). Education and self-rated health: Cumulative advantage and its rising importance. *Research on Aging, 30*, 93–122.

Morin, A. (2004). A neurocognitive and socio-ecological model of self-awareness. *Genetic, Social, and General Psychology Monographs, 130*, 197–222.

National Household Travel Survey. (2001a). *Our nation's travel: Current issues.* Retrieved September 30, 2008, from *nhts.ornl.gov/2001/pub/Issues.pdf.*

National Household Transportation Survey. (2001b). *Summary of travel trends.* Retrieved September 30, 2008, from *nhts.ornl.gov/2001/pub/STT.pdf.*

Olshansky, S. J., & Ault, B. (1987). The fourth stage of the epidemiologic transition: The age of delayed degenerative diseases. In T. A. Smeeding (Ed.), *Should medical care be rationed by age?* (pp. 11–14). Lanham, MD: Rowman & Littlefield.

O'Rand, A. M. (1996). The precious and the precocious: Understanding cumulative disadvantage and cumulative advantage over the life course. *Gerontologist, 36,* 230–238.

Pappas, G., Queen, S., Hadden, W., & Fisher, G. (1993). The increasing disparity between socioeconomic groups in the United States, 1960 and 1986. *New England Journal of Medicine, 329,* 103–109.

Philipson, T. (2001) The world-wide growth in obesity: An economic research agenda. *Health Economics, 10,* 1–7.

Pincus, T. (1996). Importance of self-care in the association between health and socioeconomic status: Implications for health policy. *The Bulletin, 40,* 5–20.

Pincus, T., Esther, R., DeWalt, D. A., & Callahan, L. F. (1998). Social conditions and self-management are more powerful determinants of health than access to care. *Annals of Internal Medicine, 129,* 406–411.

Pollan, M. (2006). *The omnivore's dilemma: A natural history of four meals.* New York: Penguin.

Rashad, I., Grossman, M., & Chou, S. Y. (2006). The super size of America: An economic estimation of body mass index and obesity in adults. *Eastern Economic Journal, 32,* 133–148.

Rogers, R. G., Hummer, R. A., & Nam, C. B. (2000). *Living and dying in the USA.* New York: Academic Press.

Rosenbaum, M., Leibel, R. L., & Hirsch, J. (1997). Obesity. *New England Journal of Medicine, 333,* 396–407.

Ross, C. E., & Mirowsky, J. (2000). Does medical insurance contribute to socioeconomic differentials in health? *Milbank Quarterly, 78,* 291–321.

Ross, C. E., & Wright, M. P. (1998). Women's work, men's work and the sense of control. *Work and Occupations, 25,* 33–55.

Ross, C. E., & Wu, C. L. (1995). The links between education and health. *American Sociological Review, 60,* 719–745.

Ross, C. E., & Wu, C. L. (1996). Education, age and the cumulative advantage in health. *Journal of Health and Social Behavior, 37,* 104–120.

Schlosser, E. (2002). *Fast food nation.* New York: HarperCollins.

Seeman, T., Singer, B., Rowe, J., Horwitz, R., & McEwen, B. (1997). Price of adaptation–allostatic load and its health consequences: MacArthur Studies of Successful Aging. *Archives of Internal Medicine, 157,* 2259–2269.

Stroebe, W. (2000). *Social psychology and health: Second edition.* Philadelphia: Open University Press.

Taylor, S. E., Repetti, R. L., & Seeman, T. (1997). Health psychology: What is an unhealthy environment and how does it get under the skin? *Annual Review of Psychology, 48,* 411–447.

Toscano, G. (1997, Summer). Dangerous jobs. *Compensation and Working Conditions,* pp. 57–60.

Toscano, G., & Windau, J. (1994, October). The changing character of fatal work injuries. *Monthly Labor Review,* pp. 17–28.

Transportation Research Board. (2005). *Does the built environment influence physical activity?: Examining the evidence* (TRB Special Report No. 282). Retrieved September 30, 2008, from *onlinepubs.trb.org/onlinepubs/trnews/trnews237activity.pdf.*

Wray, L. A., Herzog, A. R., Willis, R. J., & Wallace, R. B. (1998). The impact of education and heart attack on smoking cessation among middle-aged adults. *Journal of Health and Social Behavior, 4,* 271–294.

Wyatt, I. A., & Hecker, D. E. (2006, March). Occupational changes during the 20th century. *Monthly Labor Review,* pp. 35–57.

CHAPTER 16

How Genetics Will Change Medicine and Health Psychology

Jeanne M. McCaffery

Recent genomewide association studies have for the first time produced confirmed genetic associations with a number of common diseases of interest to health psychologists, ranging from diabetes to cardiovascular disease, to cancer, to autoimmune diseases, to gastrointestinal and neuropsychiatric disorders (Manolio, Brooks, & Collins, 2008). The number of common diseases showing confirmed genetic association and the number of linked genes identified for each disease will continue to increase with aggregated genomewide association studies and advancing technologies.

A great but largely unrealized promise of this knowledge is the potential for "personalized medicine," or tailored medical treatment based on genetic background. Personalized medicine encompasses a number of strategies to leverage genetic information to improve health and treatment. This includes the use of genetic and genomic data to provide more accurate diagnosis and prognosis of disease and tailoring of pharmaceutical treatment to genetic background to improve effectiveness and safety. Within 10 years, it would not be surprising if genetic tests aid in making diagnoses, and medicines tailored

to the genetic signature of the diagnosis are prescribed. One example of a medicine tailored to a genetic diagnosis is the breast cancer chemotherapeutic trastuzumab (Herceptin), a genetically engineered antibody that targets a protein that is overexpressed on breast cancer cells in approximately 25–30% of breast cancer patients. Thus, the incorporation of genetic information into diagnosis has clear potential to clarify the nature of the disease and, in doing so, permit more directly targeted pharmacological interventions.

The promise of personalized medicine, however, extends well beyond diagnoses and pharmacological treatments for existing disease to the prevention of disease. Many of the common diseases currently targeted by genomewide association studies have known behavioral or psychosocial predictors. In several cases, effective behavioral interventions have been demonstrated to reduce disease risk dramatically. This raises the possibility that genetic information may be used as a tool to alert people to their disease risks and motivate effective behavior change to prevent the onset of disease. Behavioral treatments tailored to genetic background are here referred to as "personalized behavioral medicine."

To illustrate the promise of personalized behavioral medicine for disease reduction, the example of Type 2 diabetes (T2D) is used. Obesity and genetic background are both known to increase risk for T2D. Figure 16.1 depicts a continuum of risk for T2D based on obesity and genetic risk. Either being overweight or having a genetic risk begins the risk continuum. When these risk factors occur together, risk substantially increases. Over time, at-risk people begin to show evidence of impaired glucose tolerance. At this point, people may already have begun to experience a substantial health impact, such as a significant increase in cardiovascular disease risk. Finally, full-blown diabetes emerges, along with substantially increased risk of heart disease, kidney disease, nervous system disease, and blindness.

Genetic testing for T2D has the potential to identify people at increased risk before they develop obesity. If people are already obese, genetic testing for T2D can identify increased risk before people develop impaired glucose tolerance and begin to experience increased health risks, some of which may be irreversible. To the extent that information on genetic testing for T2D motivates people to lose weight effectively, this genetic testing has the potential to prevent disease. Indeed, T2D may become the prototype for personalized behavioral medicine because replicated genetic associations have already been documented *and* behavioral interventions are known to be effective in disease prevention, as documented below.

TCF7L2 Predicts T2D

A microsatellite marker in the transcription factor 7–like 2 gene (*TCF7L2*), DG10S478, was initially shown to be associated with T2D in 2006 (Grant et al., 2006). For the time, this was a strong report on several accounts. First, the association followed a prior report by two groups of suggestive linkage in the region of this gene on chromosome 10q (Duggirala et al., 1999; Reynisdottir et al., 2003). Thus, there was replicated evidence of a positional candidate in the region. In addition, the initial association, first seen in a case–control study of Icelanders with and without T2D, was replicated in separate case–control studies that comprised female Danes and male and female European Americans. Replication is now the "gold standard" for documented genetic associations.

The microsatellite was in strong linkage disequilibrium (LD) with (i.e., often coinherited with) two single-nucleotide polymorphism (SNP) markers, rs12255372 and rs7903146, which were also strongly associated with T2D in the initial report. Helgason and colleagues (2007) refined the association between the *TCF7L2* gene and T2D

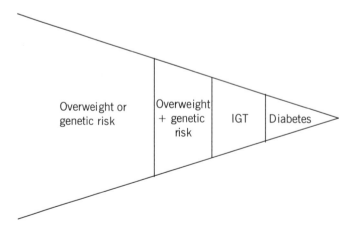

FIGURE 16.1. Continuum of risk for Type 2 diabetes based on overweight and genetic risk. Genetic testing can identify people at risk years before disease sequelae begin to emerge, as in IGT (impaired glucose tolerance).

to the T allele of rs7903146. Specifically, they found association between DG10S478, rs12255372 and rs7903146, and T2D in two populations of European descent, in which each of these markers tend to have high LD. However, haplotypes carrying risk alleles for DG10S478 and rs12255372, but not rs7903146, did not confer increased risk for T2D, implicating rs7903146 as the primary risk allele. Furthermore, in a more genetically diverse sample from West Africa, with fewer regions of strong LD, rs7903146 was strongly associated with risk for T2D, whereas the other markers were not.

The association between *TCF7L2* and T2D has now been replicated numerous times, including by our own group (Duan et al., 2007), and a recent meta-analysis by Cauchi and colleagues (2007) documents that the T allele is associated with a highly significant odds ratio of 1.46 ($p = 5.4 \times 10^{-54}$) across studies. Figure 16.2, from the meta-analysis, documents the consistency and strength of these associations. Furthermore, it documents significant associations across studies among Northern European, other Caucasian, Asian, and African populations. Thus, there is strong evidence that genetic variation within *TCF7L2* shows consistent association with risk for T2D, an effect that has been replicated across several population groups.

Behavior and Genetics in the Diabetes Prevention Program

Research by the United States Diabetes Prevention Program (DPP; Diabetes Prevention Program Research Group, 1999, 2002) has established that T2D can be prevented with lifestyle intervention involving diet, exercise, and behavior modification, even among susceptible individuals (e.g., people who are overweight and have impaired glucose tolerance). In the DPP, 3,234 overweight, nondiabetic persons with elevated fasting glucose and postload glucose were randomly assigned to a lifestyle intervention, pharmacological treatment with metformin (850 mg twice daily), or placebo. Both lifestyle intervention and metformin reduced the incidence of diabetes at 3-year follow-up; however, lifestyle intervention was more effective than metformin. Specifically, lifestyle

intervention reduced the incidence of diabetes by 58% relative to placebo, whereas metformin was associated with a 31% reduction in incidence. This suggests that behavioral intervention promoting weight loss and increased physical activity can be very effective in reducing diabetes onset, even among at-risk individuals.

In the DPP, rs7903146 in *TCF7L2* also predicted progression to diabetes at an average of 3-year follow-up (Florez et al., 2006). Participants with the TT genotypes were more likely to progress from impaired glucose tolerance to diabetes than participants with the CC genotype at rs7903146. However, this effect was stronger in the placebo group than in the metformin and lifestyle intervention groups, although the genotype × treatment arm interaction did not reach statistical significance. The impact of the genetic marker on cumulative diabetes risk by treatment arm is presented in Figure 16.3. As can be seen, participants with the TT genotype demonstrated a marked increase in diabetes risk among those randomized to a placebo. This effect appears to be mitigated somewhat in the metformin group, and no differential genetic risk based on the TT allele at rs7903146 was seen in the lifestyle intervention group. This strongly suggests that behavioral lifestyle intervention not only reduces overall risk for T2D but may also counter the genetic risk for T2D conferred by rs7903146 in *TCF7L2*. Thus, DPP demonstrated that lifestyle intervention is effective in reducing overall diabetes risk. The more recent paper by Florez and colleagues indicates that this benefit occurs in all genotype groups at *TCF7L2*; however, the TT carriers may show the greatest benefit in overall risk reduction.

Personalized Behavioral Medicine: Are We Ready?

The example from DPP provides a proof of the principle that genetic and behavioral factors combine to influence disease risk, and that behavioral intervention can be an effective means of disease prevention, even among those at highest genetic risk. These studies are clearly consistent with the notion that personalized behavioral medicine has the potential to impact the incidence of dis-

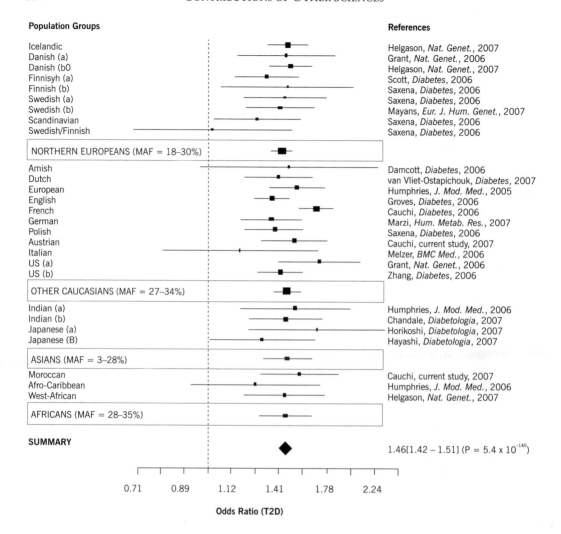

FIGURE 16.2. Association of the *TCF7L2* rs7903146 T allele with T2D. Data are shown for allelic odds ratios based on allele counts. *MAF* stands for minor allele frequency in controls. For each study, the point estimate is given by a *square* whose height is inversely proportional to the standard error of the estimate and the extent of the 95% around the estimate is given by the *horizontal line*. The summary odds ratio is drawn as a *diamond* with horizontal limits at the confidence limits and width inversely proportional to its standard error. This meta-analysis compared 29,195 control individuals with 17,202 subjects with T2D. No heterogeneity in genotypic distribution was found (Woolf test: $\chi^2 = 31.5$, $df = 26$, $p = .21$; Higgins statistic: I2 = 14.1%). No publication bias was detected using the conservative Egger's regression asymmetry test ($t = -1.6$, $df = 25$, $p = .11$). A Mantel–Haenszel (fixed effects) procedure was then performed to provide a pooled odds ratio. (See original article for references listed.) Copyright 2007 by Springer Science & Business Media. Reprinted by permission.

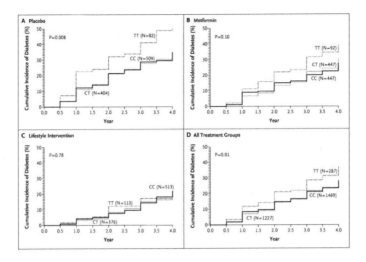

FIGURE 16.3. Incidence of diabetes according to treatment group and genotype at variant rs7903146 in the United States Diabetes Prevention Program. The *p* values were determined by the log-rank test. From Florez et al. (2006). Copyright 2006 by the Massachusetts Medical Society. Reprinted by permission.

ease. During the DPP intervention, however, participants were unaware of their genotype at *TCF7L2*. Thus, from the DPP, we know that behavioral intervention can reduce risk even in those who are genetically at risk, but we do not know what impact, if any, knowledge of genetic risk status would have had on their participation in the interventions and risk for diabetes. Implicit to the concept of personalized behavioral medicine is that the incorporation of genetic information into behavioral medicine interventions can improve outcomes.

A small number of studies have attempted to incorporate genetic markers to promote behavioral change, but with mixed results. People report that additional motivation to improve health behaviors is one of the most common reasons given for seeking genetic testing (Esplen et al., 2001; Julian-Reynier et al., 2001). In addition, it is well documented that positive tests for cancer-related variants, such as breast cancer genes *BRCA1* and *BRCA2*, can increase compliance with preventive behavior, such as yearly mammography screening (Lerman, Croyle, Tercyak, & Hamann, 2002; Meiser, 2005; Wainberg & Husted, 2004). Following genetic testing for hereditary nonpolyposis colorectal cancer (HNPCC), 65% of unaffected carriers in one study were compliant with colonoscopy screening recommendations within 1 year

(Hadley et al., 2004) and nearly 80% of unaffected carriers in another study underwent colonoscopy within 1–2 years of the test (Ponz de Leon et al., 2004). Thus, genetic feedback on cancer risk increased compliance with yearly screening.

The prior studies attempting to use genetic testing to motivate a more complex behavior change have focused primarily on smoking cessation (Carpenter et al., 2007; Lerman et al., 1997; McBride et al., 2002; Sanderson & Wardle, 2005). Positive genetic tests for variants related to lung cancer or emphysema have been successful in increasing perceived risk, perceived benefits of quitting, and fear arousal (Lerman et al., 1997); motivation to quit (Sanderson & Wardle, 2005); and quit attempts, seeking medication or a counseling program for cessation, and reducing cigarette intake by at least 50% (Carpenter et al., 2007). However, effects on cigarette abstinence have largely been disappointing, potentially due to the limited nature of the smoking cessation intervention in these studies (Carpenter et al., 2007; Lerman et al., 1997; Sanderson & Wardle, 2005). One study examined whether genetic testing for a marker within *GSTM1*, a gene involved in the metabolism of carcinogens in cigarette smoke, could heighten risk perceptions and improve smoking cessation rates relative to a smoking cessation brochure. A more intensive intervention was provided with the genetic test, including four phone calls over 12 weeks to maintain the salience of the genetic test result and to provide assistance with smoking cessation. Smoking cessation was significantly increased in the genetic testing condition 6 months after the intervention but not 12 months after treatment was withdrawn (McBride et al., 2002). These studies indicate that genetic testing can increase fear arousal and motivation for behavior change, but, based on this literature, it appears that additional considerations are likely to be needed before successful behavior change and disease reduction occurs.

Implementing Effective Personalized Behavioral Medicine

Although seemingly feasible and of strong potential public health impact, implementing effective personalized behavioral medicine requires consideration and integration of a number of factors. Enumeration of several of these issues follows.

How Is a Genetic Test Best Defined?

The knowledge base about the genetics of complex disease is evolving daily. In complex disease, it is assumed that multiple genes increase risk and that the impact of each of these genes may be small. In the case of T2D, nearly 20 genes now show replicated evidence of association. With advancing technology and the search for additional variants progressing, it is likely that the number will continue to grow, and increasingly detailed tests of genetic risk for T2D will become possible. Despite this great success in identifying a number of risk genes within a few years, the combined impact of these genes on T2D risk remains a subject of controversy. The magnitude of effect varies from an odds ratio of 4.2 between the most extreme genotype groups in one paper (Lango et al., 2008) to an odds ratio of 8.7 using a similar comparison (Cauchi et al., 2008). In addition, the majority of associations were first identified in European American samples and the extent to which individual genetic markers predict risk in non–European American populations largely remains to be determined. Thus, questions

of how many genes to include in a clinical genetic test, how to define risk based on this test, how much risk is necessary before a genetic test should be conducted, and how to define the populations for which the test is valid, quickly arise as challenging questions in the implementation of personalized behavioral medicine.

How Do Genes and Behavior Combine to Produce Disease?

The model of how genetic and behavioral factors combine to impact disease can have a substantial impact on the extent to which behavior change would be predicted to alter disease risk in the context of genetic risk. However, for the majority of genetic associations relevant to complex disease, it remains to be determined whether behavioral or psychosocial predictors show additive or interactive effects with the genetic markers identified in predicting disease. In the case of additive effects, effective behavioral interventions hold the promise to reduce disease risk attributable to the behavioral factor independent of genetic risk, resulting in an overall lower disease risk despite genetic risk. In the case of gene × environment interaction in which an environmental or behavioral risk factor is necessary for the expression of genetic effects on a disease state, it is plausible that effective behavioral intervention may not only reduce overall risk by reducing risk attributable to behavior but also mitigate genetic risk by eliminating the environmental conditions required for the genetic risk to be realized. However, in gene × environment interactions in which either genetic or behavior vulnerability is sufficient to cause disease but no additive effects of these factors occur, behavior change may not result in a reduction of individual disease risk. Thus, understanding the combined effects of genetic and behavioral factors can be critical for understanding the role of personalized behavioral medicine.

Ensuring Valid Test Results

It is critical to ensure valid genetic test results. The majority of molecular markers emerging from the genomewide association studies of T2D can be routinely characterized with basic molecular genetic equipment. Indeed, a number of genetic tests are currently available for direct purchase by consumers over the Internet, including rs7903146 at *TCF7L2*. Genotyping errors do occur, and safeguards against these errors need to be of the utmost precision, particularly when providing clinical feedback based on this information to patients or research participants. Genetic testing is not formally regulated in the United States. A voluntary listing of laboratories that meet Clinical Laboratory Improvement Amendment (CLIA) guidelines for quality control and proficiency testing standards for high-complexity laboratory tests and offer specific genetic tests is available on the GeneTests website at *www.geneclinics.org*. Additional resources for genotyping may be laboratories affiliated with well-respected universities or companies, particularly those involved in the identification of risk markers for the disease of interest.

What Is the Benefit/Risk Ratio of Conducting the Genetic Test?

The benefit–risk ratio of conducting genetic testing needs to be considered. For those who test positive, the benefits of genetic testing could include the potential for health behavior change to reduce risk and increased medical screening to identify emerging disease. Genetic testing may also help with planning for the future, such as medical and financial planning. Potential risks of genetic testing for those who test positive include a potential fatalism about their risk for disease and a negative impact on their belief that changing behavior can reduce their disease risk. A positive genetic test can also have a negative impact on psychological well-being, including increased anxiety and depression.

Assessing the benefit–risk ratio of genetic testing must also consider the impact of the genetic test on those who test negative. A negative test may be a benefit if it reaffirms commitment to behavior change. For example, in response to a negative test, a person may decide to focus on behavior change because genetic factors do not appear to play as important a role in the disease risk. However, it is also quite possible that people receiving a negative test will feel relieved about their risk, reduce their motivation for behavior change, and potentially increase their disease risk. Because many people test negative for any given genetic test, it is criti-

cal to evaluate the net impact of providing a genetic test result on behavior and, ultimately, disease risk.

A potential risk of genetic testing is discrimination based on genetic test results. In 2008, the Genetic Information Nondiscrimination Act (GINA) was signed into law. It prohibits discrimination in health insurance or employment decisions based on genetic test results. This substantially mitigates some of the most common concerns about genetic testing. However, other sources of discrimination and potential adverse consequences remain, such as the concern that a genetic sample may be used in a criminal investigation.

Complexity of Conveying the Test Result

The extent of behavior change following a genetic test result may depend on the extent to which a patient understands the result and its implications for disease risk. Even if only one marker is used as a genetic test, the communication of an individual's risk based on this result, and the potential for behavior change to reduce this risk, is relatively complex. Taking the example of *TCF7L2*, rs7903146 encompasses three genotypes with roughly additive risk for T2D. The TT genotype, which occurs in roughly 10% of European American populations, is associated with a doubling of risk relative to the lowest risk genotype CC, which occurs in roughly 50% of European American populations. The intermediate risk genotype CT occurs in roughly 40% of European American populations and is associated with 1.5 times the risk of diabetes. Based on a 10% prevalence of T2D among CC genotypes, these odds ratios imply that the CT genotype would be associated with a 15% prevalence of diabetes, and the TT genotype with a 20% prevalence. Thus, the interpretation of the results of the genetic test alone requires both basic health literacy and an understanding of mathematical concepts. The difficulty in understanding the mathematical concepts may be worsened when risk is not reflected by a relatively simple effect, such as a doubling or tripling of risk.

This picture is further complicated by quantifying the potential impact of behavior change on these risk estimates. From the DPP, we have some of the best estimates of the impact of a behavior change on a disease outcome. Specifically, it is known that weight loss of 7% or more can reduce the risk of diabetes by approximately 50% (Knowler et al., 2002), regardless of genotype. Furthermore, studies have shown that although small, nonadditive effects may be present, the effects of TCF7L2 and obesity on diabetes largely appear to be additive (Duan et al., 2007). Thus, the potential impact of weight loss on diabetes risk can be roughly approximated by halving the overall risk for diabetes in each genotype group. However, it is easy to see how strong data on the impact of behavior change interventions on disease outcomes is critical for personalized behavioral medicine.

It is also easy to see how a patient's understanding of this information may be biased in terms of educational level and comfort with health statistics. Furthermore, it is quite plausible that risk information would be experienced as confusing and reduce the likelihood that persons might be motivated to engage in the behavior change. The challenge of communicating complex risk algorithms and genetic concepts to patients will only be exaggerated by models incorporating multiple genes and potentially multiple behaviors. Research on the most effective methods to communicate complex genetic risk information is critical for the implementation of personalized behavioral medicine.

Conclusions

One of the key promises of the recent advances in identifying genes that predict complex disease is personalized medicine. Genetic or genomic information may soon be used to provide more accurate disease diagnosis and prognosis, and to develop medicines tailored to these genetic signatures. Personalized medicine also has the potential to extend beyond diagnosis and treatment to disease prevention because genotype information could potentially be used to alert people to their disease risk prior to the onset of disease, thereby promoting early healthy behavior change. An example in which genetic risk information may be used to promote health behavior change is T2D, for which replicated genetic associations have

been identified and weight loss is known to reduce risk.

Further Reading

Andreasen, C. H., & Andersen, G. (2009). Gene–environment interactions and obesity—further aspects of genomewide association studies. *Nutrition, 25*(10), 998–1003.

Cauchi, S., El Achhab, Y., Choquet, H., Dina, C., Krempler, F., Weitgasser, R., et al. (2007). TCF7L2 is reproducibly associated with type 2 diabetes in various ethnic groups: A global meta-analysis. *Journal of Molecular Medicine, 85*(7), 777–782.

Florez, J. C., Jablonski, K. A., Bayley, N., Pollin, T. I., de Bakker, P. I., Shuldiner, A. R., et al. (2006). TCF7L2 polymorphisms and progression to diabetes in the Diabetes Prevention Program. *New England Journal of Medicine, 355*(3), 241–250.

Hudson, K. L., Holohan, M. K., & Collins, F. S. (2008). Keeping pace with the times—the Genetic Information Nondiscrimination Act of 2008. *New England Journal of Medicine, 358*(25), 2661–2663.

Lerman, C., Croyle, R. T., Tercyak, K. P., & Hamann, H. (2002). Genetic testing: Psychological aspects and implications. *Journal of Consulting and Clinical Psychology, 70*(3), 784–797.

Manolio, T. A., Brooks, L. D., & Collins, F. S. (2008). A HapMap harvest of insights into the genetics of common disease. *Journal of Clinical Investigation, 118*(5), 1590–1605.

References

Carpenter, M. J., Strange, C., Jones, Y., Dickson, M. R., Carter, C., Moseley, M. A., et al. (2007). Does genetic testing result in behavioral health change?: Changes in smoking behavior following testing for alpha-1 antitrypsin deficiency. *Annals of Behavioral Medicine, 33*(1), 22–28.

Cauchi, S., El Achhab, Y., Choquet, H., Dina, C., Krempler, F., Weitgasser, R., et al. (2007). TCF7L2 is reproducibly associated with Type 2 diabetes in various ethnic groups: A global meta-analysis. *Journal of Molecular Medicine, 85*(7), 777–782.

Cauchi, S., Meyre, D., Durand, E., Proenca, C., Marre, M., Hadjadj, S., et al. (2008). Post genome-wide association studies of novel genes associated with type 2 diabetes show gene–gene interaction and high predictive value. *PLoS ONE, 3*(5), e2031.

Diabetes Prevention Program Research Group.

(1999). The Diabetes Prevention Program: Design and methods for a clinical trial in the prevention of type 2 diabetes. *Diabetes Care, 22*(4), 623–634.

Diabetes Prevention Program Research Group. (2002). Reduction in the incidence of Type 2 diabetes with lifestyle intervention or metformin. *New England Journal of Medicine, 346*(6), 393–403.

Duan, Q. L., Dube, M. P., Frasure-Smith, N., Barhdadi, A., Lesperance, F., Theroux, P., et al. (2007). Additive effects of obesity and *TCF7L2* variants on risk for Type 2 diabetes among cardiac patients. *Diabetes Care, 30*(6), 1621–1623.

Duggirala, R., Blangero, J., Almasy, L., Dyer, T. D., Williams, K. L., Leach, R. J., et al. (1999). Linkage of Type 2 diabetes mellitus and of age at onset to a genetic location on chromosome 10q in Mexican Americans. *American Journal of Human Genetics, 64*(4), 1127–1140.

Esplen, M. J., Madlensky, L., Butler, K., McKinnon, W., Bapat, B., Wong, J., et al. (2001). Motivations and psychosocial impact of genetic testing for HNPCC. *American Journal of Medical Genetics, 103*(1), 9–15.

Florez, J. C., Jablonski, K. A., Bayley, N., Pollin, T. I., de Bakker, P. I., Shuldiner, A. R., et al. (2006). *TCF7L2* polymorphisms and progression to diabetes in the Diabetes Prevention Program. *New England Journal of Medicine, 355*(3), 241–250.

Grant, S. F., Thorleifsson, G., Reynisdottir, I., Benediktsson, R., Manolescu, A., Sainz, J., et al. (2006). Variant of transcription factor 7–like 2 (*TCF7L2*) gene confers risk of Type 2 diabetes. *Nature Genetics, 38*(3), 320–323.

Hadley, D. W., Jenkins, J. F., Dimond, E., de Carvalho, M., Kirsch, I., & Palmer, C. G. (2004). Colon cancer screening practices after genetic counseling and testing for hereditary nonpolyposis colorectal cancer. *Journal of Clinical Oncology, 22*(1), 39–44.

Helgason, A., Palsson, S., Thorleifsson, G., Grant, S. F., Emilsson, V., Gunnarsdottir, S., et al. (2007). Refining the impact of *TCF7L2* gene variants on Type 2 diabetes and adaptive evolution. *Nature Genetics, 39*(2), 218–225.

Julian-Reynier, C. M., Bouchard, L. J., Evans, D. G., Eisinger, F. A., Foulkes, W. D., Kerr, B., et al. (2001). Women's attitudes toward preventive strategies for hereditary breast or ovarian carcinoma differ from one country to another: Differences among English, French, and Canadian women. *Cancer, 92*(4), 959–968.

Knowler, W. C., Barrett-Connor, E., Fowler, S. E., Hamman, R. F., Lachin, J. M., Walker, E. A., et al. (2002). Reduction in the incidence of Type 2 diabetes with lifestyle intervention or metformin. *New England Journal of Medicine, 346*(6), 393–403.

Lango, H., Palmer, C. N., Morris, A. D., Zeggini, E., Hattersley, A. T., McCarthy, M. I., et al. (2008). Assessing the combined impact of 18 common genetic variants of modest effect sizes on Type 2 diabetes risk. *Diabetes, 57*(1), 3129–3135.

Lerman, C., Croyle, R. T., Tercyak, K. P., & Hamann, H. (2002). Genetic testing: Psychological aspects and implications. *Journal of Consulting and Clinical Psychology, 70*(3), 784–797.

Lerman, C., Gold, K., Audrain, J., Lin, T. H., Boyd, N. R., Orleans, C. T., et al. (1997). Incorporating biomarkers of exposure and genetic susceptibility into smoking cessation treatment: Effects on smoking-related cognitions, emotions, and behavior change. *Health Psychology, 16*(1), 87–99.

Manolio, T. A., Brooks, L. D., & Collins, F. S. (2008). A HapMap harvest of insights into the genetics of common disease. *Journal of Clinical Investigation, 118*(5), 1590–1605.

McBride, C. M., Bepler, G., Lipkus, I. M., Lyna, P., Samsa, G., Albright, J., et al. (2002). Incorporating genetic susceptibility feedback into a smoking cessation program for African-American smokers with low income. *Cancer Epidemiology, Biomarkers and Prevention, 11*(6), 521–528.

Meiser, B. (2005). Psychological impact of genetic testing for cancer susceptibility: An update of the literature. *Psycho-Oncology, 14*(12), 1060–1074.

Ponz de Leon, M., Benatti, P., de Gregorio, C., Pedroni, M., Losi, L., Genuardi, M., et al. (2004). Genetic testing among high-risk individuals in families with hereditary nonpolyposis colorectal cancer. *British Journal of Cancer, 90*, 882–887.

Reynisdottir, I., Thorleifsson, G., Benediktsson, R., Sigurdsson, G., Emilsson, V., Einarsdottir, A. S., et al. (2003). Localization of a susceptibility gene for Type 2 diabetes to chromosome 5q34-q35.2. *American Journal of Human Genetics, 73*(2), 323–335.

Sanderson, S. C., & Wardle, J. (2005). Will genetic testing for complex diseases increase motivation to quit smoking?: Anticipated reactions in a survey of smokers. *Health Education and Behavior, 32*(5), 640–653.

Wainberg, S., & Husted, J. (2004). Utilization of screening and preventive surgery among unaffected carriers of a *BRCA1* or *BRCA2* gene mutation. *Cancer Epidemiology, Biomarkers and Prevention, 13*(12), 1989–1995.

CHAPTER 17

Nursing Science and Psychological Phenomena

Diane Lauver
Rebecca West
Jean E. Johnson

As disciplines, nursing and psychology share some similarities. Both disciplines espouse a holistic view of health (e.g., biopsychosocial–environmental perspective) and of people (e.g., in a body–mind–spirit perspective) rather than a biomedical perspective. The two disciplines address prevention and management of illness or disease from multidimensional perspectives. As researchers, both nurses and psychologists are theory-based. Nurse-scientists often have used, revised, and expanded upon existing psychological theories (e.g., health belief model, social cognitive theory).

Nurse-scientists have an intimate understanding of how people cope with actual and potential threats to health within the complexities of their lives. Thus, typically, nursing science is practice-driven and has the ultimate purpose of developing efficacious interventions to improve people's health status. For example, nurse-scientists have improved how young children navigate adolescence and deal with having diabetes (Grey, Boland, Davidson, Li, & Tamborlane, 2000), how teenage mothers from disadvantaged environments deal with pregnancy and mothering (Olds et al., 2007), and how older men cope with prostate cancer to maintain their usual activities (Johnson, Nail, Lauver, King, & Keys, 1988).

One major focus of nursing research has involved the psychological and behavioral aspects of health and illness. Some research by nurse-scientists on behavioral aspects of health and illness predates the establishment of the Division of Health Psychology in the American Psychological Association. To clarify, nurse-scientists also study aspects of health and illness from many other disciplinary perspectives, such as basic physiological processes, sociological phenomena, improvement of health care systems, and informational technologies.

In this chapter, *our primary purpose is to offer selected examples of nursing research that are especially relevant to health psychology. Our secondary purpose is to describe briefly some considerations for understanding more about science in the context of the discipline of nursing.* By highlighting examples of research by nurse-scientists that are of interest to psychologists, this chapter cannot be exhaustive. We selected research programs to illustrate a breadth of clinical phenomena studied, theories drawn upon, questions asked, populations sampled, and settings utilized. We hope that readers gain a greater understanding of not only the richness of nursing science but also its impact on health outcomes, and testing and refining of theories relevant to psychology.

The Discipline of Nursing

In this section, we briefly describe considerations for understanding nursing science. We present *philosophical assumptions in the nursing profession* that define the discipline of nursing and share elements of a working philosophy of nursing. We clarify *educational pathways to nursing*, including doctoral education among nurses. Also, we summarize concisely the *history of funding for nursing science.*

Defining the Discipline of Nursing

A practice-based discipline, "nursing" is defined in the American Nurses Association (ANA) *Nursing's Social Policy Statement* (2003) as the "protection, promotion, and optimization of health and abilities, prevention of illness and injury, alleviation of suffering through diagnosis and treatment of human response, and advocacy in the care of individuals, families, communities, and populations" (pp. 4–5). However, nursing involves not only attending to the breadth of human experiences and responses to health and illness in diverse physical and social environments but also influencing social and public policy for social justice, as well as advancing knowledge through scientific inquiry.

The ANA (2003) Social Policy Statement includes the following assumptions that are central to a philosophy of nursing: Quality health care is a human right; the nursing profession is responsible to society; and nursing has the responsibility to regulate itself to ensure quality performance. Although some may think of nursing as focusing exclusively on the care of individuals, nursing also focuses on social concerns related to health care. These social concerns include, but are not limited to, the development of knowledge, policies, and resources for improving health care, as well as the provision of services for maintaining and promoting the health of the public.

Educational Pathways to Nursing

Because the type of educational preparation influences the scholarship in a discipline, we summarize briefly the educational preparation of nurses. Registered nurses are currently prepared at three different levels. The ANA considers the primary preparation for professional nurses to be the 4-year bachelor's degree. Technical level nurses are educated mostly in 2-year associate degree programs and less often in 3-year hospital-based diploma programs. Graduates of state-approved nursing programs sit for a national licensing exam and are licensed by their states.

Increasing demands for high-quality and cost-effective health care drives a need for nurses with advanced practice education and skills. Advanced practice nurses (APNs) include nurse practitioners, clinical nurse specialists, nurse midwives, and nurse anesthetists. These advanced practitioners typically hold a master's degree in nursing and are board-certified in a given population (e.g., family or adult health, pediatrics, women's health, or geriatrics) or specialty area (e.g., acute care, psychiatric-mental health, emergency, or anesthesia).

The Doctor of Nursing Practice (DNP) is in the process of replacing the Master of Science degree as the entry-level preparation for APNs. This practice doctorate degree continues the tradition of expert clinical knowledge and skills currently provided by APNs. The DNP provides additional training and expertise in leadership skills in the delivery of health care in complex organizations, evaluation of systems, and policymaking. In collaborative relationships with PhD-prepared nurse-researchers, DNPs can facilitate translational research to improve health care outcomes.

History of Doctoral Education for Nurses as Researchers

Before World War II, nurses who sought advanced educational degrees studied at schools of education. Graduates of these programs studied nurses, their delivery of care, and their working environment. This focus dominated nursing scholarship for several decades.

After World War II, health care changed. With the discovery of penicillin as an antibiotic, many infections were well controlled, and deaths due to infections declined. As people recovered more often from major health crises, they began to live with chronic illnesses. With the development of increasingly complex surgeries, such as open heart surgery, accompanying postoperative complications arose (e.g., respiratory failure and shock).

Nurses realized they did not have sufficient knowledge to care for patients with particularly complex needs. Nurses wanted to be knowledgeable about not only the technical aspects of patient care but also about how patients made decisions, behaved in certain ways, and reacted emotionally (Fairman, 2008). Nurses interested in studying psychological aspects of health and illness had few opportunities to pursue education and training as scientists.

History of Funding for Nurse-Scientists and Nursing Science

Although nursing practice has been well established, nursing science is relatively young. In the mid-1950s, a Federal program for funding pre- and postdoctoral education and research for nurses was established in the Division of Nursing Resources, Bureau of Medical Services. In 1962, a Federal program provided support to universities that opened their graduate science programs to qualified nurses. Although both social and biological science departments participated in this program, the most popular departments among nurses were the social sciences, including psychology. With these educational opportunities, nurses became scientists and investigated clinical problems from their practices.

In the 1970s, with a cadre of PhD-prepared nurse-scientists, schools of nursing began programs for the PhD in nursing. PhD-prepared nurses are professors in universities, researchers engaged in scholarly inquiry, leaders in nursing and health care, and activists who work to influence policy. As doctoral programs in nursing grew in the 1980s, some offered Doctorate in Nursing Science (DNS) degrees; others offered PhDs. Conceptually, the DNS degree was more clinically focused, and the PhD, more research focused.

In the 1980s, an existing Federal program for nursing education and research was moved to the National Institutes of Health (NIH), and a National Center for Nursing Research was activated. The Center has funded pre- and postdoctoral education to prepare nurses as scientists to develop knowledge in the discipline further.

In the early 1990s, the Institute of Medicine recommended that the Center be elevated to the status of an Institute within NIH, so that nursing would be included more directly in behavioral and biomedical sciences. The Center was promoted to the National Institute for Nursing Research (NINR) in 1993. Thus, the Federal government has been the primary source of funding for nurses in their pre- and postdoctoral education (NINR, 2009).

Exemplars of Nursing Research and Psychological Phenomena

Promoting Health and Preventing Problems among Vulnerable Families

In the following sections we share exemplars of research that have contributed to nursing science and are relevant to psychology. In this particular section we discuss research on one long-standing social issue that has been intertwined with health issues, that is, teenage pregnancy among women from socially disadvantaged populations. Kitzman, with a PhD in Nursing and experience as a pediatric nurse, and Olds, with a PhD in Human Development and Family Studies, wanted to prevent problems experienced by disadvantaged pregnant teens. This team designed interventions to answer the overall question, "Will intensive prenatal and postnatal nurse home visits improve outcomes of pregnancy, early childhood, and life course development among teenage, unmarried, and/or poor women bearing their first children?"

Because of the multiple influences on maternal and child behavior, Kitzman's and Olds' research was based on a combination of theories about individual adaptation, such as attachment theory (Bowlby, 1969) and self-efficacy theory (Bandura, 1977), as well as about environmental context, such as human ecology theory (Bronfenbrenner, 1979). Kitzman and Olds conceptualized a person–process–context model that simultaneously incorporates behavioral, biological, sociological, and economic factors, and their interactions, to account for the system of influences on maternal and child functioning (Olds, Kitzman, Cole, & Robinson, 1997). A combination of nursing competence and knowledge of human development across the lifespan, family function, and psychological theories, as well as expertise in program design, was brought to bear on this program of research.

Randomized controlled trials (RCTs) were used throughout the research program. Various control groups were used for comparison purposes and to rule out alternative hypothesis in three RCTs (Kitzman et al., 1997; Olds, Henderson, Tatelbaum, & Chamberlin, 1986; Olds et al., 2002). Data were collected from families when the children of teenage mothers were 3, 4, 6, 9, and 15 years old (Kitzman et al., 2000; Olds, Eckenrode, et al., 1997; Olds, Kitzman, et al., 2004; Olds, Robinson, et al., 2004; Olds et al., 2007); data collection has continued. Participants have been from semirural and urban settings, and from different racial and ethnic backgrounds (e.g., African American, Mexican American, and European American).

Specially trained nurses delivered the intervention during home visits. These visits occurred every 2 weeks during the women's pregnancies, once a week for 1 month after birth, and with diminishing frequency until their children were 2 years old. The central aspect of the intervention was to emphasize the coping skills of the women and their families. Using a strengths-based approach, nurses provided (1) parents with education about positive, health-related behaviors during pregnancy and competent care of their children, and (2) pregnant women/mothers with education and skills for their personal development (family planning, educational achievement and participation in the workforce). Nurses also facilitated women in building resources; they encouraged them to involve other family members and friends in the pregnancy, birth, and early care of the child. Nurses also linked families with needed health care and human services (Kitzman et al., 1997).

Consistent with their person–process–context model, Kitzman and Olds used a breadth of outcome measures in their studies. Across their trials they consistently observed the following: Among the families, there were increases in fathers' involvement,

reductions in welfare and food stamp use, and increased employment; among the children, there were reductions in injuries and improvements in school readiness; among mothers, there was increased prenatal health and a reduction in closely spaced subsequent pregnancies. At 15-year follow-up, mothers who received nurse visitations had lower rates of arrest, alcohol and other drug use, and abuse and neglect of their children when compared to mothers in the control group (Olds, Eckenrode, et al., 1997).

To manage national replications of this impressive program, a nonprofit organization, the Nurse–Family Partnership National Service Office (*www.nursefamilypartnership.org*) was formed. The purpose of the organization is to build community capacity, provide training and assistance to nurses to deliver the program, maintain the fidelity of the intervention, and make the program available to a large portion of low-income pregnant women in the United States. In a cost–benefit analysis, the Nurse–Family Partnership program yielded a $17,189 benefit over cost for each family enrolled (Washington State Institute for Public Policy, 2004). Having extensive national impact, the program serves over 13,500 families a day in over 310 counties in 23 states. The program is being tested in five additional countries: England, Australia, Canada, the Netherlands, and Germany.

Minimizing Distress and Promoting Function by Facilitating Coping with Novel Health Events

In the 1960s, most clinicians believed that patients should be given only limited information about their clinical situation, assuming that detailed information would make patients more anxious and less able to cope. For example, people with cancer often were not told their actual diagnoses. From her clinical experience as a nurse, Jean Johnson had the hunch that patients were overly anxious because they had *not* been told what to expect would happen to them during a new procedure or treatment.

Johnson combined her hunch from nursing practice with Leventhal's developing common sense theory about coping with illness (Leventhal, Meyer, & Nerenz, 1980). Leventhal proposed that peoples' cognitive representation of illness drives their responses to illness. Johnson reasoned that if people were given an accurate description about upcoming events, then they would form an accurate cognitive representation, have greater understanding about what to expect, and cope more effectively regarding such events. Johnson proposed that if nurses gave patients concrete, objective information about likely sensations they could experience during a novel event, then this concrete–objective content would replace vague ideas and/or emotionally focused content in patients' cognitive representation.

Johnson also proposed that there were types of information *not* to share with patients. If nurses told patients about possible emotional reactions and subjective evaluations, then this information would likely focus patients' attention, expectations, and experiences on subjective responses, and they could be more upset. Instruction in coping strategies without the contextual concrete–objective descriptions of the impending experience could cause patients to rely unduly on care providers for how to cope and undermine their confidence in their own abilities to cope. When cognitive representations contain familiar sensations, then patients could choose to use whatever coping strategies they prefer. With concrete–objective information about a novel event, patients could be self-regulating rather than dependent on clinicians' directions for coping.

The first tests of Johnson's hypothesis were done in the laboratory because of clinicians' concerns about providing patients with relevant, detailed clinical information. In an experiment, participants were either given preparatory information or not. The information consisted of descriptions of typical physical sensations they could experience (i.e., see, hear, feel) and used concrete, objective terms that were emotionally neutral. As expected, participants who received the preparatory information found the stimuli less distressing than participants who did not (Johnson, 1973). This research also showed that participants cognitively could separate the intensity of their physical sensations and their distress from these sensations. Based on findings from laboratory studies, research was extended to clinical settings.

Because clinical procedures and treatments are more complex than laboratory situations, the content of Johnson's interventions was expanded. In addition to descriptions of sensations, she included temporal characteristics, environmental features, and causes of sensations regarding the event. To generate accurate, concrete, and objective descriptions of what patients experienced with clinical events, Johnson and her colleagues (McHugh, Christman, & Johnson, 1982) interviewed patients who had undergone such events. The typical words patients used to describe what they experienced (e.g., saw, heard, felt) and their observations of events (i.e., procedure or treatment) were used to construct subsequent interventions.

Johnson's first RCT in a clinical setting was conducted with patients undergoing their first gastroendoscopy (Johnson, Morrissey, & Leventhal, 1973). Patients who received the audiotaped, concrete objective descriptions prior to gastroendoscopy were better able to cope (i.e., required less tranquilizing drugs) than patients who received usual care. Johnson conducted RCTs to replicate and extend this research with surgical patients (Johnson, Rice, Fuller, & Endress, 1978) and cancer patients receiving radiation therapy (Johnson et al., 1988). In all trials, patients received concrete–objective descriptions of their expected events by audiotape.

The most consistent finding was that providing concrete–objective information about novel clinical events increased patients' abilities to cope with such events. This was indicated by patients' ability to regain or maintain usual activities. Johnson proposed that the effect of such informational interventions on coping was mediated by participants' degree of knowledge about what to expect and their level of understanding about what was happening to them.

Johnson's hypothesis about mediation was supported in a study of cancer patients. The effect of preparatory information on patients' functional outcomes was mediated by participants' reports of their (1) predictions of impending experiences and (2) understanding of that experience (Johnson, Lauver, & Nail, 1989). Melnyk (1995) tested this mediation hypothesis with mothers who faced their children's unexpected hospitalization. As expected, she found that the effect of preparatory information about children's hospitalization on mothers' subsequent coping was mediated by predictability and understanding of their children's responses and behaviors.

The culmination of these studies was Johnson's development of a theory of self-regulation about information and coping in novel health care situations (Johnson, 1999). A basic premise of her theory of self-regulation is consistent with Leventhal's common sense theory of coping. In both theories, cognitive representations guide people's responses to and coping with novel situations.

Johnson's program of research has influenced clinical practice substantially in the United States. It contributed to the abolishment of the practice of withholding information from patients. In many health care settings, nurses and other clinicians routinely provide their patients with neutral, concrete–objective descriptions of what to expect during new procedures and novel treatments. Now it is difficult to find a clinical setting in the United States to test the theory further. Because Johnson's self-regulation theory rests heavily upon cognitions and was developed in the United States, one could hypothesize that it is not applicable in other cultures. However, investigators in Germany, Korea, Taiwan, Austria, the United Kingdom, Australia, Ireland, Sweden, and Canada have found that informational interventions—based on self-regulation theory—enhance coping with health care experiences.

Promoting Cancer Screening with Tailored Interventions: Guided by the Health Belief Model

As part of their role, nurses may encourage people to engage in screening for potentially serious conditions. Nurses can be challenged when people do not engage in such screening. As researchers, nurses have identified theories to guide research on interventions to promote greater engagement in recommended screenings.

With a long-standing interest in oncology nursing, Champion has studied ways to improve early cancer detection (e.g., breast and colon). Champion (1983) identified the health belief model (HBM) as promising to guide research on breast cancer screening. She developed reliable and valid instruments to measure the concepts of the HBM and has revised these scales over time (Champion, 1999; Champion, Skinner, & Menon, 2005). Guided by the HBM, Champion conducted RCTs to promote breast cancer screening. She was one of the first nurses to conduct a tailored intervention. A tailored intervention is one that involves an assessment of participants on a limited number of

key characteristics, and customization of the intervention delivery based on those characteristics (Lauver et al., 2002).

In an RCT, Champion and Huster (1995) tested tailored interventions guided by the HBM on mammography use. Nurse interveners obtained participants' baseline data on perceived susceptibility of breast cancer, and perceived benefits and barriers to mammography. If participants' baseline beliefs on perceived susceptibility or benefits were low, then interveners provided information designed to improve these beliefs, using predetermined text. And if participants' baseline perceived barriers were high, then the nurse shared information designed to reduce these perceptions. As expected, mammography use was higher among women in the intervention group than among those in the usual care group.

Champion added complexity to her research by using both the HBM and the transtheoretical model (TTM) to guide her interventions. For example, Champion, Skinner, and Foster (2000) designed intervention messages tailored on not only perceived susceptibility, benefits, and barriers but also stage of adoption of mammography. In this RCT, there were three groups: (1) The first group received tailored messages by phone; (2) the second group received tailored messages in person; and (3) the third group received usual care. Both intervention groups had higher rates of mammography use than did the usual care group. The odds of having mammography among participants who had tailored phone messages were double that for those who had usual care. The odds of having mammography among participants who had tailored messages in person were almost three times that for those who had usual care. When researchers controlled for baseline scores, participants who had either type of message had improved scores on knowledge, perceived susceptibility, and benefits, as well as lower barriers scores.

In another RCT, Champion and colleagues (2003) compared effects of mode of delivery and of tailored informational messages on mammography use. In this study of participants who had not had recent mammograms, five informational messages were compared (e.g., tailored print, nontailored print, or phone). All message groups had higher mammography use compared to the usual care group; participants who had been precontemplators at baseline had the highest rates of mammography adoption.

Champion has replicated and extended her tailored interventions to promote mammography in numerous ways. Partnering with interdisciplinary colleagues, Champion has recruited participants from different geographic and clinical settings (e.g., health maintenance organizations [HMOs] and clinics) and in different populations (e.g., African Americans). In summary, Champion has demonstrated that the HBM and TTM can guide screening research well, and that tailored informational messages are effective in promoting breast cancer screening.

Promoting Cancer Screening with Tailored Interventions: Guided by a Multidimensional Theory

As a nurse practitioner (NP) in women's health, Diane Lauver knew that many clients did not engage in health practices as recommended (e.g., breast cancer screening). Whereas some scholars maintained that beliefs primarily explain health behaviors, Lauver (1987) thought that such behaviors were influenced by not only beliefs but also other variables (e.g., feelings and environmental factors regarding the behavior). In her research program on health-related behaviors among women, Lauver selected particular theories to guide studies of different types of preventive behavior because she believed that a single behavioral theory would not be applicable to a variety of different preventive health behaviors. For example, behaviors for early disease detection (e.g., screening in asymptomatic states) are characteristically different than health promotion or disease management behaviors; they inherently involve the possibility of learning one has a serious disease (Lauver, 1987). Whereas some proposed that women do not engage in screening primarily because of fear of disease, Lauver maintained that such emotions were relevant but not sufficient to explain such behavior; situational conditions of the health care system were also influences. Lauver thought that those who proposed fear as the primary barrier to women's screening behaviors were operating under the fundamental attribution error and thought that women are overly emotional.

After consulting with clinicians about challenges in their practices, Lauver focused on explaining women's search for professional care for early detection of disease (precursors to cancer or cancer). Lauver (1992) reviewed possible theories, including the HBM, and chose a multidimensional theory to guide her research on seeking care for breast cancer symptoms. In his theory of behavior, Triandis (1980) proposed that facilitating (i.e., objective–environmental) conditions and physiological arousal interacted with intentions and habit to influence the behavior of interest. Furthermore, Triandis proposed that intentions were a function of (1) affect, (2) worth or utility (i.e., subjective, expected utility = consequences × values), and (3) social factors (i.e., norms, interpersonal agreements) regarding the behavior.

When applying Triandis's theory to behaviors for early detection of disease (e.g., for cancer), Lauver (1992) maintained that physiological arousal related to the likelihood of abnormality would likely be confounded with affect (e.g., anxiety). In her revision, she did not include a variable of physiological arousal. Given a focus on explaining behavior, and given Triandis's proposal that intention could be explained by three psychosocial variables, Lauver substituted these three variables for intention in her theory and omitted a separate variable of intentions. When applying Triandis's concepts to early detection of disease behaviors, Lauver defined them in relation to this type of behavior; for example, when defining norms, she included not only peer norms but also professional recommendations regarding the behavior. In her revision of Triandis's theory, she proposed that psychosocial variables and habit influenced behavior in moderation with facilitating external conditions (e.g., affordability, accessibility of care). Although more complex than some other theories, Lauver's revised theory was valid in that it reflected what she had seen in practice, and it seemed to explain early detection behaviors more adequately.

Based on the revised theory, Lauver conducted correlational studies of women seeking evaluation for breast cancer symptoms (e.g., Lauver, 1994). Whereas beliefs about the worth of seeking care were correlated with delay, habit was associated with promptness. Affect (e.g., anxiety) explained delay in seeking care in moderation with a facilitating condition and having an identified clinician for routine health care; those with some level of anxiety who also had an identified clinician were more likely to seek care than were those who did not have an identified clinician. Lauver's theory and research have stimulated related research by other nurse-scientists (Baumann, Fontana, Brown & Cameron, 1993; Facione, 1993; Facione, Dodd, Holzemer, & Meleis, 1997; Reifenstein, 2007).

When women's underuse of mammography and clinical breast examination was a concern, Lauver and colleagues studied these behaviors also. Based on her revision of Triandis's theory, she examined existing measures (Lauver, 1996), developed new measures, and conducted descriptive correlational studies of professional breast cancer screening (Lauver, Nabholz, Scott, & Tak, 1997). Lauver then designed a patient-centered, tailored informational intervention focused on women's use of professional breast cancer screening.

In an RCT (Lauver, Settersten, Kane, & Henriques, 2003), participants were women 51–80 years old who had not had mammograms as recommended. Participants were assigned to three different groups: an observation group, a recommendation about screening group, or a recommendation about screening plus tailored discussion (on affect, beliefs, and external conditions regarding breast screening). Screening was assessed as short-term behavior at 3–6 months postintervention and as long-term behavior at 13–16 months after that. Mammography use was highest in the tailored discussion group *and* at long-term follow-up. It is noteworthy that women who had not had routine screenings previously and had received the tailored discussion were able to maintain screening behaviors over 2 years. Consistent with theory, the effect of messages was moderated by external barriers. Among participants with high external barriers, those in the message conditions (especially the tailored group) had the highest screening rates; among participants with low barriers, screening rates were similar across groups. The tailored discussions were most helpful to those who had identified high barriers to screening, women who might have been "written off" as least likely to seek screening (Lauver et al., 2003).

While Lauver was studying mammography, the TTM (Prochaska et al., 1994) gained popularity (Rakowski, Dube, & Goldstein, 1996). Lauver questioned whether the TTM variables of "pros" and "cons" adequately explained women's use of mammography because these "pros" and "cons" focused on cognitions. Lauver, Henriques, Settersten, and Bumann (2003) examined whether variables from Lauver's revision of Triandis's theory distinguished among stage of adoption of mammography defined consistently with the TTM. As expected from Triandis's theory, beliefs about utility, as well as both social influences and practitioner interactions regarding mammography, differed by stage of adoption in multivariate analyses. The scores for these three variables had an overall pattern such that the lowest scores were among those in the precontemplation stage and the highest were among those in the action stage. As expected, negative affect and external barriers regarding mammography differed by stage in multivariate analyses. The scores for these two variables had an overall pattern such that the highest scores were among precontemplators and the lowest were among those in action stage. Furthermore, after controlling for "pros" and "cons" defined by the TTM, negative affect differed by stage. If researchers incorporated the variable affect and additional dimensions of "pros" and "cons," such as measures of both social and practitioner influences regarding screening, then they could explain more variance in screening behavior than with typical prior measures of "pros" and "cons."

Lauver has contributed to nursing science by refining a psychologist's multidimensional theory about behavior and applying it to women's behaviors for early detection of cancer. From tests of this theory, consistent findings are that (1) both psychosocial variables *and* facilitating factors (i.e., situational characteristics of the health care system) can explain seeking care for abnormalities, and (2) the effect of psychosocial variables and tailored interventions in explaining and predicting care-seeking behaviors can be moderated by facilitating factors. Supporting Lauver's observations in practice, psychosocial variables can be important to early detection behaviors, but may not be sufficient. Women also need affordable, accessible, and acceptable services to engage in early detection behaviors. Public policy interventions to improve access and affordability of services are needed, as well as individual-level interventions to promote early detection of disease behaviors.

Facilitating Coping with Symptoms of Disease among Adults

Symptom management is a complex and ongoing clinical problem addressed by nurses. Major obstacles to adequate symptom management may be patients' myths and misinformation about symptoms and its treatment. For example, patients hold specific beliefs about the origin of pain, the use of pain medication, and the possible outcomes of treatment for pain. If such beliefs are inaccurate, then they can represent an important barrier to adequate pain management. Innovative patient education interventions are needed to identify and overcome these patient barriers.

Ward (Donovan & Ward, 2001; Ward et al., 2008, 2009) has led an effort to develop a middle-range theory useful in guiding the design of individualized patient education interventions. Developing an understanding of what patients know and believe about their illness enables nurses to (1) identify specific misconceptions, (2) target accurate replacement information individualized to the patient's sensibilities, and (3) select information that is believable and beneficial. People's beliefs and knowledge serve as a framework for cognitions that drive behavior. People are more likely to alter such representations when they realize that their existing representations are limited, inaccurate, and not helpful (Donovan et al., 2007; Hewson & Hewson, 1984).

Ward's representational approach (Donovan & Ward, 2001; Donovan et al., 2007) combines two complementary theories: one from psychology regarding illness cognitions (i.e., representations or beliefs) and the other from educational science related to how learning and conceptual change occur (i.e., how new knowledge is adopted). Based on Leventhal's common sense model (Leventhal & Diefenbach, 1991; Leventhal et al., 1984) people's particular tradition-based representations or experience-based beliefs about their illnesses are associated with its identity, cause, time line, consequences, and cure. These representations may be resistant to change and significant obstacles to the conceptual change needed for effective patient education interventions.

Expanding on hypotheses from contemporary philosophy of science, Posner, Strike, Hewson, and Gertzog (1982) developed a model of conceptual change processes. Based on their model, conceptual change is said to occur under specific conditions: (1) The existing concept is not satisfying or not working to solve existing problems; (2) the new concept is readily understandable; (3) the new concept must appear to be plausible, that is, to make sense or be somewhat consistent with previous knowledge; and (4) the new concept must appear to be more fruitful, that is, to be a promising option or to be seen as more beneficial. Thus, by combining these two theories, the representational approach guides both the content of the intervention and the process of delivery (Donovan & Ward, 2001; Donovan et al., 2007).

Ward and colleagues (2008) have proposed and tested a theory in which they posit that the most beneficial patient education encounter is likely to occur when patients' individual beliefs and knowledge are determined prior to offering new information. Donovan and Ward (2001) suggested that nurses engage patients in a bidirectional discussion intended to create a supportive environment, in which patients can explore and reflect upon accuracy of current illness representations and the usefulness of current coping strategies. The process is characterized by the nurses' assessment and attention to patients' illness representations, including (1) beliefs about the identity or label; (2) causal beliefs; (3) temporal beliefs (e.g., acute, chronic, or cyclical); (4) beliefs about short and long-term consequences; and (5) beliefs about cure or control. Patients' knowledge gaps, errors, and misconceptions are identified and explored. Nurses assist patients to reflect about these limitations and the consequences of their current representations and coping strategies. From this dialogue, patients may realize that they can "rethink their illness" or, in other words, change their representation. Nurses can capitalize on this opportunity to offer useful knowledge and emphasize the benefits of acting on such information.

The representational approach to patient education has been implemented and tested in several studies with promising results. Two experiments were devised to decrease pain in cancer patients by overcoming attitudinal barriers to reporting pain and using pain medication. Ward and colleagues (2008) first tested the intervention by comparing individual participants with an active control group that received standardized patient education. The intervention changed patients' barriers to pain management, beliefs about pain, and some measures of pain severity. Change in beliefs mediated long-term intervention effects on usual pain severity (but not short-term effects). Refining the prior intervention, Ward and colleagues (2009) compared a patient-only intervention group to one with dyads of patient and significant other, and to a comparison group. Participants who received the intervention (either as patient alone or as part of dyad groups) showed greater decreases in attitudinal barriers than those who did not. As expected, change in barriers mediated the intervention (either patient alone or in dyad groups) effects on pain severity, pain relief, pain interference, negative mood, and global quality of life. The dyad condition was not superior to the patient-only group.

Heidrich and colleagues (2009) also developed an intervention based on the representational approach; their aim was to reduce symptom distress and improve quality of life. This intervention expanded on previous studies by including multiple symptoms and giving participants a choice of symptoms on which to focus, including symptoms unrelated to cancer. Following a pilot study in which feasibility and short-term effects were measured, a longitudinal experimental study was conducted, incorporating reinforcement sessions and longer follow-up. Both studies demonstrated lower levels of symptom distress in the intervention than in the control group, as well as beneficial changes in self-care, symptom management, and communication with health care providers. A larger RCT is under way at this time.

One limitation of the representational approach is the amount of time needed to complete the interview process in which a clinician assesses a patient's current knowledge and beliefs, especially when trying to address a belief system for each symptom when a patient may have a multiple-symptom cluster. To address this limitation, Donovan and her team (2007) are evaluating the feasibility and acceptability of using secure Internet messaging (i.e., Written Representational Intervention to Ease Symptoms [WRITE]) to deliver their educational intervention among women with recurrent ovarian cancer who are managing multiple symptoms related to their disease. This study builds on prior research by (1) providing a secure space for participants to organize their educational materials on symptom management; (2) reducing the amount of time needed for face-to-face interviews; and (3) providing both patient and provider the time and "space" to respond thoughtfully to the questions and demands of complex information processing, thereby facilitating a supportive environment in which conceptual change processes may occur.

Although the representational approach retains the primary concept of cognitive representation from the common sense model, it has incorporated additional concepts and elements, including (1) elements of how conceptual change occurs; (2) collaboration with patients to establish goals and to develop specific strategies to achieve those goals; and (3) incorporation of follow-up contacts by the interventionist to revisit goals and strategies with participants, evaluate patients' progress, and formulate future plans. The representational approach offers an intriguing alternative to the traditional delivery of patient education.

Facilitating Coping among Children with Chronic Disease

With her background in pediatric endocrinology and as a researcher in behavioral health, Grey, PNP, DrPH, has studied how children and adolescents deal with living with diabetes. With a multidimensional view of adaptation, she has addressed not only the physiological adaptation to diabetes—metabolic control—but also psychological, social, and familial adaptations. In other words, Grey has studied adolescents' self-management of their diabetes (Grey & Berry, 2004).

With correlational designs, Grey and colleagues have described how children's coping strategies influence their psychological, social, and physiological adaptation to having insulin-dependent diabetes. Grey, Cameron, and Thurber (1991) have reported that preadolescents use more effective coping strategies and have fewer negative moods, less psychological adjustment issues, and better physiological control of their diabetes compared to adolescents. In a study with a longitudinal design, Grey, Cameron, Thurber, and Lipman (1997) sampled children at the time of their diabetes diagnosis and followed them until 1-year postdiagnosis. Patients who coped with humor or who engaged in more positive self-care had greater self-worth 1 year later. Patients' earlier engagement in self-care was associated with better psychosocial adjustment 1 year later. Patients who used avoidance to cope were more likely to have poor psychosocial adjustment and poor physiological control of their diabetes 1 year later.

Building on such studies, Grey conducted an intervention designed to build positive coping skills in children with diabetes and to promote their overall health. She proposed adding an innovative behavioral intervention—designed to improve diabetic teens' coping skills, health behaviors, and health status (Grey, Boland, Davidson, Li, & Tamborlane, 1999)—to an existing evidence-based protocol for medical management of diabetes. Her coping skills training (CST) intervention based on Bandura's (1986) research comprised forming positive coping strategies and retraining ineffective coping strategies. This CST focused on five key skills: social problem solving, communication skills training, social skills training, cognitive-behavioral modification, and conflict resolution (Grey & Berry, 2004). It included scenarios and role playing to build participants' self-efficacy with regard to their diabetes management and life in general.

In an RCT, all patients received evidenced-based medical care, but some were assigned randomly either to receive the innovative behavioral program or standard care. Both groups had reductions in their glycosylated hemoglobin (HbA1c), a marker of average blood sugar levels over the prior 2–3 months. However, the CST group had lower levels than did the standard care group; this was observed at 6-month follow-up and maintained at 1-year follow-up. Also, the

CST group had higher scores on self-efficacy and better scores regarding quality of life than did the standard care group at 1-year follow-up (Grey et al., 1999, 2000). Grey, Davidson, Boland, and Tamborlane (2001) reported on additional 1-year outcomes. Patients who received CST, and who had lower scores on the HbA1c test at baseline, had lower HbA1c levels 1 year later than participants who did not receive CST. Family participation in diabetes management also was associated with lower HbA1c. Patients who received CST, and who had had little influence on their quality of life at baseline, had less impact on their quality of life 1 year later than those who did not receive CST. Patients' baseline depression also was associated with the negative impact of diabetes 1 year later. CST can improve the physiological status as well as the psychosocial health of teens with diabetes.

Grey also observed whether patients' self-efficacy and metabolic control of diabetes changed similarly over time as a result of her CST. From Bandura's theory, one would propose that as people practice new behaviors, their self-efficacy regarding these behaviors also increases. In contrast to Bandura's hypothesis, Grey's team observed that as self-management behaviors to improve blood sugar levels increased, metabolic control also improved, but improvements in patients' self-efficacy about diabetes lagged behind patients' improvements in metabolic control. Her team proposed that adolescents' self-efficacy about disease management may take longer to develop than that for other patients, or that they may need to see the actual clinical results of their self-management behaviors prior to perceiving increases in their self-efficacy related to diabetes (Grey et al., 2000).

Grey's colleague Whittemore conducted a pilot study to translate their CST intervention into primary care settings (Whittemore et al., 2009). Delivery of the intervention by NPs was feasible, attrition of patients was low, and physiological and behavioral outcomes had positive trends. Collaborating with Grey, Whittemore (2007) developed a Web-based CST curriculum for teens with diabetes; feedback from teens has been positive.

Most recently, Grey (2009) has trained schoolteachers in an urban city in the north-east United States to conduct similar CST in classrooms. Children received either CST or general health education. At baseline, a disproportional percent were children of color, their mean body mass index (BMI) was over 30, and 30% of children reported depression. In preliminary analyses, participants who received CST had more weight loss, as well as lower insulin and glucose levels, compared to the health education group. Children who received CST also tended to make better food choices, to engage in more physical activity, and to have lower triglyceride levels compared to the health education group (Grey, 2009).

As a NP-researcher, Grey has demonstrated how nursing science can improve not only the physiological adaptation but also the psychosocial adaptation of teens with diabetes. This is especially noteworthy given that adolescence can be challenging time developmentally even without a major chronic disease that must be managed daily. And the rising incidence of diabetes is a public health concern. With interdisciplinary colleagues, Grey has shown how teens and families manage their lives with diabetes rather than manage only the disease of diabetes. Using a popular psychological theory—social cognitive theory—to guide her research, Grey observed that self-efficacy did not change as expected in a population of adolescents with diabetes, thereby revealing boundaries of this theory.

Promoting Health by Facilitating People's Coping with Life Demands

Both the external environment—whether defined physically or socially—and people's internal environment can influence their health status (Adler et al., 1994; Chida & Steptoe, 2008). In this section we discuss contemporary nursing research that has focused on people's management of their internal environment with contemplative practices, such as mindfulness meditation, and subsequent health outcomes. Nurses have tested mindfulness-based interventions and been guided often by a psychoneuroimmunology (PNI) framework (Cuellar, 2008; Starkweather, Witek-Janusek, & Mathews, 2005). The PNI field investigates the bidirectional interaction of mind and body (Ader, 1980). For instance, persistent negative

moods stimulate the hyperarousal of stress physiology, which in turn dysregulates the immune system (Glaser & Kiecolt-Glaser, 2005). Engaging in a contemplative practice such as mindfulness has been shown to decrease perceived stress and negative moods, yet increase positive mood, quality of life, and immune function (Carmody & Baer, 2008; Davidson et al., 2003). In this relatively new area of research on mindfulness, nurse-researchers have combined subjective, self-reported psychological variables with important objective biomarkers of the immune system.

"Mindfulness" is a quality of consciousness that is grounded in the present moment (Brown & Ryan, 2003) and characterized by an open awareness of all feelings, thoughts, and physical sensations (Kabat-Zinn, 1990). Being mindful, one applies a curious and nonjudgmental attitude, cultivating moment-to-moment attention to the experience at hand (Kabat-Zinn, 1990). Mindfulness practice emphasizes the avoidance of rumination on the past or forecasting into the future (Brown, Ryan, & Creswell, 2007) and is intended for practice during everyday activities and interactions in daily life. Mindfulness practices have been secularized from Buddhism and developed into a popular program in the West known as mindfulness-based stress reduction (MBSR; Kabat-Zinn, 1990). While other approaches to teaching mindfulness exist, MBSR has been (1) standardized more than other approaches, (2) empirically investigated, (3) offered to diverse clinical and community populations in a variety of settings, and (4) endorsed by many respected hospitals and universities. For these reasons, MBSR is among the most widely studied programs of mindfulness training. MBSR consists of eight weekly group meetings, daily home practice of mindfulness, additional exercises (e.g., body scan exercises or yoga), and typically includes a daylong silent retreat.

In a quasi-experimental, pre- and posttest comparison group design, Robinson, Mathews, and Witek-Janusek (2003) tested the effects of MBSR on perceived stress, mood, and endocrine and immune function biomarkers in patients living with the human immunodeficiency virus (HIV). At pretest, both the MBSR and the comparison group showed depressed natural killer (NK) cell numbers and NK cell activity (NKCA). At posttest, participation in MBSR showed an increase in immune function. There were no effects on other psychological, endocrine, or function variables measured. More recently, Witek-Janusek and colleagues (2008) tested the effects of MBSR on immune function, quality of life and dispositional coping in women with newly diagnosed breast cancer. Using a three-group, quasi-experimental design, the researchers compared three groups of women. Two groups consisted of women recently diagnosed with breast cancer: The first group comprised women who volunteered to learn MBSR, and the second group, those who declined the intervention but agreed to be assessed on study variables. The third group comprised age-matched and cancer-free women. The groups were assessed at pretest, at midpoint during the intervention, at the conclusion of the intervention, and at 4-week postintervention. The MBSR group had greater immune function (e.g., NKCA) than the assessment-only cancer group, on average and over time. In the MBSR group, immune function (NKCA and interferon-gamma), returned to levels similar to the cancer-free group, but the observation group of cancer patients did not. The MBSR group had lower cortisol levels and higher scores on quality of life and coping effectively than the non-MBSR cancer group (Witek-Janusek et al., 2008).

In an RCT, Lengacher and her team (2009) studied MBSR training among breast cancer patients in a "survivorship" transition period after the end of treatment, and at the beginning of the resumption of normal daily activities. They were randomized to receive either a shortened MBSR program (6 weeks) or usual care, and to be wait-listed to receive this MBSR later. After the program, the MBSR group had reduced fear of recurrence, less anxiety and depression, and improved quality of life in three domains (i.e., physical function, role function, energy) compared to the usual care group.

Although widely used and recognized, the MBSR program has some limitations, including lack of availability outside larger metropolitan areas, high cost of the program, and substantial time commitment required for meeting with a group. One author (West) is addressing these concerns in an NIH-funded feasibility study of patient-centered mindfulness skills training that targets a rural, low socioeconomic status (SES) working population. Low SES is correlated with chronic psychological stress and poor health outcomes (Adler et al., 1994). In addition, people of low SES are more likely to be employed in occupations with high demands and low control over time and tasks, which has also been linked to high levels of stress. Chronic stress is associated with leading causes of morbidity and mortality (Innes, Vincent, & Taylor, 2007). This study will examine the delivery of introductory mindfulness skills training on an individualized basis, using inexpensive technology (i.e., MP3 player) to facilitate accessibility, affordability and flexibility. The intervention promises to deliver mindfulness skills training to an often overlooked population (i.e., the "working poor") that is more likely to experience chronic stress and its associated detrimental health outcomes, yet less likely to have access to such resources.

Conclusions

The exemplars from nursing science reviewed here illustrate the methods and theories that nurse-scientists have used. Among the designs and interventions discussed, individualized and tailored interventions were effective in complex clinical situations (e.g., by Champion et al., 2000, 2003; Grey et al., 1999, 2000; Kitzman et al., 1997, 2000; Lauver et al., 2003; Ward et al., 2008, 2009). The exemplars included two research programs that have reached maturity and been translated into nursing practice (i.e., the interventions with pregnant teenagers and coping with novel health care events). We reviewed research programs that are positioned to guide effectiveness studies for translation into practice (e.g., pain control, women's screening behaviors, teens coping with diabetes). We also presented a new area of research for nurses and psychologists regarding PNI, which is mindfulness. There is a large body of nursing research on diverse topics relevant to health psychology in journals such as the *Journal of Nursing Scholarship*, *Nursing Research*, and *Research in Nursing and Health*. Of note, nursing literature can be accessed electronically through a database called the Cumulative Index to

Nursing and Allied Health Literature (CI-NAHL). Nurses also publish in clinical and interdisciplinary journals, as indicated in our reference list.

We have identified different psychological theories that nurse-scientists have used to guide their research. These scientists have contributed to building science by confirming a theory (e.g., the HBM; Champion, 1983), disconfirming hypotheses, (e.g., regarding when self-efficacy changes, as proposed from social cognitive theory, Grey, 2009; Grey et al., 2000); revising theories (e.g., Lauver, 1992), incorporating psychological theory into an ecological model (e.g., Olds, Kitzman, et al., 1997), and generating new theory (Johnson's [1999] self-regulation theory; Donovan and Ward's [2001] representational approach; see also Donovan et al., 2007; Ward et al., 2007, 2009). When nurse-scientists apply psychological theories to previously untested health care contexts, they advance our knowledge of how to improve health care outcomes.

We have illustrated how nurses have studied diverse health-related phenomena in a broad range of situations and populations (e.g., adolescents, young mothers, adults, and people with chronic disease or those at risk for the same). These studies document the complexity of problems that nurses have studied, as well as the real-life settings in which they have tested their ideas.

Exemplars shared here illustrate how interventions—based on psychological concepts and processes and designed by nurse-researchers—have improved the health of people of different ages and those living with potential and actual health threats (e.g., reducing problems for teenage mothers, adolescents with diabetes, pain and cancer patients, as well as improving engagement in recommended behaviors by those at risk). Some nurse-researchers (e.g., Grey et al., 2000; Kitzman et al., 2000; Lauver et al., 2003; Olds et al., 1997) have demonstrated sustained health outcomes of their interventions rather than only short-term effects. Also, we have highlighted the emerging research by nurses on mindfulness, in which improvements in physiological, psychological, and behavioral outcomes have been observed among different samples. In conclusion, this chapter has highlighted selected nurse-scientists' contributions to understanding, explaining, and predicting phenomena related to health and illness that are of interest to psychologists.

Acknowledgments

We would like to thank, in alphabetical order, Jorna Cychosz for efficient editing assistance and Betty Kaiser, Tonya Roberts, Rachel Roiland, Heather Royer, and Maria Yelle for critical suggestions that made this chapter stronger.

Further Reading

Donovan, H. S., Ward, S. E., Song, M., Heidrich, S. M., Gunnarsdottir, S., & Phillips, C. M. (2007). An update on the representational approach to patient education. *Journal of Nursing Scholarship, 39*(3), 259–265.

Grey, M., Boland, E. A., Davidson, M., Li, J., & Tamborlane, W. V. (2000). Coping skills training for youth with diabetes mellitus has long-lasting effects on metabolic control and quality of life. *Journal of Pediatrics, 137*(1), 107–113.

Hinshaw, A. S., Feetham, S., & Shaver, J. (1999). *Handbook of clinical nursing research.* Thousand Oaks, CA: Sage.

Johnson, J. E. (1999). Self-regulation theory and coping with physical illness. *Research in Nursing and Health, 22*, 435–448.

Kitzman, H., Olds, D. L., Sidora, K., Henderson, C. R., Hanks, C., & Cole, R. (2000). Enduring effects of nurse home visitation on maternal life course: A 3-year follow-up of a randomized trial. *Journal of the American Medical Association, 283*, 1983–1989.

National Institute of Nursing Research. (2006). *Changing practice, Changing lives: 10 landmark nursing studies* (U.S. Department of Health and Human Services, Publication No. 06 6094). Retrieved November 18, 2009, from *www.ninr.nih.gov/nr/rdonlyres/27F3fb10-fe62-4119-9fA9-1140B6950AFF/0/10landmarknursingresearchstudies508.pdf.*

Olds, D. L., Kitzman, H., Hanks, C., Cole, R., Anson, E., Sidora-Arcoleo, K., et al. (2007). Effects of nurse home visiting on maternal and child functioning: Age-9 follow-up of a randomized trial. *Pediatrics, 120*, 832–845.

References

Ader, R. (1980). Presidential address: Psychosomatic and psychoimmunological research. *Psychosomatic Medicine, 42*, 307–321.

Adler, N. E., Boyce, T., Chesney, M. A., Cohen, S., Folkman, S., Kahn, R. L., et al. (1994).

Socio-economic status and health: Challenge of the gradient. *American Psychologist, 49,* 15–24.

American Nurses Association. (2003). *Nursing's social policy statement.* Washington, DC: Author.

Bandura, A. (1977). Self-efficacy: Toward a unifying theory of behavioral change. *Psychological Review, 84,* 191–215.

Bandura, A. (1986). *Social foundations of thought and action: A social cognitive theory.* Englewood Cliffs, NJ: Prentice-Hall.

Baumann, L. J., Fontana, S. A., Brown, R. L., & Cameron, L. (1993). Testing a model of mammography intention. *Journal of Applied Social Psychology, 23,* 1733–1756.

Bowlby, J. (1969). *Attachment and loss: Vol. 1 Attachment.* New York: Basic Books.

Bronfenbrenner, U. (1979). *The ecology of human development: Experiments by nature and design.* Cambridge, MA: Harvard University Press.

Brown, K., & Ryan, R. (2003). The benefits of being present: Mindfulness and its role in psychological well-being. *Journal of Personality and Social Psychology, 84,* 822–848.

Brown, K. W., Ryan, R. M., & Creswell, J. D. (2007). Mindfulness: Theoretical foundations and evidence for its salutary effects. *Psychological Inquiry, 18,* 211–237.

Carmody, J., & Baer, R. A. (2008). Relationship between mindfulness practice and levels of mindfulness, medical and psychological symptoms and well-being in a mindfulness based stress reduction program. *Journal of Behavioral Health, 31,* 23–33.

Champion, V. L. (1983). Tool construction for measurement of health belief model constructs (Doctoral dissertation, Indiana University School of Nursing, 1981). *Dissertation Abstracts International, 44*(3-B), 748.

Champion, V. L. (1999). Revised susceptibility, benefits, and barriers scale for mammography screening. *Research in Nursing and Health, 22,* 341–348.

Champion, V. L., & Huster, G. (1995). Effect of interventions on stage of mammography adoption. *Journal of Behavioral Medicine, 18,* 169–186.

Champion, V. L., Maraj, M., Hui, S., Perkins, A. J., Tierney, W., Menon, U., et al. (2003). Comparison of tailored interventions to increase mammography screening in nonadherent older women. *Preventive Medicine, 36,* 150–158.

Champion, V. L., Skinner, C. S., & Foster, J. L. (2000). The effects of standard care counseling or telephone/in-person counseling on beliefs, knowledge, and behavior related to mammography screening. *Oncology Nursing Forum, 27,* 1565–1571.

Champion, V. L., Skinner, C. S., & Menon, U. (2005). Development of a self-efficacy scale for mammography. *Research in Nursing and Health, 28,* 329–336.

Chida, Y., & Steptoe, A. (2008). Positive psychological well-being and mortality: A quantitative review of prospective observational studies. *Psychosomatic Medicine, 70,* 741–756.

Cuellar, N. G. (2008). Mindfulness meditation for veterans—implications for occupational health providers. *Business and Leadership, 56,* 357–363.

Davidson, R. J., Kabat-Zinn, J., Schumacher, J., Rosenkranz, M., Muller, D., Santorelli, S. F., et al. (2003). Alterations in brain and immune function produced by mindfulness meditation. *Psychosomatic Medicine, 65,* 564–570.

Donovan, H. S., & Ward, S. (2001). A representational approach to patient education. *Journal of Nursing Scholarship, 33,* 211–216.

Donovan, H. S., Ward, S. E., Song, M., Heidrich, S. M., Gunnarsdottir, S., & Phillips, C. M. (2007). An update on the representational approach to patient education. *Journal of Nursing Scholarship, 39,* 259–265.

Facione, N. C. (1993). The Triandis model for the study of health and illness behavior: A social-behavior theory with sensitivity to diversity. *Advances in Nursing Science, 15,* 49–58.

Facione, N. C., Dodd, M. J., Holzemer, W., & Meleis, A. I. (1997). Help seeking for self-discovered breast symptoms: Implications for early detection. *Cancer Practice, 5,* 220–227.

Fairman, J. (2008). Context and contingency in the history of post World War II nursing scholarship in the United States. *Journal of Nursing Scholarship, 40,* 4–11.

Glaser, R. & Kiecolt-Glaser, J. K. (2005). Stress-induced immune dysfunction: Implications for health. *Nature Reviews Immunology, 5,* 243–251.

Grey, M. (2009, May 8). *Preventing type 2 diabetes among high-risk youth* [Lecture]. Presented at the University of Wisconsin–Madison.

Grey, M., & Berry, D. (2004). Coping skills training and problem solving in diabetes. *Current Diabetes Reports, 4,* 126–131.

Grey, M., Boland, E. A., Davidson, M., Li, J., & Tamborlane, W. V. (2000). Coping skills training for youth with diabetes mellitus has long-lasting effects on metabolic control and quality of life. *Journal of Pediatrics, 137*(1), 107–113.

Grey, M., Boland, E. A., Davidson, M., Yu, C., & Tamborlane, W. V. (1999). Coping skills training for youth with diabetes on intensive therapy. *Applied Nursing Research, 25,* 3–12.

Grey, M., Cameron, M. E., & Thurber, F. W. (1991). Coping and adaptation in children with diabetes. *Nursing Research, 40,* 144–149.

Grey, M., Cameron, M. E., Thurber, F. W., & Lipman, T. H. (1997). The contribution of coping behaviors at diagnosis to adjustment one year post diagnosis in children with diabetes. *Nursing Research, 46,* 312–317.

Grey, M., Davidson, M., Boland, E. A., & Tamborlane, W. V. (2001). Clinical and psychosocial factors associated with achievement of treatment goals in adolescents with diabetes mellitus. *Journal of Adolescent Health, 28,* 377–385.

Heidrich, S. M., Brown, R. L., Egan, J. J., Perez, P. A., Phelan, C. H., Yeom, H., et al. (2009). An individualized representational intervention to improve symptom management (IRIS) in older breast cancer survivors: Three pilot studies. *Oncology Nursing Forum, 36*(3), 133–143.

Hewson, P. W., & Hewson, M. G. (1984). The role of conceptual conflict in conceptual change and the design of instruction. *Instructional Science, 13,* 1–13.

Innes, K. E., Vincent, H. K., & Taylor, A. G. (2007). Chronic stress and indices of resistance-related indices of cardiovascular disease risk: Part I. Neurophysiological responses and pathological sequelae. *Alternative Therapies in Medicine and Health, 13,* 46–52.

Johnson, J. E. (1973). The effects of accurate expectations about sensation on the sensory and stress components of pain. *Journal of Personality and Social Psychology, 27,* 261–275.

Johnson, J. E. (1999). Self-regulation theory and coping with physical illness. *Research in Nursing and Health, 22,* 435–448.

Johnson, J. E., Lauver, D., & Nail, L. (1989). Process of coping with radiation therapy. *Journal of Consulting and Clinical Psychology, 57,* 358–364.

Johnson, J. E., Morrissey, J. F., & Leventhal, H. (1973). Psychological preparation for an endoscopic examination. *Gastrointestinal Endoscopy, 19,* 180–182.

Johnson, J. E., Nail, L. M., Lauver, D., King, K. B., & Keys, H. (1988). Reducing the negative impact of radiation therapy on functional status. *Cancer, 61,* 46–51.

Johnson, J. E., Rice, V. H., Fuller, S. S., & Endress, M. P. (1978). Sensory information, instruction in a coping strategy, and recovery from surgery. *Research in Nursing and Health, 1,* 4–17.

Kabat-Zinn, J. (1990). *Full catastrophe living: Using the wisdom of your body and mind to face stress and illness.* New York: Delta.

Kitzman, H., Olds, D. L., Henderson, C. R., Jr., Hanks, C., Cole, R., Tatelbaum, R., et al. (1997). Effects of prenatal and infancy home visitation by nurses on pregnancy outcomes, childhood injuries, and repeated childbearing: A randomized controlled trial. *Journal of the American Medical Association, 278,* 644–652.

Kitzman, H., Olds, D. L., Sidora, K., Henderson, C. R., Hanks, C., & Cole, R. (2000). Enduring effects of nurse home visitation on maternal life course: A 3-year follow-up of a randomized trial. *Journal of the American Medical Association, 283,* 1983–1989.

Lauver, D. (1987). Theoretical perspectives relevant to breast self-examination. *Advances in Nursing Science, 9,* 16–24.

Lauver, D. (1992). A theory of care-seeking behavior. *Image—Journal of Nursing Scholarship, 24,* 265–271.

Lauver, D. (1994). Care-seeking behavior with breast cancer symptoms in Caucasian and African-American women. *Research in Nursing and Health, 17,* 421–431.

Lauver, D. (1996). Understanding barriers to mammography use among women of low socioeconomic status: Comparisons from quantitative and qualitative data. *Journal of Women's Health, 5,* 473–480.

Lauver, D., Henriques, J., Settersten, L., & Bumann, M. (2003). Psychosocial variables, external barriers and stages of adoption of mammography. *Health Psychology, 22,* 649–653.

Lauver, D., Nabholz, S., Scott, K., & Tak, Y. (1997). Testing theoretical explanations of mammography use. *Nursing Research, 46,* 32–39.

Lauver, D., Settersten, L., Kane, J., & Henriques, J. (2003). Tailored messages, external barriers and women's utilization of professional breast cancer screening over time. *Cancer, 97,* 2724–35.

Lauver, D., Ward, S., Bowers, B., Brennan, P. F., Heidrich, S., Keller, M., et al. (2002). Patient-centered interventions. *Research in Nursing and Health, 25,* 246–255.

Lengacher, C. A., Johnson-Mallard, V., Post-White, J., Moscoso, M. S., Jacobsen, P. B., Klein, T. W., et al. (2009). Randomized controlled trial of mindfulness-based stress reduction (MBSR) for survivors of breast cancer. *Psycho-Oncology, 18,* 1261–12722.

Leventhal, H., & Diefenbach, M. (1991). The active side of illness cognitions. In J. Skelton & R. Croyle (Eds.), *Mental representation in health and illness* (pp. 247–272). New York: Springer-Verlag.

Leventhal, H., Meyer, D., & Nerenz, D. (1980). The common sense representation of illness danger. In S. Rachman (Ed.), *Contributions to medical psychology* (Vol. 3, pp. 7–30). New York: Pergamon Press.

Leventhal, H., Nerenz, D. R., & Steele, D. J. (1984). Illness representations and coping with health threats. In A. Baum, S. E. Taylor, & J.

E. Singer (Eds.), *Handbook of psychology and health* (pp. Vol. 4, 219–252). Hillsdale, NJ: Erlbaum.

McHugh, N., Christman, N., & Johnson, J. E. (1982). Preparatory information: What helps and why. *American Journal of Nursing, 82,* 780–782.

Melnyk, B. M. (1995). Coping with unplanned childhood hospitalization: The mediating functions of parental beliefs. *Journal of Pediatric Psychology, 20,* 299–312.

National Institute of Nursing Research (NINR). (2009). *Important events in the National Institute of Nursing Research history.* Retrieved May 15, 2009, from *www.ninr.nih.gov/About-ninr/ninrhistory.*

Olds, D. L., Eckenrode, J., Henderson, C. R., Jr., Kitzman, H., Powers, J., Cole, R., et al. (1997). Long-term effects of nurse home visitation on maternal life course and child abuse and neglect: 15-year follow-up of a randomized trial. *Journal of the American Medical Association, 278,* 637–643.

Olds, D. L., Henderson, C. R., Jr., Tatelbaum, R., & Chamberlin, R. (1986). Improving the delivery of prenatal care and outcomes of pregnancy: A randomized trial of nurse home visitation. *Pediatrics, 77,* 16–28.

Olds, D. L., Kitzman, H., Cole, R., & Robinson, J. A. (1997). Theoretical foundations of a program of home visitation for pregnant women and parents of young children. *Journal of Community Psychology, 25,* 9–25.

Olds, D. L., Kitzman, H., Cole, R., Robinson, J. A., Sidora, K., Luckey, D. W., et al. (2004). Effects of nurse home-visiting on maternal life-course and child development: Age-six follow-up results of a randomized trial. *Pediatrics, 114,* 1550–1559.

Olds, D. L., Kitzman, H., Hanks, C., Cole, R., Anson, E., Sidora-Arcoleo, K., et al. (2007). Effects of nurse home visiting on maternal and child functioning: Age-nine follow-up of a randomized trial. *Pediatrics, 120,* 832–845.

Olds, D. L., Robinson, J. A., O'Brien, R., Luckey, D. W., Pettitt, L. M., Henderson, C. R., Jr., et al. (2002). Home visiting by paraprofessionals and by nurses: A randomized controlled trial. *Pediatrics, 110,* 486–496.

Olds, D. L., Robinson, J. A., Pettitt, L., Luckey, D. W., Holmberg, J., Ng, R. K., et al. (2004). Effects of home visits by paraprofessionals and by nurses: Age-4 follow-up of a randomized trial. *Pediatrics, 114,* 1560–1568.

Posner, G. J., Strike, K. A., Hewson, P. W., & Gertzog, W. A. (1982). Accommodation of a scientific conception: Toward a theory of conceptual change. *Science Education, 66,* 211–227.

Prochaska, J., Velicer, W., Rossi, J., Goldstein,

M., Marcus, B., Rakowski, W., et al. (1994). Stages of change and decisional balance for 12 problem behaviors. *Health Psychology, 13,* 39–46.

Rakowski, W., Dube, C., & Goldstein, M. (1996). Considerations for extending the transtheoretical model of behavioral change to screening mammography. *Health Education Research: Theory and Practice, 11,* 77–96.

Reifenstein, K. (2007). Care-seeking behaviors of African American women with breast cancer symptoms. *Research in Nursing and Health, 30,* 542–557.

Robinson, F. P., Mathews, H. L., & Witek-Janusek, L. (2003). Psycho–endocrine–immune response to mindfulness-based stress reduction in individuals infected with the human immunodeficiency virus: A quasiexperimental study. *Journal of Alternative and Complementary Medicine, 9,* 683–694.

Starkweather, A., Witek-Janusek, L., & Mathews, H. L. (2005). Applying the psychoneuroimmunology framework to nursing research. *Journal of Neuroscience Nursing, 37,* 56–62.

Triandis, H. (1980). Values, attitudes and interpersonal behavior. In M. Page (Ed.), *1979 Nebraska Symposium on Motivation* (pp. 195–259). Lincoln: University of Nebraska Press.

Ward, S., Donovan, H., Gunnarsdottir, S., Serlin, R. C., Shapiro, G. R., & Hughes, S. (2008). A randomized trial of a representational intervention to decrease cancer pain (RIDcancerPain). *Health Psychology, 27,* 59–67.

Ward, S. E., Serlin, R. C., Donovan, H. S., Ameringer, S. W., Hughes, S., Pe-Ronashko, K., et al. (2009). A randomized trial of a representational intervention for cancer pain: Does targeting the dyad make a difference? *Health Psychology, 28*(5), 588–597.

Washington State Institute for Public Policy. (2004, September 17). *Benefits and costs of prevention and early intervention programs for youth.* Retrieved June 4, 2009, from *www.wsipp.wa.gov/rptfiles/04-07-3901.pdf.*

Whittemore, R. (2007). Culturally competent interventions for Hispanic adults with type 2 diabetes: A systematic review. *Journal of Transcultural Nursing, 18,* 157–166.

Whittemore, R., Melkus, G., Wagner, J., Dziura, J., Northrup, V., & Grey, M. (2009). Translating the diabetes prevention program to primary care: A pilot study. *Nursing Research, 58,* 2–12.

Witek-Janusek, L., Albuquerque, K., Chroniak, K. R., Chroniak, C., DurazoArvizu, R., & Mathews, H. L. (2008). Effect of mindfulness-based stress reduction on immune function, quality of life and coping in women newly diagnosed with early stage breast cancer. *Brain, Behavior, and Immunity, 22,* 969–981.

CHAPTER 18

Medical Anthropology

William W. Dressler

"Medical anthropology" is a topical focus in anthropology on health and healing with a cross-cultural perspective. The ways in which different societies cope with the fundamental existential issues of health have been addressed to a greater or lesser extent by ethnographers, ever since the beginning of modern anthropological fieldwork in the early 20th century. But the separate topic of medical anthropology, with a society organized by specialists in its study (the Society for Medical Anthropology), and with journals devoted to the publication of such studies (*Medical Anthropology Quarterly*; *Medical Anthropology*; *Culture, Medicine, and Psychiatry*; *Culture and Medicine*; *Ethnomedizin*; and *Social Science and Medicine*, with its associate editor in medical anthropology) came much later.

A seminal point in the development of the field came with the publication of *Health, Culture and Community*, edited by Ben Paul (1955). The years following World War II saw an expansion of North American and European global influence that included, within its mission of promoting "modernization," the delivery of health care based on scientific biomedicine. In many instances,

however, "the natives" evinced little interest in much of biomedicine. Paul's collection consisted of anthropologists and public health specialists assessing the effectiveness of health campaigns in a variety of cultural settings. These studies also laid the foundation for the importance of medical anthropology as a focus within applied anthropology, and ever since, medical anthropologists have represented a substantial proportion of the members of the Society for Applied Anthropology and have published regularly in its journal *Human Organization*.

At roughly the same time, the psychiatrist-anthropologist Alexander Leighton and his colleagues were beginning their groundbreaking epidemiological studies of psychiatric disorder, first in Stirling County (maritime Canada) and later among the Yoruba (Nigeria) (Leighton & Leighton, 1967). Drawing on anthropological studies of social change and modernization, and especially Robert Redfield's notion of a folk–urban continuum, Leighton posited a rural–urban continuum of risk for psychiatric disorder, hypothesizing that higher rates of disorder in urban and urbanizing communities were a function of the social disorganization accompanying culture change. This research set the stage for many anthropological studies of modernization and disease, especially the (then) newly emerging "epidemic" of cardiovascular disease.

In certain respects, the development of medical anthropology and its current foci stem from the elaboration of two fundamental questions:

How do cultural factors influence the risk of disease?

How do cultural factors influence the definition of illness and its resolution?

These two broad research directives, of course, generate myriad more specific research questions, so that the rapid growth and expansion of the field over the past 50 years is hardly surprising.

This brief review is of necessity selective. For more in-depth coverage of topics, the interested reader is urged to consult review papers in volumes such as the *Annual Review of Anthropology* and the two-volume *Encyclopedia of Medical Anthropology* (Ember & Ember, 2004). This review is organized around a series of basic questions that span a "natural history of disease" and illustrate how medical anthropologists have addressed them. These questions include the following:

How do cultural factors shape the risk of disease?

Within a particular ecology of disease risk, how do persons recognize and organize signs and symptoms of dysfunction into illness?

Given that an illness is recognized and labeled, how do they decide to seek care, and from whom?

How does the process of healing unfold?

Finally, how are illness episodes resolved?

Culture and the Risk of Disease

As noted earlier, the initial studies of culture and the risk of disease emphasized the effect of culture change and "modernization" on health. Work representative of this orientation includes that of Leighton and Leighton (1967) cited earlier; Scotch's (1963) examination of rural–urban differences in hy-

pertension in South Africa; Baker's (Baker, Hanna, & Baker, 1986) research on blood pressure among Samoans; and the Tokelau Island study of blood pressure (Beaglehole et al., 1977); see Dressler (1999) for a more comprehensive review of studies of modernization and disease. The basic design of these studies is to identify three or more communities along a continuum of modernization from more "traditional" to more "modernized" communities. A traditional community is usually defined as one in which there is an emphasis on subsistence production in the economy; little formal education; an emphasis on large, generationally organized kin groups that structure social relationships; and, little change in religion or belief systems. In a modernized community, economic production shifts from subsistence to wage labor; introduction of formal educational systems; emphasis on social relationships contracts from larger kin groups to the nuclear family, the household, and networks of extended kin; and, introduction of one (or more) of the global religious systems, usually by missionaries. In many of the most important studies of modernization and disease, researchers adopted blood pressure as an outcome variable, due to its importance as a precursor of many causes of mortality and its ease of measurement in difficult field situations.

There is an increase in disease risk along this continuum of modernization. For example, McGarvey and Baker (1979) found a nearly 15 mmHg (millimeters of mercury) difference in mean systolic blood pressure between the most traditional and most modernized communities in Samoa for persons age 50 and over, with a nearly 20% increase in the prevalence of hypertension. The question then becomes what contributes to this risk? One of the problems in interpreting such findings is that there are so many changes, including economic, social, political, ideological, and dietary, included under the definition of modernization, it is difficult to isolate what is causal. For example, the rise of blood pressure with modernization has been variously attributed to increasing obesity (as a result of increased caloric intake and decreased physical activity); increasing sodium consumption; and, increasing psychological and social stresses that accompany culture change. These, of course, are not mutually exclusive explanations; however, controlling for sodium intake and the body mass index (a measure of obesity) results in a relatively small reduction of the differences between communities in blood pressure. This, coupled with findings on the psychological effects of modernization, led to more focused studies of the stressful effects of culture change.

One of the challenges of this research involved adapting models of the stress process to diverse cultural contexts. There is no reason to suppose, and indeed every reason to doubt, that measures of stressors or resistance resources developed for use in North American, predominantly middle-class samples would be valid in societies in the Pacific, Africa, or South America undergoing culture change. Therefore, models of the stress process developed for North American and European samples were used for inspiration in these studies but at the same time were subjected to a rigorous ethnographic critique, to specify these models in ways appropriate for modernizing societies. For example, Dressler (1982) argued that a fundamental change occurring in modernizing societies is the exposure of local populations to nonlocal lifestyles, specifically, in the sense of material goods for domestic consumption (e.g., cars, stereo systems, televisions) and leisure time activities (e.g., going to movies or restaurants). The ability to accumulate consumer goods and adopt these leisure time activities becomes incorporated into local systems of social status, at least complementing traditional forms of social status or, in some cases, supplanting them. The problem in developing societies, however, is that the social status accorded a new lifestyle can quickly outstrip growth in the economy of the community that supplies jobs and other economic resources required to achieve that lifestyle. The likelihood is high, therefore, that some individuals will attempt to achieve and maintain a modern, high-status lifestyle, but in the context of meager economic resources in low-status jobs. This process can then be linked directly to more general theories of status inconsistency as a stressor (Dressler, 2004). Dressler (1999) and others found higher blood pressure associated with this kind of status inconsistency.

The application of this model to Samoan immigrants to northern California by Janes (1990), and to Samoans in Samoa by McDade (2002), illustrates the importance of the appropriate ethnographic specification of variables. Traditionally, Samoans lived in a redistributive economy in which all economic production flowed to leaders (called *matai*) of large corporate kin groups; production was then redistributed within the kin group by the *matai*. Other *matai* had specialized political functions, and, of course, all *matai* were of high status. With modernization and migration, despite substantial changes in economic organization, the *matai* status has persisted, albeit with different functions. Janes found that Samoan migrants to northern California with *matai* status who had lower socioeconomic status in American society (in terms of education and occupation) had higher blood pressure. Similarly, McDade found that adolescents in Samoa living in households with *matai* status, but who had lower status in terms of lifestyle, had lower immune function, as measured by cell-mediated immunity. Again, these studies point both to the chronically stressful nature of this status inconsistency and to the importance of specifying models of the stress process in terms of local cultural contexts.

The importance of specifying variable measurement in terms of local cultural context is illustrated as well by the examination of buffers against stressful circumstances, especially social support. While modernization usually entails a contraction of the range of kin in an individual's social network, kin frequently retain a special status as providers of social support. For example, among Samoan migrants to northern California, Janes (1990) found that the large descent groups that form the foundation of traditional Samoan social organization were still somewhat intact in the urban setting, but that these groups had lost much of their meaning for people. Instead, social support systems were built from networks among households of adult siblings who, traditionally, share a close affective relationship in Samoa. These kin-based networks provided a buffer against status inconsistency in this setting. Dressler (1994) has discussed the cultural construction of social support in greater detail.

There is a two-stage method implicit in cross-cultural perspective in these studies of stress and disease. The first involves an ethnographic analysis of the shared understandings within a community that define, for example, a particular lifestyle as desirable, or particular kinds of social supporters as appropriate for specific problems. Then, the epidemiological measurement strategy involves determining how closely individuals match these collective representations. Those who are less able to fulfill cultural expectations appear to be at higher risk of disease. Dressler (2007a) has formalized these insights in his theory of "cultural consonance," which is defined as the degree to which individuals approximate, in their own beliefs and behaviors, the prototypes for those beliefs and behaviors encoded in cultural models.

Cultural consonance theory is explicitly based in a cognitive theory that defines "culture" as that which one must know to function effectively in a given society. Cultural knowledge is organized and socially distributed in the form of models or schemas that define the elements of specific cultural domains (e.g., lifestyles) and how those elements are patterned. The degree of sharing of a given cultural model can then be quantified using the cultural consensus model developed by Romney, Weller, and Batchelder (1986). The cultural consensus model tests for the degree of agreement among members of society regarding the semantic structure of a given cultural domain. For example, in a cultural domain such as social support, this semantic structure may involve preferred sources of social support in relation to specific kinds of problems commonly encountered in that community. If there is a sufficient level of shared understanding within a domain, it is reasonable to infer that respondents are collectively drawing on a shared, or cultural, model of social support. If there is a shared model, a culturally best estimate of the configuration of elements in a cultural domain (e.g., Who, culturally, are the most important sources of social support collectively defined in a specific community?) can be estimated. Given this specification of a cultural model, the degree to which individuals actually enact that model in their own lives can be assessed. For example, if a particular configuration of social supports is culturally defined as appropriate, how consonant are individuals with this configuration in their own reported seeking of social support?

Using this approach, Dressler and associates have demonstrated in research in Brazil and in an African American community in the rural southern United States that low cultural consonance in several domains is associated with higher arterial blood pressure; higher psychological distress; lower immune function; higher body mass; and, prospectively, higher depressive symptoms (Dressler, 2007a; Dressler, Balieiro, Ribeiro, & dos Santos, 2005, 2007). Using similar methods, Gravlee, Dressler, and Bernard (2005), working in Puerto Rico, have shown that assignment of skin color categories on the basis of local cultural models of race is a better predictor of blood pressure than skin reflectometer measures of skin color. And Decker, Flinn, England, and Worthman (2003) have shown that West Indian men who more closely approximate the local cultural model of a "good man" have lower mean daily cortisol levels. The accumulated research findings from studies of modernization and disease, cross-cultural studies of the stress process, and studies of cultural consonance, point to the fundamental importance of the cultural milieu in shaping the risk of disease.

The Cultural Definition of Illness

The studies of culture and the risk of disease just described are clearly biocultural in orientation and are organized in part by scientific biomedical definitions of physiology and disease. In any given cultural setting, however, individuals experiencing these kinds of cultural stresses in turn experience a variety of signs and symptoms that must be collated, interpreted, and named if remedial action is going to take place. There is an imperfect overlap between biomedical definitions of disease in terms of biomedical pathophysiology, and collective and individual definitions of illness that describe the experience of dysfunction, a distinction that was elaborated most clearly by Kleinman (1980). Therefore, understanding how illness is collectively defined, and how that may or may not correspond to biomedical definitions of disease, has been an important research topic.

The most dramatic differences between biomedical and alternative understandings of disease and illness are found in the study of "culture-bound syndromes," now referred to as "cultural syndromes." These are named illnesses, with a constellation of signs and symptoms, a defined pathophysiology, and recommended treatment that are unknown in biomedicine. One widely distributed cultural syndrome in Latin America is referred to as *susto*. As its name implies, *susto* results from a sudden and severe fright of any sort. In classic definitions of the syndrome, this fright causes the soul of the person to leave the body, and this in turn leads to the symptoms of the illness, which include generalized fatigue, lack of interest in normal activities, sadness, and loss of appetite. Treatment requires both the alleviation of symptoms and that the soul be "called" back to the body, which, in some circumstances, can be quite difficult, since the wandering soul can be held captive by other spirits.

A comprehensive study of *susto* was carried out by Rubel, O'Nell, and Collado-Ardon (1991) in Oaxaca in southern Mexico. This was a case–control study of respondents who reported having been diagnosed as *assustado* (i.e., persons with *susto*) compared to age- and sex-matched controls. Rubel and colleagues were particularly interested in the kinds of cultural stresses that might increase the risk of *susto*, and they developed a measure of social stress very much like measures of cultural consonance referred to earlier, in that stress was seen to result from the failure to meet widely shared age- and sex-appropriate social expectations. *Assustados* had higher stress scores than matched controls. Additionally, measures of general health (in the form of a physical exam) and a brief (22-item) inventory of symptoms of "psychiatric impairment" were obtained, and while persons with *susto* were generally in poorer health than controls, they were not found to more psychiatrically impaired. Finally, in a 7-year follow-up, persons who reported *susto* were at higher risk of mortality than matched controls.

One explanation of cultural syndromes is that they are "real" biomedical diseases, but with another name in another setting (e.g., *susto* is "really" depression). Guarnaccia, Canino, Rubio-Stipec, and Bravo (1993) have examined this question in a study of *ataques de nervios* (nerve attacks) in Puerto Rico. *Ataques de nervios* (or *ataques*) are dramatic, panic attack–like reactions to highly stressful circumstances, such as learning of the death of a family member, attending a funeral, or being the victim of aggression. Symptoms include violent crying and shaking, and can even progress to seizure-like reactions. Once the *ataque* has subsided, supportive care by family members usually results in a return to health, although it is possible for a chronic *nervios* to develop. In an islandwide survey of nearly 1,000 respondents, Guarnaccia and colleagues found a 16% lifetime prevalence rate for *ataques*. Persons at the highest risk were older women, the less well-educated, and persons lacking social support. Furthermore, in the same survey the Diagnostic Interview Schedule (Robins, Helzer, Croughnan, & Ratcliffe, 1981) was used to generate data for psychiatric diagnoses consistent with the *Diagnostic and Statistical Manual of Mental Disorders*. Persons who reported having had an *ataque* were also more likely to reach the threshold for a DSM psychiatric diagnosis, but not in any particular diagnostic category; that is, they were more likely to have *a* diagnosis, but not any specific diagnosis. Guarnaccia and colleagues concluded that this cultural syndrome is likely a comorbid condition with other psychiatric diagnoses, but that it cannot be explained by those diagnoses.

A cultural syndrome can be viewed as an "idiom of distress" within a particular society (Nichter, 1981). An individual experiencing particular kinds of stresses that are highly salient in that community can signal that distress by developing a particular cultural syndrome that is widely understood in the community to be a result of "a life lived harshly." This signaling of distress then, it is hoped, calls forth supportive responses from others. The particular configuration of psychophysiological signs and symptoms can be to a greater or lesser extent, learned and conditioned within that community. For example, Oths (1999) examined the little-studied cultural syndrome of *debilidad* in the Andean highlands. This syndrome is characterized by weakness, fatigue and, especially, severe headaches. Oths found that it is most likely to strike victims in households with an imbalanced sex ratio because peasant households depend on a sex role balanced workforce to accomplish the many difficult tasks of high-altitude agriculture. Where the sex ratio becomes imbalanced, inappropriate workloads fall to household members, creating severe social stresses. Furthermore, cases of *debilidad* tend to cluster in households as a result of not only shared stresses but also perhaps because the configuration of signs and symptoms defining the syndrome are learned by one sufferer from another.

While cultural influences on the definition of illness stand out clearly in the study of cultural syndromes, standard biomedical labels such as "hypertension" or "heart disease" can mean quite different things in different social groups. For example, Daniulaityte (2004) examined the meaning of "diabetes" in a sample of diabetics in urban Mexico. Diabetes is a significant public health problem in Mexico, accounting for the preponderance of health care expenditures in the Mexican social security system. Using cultural consensus analysis (the technique discussed earlier to verify sharing of cultural models of specific cultural domains), Daniulaityte found that patients with diabetes shared a substantially more varied model of diabetes than their physicians, especially with respect to etiology. In addition to the usual elements of family history, diet, and physical activity, patients with diabetes attributed the onset of diabetes to factors as varied as pollution, changing quality of the food supply and *susto*; furthermore, these were not isolated and idiosyncratic responses but were shared within a sample of patients with diabetes.

Chavez, Hubbell, McMullin, Martinez, and Mishra (1995) examined the diversity in knowledge of breast and cervical cancer in a community in southern California, comparing recent Hispanic immigrant women from Mexico and San Salvador, Chicanas (Hispanic women born and raised in California), Anglo women, and physicians. These researchers were particularly interested in different understandings of the causes of these reproductive cancers, so they generated inventories of causal factors from each group using a free listing technique. Then, each group rank ordered a master list of 29 potential causes, developed by sampling from each group's list, in terms of the most to the least important causes. Using cultural consensus analysis, Chavez and colleagues found no agreement when the groups were combined. When divided by ethnicity, there

was cultural consensus within each group. But perhaps more interesting was the overlap between groups. Immigrant women agreed substantially with Chicanas but less so with Anglos, and not at all with physicians. Similarly, Chicanas agrees substantially with Anglos but less so with physicians, and Anglos agreed most with physicians. This generated, graphically, a "cultural cline" (analogous to a biological cline, in which there is a continuous geographic distribution of phenotypic traits—e.g., skin color—with no sharp points of demarcation separating groups), with overlap in agreement among all the groups, but with the two groups at either end of the continuum showing virtually no agreement. The nature of the agreement (or disagreement) is discussed further below; here, it is important to note the distributive nature of cultural knowledge of disease and illness, which is an important corrective to categorical thinking about sharp cultural edges and boundaries separating social groups.

Baer, Weller, Garcia, and Rocha (2004) conducted a similar study comparing physicians and general population samples in Texas and Mexico in terms of their cultural models of HIV/AIDS. The aim of the study was to determine the relative contributions of professional versus lay status and country of origin to cultural models of illness. Overall, they found considerable similarity in the configuration of cultural models across the four groups; however, there was greater similarity between professional and lay groups within each country than that between professional or lay groups across the two countries. Even in the case of professionally socialized, biomedically trained physicians, there is an overlay of cultural knowledge that alters the configuration of their cultural model of HIV/AIDS.

The studies reviewed here exemplify the varied ways in which illness and disease are defined, ranging from the definition of illness completely outside of biomedical nosology to the differential interpretation of biomedically defined disease.

Culture and Treatment Choice

As noted earlier, in the years following World War II there was a substantial increase in the availability of scientific biomedicine in developing countries, both through foreign aid and the expanded training of physicians in those societies. These biomedical treatment options became available alongside, and did not supplant, existing forms of medical treatment, which led developing societies to be characterized as "pluralistic medical systems." A question of both theoretical and applied significance arose in relation to these systems: How, given the experience of illness, do people decide what kind of care to seek out? Early in the study of pluralistic medical systems it became apparent that there was no single path through treatment, nor did individuals commit themselves solely to one system or the other. Rather, people tended to mix systems, based on a number of factors, including (but not limited to) the explanatory model for the etiology of the illness.

Young and Garro (1994) examined treatment choice in a highland village in Mexico and specified the factors influencing such choices in a formal decision model. The critical factors affecting choice of treatment included whether a cure was known within the household; the severity of the illness; barriers to treatment (especially expense, not necessarily of the treatment itself, but expense of transportation to treatment); and what Young and Garro refer to as "faith" in the medical system being considered. The Mexican villagers in the study had access to a variety of traditional healers, including herbalists, midwives, bonesetters, and *curanderos*, who could treat illness of both natural and supernatural etiology; lay biomedical healers, in the form of pharmacists and *practicantes* (persons with some level of biomedical training, e.g., medics retired from the army); and, biomedical physicians seen both in private practice and through the government health care system. Young and Garro developed a decision model based on intensive interviewing of a few key respondents, then tested the model with a sample of nearly 500 illness episodes collected within the village over a 6-month period. Specific decisions depended on the particular constellation of factors noted earlier, and using this decision model, Young and Garro were able to predict accurately over 90% of the treatment choices.

One advantage Young and Garro (1994) had in their study was that they were dealing with a sample of relatively young families with small children who, overall, were fairly healthy. What this meant is that many of the illnesses they encountered in their sample were episodes such as upper respiratory infections that were relatively mild and self-limiting. Mathews and Hill (1990) adapted this model to a very different setting, with different results. They conducted their research in an ethnically mixed community on the Caribbean coast of Costa Rica. In addition to the *mestizo* community (of mixed European and Indian descent), there was a large community of Afro-Caribbean laborers on local plantations. When Mathews and Hill adapted the Young–Garro model to this setting, even though they altered a number of parameters to fit the local ethnographic realities better, they found substantially lower predictive strength of the model, successfully predicting 62% of the treatment choices. The lower predictive strength of the model was found to be a function of two factors. First, Spanish language fluency allowed the *mestizo* sample to take advantage of a broader range of health care options than the Afro-Caribbean sample, most of which had only rudimentary fluency in Spanish. Second, the epidemiological profile of the two groups differed, with the treatment of chronic diseases (e.g., hypertension and diabetes) much more important in the Afro-Caribbean sample. This study reveals another layer of complexity in the treatment choice process.

Oths (1994) examined treatment choice of individuals in the Andean highlands under conditions of severe financial stress. In the late 1980s, all of South America was convulsed by a period of economic hyperinflation, during which prices were inflated as much as 100% per month. Oths happened to be collecting data on illness episodes from a sample in a highland village before and then during the onset of hyperinflation, which provided her with a kind of natural experiment for the impact of economic factors on treatment choice. Comparing preinflation and postonset of inflation decisions, she found that there was a major decline in seeking treatment for mild and moderately severe illnesses, and that the decline in seeking care from traditional sources was greater than that from biomedical providers. This was a function of not only the relative efficacy of biomedical treatment but also the cost of traditional treatments. Treatment from a *curandero* often involves repeated visits and the purchase of a variety of herbal remedies and other treatments; visiting a physician, on the other hand, while expensive, usually involved only a single visit and the receipt of an injection or the filling of a prescription. This study also demonstrates how the environment within which decisions are made can substantially alter treatment choice.

In addition to research that addresses the seeking of medical care in response to specific symptoms, some investigators have examined cultural factors influencing the decision to engage in preventative practices. In one of the more sophisticated studies in this area, Chavez, McMullin, Mishra, and Hubbell (2001) built on their investigation of ethnic variation in cultural models of reproductive cancer. As noted earlier, Chavez and colleagues (1995) found a cultural cline in models of breast and cervical cancers, from Hispanic immigrants from El Salvador and Mexico to Chicanas and Anglos, to physicians in southern California. For cervical cancer, Hispanic immigrant women emphasized physical trauma as most important with respect to etiology. Chicanas and Anglos, on the other hand, had a much more generic view of cancer risk, with family history and limited access to medical care assuming greater prominence. Physicians emphasized the importance of sexually transmitted infections, early initiation of sexual activity, and multiple sexual partners.

In their follow-up study, Chavez and colleagues (2001) examined how cultural consonance—that is, a woman incorporating one of these cultural models into her own personal beliefs regarding cervical cancer—might influence her decision to get a screening test (i.e., Pap [Papanicolaou] exam) for cervical cancer. In a survey, these investigators asked nearly 1,000 women to rank-order the importance of a subset of potential etiological factors, with representative factors drawn from each of the cultural models. They could then calculate a cultural consonance score for each woman, indicating how closely her individual beliefs aligned with

either the immigrant model, the Chicana–Anglo model, or the physician model. They then determined whether the woman had had a Pap exam in the past 2 years and, controlling for insurance status, age, education, and income, which of the measures of cultural consonance was most closely associated with having had the exam. Interestingly, they found that if a woman was culturally consonant with the immigrant model, then she was neither more nor less likely to have had a Pap exam. If a woman was consonant with the Chicana–Anglo model, then she was significantly more likely to have had an exam (odds ratio = 1.67, $p < .05$); if, however, a woman was consonant with the physician model, she was significantly *less* likely to have had an exam (odds ratio = 0.60, $p < .05$).

Chavez and colleagues (2000) linked these somewhat counterintuitive findings to the meanings that underlie consonance with one or another model:

> Associating, even unconsciously, Pap exams and cervical cancer with nonnormative and morally questionable behavior [i.e., multiple sex partners and early initiation of sexual activity] may not motivate some Latinas, especially immigrants, to proactively seek out Pap exams. On the other hand, downplaying sex-related risk factors and elevating heredity, for which no one is to "blame," and a lack of medical care, as Anglo women do, does not raise the specter of nonnormative, morally questionable behavior. (p. 1125)

It is likely, in other words, that cultural models regarding health and illness link both horizontally and vertically with other cultural models, in this case, one defining moral and proper behavior. The woman who links cancer risk to immoral and improper behavior would define seeking a Pap exam for cervical cancer as an admission of moral failure.

Seeking and utilizing health care is the result of a complex calculus that links issues of economic and geographic access to care, shared definitions of disease, and the links between cultural models in different domains. Furthermore, insights from the study of pluralistic medical systems in different societies are of clear relevance to our own society given that it is becoming more, not less, pluralistic.

Patients and Healers

A wide variety of healers are found cross-culturally. These range from practitioners trained in licensed educational settings, such as biomedical physicians, practitioners of traditional Chinese medicine, Ayurvedic doctors (trained in the professional healing tradition of South Asia), naturopaths (trained in a system of healing that emphasizes the body's intrinsic ability to heal itself with supportive care) and chiropractors to the *practicantes* noted earlier, who pick up bits of knowledge here or there, to the more exotic curers, who utilize skills in herbal preparations and supernatural intervention (Erickson, 2008). Ethnographic research on patients and healers has addressed a number of issues, including patient–healer interaction. The work of Arthur Kleinman (1980) has been perhaps the most influential in this regard. Kleinman is, in general, interested in the intersection of knowledge and belief regarding health and illness in different segments of any society. These segments include the professional sector, the popular sector (that combines some elements of professional knowledge with other sources of information for laypersons) and the folk sector (that refers to traditional medical knowledge). More specifically, Kleinman seeks to clarify how these different domains of medical knowledge might be deployed in the interaction of patient and healer.

These interests led Kleinman (1980) to develop the concept of "explanatory model." He argues that patients and healers enter into focused social interactions organized around their own explanations for why a particular health problem occurred when it did, its pathophysiology, the course it is likely to run, and the steps necessary to resolve the problem. These specialized cognitive models are referred to as "explanatory models." Problems can occur because, typically, in biomedicine, it is only the explanatory model of the healer that is privileged. At best, the patient's model is seen as a set of potential clues to what is 'really' occurring, which can only be adequately explained by the physician's explanatory model. At worst, the patient's model is seen as an obstacle of ignorance to be overcome. Kleinman argues, however, that a serious consideration of patient explanatory models can lead to a more effective therapeutic relationship between patient and healer. By highlighting points of convergence and divergence in explanatory models, a mutually satisfactory treatment plan can be negotiated, and therapy can proceed on the basis of mutually agreed-upon therapeutic goals.

Kleinman's approach immediately poses the question of how much patients and healers share in their understanding of health and illness. Some of the research reviewed earlier addresses this question. For example, Chavez and colleagues (1995) demonstrated a cultural cline in the distribution of cultural models of reproductive cancers, so that biomedical physicians and their (potential) patients could be seen to share much or little of their understanding, depending on how ethnic boundaries are drawn within the sample of patients. Also as noted earlier, Baer and colleagues (2004) found substantial sharing in the cultural models of HIV/AIDS held by physicians and laypersons in the same communities in Mexico and Texas.

Garro (1986) investigated the degree of sharing of medical knowledge between laypersons and traditional healers (*curanderas*) in a village in the highlands of Mexico. Using the cultural consensus model, she found overall agreement among *curanderas* and laypersons regarding the causes, course, and treatment of common illnesses; however, there was a clear difference in expertise between *curanderas* and laypersons. When mapped in two-dimensional space, the *curanderas* formed a tight cluster in the middle of the space. Arrayed around them in a circular pattern were older female laypersons, and arrayed in a circular pattern around them were younger female laypersons. In other words, the *curanderas* employed the same knowledge as laypersons, but they had greater cultural expertise. Older women, with their years of experience managing the health of households, were closer to the *curanderas* in expertise, while younger women, with little expertise, were more distant.

Not all ethnographic settings conform to this pattern, however. Finkler (1994) examined Mexican spiritualist healing traditions in another part of the country. While *curanderas* approach a clinical encounter in much the same way a biomedical physician would, spiritualist healers rely on trance and spirit possession to determine a patient's problem and the appropriate therapeutic steps to be taken. This changes dramatically the dynamic with respect to interaction between healer and patient. There is very little information exchanged; hence, little opportunity for healer and patient to develop either a shared understanding of the specific problem at hand or general health beliefs. In this situation, the cognitive cultural gulf between patient and healer can be as great as that between the biomedical physicians and Hispanic immigrant women in the study by Chavez and associates (1995).

The topic of recruitment and training of healers has been investigated most completely in societies with formal systems of professional licensure, such as the United States. Seligman (2005), however, examined how individuals enter into the role of spirit medium in an Afro-Brazilian syncretic form of spiritualism knows as *candomblé*. The narratives describing how *candomblé* spirit mediums enter the role conform to a cultural model involving significant social loss and trauma; that is, persons who go on to become spirit mediums are seen as having first experienced significant events, such as the death of close family members, severe economic difficulties, or abusive conjugal relationships. These eventually lead to a health crisis that is irresolvable by normal biomedical treatment and, ultimately, to spontaneous spirit possession that leads to recovery. It is this spontaneous possession that signals their fitness for the healing role.

Finally, Oths and Hinojosa (2004) have helped to complete the cross-cultural description of traditional healers with their recent survey of manual therapies. There has been somewhat of a bias toward the exotic in ethnographic descriptions of healers, placing emphasis on the supernatural and shamanistic healing. This has ignored the fact that, especially in many peasant communities, injuries to the musculoskeletal system represent a significant burden of morbidity. Manual therapy, or "bone-setting," as it is often known, although often overlooked, represents an important part of healing traditions in every society. In a survey of manual therapies, including traditional Andean bone-setters, lay Welsh massage therapists, professionally licensed manual therapists such as chiropractors, and newly developing healing traditions such as rolfing, Oths and Hinajosa enlarge our understanding of healers.

Healing and Curing

The question, as posed by Csordas and Kleinman (1996) is "How do traditional healers heal?", although the pertinent question may be "How does any healer heal?" While we in the West have a tendency to privilege the scientific basis of biomedicine, the gap between biological sciences and biomedical practice is fairly large. Evidence of that comes from Lynn Payer's (1988) journalistic (and often pithy) comparisons of biomedical healing traditions in Western Europe and North America. The ways in which cultural setting modifies the supposed science of biomedicine are quite remarkable.

A similar and more systematic demonstration of how culture intersects with biology in healing comes from Moerman's (2002) work on international variation in the placebo response. Moerman collated data from various countries on clinical trials for new pharmaceutical treatments for gastric ulcers and essential hypertension. These were all double-blind, randomized clinical trials with a placebo control group. He found quite striking variation in the placebo effect, or the proportion of patients who responded clinically to an inert substance. For example, only 10% of Brazilian ulcer patients responded to the placebo, while 59% of German patients did. At the same time, only 22% of Danish patients responded to the placebo, while nearly 50% of American patients did (Moerman, 2002, pp. 80–81). These results, coupled with other findings on the consumption of inert substances (e.g., pink placebos generate a larger stimulant response than blue placebos), led Moerman to label these a general "meaning effect," emphasizing that symbolic properties of the treatments have physiological and metabolic effects.

This is clearly one pathway in which traditional healers can heal, by manipulating symbols that are meaningful to patients with respect to curing and healing. Unfortunately, studies to evaluate meaning effects are notoriously difficult to design and carry out under typical field conditions in anthropological research. Thus, most data on traditional healing come from case studies (e.g.,

Gillin's [1948] classic study of a case of *susto*). While it is not a pure evaluation design, Finkler's (1994) study of Mexican spiritualism provides some systematic data in this regard. Finkler compared four groups: patients seeking care from local physicians; persons who were regular attendees at the spiritualist temple; persons who were only seeking consultations for health problems at the temple; and a control group. Respondents were administered the Cornell Medical Index (CMI, a count of symptoms across organ systems) before their consultations/visits and 4 weeks later. At the initial CMI, both the temple attendees and physicians' patients had the highest symptom counts. After treatment, the temple attendees' symptom counts had significantly declined at least as low as those of patients visiting physicians.

Some fundamental logical problems limit Finkler's study, most notably the problem of selection, since patients could not be randomly assigned to treatment conditions. Nevertheless, the fact that both physicians' patients and temple attendees started out at the same level of symptom expression, and both declined significantly, suggests that symbolic healing occurred with the temple treatments. While temple spirit mediums would prescribe herbal preparations and even some over-the-counter drugs to their patients, healing principally took the form of a *limpia*, or symbolic cleansing. Finkler (1994) suggests that this cleansing was particularly meaningful for temple patients, in that a major explanatory model for illness in the community emphasized pollution in the air, water, and food supply as major causes for illness in this rapidly industrializing region north of Mexico City. Kirmayer (2004) discusses symbolic healing of this nature more extensively.

Not all traditional healing, indeed, not all biomedical healing, is a function of the meaning response, however, as evidenced by the considerable investment of large pharmaceutical companies in collecting ethnomedical knowledge and ethnobotanical samples. In a focused study of ethnomedical knowledge, McDade and colleagues (2007), in a study of the Tsimane' of lowland Bolivia, found that in households in which adult family members possessed greater knowledge of traditional healing the children had lower levels of chronic inflammation, as measured by C-reactive protein. Other forms of healing, such as that of bone-setters and specialists in physical manipulation of the body, described in Oths and Hinojosa (2004), are obviously manipulating physical structures directly and providing relief in that way. Nevertheless, the data on cross-national variation in the placebo response and data evaluating the symbolic impact of traditional healing suggest that all healing proceeds as a function of both pharmacological and symbolic effects on the body, whether the health care provider is a spirit medium or a biomedically trained physician.

Conclusions

As I noted at the outset, this has been a highly selective review of research in medical anthropology, organized by the progression of the natural history of disease. It has, furthermore, emphasized research in medical anthropology that fits comfortably under a "biocultural" theoretical orientation that takes seriously both human biology and the shared and culturally constructed systems of meaning within which humans function that shape, and are shaped by, human biology.

Even a casual perusal of the literature in medical anthropology will show that this is but one of a number of theoretical orientations guiding research in the area. Among the social sciences, anthropology is perhaps the most internally heterogeneous field, in the sense that its broad orientations not only offer different hypotheses about how the world works but also entail different, and in large part incomparable, methods for investigating those differences. These other approaches include political–economic perspectives (Goodman & Leatherman, 1998), critical medical anthropology (Scheper-Hughes & Lock, 1987; Singer, 2004), and interpretative orientations (Mattingly & Garro, 2000). I have chosen to emphasize an approach that examines the intersection of culture and human biology, and that, as well, utilizes mixed qualitative and quantitative methods of research. As I have argued elsewhere (Dressler 2001, 2007b), a biocultural orientation, focusing on both the cultural construction of meaning and the constraining forces of social structure, is uniquely situated for the investigation of the intersection of culture and health.

Further Reading

Alland, A. (1970). *Adaptation in cultural evolution: An approach to medical anthropology.* New York: Columbia University Press.

Ember, C. R., & Ember, M. (Eds.). (2004). *Encyclopedia of medical anthropology.* New York: Kluwer Academic/Plenum Press.

Farmer, P. (1992). *AIDS and accusation: Haiti and the geography of blame.* Berkeley and Los Angeles: University of California Press.

Farmer, P. (1999). *Infections and inequalities: The modern plagues.* Berkeley and Los Angeles: University of California Press.

Goodman, A. H., & Leatherman, T. L. (Eds.). (1998). *Building a new biocultural synthesis: Political–economic perspectives on human biology.* Ann Arbor: University of Michigan Press.

Hahn, R. A. (1995). *Sickness and healing: An anthropological perspective.* New Haven, CT: Yale University Press.

Kleinman, A. (1980). *Patients and healers in the context of culture.* Berkeley: University of California Press.

Leslie, C. (1976). *Asian medical systems: A comparative study.* Berkeley: University of California Press.

References

Baer, R. D., Weller, S. C., Garcia, J. G., & Rocha, A. L. S. (2004). A comparison of community and physician explanatory models of AIDS in Mexico and the United States. *Medical Anthropology Quarterly, 18,* 3–22.

Baker, P. T., Hanna, J.M., & Baker, T. S. (Eds.). (1986). *The changing Samoans: Behavior and health in transition.* New York: Oxford University Press.

Beaglehole, R., Salmond, C. E., Hooper, A., Huntsman, J., Stanhope, J. M., Cassel, J. C., et al. (1977). Blood pressure and social interaction in Tokelauan migrants in New Zealand. *Journal of Chronic Diseases, 30,* 803–812.

Chavez, L., Hubbell, F. A., McMullin, J. M., Martinez, R. M., & Mishra, S. I. (1995). Structure and meaning in models of breast and cervical cancer risk factors. *Medical Anthropology Quarterly, 9,* 40–74.

Chavez, L., McMullin, J. M., Mishra, S. I., & Hubbell, F. A. (2001). Beliefs matter. *American Anthropologist, 102,* 1114–1129.

Csordas, T. J., & Kleinman, A. (1996). The therapeutic process. In C. Sargent & T. Johnson (Eds.), *Medical anthropology: A handbook of theory and method* (2nd ed., pp. 3–21). New York: Greenwood Press.

Daniulaityte, R. (2004). Making sense of diabetes. *Social Science and Medicine, 59,* 1899–1912.

Decker, S., Flinn, M., England, B. G., & Worthman, C. M. (2003). Cultural congruity and the cortisol stress response among Dominican men. In J. M. Wilce, Jr. (Ed.), *Social and cultural lives of immune systems* (pp. 147–169). London: Routledge.

Dressler, W. W. (1982). *Hypertension and culture change: Acculturation and disease in the West Indies.* South Salem, NY: Redgrave.

Dressler, W. W. (1994). Cross-cultural differences and social influences in social support and cardiovascular disease. In S. A. Shumaker & S. M. Czajkowski (Eds.), *Social support and cardiovascular disease* (pp. 167–192). New York: Plenum Press.

Dressler, W. W. (1999). Modernization, stress and blood pressure: New directions in research. *Human Biology, 71,* 583–605.

Dressler, W. W. (2001). Medical anthropology: Toward a third moment in social science? *Medical Anthropology Quarterly, 15,* 455–465.

Dressler, W. W. (2004). Social or status incongruence. In N. A. Anderson (Ed.), *The encyclopedia of health and behavior* (pp. 764–767). Thousand Oaks, CA: Sage.

Dressler, W. W. (2007a). Cultural consonance. In D. Bhugra & K. Bhui (Eds.), *Textbook of cultural psychiatry* (pp. 179–190). Cambridge, UK: Cambridge University Press.

Dressler, W. W. (2007b). Meaning and structure in research in medical anthropology. *Anthropology in Action, 14,* 30–43.

Dressler, W. W., Balieiro, M. C., Ribeiro, R. P., & dos Santos, J. E. D. (2005). Cultural consonance and arterial blood pressure in urban Brazil. *Social Science and Medicine, 61,* 527–540.

Dressler, W. W., Balieiro, M. C., Ribeiro, R. P., & dos Santos, J. E. D. (2007). A prospective study of cultural consonance and depressive symptoms in urban Brazil. *Social Science and Medicine, 65,* 2058–2069.

Ember, C. R., & Ember, M. (Eds.). (2004). *Encyclopedia of medical anthropology.* New York: Kluwer Academic/Plenum Press.

Erickson, P. I. (2008). *Ethnomedicine.* Long Grove, IL: Waveland Press.

Finkler, K. (1994). *Spiritualist healers in Mexico.* Salem, WI: Sheffield.

Garro, L. C. (1986). Intracultural variation in folk medical knowledge: A comparison between curers and noncurers. *American Anthropologist, 88,* 351–370.

Gillin, J. (1948). Magical fright. *Psychiatry, 11,* 387–400.

Goodman, A. H., & Leatherman, T. L. (Eds.). (1998). *Building a new biocultural synthesis: Political–economic perspectives on human biology.* Ann Arbor: University of Michigan Press.

Gravlee, C. C., Dressler, W. W., & Bernard, H. R. (2005). Skin color, social classification, and blood pressure in southeastern Puerto Rico. *American Journal of Public Health, 95,* 2191–2197.

Guarnaccia, P. J., Canino, G., Rubio-Stipec, M., & Bravo, M. (1993). The prevalence of *ataques de nervios* in the Puerto Rico Disaster Study. *Journal of Nervous and Mental Disease, 181,* 157–165.

Janes, C. R. (1990). *Migration, social change, and health: A Samoan community in urban California.* Stanford, CA: Stanford University Press.

Kirmayer, L. J. (2004). The cultural diversity of healing. *British Medical Bulletin, 69,* 33–48.

Kleinman, A. (1980). *Patients and healers in the context of culture.* Berkeley: University of California Press.

Leighton, A. H., & Leighton, D. C. (1967). Mental health and social factors. In A. M. Freedman & H. I. Kaplan (Eds.), *Comprehensive textbook of psychiatry* (pp. 1520–1533). Baltimore: Williams & Wilkins.

Mathews, H. F., & Hill, C. E. (1990). Applying cognitive decision theory to the study of regional patterns of illness treatment choice. *American Anthropologist, 92,* 155–170.

Mattingly, C., & Garro, L. C. (Eds.). (2000). *Narrative and the cultural construction of illness and healing.* Los Angeles and Berkeley: University of California Press.

McDade, T. W. (2002). Status incongruity in Samoan youth: A biocultural analysis of culture change, stress and immune function. *Medical Anthropology Quarterly, 16,* 123–150.

McDade, T. W., Reyes-Garcia, V., Blackinton, P., Tanner, S., Huanaca, T., & Leonard, W. R. (2007). Ethnobotanical knowledge is associated with indices of child health in the Bolivian Amazon. *Proceedings of the National Academy of Sciences USA, 104,* 6134–6139.

McGarvey, S. T., & Baker, P. T. (1979). The effects of modernization and migration on Samoan blood pressures. *Human Biology, 51,* 467–479.

Moerman, D. (2002). *Meaning, medicine and the "placebo effect."* Cambridge, UK: Cambridge University Press.

Nichter, M. (1981). Idioms of distress. *Culture, Medicine, and Psychiatry, 5,* 379–408.

Oths, K. S. (1994). Health care decisions of households in economic crisis. *Human Organization, 53,* 245–254.

Oths, K. S. (1999). *"Debilidad"*: A reproductive-related illness of the Peruvian Andes. *Medical Anthropology Quarterly, 13,* 386–315.

Oths, K. S., & Hinojosa, S. Z. (Eds.). (2004). *Healing by hand: Manual medicine and bonesetting in global perspective.* Walnut Creek, CA: Altamira Press.

Paul, B. D. (Ed.). (1955). *Health, culture, and community: Case studies of public reactions to health programs.* New York: Russell Sage Foundation.

Payer, L. (1988). *Medicine and culture.* New York: Penguin Books.

Robins, L. N., Helzer, J. E., Croughnan, J., & Ratcliffe, K. S. (1981). National Institute of Mental Health Diagnostic Interview Schedule. *Archive of General Psychiatry, 38,* 281–389.

Romney, A. K., Weller, S. C., & Batchelder, W. H. (1986). Culture as consensus: A theory of culture and informant accuracy. *American Anthropologist, 88,* 313–338.

Rubel, A. J., O'Nell, C. W., & Collado-Ardon, R. (1991). *Susto: A folk illness.* Los Angeles and Berkeley: University of California Press.

Scheper-Hughes, N., & Lock, M. (1987). The mindful body: A prolegomenon to future work in medical anthropology. *Medical Anthropology Quarterly, 1,* 6–41.

Scotch, N. A. (1963). Sociocultural factors in the epidemiology of Zulu hypertension. *American Journal of Public Health, 53,* 1205–1213.

Seligman, R. (2005). From affliction to affirmation. *Transcultural Psychiatry, 42,* 272–294.

Singer, M. (2004). Critical medical anthropology. In C. R. Ember & M. Ember (Eds.), *Encyclopedia of medical anthropology* (pp. 23–30). New York: Kluwer Academic/Plenum Press.

Young, J. C., & Garro, L. (1994). *Medical choice in a Mexican village.* Prospect Heights, IL: Waveland Press.

CHAPTER 19

Health Psychology Meets Health Economics

Yaniv Hanoch
Thomas Rice

Between 1991 and 2002 the number of smokers in New York City remained stable, with slightly more than 21% of the population identified as smokers. North Carolina reported a similar phenomenon, with the number of smokers showing very little fluctuation until 2006. In 2002, New York City (and New York State), and in 2006, the state of North Carolina increased the sales tax on tobacco. While North Carolina increased the sales tax from $0.05 to $0.35 per pack of cigarettes, the New York City increase was more dramatic, from $0.08 to $1.50 per pack (this was in addition to the New York State increase of about $0.40 during the same time period). Shortly after the sales tax increase came into effect, New York City officials reported that the number of smokers decreased by 11% (from 21.6 to 19.2%; Frieden et al., 2005), and in North Carolina, cigarette sales fell by 18%. It seems that an increase in cigarettes price has had a direct and substantial effect on the number of people who smoke and/or the number of cigarettes smoked. Such findings would come as no surprise to many economists, who have long been aware of the phenomenon of price elasticity. Derived from the law of demand (one of the fundamental laws in economics), "price elasticity" assumes that people are sensitive to product price: As price goes up,

ceteris paribus, demand goes down. Thus, the theory predicts an inverse relationship between price and consumption, creating what economists call a downward-sloping demand curve (see Rice, 2003).

Changes in smoking rates are but one example where health economics and health psychology might share a common interest. Health economics, after all, studies how economics principles (the relationship between scarce resources, e.g., time and money, consumer demand) affect, relate to, and determine health behaviors and outcomes. The range of phenomena examined by health economics encompasses topics such as smoking prevention, physician reimbursement and performance, insurance and health outcome, urban and rural utilization of health services, and health disparity. What health economics tends to lack, however, is the usage of experimental design.[1] Instead, health economists typically analyze existing

---

[1] One notable exception is the RAND Health Insurance Experiment (HIE) According to the official RAND website, "The HIE project was started in 1971 and funded by the Department of Health, Education, and Welfare (now the Department of Health and Human Services). It was a 15-year, multimillion-dollar effort that to this day remains the largest health policy study in U.S. history" (*www. rand.org/health/projects/hie*).

databases to understand and study health-related trends. Psychologists, on the other hand, tend to run controlled experiments more frequently, while database analysis is less common. In other words, although the tools and theories that economists and psychologists' employ might differ, both disciplines are interested in explaining and understanding the same phenomena. Thus, one can view economics and psychology as complementing one another.

The New York City cigarette tax increase provides a powerful demonstration regarding the relationship between changes in price and behavior. One might wonder, therefore, whether health psychologists can learn anything from health economists; that is, can health psychologists adopt and integrate economic theories and/or methodologies? Reading health psychology books and articles might give the impression that the answer to both questions is negative. Aside from the customary discussion regarding the relationship between health insurance and health status, there has been very little exchange of information and ideas between health economics and health psychology. Even the RAND Health Insurance Experiment is hardly mentioned in health psychology textbooks. Thus, despite the possible effects of price on promoting (positive) and preventing (negative) health behaviors, or on utilization of health services by minority groups (e.g., mammography), health psychologists have failed, for the most part, to integrate health economic thinking and ideas into their theories and experiments. This is surprising because psychologists have long known about the merit of incentives or rewards, dating back at least a century to the early work of the behaviorists' school of thought.

Indeed, the modus operandi in psychology has been to overlook much that has been done in economics.[2] The tides are rapidly changing, however, as a growing number of researchers in both disciplines have come to realize that they share much in common, namely, the desire to understand and (possibly) influence behavior. While the two fields might be driven by different sets of ideas and methodologies, this, we believe, should be taken as a strength rather than a weakness, for each discipline can provide a different piece of the puzzle. In this chapter we would like to bridge the existing gap by introducing to health psychologists the ideas, methodologies, and theories common among health economics. Given the wide range of problems that health economics has tackled, we restrict our discussion to three domains: consumer behavior, health disparity, and the relationship between institutions and health. Our survey is not meant to be exhaustive, but to provide health psychologists with a sense and a flavor of economic approaches and methodologies.

Health Psychology Meets Consumer Research

The Health Psychology Division of the American Psychological Association states that its aims are the "promotion and maintenance of health, . . . the study of psychological, social, emotional, and behavioural factors in physical and mental illness, the improvement of the health care system, and formulation of health policy" (American Psychological Association, 2007). It also mentions that reports by the Surgeon General's Office indicate "that the leading causes of mortality in the U.S. have substantial behavioral components. These reports recommend that behavioral risk factors (e.g., drug and alcohol use, high risk sexual behavior, smoking, diet, a sedentary lifestyle, stress) be the main focus of efforts in the area of health promotion and disease prevention." One of main roles health psychologists can play, therefore, is to promote healthy behavior (e.g., exercising) and prevent unhealthy ones (e.g., smoking). These aims are perfectly sensible because smoking, for example, is the leading cause of preventable death (Harrell, Bangdiwala, Deng, Webb, & Bradely, 1998). Thus, although few would question the merits of promoting healthy behaviors or preventing unhealthy ones, a greater debate exists concerning the best method(s) to achieve these goals; that is, although there is a consensus regarding the potential harms of smoking, drug use, and risky sexual behavior, there is less agreement regarding the best methods

---

[2]To be fair, economists, for the most part, have ignored psychology as well. Our focus in this chapter is to inform health psychologists about economic thinking, not to inform economists about psychological findings.

to (1) prevent individuals from engaging in risky health behaviors, (2) change unhealthy behaviour, and (3) promote healthy behaviors.

In the next section, we illustrate how health economics can aid psychologists to achieve their aims in one of the domains identified by the Surgeon General's Office, namely, smoking.[3] It should be clearly stated that we are not arguing that health economics should replace psychology, or that one discipline offers a better solution to these complex problems. Rather, we suggest that economic thinking and methodology could supplement and enrich methods currently employed by health psychologists. To combine findings and approaches from both fields, we believe, can provide policymakers and practitioners a richer perspective and better tools to battle these serious and important problems.

Smoking Prevention and Cessation Programs

In light of the Surgeon General's recommendations, it is no wonder that smoking has attracted much attention from economists and psychologists. However, the two fields have employed different methodologies to achieve the following goals: (1) reduce the number of people who start to smoke and (2) increase the number of smokers who quit. In what follows, we discuss how economists have used the relationship between price and behavior to suggest ways to reduce the number of people who start to smoke and increase the number of people who quit.

In the United States, smoking prevention programs tend to concentrate on the young. Indeed, many schools across the country have used such programs to increase awareness of the risks of behaviors such as smoking. California alone spent over $400 million from 1989 to 2003 to prevent teenagers from starting to smoke. One of the rationales behind school-based prevention programs is the fact that many risky behaviors emerge during young adulthood. Indeed, over 80% of adult smokers started smoking prior to their

18th birthday (Harrell et al., 1998). However, educators, policymakers, and researchers have faced various hurdles in their attempt to reduce smoking rates and increase quit rates among the young. One of the challenges they encounter is the tendency of the young to underestimate risk, as well as the probability of becoming addicted (Johnston, O'Malley, & Bachman, 2001). To date, many methods have been utilized to combat youth smoking. In addition to school-based programs, the legislative branch, for example, has passed laws prohibiting the sale of tobacco to minors (e.g., the Synar Amendment). How successful have these programs been?

A systematic review by Wiehe, Garrison, Christakis, Ebel, and Rivara (2005; see also Glantz & Mandel, 2005) questioned the merits of school-based prevention programs, and others have had reservations about the value of legislative acts in preventing youth from taking up smoking (but see Sussman, Unger, Rohrbach, & Johnson, 2005). Wiehe and colleagues analyzed randomized controlled trials to evaluate the short- and long-term effects of different school-based prevention programs. While a number of programs produced short-term success, only one of the eight reviewed studies found a significant long-term effect (i.e., a lasting reduction in the number of young smokers). If school-based programs—which are largely grounded on psychological theories, such as the theory of planned behavior (Ajzen, 1991), of triadic influence (Flay & Petraitis, 1994), and social cognitive theory (Bandura, 1997)—have little success in reducing the number of youths who smoke, what other measures might do better?

Price increase seems to be the most successful predictor in smoking prevention and reduction: It decreases the number of youths who report intention to smoke, while increasing the number who intend to quit smoking. In their seminal work, Lewit, Coate, and Grossman (1981) were among the first to examine the relationship between economic factors (price) and youths' smoking. Analyzing a national sample of close to 7,000 youths (12 to 17 years old), they found that adolescents exhibit price elasticity of −1.44. A "price elasticity"—the relationship between price and demand—of −1.44 means that an increase of 10% in cigarette price leads to a 14.4% decrease in the number of smokers. More importantly perhaps, Lewit

---

[3]Due to space limitations, we restrict our discussion to smoking. Similar findings and results, however, have been reported in relation to drug and alcohol abuse (Chaloupka, Grossman, & Saffer, 2002), as well as dieting (Horgen & Brownell, 2002).

and colleagues found that young adults (vs. older adults) are more price sensitive (U.S. Department of Health and Human Services, 1994). In other words, an increase of $1 will, on average, have a greater effect on a young person than on an older one. While some of the Lewit and colleagues findings have been challenged, the general message—that economics and behavior are connected—still stands.

Based on a series of national surveys, Chaloupka and colleagues (2002; Ross & Chaloupka, 2004) analyzed the relationship between price and youths' smoking trends. In one study, Ross and Chaloupka (2003) studied smoking behavior of a nationally representative sample of over 17,000 high school students. Similar to Lewit and colleagues (1981), Ross and Chaloupka (2004) found an inverse relationship between price and consumption: As the price of cigarettes increased, demand for cigarettes declined. In fact, their data show that a small increase of $0.50 per pack in cigarette price could lead to a substantial reduction of about 18% in smoking. Using a sample of over 200 schools (with over 17,000 participants) across the United States, Ross, Powell, Taurus, and Chaloupka (2005) examined the impact of different price increases ($0.50, $1, $2, and $4) on high school students' smoking intentions. Higher prices, as predicted, reduced the number of student who intended to smoke, and the actual number of cigarettes smoked. Higher prices also increased the number of student who planned to quit smoking.

Drawing on data from Canada's National Population Health Survey, Zhang, Cohen, Ferrence, and Rehm (2006) were also interested in exploring the impact of price on smoking behavior. Canada's National Population Health Survey allowed a comparison of 10 different Canadian provinces. Cigarette prices in five provinces were lower (due to greater tax breaks) than those in the remaining five provinces. Zhang and colleagues' data indicate that lower price was significantly associated with higher initiation of smoking (10.5 vs. 8.5%).

Given the robust data on the relationship between price and smoking behavior, Ross and Chaloupka (2003) stated that "the single most consistent conclusion from the economic literature on the demand for cigarettes is that consumers react to price changes according to economic theory principles—an increase in price leads to decrease in consumption" (p. 219). While we agree that an increase in price can reduce consumption, price alone cannot explain why people start smoking, nor can it completely deter young people from starting or continuing to smoke.

This is where psychological research can play a prominent role (see Carvajal, Hanson, Downing, Coyle, & Pederson, 2004). For example, the economic analyses we reported earlier are perfectly aligned with psychological theories, such as the theory of planned behavior (see Kiviniemi & Rothman, Chapter 5, this volume). Although Ross and colleagues (2005) used a quasi-experimental design, their research highlights how psychological theories can inform economists about what motivates behavior, and also how economic principles can motivate psychological experiments. Emery, White, and Pierce's (2001) work reveals further interesting trends for psychologists. Looking at the relationship between cigarettes use and price, the authors found that changes in price had little effect on whether youths experimented with cigarettes. This suggests that other factors, such as peer pressure, might be in play. Sussman and colleagues' (2005; see also Sussman, Sun, & Dent, 2006) cautionary note—arguing against abandonment of school-based cessation programs—should therefore receive serious attention. Indeed, the youth-focused Florida Pilot Program on Tobacco Control (Bauer, Johnson, Hopkins, & Brooks, 2000)—using multilevel approaches to fight youth smoking, none of which included price change—reported promising results: significant reduction in cigarette use and increase in intention not to smoke. Due to lack of funds, however, the program has largely been shut down. Given the complex reasons underlying smoking behavior that affect young people all over the world, bringing together economic and psychological theories might prove to be a very powerful tool in lowering the number of youths who start to smoke and/or reducing the number who already do.

Economics, Psychology, and Health Disparity

The relationship between one's racial and ethnic background, and access to health services, treatments, quality of care, and variation in health outcomes has come under the scrutiny of both health care professionals and policymakers. A reminder of this relationship comes from the state of Mississippi, which, after years of reporting a steady decline in infant mortality, announced that rates among blacks have been going up (Eckholm, 2007). A report published by the Kaiser Family Foundation (KFF; 2007) reveals further disparities between whites' and blacks' health status. Blacks have a much higher rate of infant mortality than whites (in Wisconsin, the rate is 17.5 vs. 5.6 deaths per 1,000 live births, respectively), diabetes-related mortality (in Washington, the rate is 24.5 vs. 71.7 deaths per 100,000 population among whites and blacks, respectively), and annual AIDS case rate (in New York, the rate is 11.1 vs. 131.2 per 100,000 population among whites and blacks, respectively).

While the reasons underlying health disparities are multifaceted, a report to Michael O. Leavitt, then Secretary of the U.S. Department of Health and Human Services, states that "compelling evidence exists that differences in health status, access to care, and the provision of physical and mental health services are significantly related to race, ethnicity, primary language, geography, and various measures of socioeconomic position, such as educational status, income, wealth, and conditions in childhood" (National Committee on Vital and Health Statistic, 2005, p. 8). As the report to Leavitt indicates, socioeconomic factors are among the leading reasons behind heath disparities. It is not surprising, therefore, that the KFF study (2007) found that higher rates of blacks than whites live in poverty (in Iowa, 49.6 vs. 10.2%, respectively), rely on Medicaid (in Rhode Island, 37.3 vs. 12.2%, respectively), and are uninsured (in Louisiana, 27.0 vs. 16.3%, respectively).[4]

One health domain that has garnered much attention has been racial and ethnic disparities in cancer screening, treatment, and outcome. In the United States, over 1 million Americans are diagnosed with can-

cer each year (National Center for Health Statistics, 2006). Not only are many types of cancers are more prevalent among blacks (National Center for Health Statistics, 2006), but a greater percentage of blacks than of any other racial group die of cancer. They have, for example, 12% higher incidence of colorectal cancer than do whites. Mortality rates among blacks, however, are 36% higher than those of white (Ries et al., 2002). In fact, blacks are over 30% more likely than whites to die from cancer (Shavers & Brown, 2002).[5] Why are mortality rates different among various ethnic and racial groups? And how can economic factors aid in explaining this issue, as well as close the health gap?

In their review of the literature, Shavers and Brown (2002) provided a useful model that can help to elucidate racial and ethnic disparities in the receipt of cancer treatment (see also Krieger, 1999). Three general themes are identified as playing a key role in racial and ethnic disparity: (1) patient factors (e.g., socioeconomic), (2) physician/clinical factors (physician recommendation), and (3) structural factors (e.g., type of hospital in which one is treated). Shavers and Brown further subdivide these three main themes into subcategories that include topics such as status of health insurance and type of insurance (under the structural barriers), clinical stage and comorbidity (under the physician barriers), and transportation and family support (under the patient barriers). While not all three factors and their subcategories are relevant for our discussion, the model helps to disentangle the economic and psychological issues. We briefly discuss, below, a few of themes identified by Shavers and Brown.

The National Health Interview Survey (Breen, Wagener, Brown, Davis, & Ballard-Barbash, 2001) conducted in 1987, 1992, and 1998 reveals that rates of breast and cervical cancer screening among blacks, Hispanics, and whites have been closing.

[4]The relationship between economic state and health status among other minority groups is not always straightforward. Infant mortality rates among Hispanics, for example, are closer to those of the white population, while their economic status is closer to that of the black population.

[5]Blacks are not the only minority group to show disproportionate incidence of cancer, yet the gap between whites and blacks is the most pronounced. Hispanics, for example, are more likely than whites or blacks to have cervical cancer, while Asians and Pacific Islanders tend to have a higher rate of stomach cancer.

Unfortunately, similar trends have not been found when we examine survival rates from breast or cervical cancer (for similar trends in cardiovascular disease, see National Center for Health Statistics, 2006). Despite having lower rates of breast cancer (Peek & Han, 2004), blacks are still more likely than whites to die from breast cancer (see Breen et al., 2001, Table 1, p. 1706).

Why do lower cancer rates not translate into lower mortality rates among blacks? One possibility for the discrepancy between low prevalence rates and relatively high mortality rates—a gap that is most pronounced between whites and blacks—is the fact that minority groups are far more likely to be diagnosed with breast cancer at a later stage than their white counterparts (Lantz et al., 2006). Stage of detection, after all, is one of the best predictors for survival rate and cure (Kosary et al., 1995). Therefore, *when* cancer is detected plays a major role is one's prognosis. Stage of detection, however, is not the only factor that contributes to the mortality rate difference between ethnic and racial groups. Aside from early detection, rapid and accurate access to treatment are key ingredients in lowering morbidity and mortality rates. Blacks, unfortunately, fall short on every facet of the process, from late diagnosis to relatively poor access to state-of-the-art treatments.

Access to mammography screening is one of the main methods for early detection of breast cancer, and regular Papanicolaou (Pap) smears are known to help reduce the chance of developing cervical cancer (Kosary et al., 1995). However, despite improvement in black women's rates of mammography screening, white women are still more likely to undergo mammography screening and Pap smears. Elmore and colleagues (2005)—who looked at medical records of 400 women diagnosed with breast cancer between 1985 and 1993, and followed up to 2001, revealed disparities between racial and ethnic groups at a number of important junctures. First, the method of detection varied among the various groups. For example, among white women, breast cancer was more likely to be diagnosed after mammographic screening or clinical breast examination, whereas black women were more likely to be diagnosed after they noticed abnormalities—a method that typically detects cancer at more advance stages. Mammographic screening and clinical breast examination, for example, tend to reveal abnormalities earlier than do self-diagnosis, and are correlated with reduced breast cancer recurrence and mortality. Second, black women experience significantly longer times to complete the entire diagnostic procedure, whether breast abnormalities were self-detected or found via mammographic screening. Finally, white women received treatment in less time than their black counterparts. As in earlier studies (Lannin et al., 1998), Elmore et al. (2005) believe that "being underinsured and/or uninsured and having low income may be risk factors for late-stage diagnosis" (p. 145).

In an earlier study, Roetzheim and colleagues (1999) examined the data of over 28,000 Florida patients diagnosed with one of four types of cancer for which early screening was available (e.g., mammography). Their analysis revealed that patients insured by Medicaid or those who lacked insurance were more likely to be diagnosed with late-stage cancer. Blacks, who were overly represented among those who relied on Medicaid or lacked insurance, were significantly more likely to be diagnosed with late-stage breast cancer. Furthermore, when the authors compared white and black patients on Medicaid or those who lacked insurance, similar results emerged. Blacks received worse cancer diagnoses.

Relying on a different dataset, Friedman and colleagues (2002) demonstrated a relationship between insurance and access to preventive medicine. Looking at over 1 million records of General Motors employees and their families, Friedman and colleagues found that access to cancer screening procedures is dependent on whether one has health insurance, but more importantly, on what kind of health insurance one has (whether it charges for or covers cancer screening procedures). Women, for example, whose insurance covered cancer screening were significantly more likely to undergo mammography screening than those who had to pay for the procedure out of their own pockets. Thus, to answer the question of what determines a woman's likelihood to receive cancer screening, one needs to remember that "low socioeconomic status [SES] is a consistent marker for mammography underuse" (Peek & Han, 2004, p. 185).

Low-income women are deemed to be the furthest away from the goals set by Healthy People 2010 (HP 2010; see *www.healthy-people.gov*). One of the goals of HP 2010 is to have 70% of low-income women undergo mammography screening. As of 2004, the rate of uninsured women who had mammographies was only 50%, while over 70% of insured women had mammographies (Peek & Han, 2004). Moreover, women who have no usual care are less than half as likely to have a mammography, 34.6 vs. 73.0%, than women who have a stable source of medical care (Swan, Breen, Coates, Rimer, & Lee, 2003), and women with higher income are 20% more likely to have a mammogram than low-income women (Blackman, Bennett, & Miller, 1999). Living in rural areas has also been shown to correlate with lower utilization of mammography screening (Coughlin, Thompson, Hall, Logan, & Uhler, 2002). Living in a rural area, it should be noted, typically means longer travel time to the health facilities where women have access to mammography screening. Longer travel time is financially costly for at least two reasons. First, it forces women to lose working hours or days due to travel. Second, travel by itself is costly, whether women use their own or public transportation.

These findings resonate well with Haitt, Klabunde, Breen, Swan, and Ballard-Barbash's (2002) work. After reviewing 73 studies based on the National Health Interview Survey between 1980 and 2001, they concluded that high SES and a usual source of health care and insurance coverage were the strongest predictors of whether a woman would undergo breast and cervical screening. Examining the responses of over 50,000 women enrolled in the Women's Health Initiative Observational Study, Hsia and colleagues (2000) found that having health insurance was the best predictor that a woman would undergo cancer screening. It should be noted that having health insurance has been linked to having a usual source of health care. Perhaps expectedly, therefore, some researchers (e.g., Selvin & Brett, 2003) found that the best predictor of having breast and cervical screening is to have usual access to healthy care. Furthermore, Selvin and Brett (2003) argue that this association is particularly strong among black women, who are more likely to be uninsured, to live in poverty, and to lack usual access to health services.

Another question is what would be the best method to increase screening among minorities and low-income women? Economists suggest that one method to tackle some of these issues is lowering the cost of cancer screening. Even before President Clinton signed into law the Breast and Cervical Cancer Prevention and Treatment Act of 2000 (Public Law 106-354), which provides uninsured and underserved women free access to breast or cervical cancer screening and treatment, the National Breast and Cervical Cancer Early Detection Program has been able to increase the rate of low-income women who undergo cancer screening and receive treatment by simply offering it free of charge (May, Lee, Nadel, Henson, & Miller, 1998). Lowering the costs of screening procedures is one step in reducing health inequities, though it cannot serve as a universal panacea. As studies comparing Canadian and U.S. health care systems have shown, universal coverage does help to reduce health disparities, though it is unable to eliminate them (Lasser, Himmelstein, & Woolhandler, 2006).

Despite the complex web of reasons that contribute to health disparities, understanding factors underlying the phenomenon is the first step toward tackling and solving the problem. While psychologists have traditionally focused on health education and communication between health care professionals and patients, economists have been continuously charting the dynamics between economic factors, such as health insurance status, transportation, and SES, and health status. While economic factors, no doubt, play an important role in maintaining (and even widening) health disparities, it seems that they cannot explain the entire variance. A number of psychological issues still remain elusive and troubling, placing a barrier between ethnic/minority groups and better health.

Economics, Public Programs, and Older Adults' Health

In the previous two sections we illustrated how economists and psychologists approach health concerns—such as smoking and health disparity—by employing different set of tools and methodologies. In this final section we would like to concentrate on a domain that has been dominated almost exclusively by economists—the design of national health programs. We use the new Medicare drug benefit as an illustrative case, although other national programs—such as Medicare Parts A and B and Medicaid—have also been designed largely by economists. We believe that this domain might offer a great opportunity for psychologists to share insights with policymakers and encourage greater emphasis on the relationship between institutional design and health. Despite the impact of various public policies on health (from allocation of scarce resources to promotion of health behaviors), psychologists have contributed relatively little to their design. Given the large scope of this topic, we are able to touch only briefly on the relationship between policy design and health.

We focus our discussion, therefore, on the new Medicare Modernization Act (MMA; also known as Part D), which came into effect in January 2006. The 2003 legislation, according to the Centers for Medicare and Medicaid Services, "provides seniors and individuals with disabilities with a prescription drug benefit, more choices, and better benefits under Medicare" (see *www.cms. hhs.gov/mmaupdate*). The MMA is one of the biggest health policy changes to take place since the birth of Medicare and Medicaid in the mid-1960s. However, from its inception, Medicare Part D has drawn much criticism. While some of it is irrelevant for our current discussion, two points in particular do concern us: (1) the large number of plans available to beneficiaries (Hanoch & Rice, 2006), and (2) the amount of information and presentation formats used to educate consumers.

We believe that psychologists could have played a more prominent role in the design of the program by contributing their extensive knowledge of older adults' decision-making styles and cognitive abilities. They could have also formed closer ties with policymakers because some of the concerns about the program are psychological rather than economical in nature. It is possible that more active involvement of psychologists could have averted some of the problems with the design of the program.

Given the evidence on older adults' cognitive and decision-making capacities, one might wonder about the rationale behind the design of the Medicare program. Not only must older adults face extremely complex information, they need to do so in an environment that contains over 50 different plans. The current design of Medicare Part D can be attributed, in part, to economists' belief that more choices are better than fewer choices. A number of assumptions are implicit in the idea that more choices are useful rather than harmful to individuals: (1) People possess enough information about the alternatives available to them; (2) they have the cognitive ability to evaluate the various options available and to choose the one that will maximize the plan's utility; (3) consumers will not regret the options not chosen; (4) they do not think (too much) about what other individuals possess; and (5) market competition does not lead to excessive waste. Following the dictates of rational choice theory, the U.S. health care system has always championed choice, as is apparent in the plenitude of health insurers, hospitals, and specialists. The design of the Medicare drug benefit can be seen as a natural extension of this line of thought. The legislative branch, after all, could have designed the program in many different ways. However, it decided to adhere to traditional economic thinking—let too many firms compete in the market.

Psychologists have long been aware of, and interested in, people's cognitive limitations. Starting with the pioneering work of Herbert Simon in the late 1940s (1947, 1955), the idea that people's rationality is bounded has been largely supported by a range of experiments and findings (for reviews, see Conlisk, 1996; Kahneman, 2003; Rabin, 1998). Simon's notion of bounded rationality was a reaction to rational choice theory—one of the pillars of economic theory. Rational choice theory, Simon argued, ignores how real people behave and make decisions. In addition, Simon (1956) was interested in the relationship between environmental properties and cognitive architecture. One of his great insights was to show that how an environment is constructed—for example, whether it is rich or poor in information—has a direct influence on an agent's cognitive capacities and, more remarkably, on its cognitive architecture. To the best of our knowledge, most health economists and health psychologists have been oblivious to Simon's work and the need to study how environmental structures (e.g., institutions) affect people's health and access to health services. (To be fair, economists and psychologists have been interested in how certain environmental factors, such as living in an urban or rural area, affect health.)

An area that has garnered much attention is the relationship between old age and executive functioning; that is, while young people show some cognitive limitations, these cognitive abilities tend to decline even further with age. A growing corpus of data, for example, has shown an inverse relationship between age and decision-making abilities (for a review, see Thornton & Dumke, 2005). Researchers (e.g., MacPherson, Phillips, & Della-Sala, 2002) have demonstrated that an increase in age is related to lower scores on executive function tests, working memory functioning, dual tasking (Korteling, 1991), and even routine daily tasks, such as remembering bus schedules or navigating menus. Researchers (e.g., Beisecker, 1988) have argued that even in important areas related to their own health, older adults tend to be less engaged and involved in making decisions, to encounter more difficulties recalling medically related information (Brown & Park, 2002) and treatment recommendations (Meyer, Russo, & Talbot, 1995), and generally to score lower on comprehension tests (Morrell, Park, & Poon, 1989). In a series of studies, Johnson (1990, 1993), found that older (vs. younger) adults tend to examine less information before choosing to rent an apartment, to require more time to process information, to use less information, and to reevaluate information more frequently when making a hypothetical car purchase decision.

Older adults face other obstacles in making health-related decisions. Many have poor reading or mathematical abilities. These skills, however, are necessary to comprehend fully the intricacies of insurance plans or treatment options (Hibbard, Jewett, Engelmann, & Tusler, 1998). For example, a study by Finucane and colleagues (2002) examined older and younger adults' decision-making capacities by measuring their comprehension of health plan information. Older adults' scores (compared to those of younger adults) were much lower on a number of tasks that required the use of tables or graphs.

While thinking about the merits of having a wide range of choices (e.g., it leads to market efficiency), economists, for the most part, have failed to consider the psychological price that choice might carry (see Schwartz, 2004). Indeed, policymakers have neglected, for the most part, to investigate what Medicare beneficiaries think about its intended structure. Would they prefer to encounter more or less choice? And, more importantly, does more choice hamper older adults' ability to make decisions? Economists might be surprised by the answers.

Recent psychological work has challenged the idea that having more choice is necessarily better. Schwartz (2004) suggested, in contrast to what many economists think, that having more choices does not necessarily lead to greater satisfaction. He found that "aspiration to self-determination, presumably through processes resembling those of rational choice, is a mistake, both as an empirical description of how people act and as a normative ideal" (Schwartz, 2000, p. 80). Earlier studies by Beattie, Baron, Hershey, and Spranca (1994) demonstrated that when faced with difficult medical decisions, people prefer to transfer the decision to their health caretaker rather than make the decision on their own.

Further support for the idea that more choice does not necessarily translates into better decisions emerges from the work of Iyengar and Lepper (2000). In a number of experiments, they showed that facing a large (vs. small) choice set (6 vs. 24 choices of chocolate, exams, or jams) can have negative effects on the decision maker. For example, those who faced greater choice size reported lower satisfaction with their decisions, an increased sense of regret over their choices, as well as a greater likelihood of avoidance of making a decision. In another study, Iyengar and Jiang (2005) demonstrated that having a larger array of investment options can discourage consumers from investing their money wisely. Iyengar and colleagues' studies follow earlier research by Shafir, Simonson, and Tversky (1993; see also Tversky & Shafir, 1992), which suggests that one of the main sources of decision conflict comes from consumers being faced with competing options and feel incapable of weighing the trade-offs of one option attribute against another, when no dominate alternative exists.

The ideas developed by Simon on older adults' cognitive capacities and research into the harmful effects of too much choice should have influenced policymakers. As is evident from the design of the new Medicare Part D, policymakers have largely been unaware of this body of work and have relied almost exclusively on traditional economic thinking. Why did they fail to incorporate psychological findings? As we indicated earlier, old age is associated with decline in cognitive capabilities. Furthermore, recent research has shown that increasing the number of available choices also raises the demands on the cognitive system while reducing satisfaction levels. Nonetheless, instead of constructing a program that beneficiaries could easily navigate and understand, policymakers opted for a complex program. Indeed, the KFF's (2006) National Survey of Physicians and National Survey of Pharmacists found that doctors, pharmacists, and older adults alike deemed the program too complicated to understand. Their surveys also found that many pharmacists believe that many Medicare beneficiaries do not comprehend the new program well, if at all.

That most seniors think the new Medicare drug benefit is too complicated would not surprise many psychologists. Had they been consulted at an early stage of the program's development, they would have been in the position to alert policymakers to the possible obstacles that older adults might encounter in such a complex program. In addition, psychologists could have suggested decision-making aids to help older adults better understand the nature of the program, as well as contributed to the development of the various websites to help beneficiaries make informed decisions. For example, much of the information older adults encounter—whether in print or over the Internet—is far from ideal. Many websites, including the official site of the Centers for Medicare and Medicaid Services, which administers the program, are written in too small a font. It seems to us that the structure of the environment and how information is provided are precisely the areas in which psychologists could have contributed to make the program both more cognitively accessible and better formulated to meet the needs of older adults.

Conclusions

A survey by the KFF/Harvard School of Public Health (2007) found that one of the top issues in the 2006 congressional election was the public concern about health care. When asked what they would like the 2008 presidential candidates to talk about, 20% of the participants mentioned health care issues, with insurance as one of the main sub-themes. On May 30, 2007, Senator Barack Obama unveiled his health care policy, declaring that he would make health coverage accessible to all, as well as reduce its costs (Toner, 2007). Whether President Obama will be able to implement a new health policy program remains to be seen; however, to do so would mark one of the most profound shifts in the history of the U.S. health care system. While we would not like to prophesy what will take place, it is clear that health economists should play a crucial role in its design and implementations. Indeed, three of Obama's top advisors are economists, while not a single psychologist (to our knowledge) has been involved in the health policy design. Yet economists and psychologists share a common interest and goal—to promote healthy behavior and reduce unhealthy behavior. How economists and psychologists approach these important problems—reducing smoking prevalence, increasing access to screening procedures, or designing institutions—is, however, fundamentally different. As we have argued throughout the chapter, both disciplines have much to contribute because neither field holds the panacea to solve the complex, myriad problems that prevail within the health care system. While access to health care does improve the chances that a woman would have mammography screening, and increasing cigarettes prices does reduce smoking prevalence, neither factor—as some economists might like to believe—is sufficient to solve the problem. At the same time, it would be wise for health psychologists to learn the tools of the trade that economists have been using, if they are ever interested in influencing policymakers and helping to design health-related institutions—as in the case of Medicare Part D.

Acknowledgment

Parts of this chapter previously appeared in Hanoch, Y., & Gummerum, M. (2008). What can health psychologists learn from health economics?: From monetary incentives to health policy programs. *Health Psychology Review, 2*, 2–19. Copyright 2008 by the European Health Psychology Society. Reprinted with permission from Taylor & Francis (*www.informaworld.com*).

Further Reading

Friedman, C., Ahmed, F., Franks, A., Weatherup, T., Manning, M., Vance, A., et al. (2002). Association between health insurance coverage of office visit and cancer screening among women. *Medical Care, 40*, 1060–1067.

Horgen, K. B., & Brownell, K. D. (2002). Comparison of price change and health message interventions in promoting healthy food choice. *Health Psychology, 21*, 505–512.

Marteau, T. M., Ashcroft, R. E., & Oliver, A. (2009). Using financial incentives to achieve healthy behaviour. *British Medical Journal, 338*, 983–985.

Rice, T. (2003). *The economics of health reconsidered* (2nd ed.). Chicago: Health Administration Press.

Ross, H., & Chaloupka, F. J. (2004). The effect of public policies and prices on youth smoking. *Southern Economic Journal, 70*, 796–815.

Volpp, K. G., John, L. K., Troxel, A. B., Norton, L., Fassbender, J., & Loewenstein, G. (2008). Financial incentive-based approaches for weight loss: A randomized trial. *Journal of the American Medical Association, 300*, 2631–2637.

References

Ajzen, I. (1991). The theory of planned behaviour. *Organizational Behavior and Human Decision Process, 50*, 179–211.

American Psychological Association, Health Psychology, Division 38. (2007). *Mission statement.* Retrieved May 5, 2007, from *www.health-psych.org/mission.php.*

Bandura, A. (1997). *The exercise of control.* New York: Freeman.

Bauer, U. E., Johnson, T. M., Hopkins, R. S., & Brooks, R. G. (2000). Changes in youth cigarettes use and intention following implementation of a tobacco control program: Findings from the Florida Youth Tobacco survey, 1999–2000. *Journal of the American Medical Association, 284*, 723–728.

Beattie, J. J., Baron, J., Hershey, J. C., & Spranca, M. (1994). Determinants of decision attitude. *Journal of Behavioral Decision Making, 7*, 129–144.

Beisecker, A. E. (1988). Aging and the desire for information and input in medical decisions: Patient consumerism in medical encounter. *Gerontologist, 28*, 330–335.

Blackman, D. K., Bennett, E. M., & Miller, D. S. (1999). Trends in self-reported use of mammograms (1989–97) and Papanicolaou tests (1991–97—Behavioral Risk Factors Surveillance System. *Morbidity and Mortality Weekly Report, 48*, 1–22.

Breen, N., Wagener, D. K., Brown, M. L., Davis, W. W., & Ballard-Barbash, R. (2001). Progress in cancer screening over a decade: Results of cancer screening from 1987, 1992, and 1998 National Health Interview Survey. *Journal of the National Cancer Institute, 93*, 1704–1713.

Brown, S. C., & Park, D. C. (2002). Roles of age and familiarity in learning health information. *Educational Gerontology, 28*, 695–710.

Carvajal, S. C., Hanson, C., Downing, R. A., Coyle, K. K., & Pederson, L. L. (2004). Theory-based determinants of youth smoking: A multiple influence approach. *Journal of Applied Social Psychology, 34*, 59–84.

Chaloupka, F. J., Grossman, M., & Saffer, H. (2002). The effects of price on alcohol consumption and alcohol-related problems. *Alcohol Research and Health, 26*, 22–34.

Conlisk, J. (1996). Why bounded rationality? *Journal of Economic Literature, 34*, 669–700.

Coughlin, S. S., Thompson, T. D., Hall, H. I., Logan, P., & Uhler, R. J. (2002). Breast and cervical carcinoma screening practices among women in rural and nonrural areas of the United States. *Cancer, 94*, 2801–2812.

Eckholm, E. (2007). In turnabout, infant deaths climb in South. *New York Times.* Retrieved April 22, 2007, from *www.nytimes.com/2007/04/22/health/22infant.html?ex=1180584000&en=5b29704d014b531b&ei=5070.*

Elmore, J. G., Nakano, C. Y., Linden, H. M., Reisch, L. M., Ayanian, J. Z., & Larson, E. B. (2005). Racial inequities in the timing of breast cancer detection, diagnosis, and initiation of treatment. *Medical Care, 43*, 141–148.

Emery, S., White, M. M., & Pierce, J. P. (2001). Does cigarette price influence adolescent experimentation? *Journal of Health Economics, 20*, 261–270.

Finucane, M. L., Slovic, P., Hibbard, J. D., Peters, E., Mertz, C. K., & Macgregor, D. G. (2002). Aging and decision-making competence: An analysis of comprehension and consistency skills in older versus younger adults considering health-plan options. *Journal of Behavioral Decision Making, 15*, 141–164.

Flay, B. R., & Petraitis, J. (1994). The theory of triadic influence: A new theory of health behaviour with implications for preventive interventions. In G. L. Albrecht (Ed.), *Advances in medical sociology* (Vol. IV, pp. 19–44). Greenwich, CT: JAI Pres.

Frieden, T. R., Mostashari, F., Kerker, B. D., Miller, N., Hajat, A., & Frankel, M. (2005). Adult tobacco use levels after intensive tobacco control measures: New York City, 2002–2003. *American Journal of Public Health, 95,* 1016–1023.

Friedman, C., Ahmed, F., Franks, A., Weatherup, T., Manning, M., Vance, A., et al. (2002). Association between health insurance coverage of office visit and cancer screening among women. *Medical Care, 40,* 1060–1067.

Glantz, S. A., & Mandel, L. L. (2005). Since school-based smoking prevention programs do not work, what should we do? *Journal of Adolescent Health, 36,* 157–159.

Haitt, R. A., Klabunde, K., Breen, N., Swan, J., & Ballard-Barbash, R. (2002). Cancer screening practices from National Health Interview Surveys: Past, present, and future. *Journal of the National Cancer Institute, 94,* 1837–1846.

Hanoch, Y., & Rice, T. (2006). Can limiting choice increase social welfare?: The elderly and health insurance choice. *Milbank Quarterly, 84,* 37–73.

Harrell, J. S., Bangdiwala, S. I., Deng, S., Webb, J. P., & Bradely, C. (1998). Smoking initiation in youth: The role of gender, race, socioeconomics, and developmental status. *Journal of Adolescent Health, 23,* 271–279.

Hibbard, J. H., Jewett, J. J., Engelmann, S., & Tusler, M. (1998). Can Medicare beneficiaries make informed choices? *Health Affairs, 17,* 181–193.

Horgen, K. B., & Brownell, K. D. (2002). Comparison of price change and health message interventions in promoting healthy food choice. *Health Psychology, 21,* 505–512.

Hsia, J., Kemper, E., Kiefe, C., Zapka, J., Sofaer, S., Pettinger, M., et al. (2000). The importance of health insurance as a determinant of cancer screening: Evidence from women's health initiative. *Preventive Medicine, 31,* 261–270.

Iyengar, S. S., & Jiang, W. (2005). *The psychological costs of ever increasing choice: A fallback to the sure bet.* Manuscript submitted for publication.

Iyengar, S. S., & Lepper, M. R. (2000). When choice is demotivating: Can one desire too much of a good thing? *Journal of Personality and Social Psychology, 79,* 995–1006.

Johnson, M. M. S. (1990). Age differences in decision making: A process methodology for examining strategic information processing. *Journal of Gerontology, 45,* P75–P78.

Johnson, M. M. S. (1993). Thinking about strategies during, before, and after making a decision. *Psychology and Aging, 8,* 231–241.

Johnston, L. D., O'Malley, P. M., & Bachman, J. D. (2001). *Monitoring the future: National survey results on drug use, 1975–2000: Vol. I. Secondary school students.* Bethesda, MD: National Institute on Drug Abuse.

Kahneman, D. (2003). Maps of bounded rationality: Psychology for behavioral economics. *American Economic Review, 93,* 1449–1475.

Kaiser Family Foundation. (2006). *National Survey of Pharmacists and National Survey of Physician.* Retrieved April 10, 2007, from *www.kff.org/kaiserpolls/upload/7556.pdf.*

Kaiser Family Foundation. (2007). *Key health and health care indicators by race/ethnicity and state.* Retrieved May 4, 2007, from *www.kff.org/minorityhealth/upload/7633.pdf.*

Kaiser Family Foundation/Harvard School of Public Health. (2007). *The public's health care agenda for the new congress and presidential campaign.* Retrieved February 8, 2007, from *www.kff.org/kaiserpolls/upload/7597.pdf.*

Korteling, J. E. (1991). Effects of skill integration and perceptual competition on age-related differences in dual-task performance. *Human Factors, 33,* 35–44. ·

Kosary, C. L., Reis, L. A. G., Miller, B. A., Hankey, B. F., Harras, A., & Edwards, B. K. (Eds.). (1995). *SEER Cancer Statistics Review, 1973–1992: Tables and graphs* (NIH Publication No. 96-2789). Bethesda, MD: National Institutes of Health.

Krieger, N. (1999). Embodying inequality: A review of concepts, measures, and methods for studying health consequences of discrimination. *International Journal of Health Services, 29,* 295–352.

Lannin, D. R., Matthews, H. F., Mitchell, J., Swanson, M., Swanson, F., & Edwards, M. (1998). The influence of race, socioeconomic factors, and cultural factors on breast cancer stage in the rural southern United States. *Journal of the American Medical Association, 279,* 1801–1807.

Lantz, P. M., Mujahid, M., Schwartz, K., Janz, N. K., Fagerlin, A., Salem, B., et al. (2006). The influence of race, ethnicity, and individual socioeconomic factors on breast cancer stage of detection. *American Journal of Public Health, 96,* 2173–2178.

Lasser, K. E., Himmelstein, D. U., & Woolhandler, S. (2006). Access to care, health status, and health disparities in the United States and Canada: Results of a cross-national population-based survey. *American Journal of Public Health, 96,* 1300–1307.

Lewit, E. M., Coate, D., & Grossman, M. (1981). The effects of government regulation on teenage smoking. *Journal of Law and Economics, 24,* 545–569.

MacPherson, S. E., Phillips, L. H., & Della-Sala, S. (2002). Age, executive function, and social decision making: A dorsolateral prefrontal theory of cognitive aging. *Psychology and Aging, 17,* 598–609.

May, D. S., Lee, N. C., Nadel, M. R., Henson, R. M., & Miller, D. S. (1998). The National Breast and Cervical Cancer Early Detection Program: Report on the first 4 years of mammography provided to medically underserved women. *American Journal of Roentegenology, 170,* 97–104.

Meyer, B. J. F., Russo, C., & Talbot, A. (1995). Discourse comprehension and problem solving: Decisions about the treatment of breast cancer by women across the life span. *Psychology and Aging, 10,* 84–103.

Morrell, R. W., Park, D. C., & Poon, L. W. (1989). Quality of instructions on prescription drug labels: Effects on memory and comprehension in young and old adults. *Gerontologist, 29,* 345–354.

National Center for Health Statistics. (2006). Health, United States, 2006. Retrieved May 30, 2007, from *www.cdc.gov/nchs/data/hus/hus06.pdf.*

National Committee on Vital and Health Statistics. (2005). *Eliminating health disparities: Strengthening data on race, ethnicity, language in the U.S.* Retrieved May 15, 2007, from *www.ncvhs.hhs.gov/051107rpt.pdf.*

Peek, M. E., & Han, J. H. (2004). Disparities in screening mammography: Current status, interventions, and implications. *Journal of General Internal Medicine, 19,* 184–194.

Rabin, M. (1998). Psychology and economics. *Journal of Economic Literature, 36,* 11–46.

Rice, T. (2003). *The economics of health reconsidered* (2nd ed.). Chicago: Health Administration Press.

Ries, L. A. G., Eisner, P., Kosary, C. L., Hankey, B. F., Miller, B. A., Clegg, L., et al. (2002). *SEER Cancer Statistics Review, 1973–1999.* Bethesda, MD: National Cancer Institute. Retrieved from *seer.cancer.gov/csr/1973-1999.*

Roetzheim, R. G., Pal, N., Tennat, C., Voti, L., Ayanian, J. Z., Schawbe, A., et al. (1999). Effects of health insurance and race on early detection of cancer. *Journal of the National Cancer Institute, 91,* 1409–1415.

Ross, H., & Chaloupka, F. J. (2003). The effect of cigarette prices on youth smoking. *Health Economics, 12,* 217–230.

Ross, H., & Chaloupka, F. J. (2004). The effect of public policies and prices on youth smoking. *Southern Economic Journal, 70,* 796–815.

Ross, H., Powell, L. M., Taurus, J. A., & Chaloupka, F. J. (2005). New evidence on youth smoking behaviour based on experimental price increase. *Contemporary Economic Policy, 23,* 195–210.

Schwartz, B. (2000). Self-determination: The tyranny of freedom. *American Psychologist, 55,* 79–88.

Schwartz, B. (2004). *The paradox of choice: Why more is less.* New York: HarperCollins.

Selvin, E., & Brett, K. M. (2003). Breast and cervical cancer screening: Sociodemographic predictors among white, black, and Hispanic women. *American Journal of Public Health, 93,* 618–623.

Shafir, E., Simonson, I., & Tversky, A. (1993). Reasoned-based choice. *Cognition, 49,* 11–36.

Shavers, V. C., & Brown, M. L. (2002). Racial and ethnic disparities in the receipt of cancer treatment. *Journal of the National Cancer Institute, 94,* 334–357.

Simon, H. A. (1947). *Administrative behavior.* New York: Macmillan.

Simon, H. A. (1955). A behavioral model of rational choice. *Quarterly Journal of Economics, 69,* 99–118.

Simon, H. A. (1956). Rational choice, and the structure of the environment. *Psychological Review, 63,* 129–138.

Sussman, S., Sun, P., & Dent, C. W. (2006). A meta-analysis of teen cigarettes smoking cessation. *Health Psychology, 25,* 549–557.

Sussman, S., Unger, J., Rohrbach, L. A., & Johnson, A. C. (2005). School-based smoking prevention research. *Journal of Adolescent Health, 37,* 4.

Swan, J., Breen, N., Coates, R. J., Rimer, B. K., & Lee, N. C. (2003). Progress in cancer screening practices in the United States: Results from the 2000 National Health Interview Survey. *Cancer, 97,* 1528–1540.

Thornton, W. J. L., & Dumke, H. A. (2005). Age differences in everyday problem-solving and decision-making effectiveness: A meta-analytic review. *Psychology and Aging, 20,* 85–99.

Toner, R. (2007). Obama calls for wider and less costly health care coverage. *New York Times.* Retrieved May 30, 2007, from *www.nytimes.com/2007/05/30/us/politics/30obama.html?ref=health.*

Tversky, A., & Shafir, E. (1992). Choice under conflict: The dynamics of deferred decision. *Psychological Science, 3,* 358–361.

U.S. Department of Health and Human Services. (1994). *Preventing tobacco use among yang people. A report of the Surgeon General.* Atlanta, GA: Centers for Disease Control, Office on Smoking and Health.

Wiehe, S. E., Garrison, M. M., Christakis, D. A., Ebel, B. E., & Rivara, F. P. (2005). A systematic review of school-based smoking prevention trials with long-term follow-up. *Journal of Adolescent Health, 36,* 162–169.

Zhang, B., Cohen, J., Ferrence, R., & Rehm, J. (2006). The impact of tobacco tax cuts on smoking initiation among Canadian young adults. *American Journal of Preventive Medicine, 30,* 474–479.

CHAPTER 20

The Evidence-Based Movement in Health Psychology

Maya Rom Korin
Robert M. Kaplan
Karina W. Davidson

Improving the quality of health care requires systematic reviews of evidence. Evidence-based advances in health psychology, the foci of this chapter, help us understand how biology, behavior, and social context can improve health and illness. Health psychology is practiced by a diverse group of professionals that includes not only psychologists but also nurses, physicians, physical therapists, occupational therapists, social workers, and nutritionists. Still, the dissemination of health psychology practices with evidence to support their use is not yet efficient or routine (e.g., Committee on Quality Health Care in America, 2001; Kerner, Guirguis-Blake, et al., 2005; Kerner, Rimer, & Emmons, 2005). Whereas paths have been forged to move other sciences quickly into medical practice (e.g., Mosca et al., 2005), health psychology scientists and practitioners still struggle to implement research findings, and clinicians do not always benefit from advances in research (e.g., Addis & Hatgis, 2000; Montgomery & Ayllon, 1995; Sogg, Read, Bollinger, & Berger, 2001; Spring et al., 2005). In this chapter, we review evidence-based principles, particularly as they originated in medicine, and provide a brief historical overview of evidence-based medicine (EBM). We then provide stages that are typically encountered as an assessment or intervention practice moves to standard of care, and conclude with an example from preventive cardiology, to illustrate the advantages of EBM principles and practices.

What Is Evidence-Based Medicine?

The evidence-based movement or process is defined as

the conscientious, explicit, and judicious use of current best evidence in making decisions about the care of individual patients. The practice of evidence-based medicine means integrating individual clinical expertise with the best available external clinical evidence from systematic research. By individual clinical expertise we mean the proficiency and judgment that individual clinicians acquire through clinical experience and clinical practice. Increased expertise is reflected in many ways, but especially in more effective and efficient diagnosis and in the more thoughtful identification and compassionate use of individual patients' predicaments, rights, and preferences in making clinical decisions about their care. By best available external clinical evidence we mean clinically relevant research, often from the basic sciences of medicine, but especially from patient centered clinical research. . . . (Sackett, Rosenberg, Gray, Haynes, & Richardson, 1996, p. 71)

EBM emphasizes scientific evidence rather than expert opinion alone as a basis for clinical practice. By providing a coherent scientific approach to clinical decision making, clinicians are equipped to choose how to care for a patient with a greater degree of confidence that their interventions will produce greater benefit and less harm.

The first requirement of evidence-based practice is the systematic accumulation of evidence on many aspects or perspectives of a public health problem. This accumulated information, commonly known as the "evidence base," is then paired with an evidence-based process that usually involves input from practitioners and evaluation by regulatory bureaus, policymakers, and reimbursement agencies. This process leads to the creation of clinical standards of care, reimbursement for certain practices, and improved outcomes for clients, patients, or other targets. The evidence-based movement is mindful and respectful of the professional acuity of practitioners, since they evaluate the relevance of the evidence to the client who requires care.

Practitioners need to make difficult decisions about treatment types, duration, and intensity, often without any practical research guidance or information about what helps or what harms. The evidence-based movement aids practitioners by providing systematic tools to draw inferences from data that are relevant to individual practice in ways that were not possible before such an approach existed.

History of Evidence-Based Medicine

Although references to EBM can be traced back to biblical times (Claridge & Fabian, 2005), it was only in the 1970s that the evidence-based movement in its current form was developed. Medicine at that time focused on the clinical aspect of patient management. While basic science provided the foundation for medical practice, there was no formal iterative process that addressed the application of new scientific advances to clinical decision making (Daly, 2005).

To address this gap, a group of clinical epidemiologists at McMaster University published a series of articles on how to read clinical journals in the *Canadian Medical Association Journal*. They coined the term "clinical appraisal" to describe the application of basic rules of evaluating evidence. Yet the researchers, led by David Sackett, encountered barriers in motivating clinicians not only to browse the journals but also actually apply the information to their daily practice. To this end, McMaster developed a residency program that would be fundamentally different philosophically from the other residency programs. The program taught that each clinical decision would be supported by medical expertise and findings from the scientific literature. Gordon Guyatt, the residency director, termed the new medical philosophy "evidence-based medicine" (Guyatt & Rennie, 2002).

Meanwhile, in the United Kingdom, Archie Cochrane published his classic text *Effectiveness and Efficiency: Random Reflections on Health Services* in 1972. This, too, had a profound influence on reshaping medical philosophy, setting out the importance of randomized controlled trials for evaluating treatments. Cochrane's work led to setting up the Cochrane Center, now known as the Cochrane Collaboration, a worldwide project designed to collect, evaluate, and synthesize randomized control trials from all areas of medicine and to disseminate the findings (Claridge & Fabian, 2005).

In 1993, the *Journal of the American Medical Association* (JAMA) began publishing a 25-part series called "Users' Guide to the Medical Literature," which sought to provide clinicians with "strategies and tools to interpret and integrate evidence form published research in their care of patients" (Guyatt et al., 2000, p. 1291). These articles provided the basis for the shift from a medical paradigm that relied on clinical intuition and experience to one based on a formal set of rules that worked with medical training to understand and integrate clinical research.

Currently, the influence of EBM can be found throughout medicine, as well as the lay media. The Internet has aided in locating and accessing original scientific findings, making it easier for practitioners to gather evidence and make informed clinical decisions. The massive undertaking of the National Library of Medicine to develop and maintain a digital archive on the PubMed database is emblematic of the shift toward EBM. Additionally, systematic reviews are gaining momentum, integrating all the best available evidence to address a particular clinical problem.

Principles of Evidence-Based Medicine

While evidence is essential in making informed clinical decisions, it is never enough without trained, expert clinical judgment. Clinical expertise is essential for identifying and integrating the best research evidence with clinical data (e.g., information about the patient obtained over the course of assessment) in the context of the patient's characteristics and preferences to deliver services that have the highest probability of achieving the goals of treatment. Clinical expertise encompasses a number of competencies that promote positive therapeutic outcomes. As the American Psychological Association (2006) outlines, these include (1) assessment, diagnostic judgment, systematic case formulation, and treatment planning; (2) clinical decision making, treatment implementation, and monitoring of patient progress; (3) interpersonal expertise; (4) continual self-reflection and acquisition of skills; (5) appropriate evaluation and use of research evidence in both basic and applied psychological science; (6) understanding the influence of individual and cultural differences on treatment; (7) seeking available resources (e.g., consultation, adjunctive or alternative services) as needed; and (8) having a cogent rationale for clinical strategies. This expertise develops from not only clinical and scientific training but also an understanding of theory and knowledge of research, as well as the ability to self-reflect and engage in continuing professional education and training. It is manifested in all clinical activities and includes but is not limited to forming therapeutic alliances; assessing patients and developing systematic case formulations, planning treatment, and setting goals; selecting and applying interventions skillfully; monitoring

patient progress and adjusting practices accordingly; attending to patients' individual, social, and cultural contexts; and seeking available resources as needed (e.g., consultation, adjunctive or alternative services).

Thus, evidence by itself is not sufficient without an understanding one's own skills, heuristics, and biases, as well as an understanding of the patient being treated. Understanding and weighing available options for patients, and taking into consideration their relative benefits, harms, costs, and barriers is critical in clinical decision making. Evidence can aid in clinical judgment but is neither enough to replace it nor to guarantee proper treatment observance by the physician or the patient (Hamer, 1999).

There is another side to this argument. Clinical psychology is a very individualized art, and it is appealing to use the nature of the practice to dismiss the justification for evidence-based health care. The basis for evidence-based health care should not be so easily disregarded. For example, psychodynamic approaches to therapy dominated clinical practice for many years. It was not until experimental trials entered the literature that new approaches, such as cognitive-behavioral therapy, gained a foothold. Clinicians in all areas of health care are being forced to justify their practice with sound scientific data, and psychologists should be no different. The available evidence supports the value of some, but not all, behavioral intervention practices. Perhaps most importantly, by ignoring calls for evidence, rather than clinical opinion, to justify practice, psychologists may risk being excluded from decisions about reimbursement.

Hierarchy of Evidence

Because a sizable amount of scientific evidence derives from various research designs and methodologies, the *JAMA* working group on EBM (Guyatt et al., 2000) suggested a hierarchy of evidence to address the limitations of unsystematic clinical observations and physiological rationale. The hierarchy is based on minimizing bias and guarding against misleading results when interpreting treatment efficacy and clinical utility, as is shown in Table 20.1. Additionally, the American Psychological Associa-

TABLE 20.1. A Hierarchy of Strength of Evidence for Treatment Decisions

- Systematic reviews of randomized trials.
- Single randomized trial.
- Systematic review of observational studies addressing patient-important outcomes.
- Physiological studies (blood pressure, cardiac output, exercise capacity, bone density, etc.).
- Unsystematic clinical observations.

Note. From Guyatt et al. (2000). Copyright 2000 by the American Medical Association. Reprinted by permission. All rights reserved.

tion ranked intervention research in ascending order for its contribution to conclusions about efficacy: "clinical opinion, observation, and consensus among recognized experts representing the range of use in the field" (Criterion 2.1); "systematized clinical observation" (Criterion 2.2); and "sophisticated empirical methodologies, including quasi - experiments and randomized controlled experiments or their logical equivalents" (Criterion 2.3; American Psychological Association, 2002, p. 1054). Yet these hierarchies are meant to serve as guidelines and are not absolute. To practice EBM, it is important to know how rigorous the process was in which the evidence was collected on the health psychology practice under question, and how feasible is the intervention in the situation in which it is to be offered.

Significant Impact of Evidence-Based Medicine: The Case of Cardiovascular Disease Prevention in Women

We review an example of progress (and setbacks) from medicine to elucidate the process likely to be encountered when EBM principles are practiced in health psychology. Specifically, we review the history of the creation of evidence-based guidelines for cardiologists and illustrate an evidence-informed practice that has irrefutably benefited patients.

Defining the Problem

In 1999, a group of researchers led by Dr. Lori Mosca realized that women were receiving subpar care in cardiovascular disease (CVD) prevention. A 1998 Centers for Disease Control and Prevention (CDC) study of over 29,000 office visits indicated that women were counseled less often than men about exercise, diet, and weight reduction. Additionally, women were not being enrolled at the same rate as men in cardiac rehabilitation after an acute myocardial infarction (MI) or bypass surgery. Evidence emerged that women had several more severe levels of risk factors than did men, such as higher presence of diabetes and lower levels of high-density lipoprotein (HDL) cholesterol, yet they were being treated less aggressively than men. And although coronary heart disease (CHD) causes more than 250,000 deaths in women each year, much of the CHD research in the last 20 years has either excluded women or included very few women. As a result, many of the tests and therapies to treat women for CHD were based on studies conducted predominantly in men. It became increasingly clear that clinicians needed a set of evidence-based guidelines for preventive cardiology for women.

Gathering Evidence

The leadership of the American Heart Association nominated experts in each scientific council with particular knowledge on women and CVD prevention. Other members were appointed to fill in gaps of expertise, and other organizations with similar mission statements were recruited to serve as cosponsors and to nominate representatives for the expert panel. The expert panel reviewed and decided upon a set of timely topics for further systematic literature review.

The first part of gathering evidence was to decide on inclusion and exclusion criteria. Because the goal of the evidence-based clinical guidelines was to provide recommendations on prevention strategies, the panel selected studies that focused on interventions rather than on the etiology of CVD. The expert panel only included randomized clinical trials or large prospective cohort studies with more than 1,000 subjects, as well as meta-analyses.

The panel utilized the Duke Center for Clinical Health Policy Research to conduct the systematic search, in which search terms were expanded to include related articles on Ovid, MEDLINE, Cumulative Index to Nursing and Allied Health Literature (CINAHL), and PsycINFO. In the first set of guidelines, out of the 6,819 articles initially identified, more than 1,200 went on for a full-text screening, and an abstraction form was completed to document the study design, conclusion, and the decision to include or exclude.

Assessment and Consensus of Evidence

An evidence rating system was established to classify the strength of the recommendation and the level of evidence. Studies were first classified by the usefulness and efficacy of the intervention under study, then by level of evidence based on the type and strength of studies, and finally by the generalizability of the study results to women. The panel grouped recommendations by lifestyle interventions, atrial fibrillation/stroke prevention, preventive drug interventions, and a Class III category, in which routine intervention for CVD is not recommended. The expert panel tried to simplify the guidelines as much as possible while still upholding the evidence-based process.

Further Investigation

The panel originally found that although 75% of the studies included female subjects in their analysis, few presented results separately for men and women, and very few studies included women over 80 years of age. Thus, there remained a research gap in which studies did not provide the subgroup analyses needed so that guidelines could be better tailored. The group requested subgroup analyses from a number of existing studies, and with this new evidence expanded recommendations tailored for women as new studies emerged and filled gaps in evidence. For example, in the 2004 guidelines, when clinical trials on hormone replacement therapy showed no benefit for CVD prevention, they were added to the Class III category (interventions with no evidence of benefit or with some indication of harm). The 2007 guidelines highlighted a need for better understanding of the role of genetics in risk stratification and responsiveness to preventive interventions. Some differences in benefits of men and women were also noted in

the 2007 guidelines; for example, closer examination by meta-analysis suggested that aspirin therapy for MI prevention was *not* beneficial for women (Class III recommendation), although aspirin as a MI prevention strategy was still recommended for men at that time (Berger et al., 2006; Mosca et al., 2005). Later evidence called into question the value of aspirin therapy for both men and women (Belch et al., 2008; Hiatt, 2008).

The latest guidelines, released in 2007, focused on the need for populationwide strategies to combat the pandemic of CVD in women because individually tailored interventions alone are likely insufficient for maximal prevention and control of CVD. Thus, public policy must also become an integral strategy in reducing the burden of gender-based disparities in CVD and improving cardiovascular outcomes among women (Mosca et al., 2005).

Guidelines and Dissemination of Results

Since the guidelines were established, they have been updated every 3 years, and results have been disseminated through various means. Dr. Mosca established regular continuing medical education (CME) activities to inform clinicians of the newest guidelines and preventive measures that are imperative for women at risk of CVD. Patient education materials that were created clearly outlined the recommendations of the guidelines in a user-friendly format.

Additionally, there needed to be rigorous testing of the impact of guidelines themselves in preventing and slowing the progression of risk factors, and reducing the burden of CVD. Research is also needed on effective methods to disseminate and implement the guidelines in diverse health care settings and communities. A study by Mosca and colleagues (2005) showed that there were still barriers to implementation of guidelines that varied by type of physician, showing a need to raise awareness among not only patients, but also health care providers.

In summary, following a process such as the one we have described can build an evidence base in health psychology and help health psychology join the evidence-based movement. Although our example was from medicine, many of these lessons can be applied to health psychology.

How Can Health Psychology Use Evidence-Based Medicine?

To provide further details on how health psychology can employ evidence-based processes, the following five stages are outlined (McKibbon, Eady, & Marks 1999; Sackett, Richardson, Rosenberg, & Haynes, 2000). In Stage 1, the definitional stage, disagreement about basic concepts in research, such as how to assess and what to name the underlying construct, is the foremost issue. Arguments and controversies emerge during the definitional stage, and not until someone demands standardization of terms and concepts can the creation of an evidence base truly begin. As shown in the Mosca and colleagues (2005) example, the first step was to define what was problematic and missing in women's CVD prevention. Some similar areas in health psychology include moderating effects of cognition and coping in stress (Folkman & Lazarus, 1985), the effect of illness on quality of life (Kaplan, 1990; Littlewood et al., 2001), and the effect of psychological intervention in medical conditions (Dusseldorp, van Elderen, Maes, Meulman, & Kraaij, 1999; Fawzy et al. 1993; Friedman et al., 1986). In all of these examples, the underlying tenets required to build an evidence base are that there be a consensus on the construct and an understanding of phenomena that have yet to be established.

In Stage 2, evidence is gathered in a standard fashion, uniform nomenclature is proposed, and reasonable assessment techniques and the need for risk categorization and prevalence estimates for real-world patients emerge as resolvable. In this stage, there is accumulation of all scientific evidence available to answer the question of interest. Often an expert panel, like that in the Mosca and colleagues (2005) example, is utilized to form a coherent set of criteria in sifting through and comparing outcomes between studies. This stage is crucial in preparing for Stage 3, the analysis of the evidence.

Stage 3 involves a critical appraisal of the evidence accumulated in Stage 2, looking at issues of validity, impact, and applicability. The expert panel working on the Mosca and colleagues (2005) guidelines created an evidence rating system to sift through the studies in a methodical fashion. Others conduct meta-analyses to combine the data from different studies (Dickson, 1999). The final part of Stage 3 is achieving consensus about what is known and not known, and to synthesize what is known in a meaningful way.

In Stage 4, practical issues come to light in integrating the results from Stage 3 with clinical expertise, as well as figuring out what gaps still remain in the evidence. This stage is crucial in understanding the limitations of the current evidence and how it will impact on clinical practice (Sackett et al., 2000).

Finally, Stage 5 involves dissemination and implementation of the evidence base, by translating research findings into practical and sustainable standards of care. Dr. Mosca's group (2005) worked with the American Heart Association to establish guidelines that were taught to both patients and clinicians, and endorsed by many medical organizations. By establishing a concrete framework for clinical recommendations, Mosca's group was able to give clinicians and patients a strong, evidence-based approach to tackling CVD prevention in women. The hallmark of Stage 5 is that guidelines are updated in much less contentious ways because the groundwork has already been laid. In contemporary heath care, "quality" is often defined as adherence to guidelines (McGlynn et al., 2003). Furthermore, some organizations "pay for performance," which means that clinicians are incentivized to offer the evidence-based service (Bremer, Scholle, Keyser, Houtsinger, & Pincus, 2008). Results clearly suggest that use of the evidence-based service significantly increases when clinicians are given this extra payment (Rosof, Sirio, & Kmetik, 2008). Thus, setting a guideline may have a big impact on what care gets delivered.

Yet the question remains: How can this methodology be translated into health psychology? Currently, a sizable body of scientific evidence, drawn from a variety of research designs and methodologies, attests to the effectiveness of psychological practices and their effects on a health condition. Health psychologists are well equipped in designing, conducting, and interpreting research studies that can guide evidence-based practice. Furthermore, health psychology is distinctive as an interdisciplinary field that seeks to combine scientifically validated treatments with an emphasis on human relationships and individual differences in understanding physical health. Thus, health psychology is perfectly positioned to develop, broaden, and improve the research base for evidence-based practice.

Conclusions

Since health psychology encompasses both behavioral science and medicine, the connection between evidence and practice is all the more important. As health psychology expands and includes more diverse topics of study and intervention, additional consensus in both evaluation and treatment is needed for the field to be properly utilized. Although meta-analytic investigations since the 1970s have shown that most therapeutic practices in widespread clinical use are generally effective for treating a range of problems (Lambert & Ogles, 2004; Wampold, 2001), and the effect sizes often rival or exceed those of widely accepted medical treatments (Barlow, 2004; Lipsey & Wilson, 2001; Rosenthal, 1990; Weisz, Jensen, & McLeod, 2005), there still remains a gap in applying evidence specifically in the field of health psychology. There needs to be an integration of widely used psychological practices, as well as innovations developed in the field or laboratory, and barriers to conducting this evidence-based process should be identified and addressed.

With time, as the evidence-based process becomes more widely accepted in health psychology, the promise of insurer reimbursement and evidence-based standards of care for health psychology assessments and practices can be fulfilled. Additionally clinical exceptions, empirical reasons for variations in clinical practice, and further explanations of the mechanisms by which risk is conferred can be rigorously tested. This will be central as the field of health psychology moves forward, enhancing its acceptance by other medical professions (Gidron 2002). For example, in recent international data on the risk factors for CHD, psychosocial factors constitute one of the greatest risk factors for MI, and the other major risk factors are almost exclusively behavioral (Yusuf et al., 2004). Thus, there is important work to be done in this discipline, and evidence-based practice can greatly improve the understand-

ing and efficacy in recommendations. Herein we have outlined the benefits of creating an evidence-based movement for health psychology and have suggested how health psychologists can learn from and influence the overall movement. We conclude by offering advice on improvements in health psychology research that would accelerate the pace at which we join the evidence-based movement.

We have few systematic reviews of randomized controlled trials for our interventions or assessments. In stark comparison to medicine, where practitioners can easily locate a number of accessible systematic reviews of practices for any presenting problem, practicing psychologists are still faced with the daunting task of reading, critiquing, and synthesizing the primary reports of randomized controlled trials. This is an unacceptable and unreasonable barrier to actual use of the evidence we have already obtained. We need more easily available, widely disseminated, systematic reviews.

We have few health psychology randomized controlled trials of high methodological quality. Unfortunately, to accomplish the first task of offering high-quality systematic reviews of our interventions and assessments, we need to have high-quality primary studies. Although clearly some exist, we actually require a body of high-quality studies, all addressing the same psychological practice. Without the generation of high-quality primary studies, syntheses are useless at best, and misrepresentative at worst.

We have few clearly reported, high-quality health psychology studies. When we do have a high-quality study, often its reporting leaves so many basic questions unaddressed that neither the systematic reviewer nor the practitioner can use the study in any meaningful way. Clear reports of what was done, to whom, and by whom are not yet the standard in our field. Guidelines for reporting findings clearly and effectively exist (e.g., Consolidated Standards of Reporting Trials [CONSORT]: Zwarenstein et al., 2008; Meta-Analysis of Observational Studies in Epidemiology [MOOSE]: Stroup et al., 2000), and we need to incorporate adherence to these guidelines into every report of a study. Until we more actively engage in these three behaviors—generating higher quality evidence, reporting those data accurately and completely, and synthesizing the evidence in a way that is meaningful to our clinicians—we do not offer our patients the highest quality health psychology care. Closer interaction between researchers and clinicians, and training in evidence-based principles for both types of psychologists, can quickly close these quality gaps.

Further Reading

American Psychological Association. (2006). Evidence-based practice in psychology. *American Psychologist, 61*(4), 271–283.

Barlow, D. H. (2004). Psychological treatments. *American Psychologist, 59,* 869–879.

Bremer, R. W., Scholle, S. H., Keyser, D., Houtsinger, J. V., & Pincus, H. A. (2008). Pay for performance in behavioral health. *Psychiatric Services, 59*(12), 1419–1429.

Davidson, K. W., Goldstein, M., Kaplan, R. M., Kaufmann, P. G., Knatterud, G. L., Orleans, C. T., et al. (2003). Evidence-based behavioral medicine: What is it, and how do we achieve it? *Annals of Behavioral Medicine, 26*(3), 161–171.

Stroup, D. F., Berlin, J. A., Morton, S. C., Olkin, I., Williamson, G. D., Rennie, D., et al. (2000). Meta-Analysis of Observational Studies in Epidemiology: A proposal for reporting. *Journal of the American Medical Association, 283*(15), 2008–2012.

Zwarenstein, M., Treweek, S., Gagnier, J. J., Altman, D. G., Tunis, S., Haynes, B., et al. (2008). Improving the reporting of pragmatic trials: An extension of the CONSORT statement. *British Medical Journal, 337,* 1223–1226.

References

Addis, M. E., & Hatgis, C. (2000). Values, practices, and the utilization of empirical critiques in the clinical trial. *Clinical Psychology: Science and Practice, 7*(1), 120–124.

American Psychological Association. (2002). Criteria for evaluating treatment guidelines. *American Psychologist, 57,* 1052–1059.

American Psychological Association. (2006). Evidence-based practice is psychology. *American Psychologist, 61*(4), 271–283.

Barlow, D. H. (2004). Psychological treatments. *American Psychologist, 59,* 869–879.

Belch, J., MacCuish, A., Campbell, I., Cobbe, S., Taylor, R., Prescott, R., et al. (2008). The Prevention of Progression of Arterial Disease and Diabetes (POPADAD) trial: Factorial randomised placebo controlled trial of aspirin and antioxidants in patients with diabetes and asymptomatic peripheral arterial disease. *British Medical Journal, 337,* a1840.

Berger, J. S., Roncaglioni, M. C., Avanzini, F., Pangrazzi, I., Tognoni, G., & Brown, D. L. (2006). Aspirin for the primary prevention of cardiovascular events in women and men: A sex-specific meta-analysis of randomized controlled trials. *Journal of the American Medical Association, 295,* 306–313.

Bremer, R. W., Scholle, S. H., Keyser, D., Houtsinger, J. V., & Pincus, H. A. (2008). Pay for performance in behavioral health. *Psychiatric Services, 59*(12), 1419–1429.

Claridge, J. A., & Fabian, T. C. (2005). History and development of evidence-based medicine. *World Journal of Surgery, 29,* 547–553.

Cochrane, A. L. (1972). *Effectiveness and efficiency: Random reflections on health services.* London: Nuffield Provincial Hospitals Trust.

Committee on Quality Health Care in America. (2001). *Crossing the quality chasm: A new health system for the 21st century.* Washington, DC: National Academy Press.

Daly, J. (2005). *Evidence-based medicine and the search for a science of clinical care.* Berkeley: University of California Press.

Dickson, R. (1999). Systematic reviews. In S. Hamer & G. Collinson (Eds.), *Achieving evidence-based practice* (pp. 41–60). London: Bailliere Tindall.

Dusseldorp, E., van Elderen, T., Maes, S., Meulman, J., & Kraaij, V. (1999). A meta-analysis of psychoeducational programs for coronary heart disease patients. *Health Psychology, 18,* 506–519.

Fawzy, F. I., Fawzy, N. W., Hyun, C. S., Elashoff, R., Guthrie, D., Fahey, J. L., et al. (1993). Malignant melanoma: Effects of an early structured psychiatric intervention, coping and affective state, on recurrence and survival 6 years later. *Archives of General Psychiatry, 50,* 681–689.

Folkman, S., & Lazarus, R. S. (1985). If it changes it must be a process: Study of emotion and coping during the tree stages of a college examination. *Journal of Personality and Social Psychology, 48,* 150–170.

Friedman, M., Thoresen, C. E., Gill, J. J., Ulmer, D., Powell, L. H., Price, V. A., et al. (1986). Alteration of type A behavior and its effect on cardiac recurrences in post myocardial infarction patients: Summary results of the recurrent coronary prevention project. *American Hearth Journal, 112,* 653–665.

Gidron, Y. (2002). Evidence-based health psychology: Rationale and support. *Psicologia: Saúde & Doenças, 3*(1), 3–10.

Guyatt, G., Haynes, R. B., Jaeschke, R. Z., Cook, D. J., Green, L., Naylor, C. D., et al. (2000). Users' guide to the medical literature: XXV. Evidence-based medicine: Principles for applying the users' guide to patient care. *Journal of the American Medical Association, 284*(10), 1290—1296.

Guyatt, G., & Rennie, D. (Eds.). (2002). *User's guides to the medical literature: A manual for evidence-based clinical practice.* Chicago: American Medical Association Press.

Hamer, S. (1999). Evidence-based practice. In S. Hamer & G. Collinson (Eds.), *Achieving evidence-based practice: A handbook for practitioners* (pp. 3–12). London: Harcourt.

Hiatt, W. R. (2008). Aspirin for prevention of cardiovascular events. *British Medical Journal, 337,* a1806.

Kaplan, R. M. (1990). Behavior as the central outcome in healthcare. *American Psychologist, 45,* 1211–1220.

Kerner, J., Rimer, R., & Emmons, K. (2005). Introduction to the special section on dissemination: Dissemination research and research dissemination: How can we close the gap? *Health Psychology, 24*(5), 443–446.

Kerner, J. F., Guirguis-Blake, J., Hennessy, K. D., Brounstein, P. J., Vinson, C., Schwartz, R. H., et al. (2005). Translating research into improved outcomes in comprehensive cancer control. *Cancer Causes and Control, 16*(Suppl. 1), 27–40.

Lambert, M. J., & Ogles, B. M. (2004). The efficacy and effectiveness of psychotherapy. In M. J. Lambert (Ed.), *Bergin and Garfield's handbook of psychotherapy and behavior change* (5th ed., pp. 139–193). New York: Wiley.

Lipsey, M. W., & Wilson, D. B. (2001). The way in which intervention studies have "personality" and why it is important to meta-analysis. *Evaluation and the Health Professions, 24,* 236–254.

Littlewood, T. J., Bajetta, E., Nortier, J. W., Vercammen, E., Rapoport, B., and the Epoetin Alpha Study Group. (2001). Effects of epoetin alpha on hemotologic parameters and quality of life in cancer patients receiving nonplatinum chemotherapy: Results of a randomized, double-blind, placebo-controlled trial. *Journal of Clinical Oncology, 19*(11), 2865–2874.

McGlynn, E. A., Asch, S. M., Adams, J., Keesey, J., Hicks, J., DeCristofaro, A., et al. (2003). The quality of health care delivered to adults in the United States. *New England Journal of Medicine, 348*(26), 2635–2645.

McKibbon, A., Eady, A., & Marks, S. (1999). *PDQ: Evidence-based principles and practice.* Hamilton, ON, Canada: Decker.

Montgomery, R. W., & Ayllon, T. (1995). Matching verbal repertoires: Understanding the contingencies of practice in order to functionally communicate with clinicians. *Journal of Behavior Therapy and Experimental Psychiatry, 26*(2), 99–105.

Mosca, L., Linfante, A. H., Benjamin, E. J.,

Berra, K., Hayes, S. N., Walsh, B. W., et al. (2005). National study of physician awareness and adherence to cardiovascular disease prevention guidelines. *Circulation, 111*(4), 499–510.

Rosenthal, R. (1990). How are we doing in soft psychology? *American Psychologist, 45,* 775–777.

Rosof, B. M., Sirio, C. A., & Kmetik, K. S. (2008). Pay-for-performance system for English physicians. *New England Journal of Medicine, 359*(20), 2176–2177.

Sackett, D. L., Richardson, W. S., Rosenberg, W., & Haynes, R. B. (2000). *Evidence-based medicine: How to practice and teach EBM.* London: Churchill Livingstone.

Sackett, D. L., Rosenberg, W. M., Gray, J. A., Haynes, R. B., & Richardson, W. S. (1996). Evidence-based medicine: What it is and what it isn't. *British Medical Journal, 312*(7023), 71–72.

Sogg, S., Read, J., Bollinger, A., & Berger, J. (2001). Clinical sensibilities and research practicalities: Meeting at the crossroads. *Behavior Therapist, 24*(6), 122–126, 133.

Spring, B., Pagoto, S., Kaufmann, P. G., Whitlock, E. P., Glasgow, R. E., Smith, T. W., et al. (2005). Invitation to a dialogue between researchers and clinicians about evidence-based behavioral medicine. *Annals of Behavioral Medicine, 30*(2), 125–137.

Stroup, D. F., Berlin, J. A., Morton, S. C., Olkin, I., Williamson, G. D., Rennie, D., et al. (2000). Meta-Analysis of Observational Studies in Epidemiology: A proposal for reporting. *Journal of the American Medical Association, 283*(15), 2008–2012.

Wampold, B. E. (2001). *The great psychotherapy debate: Models, methods, and findings.* Mahwah, NJ: Erlbaum.

Weisz, J. R., Jensen, A. L., & McLeod, B. D. (2005). Development and dissemination of child and adolescent psychotherapies: Milestones, methods, and a new deployment-focused model. In E. D. Hibbs & P. S. Jensen (Eds.), *Psychosocial treatments for child and adolescent disorders: Empirically based strategies for clinical practice* (2nd ed., pp. 9–39). Washington, DC: American Psychological Association.

Yusuf, S., Hawken, S., Ounpuu, S., Dans, T., Avezum, A., Lanas, F., et al. (2004). Effect of potentially modifiable risk factors associated with myocardial infarction in 52 countries (the INTERHEART study): Case–control study. *Lancet, 364,* 937–952.

Zwarenstein, M., Treweek, S., Gagnier, J. J., Altman, D. G., Tunis, S., Haynes, B., et al. (2008). Improving the reporting of pragmatic trials: An extension of the CONSORT statement. *British Medical Journal, 337,* 1223–1226.

PART IV

HEALTH PSYCHOLOGY, PUBLIC HEALTH, AND PREVENTION

CHAPTER 21

Impacts of Being Uninsured

Dylan Habeeb Roby

Insurance Status in the United States

To understand the impact of being uninsured in the U.S. health care system, one needs to understand the scope and nature of health insurance, and who is left out of that system. In the United States, health insurance coverage and health care services can come from a variety of sources—employers, the federal government, state and county governments, as well as people who purchase insurance on their own, in the individual market. The passage of the Patient Protection and Affordable Care Act (PPACA) and the Health Care and Education Reconciliation Act in 2010 maintains the current system of health insurance. However, the new law is expected to allow 32 million more residents of the United States to receive health insurance through their employers, the individual market, or public programs such as Medicaid by 2019 (Congressional Budget Office, 2010).

The primary source of health insurance in the United States is through an employment-based benefit package (61%), which is provided to many workers in the labor market and their families (Kaiser Commission on Medicaid and the Uninsured, 2006). Often, these benefit packages include retirement plans and other incentives, in addition to health insurance coverage. In most cases, the employer does not pay for the entire health insurance premium; instead, the employer and employee share that responsibility. An employee might pay 10% of the monthly premium rate (which is negotiated by the employer and the insurance companies it chooses), while the employer pays the rest. Employees are often allowed to add their dependents and spouses to the same health insurance plan for an additional premium. Many U.S. residents obtain health insurance through the employers of their parents or spouses. Due to the passage of the PPACA, children of insured employees are now allowed to remain on their parents' health insurance plans until the child turns age 26 (Kaiser Family Foundation, 2010).

Individuals and families that do not obtain health insurance coverage through an employer, yet do not qualify for governmental insurance programs (e.g., Medicaid,

Medicare, or the Children's Health Insurance Program [CHIP]) have to join the insurance market on their own, by purchasing insurance directly from a health insurance company or insurance broker. Otherwise, the individual and his or her family may be uninsured. According to the Kaiser Commission on Medicaid and the Uninsured (2006), approximately 5% of people other than older adults (age 65 and older) purchase insurance on their own. Privately purchasing coverage can be an expensive proposition for many families: The premium costs are not subsidized by an employer, and in addition, they are not pooling their risk with other beneficiaries, resulting in more volatile premium rates and the likelihood that their coverage could be dropped if their health insurance costs are too high or if they develop an uninsurable condition.[1] While Medicaid or other public programs such as CHIP and Medicare cover about 16% of persons other than older adults, there are still 18% (47 million) uninsured adults and young adults in the United States (Kaiser Commission on Medicaid and the Uninsured, 2006). The older adult population, due to eligibility for Medicare, is not as likely to include uninsured people.

While having health insurance is not a prerequisite for seeking and receiving health care, being uninsured represents a barrier to health care access (Hadley & Cunningham, 2004). Uninsured people often must seek care in safety net clinics (e.g., community health centers and free clinics) or in hospital emergency departments when they need afterhours care, specialty care, or are suffering from an acute condition (Holohan & Spillman, 2002). While the providers that make up the health care safety net strive to provide quality health care to their uninsured patients, it is often difficult because of financial constraints, lack of ability to refer for specialty care, and overcrowding due to a high demand for services (Cook et al., 2007; Cunningham, Bazzoli, & Katz, 2008).

---

[1]The passage of PPACA will remove the ability of insurers to deny children health insurance coverage due to preexisting conditions and to rescind anyone's coverage (except in cases of fraud) by September 2010. On January 1, 2014, insurers will be unable to deny coverage to adults due to preexisting conditions.

The Andersen Model and Access to Care

To understand the problems that can result from lack of access to health care, I refer to a seminal model of health care access and use of health services. This model, Andersen's behavioral model of health services use, attempts to explain individual-level health services use. The model states that both contextual and individual characteristics predict health services use. Both the contextual and individual factors include three main predictors of use of health care: (1) predisposing, (2) enabling, and (3) needs determinants (Andersen & Davidson, 2007). Predisposing determinants of health services use include demographic characteristics, such as marital status, ethnicity, language spoken, educational level, and age at an aggregate (contextual) or individual level. Enabling determinants include insurance status or having a nearby clinic that offers services in one's language. Needs determinants include both perceived health problems and realized needs—acute illness, exacerbation of chronic conditions, and injury. Using Andersen's model in the context of the U.S. health care system, we may determine that a white, college-educated male diabetic with health insurance is more likely to use health services than a minority, high school–educated diabetic female without insurance. In addition, contextual factors such as the health of a larger community or lack of primary care providers impact health services use. It is likely, in this hypothetical scenario, that one of the major barriers to health services use is lack of insurance. In the U.S. health care system, insurance acts as an enabling factor in predicting the ability of an individual to access and use health care. I explain the reasons for this in the next section.

The Function of Health Insurance

In the U.S. healthcare system, intentionally or unintentionally, insurance serves to increase access to health care for people who have it. Conversely, those who are uninsured face barriers in accessing care, receiving the care they need, and paying for the care they do receive.

Traditionally, insurance was designed to mitigate risk and protect an individual's assets in the event of an unforeseen circumstance or occurrence. By thinking about life insurance, auto insurance, or homeowners insurance, it is generally easy to understand the intent of insurance. It protects policyholders and all or part of their belongings from catastrophe or other events that could cause a loss (Mehr, Cammack, & Rose, 1985). Insurance function is based on the idea of risk being spread out over a larger group of people or assets (Dionne & Harrington, 1991). An insurance company can meet its obligations to pay claims to its policyholders because it does not expect all policyholders to file a claim due a loss at the same time.

Health insurance in the United States is not yet a century old. In 1929, the first organized health insurance plan began in Texas at Baylor University. Later, during World War II and immediately after the war ended in 1945, health insurance coverage became a popular part of employee benefit plans offered by postwar employers. Over those 80 years, health insurance has changed from a system to protect families from major, catastrophic medical costs to a much more comprehensive part of the health care system that allows families to obtain preventive care and a much more robust set of health benefits.

Employer-based insurance coverage requires individual employers to offer their employees the ability to choose (or to "take up") insurance coverage through the company. The employer enters into contracts with insurance companies, paying a negotiated amount for premiums on employees' behalf. The employer may then choose either to ask the employee to pay a portion of the premium or provide health insurance with no employee contribution. Currently, any premium payments by the employer or employee are not taxable.[2] This tax benefit provides both a monetary incentive for the employer to offer health insurance coverage, and health-related and monetary incentives

for the employee to accept that health insurance coverage.

In addition to negotiating the premium amount with insurance companies, the employer also negotiates other specific components of the insurance policy choices. These include benefit packages (i.e., medical, dental, mental health and substance abuse, or vision coverage), as well as cost sharing (e.g., deductibles and copayments for office visits, prescriptions, emergency department visits, and inpatient hospital stays). As the RAND Health Insurance Experiment showed, use of health services is linked to lower cost sharing and less out-of-pocket spending on the part of the policyholder (Manning et al., 1987).

Insurance coverage enables individuals to access health care, as indicated by previous research showing differential levels of health services use for the insured compared to the uninsured. In addition, more generous benefit packages allow the insured to use services that may not be readily available to the uninsured.

How Payments Impact Health Care Access

In the modern U.S. health care system, insurance coverage plays a much larger role in physician payment than it did in the past. Until the early 1990s, many health insurance companies did not have contracts with individual physicians. Physicians were paid on a fee-for-service basis for each service they provided (Iglehart, 1994). This provided an incentive for physicians to provide more services than were necessary, in order to earn more money (Leibowitz & Schlackman, 1996). This resulted in unnecessary overuse of health care services and a cost crisis in the U.S. health care system (Levit et al., 1994). To rein in the perceived out-of-control costs, many insurers moved toward tenets of managed care as a mechanism to reduce payments to physicians and unnecessary utilization. Managed care delivery systems often used the idea of a primary care provider to act as a gatekeeper in regulating the unnecessary physician payments, specialty visits, second opinions, and elective surgeries driving up health care costs until the early 1990s (Zwanziger & Melnick, 1996).

___
[2]The PPACA of 2010 will introduce a new excise tax on high-cost plans, commonly called the "Cadillac Tax." This excise tax will be introduced in 2018 and will result in a 40% tax on any portion of health insurance plan premiums over $10,200 for an individual or $27,500 for a family. This tax is designed to encourage insurers to offer and employers and employees to choose less costly health insurance plans.

Managed care, through health maintenance organizations (HMO) or preferred provider organizations (PPO), has resulted in physicians being contracted to different insurers as part of their provider network and being paid discounted or capitated rates per visit or per person, based on the types of services delivered during those visits (Isenberg, 1998). For example, under a fee-for-service arrangement, a physician may have been paid $50 for providing a cancer screening, $25 for a blood test, and $25 to counsel a patient about weight management—all in the same visit. In today's managed care–based environment, a physician may provide all of those services in one visit but would be paid a bundled or discounted fee of $60 per visit or 80% of the rate for each service based on an existing contract between the network provider and the insurance company. In a capitated contract, a physician may be paid $100 per member per month to care for a patient, regardless of actual service use. If a patient does not use the physician all year, the doctor is still paid $1,200. However, if a patient uses more than $1,200 worth of services, the burden of risk for those costs is on the physician.

As depicted in Figure 21.1, the flow of money in the U.S. health care system can be very complex. Although insurance companies and government agencies fund most of

the health care provided in the United States by paying physicians for services provided, individuals also fund some health care use from their own pockets. The uninsured spend much more on average (35%) as a percentage of family income, out-of-pocket (not including premiums), than their insured counterparts (20%) over a full year (Hadley & Holohan, 2004). However, to share in the overall cost, the commercially insured and the publicly insured (Medicare, Medicaid, and CHIP) also pay into the system in the form of copays, deductibles, and premiums. Insurance status impacts the level of out-of-pocket (including premiums) medical expenditures made by families in the United States. While publicly and commercially insured families spend more than $6,400 on health care a year on average, the uninsured only spend $1,208 (Bernard & Banthin, 2007). This confirms that when premiums are included in aggregate medical out-of-pocket spending, the insured spend more than the uninsured on premiums and other out-of-pocket costs. The increased access experienced by insured individuals enhances their ability to obtain needed care, assuming that their benefits and cost-sharing requirements do not significantly limit care.

The way in which physicians are paid for medical care can be a disadvantage for the uninsured. Previously, hospitals, clinics, and

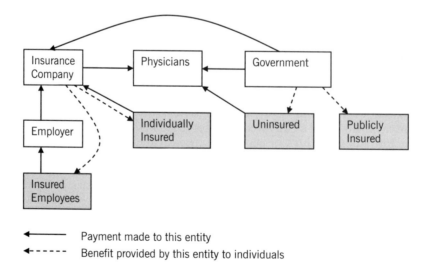

FIGURE 21.1. The flow of money in the U.S. health care system. Depending on the insurance plan and source, there could be some payment going directly to the physician from the four groups representing individuals seeking health care (highlighted in gray).

other providers were able to subsidize their uncompensated care (i.e., care provided to the uninsured that was not paid for) by relying on the more generous payments they received from commercial insurance reimbursement. This activity is called "cost shifting," and its presence in the health care market has been supported by various studies (Dobson, DaVanzo, & Sen, 2006). However, more recently, due to decreasing reimbursement from commercial insurers, as well as Medicaid and Medicare, and the presence of managed care, researchers have identified a new cost shifting method. Because hospitals and other providers cannot obtain reimbursement of full charges from traditional payers, they instead charge their uninsured patients that rate. The insurers are able to negotiate lower rates on behalf of their plan members, as is the federal government. However, the uninsured are not privy to the underlying cost or negotiated rates between providers and insurers, and they are asked to pay the full amount for their care (Anderson, 2007). According to Anderson (2007), the uninsured were often charged 250% of what most commercial health insurers paid for the same service.

Understanding the way the health system is structured, as well as how payments are made to providers, allows one to realize some of the problems faced by the uninsured. They are likely to have a hard time finding a physician who will care for them without payment, and when they do find a physician, they may be charged higher rates than a commercially insured patient would be charged. In the following sections, I explore specific problems faced by the uninsured, including medical bankruptcy, disparities in access and quality of care, and lack of access to specialty care.

Medical Bankruptcy

The uninsured are likely to face significant financial problems due to medical costs, which include facing medical bankruptcy and forgoing other needs (Seifert & Rukavina, 2006). A recent Harvard study found that medical debt contributed to slightly more than half of all bankruptcies in the United States, with over 46% of all bankruptcies qualifying as major medical bank-

ruptcies (Himmelstein, Warren, Thorne, & Woolhandler, 2005). Other studies found that half of the uninsured had problems paying for their health care, with one-third having medical debt in collections (Duchon et al., 2001).

Although the Emergency Medical Treatment and Active Labor Act (EMTALA) requires hospital emergency departments to assess and stabilize all patients, regardless of health insurance status, it does not require them to provide free health care to the uninsured. Uninsured individuals, who can only receive affordable care at community health centers or other safety net clinics, are often forced to seek emergency care when they cannot get an appointment with a specialist or when urgent situations call for basic primary care. This is much more expensive than a visit to a private physician's office. One office visit might cost an uninsured individual between $80 and $120. A 2003 analysis by the Agency for Healthcare Research and Quality determined that the average emergency room visit cost $560 (or $660 in 2010 dollars) (Machlin, 2006). Often, when the uninsured are billed for this service and cannot pay, the bill is sent to a collections agency.

Not being able to pay for incurred health care costs, the uninsured are likely to avoid seeing the doctor and to delay treatment until it becomes a serious issue that is more expensive and potentially creates more financial trouble for them, or for the providers who are not able to recover the cost of the care (Weissman, 2005). Local, state, and federal programs may enable certain low-income members of the uninsured population to benefit from free care; however, many of the uninsured do not know about these programs, and are still likely to avoid seeking needed care (Weissman, Dryfoos, & London, 1999).

Health Disparities

The uninsured are not only less likely than their insured counterparts to receive appropriate immunizations and other preventive care, but they are also likely to delay care due to cost or other issues, such as child care and distance to a doctor (which also are linked to having a low income). Because of this lack of health care, uninsured individuals may not know about their own health conditions (i.e., hypertension or high cholesterol) or treatable cancers that would have been diagnosed through a routine screening by a primary care physician (Ayanian, Kohler, Abe, & Epstein, 1993; Ayanian, Zaslavsky, Weissman, Schneider, & Ginsburg, 2003).

While much of the disparities discussion focuses on socioeconomic differences related to ethnic and income-based factors, many argue that access to health care is the most limiting factor, and that health insurance would provide better access for groups that suffer from disparities in health status (Andrulis, 1998). One would expect that if given health insurance coverage through a public program (Medicaid, Medicare, or CHIP) or through an employer, a low-income, uninsured individual would have better access to care and be more likely to use health services as predicted in Andersen's behavioral model of health services use (Lasser, Himmelstein, & Woolhandler, 2006).

Health disparities are persistent in certain ethnic groups in terms of both access and outcomes. Ethnic minorities are less likely to receive appropriate medications for heart problems, transplants, and necessary surgeries in comparison to their white counterparts (Institute of Medicine, 2002a). However, the minority uninsured are at an even greater disadvantage due to poor access and health outcomes than minorities with insurance coverage (McWilliams, Meara, Zaslavsky, & Ayanian, 2007b). To further demonstrate the impact of insurance on the reduction of health disparities, several studies have used Medicare, which provides insurance to U.S. residents over the age of 65, as a natural experiment. Previously uninsured individuals who enrolled in Medicare experienced better heart disease- and diabetes-related outcomes compared to uninsured individuals with similar characteristics who were not yet eligible for Medicare due to their age (McWilliams et al., 2007a).

Delaying Care

The uninsured, due to cost, are more likely not to see a doctor when they have a health problem, obtain a prescription, or see a specialist than their insured counterparts (Du-chon et al., 2001). Even when researchers look at two groups that rate themselves as having poor health status, the uninsured are about three times more likely to go without needed care than their insured counterparts (Ayanian, Weissman, Schneider, Ginsburg, & Zaslavsky, 2000).

When comparing duration of insurance status, those with longer periods of being uninsured are at higher risk than those with shorter periods of uninsurance, although people with short periods without insurance (less than 1 year) still use less care and are less likely than the insured to receive routine care. U.S. residents who are uninsured more than 1 year are more likely to forgo recommended (every 2 years) routine checkups (43%) compared to the insured (18%) and those who were uninsured less than 1 year (22%). They are also less likely to obtain appropriate cancer screenings, diabetes care, and heart disease prevention care (Ayanian et al., 2000).

Delaying health care can contribute to higher medical costs once a medical need is realized, premature mortality, and worse health outcomes once care is received (Lurie, Ward, Shapiro, & Brook, 1984). The uninsured are at great risk of all three of these problems because of their likelihood of not being able to afford care, and to forgo or delay necessary care.

Medical Home

The main goals of managed care are to reduce unnecessary health care utilization, improve health status, and reduce costs. One of the ways managed care firms, especially HMOs, do this is through the assignment of a "medical home," which is designed to give individuals a usual source of care, where they can comfortably seek follow-up care and medical advice, obtain refills of medications, and get referrals to specialty care as appropriate (American College of Physicians, 2007). On the insurance side, that medical home also acts as an effective gatekeeper and navigator of the insurance company's network and system of referrals, treatment choices, and utilization controls. The Commonwealth Fund describes the medical home as "a health care setting that provides patients with timely, well-organized care, and enhanced access to providers" (Beal, Doty, Hernandez, Shea, & Davis, 2007, p. ix).

Having health insurance coverage along with a medical home decreases racial and ethnic disparities in minority adults. The presence of a medical home appears to improve access to necessary care, and use of routine preventive care and screenings, and chronic disease management. However, according to the 2006 Health Care Quality Survey, only 16% of the uninsured reported a medical home, while another 39% reported a usual source of care (that did not serve as a medical home)—a total of 55%. (In this report, having a "medical home" was defined as having a regular provider or place of care, reporting no difficulty contacting the provider by phone or getting advice and medical care on weekends or evenings, and always or often finding office visits well organized and running on time.) In comparison, close to 90% of the insured population has a medical home or usual source of care (Beal et al., 2007).

Lack of insurance is strongly linked to lacking a medical home, which translates to an inability to receive timely and appropriate primary care and specialty physician visits, needed prescriptions, and assistance in managing chronic illnesses. Having health insurance would greatly increase the ability of previously uninsured individuals to find and take advantage of a medical home in managing their health needs, to limit disparities, and to improve health outcomes.

Chronic Conditions

Lack of primary care for the uninsured can be a serious problem, especially if the uninsured individual has a chronic condition such as diabetes, hypertension, or asthma. All of these diseases can be managed through primary care, self-management, and proper medication. However, lack of access to health care can result in hospitalizations and emergency department visits that could have been prevented by primary care.

Recent studies indicate that the prevalence of chronic disease in American adults is increasing. However, at the same time, the number of the uninsured adults is increasing. Approximately 11.4 million adult and young adult U.S. residents with chronic disease are uninsured—representing between 15 and 16% of all adults and young adults with diabetes, hypertension, and cardiovascular disease in the country. These uninsured U.S. residents are not only chronically ill, but they also have much lower rates of utilization of health care than their insured counterparts. Almost 23% (1 in 4) of the uninsured had not visited a health professional, compared to 6% of the insured (1 in 16), and uninsured were seven times as likely to report their usual source of care as the hospital emergency department (Wilper et al., 2008).

An emergency department certainly does not meet the definition of a medical home as described by the Commonwealth Fund. Using an emergency department for a usual source of care could result in the inability of physicians to assess medical records, sporadic preventive and chronic care management, excessive patient diagnostic testing, and lack of a relationship with the physician. While emergency department physicians are well trained to deal with episodic, acute exacerbations of chronic disease, they do not provide the primary care home that allows chronically ill patients to manage their disease actively in collaboration with a primary care provider, as prescribed by the chronic care model and other patient-centered strategies to deal with chronic diseases (Wagner et al., 2001).

Without receiving help from a primary care provider and having access to specialty services when necessary, it is very difficult for chronically ill individuals to manage their diseases, obtain the appropriate medications and treatment, and experience positive health outcomes. As I mentioned in previous sections, the uninsured are more likely to lack access to primary care and chronic care management, which could result in premature death, disability, more inpatient hospitalizations and avoidable emergency department visits, and increased health care costs.

Continuity of Care

Although obtaining care through competent primary care clinics that target the uninsured can be instrumental in improving the health status of the uninsured, there are still barriers to care faced by the uninsured. Often, primary care clinics do not have specialists on staff, and clinic physicians have a difficult time referring their patients to community-based specialty providers or hospitals that do provide those specialty services, especially for uninsured patients (Cook et al., 2007; Skinner & Mayer, 2007).

Without proper access to specialists (i.e., oncologists, cardiologists, urologists), the uninsured may potentially face complications that worsen over time related to cancer, diabetes, heart disease, and other conditions that may require specialty care. Without a medical home or an active primary care provider to coordinate services, make specialty referrals, and manage the treatment provided by all sources of care, it can be difficult for uninsured individuals to take advantage of the health care to which they do have access. One way for an uninsured person to have that medical home with actively coordinated care is to obtain health care from a community health center or other community primary care clinic that has extensive relationships with local specialists and academic medical centers. However, it is still likely that uninsured patients will face longer wait times (more than 3 months) and prohibitive cost barriers when seeking specialty care.

The Fragile Safety Net

The health care safety net in the United States is always under significant pressure to care for the uninsured, as well as low-income Medicaid and CHIP beneficiaries, and the commercially insured in rural areas or areas with no usual source of care. The "safety net" in the United States is made up primarily of nonprofit, mission-driven hospitals (like religiously affiliated and children's hospitals), public or teaching hospitals, community health centers and other community clinics, county government public health and primary care clinics, rural health centers, and community-based physicians who provide free or discounted care to uninsured patients (Forrest & Whelan, 2000).

The major funding for safety net services in local areas comes from two sources: disproportionate share hospital (DSH) payments and Bureau of Primary Health Care Federally Qualified Health Center (FQHC)

grants. DSH payments are made mainly to a small number of teaching and public hospitals that provide a large amount of care to uninsured patients and Medicaid beneficiaries, while FQHC grants target nonprofit, mission-driven clinics that provide significant levels of care to the same two groups. While DSH hospitals and FQHCs count on these subsidies to be able to take care of their uninsured patients, they often represent less than one-fourth of their overall revenues. These safety net facilities also obtain revenue from reimbursement for insured patients, self-pay patients, and other sources of grants and funds—including county appropriations. All of these funding sources are necessary to maintain operations of safety net hospitals and clinics, which are often overcrowded, understaffed, and under constant pressure to care for the uninsured. Historically, DSH funding is often the source of political debate, and safety net hospitals that rely on the revenue to care for the uninsured and Medicaid beneficiaries face pressures due to DSH funding reductions, like those in the Balanced Budget Act of 1997 (Guterman, 1998). FQHCs also face pressures due to stagnant federal grants, Medicaid policy changes, low reimbursement rates, and the rising number of uninsured. Financial pressures can force FQHCs to close or reduce the provision of services (Roby, 2006).

Many urban centers have multiple public hospitals and community health centers to meet the needs of the uninsured. However, in rural or suburban areas, there may be no public hospital, and the closest community health center may be hours away. In these areas, it can be very difficult for uninsured patients to obtain primary and specialty care due to the lack of facilities able to handle their needs while also providing low cost or free health care.

Premature Death

Previous studies have explained that uninsured adults have a higher likelihood of dying at a younger age than insured adults (Franks, Clancy, & Gold, 1993; Institute of Medicine, 2002a). Recently, the Urban Institute stated that 22,000 U.S. residents died prematurely due to lack of insurance in 2006. The report went on to say that between 2000 and 2006, approximately 137,000 U.S. residents died early due to being uninsured (Dorn, 2008). Premature death, it is hypothesized, is linked to lack of primary care, lack of appropriate screening for treatable cancers, and lack of knowledge about existing conditions that could be prevented or managed.

The pre-Medicare, low-income adult population is likely to experience the most health problems while being uninsured. It was determined that uninsured, middle-aged (under 65) individuals are 40% more likely to die early compared to their insured counterparts (McWilliams, Zaslavsky, Meara, Ayanian, 2004).

Conclusions: How Do We Solve the Problem of the Uninsured?

Universal health insurance, while popular among much of the population, faces a difficult battle in our current political and health care environment (Blendon & Benson, 2009). The last failed attempt at national reform occurred in 1994, under President Bill Clinton (Hacker, 1997). Recently, debates raged across the country about whether to enact health care reform, and how it should deal with the problem of the uninsured. The Democratic proposal that was passed in March 2010 as the Patient Protection and Affordable Care Act and Health Care and Education Reconciliation Act is based on the idea of an individual mandate, in addition to expansions of state Medicaid programs and requirements for employers with 50 or more employees offer insurance coverage or pay fees. Under this mandate, which will take effect on January 1, 2014, individuals will be required to purchase insurance coverage unless they meet certain conditions (Kaiser Family Foundation, 2010). If individuals are uninsured and do not qualify for financial hardship exemptions, have religious objections, are uninsured for more than 3 months, or meet other exemption criteria, they will be responsible for paying an income tax penalty of $695 per person (up to a family maximum of $2,085) or 2.5% of their income starting in 2016. Under the statute, undocumented immigrants would not be required to purchase coverage and would not be allowed to receive any subsidies or purchase insurance through a new Health Insurance Ex-

change designed to allow legal residents and citizens to buy individual and small group insurance coverage. The removal of undocumented immigrants from the individual and small group insurance market, along with noncompliance with the individual mandate by legal residents and citizens, will leave a number of individuals uninsured despite enactment of the health care reform law. The Congressional Budget Office estimates that by the time the law is fully implemented in 2019, the United States will still have 22 million uninsured people, including undocumented immigrants and those who are not subject to the law due to religious objections and financial hardship (Kaiser Family Foundation, 2010).

The enactment of PPACA is not only designed to provide insurance to the uninsured. Many of the reforms focus on delivery system changes, insurance regulation, and other efforts to make health insurance accessible and premiums affordable. While the 32 million newly insured residents and citizens will benefit from health insurance subsidies and new insurance regulations, the 22 million expected to remain uninsured in 2019 will still face barriers to receiving timely, high-quality health care.

Even with access to care from community health centers dedicated to the medical home model, and specialty services available at local public hospitals, the uninsured face barriers in accessing care in a timely, coordinated, and affordable manner. Until these barriers are removed, the uninsured will continue to have lower health care use rates, lower rates of having a medical home or usual source of care, lack continuity of care, and have a higher likelihood of premature death.

Further Reading

Andersen, R. M., Rice, T. H., & Kominski, G. F. (2007). *Changing the U.S. health care system: Key issues in health services policy and management* (3rd ed.). San Francisco: Jossey-Bass.

Ayanian, J. Z., Weissman, J. S., Schneider, E. C., Ginsburg, J. A., & Zaslavsky, A. M. (2000). Unmet health needs of uninsured adults in the United States. *Journal of the American Medical Association, 284*(16), 2061–2069.

Dobson, A., DaVanzo, J., & Sen, N. (2006).

The cost shift payment "hydraulic": Foundation, history, and implications. *Health Affairs, 25*(1), 22–33.

Hadley, J., & Cunningham, P. (2004). Availability of safety net providers and access to care of uninsured persons. *Health Services Research, 39*(5), 1527–1546.

Hadley, J., & Holahan, J. (2004). *The cost of care for the uninsured: What do we spend, who pays, and what would full coverage add to medical spending?* Washington, DC: Kaiser Commission on Medicaid and the Uninsured. Retrieved September 19, 2008, from *www.kff.org/uninsured/upload/the-cost-of-care-for-the-uninsured-what-do-we-spend-who-pays-and-what-would-full-coverage-add-to-medical-spending.pdf.*

Rice, T., & Unruh, L. (2009). *The economics of health reconsidered* (3rd ed.). Chicago: Health Administration Press.

References

Andersen, R. M., & Davidson, P. L. (2007). Improving access to care in America: Individual and contextual indicators. In R. M. Andersen, T. H. Rice, & G. F. Kominski (Eds.), *Changing the U.S. health care system* (3rd ed., pp. 3–32). San Francisco: Jossey-Bass.

Anderson, G. F. (2007). From "soak the rich" to "soak the poor": Recent trends in hospital pricing. *Health Affairs, 26*, 780–789.

Andrulis, D. P. (1998). Access to care is the centerpiece in the elimination of socioeconomic disparities in health. *Annals of Internal Medicine, 129*, 412–416.

Ayanian, J. Z., Kohler, B. A., Abe, T., & Epstein, A. M. (1993). The relation between health insurance coverage and clinical outcomes among women with breast cancer. *New England Journal of Medicine, 329*, 326–331.

Ayanian, J. Z., Weissman, J. S., Schneider, E. C., Ginsburg, J. A., & Zaslavsky, A. M. (2000). Unmet health needs of uninsured adults in the United States. *Journal of the American Medical Association, 284*, 2061–2069.

Ayanian, J. Z., Zaslavsky, A. M., Weissman, J. S., Schneider, E. C., & Ginsburg, J. A. (2003). Undiagnosed hypertension and hypercholesterolemia among uninsured and insured adults in the Third National Health and Nutrition Examination Survey. *American Journal of Public Health, 93*, 2051–2054.

Beal, A. C., Doty, M. M., Hernandez, S. E., Shea, K. K., & Davis, K. (2007). *Closing the divide: How medical homes promote equity in health care.* New York: Commonwealth Fund.

Bernard, D., & Banthin, J. (2007). *Family-level expenditures on health care and insurance premiums among the U.S. nonelderly population, 2004.* Rockville, MD: Agency for Healthcare Research and Quality.

Blendon, R. J., & Benson, J. M. (2009). Understanding how Americans view health care reform. *New England Journal of Medicine, 361*, e131–e134.

Cook, N. L., Hicks, L. S., O'Malley, J., Keegan, T., Guadagnoli, E., & Landon, B. E. (2007). Access to specialty care and medical services in community health centers. *Health Affairs, 26*, 1459–1468.

Cunningham, P. J., Bazzoli, G. J., & Katz, A. (2008). Caught in the competitive crossfire: Safety-net providers balance margin and mission in a profit-driven health care market. *Health Affairs, 27*, w374–w382.

Dionne, G., & Harrington, S. E. (1991). *Foundations of insurance economics: Readings in economics and finance.* Boston: Kluwer Academic.

Dobson, A., DaVanzo, J., & Sen, N. (2006). The cost shift payment "hydraulic": Foundation, history, and implications. *Health Affairs, 25*, 22–33.

Dorn, S. (2008). *Uninsured and dying because of it: Updating the Institute of Medicine analysis on the impact of uninsurance on mortality.* Washington, DC: Urban Institute.

Duchon, L., Schoen, C., Doty, M. M., Davis, K., Strumpf, E., & Bruegman, S. (2001). *Security matters: How instability in health insurance puts U.S. workers at risk.* New York: Commonwealth Fund.

Felt-Lisk, S., McHugh, M., & Howell, E. (2001). *Study of safety net provider capacity to care for low-income uninsured patients.* Washington, DC: Mathematica Policy Research, Inc.

Forrest, C. B., & Whelan, E. M. (2000). Primary care safety-net delivery sites in the United States: A comparison of community health centers, hospital outpatient departments, and physicians' offices. *Journal of the American Medical Association, 284*, 2077–2083.

Franks, P., Clancy, C. M., & Gold, M. R. (1993). Health insurance and mortality. Evidence from a national cohort. *Journal of the American Medical Association, 270*, 737–741.

Guterman, S. (1998). The Balanced Budget Act of 1997: Will hospitals take a hit on their PPS margins? *Health Affairs, 17*, 159–166.

Hacker, J. S. (1997). *The road to nowhere.* Princeton, NJ: Princeton University Press.

Hadley, J., & Cunningham, P. (2004). Availability of safety net providers and access to care of uninsured persons. *Health Services Research, 39*(5), 1527–1546.

Hadley, J., & Holahan, J. (2004). *The cost of care for the uninsured: What do we spend, who pays, and what would full coverage add to medical spending?* Washington, DC: Kaiser Commission on Medicaid and the Uninsured.

Health Care and Education Affordability Reconciliation Act of 2010, H.R. 4872, 111th Cong. 2nd Sess. (2010). Retrieved March 30, 2010, from *docs.house/gov/rules/hr4872/111_hr4872_amndsub.pdf.*

Himmelstein, D. U., Warren, E., Thorne, D., & Woolhandler, S. (2005). MarketWatch: Illness and injury as contributors to bankruptcy. *Health Affairs, 25,* 63–73.

Holohan, J., & Spillman, B. (2002). *Health care access for uninsured adults: A strong safety net is not the same as insurance.* Washington, DC: Urban Institute.

Iglehart, J. K. (1994). Physicians and the growth of managed care. *New England Journal of Medicine, 331,* 1167–1171.

Institute of Medicine. (2002a). *Care without coverage: Too little, too late.* Washington, DC: National Academy Press.

Institute of Medicine. (2002b). *Unequal treatment: Confronting racial and ethnic disparities in health care.* Washington, DC: National Academy of Sciences.

Isenberg, S. F. (1998). *Managed care, outcomes, and quality: A practical guide.* New York: Thieme Medical Publishers.

Kaiser Commission on Medicaid and the Uninsured. (2006). *Health insurance coverage in America, 2006.* San Francisco: Author.

Kaiser Family Foundation. (2010). *Summary of new health reform law.* San Francisco: Author. Retrieved May 17, 2010, from *www.kff.org/healthreform/upload/8061.pdf.*

Lasser, K. E., Himmelstein, D. U., & Woolhandler, S. (2006). Access to care, health status, and health disparities in the United States and Canada: Results of a cross-national population-based survey. *American Journal of Public Health, 96,* 1300–1307.

Leibowitz, A., & Schlackman, N. (1996). Corporate managed care. *New England Journal of Medicine, 334,* 1060–1063.

Levit, K. R., Sensenig, A. L., Cowan, C. A., Lazenby, H. C., McDonnell, P. A., Won, D. K., et al. (1994). National health expenditures, 1993. *Health Care Financing Review, 16,* 247–294.

Lurie, N., Ward, N. B., Shapiro, M. F., & Brook, R. H. (1984). Termination from Medi-Cal: Does it affect health? *New England Journal of Medicine, 311,* 480–484.

Machlin, S. R. (2006). *Expenses for a hospital emergency room visit, 2003* (Statistical Brief No. 111). Rockville, MD: Agency for Healthcare Research and Quality.

Manning, W. G., Newhouse, J. P., Duan, N., Keeler, E. B., Leibowitz, A., & Marquis, M. S. (1987). Health insurance and the demand for medical care: Evidence from a randomized experiment. *American Economic Review, 77,* 251–277.

McWilliams, J. M., Meara, E., Zaslavsky, A. M., & Ayanian, J. Z. (2007a). Health of previously uninsured adults after acquiring Medicare coverage. *Journal of the American Medical Association, 298,* 2886–2894.

McWilliams, J. M., Meara, E., Zaslavsky, A. M., & Ayanian, J. Z. (2007b). Use of health services by previously uninsured Medicare beneficiaries. *New England Journal of Medicine, 357,* 143–153.

McWilliams, J. M., Zaslavsky, A. M., Meara, E., & Ayanian, J. Z. (2004). Health insurance coverage and mortality among the near-elderly. *Health Affairs, 23,* 223–233.

Mehr, R. I., Cammack, E., & Rose, T. (1985). *Principles of insurance* (8th ed.). Scarborough, ON, Canada: Richard D. Irwin.

Roby, D. H. (2006). *An analysis of the characteristics of health centers facing financial deficits.* Doctoral dissertation, George Washington University, Washington, DC.

Seifert, R. W., & Rukavina, M. (2006). Bankruptcy is the tip of a medical-debt iceberg. *Health Affairs, 25*(2), w89–w92.

Skinner, A. C., & Mayer, M. L. (2007). Effects of insurance status on children's access to specialty care: A systematic review of the literature. *BMC Health Services Research, 7,* 194. Retrieved March 30, 2010, from *www.biomedcentral.com/content/odf/1472-6963-7-194.pdf.*

United States Congressional Budget Office. (2010, March 18). Analysis of HR 4872 Reconciliation Act of 2010 for Speaker of the House Nancy Pelosi. Retrieved March 30, 2010, from *www.cbo.gov/ftpdcos/113xx/doc11355/hr4872.pdf.*

Wagner, E. H., Austin, B. T., Davis, C., Hindmarsh, M., Schaefer, J., & Bonomi, A. (2001). Improving chronic illness care: Translating evidence into action. *Health Affairs, 20,* 64–78.

Weissman, J. S. (2005). The trouble with uncompensated hospital care. *New England Journal of Medicine, 353,* 1171–1173.

Weissman, J. S., Dryfoos, P., & London, K. (1999). Income levels of bad-debt and free-care patients in Massachusetts hospitals. *Health Affairs, 18,* 156–166.

Wilper, A. P., Woolhandler, S., Lasser, K. E., McCormick, D., Bor, D. H., & Himmelstein, D. U. (2008). A national study of chronic disease prevalence and access to care in uninsured U.S. adults. *Annals of Internal Medicine, 149,* 170–176.

Zwanziger, J., & Melnick, G. A. (1996). Can managed care plans control health care costs? *Health Affairs, 15,* 185–199.

CHAPTER 22

Health Services Research

Alison K. Herrmann

Health services research is a multidisciplinary field concerned with the delivery of health care and the effects of care on individuals and communities. AcademyHealth, the primary organization bridging health research and policy, defines "health services research" as

> the multidisciplinary field of scientific investigation that studies how social factors, financing systems, organizational structures and processes, health technologies, and personal behaviors affect access to health care, the quality and cost of health care, and ultimately our health and well-being. Its research domains are individuals, families, organizations, institutions, communities, and populations. (2009; *www.academyhealth.org*)

The Agency for Healthcare Quality and Research (AHRQ) is the government agency most clearly aligned with health services research. It was originally established as the Agency for Healthcare Policy and Research (AHCPR) within the U.S. Department of Health and Human Services (DHHS) in 1989. The agency was reauthorized, in 1999, as AHRQ. The official mission of AHRQ is to support research designed to improve the quality, safety, efficiency, and effectiveness of health care for all Americans. The research sponsored, conducted, and disseminated by AHRQ provides information that helps people make better decisions about health care. (2001)

The main goals of health services research are to identify the most effective ways to organize, manage, finance, and deliver high-quality care, reduce medical errors, and improve patient safety (AHRQ, 2002). To achieve these goals, health services researchers conduct both basic and applied investigations of organization, delivery, financing, access, use, quality, costs, and outcomes of health care services. In addition to physical health, health services researchers aim to understand mental and dental health. As such, health services research encompasses the full range of the health care spectrum, increasing knowledge and understanding of the structure, processes, and effects of health services for individuals and populations (Institute of Medicine [IOM], 1994).

Health services research is multidisciplinary. Investigations are guided by theories, instruments, methods, and conceptual models from a range of disciplines, including social and behavioral epidemiology, sociology, political science, economics, management, medicine, nursing, psychology, and biostatistics. Researchers use a wide variety of experimental and quasi-experimental designs to analyze information obtained from large epidemiological datasets, administrative data, and primary data collection. Investigations focus on personal behaviors, social factors, and organizational structures and processes. Findings inform both health care practice and health policy. Health services researchers work in diverse settings, including academia, government agencies, policy consortiums, and clinical settings.

The field of health services research has grown tremendously in recent years. The National Center for Health Services Research (NCHSR) was established less than 50 years ago, in 1968. In 1970, the IOM was established to examine issues affecting public health, and today the IOM is perhaps the most important voice for studies relevant to health services issues.

This chapter provides a broad introduction to health services research, offering an overview of the structural factors of the health care system evaluated in health services research. Four major focus areas of health services research are reviewed: access, quality, cost, and outcomes. Health care access is addressed first, including a discussion of Andersen's behavioral model of health services. Next, issues related to health care quality are considered, including a brief review of the classic Donabedian model, followed by a focus on the issue of health care cost, along with an overview of cost-effectiveness analysis. Finally, the study of health care outcomes is reviewed, including an introduction to the emerging field of comparative effectiveness research. Examples of published research relevant to each area are provided. For explanatory purposes, these major focus areas within health services research are addressed in turn. However, as described previously, health services research is actually conducted in an effort to understand the relationships among structure, access, quality, cost, and outcomes in the health care system. While this chapter focuses on the U.S. health care system, health services research takes place in a global context, with many investigations targeting issues related to international health systems, global health, and health in the developing world.

Structure of the Health Care System

Structural factors of the health care system include health care service providers and health care facilities. Health care financing mechanisms can also be thought of as a structural factor of the larger health care system. Health service research considers the impact of structural factors on health care access, quality, cost, and outcomes.

Health services researchers consider the influence that different types of health care providers, or groups of providers, have on health care. The DHHS identified major shortages in the health care workforce and projected that shortages will continue to increase. Health services researchers investigate the impact of these shortages on health care and health outcomes. Examples include study of the implications of shortages of medical personnel at community health centers in relation to capacity to provide health services to underserved populations (Rosenblatt, Andrilla, Curtin, & Hart, 2006) and investigation of the relationship between nursing home staffing levels and state Medicaid reimbursement rates (Harrington, Swan, & Carrillo, 2007). General examples of the types of health services research conducted in relation to health care providers include investigations of quality and outcomes of care provided by physicians versus nurse practitioners; the cost, quality, and outcomes of care provided by specialists versus generalists; patients' access to quality care, and their health care outcomes, in relation to the demographic characteristics of health care providers.

Health care facilities are another important structural factor considered by health services researchers. For example, differences in access, quality, cost, and outcomes of care provided at for-profit versus not-for-profit hospitals are foci of health services research. Other examples of health services research focused on health care facilities include investigations of the prevalence of community clinics and community health centers in relation to the health of community members; the influence of hospital and emergency room closures on the health status of communities; the geographic distribution of veterans' health care facilities; and the health of veterans in urban versus rural areas. Investigations of the influence of major policy changes on the health care system are another example of health services research related to health care facilities (e.g., see the Bazzoli, Lindrooth, Kang, & Hasnain-Wynia [2006] study of the impact of the Balanced Budget Act of 1997 on the function of the health care safety net).

A large proportion of health services research is focused on health services financing structure. The three most important federally funded programs include Medicare, a program administered by the federal government that focuses on people 65 and older; Medicaid, a program administered by states that concentrates on the blind, the disabled, and families with dependent children; and the Children's Health Insurance Program (CHIP). These programs are continuously evaluated by health services researchers. Managed care versus fee-for-service health care providers and health systems are evaluated in relation to health care access, quality, cost, and outcomes. Variations in publicly funded versus individually purchased versus employer-provided insurance coverage are widely investigated. Research related to health services financing structures frequently is used to inform political debates regarding health care reform.

In addition to evaluating the influence of individual structural components of the health care system, health services researchers conduct important investigations related to the coordination of care across the health care system. Investigations have demonstrated that the current structure of the U.S. health care system is generally associated with fragmented care, which results in low efficiency, high cost, poor quality, and poor outcomes. Evaluations of potential solutions to discontinuities in the health care system, such as improved health information technology systems, are also the domain of health services researchers.

Health services research commonly addresses relationships among structures of the health care system. In the next sections we consider the core areas of health services research: access, quality, cost, and outcomes. The discussion begins with a consideration of health care access.

Access

Access to health care includes everything that facilitates or impedes the use of health care services, as well as the actual use of services (Andersen & Davidson, 2007). "Access" is commonly defined in terms of potential, as well as actual, entry of a population into the health care system. Utilization is an important component of access, and utilization rates are often the focus of investigations of health services access. A comprehensive evaluation of access however, considers the correlation among need, demand, and utilization (Williams & Torrens, 2002).

Health services researchers commonly ask questions related to trends in access. Many large, national probability surveys, such as the National Health Interview Survey (NHIS), collect valuable information that enables health services researchers to investigate trends in access. Such trends serve as key indicators of changes in the ability of the health care system to meet the needs of the population (Andersen & Davidson, 1996).

Need, demand, and utilization of health services vary in relation to the characteristics of the population. At present, the U.S. population is becoming both older and more racially and ethnically diverse. These changes in population characteristics are important in the context of health services access. Hence, much health services research focuses on the relationship between demographic trends and their influence on health services access. Research along these lines informs decisions related to the structure of the health care system, as well as health care policy. In recent years, a significant amount of attention has focused on disparities in access experienced by diverse population groups, as described in the seminal IOM report *Unequal Treatment* (Smedley, Stith, & Nelson, 2002).

A common overall measure of health services access included in much health services research is whether an individual has a usual source of care (i.e., a relationship with a health care provider or some other connection to the health care system). Health services researchers most commonly measure this by asking individuals whether there is a place they usually go when they are sick or in need of advice about their health. Those who report having a usual source of care have better access to health care services

(Andersen, 1995). This single-item measure has been demonstrated to be a robust predictor of health status (Breslow, 2007).

Health insurance coverage also plays an important role in health services research because it enables utilization by providing financial access to health services (IOM, 2001a). Additionally, it is widely recognized that individuals' resources, wants, and needs influence potential and actual access to health services. System-level factors, such as waiting time, business hours, and cultural competency of care, also influence health services access.

Multiple complex models of access to health care, most with economic and behavioral components, have been developed by researchers. Models generally include individual- and community-level variables such as health beliefs, behaviors, knowledge, and resource availability, as well as population-level characteristics. The most widely cited framework for the study of health services access is the Andersen (1995) behavioral model of health services use. The multivariate model originally proposed by Andersen (1968), has undergone multiple modifications, with increasing recognition of the influence of the health care system and the health care environment. The version of the model presented by Andersen in 1995 is most commonly cited.

The Andersen model enables researchers to consider access in accordance with its multidimensional nature. The four major components of the model are predisposing characteristics, enabling resources, perceived need, and use of services. Potential access is measured by the enabling resources, which include contextual factors such as policy and financing, as well as individual-level factors such as insurance status, income, and regular source of care. Actual use of services is measured in terms of utilization. Predisposing characteristics and perceived need give recognition to the importance of individual- and community-level behavioral factors.

Access to health care has posed a challenge to our national health care system for many years. Currently, the lack of health insurance in nearly 15% of the U.S. population (nearly 47 million people) is a major driver in the political debate on health care reform. Using data from the Medical Expenditure Panel Surveys (MEPS), Hadley (2007) demonstrated that uninsured individuals receive less medical care and have poorer short-term changes in health than those with insurance following a new diagnosis or unintentional injury. Population characteristics associated with differential access to care have informed the policy debate, and much current research considers equity of health services access. Changes in policy, such as welfare reform, are also evaluated in relation to the impact of insurance coverage on specific population groups (e.g., Cawley, Schroeder, & Simon, 2006).

At previous points in our nation's history, federal legislation has been passed, and programs developed, to ensure health services access for particular population groups. Inasmuch as health insurance coverage ensures access to care, Medicare ensures access for older adult Americans and Medicaid ensures access for disabled Americans. Since the inception of these programs, health services researchers have been involved in their evaluation and the determination of whether the programs are achieving their goals, in terms of access and otherwise. In this way, health services research informs ongoing program development and change. Health services researchers will evaluate the impact of the changes introduced by national health care reform.

Research related to health services access enables prediction of the use of health services and promotion of social justice, and informs efforts to improve effectiveness and efficiency in health services delivery (Andersen & Davidson, 2007). It is recognized that access in and of itself is only one component of health services. To get a real sense of the value of health services access and to determine whether equity exists, quality must also be considered. The discussion now turns to a consideration of quality in health services research.

Quality

The IOM defines quality as "the degree to which health services for individuals and populations increase the likelihood of desired health outcomes and are consistent with current professional knowledge" (Lohr, 1990, p. 4). In keeping with this definition, good quality is understood to involve the provision of appropriate health services in a technically competent manner, with good communication, shared decision making, and cultural sensitivity. Poor quality, on the other hand, is understood to refer to both underuse and overuse of health care (Schuster, McGlynn, & Brook, 2005). Both implicit and explicit methods are important for the assessment of quality in health services (Brook, McGlynn, & Shekelle, 2000).

Health services are considered appropriate when expected health benefits exceed expected health risks by a wide enough margin to make the intervention or service worth doing. Appropriateness is generally considered in relation to particular clinical and/or personal characteristics. Health services are considered necessary when there is a reasonable chance of a nontrivial benefit to the recipient of services, and when it would be ethically unacceptable not to provide the service (Schuster et al., 2005).

Donabedian (1980) developed the classic paradigm for investigations of health care quality. The Donabedian model evaluates quality in terms of the structure, process, and outcomes of health care. Characteristics of physicians and hospitals are structural, whereas process includes the components of the health care encounter, and outcomes refer to changes in health status. Studies of process in relation to quality appear most frequently in the published literature (Schuster et al., 2005). Examples of this type of research include prospective investigation of the association between ambulatory process of care and health-related quality of life (Kahn et al., 2007); evaluation of adherence to clinical practice guidelines for depression using patient self-report data (Hepner et al., 2007); and analysis of videotaped office visits with primary care providers to evaluate visit length in relation to health issues presented (Tai-Seale, McGuire, & Zhang, 2007). Health services researchers also evaluate the impact of changes to the healthcare delivery and financing system on quality of care.

Quality issues have been a major focus area of the IOM over the past decade. Health service research informed the conclusions and recommendations included in the seminal report *Crossing the Quality Chasm* (IOM, 2001b), as well as the report (Adams & Corrigan, 2003) entitled *Priority Areas for National Action: Transforming Health Care Quality*. The IOM report considers how the health system could be reformed through innovation to improve the delivery of care, and the 2003 report by Adams and Corrigan recommends priority focus areas for overall improvement of quality of health care in the United States.

Health services research related to quality includes investigations of the level of quality of care provided at particular facilities, in specific service groups, within a geographic region, or to a particular population. In 2003, McGlynn and colleagues concluded that adult patients in the United States were receiving only 55% of recommended care. Studies on quality often produce results that those outside of the health care field do not expect. For example, pubic health care systems such as the Veterans Health Administration (VA) are often assumed to be of lower quality than private facilities. But systematic analysis has demonstrated that VA patients are more likely to receive recommended care than other patients in the national sample (Asch et al., 2004).

In a now famous study, Schulman and colleagues (1999) demonstrated that physicians' recommendations vary in relation to patients' gender and race. More recently, variations both between and within physicians recommending cancer screening depend on patient race/ethnicity and socioeconomic characteristics, with the largest differences observed within physicians (Bao, Fox, & Escarce, 2007). Little relationship was found however, between racial disparities and overall quality of care delivered through Medicare health plans, based on Health Plan Employer and Data Information Set (HEDIS) measures (Trivedi, Zaslavsky, Schneider, & Ayanian, 2006).

The widely recognized work of John Wennberg (2008) and his colleagues at the Dartmouth Atlas Project has demonstrated that the amount and cost of health care delivered varies widely across the United States, and that neither more care nor more expensive care is associated with higher quality care. A recent study of care provided within the United States illustrated wide regional- and state-level variations in both the amount and cost of care provided for the same health conditions, and revealed care to be as good, or better, in the lower cost areas. Patients in areas where less is spent fare about as well as patients in areas where more money is spent, and there is some suggestive evidence that people living in areas where health care is more expensive have poorer health outcomes. These results are systematically adjusted for disease burden, age, race, and socioeconomic status (Fisher, Bynum, & Skinner, 2009).

The association between quality and cost of care is a major focus of health services research. Quality-based payment strategies, such as pay for performance targeting both individual physicians and medical groups, have been evaluated by health services researchers as a means of bridging the quality and cost gap (e.g., Robinson et al., 2009). Aaron and Ginsburg (2009) highlight the complexities inherent in reducing spending without sacrificing the current state of quality. Having addressed the issue of quality of care, the discussion now turns to the topic of research related to health care cost.

Cost

Measurement of health care costs and expenditures, evaluation of trends in costs and spending, and projections related to future spending play an important role in much of health services research. The high, and rising, cost of health care in the United States is believed by many to threaten the future of the health care system, as well as the larger national economy. Both within the United States, and in international comparisons, it

is recognized, as noted earlier, that the most expensive care is not the best care. Health services researchers lead efforts to understand the drivers and consequences of health care costs, as well as to evaluate potentially viable methods for widespread cost control in the health care system.

In 2009, health care spending is expected to account for nearly 18% of the U.S. gross domestic product (GDP) (Siska et al., 2009). Spending on health care more than tripled between 1990 and 2007 (Centers for Medicare and Medicaid Services [CMS], 2009) and is higher in the United States than in all other industrialized countries (Organisation for Economic Co-operation and Development [OECD], 2009). The trend in U.S. health care spending as a percentage of GDP is depicted, from 1960 to 2005, and in relation to other industrialized countries in Figure 22.1. Efforts to control the growth of costs is a major political priority, fueled by concerns that individuals, employers, and the government are not capable of keeping pace with rising costs.

Health services researchers have demonstrated a significant association between rising health care costs and diminished insurance coverage (Kaiser Family Foundation [KFF], 2009b). The primary reason cited for a lack of insurance coverage in national surveys is the cost of coverage (KFF, 2009b). Over the last decade, employer-sponsored

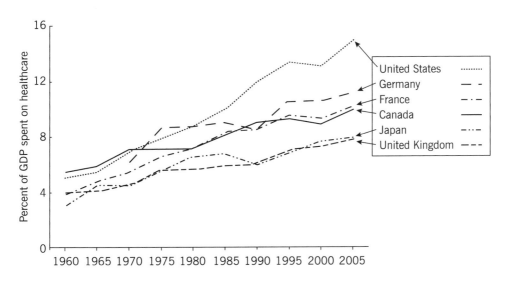

FIGURE 22.1. Health care spending as a percentage of gross domestic product: Selected countries, 1960–2005. From Garber and Skinner (2008). Copyright 2008 by the American Economic Association. Reprinted by permission.

health insurance premiums increased at four times the rates of inflation and wages (KFF, 2009a). These increases have made it challenging for many employers to provide insurance, resulting in increases in employees' share of spending or discontinuation of coverage altogether. Figure 22.2 illustrates the relationship between trends in health care spending and uninsured rates among workers. Per capita health spending is divided by the median income as a rough adjustment for inflation. Between 1979 and 2007, these two variables tracked almost perfectly. The most likely explanation is that employers, when faced with rising health care costs, may choose to abandon providing coverage for their employees. When significant portions of premiums are used to cover ineffective services, there may be little effect in terms of health outcomes. Yet costs increase, and as shown in Figure 22.2, the uninsured rate goes up. Thus, the end result of higher health care costs might be reduced population health status.

Even among insured individuals, the high cost of health care is cause for concern. Recent findings demonstrated that 62% of 2007 bankruptcies could be linked to medi-

cal expenses, and almost 80% of those who filed had health insurance coverage (Himmelstein, Thorne, Warren, & Woolhander, 2009).

Among the major sources of high and increasing health care costs considered by health services researchers are prescription drugs and technology, chronic disease rates, the increasing age of the national population, and administrative costs. Some health services researchers argue that the cost of developing new prescription drugs and health care technologies, and the high consumer demand for these costly new products drive the overall cost of care (Congressional Budget Office, 2008). A more significant body of research, however, supports the view that chronic disease rates are driving increasing health care costs.

The U.S. health care system was developed to treat acute illness, and increasing rates of chronic disease witnessed over the course of the past century have significantly challenged the system. It is estimated that health care costs associated with the treatment of chronic disease account for over 75% of national health expenditures (Centers for Disease Control and Prevention

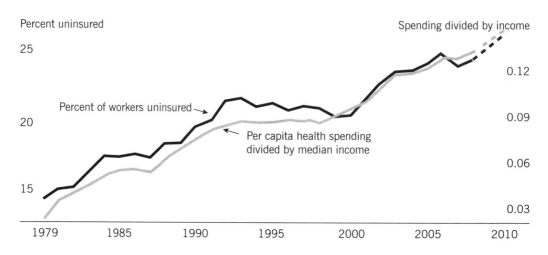

FIGURE 22.2. Uninsurance rate (%) among workers and per capita health spending divided by median income, 1979–2007, and projected, 2008–2010. From Gilmer and Kronick (2009). Copyright 2009 by Project HOPE/*Health Affairs*. Reprinted by permission. The figure presents Gilmer and Kronick's analysis of data from the Current Population Survey, March supplements; Annual Demographics Files, 1980–2008; and Centers for Medicare and Medicaid Services, National Health Accounts, 1979–2007. Percentage uninsured (black line) relates to the left-hand y axis. Per capita spending divided by median income (gray line) relates to the right-hand y axis. The series for workers is restricted to those not covered as a dependent or by a public program. Projected uninsurance and spending divided by income are denoted by dashed lines. Data for 1980 were not available.

[CDC], 2009). Finkelstein, Trogdon, Cohen, and Dietz (2009) estimated that increased prevalence of obesity alone is responsible for almost $40 billion increased medical spending in the United States through 2006, and argue that large, systemwide savings could be realized through reduction of obesity and related health risk factors.

The aging of the national population contributes to both the demand for new prescription drugs and health care technology and increasing rates of chronic disease. It is understood that health care expenses rise with age. Yet experts generally agree that aging of the population contributes only minimally to high rates of growth in health care spending (Orszag, 2008). A significant amount of health services research focuses, however, on issues associated with shifting costs from the private to the public sector as an increasing proportion of the population is eligible for Medicare. Health services researchers at the Social Security and Medicare Board of Trustees (2009) correctly estimated that expenditures in 2009 would exceed revenues of Medicare's Hospital Insurance Trust Fund.

Fortunately, public programs, including Medicare, demonstrate better administrative cost control than that demonstrated in the private sector. Over 7% of all private health care expenditures are estimated to be administrative, compared with less than 2% in the public sector (KFF, 2005). Health services researchers at McKinsey and Company (2008) estimated that $186 billion of the excess health care spending in the United States, as compared with other industrialized nations, is due to high administrative costs. Overall, the role of administrative costs associated with the combined public–private health care system is an important consideration for health services researchers.

A major challenge inherent to investigations of health care costs in the United States is that the private insurers are not required to collect or release information about their expenditures. The primary data source for U.S. health care spending is produced by the Office of the Actuary of the CMS at the DHHS. Data on developed and developing nations also are frequently used to further efforts better to understand U.S. health care spending in relation to other countries. The OECD collects and reports international health care cost data.

Health services researchers use these and other data, such as hospital discharge records, to evaluate the effectiveness of different cost containment mechanisms. For example, costs incurred via the traditional fee-for-service system might be compared with costs incurred under managed care or other capitated service mechanisms. Miller (2009) suggested that bundling services would increase providers' ability to control costs compared with traditional fee-for-service billing. "Bundling" groups related health care services for billing as a single episode of care as opposed to billing separately for each distinct component of service provided (Luft, 2009). Both capitation and bundled billing are key components of major national health care reform proposals currently considered by Congress.

As the need to contain health care costs in the United States has become more readily apparent, the promise of cost-effectiveness analysis (CEA) as a rational way of allocating limited health care resources has gained increased attention and support. One of the major health care problems is that there are so many attractive alternatives. All providers want payment for the services they offer. The difficulty is that there is simply not enough money to pay for all of the alternatives. On the other hand, many of the services offer little benefit. The Congressional Budget Office, for example, estimates that about one-third of the services for which Medicare pays have little or no benefit (Orszag, 2008). That amounts to expenditures of about $700 billion each year in the United States! CEA uses economic principles to consider competing alternatives and to compare their relative costs and effectiveness. While many countries incorporate this economic approach in their efforts to maximize population health, the idea has traditionally met with strong opposition in the United States.

CEA can be used to inform health care decision making, specifically with regard to which care should be provided. The method compares the costs and effectiveness of treatment alternatives to produce a ratio of the change in cost divided by the change in effectiveness: the incremental cost-effectiveness ratio (ICER). Treatment alternatives that produce the greatest efficacy for the least cost, or the smallest ICER, are favored.

A standard measure of intervention effectiveness, the quality-adjusted life year

(QALY), compares interventions across different health conditions. QALYs are an adaptation of traditional survival analysis that considers how long people live. In survival analysis, each year of completed life is scored as 1.0. One essentially gets a point for each year one lives. In adjusted survival analysis, survival time is adjusted for lost quality of life. A year spent in pain might be scored as a half-year to account for the loss in life quality. To derive the QALY associated with a particular health condition, a utility rating that represents quality of life is ascribed to the health state. The convention in determining utility ratings for healthy individuals is to rate different health states on a scale of 0 (death) to 1 (perfect health). Utility ratings are adjusted for the amount of time spent in the health state to produce the final QALY rating for use in the cost-effectiveness equation. QALYs are the product that results from multiplying the utility rating ascribed to a health state by the amount of time spent in that state.

QALYs are used to describe the effect of a health intervention in terms of the number of quality-adjusted life years it provides. The ICER is derived by dividing differences in intervention costs by the difference in QALYs produced by the intervention. Therefore, the ICER presents a means of comparing the cost-effectiveness of interventions across health conditions. When a societal perspective is taken in determining the costs that enter into the equation, CEA provides a rational means of determining how best to allocate health care resources to ensure that the greatest amount of societal health is obtained for the investment.

QALYs are one means of measuring health care outcomes. CEA involves consideration of the relationships between health care costs and outcomes. The discussion now turns from cost to focus on outcomes in health services research.

Outcomes

Outcomes include everything that happens as a result of receipt of health care. Outcomes considered by health services researchers include mortality and clinical variables, as well as health-related quality of life (HRQL). In comparative effectiveness, an emerging field of health services research, outcomes obtained in association with different interventions or treatments are compared. The breadth of health care outcomes research corresponds to the World Health Organization's (WHO; 1948) definition that specifies "health" as more than the mere absence of disease, but rather as complete physical, mental, and social well-being.

The Donabedian (1980) model is commonly used to understand how structure and process of care are associated with health care outcomes. Many of the large epidemiological studies by health services researchers focus on mortality outcomes and other clinical variables, both generally and in relation to specific health conditions. HRQL measures are used by health services researchers for observational studies, clinical trials, clinical practice, as well as population and population subgroup monitoring.

HRQL describes well-being, health, and ability to perform functions of daily living from an individual's own perspective, taking into account his or her health status (Ganz, Litwin, Hays, & Kaplan, 2007). The QALY, which combines length and quality of life, is one of many mechanisms available to health services researchers for the study of HRQL. Various decision mechanisms are available for calculating HRQL ratings; many health services researchers use direct preference measures, such as standard gambles and time trade-offs, while others prefer indirect preference measures, such as the Quality of Well-Being Scale (QWB; Kaplan, Ganiats, Sieber, & Anderson, 1998). The "standard gamble" is the classic method of assessing preferences; it conforms to economic utility theory and incorporates uncertainty by asking respondents to choose between a certain outcome and a gamble. In a "time trade-off" paradigm, individuals choose between two certain outcomes, trading years of life for quality of life. The time trade-off is often selected due to its ease of administration in comparison to the standard gamble. The QWB summarizes HRQL in QALYs, incorporating individuals' ratings of their abilities related to physical activity, mobility, and social activity, as well as their health symptoms or problems.

Health services research focused on outcomes provides important information related to health disparities, efficacy of health interventions, and the impact of policy changes on health status. In 1985, health services researchers working on the DHHS Task Force on Black and Minority Health identified a significant excess in deaths among racial/ethnic minority populations in the United States after controlling for age and gender, as well as significant, large, and persistent gaps in the health status of Americans in relation to race/ethnicity (CDC, 1986). This early work led to widespread efforts to eliminate racial/ethnic health disparities in the United States. Today, health services researchers continue to evaluate overall levels of mortality and morbidity in relation to race/ethnicity. In addition, researchers evaluate the complex relationships associated with disparities in health outcomes, such as the relationship between education and race/ethnicity and all-cause mortality (Jemal, Thun, Ward, et al., 2008), and with cancer mortality (Albano et al., 2007). Other investigations consider disparities in outcomes associated with specific health conditions (e.g., Spertus, Safley, Garg, Jones, & Peterson, 2005).

Beyond determining the factors associated with various health outcomes, health services researchers evaluate the efficacy of interventions targeting health outcomes. The Diabetes Prevention Program (DPP) provides an example of health services research that evaluates a health outcome in relation to an intervention (see Ratner, 2006, for a complete DPP summary). At the onset of the intervention, the DPP randomized 3,800 participants at risk of developing diabetes to intensive lifestyle changes, standard lifestyle plus drug treatment, or standard lifestyle plus placebo. Researchers determined that both intensive lifestyle change and drug treatment were associated with a significant reduction in risk of developing diabetes compared with placebo. Additionally, it was determined that the intensive lifestyle change was associated with a comparably greater risk reduction than drug treatment. Outcome evaluation of the DPP also included CEA, and both intensive lifestyle change and drug treatment were found to be cost-effective methods for delaying or preventing the onset of diabetes.

Policy changes can also function as health interventions. Health services researchers are often called upon to support advocacy efforts and, subsequently, to evaluate the impact of policy changes on health outcomes. Major policy changes related to tobacco as a result of the Master Settlement Agreement signed by the tobacco industry in 1998 are examples of health services outcome research related to policy changes.

Health services researchers were instrumental in providing data related to poor health outcomes associated with tobacco use that fueled the policy process, ultimately leading to widespread policy change. Today, the work of health services researchers continues to inform tobacco control policy. Researchers at the American Cancer Society, the CDC, the National Cancer Institute, and the North American Association of Cancer Registries collaborate to report yearly on trends in tobacco use, tobacco control, and lung cancer (Jemal, Thun, Ries, et al., 2008). Other researchers conduct investigations of tobacco policies' impact on health outcomes. For example, Tengs, Osgood, and Lin (2001) evaluated the public health impact of changes in smoking behavior associated with tobacco policy, while Rodu and Cole (2001) evaluated lung cancer mortality in relation to antismoking campaigns. The work of health services researchers will continue to be important in evaluating the health impact of past and future tobacco control policies enacted at local, state, and national levels.

As researchers work to evaluate health outcomes, increasing recognition has been given to the importance of knowing which treatments and interventions are associated with the best outcomes. When competing alternatives are evaluated, and the results of these investigations are widely disseminated, evidence-based treatments with the best possible outcomes can be advocated by individuals, organizations, and policymakers. The recognized value of this type of information has generated support for comparative effectiveness research.

Comparative Effectiveness Research

The United States leads the world in investing in biomedical research and health care, but the pace of translating new knowledge into actual clinical care and improvements in human health too often lags behind the pace of gains in new knowledge. Despite advances in knowledge and treatments for many conditions, recent reports suggest substantial gaps in available knowledge on the comparative effectiveness of many common practices in health care, and even where evidence is well-documented, only a small amount of that knowledge is consistently applied in actual practice.

The IOM of the National Academies of Science suggests that between one-third and one-half of all expenditures on health care do not contribute to better health. In 2008, the Congressional Budget Office released a report suggesting that health care is the most inefficient sector in our economy. We spend over $2 trillion per year on health care, and about $700 billion is spent on services that have little or no effect. If we could eliminate these services, we could pay for the Wall Street bail out every year!

Included in President Obama's 2009 stimulus package was $1.1 billion for comparative effectiveness research. The money will be used for a federal coordinating Council for Comparative Clinical Effectiveness Research. This group will oversee studies on health outcomes, review medical literature, and evaluate the effectiveness of treatments. The AHRQ defines comparative effectiveness research (CER) as "the conduct and synthesis of research comparing the benefits and harms of different interventions and strategies to prevent, diagnose, treat and monitor health conditions in 'real world' settings."

Comparative effectiveness studies might compare the effects of similar treatments, such as competing drugs, or analyze very different approaches, such as medical versus behavioral treatment of depression. CER compares a wide range of interventions, including any potential medical or behavioral interventions. These can be prognostic, preventive, diagnostic, therapeutic, or palliative.

It is widely known that much of what is done in medicine does not make patients better. CER systematically compares the efficacy and value of different treatment alternatives. It will allow us to identify services that do good and separate them from services that produce little benefit or even produce harm.

Unfortunately, we do not always get value for the money we spend on health care. For each dollar we spend on health care, the United Kingdom spends the equivalent of $.40. Yet people in the United Kingdom live longer than those in the United States, the British have a lower infant mortality rate, and all other indicators suggest that they are at least as healthy, if not healthier, than Americans. In fact, our excessive health care spending may be making us less healthy.

Not everyone likes the idea of comparative effectiveness. In particular, many fear that this type of research could affect the way health care is delivered and, of course, the income of providers. The American Heart Association, for example, expressed concern that CER could be used to control costs. The Pharmaceutical Research and Manufacturers of America Association argued that the bill that authorized CER had offending language that would limit "patient choice." What they really mean is not patient choice, but rather "doctor choice." In the current practice of medicine, many patients have little say in the selection of their treatments. Comparative effectiveness analysis might limit doctors choices of more expensive but less effective medications for their patients. However, a central tenet is that information be made available to both providers and patients, and that better-informed patients can play a greater role in selecting the treatments they receive.

CER has also been attacked as "rationing." Opponents argue that economically attractive alternatives will be rationed over the preferred products. The rationing argument fails to recognize that we are currently rationing health care. We do not necessarily ration services. Instead, we ration people by allowing the system to exclude nearly 50 million individuals.

CER, then, is associated with not only health care outcomes, but also access to health care. It also has been demonstrated that CER is associated with issues related to cost and quality of health services. As such, CER is an excellent example of health services research; CER is conducted in an effort to clarify relationships among access, quality, cost, and outcomes in the health care system.

Conclusions

This chapter has provided an introduction to the multidisciplinary field of health services research. Structural factors of the health system were reviewed, including providers, facilities, and financing. Major focus areas within the field of health services research were then described in some detail, including access, quality, cost, and outcomes. An overview was provided of the most commonly referenced theoretical frameworks in health services research: The Andersen behavioral model of health services use (1995) and the Donabedian model (1980). CEA and CER were also introduced.

As demonstrated in the examples provided, health services investigations focus on personal behaviors, social factors, and organizational structures and processes. Health services researchers seek to understand the nature of the relationships among the structure of the health care system, access to care, quality of care, cost of care, and outcomes of care. The findings of health services investigations are used to guide health care practice and policy. Results of health services investigations promise to serve as a valuable tool as we embark upon national health care reform.

Further Reading

Andersen, R. M., Rice, T. H., & Komiski, G. F. (Eds.). (2007). *Changing the U.S. health care system* (3rd ed.). San Francisco: Jossey-Bass.

Kennedy P. (2003). *A guide to econometrics* (5th ed.). Malden, MA: Blackwell.

Long, J. S. (1997). *Advanced quantitative techniques in the social sciences: Vol. 7. Regression models for categorical and limited dependent variables.* Thousand Oaks, CA: Sage.

Shi, L. (2008). *Health services research methods* (2nd ed.). Clifton Park, NY: Thomson/Delmar Learning.

Williams, J., & Torrens, P. (2002). *Introduction to health services* (6th ed.). Albany, NY: Delmar.

Wooldridge, J. M. (2006). *Introductory econometrics: A modern approach* (3rd ed.). Mason, OH: Thomson/South-Western.

The following leading health services journals are available online:

Health Affairs (available at *www.healthaffairs.org*)

Health Services Research (available at *www.hsr.org*)

Additional online resources:

AcademyHealth (*www.academyhealth.org*)
Commonwealth Fund (*www.commonwealthfund.org*)
Kaiser Family Foundation (*www.kff.org*)

References

Aaron, H. J., & Ginsburg, P. B. (2009). Is health care spending excessive?: If so, what can we do about it? *Health Affairs, 28*(5), 1260–1275.

AcademyHealth. (2009). What is health services research? Retrieved October 10, 2009, from *www.academyhealth.org.*

Adams, K., & Corrigan, J. M. (Eds.). (2003). *Priority areas for national action: Transforming health care quality* (Institute of Medicine Committee on Identifying Priority Areas for Quality Improvement, Board on Health Care Services). Washington, DC: National Academies Press.

Agency for Healthcare Research and Quality (AHRQ). (2001). *AHRQ profile.* Retrieved October 9, 2009, from *www.ahrq.gov/about/profile.htm.*

Agency for Healthcare Research and Quality (AHRQ). (2002). *Helping the nation with health services research* (Fact sheet, AHRQ Publication No. 02-P014). Washington, DC: U.S. Department of Health and Human Services.

Albano, J. D., Ward, E., Jemal, A., Anderson, R., Cokkinides, V. E., Murray, T., et al. (2007). Cancer mortality in the United States by education and race. *Journal of the National Cancer Institute, 99*(18), 1384–1394.

Andersen, R. M. (1968). *Behavioral model of families' use of health services* (Research Series No. 25). Chicago: Center for Health Administration Studies, University of Chicago.

Andersen, R. M. (1995). Revisiting the behavioral model and access to medical care: Does it matter? *Journal of Health and Social Behavior, 36,* 1–10.

Andersen, R. M., & Davidson, P. (1996). Measuring access and trends. In R. M. Andersen, T. H. Rice, & G. F. Kominiski (Eds.), *Changing the U.S. health care system* (pp. 13–40). San Francisco: Jossey-Bass.

Andersen, R. M., & Davidson, P. L. (2007). Improving access to care in America: Individual contextual indicators. In R. M. Andersen, T. H. Rice, & G. F. Komiski (Eds.), *Changing the U.S. health care system* (3rd ed., pp. 3–32). San Francisco: Jossey-Bass.

Asch, S. M., McGlynn, E. A., Hogan, M. M., Hayward, R. A., Shekelle, P., Rubenstein, L., et al. (2004). Comparison of quality of care for patients in the Veterans Health Administration and patients in a national sample. *Annals of Internal Medicine, 141*(2), 938–945.

Bao, Y., Fox, S. A., & Escarce, J. J. (2007). Socioeconomic and racial/ethnic differences in the discussion of cancer screening: "Between-" versus "within-" physician differences. *Health Services Research, 42*(3), 950–970.

Bazzoli, G. J., Lindrooth, R. C., Kang, R., & Hasnain-Wynia, R. (2006). The influence of health policy and market factors on the hospital safety net. *Health Services Research, 41*(4), 1159–1179.

Breslow, L. (2007, October 5). *A public health perspective on health.* Presentation at UCLA School of Public Health, Los Angeles, CA.

Brook, R. H., McGlynn, E. A., & Shekelle, P. G. (2000). Defining and measuring quality of care: A perspective from U.S. researchers. *International Journal for Quality in Health Care, 12,* 281–295.

Cawley, J., Schroeder, M., & Simon, K. I. (2006). How did welfare reform affect the health insurance coverage of women and children? *Health Services Research, 41*(2), 486–506.

Centers for Disease Control and Prevention. (1986). Perspectives in disease prevention and health promotion: Report of the Secretary's Task Force on Black and Minority Health. *Morbidity and Mortality Weekly Report, 35*(8), 109–112.

Centers for Disease Control and Prevention. (2009). *Chronic disease overview.* Atlanta, GA: Author. Retrieved October 17, 2009, from *www.cdc.gov/nccdphp/overview.htm.*

Centers for Medicare and Medicaid Services (CMS). (2009). *2007 National health care expenditures data.* (Office of the Actuary, National Health Statistics Group). Retrieved October 17, 2009, from *www.cms.hhs.gov/nationalhealthexpenddata/01_overview.asp?.*

Congressional Budget Office. (2008). *Technological change and the growth of health care spending* (Publication no. 2764). Washington, DC: Author.

Donabedian, A. (1980). *Exploration in quality assessment and monitoring: Vol. 1. The definition of quality and approaches to its assessment.* Ann Arbor, MI: Health Administration Press.

Finkelstein, E. A., Trogdon, J. G., Cohen, J. W., & Dietz, W. (2009). Annual medical spending attributable to obesity: Payer and service-specific estimates. *Health Affairs, 28*(5), w22–w831.

Fisher, E. S., Bynum, J. P., & Skinner, J. S. (2009). Slowing the growth of healthcare costs: Lessons from regional variation. *New England Journal of Medicine, 360*(9), 849–852.

Ganz, P. A., Litwin, M. S., Hays, R. D., & Kaplan, R. M. (2007). Measuring outcomes and health-related quality of life. In R. M. Andersen, T. H. Rice, & G. F. Komiski (Eds.), *Changing the U.S. health care system* (3rd ed.), pp. 185–212). San Francisco: Jossey-Bass.

Garber, A. M., & Skinner, J. (2008). Is American health care uniquely inefficient? *Journal of Economic Perspectives, 22*(4), 27–50.

Gilmer, T. P., & Kronick, R. G. (2009). Hard times and health insurance: How many Americans will be uninsured by 2010? *Health Affairs, 28*(4), w573–w577.

Hadley, J. (2007). Insurance coverage, medical care use, and short-term health changes following an unintentional injury or the onset of a chronic condition. *Journal of the American Medical Association, 297*(10), 1073–1084.

Harrington, C., Swan, J. H., & Carrillo, H. (2007). Nurse staffing levels and Medicaid reimbursement rates in nursing facilities. *Health Services Research, 42*(3), 1105–1129.

Hepner, K. A., Rowe, M., Rost, K., Hickey, S. C., Sherbourne, C. D., Ford, D. E., et al. (2007). The effect of adherence to practice guidelines on depression outcomes. *Annals of Internal Medicine, 147,* 320–329.

Himmelstein, D. U., Thorne, D., Warren, E., & Woolhander, S. (2009). Medical bankruptcy in the United States, 2007: Results of a national study. *American Journal of Medicine, 122,* 741–746. Retrieved October 15, 2009, from *www.pnhp.org/new_bankruptcy_study/Bankruptcy-2009.pdf.*

Institute of Medicine (IOM). (1994). *Health services research: Opportunities for an expanding field of inquiry—an interim statement.* Washington, DC: National Academy Press. Retrieved October 15, 2009, from *www.nap.edu/openbook.php?record_id=9242.*

Institute of Medicine (IOM). (2001a). *Committee on the Consequences of Uninsurance: Coverage matters: Insurance and health care.* Washington, DC: National Academy Press.

Institute of Medicine (IOM). (2001b). *Committee on Quality of Health Care in America: Crossing the quality chasm: A new health system for the 21st century.* Washington, DC: National Academy Press.

Jemal., A., Thun, M. J., Ries, L. A. G., Howe, H. L., Weir, H. K., Center, M. M., et al. (2008). Annual report to the nation on the status of cancer, 1975–2005, featuring trends in lung cancer, tobacco use, and tobacco control. *Journal of the National Cancer Institute, 100,* 1672–1694.

Jemal, A., Thun, M. J., Ward, E. E., Henley, S. J., Cokkinides, V. E., & Taylor, T. E. (2008). Mortality from leading causes by education and race in the United States, 2001. *American Journal of Preventive Medicine, 43*(1), 1–8.

Kahn, K. L., Tisnado, D. M., Adams, J. L., Liu, H., Chen, W., Hu, F. A., et al. (2007). Does ambulatory process of care predict health-related quality of life outcomes for patients with chronic disease? *Health Services Research, 42*(1), 63–83.

Kaiser Family Foundation (KFF). (2005). *Medicare Chart Book.* Retrieved October 15, 2009, from *www.kff.org/medicare/7284.cfm.*

Kaiser Family Foundation (KFF). (2009a). *Employee Health Benefits: 2009 Annual Survey.* Retrieved October 15, 2009, from *ehbs.kff.org.*

Kaiser Family Foundation (KFF). (2009b). *The uninsured: A primer, key facts about Americans without health insurance.* Retrieved October 15, 2009, from *www.kff.org/uninsured/upload/7451.pdf.*

Kaplan, R. M., Ganiats, T. G., Sieber, W. J., & Anderson, J. P. (1998). The Quality of Well-Being Scale: Critical similarities and differences with SF-36. *International Journal for Quality in Health Care, 10,* 509–520.

Lohr, K. N. (Ed.). (1990). *Medicare: A strategy for quality assurance.* Washington, DC: National Academy Press.

Luft, H. S. (2009). Health care reform: Toward more freedom, and responsibility, for physicians. *New England Journal of Medicine, 361,* 623–628.

McGlynn, E. A., Asch, S. M., Adams, J., Keesey, J., Hicks, J., DeCristofaro, A., et al. (2003). The quality of healthcare delivered to adults in the United States. *New England Journal of Medicine, 348*(26), 2635–2645.

McKinsey & Company. (2008). *Accounting for the cost of U.S. health care: A new look on why Americans spend more.* Retrieved October 18, 2009, from *www.mckinsey.com/mgi/publications/us_healthcare.*

Miller, H. D. (2009). From volume to value: Better ways to pay for health care. *Health Affairs, 28*(5), 1418–1428.

Organization for Economic Co-operation and Development (OECD). (2009). *Directorate for Employment, Labour, and Social Affairs: OECD Health Data, June 2009.* Retrieved October 27, 2009, from *www.oecd.org.*

Orszag, P. (2008, January 31). *Congressional Budget Office testimony: Growth in health care costs.* Delivered before the Committee on the Budget, United States Senate, Washington, DC.

Ratner, R. E. (2006). An update on the diabetes prevention program. *Endocrine Practice, 12*(1), 20–24.

Robinson, J. C., Shortell, S. M., Rittenhouse, D. R., Fernandes-Taylor, S., Gillies, R. R., & Casalino, L. P. (2009). Quality-based payment for medical groups and individual physicians. *Inquiry, 46,* 172–181.

Rodu, B., & Cole, P. (2001). Impact of the American anti-smoking campaign on lung cancer mortality. *International Journal of Cancer, 97*(6), 804–806.

Rosenblatt, R. A., Andrilla, H. A., Curtin, T., & Hart, G. (2006). Shortages of medical personnel at community health centers: Implications for planned expansion. *Journal of the American Medical Association, 295*(9), 1042–1049.

Schulman, K. A., Berlin, J. A., Harless, W., Kerner, J. F., Sistrunk, S., Gersh, B. J., et al. (1999). The effect of race and sex on physicians recommendations for cardiac catheterization. *New England Journal of Medicine, 340*(14), 618–626.

Schuster, M. A., McGlynn, E. A., & Brook, R. H. (2005). How good is the quality of health care in the United States? *Millbank Quarterly, 83*(4), 843–895.

Siska, A., Truffer, C., Smith, S., Keehan, S., Cylus, J., Poisal, J. A., et al. (2009). Health spending projections through 2018: Recession effects add uncertainty to the outlook. *Health Affairs, 28*(2), w346–w357.

Smedley, B. D., Stith, A. Y., & Nelson, A. R. (Eds.). (2002). *Unequal treatment: Confronting racial and ethnic disparities in health care.* Washington, DC: National Academy Press.

Social Security and Medicare Board of Trustees. (2009). A summary of the 2009 annual reports. Retrieved October 17, 2009, from *www.ssa.gov/oact/trsum/index.html.*

Spertus, J., Safley, D., Garg, M., Jones, P., & Peterson, E. D. (2005). The influence of race on health status outcomes one year after an acute coronary syndrome. *Journal of the American College of Cardiology, 46*(10), 1838–1844.

Tai-Seale, M., McGuire, T. G., & Zhang, W. (2007). Time allocation in primary care office visits. *Health Services Research, 42*(5), 1871–1894.

Tengs, T. O., Osgood, N. D., & Lin, T. H. (2001). Public health impact of changes in smoking behavior: Results from the tobacco policy model. *Medical Care, 39*(10), 1131–1141.

Trivedi, A. N., Zaslavsky, A. M., Schneider, E. C., & Ayanian, J. Z. (2006). Relationship between quality of care and racial disparities in Medicare health plans. *Journal of the American Medical Association, 296*(16), 1998–2004.

Wennberg, J. E. (2008). *Tracking the care of patients with severe chronic illness: The Dartmouth Atlas of Health Care.* Lebanon, NH: Trustees of Dartmouth College.

Williams, J., & Torrens, P. (2002). *Introduction to health services* (6th ed.). Albany, NY: Delmar.

World Health Organization [WHO]. (1948). *Constitution of the World Health Organization: Basic documents.* Geneva: Author.

CHAPTER 23

Primary Care and Prevention

JoEllen Patterson
Joseph E. Scherger
Ann Marie Smith

According to the Institute of Medicine (1996), most Americans initially seek health services from their primary care providers. Primary care is often thought of as first-contact care, including care administered in an emergency room, but the full definition extends further. *Primary care* consists of preventive services, treatment of common problems, and management of chronic disease. Primary care also includes continuity of care, or responsibility for the whole person over time. The providers of primary care address a range of physical and mental health care needs in an individual, and as such, these providers include family physicians, internists, pediatricians, obstetricians/gynecologists (OB/GYNs), nurse practitioners, physician assistants, and mental health clinicians.

Primary care is an important foundation of any organized health care system. Most industrialized countries endorse primary care, and primary care providers constitute at least 50% of all health care providers. In the United States, where specialization is emphasized, primary care providers represent only 35% of the health care workforce (Phillips, 2005). Due to the shortage

of primary care providers relative to patient demands, Americans often utilize specialists for certain health concerns rather than depend on their primary care physicians. Starfield, Shi, and Macinko (2005) argue that, for this reason, health care in the United States is far more expensive per capita than in other countries and yields inferior health outcomes.

Primary care in the United States is in trouble because fewer graduates of medical schools and other health professions schools choose to practice primary care due to low reimbursement and stressful work lives. High caseloads result in less time with patients, compounding the problem. In 2006, the American College of Physicians, representing internists, warned that primary care in the United States is at grave risk of collapse.

Numerous studies demonstrate the critical importance and value of primary care to any health system. Franks and Fiscella (1998) showed that a nationally representative sample of adults cared for by primary care physicians had thirty-three percent lower annual health care costs and lower mortality than people cared for only by specialists. The data were adjusted for demographic and health problems. Areas of the U.S. and other countries with more primary care physicians per capita have lower hospitalization rates and improved health outcomes than areas and countries with fewer primary care physicians. Of concern, multiple investigators have shown that a higher number of specialists per capita not only results in higher costs of care but also results in lower health outcomes (Starfield, Shi, Grover, & Macinko, 2005).

Leading primary care professional organizations have come together to propose a redefinition of the role of primary care as the personal medical home for patients (American Academy of Family Physicians [AAFP], 2008). The medical home model is much preferred over the "gatekeeper" concept used in managed care, which implies restriction of services. A "medical home" is a place patients can receive comprehensive, high-quality care, with the use of specialists as needed. In 2007, the American Academy of Family Physicians (AAFP), the American College of Physicians (ACP), the American Academy of Pediatrics (AAP), and the American Osteopathic Association (AOA) proposed reimbursement for the coordination of care over and above the provision of primary care services. Such increased reimbursement would come from savings achieved by having care coordinated by the medical home rather than the patient bouncing from one specialist to another. In addition, the stressful work life in primary care can be improved through the use of health information technology and team models of care, described in more detail below.

A large number of patient complaints seen in primary care have major psychosocial components. According to Petterson and colleagues (2008), studies have shown that up to 75% of patients treated in primary care have unrecognized psychosocial complaints that should be addressed. For approximately 50% of patients, the psychosocial issues are dominant. Thus, incorporating mental health providers into the primary care team enhances patient care and reduces costs (Petterson et al., 2008). The integration of mental health providers into primary care settings, called "collaborative primary care," would make generalist mental health providers a vital part of the primary medical home.

In spite of advocacy for collaborative mental health services, payment policy barriers currently prevent the full integration of mental health services. This is surprising because research by Petterson and colleagues (2008) suggests that patients with severe mental illnesses are at greater risk of developing life-threatening physical ailments. Colton indicates that public mental health patients die 25 years earlier than expected because they lack appropriate primary care (as cited in Petterson et al., 2008, p. 757). Failure to treat both physical and mental health illnesses results in poorer outcomes and higher costs. For example, the typical adult's medical care costs $1,913 annually. For this same adult, with a mental health condition, the cost would be approximately $3,545 per year (Petterson et al., 2008).

Prevention is a major component of primary care and speaks to the World Health Organization (WHO; 2007) definition of "health" as not just the absence of disease but a state of physical and emotional well-being. The role of preventive medicine is keeping people healthy. There is a dual focus to preventive care: promoting healthy lifestyle behaviors and early detection of problems, or health screening, to prevent more advanced disease. Immunizations are a third dimension of prevention.

From a public health perspective, prevention is divided into primary, secondary, and tertiary types. "Primary prevention" is preventing disease and illness from ever happening. Examples of primary prevention are efforts to promote a healthy lifestyle, such as not smoking, maintaining good nutrition and physical activity, and reducing stress. Immunizations are a means of primary prevention. Healthy relationships and pleasure at work also contribute to primary prevention.

"Secondary prevention" is early detection to prevent disease or illness from progressing. Examples include mammography for breast cancer, Papanicolaou (Pap) smears for cervical cancer, prostate-specific antigen (PSA) tests for prostate cancer, and blood pressure and lipid screenings for heart disease risk. Screening for depression, alcoholism, and other psychosocial problems would also be secondary prevention.

"Tertiary prevention" in patients with chronic illness prevents complications or progression of the disease. For example, in patients with diabetes, preventive efforts target avoiding eye disease, kidney failure, neuropathy, and vascular problems. Good tertiary prevention keeps people with chronic diseases as healthy as their disease permits. This includes psychosocial interventions.

Biology has only a small influence on prevention compared to other influences, for example, lifestyle behaviors. Indeed, Mokdad, Marks, Stroup, and Gerberding (2004) argued that 50–60% of premature disease and death is related to lifestyle behaviors. Funding, government policy, physician and patient knowledge and motivation, and business practices also play important roles. Many current initiatives to overhaul health care focus on these variables.

In fact, prevention resources and barriers to effective prevention in primary care may be quite different in the next few years because of changes in the U.S. health care system. A multitude of forces created the current U.S. system, one that focuses on disease, not illness; treatment, not prevention; and procedures, not education. As a result, the United States currently has one of the most expensive health care systems in the world, with mediocre health outcomes (Woolf, 2008). In addition, health care costs continue to rise each year. To ameliorate the situation, the National Committee for Quality Assurance (NCQA) created the new paradigm mentioned earlier, the patient-centered medical home, to promote comprehensive and coordinated care that includes a strong focus on prevention in conjunction with continuity of care (AAFP, 2008).

In addition to the primary medical home movement, numerous other initiatives have also focused on prevention. Funders and policymakers want to know whether evidence suggests that preventive measures make a difference in the health of patients. Usually these preventive measures include screening for illness, counseling for lifestyle decisions, and recommendations for use of supplements, such as vitamins or fluoride. Consequently, two different questions emerge:

1. Will the effort of the preventive intervention lead to positive outcomes?
2. Do we have evidence demonstrating the benefit?

The U.S. Preventive Services Task Force (USPSTF), now under the federal Agency for Healthcare Research and Quality (AHRQ), has been working since 1984 to answer these questions. Answers are necessary because, in some cases, a physician might hope that an intervention helps but have no systematic data on the question. As a result, the USPSTF is trying to create a more systematic approach to prevention.

The USPSTF, an independent panel of experts in primary care and prevention, systematically reviews the evidence of effectiveness and develops recommendations for preventive services.

> The USPSTF conducts rigorous, impartial assessments of the scientific evidence for the effectiveness of a broad range of clinical preventive services, including screening, counseling, and preventive medications. Its recommendations are considered the "gold standard" for clinical preventive services. (AHRQ, 2006, paragraph 1)

The recommendations from the USPSTF have formed the basis of the clinical standards for many health organizations and medical quality review groups. In addition to establishing the importance of prevention in primary care, the task force works to ensure insurance coverage for preventive services and supports primary care providers as they attempt to deliver effective care. For example, the task force publishes specific recommendations. Thus, an individual physician who wonders about a specific issue, such as screening for osteoporosis in women, can find easily accessible recommendations based on current evidence.

The USPSTF has made extensive use of technology and evidence-based guidelines. Technologies such as e-mail, video conferencing, and text messaging are being used to share recommendations with providers and to educate patients. In addition, novel uses of technology, such as sending reminders for routine screening, are currently being used. The first step of the process is to review the evidence about the value of a specific preventive intervention, including evaluation of risk. Recommendations are formed. Then, technology helps to educate providers and patients about specific recommendations.

Evidence-Based Practice Centers

Since 1997 the AHRQ has promoted evidence-based practice in everyday care. AHRQ established evidence-based practice centers (EPCs) that develop reports and technology assessments on preventive practices. Special focus is given to questions about costs and efficacy. The quality of evidence is evaluated as *Good, Fair,* or *Poor.* Goals of the AHRQ include synthesizing the evidence and facilitating the translation of evidence-based research into practical recommendations for prevention. Prevention topics can be suggested by both government and non-government partners, such as private insurers, medical groups, and health advocacy groups. Evidence-based findings are used to inform practice guidelines, quality assessment measures, educational materials, and future research agendas.

Once the evidence has been compiled, the USPSTF makes its recommendations based on explicit criteria. In essence, the task force evaluates the risk–benefit ratio of preventive care decisions. The evidence is graded on a continuum, so that recommendations range from *Strongly recommends* to *Recommends against.* There is also a category for insufficient evidence (Harris et al., 2001). Preventive recommendations are made in partnership with other federal agencies, such as the Centers for Disease Control and Prevention (CDC), and primary care organizations, such as the AAFP.

Health Information Technology and the Redesign of Primary Care

In July 2005, Michael Leavitt, Secretary of Health and Human Services in the U.S. declared the decade of health information technology (HIT). By 2014, all people should have an electronic health record (EHR). The entire health system is moving from paper-based systems to electronic systems capable of sharing patient records among providers and patients. The patient version of the EHR is the personal health record (PHR), and major digital companies such as WebMD, Revolution Health, Microsoft, and Google are racing to become the Web-based "medical home" for patients.

The developments in HIT have enormous implications for primary care and prevention. Knowledge of recommended preventive services is now readily available to everyone. As patients develop Web-based medical homes connected to their primary care medical homes, their customized preventive care recommendations will be on their home pages. Large medical groups, such as Kaiser, are having people coordinate their own preventive services and use reminders if they do not follow recommendations. As for behavior modification and lifestyle change, links to online services can be added to the medical home as well.

For the past 40 years, primary care has been delivered by a "make an appointment, come in for a visit" model of care. With HIT, a new "first tier" of health care interaction is emerging, in which patients communicate with their caregivers online. This new communication has been shown in pilot applications to reduce office visits by 20–25% (Lawrence, 2002). Innovative primary care practices such as GreenField Health (2008) in Portland, Oregon, encourage both online and telephone visits, and conduct 40–60% of patient care without visits. The primary care physicians and other providers see patients in the office selectively and have more time for these visits. Longer visits should result in greater satisfaction for both the provider and patient, and higher quality of service.

Another important component of HIT is clinical decision support (CDS). Physicians and other caregivers have mostly been working "off the top of their heads," only occasionally looking things up at the point of patient care. McGlynn and colleagues (2003) at the RAND Corporation showed that such care results in only about 55% of patients receiving current recommended care. As David Eddy has said, "The complexity of modern medicine exceeds the inherent limitations of an unaided human mind" (quoted in Millenson, 1997, p. 75). More advanced EHR systems are embedding CDS into the record to be available at the point of patient care. Such CDS systems include links to clinical guidelines each time a new problem is entered into the record, drug–drug and drug–disease interactions, electronic prescribing to avoid medication errors, and automatically completed prevention schedules, with reminders for each patient. HIT will soon be guiding the patient care process, and providers will not have to worry as much about memorizing medical knowledge.

Advanced EHR systems also have portals for secure and automatically documented communication for patients and for providers. Health care will be revolutionized in the 21st century when patients and all their providers share a common health record and communicate together regarding care. This is the new platform of communication and care, and face-to-face visits become selective rather than the dominant means of providing care.

Financially, models need to be developed to support online communication and care, and this is possible with the greater efficiency and higher quality of a continuous platform of care. Kaiser Health System, one of a few prepaid care plans, has launched just such a platform of care in nine states. Similarly, all of the major medical groups in the Minneapolis–St. Paul area offer "eVisits" as a new platform of care built into the EHR. There are now current procedural terminology (CPT) codes for online care, such as code 99444, which refers to a physician's online evaluation and management of a patient. Many major health insurers now cover this care. One study using online care showed that overall patient costs were reduced by more then $3.50 per member per month, with about two-thirds of the reduction being lower costs for the primary care visit (RelayHealth, 2002). To a health insurer, these are major savings, and primary care providers can be reimbursed for providing these savings.

The first rule of the redesign of care in the Institute of Medicine report *Crossing the Quality Chasm* (2001) states that care should be based on a continuous healing relationship and not on visits. HIT, with an online platform of communication and care, helps make patient care continuous as opposed to the late 20th century episodic "make an appointment, come and get it"

model of care. Technology in medicine can enhance doctor–patient relationships, not eliminate them.

Modern EHR systems have embedded CDS to help guide care. Guidelines for preventive medicine, including risk factors, are well known for children and adults of any age. Personalized clinical guidelines with reminders will become part of the medical record, shared by the patient and the care team. Thus, using these guidelines, people can coordinate their own preventive services and arrange for their own care.

Fortunately, numerous websites have organized preventive guidelines and education because looking for individual recommendations by reviewing the vast literature is not practical for the typical, busy primary care provider who sees approximately 20–25 patients per day. In addition, as the public has become more adept at searching the Internet, health educators have created user-friendly websites for patient education. Figure 23.1 shows a list of Internet resources recommended by the AHRQ. Nevertheless, primary care providers and expert panels need some categories to synthesize the vast literature. In general, recommendations for prevention are organized by the following categories: age, gender, ethnicity, pregnancy, sexual activity, and tobacco use. While the first three categories apply to all people, pregnancy, of course, is unique to women. Sexual activity and tobacco use are behavioral choices. In addition to these main categories, prevention research has also focused on the unique needs of special populations, including minorities, gays and lesbians, immigrants, rural patients, veterans, and others.

While it is beyond the scope of this discussion to cover every topic on prevention, the rest of this chapter utilizes the category of age to summarize the prevention literature. In addition, we briefly touch on other categories, such as current screening guidelines and healthy behaviors. The most important lifestyle factors relative to health are avoidance of tobacco use, good nutrition, physical activity, stress management, and pregnancy. In general, two questions are considered. At present, what critical areas of prevention have emerged based on the evidence-based guidelines? And, within a specific category, what recommendations, questions, imple-

Preventive Services Resource Links

Put Prevention into Practice

Tools and resources for implementing preventive services in clinical practice to help health care providers determine appropriate services and patients keep track of their preventive care.

Guide to Community Preventive Services

Evidence-based recommendations on the effectiveness and cost-effectiveness of essential community preventive health services.

Healthy People 2010

Continuation of the national prevention initiative Healthy People 2000.

National Guideline Clearinghouse™

Comprehensive database of evidence-based clinical practice guidelines and related documents.

Canadian Task Force on Preventive Health Care

Evidence-based recommendations on a wide variety of preventive health interventions.

Cancer Control P.L.A.N.E.T.

Web portal collaborative providing data and resources for evidence-based cancer control programs.

Steps to a Healthier U.S.

An initiative that advances the goal of helping Americans live longer, better, and healthier lives.

FIGURE 23.1. List of Internet resources from the AHRQ for health care providers and patients (current as of January 2006).

mentation barriers, and other related issues exist?

Prevention for Adults

Using the best available evidence, the USP-STF has developed recommendations for preventive care at different ages. Figures 23.2 and 23.3 show preventive recommendations from the AAFP for men and women. Noticeably absent from these recommendations is the "complete physical." No evidence supports having a healthy person go annually to his or her primary care provider for this time-honored physical exam. Rather, people

should be aware of recommended health behaviors, immunizations and screening tests, and receive these according to schedules based on the best available evidence. This does result in a sexually active woman using birth control having an annual exam. Men and women age 50 and over should visit their primary care providers annually for heart disease and cancer screening tests. People with high-risk family histories of heart disease or cancer usually start such screening at age 40. With HIT and Web-based medical homes for patients, more preventive care will be coordinated by the patient, with visits to receive recommended services becoming more efficient.

Since lifestyle behavior causes about 60% of premature disease and death (Mokdad et al., 2004), counseling for healthy behaviors is a major part of preventive care. A health team including the medical provider, a behaviorist, a nutrition counselor, and even a personal trainer could contribute to high-level wellness. These providers may all be available to a patient online to provide continuous access to behavioral coaching.

The transtheoretical model (TTM) of behavior change, developed by Prochaska and DiClemente (1992), is useful when working with adults. At every encounter, an effort is made to move the patient along the stages of precontemplation, contemplation, preparation, action, and maintenance. Doing this effectively often requires a team that comprises the primary care provider and a mental health counselor, both using resources such as classes and written material. To help smokers quit, the U.S. Department of Health and Human Services (2008a) teamed with the American Medical Association (AMA) to promote a reworded version of the TTM model: Ask about tobacco use at every visit; advise tobacco users to stop; assess readiness to quit; assist tobacco users with a quit plan; and arrange follow-up visits (U.S. Department of Health and Human Services, 2008b).

Prevention for adults is a blend of promoting healthy lifestyle behaviors and providing important screening tests and immunizations. In the past, these activities depended on a physician or other delivery site to provide the information and services to patients. In the future, patients will be armed with all the information for their preventive

RECOMMENDED CLINICAL PREVENTIVE SERVICES FOR ADULT MEN

Clinical preventive services for adults, based on the AAFP Summary of Recommendations for Clinical Preventive Services

UPPER AGE LIMITS SHOULD BE INDIVIDUALIZED FOR EACH PATIENT

	18	25	30	35	40	45	50	55	60	65	70	75
ACCIDENTAL INJURY	(R) Counsel as appropriate for age											
ALCOHOL MISUSE	(R) Screen and counsel behavior to reduce misuse											
AORTIC ANEURYSM, ABDOMINAL										(R) One-time screening by ultrasonography[1]		
COLORECTAL CANCER							(SR) Screen for colorectal cancer					
CORONARY HEART DISEASE	(SR) Counsel adults at increased risk regarding benefits and risks of aspirin prophylaxis											
DEPRESSION	(R) Screen for depression											
HEARING DIFFICULTIES										(R) Screen and counsel		
HYPERTENSION	(SR) Screen for high blood pressure											
LIPID DISORDERS				(SR) Screen with fasting lipid profile or nonfasting total and HDL cholesterol								
OBESITY	(R) Screen for obesity by measuring height and weight periodically											
	(R) Intensive counseling and behavioral interventions to promote sustained weight loss for obese adults[2]											
PHYSICAL ACTIVITY	(HB) Recognize that physical activity is desirable and provide advice accordingly											
SECONDHAND SMOKE	(SR) Counsel patients who smoke regarding harmful effects of smoking on children's health											
STDs	(R) Counsel regarding the risks for STDs and how to prevent them											
TOBACCO USE	(SR) Screen for tobacco use and provide tobacco cessation interventions as appropriate											
VIOLENCE, FAMILY AND PARTNER	(HB) Be alert to physical and behavioral signs and symptoms associated with abuse or neglect											
VISUAL DIFFICULTIES										(R) Screen with Snellen acuity		

1. In men who have ever smoked
2. Intensive counseling involves more than 1 session per month for at least 3 months

(SR) **Strongly Recommend:** Good quality evidence exists which demonstrates substantial net benefit over harm; the intervention is perceived to be cost effective and acceptable to nearly all patients.

(R) **Recommend:** Although evidence exists which demonstrates net benefit, either the benefit is only moderate in magnitude or the evidence supporting a substantial benefit is only fair. The intervention is perceived to be cost effective and acceptable to most patients

(HB) **Healthy Behavior:** Healthy Behavior is identified as desirable but the effectiveness of physician's advice and counseling is uncertain

AAFP Age Charts for Clinical Preventive Services are based on the AAFP Summary of Recommendations for Clinical Preventive Services. These charts include only positive recommendations. For negative recommendations; detailed language and further information, consult the Recommendations. For immunization information, you may also consult the Adult Immunization Schedule. These age charts are provided only as an assistance for physicians making clinical decisions regarding the care of their patients. They cannot substitute for the individual situation by the patient's family physician. Based on AAFP Policy Action November 1996, Revision 6.1, April 2006.

FIGURE 23.2. Recommended clinical preventive services for adult men. Adapted with permission from .pdf files of the Recommended Clinical Preventive Services for Adult Men, Women, and High-Risk Adults. *www.aafp.org.* Copyright 2006 by the American Academy of Family Physicians. All rights reserved.

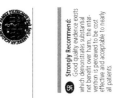

RECOMMENDED CLINICAL PREVENTIVE SERVICES FOR ADULT WOMEN

Clinical preventive services for adults, based on the AAFP Summary of Recommendations for Clinical Preventive Services

UPPER AGE LIMITS SHOULD BE INDIVIDUALIZED FOR EACH PATIENT

Age columns: 18 25 30 35 40 45 50 55 60 65 70 75

- **ACCIDENTAL INJURY** — (R) Counsel as appropriate for age
- **ALCOHOL MISUSE** — (R) Screen and counsel behavior to reduce misuse
- **BREAST CANCER** — (R) Screen with mammography every 1–2 years after counseling about risks and benefits
- **BREASTFEEDING** — (HB) Provide structured breastfeeding education and counsel behavior to promote benefits
  - (HB) Recognize that breastfeeding is desirable and provide advice accordingly
- **CERVICAL CANCER** — (SR) Screen women who have a cervix and have had sex with Pap smear at least once every 3 years
- **CHLAMYDIA** — (SR) Screen sexually active women
- **COLORECTAL CANCER** — (SR) Screen for colorectal cancer
- **CONGENITAL RUBELLA SYNDROME** — (R) Screen by assuring immunity by history, serology, or vaccination
- **CORONARY HEART DISEASE** — (R) Counsel adults at increased risk regarding benefits and risks of aspirin prophylaxis
- **DEPRESSION** — (R) Screen for depression
- **HEARING DIFFICULTIES** — (R) Screen and counsel
- **HYPERTENSION** — (SR) Screen for high blood pressure
- **LIPID DISORDERS** — (SR) Screen with fasting lipid profile or nonfasting total and HDL cholesterol
- **OBESITY** — (R) Screen for obesity by measuring height and weight periodically
  - (R) Intensive counseling and behavioral interventions to promote sustained weight loss for obese adults[1]
- **OSTEOPOROSIS** — (R) Screen women at risk for fractures / (R) Screen for osteoporosis
- **PHYSICAL ACTIVITY** — (R) Counsel to maintain adequate calcium intake to prevent osteoporosis
  - (HB) Recognize that physical activity is desirable and provide advice accordingly
- **PREGNANCY**
- **BACTERIURIA, ASYMPTOMATIC** — (SR) Screen pregnant women with urine culture at 12–16 weeks' gestation or first prenatal visit
- **CHLAMYDIA** — (R) Screen asymptomatic pregnant women
- **HEPATITIS B VIRUS INFECTION** — (SR) Screen pregnant women at first prenatal visit
- **HIV INFECTION** — (R) Screen pregnant women
- **IRON DEFICIENCY ANEMIA** — (R) Screen asymptomatic pregnant women
- **NEURAL TUBE DEFECTS** — (R) Prescribe 0.4–0.8 mg per day of folic acid from 1 month prior to conception through first trimester of pregnancy[2]
  - (SR) Prescribe 4 mg per day of folic acid from 1 to 3 months prior to conception through first trimester of pregnancy[3]
  - (R) Prescribe 0.4 mg of folate supplementation[4]
- **RH(D) INCOMPATIBILITY** — (SR) Rh(D) blood typing and antibody testing for all pregnant women at first prenatal visit
  - (R) Repeated antibody testing for all unsensitized Rh(D)-negative women at 24–28 weeks' gestation
- **SYPHILIS** — (SR) Screen as pregnant women for syphilis infection
- **TOBACCO USE** — (R) Provide 5–15 minutes of smoking cessation counseling to all pregnant women
- **SECONDHAND SMOKE** — (SR) Counsel parents who smoke regarding harmful effects of smoking on children's health
- **STDs** — (R) Counsel regarding the risks for STDs and how to prevent them
- **TOBACCO USE** — (SR) Screen for tobacco use and provide tobacco cessation interventions as appropriate
- **VIOLENCE, FAMILY AND PARTNER** — (HB) Be alert to physical and behavioral signs and symptoms associated with abuse or neglect
- **VISUAL DIFFICULTIES** — (R) Screen with Snellen acuity

(SR) Strongly Recommend: Good quality evidence exists which demonstrates substantial net benefit over harm, the intervention is perceived to be cost effective and acceptable to nearly all patients.

(R) Recommend: Although evidence exists which demonstrates net benefit, either the benefit is only moderate in magnitude or the evidence supporting a substantial benefit is only fair. The intervention is perceived to be cost effective and acceptable to most patients.

(HB) Healthy Behavior: Healthy Behavior is identified as desirable but the effectiveness of physician's advice and counseling is uncertain.

AAFP Age Charts for Clinical Preventive Services are based on the AAFP Summary of Recommendations for Clinical Preventive Services. These charts include only positive recommendations. For negative recommendations, detailed language, and further information, consult the Recommendations. For immunization information, you may also consult the Adult Immunization Schedule. These age charts are provided only as an assistance to physicians making clinical decisions regarding the care of their patients. They cannot substitute for the individual judgment brought to each clinical situation by the patient's family physician. Based on AAFP Policy Action November 1996, Revision 6.1, April 2006, March 2007.

Footnotes:

1 Intensive counseling involves more than 1 session per month for at least 3 months

2 To women planning a pregnancy who have not had a previous pregnancy affected by a neural tube defect

3 To women who are planning a pregnancy and had a pregnancy affected by a neural tube defect

4 To women not planning a pregnancy but of childbearing potential who have not had a baby with a neural tube defect

FIGURE 23.3. Recommended clinical preventive services for adult women. Adapted with permission from .pdf files of the Recommended Clinical Preventive Services for Adult Men, Women, and High-Risk Adults. *www.aafp.org.* Copyright 2007 by the American Academy of Family Physicians. All rights reserved.

needs and be proactively obtaining services. A multidisciplinary care team remains vital to working with patients in the hard work of staying healthy.

Prevention for Children

Well-child care is a time-honored tradition in medicine, and there is ample evidence to support a regular schedule of screenings, immunizations, and health guidance. Parents are an integral part of child health, and counseling of parents regarding childhood behaviors is vitally important. Primary care providers need to be on the lookout for depression in the parent or child, and for evidence of abuse or neglect. Mental health providers in the primary care setting who help with such care early help to avoid later complications and tragic outcomes.

Pregnancy, Birth, Development, and Growth

Prevention practices for children begin during their mothers' pregnancies. Risk indicators for both the pregnant mother and the growing fetus include poor pregnancy weight gain and low prepregnancy weight. Protective factors for mother and fetus include cessation of drug, alcohol, and tobacco use during pregnancy. Zinc and folic acid supplements are also associated with a healthy pregnancy and the birth of a healthy child.

Prevention researchers point out that child and adolescent development present unique challenges and opportunities for prevention. Children and teens are usually dependent on parents and other adults for access to care. Children's health and lifestyle choices are strongly influenced by context, primarily their home environment. Recognizing children's dependence on the adults in their lives has led to specific recommendations for child-focused preventive research (Forrest, Simpson, & Clancy, 1997). These recommendations include the following:

- Expanding the disease orientation of health services research to include a focus on child development.
- Establishing child-sensitive standards for setting research priorities.
- Supporting more child-focused research.

- Developing appropriate laboratories to study child health.
- Improving coordination of research funding between various funding sources.
- Enhancing research in the private sector.

Compared to adults, children develop and change significantly each year. In addition, children and teens are seen by physicians more frequently, and the purpose of visits may be a focus on wellness, not illness. These office visits, which often include tests, immunizations, and developmental evaluations, are an excellent time to focus on prevention. During infancy, most infants are checked for phenylketonuria (PKU), thyroid disease, and sickle-cell disease. A regular schedule of required immunizations is part of every child's health plan. This form of standard primary prevention has already been successfully implemented in child care (AHRQ, 2002).

Even if a child does not have regularly scheduled appointments with a physician, schools and athletic teams require immunizations for participation, so parents are prompted to take their child to a physician. Besides immunizations, physicians often focus on vision, dental, and hearing exams, screening for lead poisoning and tuberculosis, acquisition of developmental milestones, and parent education. Parent education may cover topics including nutrition, physical exercise, sleep, and injury prevention. It is evident that plenty of opportunity exists to implement prevention strategies in child primary care.

Abuse and Injuries

Many physician visits by children and their caregivers are for injuries, and injuries are the leading cause of death among young people in the United States (AHRQ, 2002). Unfortunately, 1 in 5 childhood injuries may be caused by abuse (Flaherty, Sege, Mattson, & Binns, 2002). Often, the physician may suspect abuse but not be certain. Initiatives to prevent these dangerous problems focus on modifying parent behavior and parent education. For example, research has documented that small changes can lead to significant outcomes. Thus, parent education should focus on the following:

- Teaching parents to put infants on their back for sleeping to protect against sudden infant death syndrome.
- Encouraging and instructing parents to use car seats and seat belts properly.
- Keeping medicines, cleaning solutions and other dangerous substances away from children.
- Using fences, gates, locks and other barriers to protect young children from risk including stairs, boiling water, animals, fire, electrical outlets, guns, and pools.
- Keeping drugs, tobacco, and alcohol away from children and teens.
- Protecting children during athletics by ensuring that they have proper equipment and clothing in addition to following safe practices.
- Encouraging conversations at home about sex and sexually transmitted diseases.

The CDC (2008a) estimated that in 2006, Child Protective Services investigated 3.6 million children in the United States. The majority of these cases had no previous history of victimization (CDC, 2008b). Sixty-three percent of these children were classified as victims of neglect, 17% as victims of physical abuse, 9% as victims of sexual abuse, and 7% as victims of emotional abuse (CDC, 2008a). In general, African American children, American Indian, Alaska Native, and Pacific Islander children are more at risk for child abuse (CDC, 2008b). Girls are slightly more at risk than boys (CDC, 2008b).

Interestingly, more women than men are perpetrators of child maltreatment. These women, mostly mothers, are typically younger than male perpetrators, most of whom are fathers. Parents with some or all of the following characteristics are more likely to abuse their children: drug and alcohol abuse problems, mental illness, disabilities, and a history of intimate partner violence. In addition, homes in which there is a great deal of stress, often resulting from poverty, chronic illness, and social isolation, are more at risk for child abuse. Young children, younger than 4 years, are most at risk for abuse, especially if they are growing up in an environment where child abuse is accepted (CDC, 2008b).

While primary care physicians are mandated reporters, they are often unaware of abuse unless it reaches such significant levels that the child's life is at risk. In addition, physicians may be unsure of how to bring up abuse in an otherwise regular office visit. Besides schools, primary care offices are the most common setting for families to interact with child care professionals. Thus, physician education about abuse, especially risk factors and warning signs in parents (e.g., drug and alcohol abuse, mental illness, disabilities, partner violence, poverty, chronic illness, and social isolation), is a critical part of a comprehensive prevention strategy. In addition, screening and charting tools that can be used easily and quickly by the busy primary care provider help to prevent abuse.

Chronic Illness and Common Childhood Health Problems

Many children suffer from one or more chronic health conditions. Some of the most common chronic conditions and disabilities that affect young people include diabetes, cerebral palsy, respiratory problems, and traumatic brain injury. Other common chronic illnesses of young people include asthma, attention-deficit/hyperactivity disorder (ADHD), and mental health problems. Many of these chronic health issues intersect with normal development, and some illnesses mean that children and teens must live with an ever-present risk of serious illness or even death. Children with chronic health problems, especially poor children, receive the majority of their health care from primary care physicians. In addition, children's illnesses pose special challenges for their families, often resulting in overwhelmed families trying to balance multiple stressors, including the financial strain of the illnesses.

Two common childhood illnesses on which prevention researchers have focused are asthma and ADHD. Asthma is the most common chronic disease of childhood, and about one-fourth of those affected are less than 5 years old (AHRQ, 2002). Unfortunately, illnesses associated with asthma, such as allergies, sinusitis, and eczema, are increasing (Finkelstein et al., 2002). Preventing morbidity related to asthma or asthma-related conditions is a major objective for health care researchers.

ADHD, another common childhood problem, is characterized by symptoms of inattention, hyperactivity, and impulsivity. ADHD is frequently comorbid with learning disabilities, depression, anxiety, conduct disorder, and oppositional behaviors. Prevention research on ADHD has focused on the development of new tools, such as computer programs for children with ADHD and their families. In addition, researchers continue to explore the effectiveness and risks of pharmacological and nonpharmacological treatments for ADHD. Finally, researchers are interested in developing more effective screening tools for ADHD. Effective screening for both schools and primary care offices are especially important because these are the two settings in which at-risk children appear for services.

Barriers to Prevention

Excellent guidelines supported by research and recommendations for prevention exist in the United States. Still, according to Nash, "The US healthcare delivery systems continue to fall woefully short of its prevention targets. On the international scene, the United States lags behinds countries with less wealth and less technological savvy" (as cited in Clarke & Meiris, 2006, p. S2).

As mentioned earlier, prevention is divided into levels. Primary prevention addresses prevention of disease or injury and may focus on an individual or an environment. Educating the public about both healthy behaviors and specific protective measures is part of primary prevention. In addition, prevention can focus on changing the environment, such as providing clean water (Cassens, 1992). Secondary prevention focuses on amelioration of specific threats. Historically, the foundation of prevention efforts has occurred in primary care. Most prevention health care dollars target changes in primary care (Cassens, 1992).

Provider Barriers

Primary care physicians often lament that they are increasingly asked to do "more with less." In a 15-minute office visit, physicians are expected to screen for all risk areas, educate the patient, and address the patient's chief complaint. Physicians can easily feel overwhelmed with the demands they face and instead focus solely on the patient's chief complaint for a specific office visit. At times, physicians are unaware of the current evidence summarizing effective preventive measures, and they may even wonder whether specific measures make a difference. In addition, prevention and education are poorly reimbursed compared to other treatments, such as medical procedures and outpatient surgeries, so few financial incentives exist to practice prevention (American College of Physicians, 2006).

Patient Barriers

In addition to the hindrance of provider barriers, patients also hinder their own health. Despite revolutionizing patient health care through EHRs and interactive primary care websites, patients risk poor health outcomes by not utilizing these resources, For example, diabetes, heart disease, lung disease, and some cancers are detectable and, at times, preventable. What keeps patients from practicing prevention? Responses to this question vary depending on race, income, location, and a host of other factors (AHRQ, 2008). But, in general, patients with fewer resources including lack of private insurance, are most at risk for preventable illnesses. In addition, many at-risk populations such as the disabled, older adults, children, and others do not make their own health care decisions. Family members decide for them.

A host of individual forces also deter prevention. Fear of illness, fear of financial strain, or other fears often keep patients from seeking care. In addition, lack of knowledge about preventive measures means that individuals might not recognize personal risk. Feeling overwhelmed with the stresses and demands of daily life, and lack of motivation may keep individuals from taking basic steps (e.g., a healthy diet, regular exercise, and smoking cessation). Patients may need extra support to make needed changes, and that support may not be available from their health care providers or their families. Finally, patients may worry about the extra costs of preventive services, such as "extra" lab work or other screening tests. Research by the AHRQ (2008) suggests that patients may not be willing to invest the time, energy, or money for a test they consider optional.

Health Care System Barriers

The U.S. health care system is not designed to deliver consistent preventive services across a population. The episodic brief visit model of care is an acute care model best designed for people who become sick. Prenatal care and well-child care have found their way into common usage. Women are well motivated most of the time to receive preventive services for a healthy pregnancy and birth. Children are required to receive their immunizations to start school, and well-child visits are scheduled around immunization schedules. Adult prevention depends largely on patients' cooperation and their own volition, and prevention rates across the population usually show that usage rates for tests and procedures are well below target levels.

Additionally, most health insurance plans do not cover many preventive procedures. Traditional health insurance was designed to protect a person and family from a major medical expense due to an injury or a major disease. Even some comprehensive coverage health plans, such as Medicare, have covered preventive services mammography or colonoscopy reluctantly, and only after special legislation. When there are cost barriers to preventive services, usage rates are very low.

New platforms of care with HIT offer an opportunity to improve the population rates of prevention. Reminders through the mail or by telephone increase the use of preventive services. When people have their preventive schedules on their personal medical home pages, with automated reminders and the ability to schedule and receive their own preventive care, rates of use may go up considerably. Lifestyle change for health preventive behaviors are complex and require genuine incentives such as personal and financial rewards (e.g., lower insurance rates for not smoking and maintaining a healthy weight).

Lessons Learned

At present, research summarizing outcomes about prevention initiatives have led to humble findings. For example, researchers at the AHRQ have summarized lessons learned to date, stating,

> More experience has also confirmed that changing practice and realizing savings in health care are not easily achieved. ... Development and dissemination of even high quality, highly credible information is often insufficient to alter practices. Enhanced knowledge must be linked with supportive practice environments and incentives for change. And while it had been hoped that reduction of inappropriate, high-cost care would represent savings of hundreds of billions of dollars through outcome studies, actual success has been more modest. (1999, paragraph 3)

In addition, several years ago, principal investigators of government-funded prevention trials summarized their experiences. As a group, they felt that they had been most successful in providing accurate descriptions of what actually occurs in health care, developing tools for measuring costs of care and patient-reported outcomes, and identifying topics for future research. However, few principal investigators reported findings that definitively suggest one prevention approach is superior to another strategy. In addition, there were few findings that had been incorporated into policy or clinical decision, or interventions that measurably improved quality or significantly decrease costs. Thus, future prevention researchers should focus on problem solving and actual implementation of guidelines for quality improvement instead of focusing primarily on measurement and description (AHRQ, 1999).

One way that the AHRQ had adapted the suggestions for focusing on change/impact instead of description/methods is by creating a program focused on implementation. The Put Prevention into Practice (PPIP) program's goals include the following:

- Providing a systematic approach for delivering clinical preventive services.
- Helping providers and patients track preventive care.
- Educating providers, office staff, and patients about what services should be delivered.

Other private initiatives that affect intervention/impact are also occurring. For example, the private company U.S. Preventive Medicine, Inc. (USPM) has been harnessing the power of television and the entertainment industry to encourage consumer health behaviors such as fitness, healthy aging, and wellness, and using the Internet for prevention services. USPM wants to serve as a catalyst in focusing divergent groups (e.g., employers, consumers, and others) to create together a culture of prevention (Clarke & Meiris, 2006).

Conclusions

Prevention in health care operates at multiple levels, from public health to family and cultural practices, to individual behavior. Achieving preventive care in a population requires activities and interventions at all these levels. A community with limited parking space and no trails for biking, running, or walking, is much less likely to promote physical activity. When unhealthy fast-food restaurants dominate the environment, obesity rates soar. The preventive practices of healthy lifestyle, immunizations, and screening tests all require a concerted effort based on schedules and measurement of success. In the future, people will be better able to coordinate and receive their own preventive services rather than rely on a health care facility to remember what to do. Ultimately, prevention happens when people have incentives, and good health alone is not generally adequate. The health care system in a society must value prevention highly and make preventive behaviors an enjoyable expectation of its citizens. Achieving high levels of prevention requires a team of multidisciplinary professionals engaging with a prepared and proactive public.

Further Reading

Agency for Healthcare Research and Quality. (1999). *The outcome of outcomes research at AHCPR: Final report* [Summary]. Online resource: *www.ahrq.gov/clinic/outcosum.htm.*

American College of Preventive Medicine. (n.d.). *Clinical preventive services.* Online resource: *www.acpm.org/clinical2.htm.*

Goroll, A. H., & Mulley, A. G., Jr. (2006). *Primary care medicine* (5th ed.). Philadelphia: Lippincott/Williams & Wilkins.

Jones, R., Britten, N., Cullpepper, L., Gass, D.

A., Grol, R., Mant, D., et al. (2003). *Oxford textbook of primary medical care.* Oxford, UK: Oxford University Press.

Noble, J. (Ed.). (2001). *Textbook of primary care medicine* (3rd ed.). St. Louis, MO: Mosby.

U.S. Preventive Services Task Force. (2008). *The guide to clinical preventive services* (AHRQ Publication No. 08-05122). Online resource: *ahrq.hhs.gov.*

References

Agency for Healthcare Research and Quality (AHRQ). (1999). *The outcome of outcomes research at AHCPR: Final report* [Summary]. Rockville, MD: Author. Retrieved from *www.ahrq.gov/clinic/outcosum.htm.*

Agency for Healthcare Research and Quality (AHRQ). (2002). *Program brief: Children's health highlights.* Rockville, MD: Author. Retrieved July 15, 2008, from *www.ahrq.gov/child/highlts/chhigh.pdf.*

Agency for Healthcare Research and Quality (AHRQ). (2006). *Preventive services resource links* [U.S. Preventive Services Task Force]. Rockville, MD: Author. Retrieved July 15, 2008, from *www.ahrq.gov/clinic/uspstf/resource.htm.*

Agency for Healthcare Research and Quality (AHRQ). (2008). *Put prevention into practice* [PowerPoint slides]. Rockville, MD: Author. Retrieved from *www.ahrq.gov/ppip/manual/appenda.ppt.*

American Academy of Family Physicians (AAFP). (2008). *Patient-centered medical home questions and answers.* Leawood, KS: Author. Retrieved July 15, 2008, from *www.aafp.org/online/en/home/membership/initiatives/pcmh/brief.html.*

American Academy of Family Physicians, American Academy of Pediatrics, American College of Physicians, & American Osteopathic Association. (2007). *Joint principles of the patient-centered medical home.* Retrieved from *www.aafp.org/online/etc/medialib/aafp_org/documents/policy/fed/jointprinciplespcmh0207.par.0001.file.tmp/022107medicalhome.pdf.*

American College of Physicians. (2006). *The impending collapse of primary care medicine and its implications for the state of the nation's health care.* Retrieved from *www.acponline.org/advocacy/events/state_of_healthcare/statehc06_1.pdf.*

Cassens, B. J. (1992). *Preventive medicine and public health.* Philadelphia: Lippincott/Williams & Wilkins.

Centers for Disease Control and Prevention (CDC). (2008a). *Child maltreatment: Facts at a glance.* Atlanta, GA: Author. Retrieved from *www.cdc.gov/ncipc/dvp/cm_data_sheet.pdf.*

Centers for Disease Control and Prevention (CDC). (2008b). *Child maltreatment prevention scientific information: Risk and protective factors.* Atlanta, GA: Author. Retrieved July 15, 2008, from *www.cdc.gov/ncipc/dvp/CMP/CMP-risk-p-factors.htm.*

Clarke, J. L., & Meiris, D. C. (2006). Preventive medicine: A "cure" for the healthcare crisis. *Disease Management, 9*(1), S1–S16.

Finkelstein, J. A., Fuhlbrigge, A., Lozano, P., Grant, E. N., Shulruff, R., Arduino, K. E., et al. (2002). Parent-reported environmental exposures and environmental control measures for children with asthma. *Archives of Pediatric and Adolescent Medicine, 156*(3), 258–264.

Flaherty, E., Sege, R., Mattson, C., & Binns, H. (2002). Assessment of suspicion of abuse in the primary care setting. *Ambulatory Pediatrics, 2*(2), 120–126.

Forrest, C. B., Simpson, L., & Clancy, C. (1997). Child health services research: Challenges and opportunities. *Journal of the American Medical Association, 277*(22), 1787–1793.

Franks, P., & Fiscella, K. (1998). Primary care physicians and specialists as personal physicians: Health care expenditures and mortality experience. *Journal of Family Practice, 47*(2), 105–109.

GreenField Health. (2008). Welcome to GreenField Health. Portland, OR: Author. Retrieved July 15, 2008, from *www.greenfieldhealth.com/portal.*

Harris, R. P., Helfand, M., Woolf, S. H., Lohr, K. N., Mulrow, C. D., Teutsch, S. M., et al. (2001). Current methods of the U.S. Preventive Services Task Force: A review of the process. *American Journal of Preventive Medicine, 20*(Suppl. 3), 21–35.

Institute of Medicine. (1996). *Primary care: America's health in a new era.* Washington, DC: National Academy Press.

Institute of Medicine. (2001). *Crossing the quality chasm: A new health system for the 21st century.* Washington, DC: National Academy Press.

Lawrence, D. (2002). Integrating care: A talk with Kaiser Permanente's David Lawrence. *Health Affairs, 21*, 39–48.

McGlynn, E. A., Asch, S. M., Adams, J., Keesey, J., Hicks, J., DeCristofaro, A., et al. (2003). The quality of health care delivered to adults in the United States. *New England Journal of Medicine, 26*, 2635–2645.

Millenson, M. L. (1997). *Demanding medical excellence.* Chicago: University of Chicago Press.

Mokdad, A. H., Marks, J. S., Stroup, D. F., & Gerberding, J. L. (2004). Actual causes of death in the United States, 2000. *Journal of the American Medical Association, 291*, 1238–1245.

Petterson, S. M., Phillips, R. L., Bazemore, A. W., Dodoo, M. S., Zhang, X., & Green, L. A. (2008). Why there must be room for mental health in the medical home. *American Family Physician, 77*(6), 757.

Phillips, R. L. (2005). Primary care in the United States: Problems and possibilities. *British Medical Journal, 331*, 1400–1402.

Prochaska, J. O., & DiClemente, C. C. (1992). Stages of change in the modification of problem behaviors. *Progressive Behavior Modification, 28*, 183–218.

RelayHealth. (2002). RelayHealth webVisit Study. Atlanta, GA: Author. Retrieved July 15, 2008, from *www.relayhealth.com/general/news/studyfacts.aspx.*

Starfield, B., Shi, L., Grover, A., & Macinko, J. (2005). The effects of specialist supply on populations' health: Assessing the evidence. *Health Affairs, 10*. Retrieved July 15, 2008, from *content.healthaffairs.org/cgi/content/abstract/hlthaff.w5.97.*

Starfield, B., Shi, L., & Macinko, J. (2005). Contribution of primary care to health systems and health. *Milbank Quarterly, 83*(3), 457–502.

U.S. Department of Health and Human Services. (2008a). *About United States Preventive Services Task Force.* Retrieved July 15, 2008, from *www.ahrq.gov/clinic/uspstfab.htm.*

U.S. Department of Health and Human Services. (2008b). *Helping smokers quit: A guide for clinicians.* Retrieved July 15, 2008, from *www.ahrq.gov/clinic/tobacco/clinhlpsmksqt.htm.*

Woolf, S. H. (2008). The power of prevention and what it requires. *Journal of the American Medical Association, 299*, 2437–2439.

World Health Organization. (2007). *Working for health: An introduction to the World Health Organization.* Retrieved from *www.who.int/about/brochure_en.pdf.*

CHAPTER 24

Prevention of Coronary Heart Disease

Gerdi Weidner
Friederike Kendel

Coronary heart disease (CHD) remains a leading cause of death in the world. The disease results from an accumulation of atheromatous plaques on the walls of the arteries that supply the myocardium with oxygen (Hansson & Nilsson, 2004). It is chronic, presenting with symptoms that range from chest pain (angina pectoris) to myocardial infarction (MI) and sudden cardiac death, often co-occurring with other diseases, such as dyslipidemia, hypertension, and diabetes (see Harlapur, Abraham, & Shimbo, Chapter 28, this volume). Due to the rapidly increasing prevalence of Type 2 diabetes (Narayan, Boyle, Geiss, Saaddine, & Thompson, 2006), CHD is also likely to increase, producing considerable costs for both the individual and the society. Thus, the prevention of CHD has become one of the greatest challenges to public health.

To date, the largest global study on risk of MI is the INTERHEART Study (Yusuf et al., 2004), which compared over 15,152 cases with 14,820 sex- and age-matched controls in 52 countries on all continents. Findings from the study confirmed the importance of smoking, diabetes, dyslipidemia, hypertension, and abdominal obesity for MI, and also pointed to the significance of lifestyle factors, such as regular consumption of fruits and vegetables, exercise, and a "psychosocial stress index," consisting of depression, stress at work or at home, financial stress, major life events, and low locus of control. Interestingly, this index, adjusted for age and region, accounted for 25.3% of the population attributable risk (PAR) for acute MI in men and 40% in women. All risk factors together accounted for over 90% of the PAR (i.e., the reduction in incidence that would be observed if the population were unexposed to these factors). Yusuf and colleagues (2004) concluded that "nine easily measured and potentially modifiable risk factors account for an overwhelmingly large proportion of the risk of an initial acute MI. The effect of these risk factors is consistent in men and women, across different geographic regions, and by ethnic group, making the study applicable worldwide" (p. 945). They further stated that "lifestyle modification is of substantial importance" (p. 951).

To achieve and maintain comprehensive lifestyle changes to slow the development and progression of CHD, behavioral intervention programs are clearly needed. In this chapter, we briefly review CHD risk factors and their interdependencies. We then discuss the inclusion of these lifestyle factors in intervention programs and conclude with an example of a comprehensive lifestyle program that targets diet, exercise, and psychosocial stress.

Risk Factors for CHD

Biological Predispositions

In addition to age and family history, the male sex is considered a biological predisposition for CHD development. However, men's greater risk for CHD also appears to be influenced by elevated behavioral and psychological risk factors, such as smoking and maladaptive coping styles (Weidner, 2000; Weidner & Cain, 2003; Weidner, Kopp, & Kristenson, 2002). While men develop CHD about 10 years earlier in life, women typically have a poorer prognosis after MI (Vaccarino, Parsons, Every, Barron, & Krumholz, 1999) and after bypass surgery (Regitz-Zagrosek et al., 2004; Vaccarino, Abramson, Veledar, & Weintraub, 2002).

Clinical Risk Factors

There is general consensus that clinical risk factors such as hypertension, dyslipidemia, obesity, and diabetes are associated with higher risk of developing atherosclerotic disease (Jamrozik, 2004). The INTERHEART Study (Yusuf et al., 2004) confirmed the importance of several well-studied clinical risk factors for MI across different continents. The ratio of apolipoprotein B (ApoB) to apolipoprotein A1 (ApoA1), an index of abnormal lipids, showed a graded relation with the odds of an MI and appeared to be the most important clinical risk factor in the study, with a PAR of 52.1% in women and 53.8% in men. This risk factor was followed by abdominal obesity (PAR of 35.9% in women and 32.1% in men), hypertension (PAR of 35.8% in women and 19.5% in men), and diabetes (PAR of 19.1% in women and 10.1% in men), with all PARs adjusted for age and region.

Lifestyle Factors

The third group of risk factors constitutes the modifiable *behavioral* risk factors: smoking, physical inactivity, and unhealthy eating patterns. It has long been known that smoking contributes to the development and progression of atherosclerosis, and also appears to play a role in triggering acute coronary events (Jamrozik, 2004). In the INTERHEART Study, smoking yielded a PAR of 15.8% for women and 44% for men. Smoking cessation has long been regarded as a key predictor of treatment success after MI. Consequently, smoking cessation programs are now a standard component of cardiac rehabilitation.

Another well-studied behavioral risk factor is physical activity. The relative risk of CHD is twice as high in persons who are physically inactive compared to those who are physically active. Even moderate physical activity is thought to have a protective effect, even in patients with manifest CHD (Miller, Balady, & Fletcher, 1997). The potential of physical activity to prevent MI is also evident in the INTERHEART Study. The PAR for physically inactive women was 37.3% compared to 22.9% for men. In addition to smoking, physical activity is the second major component of traditional cardiac rehabilitation.

The importance of healthy eating patterns has been confirmed in the INTERHEART Study: Consuming fruits and vegetables on a regular basis decreased the PAR for MI by 17.8% in women and 10.3% in men. Additionally, reducing dietary fat and cholesterol, as well as trans fatty acids has been recommended. With regard to the latter, a meta-analysis of available studies showed that the pooled relative risk of CHD decreased 25% for every 2% decrease in trans fatty acid intake as a proportion of total energy (Hu & Willett, 2002). In spite of this evidence, the adoption of healthier eating patterns is not a major focus of traditional cardiac rehabilitation.

The clinical and lifestyle factors discussed earlier are not independent but are influenced by each other. For example, unhealthy eating patterns are associated with obesity, dyslipidemia, hypertension, and diabetes. Both obesity and diabetes are associated with a lack of exercise. Thus, clinical risk factors are clearly modifiable, suggesting that a large percentage of MI can be prevented by changing behavior.

Psychosocial Factors

A growing body of evidence shows that not only clinical but also psychosocial risk factors play a role in the development and progression of CHD. Research in this field falls into four domains: emotional factors, psychosocial stress, social support, and socioeconomic status (Orth-Gomér, Weidner, Anderson, & Chesney, 2010).

Emotional Factors

Since the second half of the 20th century, large epidemiological studies identified emotional reactions to stress or psychological characteristics, such as hostility and depression, as independent risk factors for CHD (Kuper, Marmot, & Hemingway, 2002). Early attempts to link emotional factors to CHD focused on the "Type A behavior pattern" (TABP). Type A people are considered hard-driving, aggressive, competitive and hostile, and prone to develop CHD. However, a meta-analysis of 25 prospective studies of TABP as a predictor of CHD yielded a nonsignificant population effect size (Myrtek, 2001). The construct is now seen as rather historical. More recent studies have indicated that it was the anger/hostility component of the original Type A construct that accounted for the increased risk for the development of CHD (e.g., Orth-Gomér et al., 2010; Player, King, Mainous, & Geesey, 2007).

In recent years, depression as a risk factor for CHD has gained increasing attention. A meta-analysis of 11 studies concluded that depression was related to a 1.64-fold increase in CHD risk in initially healthy people (Rugulies, 2002). After an acute MI, depression is a frequent condition, with a prevalence rate exceeding that of the healthy population threefold (Thombs et al., 2006). Depression is also associated with worse prognosis after MI (e.g., Frasure-Smith, Lespérance, Juneau, Talajic, & Bourassa, 1999), after bypass surgery (Blumenthal et al., 2003; Kendel, 2008), and decreases the chance of clinical improvement in socially isolated patients wait-listed for a heart transplant (Spaderna et al., 2010). The link between depression and CHD has been explained by both biological and behavioral pathways. A recent science advisory statement, issued by the American Heart Association (Lichtman et al., 2008) indicates that compared to nondepressed patients, depressed patients engage more in health-damaging behaviors and have higher levels of pathogenic biomarkers and reduced heart rate variability, known to influence cardiac events or increase atherosclerosis. Given that depression is not necessarily an epiphenomenon of cardiac disease, Lichtman and colleagues (2008) recommend routinely screening for depression in heart patients, with the goal of identifying those in need of treatment.

Psychosocial Stress

When patients with CHD are asked about the reason for their illness, "stress" is often their first response (Aalto, Heijmans, Weinman, & Aro, 2005). Generally, a distinction is made between acute stress and chronic stress. One example of acute stress may be World Cup Soccer, which was held in Germany in the summer of 2006. On days involving the German team, the incidence of cardiac emergencies was 1.82 and 3.26 times higher in German women and men, respectively, compared to a control period (Wilbert-Lampen et al., 2008). More severe acute life stressors, such as terrorist attacks or earthquakes, are also known to increase the rates of sudden cardiac death (for a review, see Everson-Rose & Lewis, 2005).

Chronic stressors have also been shown to increase the risk of CHD. Most studies that have examined the influence of work stress found consistent results indicating that work stress predicts CHD risk and MI (Kuper & Marmot, 2003). Interestingly, occupational stressors appear to affect outcomes more strongly in men, whereas caregiving and marital stress may increase CHD risk more strongly in women (Everson-Rose & Lewis, 2005; Lee, Colditz, Berkman, & Kawachi, 2003; Orth-Gomér et al., 2000).

These findings are also reflected in the INTERHEART Study (Yusuf et al., 2004). Psychosocial stress was related to acute MI in women (PAR = 40.0) and men (PAR = 25.3). More detailed analyses (Rosengren et al., 2004) revealed a higher prevalence of all four stress factors—stress at work and at home, financial stress, and major life events—in people with MI. Odds ratios were 2.14 for stress at work, 2.12 for stress at home, 1.33 for severe financial stress, and

1.48 for stressful life events. All these associations were observed across regions, ethnic groups, and gender, with one exception: Work stress was not associated with MI in women.

While the evidence linking psychosocial stress to CHD is strong, the underlying pathways are still unclear. Chronic stress appears to have an effect on blood pressure, as well as inflammatory and procoagulant markers (for a review, see Dimsdale, 2008). Chronic stress is also associated with unfavorable health behaviors, namely, smoking and sedentary lifestyle. Thus, effective prevention has to consider these pathways when addressing coronary risk reduction.

Social Support

It is important to draw a distinction between qualitative and quantitative aspects of social support. "Qualitative social support" refers to emotional and instrumental support, whereas "quantitative social support" refers to social integration (i.e., the number and frequency of available relationships and contacts). Cardiac events occur more frequently in individuals who are socially isolated and have little social support (for a review, see Schwarzer & Rieckmann, 2002). Being socially isolated decreases the chance of clinical improvement in patients wait-listed for a heart transplant (Spaderna et al., 2010). Also, social support is an important predictor for recovery. Kulik and Mahler (1989) measured the length of hospitalization of male CHD patients with and without a partner. Patients without a partner (low social support) were hospitalized longer than patients with a partner (more social support). Social support also plays an important role in facilitating protective health behaviors. For instance, people who live alone are less likely to receive assistance with complex drug treatment regimens, which may be of great importance to older patients. Moreover, survival following MI can also depend on whether someone is nearby and can call for immediate help.

Socioeconomic Status

CHD risk appears to vary with socioeconomic status (SES), which is defined by education, income and/or occupational status.

In the Whitehall Study, men in the lowest occupational groups carried a four times higher risk of CHD than men in upper positions (Marmot et al., 1991). A similarly elevated risk for MI in women with low SES was observed in the Stockholm Female Coronary Risk Study (Wamala, Mittleman, Horsten, Schenck-Gustafsson, & Orth-Gomér, 2000).

Low SES is also associated with more unfavorable health behaviors and elevated coronary risk factors. For example, in the Stockholm Female Coronary Risk Study, women with low SES were more likely to smoke, to exercise less, and to have unhealthier eating patterns than women with higher SES. The SES gradient was also associated with elevated levels of coronary risk factors (e.g., blood pressure, low-density lipoprotein cholesterol; Wamala et al., 2000). Similarly, in the Multisite Cardiac Lifestyle Intervention Program (MCLIP), low-SES participants were more likely to be obese, depressed, to have a smoking history, and to lead a sedentary life at program entry (Govil, Weidner, Merritt-Worden, & Ornish, 2008).

Prevention of CHD

In medicine, "prevention" is any activity that reduces the burden of mortality or morbidity from disease. The distinction of primary, secondary, and tertiary prevention goes back to the work of Caplan (1964) and can be ascribed according to the goal. With respect to CHD, primary prevention aims at detecting risk factors and changing risk behaviors as soon as possible to avoid the development of the disease. Secondary prevention aims at early detection of CHD, thereby increasing opportunities for intervention to prevent progression of the disease. Tertiary prevention reduces the negative impact of manifest CHD. For example, coronary bypass artery surgery is performed to relieve angina pectoris and to reduce the risk of death. After cardiac surgery, rehabilitation of patients aims at preventing rehospitalization and worsening of disease. Measures of successful rehabilitation center on (1) the social context (e.g., return to work and resumption of household activities), (2) the psychological context (i.e., improving well-being and quality of life), and (3) the somatic context (e.g., lowering risk of reinfarction, relieving angina pectoris, and reducing classical risk factors). It should be noted that in clinical practice, the differentiation between secondary and tertiary prevention is rarely made.

Primary Prevention Focusing on Risk Factor Reduction

Starting in the early 1970s, identification of CHD risk factors was followed by efforts to lower these factors in the population. Early interventions such as the North Karelia Youth Project (Puska et al., 1981) and the Stanford Heart Disease Prevention Program (Fortmann, Taylor, Flora, & Jatulis, 1993) suggested that multiple risk factor intervention via educational methods was effective and should be expanded. However, trends in both risk factors and CHD mortality observed in North Karelia, for example, were similar to those observed in the comparison regions (Ebrahim, Beswick, Burke, & Davey Smith, 2006). Ebrahim and colleagues (2006) reviewed 39 trials on this issue, concluding that multiple risk factor intervention in the general population results in only small reductions in blood pressure, cholesterol, salt intake, and weight loss, and has little or no impact on the risk of heart attack or death. The authors suggest that "the North Karelia and similar projects may be viewed as effects, or epiphenomena, of the very high CHD mortality rates experienced in many countries in the 1960s" (p. 7), and conclude that the educational interventions were not responsible for the observed improvements in risk factors.

One reason for the disappointing results of primary prevention programs might be that the motivation for health behavior change in disease-free groups is not as high as that in people who already confront the consequences of their lifestyle, for example, in people who have already experienced an MI. Also, a possible statistical reason is the difference in event rates: Because event rates are higher in high-risk groups than in the general population, finding proof for the effectiveness of primary prevention is generally more difficult in the general population.

On the basis of these results, the authors write,

> Our methods of attempting behavior change in the general population are very limited.

Different approaches to behavior change are needed and should be tested empirically before being widely promoted. For example, the availability of healthier foods and better access to recreational and sporting facilities may have a greater impact on dietary and exercise patterns respectively, than health professional advice. (Ebrahim et al., 2006, p. 2)

Thus, actions at the policy level, such as menu-labeling laws (Pomeranz & Brownell, 2008), restrictions on health claims on food packages, marketing, and advertising (Nestle, 2006), may lead to better health outcomes in the population.

Secondary and Tertiary Prevention

Secondary and tertiary prevention trials include people at high risk and patients with manifest CHD. These trials generally yield more favorable results than primary prevention trials. One of the major problems of cardiac rehabilitation to date, however, is low participation. In a review of the literature, Jackson, Leclerc, Erskine, and Linden (2004, p. 10) noted that cardiac rehabilitation is utilized by "only a fraction of eligible patients." Patient characteristics affecting participation include female gender, extent of medical insurance coverage, education, and ease of access to rehabilitation. Moreover, the physician's opinion regarding the effectiveness of rehabilitation is a major factor in the referral of patients (Jackson et al., 2004). Not all obstacles to participation can be changed, but most of the barriers seem modifiable.

Interventions Focusing on Smoking, Exercise, and Diet

Although smoking cessation is a key predictor for rehabilitation success, many patients continue to smoke after a cardiac event. Even in patients waiting for a heart transplant, 4% admitted that they were still smoking (Spaderna, Weidner, Zahn, & Smits, 2009). The Cochrane Collaboration reviewed 16 randomized smoking cessation clinical trials, employing a range of behavioral approaches (Barth, Critchley, & Bengel, 2008). Regardless of approach, the effect on abstinence after 6 or 12 months did not differ from usual care. However, duration of intervention seemed to be important, suggesting that brief interventions with no follow-up, or a follow-up within 4 weeks after the initial intervention, were least effective.

The effectiveness of exercise programs on mortality and morbidity was evaluated in a systematic review based on 8,440 patients with CHD. The effect estimate showed a 27% reduction in all-cause mortality (Jolliffe et al., 2001). The effectiveness of exercise was also confirmed by a review and meta-analysis of 48 trials, indicating that exercise-based cardiac rehabilitation reduced both cardiac and all-cause mortality, but not the risk of cardiac events (Taylor et al., 2004). Exercise dose or duration of follow-up did not appear to influence the outcome.

Most traditional cardiac rehabilitation focuses on smoking cessation and improving exercise but rarely includes a dietary component. Although the influence of healthy eating patterns on the development of CHD is undisputed, only a small number of trials with CHD end points have been conducted on this issue (Hu & Willett, 2002). The systematic review by Hooper and colleagues (2001) on dietary intervention included 27 studies and showed that alteration of dietary fat intake had no effects on all-cause mortality. However, the incidence of combined cardiovascular events was reduced by 16%, and cardiovascular mortality by 9%. Subgroup analyses suggested that in trials with follow-up longer than 2 years, the evidence of protection from cardiovascular events was much stronger than that for shorter follow-up periods. The reduction in event rates in the treatment groups was only 4%, with mean follow-up of 2 years, whereas reductions of up to 24% emerged with longer follow-ups. Because exclusion of data from one study that used a fish oil supplement in addition to dietary advice attenuated the effects on cardiovascular events, Hooper and colleagues conclude that the benefits of dietary fat reduction remain inconclusive. Given that most of the included studies did "not meet the criteria pharmacological interventions must satisfy to be considered definitive" (Yancy, Westman, French, & Califf, 2003, p. 12), this conclusion may not be surprising.

Unfortunately, most dietary interventions focus on dietary cholesterol and fat reduction rather than emphasizing healthy dietary patterns. In an analysis of INTERHEART Study data, the prudent diet that was high in fruit and vegetables showed an inverse association to MI worldwide (Iqbal et al., 2008). Thus, interventions aiming to increase protective dietary factors may present a more promising venue to reduce coronary risk (see also Connor, Ojeda, Sexton, Weidner, & Connor, 2004; Dewell, Weidner, Sumner, Chi, & Ornish, 2008).

Psychological Interventions

Although the influence of psychosocial risk factors on CHD is undisputed, this knowledge has not yet translated into clinical praxis, and risk scores are calculated solely on the basis of clinical variables and smoking (e.g., Framingham Risk Score; D'Agostino, Grundy, Sullivan, & Wilson, 2001). This may be due to the fact that, compared to treatments targeting clinical risk factors, relatively little is known about the effectiveness of psychological treatment with respect to cardiac events and mortality. A few recent meta-analyses have shown significant reductions in mortality and morbidity for psychological treatment compared to usual care (e.g., Dusseldorp, van Elderen, Maes, Meulman, & Kraaij, 1999; Linden, Stossel, & Maurice, 1996). Single reduction of mortality rates differed considerably from 3 to 71%, which is explicable considering the broad range of psychological treatments employed.

The latest meta-analysis on this issue revealed psychological treatment to be effective in reducing 2-year mortality by 27% (Linden, Phillips, & Leclerc, 2007). This benefit was moderated by gender, perceived stress, and timing of treatment. First, there was no mortality benefit for women. Second, beneficial outcomes were observed only when perceived stress reductions occurred. Third, psychological treatment initiated right after the cardiac event (less than 2 months) was not effective in reducing mortality. When psychological treatment was started at least 2 months after the event, mortality reductions of 72% were observed. The fact that the timing of an intervention seems to be an important moderator could also explain the lack of findings among women. A large percentage of patients included in the meta-analysis came from the Enhancing Recovery in Coronary Heart Disease (ENRICHD) study (Writing Group for the ENRICHD Investigators, 2003). Given the fact that the intervention in this study was initiated within 2 months after the cardiac event, the discouraging results with respect to women may not be surprising.[1]

Alternatively, as suggested by Linden and colleagues (2007), psychological treatments may have to be tailored to women's unique needs. This reasoning received some support from a study aiming to reduce stress in male and female post-MI patients (Cossette, Frasure-Smith, & Lespérance, 2001). Significant gender differences were observed: Psychological treatments based on direct advice about recommended lifestyle changes seemed helpful for men, whereas listening to worries reduced stress in female patients (see also Orth-Gomér et al., 2009).

In summary, a relatively small investment in psychological treatment may lead to reductions in morbidity and mortality. Screening for depression and distress throughout the rehabilitation process and offering psychological treatment to those who need it most 2 months after the cardiac event is advisable (Linden et al., 2007).

Comprehensive Lifestyle Changes

Our brief review of psychosocial and behavioral factors, and their role in the etiology and progression of CHD clearly suggests that cardiac rehabilitation might benefit from targeting as many of these factors as possible. Unfortunately, most of the existing programs still focus on smoking cessation and improving physical activity, with little attention to diet, often ignoring psychosocial risk factors altogether. In a similar vein, the few interventions that do focus on psychosocial risk factors exclude other important established risk factors (e.g., diet, exercise). In the following section, we present a program of research conducted within a clinical trials framework that employs an intervention that, in addition to the traditional modalities (smoking cessation, exercise) also pays close attention to diet, social support, stress reduction, depression, and hostility.

The clinical trial has become the preferred method in the evaluation of medical treatments (Friedman, Furberg, & DeMets, 1998). In their classic text titled *Fundamentals of Clinical Trials*, Friedman and colleagues (1998) distinguish among four phases of clinical trial research: Phase I tests the treatment for tolerability; Phase II establishes its safety; Phase III comprises "randomized trials, comparing the effectiveness of one or more interventions with a control" (Friedman et al., 1998, p. 3); and Phase IV long-term surveillance (no control group necessary) of an intervention found to be effective in Phase III. Similar phases have been suggested for the evaluation of behavioral interventions (Glasgow, Lichtenstein, & Marcus, 2003).

One comprehensive lifestyle intervention conducted within this framework is the well-known "Ornish Program," designed to prevent the progression of CHD by encouraging patients to follow a low-fat, whole foods diet (whole grains, fruits, vegetables), engage in moderate exercise, practice stress management, and attend support groups (Billings, 2000). All patients enrolling in this program are required to be smoke-free by the start of the program. As smoking cessation programs are now a well-integrated component of cardiac rehabilitation, the Ornish program concentrates on achieving intensive behavior change in the other components.

Research on this program spans three decades, starting with a pilot study of 11 patients. Results from this study indicated that patients were able to follow the program and showed improvements in coronary risk factors and myocardial perfusion (Ornish et al., 1979; Table 24.1).

Subsequent Phase III and Phase IV research is also shown in Table 24.1. As can be seen, results from the two Phase III clinical trials demonstrated significant medical and psychosocial benefits in intervention patients compared to controls. Based on these findings, major health plans across the United States have started to include this program as an alternative treatment of CHD. The adoption by health plans allowed for Phase IV surveillance (the Multicenter Lifestyle Demonstration Project [MLDP] and the Multisite Cardiac Lifestyle Intervention Program [MCLIP]) to help answer questions about the program's feasibility and generalizability.

---

[1]The ENRICHD Study evaluated cognitive-behavioral therapy and group support sessions in an attempt to reduce depression and social isolation. Its results with respect to the main outcomes were discouraging (Writing Group for the ENRICHD Investigators, 2003).

TABLE 24.1. The Ornish Program of Research by Clinical Trial Phase

Study	Reference	Follow-up	Outcomes	Results
Phases I and II research				
Pilot Study; pre–post; $N = 11$	Ornish et al. (1979)	9 months	Coronary risk factors; myocardial perfusion	• Significant improvements in plasma cholesterol, triglycerides, blood pressure, angina, exercise capacity, and myocardial perfusion.
Phase III research				
First Lifestyle Trial; randomized clinical trial; $N = 46$ (21% female); 23 experimental, 23 control	Ornish et al. (1983)	24 days	Coronary risk factors; angina; exercise capacity; left ventricular ejection fraction	• Significant improvements in plasma cholesterol levels (20.5% decrease), triglycerides, angina (91% reduction angina episodes), exercise capacity, and left ventricular ejection fraction favoring the experimental group.
Lifestyle Heart Trial; randomized clinical trial; $N = 48$; 28 experimental (4% female), 20 control, (20% female)	Ornish et al. (1990)	1 year	Coronary artery stenosis; coronary risk factors; angina	• There were significant improvements in percent diameter stenosis, angina severity, frequency, and duration, total and low-density lipoprotein (LDL) cholesterol, apolipoprotein B, low-density lipo-protein/high-density lipoprotein (HDL) ratio, and weight favoring the experimental group.
	Gould et al. (1992)	1 year	Stenosis dimensions, shape, and severity	• In the experimental group, complex shape change and stenosis molding characteristic of significant regressing severity was observed with improved stenosis flow reserve. The opposite pattern was observed among the controls.
	Gould et al. (1995)	5 years	Myocardial perfusion positron emission tomography [PET]; coronary risk factors	• Size and severity of perfusion abnormalities on dipyridamole PET images improved in the experimental group and worsened in the controls. There also were significant between group differences in coronary risk factors, favoring the experimental group.
	Ornish et al. (1998)	5 years	Coronary artery stenosis; cardiac events; coronary risk factors	• In the experimental group, percent diameter stenosis at baseline decreased after 1 year and continued to improve after 5 years. In the control group, stenosis increased after 1 year and continued to increase after 5 years. Significant between-group differences were observed in coronary risk factors and cardiac events, favoring the experimental group.
	Pischke, Weidner, Scherwitz, & Ornish (2008)	1, 5 years	General well-being; sense of coherence; state and trait anger; social support; health behaviors; stenosis	• After 1 year, psychological stress was significantly reduced in the experimental group compared to controls. By 5 years, improvements in hostility were maintained relative to the control group, but reduction in other stress measures were only reported by those with high 5-year program adherence. Improvements in diet were related to weight reduction and to decreases in stenosis, and improvements in stress management to decreases in stenosis at both follow-ups.

(cont.)

361

TABLE 24.1. (*cont.*)

Study	Reference	Follow-up	Outcomes	Results
Phase IV research				
Multicenter Lifestyle Demonstration Project; N = 579 (21% female). Group 1: 194 patients with coronary artery disease eligible for revascularization, but changing lifestyle instead; 139 matched controls receiving surgical procedure; Group 2: patients with previous revascularization; 8 sites	Ornish (1998)	3 years; Group 1 intervention participants; matched control group	Cardiac events; cardiac morbidity; mortality	• Intervention patients who were eligible for revascularization were able to safely avoid it for at least 3 years without increasing cardiac morbidity and mortality. Compared to the control group, the average savings per patient in the intervention group were $29,529. Reduction in angina in the intervention group was comparable to that achieved by revascularization.
	Pischke, Elliott-Eller, et al. (in press)	3 years; Group 1 intervention participants with left ventricular ejection fraction (LVEF) ≤40; matched to control group participants with LVEF ≤40	Clinical events	• Intervention patients with asymptomatic reduced LVEF who were eligible for revascularization had fewer clinical events than a usual care group that had received revascularization at study entry.
	Koertge et al. (2003)	3 months; 1 year; Group 1 and Group 2 intervention participants	Coronary risk factors; health behaviors; quality of life; by gender	• Regardless of sex, patients showed significant improvements in health behaviors, coronary risk factors, and quality of life by 3 months and maintained most improvements over 1 year.
	Pischke et al. (2006)	3 months; 1 year; Group 1 and Group 2 intervention participants; 347 men, 15.9% with diabetes; 93 women, 38.7% with diabetes	Coronary risk factors; exercise capacity; health behaviors; quality of life; by diabetic status	• Regardless of diabetic status, patients showed significant improvements in lifestyle behaviors, coronary risk factors, and quality of life by 3 months and maintained most improvements over 1 year. By the end of 1 year, reductions in glucose-lowering medications were noted for 19.8% of patients with diabetes.
	Pischke, Weidner, Elliot-Eller, & Ornish (2007)	3 months; 1 year; Group 1 and 2 intervention patients (LVEF ≤ 40, N = 50; LVEF > 40, N = 185)	Coronary risk factors; health behaviors; quality of life; by LVEF group	• Regardless of LVEF, patients showed significant improvements in health behaviors, coronary risk factors, and quality of life by 3 months and maintained most improvements over 1 year.
	Schulz et al. (2008)	12 months; Group 1, Group 2 intervention groups	Support group attendance; health behaviors; coronary risk factors; quality of life	• Improvements in all outcomes were observed; several were related to social support group attendance, favoring those who attended more sessions over 1 year. The associations of group attendance with blood pressure and quality of life remained significant when controlling for changes in health behaviors, suggesting an independent relationship. Improvements in quality of life may be in part due to improved health behaviors.

362

Program	Authors	Duration; sample	Outcomes	Findings
Multisite Cardiac Lifestyle Intervention Program; 1998–ongoing (ca. 50% female): coronary heart disease (CHD) patients and patients with ≥3 cardiac risk factors; 22 sites	Daubenmier et al. (2007)	3 months; 869 nonsmoking CHD patients (34% female)	Coronary risk factors; health behaviors; quality of life; by gender	• Improvements in outcomes were observed in both sexes. Reductions in dietary fat predicted reductions in weight, total cholesterol, LDL cholesterol, and interacted with exercise to predict reductions in perceived stress. Increases in exercise predicted improvements in total cholesterol and exercise capacity. Increases in stress management were related to reductions in hostility, weight, total cholesterol/HDL cholesterol, triglycerides, glycosylated hemoglobin (A1c).
	Frattaroli, Weidner, Merritt-Worden, Frenda, & Ornish (2008)	3 months; 1,152 nonsmoking CHD patients (34% female)	Angina; coronary risk factors; quality of life; health behaviors	• At baseline, 108 patients (43% women) reported mild angina and 174 patients (37% women) reported limiting angina. By 3 months, 74% of these patients were angina free, and an additional 9% moved from limiting to mild angina. Improvements were observed in all outcomes. Patients with angina who became angina free showed the greatest improvements.
	Govil, Weidner, Merritt-Worden, & Ornish (2009)	3 months; 869 nonsmoking CHD patients (34% female)	Coronary risk factors; health behaviors; quality of life; by education and income	• Low-SES patients were more likely to be female, not working, past smokers, to exercise less, to consume a higher fat diet, and to have less favorable risk factor profiles than those with higher SES. By 3 months, patients at all socioeconomic levels consumed a diet with 10% fat, exercised > 3 hours/week, practiced stress management > 5½ hours/week, and experienced significant improvements in outcomes.
	Pischke, Frenda, Ornish, & Weidner (in press)	3 months; 997 nonsmoking patients with elevated coronary risk factors (69% female), stratified by depression	Depressive symptoms; health behaviors; coronary risk factors; quality of life	• Depressed persons had more adverse medical status and health behaviors than nondepressed persons. To examine 3-month changes, three groups were formed: (1) depressed persons who became nondepressed; (2) persons who remained or became depressed; and (3) nondepressed persons who remained nondepressed. All persons met program goals. The greatest improvements in outcomes were observed in Group 1. Lifestyle changes are feasible and beneficial for depressed persons at high risk for CHD.

Findings from the MLDP indicated that patients with CHD in different regions of the United States can make changes in lifestyle and achieve improvements similar to those observed in the experimental arm of the Phase III trials. The MLDP also extended these findings to women (Koertge et al., 2003) and to patients differing in disease severity (e.g., CHD patients with diabetes [Pischke et al., 2006] and patients at risk for heart failure [Pischke et al., 2007]).

The MLDP also examined the benefits of social support group attendance for quality-of-life and clinical outcomes over 1 year (Schulz et al., 2008). Findings from these studies are described in more detail in Table 24.1. Additionally, a group of MLDP patients who were eligible to receive an invasive medical procedure (coronary artery bypass graft [CABG]; percutaneous transluminal coronary angioplasty [PTCA]), but opted for the lifestyle program instead were matched to a control group of similar disease status and procedure eligibility, and followed for 3 years. Almost 80% of the patients participating in the lifestyle program were safely able to avoid invasive procedures for at least 3 years by making comprehensive lifestyle changes without increasing cardiac morbidity and mortality. These benefits were even observed for patients with elevated risk for heart failure (Pischke, Elliott-Eller, et al., in press). The MLDP also provided valuable information about associated cost savings (Ornish, 1998; Pischke, Elliott-Eller, et al., in press).

The second Phase IV program (MCLIP) was covered by major health plans, which included the program as a defined benefit. There were 22 program sites with extended insurance coverage for patients with at least three cardiac risk factors but without established CHD. Enrollment in the MCLIP exceeded 2,500 patients, allowing analysis of the relative importance of each program component for improvements in risk factors and quality of life (Daubenmier et al., 2007), evaluation of changes in angina pectoris (Frattaroli, Weidner, Merritt-Worden, Frenda, & Ornish, 2008), and examination of program feasibility for patients differing in SES (Govil et al., 2009) and those presenting with symptoms of depression in the clinical range (Pischke, Frenda, Ornish, & Weidner, in press). Results from these studies are also presented in Table 24.1.

Other Phase IV findings (not shown) indicate that participation in this lifestyle intervention is associated with significant reductions in perceived stress, and that these reductions are associated with improvements in coronary risk factor profile (Campo, Weidner, Frenda, & Ornish, 2008).

The increasing interest by health insurance providers to include this program as an alternative treatment for CHD may in part be influenced by the rising costs of traditional, invasive treatment procedures. For example, in 2000, the costs for CABG were $57,140; in 2004, they were $85,653. The costs for PTCA show a similar increase (from $27,622 in 2000 to $44,110 in 2004) (National Healthcare Cost and Utilization Project, 2005). The costs for the 3-month Ornish program have remained stable over the same time period ($3,600).

Thus, programmatic research on lifestyle interventions targeting both traditional modalities (smoking cessation and exercise) and diet and psychosocial factors (social support, stress, depression, hostility) within a clinical trial framework clearly contributes to the evidence base of behavioral interventions shown to have an impact on cardiovascular health.[2] However, the benefit of any intervention is determined by not only its effectiveness but also the extent to which it is implemented into the health care system (cf. Glasgow & Emmons, 2007). The programmatic approach of the Ornish Program, spanning several decades of research, has been shown to facilitate financing and reimbursement of such interventions by not only private insurance carriers but also the U.S. Centers for Medicare and Medicaid Services (2009), which have included this program as a defined cardiac rehabilitation benefit for Medicare beneficiaries with CHD.

Future Prospects

The results of the INTERHEART Study have shown that more than 90% of MI

---

[2] Significant beneficial cardiovascular effects of this program have also been reported by others (e.g., Aldana et al., 2006; Ellsworth et al., 2004; Vizza, Neatrour, Felton, & Ellsworth, 2007) as well as in research with early-stage prostate cancer, which targets the same lifestyle behaviors as the cardiovascular intervention programs (e.g., Ornish, Lin, et al., 2008; Ornish, Magbanua, et al., 2008; Ornish et al., 2005).

worldwide may be preventable by behavioral means. In spite of this knowledge, CHD remains the leading cause of death, with diabetes and obesity on the rise. The latter has been referred to as a "ticking time bomb" that may result in an unbearable burden for our health care system. With regard to primary prevention, attempts to change health behavior of individuals have largely been disappointing. Instead, changes in policy appear to hold more promise. For example, in the United States, which has restricted smoking in public places, smoking rates have declined. With the recent adoption of laws implementing similar restrictions in Europe, a reduction in smoking may be observed there in the future as well. While the United States has a longer history of regulating smoking in public places, it still lags behind Europe with respect to bills curbing unhealthy food marketing, especially to children (Nestle, 2006). Preventive health actions at the policy level are likely to impact the health of the population at large (Nestle, 2006).

With regard to secondary prevention, efforts to change individual behavior have been somewhat more successful, but still remain challenging. For example, European surveys of MI patients (e.g., EUROSPIRE II) showed that the prevalence of smoking hardly changed within 6 months after patients' discharge from the hospital. Furthermore, rates of obesity increased during this time period. Clearly, awareness of risk factors and information on cardiac health do not necessarily influence health-related behaviors (Shepard et al., 1997). This may be due partly to psychological mechanisms such as "cognitive dissonance" (cf. Cohen, 2001; Festinger, 1957): It seems much easier to change cognitions than to change one's behavior. On the physician's side, too, concerning the implementation of guidelines, there is "a wide gap between our knowledge and our understanding of the benefits of treatment and the clinical reality" (Cohen, 2001, p. 972). This gap pertains not only to the prevention of clinical risk factors but also to implementation of psychological interventions.

Conclusions

Our review of CHD risk factors has shown the interdependencies of traditional, clinical, behavioral, and psychosocial risk factors. Thus, instead of implementing interventions aimed at the reduction of each factor alone, interventions targeting as many of these factors as possible are likely to achieve the best results at both individual and population levels.

Recent trials have posed several questions. How should interventions be tailored to the needs of men and women? What is the best timing and duration of the intervention? How many risk factors should be targeted? How can the intervention team be trained to achieve enduring health behavior change and increase participation rates in cardiac rehabilitation programs? Last, but not least, the inclusion of quality-of-life measures as outcomes, in addition to mortality and morbidity, is necessary to grasp the full relevance of treatment efforts. Given the growing population of people with chronic illnesses and the enormous increase in costs of medical care, prevention of CHD seems to be an important and worthwhile research area for health psychologists.

Acknowledgments

Preparation of this article was supported in part by grants from The Alexander von Humboldt Foundation; the German Academic Exchange Service (DAAD); the German Research Foundation (Grant No. MA 155/75-1). We thank the Medical University Charité-Universitätsmedizin Berlin for granting a visiting scholarship to F. Kendel, and Daniel Purnell for his assistance in the preparation of this article.

Further Reading

Kuper, H., Marmot, M., & Hemingway, H. (2002). Systematic review of prospective cohort studies of psychosocial factors in the etiology and prognosis of coronary heart disease. *Seminars in Vascular Medicine, 2,* 267–314.

Linden, W., Phillips, M. J., & Leclerc, J. (2007). Psychological treatment of cardiac patients: A meta-analysis. *European Heart Journal, 28,* 2972–2984.

Nestle, M. (2006). Food marketing and childhood obesity—a matter of policy. *New England Journal of Medicine, 354,* 2527–2529.

Yusuf, S., Hawken, S., Ounpuu, S., Dans, T., Avezum, A., Lanas, F., et al. (2004). Effect of potentially modifiable risk factors associated with myocardial infarction in 52 countries (the INTERHEART Study): Case–control study. *Lancet, 364*, 937–952.

References

Aalto, A. M., Heijmans, M., Weinman, J., & Aro, A. R. (2005). Illness perceptions in coronary heart disease: Sociodemographic, illness-related, and psychosocial correlates. *Journal of Psychosomatic Research, 58*, 393–402.

Aldana, S. G., Whitmer, W. R., Greenlaw, R., Avins, A. L., Thomas, D., Salberg, A., et al. (2006). Effect of intense lifestyle modification and cardiac rehabilitation on psychosocial cardiovascular disease risk factors and quality of life. *Behavior Modification, 30*, 507–525.

Barth, J., Critchley, J., & Bengel, J. (2008). Psychosocial interventions for smoking cessation in patients with coronary heart disease. *Cochrane Database of Systematic Reviews*, Issue 1 (Article No. CD006886), DOI: 10.1002/14651858.CD006886.

Billings, J. H. (2000). Maintenance of behavior changes in cardiorespiratory risk reduction: A clinical perspective from the Ornish Program for Reversing Heart Disease. *Health Psychology, 19*, 70–75.

Blumenthal, J. A., Lett, H. S., Babyak, M. A., White, W., Smith, P. K., Mark, D. B., et al. (2003). Depression as a risk factor for mortality after coronary artery bypass surgery. *Lancet, 362*, 604–609.

Campo, R. A., Weidner, G., Frenda, S., & Ornish, D. (2008). Gender differences in associations of perceived stress improvements with changes in coronary risk factors and health behaviors: The Multisite Cardiac Intervention Lifestyle Program (MCLIP). *Annals of Behavioral Medicine, 35*(Suppl.), S79.

Caplan, G. (1964). *An approach to community mental health*. London: Tavistock.

Cohen, J. D. (2001). ABCs of secondary prevention of CHD: Easier said than done. *Lancet, 357*, 972–973.

Connor, S. L., Ojeda, L. S., Sexton, G., Weidner, G., & Connor, W. E. (2004). Diets lower in folic acid and carotenoids are associated with the coronary disease epidemic in Central and Eastern Europe. *Journal of the American Dietetic Association, 104*, 1793–1799.

Cossette, S., Frasure-Smith, N., & Lespérance, F. (2001). Clinical implications of a reduction in psychological distress on cardiac prognosis in patients participating in a psychosocial intervention program. *Psychosomatic Medicine, 63*, 257–266.

D'Agostino, R. B., Grundy, S., Sullivan, L. M., & Wilson, P. (2001). CHD Risk Prediction Group. *Journal of the American Medical Association, 286*, 180–187.

Daubenmier, J. J., Weidner, G., Sumner, M. D., Mendell, N., Merritt-Worden, T., Studley, J., et al. (2007). The contribution of changes in diet, exercise, and stress management to changes in coronary risk in women and men in the Multisite Cardiac Lifestyle Intervention Program. *Annals of Behavioral Medicine, 33*, 57–68.

Dewell, A., Weidner, G., Sumner, M. D., Chi, C. S., & Ornish, D. (2008). A very-low-fat vegan diet increases intake of protective dietary factors and decreases intake of pathogenic dietary factors. *Journal of the American Dietetic Association, 108*, 347–356.

Dimsdale, J. (2008). Psychological stress and cardiovascular disease. *Journal of the American College of Cardiology, 51*, 1237–1246.

Dusseldorp, E., van Elderen, T., Maes, S., Meulman, J., & Kraaij, V. (1999). A meta-analysis of psychoeduational programs for coronary heart disease patients. *Health Psychology, 18*, 506–519.

Ebrahim, S., Beswick, A., Burke, M., & Davey Smith, G. (2006). Multiple risk factor interventions for primary prevention of coronary heart disease. *Cochrane Database of Systematic Reviews*, Issue 4 (Article No. CD001561), DOI: 10.1002/14651858.CD001561.pub2.

Ebrahim, S., & Davey Smith, G. D. (2001). Exporting failure?: Coronary heart disease and stroke in developing countries. *International Journal of Epidemiology, 30*, 201–205.

Ellsworth, D. L., O'Dowd, S. C., Salami, B., Hochberg, A., Vernalis, M. N., Marshall, D., et al. (2004). Intensive lifestyle modification: Impact on cardiovascular disease risk factors in subjects with and without clinical cardiovascular disease. *Preventive Cardiology, 7*, 168–175.

Everson-Rose, S. A., & Lewis, T. T. (2005). Psychosocial factors and cardiovascular diseases. *Annual Review of Public Health, 26*, 469–500.

Festinger, L. (1957). *A theory of cognitive dissonance*. Stanford, CA: Stanford University Press.

Fortmann, S. P., Taylor, C. B., Flora, J. A., & Jatulis, D. E. (1993). Changes in adult cigarette smoking prevalence after 5 years of community health education: The Stanford Five-City Project. *American Journal of Epidemiology, 137*, 82–96.

Frasure-Smith, N., Lespérance, F., Juneau, M., Talajic, M., & Bourassa, M. G. (1999). Gender, depression, and one-year prognosis after myocardial infarction. *Psychosomatic Medicine, 61*, 26–37.

Frattaroli, J., Weidner, G., Merritt-Worden, T. A., Frenda, S., & Ornish, D. (2008). Angina pectoris and atherosclerotic risk factors in the Multisite Cardiac Lifestyle Intervention Program. *American Journal of Cardiology, 101*, 911–918.

Friedman, L. M., Furberg, C. D., & DeMets, D. L. (1998). *Fundamentals of clinical trials* (3rd ed.). New York: Springer-Verlag.

Glasgow, R. E., & Emmons, K. M. (2007). How can we increase translation of research into practice?: Types of evidence needed. *Annual Review of Public Health, 28,* 413–433.

Glasgow, R. E., Lichtenstein, E., & Marcus, A. C. (2003). Why don't we see more translation of health promotion research into practice?: Rethinking the efficacy-to-effectiveness transition. *American Journal of Public Health, 93,* 1261–1267.

Gould, K. L., Ornish, D., Kirkeeide, R., Brown, S., Stuart, Y., Buchi, M., et al. (1992). Improved stenosis geometry by quantitative coronary arteriography after vigorous risk factor modification. *American Journal of Cardiology, 69,* 845–853.

Gould, K. L., Ornish, D., Scherwitz, L., Brown, S., Edens, R. P., Hess, M. J., et al. (1995). Changes in myocardial perfusion abnormalities by positron emission tomography after long-term, intense risk factor modification. *Journal of the American Medical Association, 274,* 894–901.

Govil, S. R., Weidner, G., Merritt-Worden, T. A., & Ornish, D. (2009). Socioeconomic status and improvements in lifestyle, coronary risk factors, and quality of life: The Multisite Cardiac Lifestyle Intervention Program. *American Journal of Public Health, 99,* 1263–1270.

Hansson, G., & Nilsson, J. (2004). Epidemiology of cardiovascular diseases. In M. H. Crawford, J. P. DiMarco, & W. J. Paulus (Eds.), *Cardiology* (2nd ed., pp. 3–14). Edinburgh, UK: Mosby.

Hooper, L., Summerbell, C. D., Higgins, J. P., Thompson, R. L., Capps, N. E., Smith, G. D., et al. (2001). Dietary fat intake and prevention of cardiovascular disease: Systematic review. *British Medical Journal, 322,* 757–763.

Hu, F. B., & Willett, W. C. (2002). Optimal diets for prevention of coronary heart disease. *Journal of the American Medical Association, 288,* 2569–2578.

Iqbal, R., Anand, S., Ounpuu, S., Islam, S., Zhang, X., Rangarajan, S., et al. (2008). Dietary patterns and the risk of acute myocardial infarction in 52 countries: Results of the INTERHEART Study. *Circulation, 118,* 1929–1937.

Jackson, L., Leclerc, J., Erskine, Y., & Linden, W. (2004). Getting the most out of cardiac rehabilitation: A review of referral and adherence predictors. *Heart, 91,* 10–14.

Jamrozik, K. (2004). Risk factors for atherosclerotic disease. In M. H. Crawford, J. P. DiMarco ,& W. J. Paulus (Eds.), *Cardiology* (2nd ed., pp. 23–32). Edinburgh, UK: Mosby.

Jolliffe, J. A., Rees, K., Taylor, R. S., Thompson, D., Oldridge, N., & Ebrahim, S. (2001). Exercise-based rehabilitation for coronary heart disease. *Cochrane Database of Systematic Reviews,* Issue 1 (Article No. CD001800), DOI: 10.1002/14651858.CD001800.

Kendel, F. (2008). *Gender and recovery from bypass surgery.* Heidelberg: Steinkopff.

Koertge, J., Weidner, G., Elliot-Eller, M., Scherwitz, L., Merritt-Worden, T. A., Marlin, R., et al. (2003). Improvement in medical risk factors and quality of life in women and men with coronary artery disease in the Multicenter Lifestyle Demonstration Project. *American Journal of Cardiology, 91,* 1316–1322.

Kulik, J. A., & Mahler, H. I. M. (1989). Social support and recovery from surgery. *Health Psychology, 8,* 221–238.

Kuper, H., & Marmot, M. (2003). Job strain, job demands, decision latitude, and risk of coronary heart disease within the Whitehall II Study. *Journal of Epidemiology and Community Health, 57,* 147–153.

Kuper, H., Marmot, M., & Hemingway, H. (2002). Systematic review of prospective cohort studies of psychosocial factors in the etiology and prognosis of coronary heart disease. *Seminars in Vascular Medicine, 2,* 267–314.

Lee, S., Colditz, G., Berkman, L., & Kawachi, I. (2003). Caregiving to children and grandchildren and risk of coronary heart disease in women. *American Journal of Public Health, 93,* 1939–1944.

Lichtman, J. H., Bigger, J. T., Jr., Blumenthal, J. A., Frasure-Smith, N., Kaufmann, P. G., Lespérance, F., et al. (2008). Depression and coronary heart disease: Recommendations for screening, referral, and treatment: A science advisory from the American Heart Association Prevention Committee of the Council on Cardiovascular Nursing, Council on Clinical Cardiology, Council on Epidemiology and Prevention, and Interdisciplinary Council on Quality of Care and Outcomes Research. *Circulation, 118,* 1768–1775.

Linden, W., Phillips, M. J., & Leclerc, J. (2007). Psychological treatment of cardiac patients: A meta-analysis. *European Heart Journal, 28,* 2972–2984.

Linden, W., Stossel, C., & Maurice, J. (1996). Psychosocial interventions for patients with coronary artery disease: A meta-analysis. *Archives of Internal Medicine, 156,* 745–752.

Marmot, M. G., Smith, G. D., Stansfeld, S., Patel, C., North, F., Head, J., et al. (1991). Health inequalities among British civil servants: The Whitehall II Study. *Lancet, 337,* 1387–1393.

Miller, T. D., Balady, G. J., & Fletcher, G. F. (1997). Exercise and its role in the prevention and rehabilitation of cardiovascular disease. *Annals of Behavioral Medicine, 19,* 220–229.

Myrtek, M. (2001). Meta-analyses of prospective studies on coronary heart disease, Type A personality, and hostility. *International Journal of Cardiology, 79,* 245–251.

Narayan, K. M. V., Boyle, J. P., Geiss, L. S., Saaddine, J. B., & Thompson, T. J. (2006). Impact of recent increase in incidence on future diabetes burden. *Diabetes Care, 29,* 2114–2116.

National Healthcare Cost and Utilization Project. (2005). *National and regional estimates on hospital use for all patients from the HCUP Nationwide Inpatient sample.* Retrieved October 30, 2006, from *hcup.ahrq.gov.*

Nestle, M. (2006). Food marketing and childhood obesity—a matter of policy. *New England Journal of Medicine, 354,* 2527–2529.

Ornish, D. (1998). Avoiding revascularization with lifestyle changes: The Multicenter Lifestyle Demonstration Project. *American Journal of Cardiology, 82,* 72T–76T.

Ornish, D., Brown, S. E., Scherwitz, L. W., Billings, J. H., Armstrong, W. T., Ports, T. A., et al. (1990). Can lifestyle changes reverse coronary heart disease?: The Lifestyle Heart Trial. *Lancet, 336,* 129–133.

Ornish, D., Gotto, A. M., Miller, R. R., Rochelle, D., McAllister, G., et al. (1979). Effects of a vegetarian diet and selected yoga techniques in the treatment of coronary heart disease. *Clinical Research, 27,* 720A.

Ornish, D., Lin, J., Daubenmier, J., Weidner, G., Epel, E., Kemp, C., et al. (2008). Increased telomerase activity and comprehensive lifestyle changes: A pilot study. *Lancet Oncology, 9,* 1048–1057.

Ornish, D., Magbanua, M. J. M., Weidner, G., Weinberg, V., Kemp, C., Green, C., et al. (2008). Changes in prostate gene expression in men undergoing an intensive nutrition and lifestyle intervention. *Proceedings of the National Academy of Sciences USA, 105,* 8369–8374.

Ornish, D., Scherwitz, L. W., Billings, J. H., Gould, K. L., Merritt, T. A., Sparler, S., et al. (1998). Intensive lifestyle changes for reversal of coronary heart disease. *Journal of the American Medical Association, 280,* 2001–2007.

Ornish, D., Scherwitz, L. W., Doody, R. S., Kesten, D., McLanahan, S. M., Brown, S. E., et al. (1983). Effects of stress management training and dietary changes in treating ischemic heart disease. *Journal of the American Medical Association, 249,* 54–59.

Ornish, D., Weidner, G., Fair, W. R., Marlin, R., Pettengill, E. B., Raisin, C. J., et al. (2005). Intensive lifestyle changes may affect the progression of prostate cancer. *Journal of Urology, 174,* 1065–1070.

Orth-Gomér, K., Schneiderman, N., Hui-Xin, W., Walldin, C., Blom, M., & Jernberg, T. (2009). Stress reduction prolongs life in women with coronary disease: The Stockholm Women's Intervention Trial for Coronary Heart Disease (SWITCHD). *Circulation: Cardiovascular Quality and Outcomes, 2,* 25–32.

Orth-Gomér, K., Wamala, S. P., Horsten, M., Schenck-Gustafsson, K., Schneiderman, N., & Mittleman, M. A. (2000). Marital stress worsens prognosis in women with coronary heart disease: the Stockholm Female Coronary Risk Study. *Journal of the American Medical Association, 284,* 3008–3014.

Orth-Gomér, K., Weidner, G., Anderson, D. E., & Chesney, M. A. (2010). Psychosocial influences on the heart: Epidemiology of cardiovascular diseases. In M. H. Crawford, J. P. DiMarco, & W. J. Paulus (Eds.), *Cardiology* (3rd ed., pp. 1819–1824). Edinburgh, UK: Mosby.

Pischke, C. R., Elliott-Eller, M., Li, M., Mendell, N. R., Ornish, D., & Weidner, G. (in press). Clinical events in heart disease patients with an ejection fraction of ≤40%: 3 year follow-up results. *Journal of Cardiovascular Nursing.*

Pischke, C. R., Frenda, S., Ornish, D., & Weidner, G. (in press). Lifestyle changes are related to reductions in depression in persons with elevated coronary risk factors. *Psychology and Health.*

Pischke, C. R., Weidner, G., Elliot-Eller, M., & Ornish, D. (2007). Lifestyle changes and clinical profile in CHD patients with ejections fraction < 40% and > 40% in the Multicenter Lifestyle Demonstration Project. *European Journal of Heart Failure, 9,* 928–934.

Pischke, C. R., Weidner, G., Elliot-Eller, M., Scherwitz, L., Merritt-Worden, T. A., Marlin, R., et al. (2006). Comparison of coronary risk factors and quality of life in coronary artery disease patients with versus without diabetes mellitus. *American Journal of Cardiology, 97,* 1267–1273.

Pischke, C. R., Weidner, G., Scherwitz, L., & Ornish, D. (2008). Long-term effects of lifestyle changes on well-being and cardiac variables among CHD patients. *Health Psychology, 27*(5), 584–592.

Player, M. S., King, D. E., Mainous, A. G., & Geesey, M. E. (2007). Psychosocial factors and progression from prehypertension to hypertension to coronary heart disease. *Annals of Family Medicine, 5,* 403–411.

Pomeranz, J. L., & Brownell, K. D. (2008). Legal and public health considerations affecting success, reach, and impact of menu-labeling laws. *American Journal of Public Health, 98,* 1578–1583.

Puska, P., Vartiainen, E., Pallonen, U., Ruotsalainen, P., Tuomilehto, J., Koskela, K., et al. (1981). The North Karelia Youth Project: A community-based intervention study on CVD risk factors among 13 to 15-year-old children: Study design and preliminary findings. *Preventive Medicine, 10,* 133–148.

Regitz-Zagrosek, V., Lehmkuhl, E., Hocher, B., Goesmann, D., Lehmkuhl, H. B., Hausmann, H., et al. (2004). Gender as a risk factor in young, not in old, women undergoing coronary artery bypass grafting. *Journal of the American College of Cardiology, 44,* 2413–2414.

Rosengren, A., Hawken, S., Ounpuu, S., Sliwa, K., Zubaid, M., Almahmeed, W. A., et al. (2004). Association of psychosocial risk factors with risk of acute myocardial infarction in 11119 cases and 13648 controls from 52 countries (the INTERHEART Study): Case–control study. *Lancet, 364,* 953–962.

Rugulies, R. (2002). Depression as a predictor for coronary heart disease: A review and meta-analysis. *American Journal of Preventive Medicine, 23,* 51–61.

Schulz, U., Pischke, C. R., Weidner, G., Daubenmier, J. J., Elliott-Eller, M., Scherwitz, L., et al. (2008). Social support group attendance is related to blood pressure, health behaviors, and quality of life in the Multicenter Lifestyle Demonstration Project. *Psychology, Health and Medicine, 13,* 423–437.

Schwarzer, R., & Rieckmann, N. (2002). Social support, cardiovascular disease, and mortality. In G. Weidner, M. S. Kopp, & M. Kristenson (Eds.), *Heart disease: Environment, stress and gender* (pp. 185–194). Amsterdam: IOS Press.

Shepard, J., Alcalde, V., Befort, P. A., Boucher, B., Erdmann, E., Gutzwiller, G., et al. (1997). International comparison of awareness and attitudes toward coronary risk factor reduction: The HELP Study. *Journal of Cardiovascular Risk, 4,* 373–384.

Spaderna, H., Mendel, N. R., Zahn, D., Wang, Y., Kahn, J., Smis, J. M. A., et al. (2010). Social isolation and depression predict 12 month outcomes in the Waiting for a New Heart Study. *Journal of Heart and Lung Transplantation, 29,* 247–252.

Spaderna, H., Weidner, G., Zahn, D., Smits, J. M. A. (2009). Psychological characteristics and social integration of patients with ischemic and non-ischemic heart failure newly listed for heart transplantation: The Waiting for a New Heart Study. *Applied Psychology: Health and Well-Being, 1,* 188–210.

Taylor, R. S., Brown, A., Ebrahim, S., Jolliffe, J., Noorani, H., Rees, K., et al. (2004). Exercise-based rehabilitation for patients with coronary heart disease: Systematic review and meta-analysis of randomized controlled trials. *American Journal of Medicine, 116,* 682–692.

Thombs, B. D., Bass, E. B., Ford, D. E., Stewart, K. J., Tsilidis, K. K., Patel, U., et al. (2006). Prevalence of depression in survivors of acute myocardial infarction. *Journal of General Internal Medicine, 21,* 30–38.

U. S., Department of Health and Human Services, Centers for Medicare and Medicaid Services. (2009). *Proposed Decision Memo for Intensive Cardiac Rehabilitation (ICR) Program— Dr. Ornish's Program for Reversing Heart Disease (GAG-00491N).* Retrieved from *http://www.cms.gov/mcd/viewdraftdecisionmemo.asp?from2=viewdraftdecisionmemo.asp&id=240&.html*

Vaccarino, V., Abramson, J. L., Veledar, E., & Weintraub, W. S. (2002). Sex differences in hospital mortality after coronary artery bypass surgery. *Circulation, 105,* 1176–1181.

Vaccarino, V., Parsons, L., Every, N. R., Barron, H. V., & Krumholz, H. M. (1999). Sex-based differences in early mortality after myocardial infarction. *New England Journal of Medicine, 341,* 217–225.

Vizza, J., Neatrour, D. M., Felton, P. M., & Ellsworth, D. L. (2007). Improvement in psychosocial functioning during an intensive cardiovascular lifestyle modification program. *Journal of Cardiopulmonary Rehabilitation and Prevention, 27,* 376–383.

Wamala, S. P., Mittleman, M. A., Horsten, M., Schenck-Gustafsson, K., & Orth-Gomér, K. (2000). Job stress and the occupational gradient in coronary heart disease risk in women: The Stockholm Female Coronary Risk Study. *Social Science and Medicine, 51,* 481–489.

Weidner, G. (2000). Why do men get more heart disease than women?: An international perspective. *Journal of American College Health, 48,* 291–294.

Weidner, G., & Cain, V. (2003). Gender gap in heart disease: Lessons from Eastern Europe. *American Journal of Public Health, 93,* 768–770.

Weidner, G., Kopp, M., & Kristenson, M. (2002). *Heart disease: Environment, stress and gender.* Amsterdam: IOS Press.

Wilbert-Lampen, U., Leistner, D., Greven, S., Pohl, T., Sper, S., Volker, C., et al. (2008). Cardiovascular events during World Cup soccer. *New England Journal of Medicine, 358,* 475–483.

Writing Group for the ENRICHD Investigators. (2003). Effects of treating depression and low perceived social support on clinical events after myocardial infarction: The Enhancing Recovery in Coronary Heart Disease Patients (ENRICHD) randomized trial. *Journal of the American Medical Association, 289,* 3106–3116.

Yancy, W. S., Westman, E. C., French, P. A., & Califf, R. M. (2003). Diets and clinical coronary events: The truth is out there. *Circulation, 107,* 10–16.

Yusuf, S., Hawken, S., Ounpuu, S., Dans, T., Avezum, A., Lanas, F., et al. (2004). Effect of potentially modifiable risk factors associated with myocardial infarction in 52 countries (the INTERHEART Study): Case–control study. *Lancet, 364,* 937–952.

CHAPTER 25

The Role of Behavior in Cancer Prevention

Deborah Bowen
Ulrike Boehmer

The field of cancer prevention has been filled with behavioral and social scientists since its formal creation just over 30 years ago. In fact, some of the first research in the area of cancer prevention was on tobacco use reduction, coming on the heels of the large-scale findings in the mid-20th century that tobacco was the behavioral and primary cause of the new epidemic of lung cancer. This single behavioral cause led a struggle first to identify the components of the risk, then on to the individual, and finally to public health methods of reducing tobacco exposure through clinical behavior change programs and public health reinforcements to quit using tobacco or never to become addicted in the first place. National reductions in smoking have given us a clear sense of success. However, the success has not always been linear, and it is not complete. In some ways many of the lessons were learned first in the tobacco trenches, giving us a model of social and behavioral causality, and solution to the cause of one of the major diseases of modern day. Intimate involvement and leadership of modern disease prevention studies, like the Women's Health Initiative (Backinger, Fagan, Matthews, & Grana, 2003), indicate the value of behavioral and social science in cancer prevention efforts. In this chapter we discuss the current role of social and behavioral research in cancer prevention and control, providing a focus for future research in these areas.

Overview of Cancer Prevention

A broad, public health analysis of the prevention of mortality due to cancer divides the field into four areas: primary, secondary, tertiary, and quaternary prevention. Figure 25.1 details these areas. "Primary prevention" is not to allow cancer ever to reach clinical significance. Many cite the common finding that prostate cancer is relatively common in older men, who die of many other things first, including accidents, heart disease, and stroke. This means that for many, prevention is reducing initial risk of cancer becoming the invasive killer that we all think of when we hear the word "cancer." Recent reviews point to tobacco use and obesity-related behaviors as causing a majority of the new cancer cases in the United States (Mermelstein & Wahl, 2008; Stein & Colditz, 2008). This

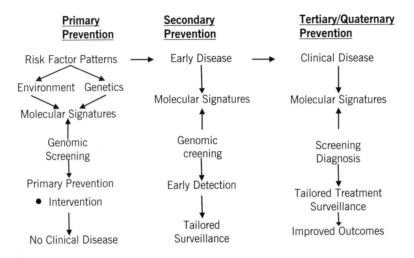

FIGURE 25.1. An overview of cancer prevention and control strategies.

enormous contribution to the cancer burden in this country points directly to the role of behavior in primary prevention. "Secondary prevention" is identification of cancer at an early stage, early enough to treat it efficaciously. Screening tests of many types have been designed with this identification process in mind. The identification of these tests and their relative clinical utility (acceptability to the general public, ability to be delivered in many different types of health or clinical settings, etc.) is a key area for research by social and behavioral scientists. "Tertiary prevention" (reducing the harm and invasiveness of cancer treatment) and "quaternary prevention" (improving the experience of dying from cancer), covered in another chapter (Diefenbach, Mohamed, Turner, & Diefenbach, Chapter 31, this volume), are areas rich with contributions of behavioral and social science to both treatment of and long-term coping with cancer.

Key Findings in the Field

Primary Prevention of Cancer

One of the key areas of growth over the past two decades has been the primary prevention of cancer. By far the most voluminous research has been in the area of tobacco use, judging from the number of well-cited reports from the Surgeon General on research into tobacco use. Indeed, tobacco use reduction is

often the model used when considering next steps in changing other behavioral targets. Moving from basic research on smoking as a behavior to interventions that help addicted smokers reduce their consumption, to policy and international law supporting cessation will reduce the burden of chronic disease across the world. New research is clarifying the genetic, pharmacological, and behavioral determinants of smoking cessation and nicotine dependence. For example, new studies indicate that small genetic differences can lead to individual differences in genetic risk of relapse among smokers (Baker et al., 2009). New behavioral strategies include delivering programs for both youth and adults using the Internet (Myung, McDonnell, Kazinets, Seo, & Moskowitz, 2009).

Findings from multidisciplinary studies will likely improve the understanding of smoking behavior change and maintenance, and allow for tailoring of smoking cessation assistance to a smoker's biological, behavioral, and social patterns. Current quit rates differ widely across population subgroups and are lower among those with psychiatric comorbidity, alcohol and substance abuse disorders, low socioeconomic status, and specific ethnic/racial backgrounds (Dhingra & Ostroff, 2008). One demographic group that has rates of adult smoking almost triple those of the general population is the lesbian, gay, bisexual, and transgendered population (The President's Cancer Panel, 2007).

Data suggest that most smokers quit without assistance and prefer not to enroll in formal treatment programs (Fiore et al., 1990). Unfortunately, the majority of ex-smokers relapse 1 year after quitting, with self-quitters relapsing at higher rates than treated smokers (Ockene et al., 2000). Needed are changes in the environment that reduce the attractiveness of smoking, combined with multiple opportunities to quit. To this end, previous research has emphasized the critical importance of improving treatment access to reach those smokers who are motivated to quit, and boosting engagement in cost-effective tobacco interventions at the public health level. Dissemination of efficacious cessation strategies is a major focus of research, along with targeting the few groups in the population that have high smoking rates.

Smoking initiation and uptake is often conceptualized as progression through a series of stages (Department of Health and Human Services, 1994). Most youths go beyond the contemplation state to trying out smoking, but far fewer move on to the subsequent stages of experimentation, regular use, and dependence. Although we know a great deal about predictors of initially trying out smoking, we know much less about what predicts progression to dependence (Turner, Mermelstein, & Flay, 2004). Predictors of initiation or of ever smoking are multilayered and multifaceted, and include individual factors (e.g., age, family socioeconomic status), social contexts (e.g., smoking peers and family), and broad policy and macroenvironmental factors (e.g., smoking access and sales policies) (Department of Health and Human Services, 1994). Early interventions for smoking prevention were often based on the assumption that finding a strong relationship between a given predictor variable and smoking would sufficiently translate into a strong intervention. For example, the finding that youth smokers reported feeling pressured to use tobacco led to early school-based smoking prevention programs that used social interactions as the intervention targets, and were not successful in preventing youths' long-term smoking behaviors. A critical link in moving from theory to intervention is understanding the causal relationships among variables, both over time and in intervention studies. Recognizing that there were broader domains

of influence on adolescents' tobacco use, researchers began supplementing school-based programs with parent involvement, media, and community-based components as well. More recently, researchers have taken a more macro-level view of changing population rates of tobacco use by attempting to influence policy change and the broader social culture of youths through tobacco countermarketing campaigns (Mermelstein & Wahl, 2008).

Dietary change is an area that has benefited from the research in smoking (Ammerman, Lindquist, Lohr, & Hersey, 2002; Bowen & Beresford, 2002). Eating habits and patterns are complex and notoriously difficult to change. Dietary patterns and food preferences are established in early childhood, and research suggests that parental feeding practices and restrictions may influence later body weight and ability to modify dietary consumption (Neumark-Sztainer et al., 2006). Among adults, studies indicate that a variety of factors may influence dietary habits. Understanding the psychosocial determinants of dietary behavior is an important step in the process. There has been a plethora of human laboratory and psychosocial research studies into the determinants of dietary behaviors and choices; this research provides the basis of intervention design to improve dietary behaviors. Changing eating habits is especially complex because it involves continuing the overall behavior (eating) while making multiple daily decisions in a variety of subbehavioral domains and settings. Clearly, there is a need for more basic theoretical research to understand how and why people change their eating habits and how best to promote these changes.

Evidence review has examined characteristics and findings across dietary intervention studies to identify common intervention components that may be most efficacious (Ammerman, et al., 2002; Bowen & Beresford, 2002). Not surprisingly, interventions focused on high-risk populations in more intensive clinical settings tended to have larger effects compared to population-based programs with average-risk individuals. Unfortunately, because of the broad diversity of study populations, methods, intervention approaches, and the requirements for inclusion in an evidence review, few conclusions could be drawn regarding efficacy of specific intervention strategies. Despite evidence that cancer disproportionately affects certain populations, relatively few dietary intervention studies have been designed for specific ethnic populations (Pignone et al., 2003). Clearly, issues of cultural, ethnic, and socioeconomic diversity are key to include in the design and evaluation of effective interventions to improve diet and reduce health disparities. There is a growing body of evidence that human–environment interactions are essential components of dietary practices and that a social-ecological approach may be effective in dietary and other health promotion interventions. The Institute of Medicine (IOM), therefore, has recommended the use of a social ecological model, which provides a framework for intervening at multiple levels of influence, including individual, interpersonal, institutional, community, and policy levels that use multiple approaches for improving public health (Smedley & Syme, 2000). Health promotion programs that take into account the complexity of health problems influenced by multiple levels are more complex to conceptualize and implement but also more likely to result in lasting behavior change.

Primary prevention of skin cancer by reducing sun exposure has received research attention in different streams of research. There have been multiple studies, including intervention studies, aimed at reduction of sun exposure in children (Buller, 2008; Saraiya et al., 2004). These have been mostly school-based interventions, or interventions targeting children and adolescents in recreational areas, such as pools, and swimming and ski settings. Most have shown improvements in sun protection behaviors, although tanning and the use of tanning facilities have been on the rise in the past several years. Mass media and mass communication interventions have also shown effects in increasing sun protection. Another stream of research has tested interventions to reduce cumulative sun exposure in adults, focusing on parents and caregivers of children, individuals from families in which melanoma is present, and occupational protection at workplaces. These programs also have reduced sun exposure, although the behavioral effects are less clear for adults than for children and adolescents.

Secondary Prevention of Cancer

Screening to detect cancer in a treatable stage has been well researched and reviewed in the field (see *www.thecommunityguide. org* for reviews and state of the science). Cancer screenings identified by the U.S. Preventive Services Task Force (USPSTF) that are recommended for use in primary care practice include breast screening via mammography, colon screening using multiple screening tests at multiple intervals, and cervical cancer screening via Pap (Papanicolaou) smears. The enormous research literature, aptly summarized in multiple reviews (Baron et al., 2008; Sabatino et al., 2008), has identified not only multiple successful interventions to improve the use of these tests but also areas for improvement, such as those revealed by measurement of behaviors. For example, colorectal cancer screening has received recent attention because the complexities of measuring frequency and type of colorectal cancer are deceptively simple, yet they have proven to be amenable to improvement through behavioral research that has prepared better questions and structures for wide use (McQueen, Tiro, & Vernon, 2008). The Community Guide (*www.thecommunityguide.org*) review of interventions to improve screening behavior by category of intervention (one-on-one, community, etc.) has successfully improved screening in diverse populations.

Screening tests for breast, cervical, and colorectal cancer are recommended due to their proven effectiveness in detecting these cancers at an early stage and, in combination with appropriate treatment, their likelihood of reducing mortality (Task Force on Community Preventive Services, 2005). A report from the 2005 National Health Interview Survey of U.S. adults indicated that whereas 67% of women 40 years of age or older reported having mammograms within the previous 2 years, 78% of women age 18 or older reported having Pap tests within the previous 3 years, and 50% of adults age 50 years reported ever having screening endoscopies, only 17% of adults age 50 years and older reported having a fecal occult blood test within the previous 2 years. Rates are even lower for persons with no usual source of health care, those with no health insurance, or those who immigrated to the

United States within the previous 10 years (13–20% for colorectal cancer, 61–67% for breast cancer, and 58–62% for cervical cancer) (Task Force on Community Preventive Services, 2005). Because screening does not occur as recommended, effective interventions to address barriers to screening have been developed and subsequently reviewed by the independent Task Force on Community Preventive Services reviewed their effectiveness. Effective interventions focus either on providers or patients (see the *www.communityguide.org* for summaries of interventions). Provider-focused interventions consist of provider reminders that have been shown to increase breast and cervical cancer screening rates, yet are not effective in increasing patients' colorectal cancer screening with colonoscopy or double-contrast barium enema (Sabatino et al., 2008). Similarly, provider assessment and feedback, which evaluates provider performance with respect to cancer screening, then informs providers about their performance, has been shown to be effective in increasing breast and cervical cancer but not colorectal cancer screening (see *www.thecommunityguide.org* for evidence-based reviews; Sabatino et al., 2008).

Interventions that focused on patients consist of reminders for screening; informational materials about screening, such as leaflets, brochures, and so forth; as well as one-on-one education, in which a health professional communicates with the patient about screening. In addition, interventions that target patients' access by reducing either out-of-pocket costs or structural barriers (scheduling of screening appointments, etc.) have been shown to be effective (Baron et al., 2008).

Several areas of newer research are ongoing in the area of screening or secondary prevention. The thoughtful research by Miles, Waller, and Wardle (2008) on the consequences of screening, identified the complexity of introducing a technology into public use to improve health; because the standard for prevention activities to do no harm is high, we should consider these findings as we move forward with new intervention opportunities. This overview documented that false-positive findings in cancer screening produce distress and anxiety in patients who first receive the notice of

positive cancer, then an all clear from the provider. Because the frequency of false-positive findings for some screening tests is relatively high, measurable distress due to this false-positive rate occurs in the population. New screening tests are entering the marketplace with little in the way of acceptability or usability testing to support their selection over existing tests. Given research findings to date, gynecological cancer secondary prevention (Wenzel, Reina-Patton, & De Alba, 2008), in which more new multistep tests are being created and implemented in research settings, is one of future research growth areas.

Overarching Issues to Consider

This research has identified some of the richness and complexity of cancer prevention and control. For example, reviews of the literature on screening indicate that we do have successful screening interventions that we can promote successfully in the population, as cited earlier. However, the use of these screening interventions is not without cost to individuals, and the costs need to be considered in future innovative technological solutions. These monetary costs may also be emotional costs in terms of distress about false-positive findings, effects on family members, and so forth. How we balance screening monetary costs with social and behavioral costs, and also the cost of lives saved, is still not clear. However, all of this must be taken into account before we release a screening test for use with the general public. The current controversy over prostate cancer screening, a screening test released into clinical practice that frequently is recommended and selected in provider settings but for which there are few or no recommendations for use with the entire population, is only one example of such a misstep that did not take all the issues into account before making the test clinically available.

Disparities exist, in that certain subpopulations bear an undue burden regardless of whether we focus on primary, secondary, tertiary, or quaternary prevention and control. Health disparities refer to more than differences. Rather, disparities are inequities resulting from economic, political, social, and psychological processes (Braveman, 2006). The subpopulations that carry the burden of disparities are the subgroups that persistently experience social disadvantage and discrimination. For example, with respect to primary prevention, tobacco use rates are higher among disadvantaged populations, such as racial and ethnic groups, American Indians, Alaska Natives, African Americans, and Southeast Asians; people with low socioeconomic status; and those who are gay, lesbian, and bisexual (The President's Cancer Panel, 2008). Or disparities in secondary prevention consist of lower colorectal and breast cancer screening rates in African Americans, Hispanics, and those with low socioeconomic status (Kelley, Moy, Stryer, Burstin, & Clancy, 2005). Social and behavioral scientists are central to the task of reducing these disparities by designing and developing interventions that are culturally appropriate for these underserved population groups (Marion & Schover, 2006).

One of the new areas of research in the field is the encouragement of physical activity and dietary change to reduce obesity. Identification of obesity as a risk factor for cancer has stimulated new research into obesity reduction and prevention. Moving from the biomedical or clinical model of "weight loss" will mean focusing on energy balance, calories in and calories out, which requires a more thoughtful look at dietary and physical activity change. Moving back and forth between the well-researched and documented individual causes of eating and activity, and to the social and environmental causes still being explored will provide a more complete picture of what drives these key behaviors and prepare us better for public health behavior change.

There is growing recognition that social determinants, the economic, social, and political conditions under which people live, determine their *health* behaviors. Figure 25.2 presents a model (Warnecke et al., 2008) that considers the larger world and how it might impact health disparities. Using multilevel analyses, health outcomes research has demonstrated the complex interactions between individual and environmental factors that result in cardiovascular disease, for example (Cozier et al., 2007). The same complex interactions apply to cancer prevention and control behaviors, in that research early on indicated that the social environment serves as a source for learning and reinforcing health maintenance behaviors, such as undergoing cancer screening, or risk behaviors, such as smoking (Taylor, Repetti, & Seeman, 1997). Therefore, only multilevel, transdisciplinary researchers that identify larger social determinants, in addition to individual-level factors of behaviors, and subsequently have the ability to design interventions that address population- and individual-level factors, will effectively improve cancer-related outcomes.

One of the key advances in cancer prevention has been in the area of methodology. As Colditz and others have argued, a shift from considering only traditional epidemiology, with its focus on individual risk factors, to a populationwide policy focus to consider the effects of health promotion interventions and the community, country, and indeed, even the world, is key (Stein & Colditz, 2008). If the causes of cancer are primarily social in nature, or socially determined, then the solutions, by definition, will likely contain social and behavioral change. Tracking these types of changes is important, whether through classic public health surveillance or more innovative mechanisms, such as the surveillance opportunities presented by the Health Information National Trends Survey (HINTS) conducted by the National Cancer Institute. This survey measures the country's communications about cancer by monitoring key communication variables across the population every few years, and helps to ensure that we stay on top of changes in what the public is doing and not doing. This will allow us to target changing disease rates by measuring shifts in population behavior levels, norms, and patterns. Focusing on theoretical models to drive behavior change will produce better, more effective, more reproducible interventions over time, and allow us to understand the overall simple human behavior patterns that likely exist. Improvements in the methodologies for individual and group randomized trials are important because randomized trials set the standard for evidence in review. Both types of methodologies are well reviewed and organized by several colleagues (e.g., Curry, Wetter, Grothaus, McClure, & Taplin, 2008; Glasgow & Emmons, 2007; Murray, Pals, & Blitstein, 2008).

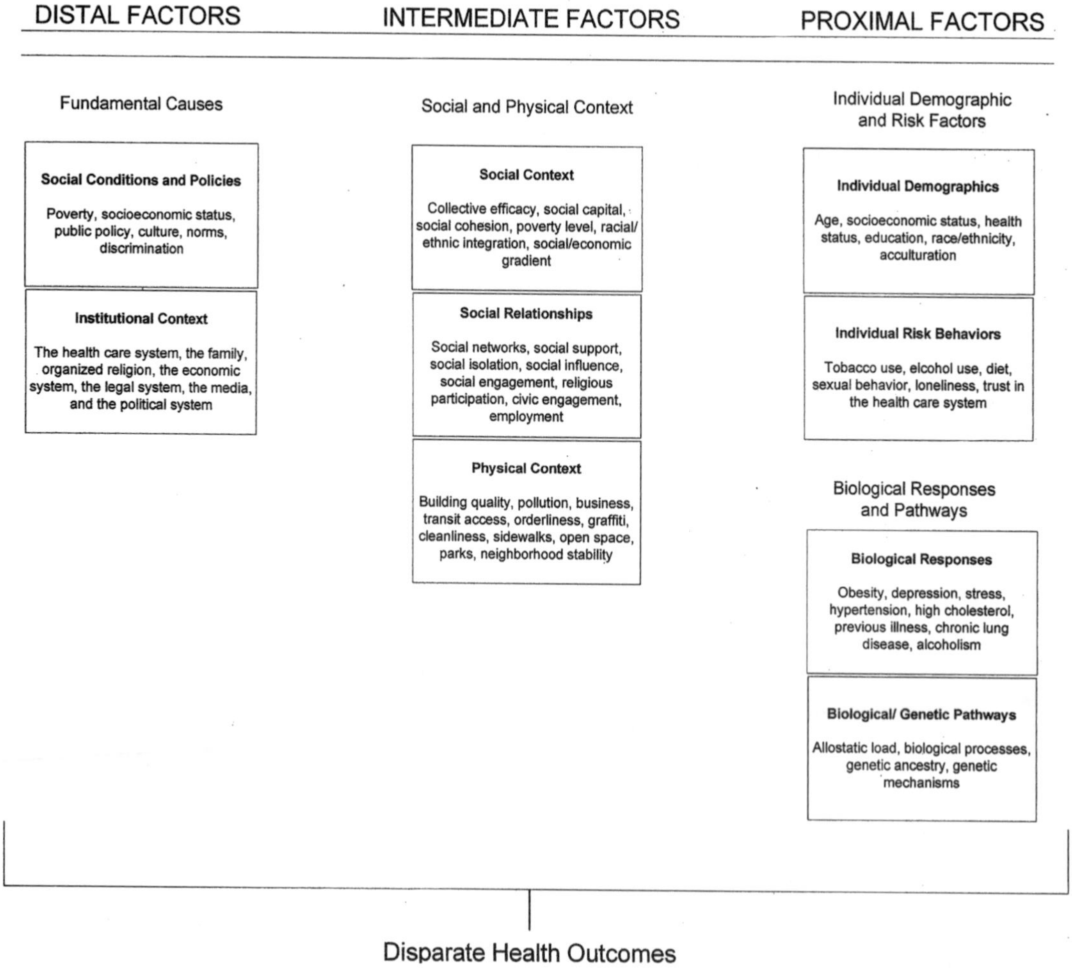

DISTAL FACTORS	INTERMEDIATE FACTORS	PROXIMAL FACTORS

Fundamental Causes

Social Conditions and Policies

Poverty, socioeconomic status, public policy, culture, norms, discrimination

Institutional Context

The health care system, the family, organized religion, the economic system, the legal system, the media, and the political system

Social and Physical Context

Social Context

Collective efficacy, social capital, social cohesion, poverty level, racial/ethnic integration, social/economic gradient

Social Relationships

Social networks, social support, social isolation, social influence, social engagement, religious participation, civic engagement, employment

Physical Context

Building quality, pollution, business, transit access, orderliness, graffiti, cleanliness, sidewalks, open space, parks, neighborhood stability

Individual Demographic and Risk Factors

Individual Demographics

Age, socioeconomic status, health status, education, race/ethnicity, acculturation

Individual Risk Behaviors

Tobacco use, alcohol use, diet, sexual behavior, loneliness, trust in the health care system

Biological Responses and Pathways

Biological Responses

Obesity, depression, stress, hypertension, high cholesterol, previous illness, chronic lung disease, alcoholism

Biological/ Genetic Pathways

Allostatic load, biological processes, genetic ancestry, genetic mechanisms

Disparate Health Outcomes

FIGURE 25.2. Levels of approach to identify and eliminate health disparities.

Future Areas of Research

How, then, shall we prevent mortality and reduce morbidity, improve quality of life, and reduce health disparities associated with cancer in patients, families, and the public? One thing is clear: Change is an inherent part of the effort, and social and behavioral changes are the key ones. Data presented in Figures 25.1 and 25.2 also allow us to consider where to focus our efforts on change using the social and behavioral approaches and methods. At each of these phases we include cultural, social, and behavioral variables as central to the solution; any new strategy for cancer control must recognize that human behavior is a major determinant of cancer incidence and outcomes (Hiatt & Rimer, 1999). A recent IOM report estimat-ed that lifestyle changes account for considerable preventable deaths (Committee on Health and Behavior: Research and Health, 2002), and a recent position paper by the Centers for Disease Control and Prevention called for action to reduce the burden of chronic disease through lifestyle changes (Gerberding, 2005). Social and behavioral science research is critical to cancer prevention and control because translating knowledge into practice at the population level requires new methods for promoting social and behavioral change (including identifying cultural barriers to change), improved cancer communications, and continuous evaluation of the outcomes of cancer interventions. The recent focus on the social and structural causes of chronic disease also calls for increased research and training on the social epidemiology of cancer and societal interventions to reduce disparities.

Cancer survivorship is important to improving overall burden of cancer. The American Cancer Society estimated that in 2000, 9.6 million Americans had a history of cancer. The 5-year relative survival rate for all cancers combined is 63%. The human toll of cancer, beyond reduced survival, is repeatedly documented in quality-of-life and other outcome studies, in ethnographic and qualitative research, and in the popular media. Almost every U.S. family is touched at one time or another by the prospect of a family member receiving a cancer diagnosis, dealing with symptoms, undergoing treatment, surviving cancer, or moving through end-of-life stages and care. Do cancer survivors move past their cancer experience, with the result that the drivers of health behavior in long-term cancer survivors look a lot like primary prevention? Although the impact of cancer screening, diagnosis, and treatment on children and adults is well known, scientific understanding of these outcomes, their social sequelae, and evidence-based studies of care are relatively sparse.

The National Institutes of Health estimated overall 2003 annual costs for cancer at $189.5 billion ($64 for direct medical costs, $16 for indirect morbidity costs, and $109 for indirect mortality costs). Treatment of breast, lung, and prostate cancers accounts for over half of direct medical costs. Thus, cancer takes a high economic toll directly and is responsible for much lost productivity and distress. Without a universal health insurance plan in the United States, some Americans are at high risk for not having access to high-quality cancer care or cancer screening opportunities. The relative expense of some cancer screening also increasingly demands evidence of outcomes in relation to cost to encourage insurance and managed care providers to include cost-effective cancer screening as routine benefits.

In addition to cultural influences, behaviors and behavior change are central to improving cancer prevention and control efforts. It is estimated that as much as 50% or more of cancer can be prevented through smoking cessation and improved dietary habits, such as increasing fruit and vegetable consumption and reducing consumption of fats, both of which are difficult changes in behavior to achieve (Stein & Colditz, 2008).

Adherence to screening recommendations can reduce breast, cervical, and colon cancer, and requires good information, culturally sensitive interventions, and motivational science-based interventions. In some cases, social and behavioral science research is needed to help resolve current dilemmas in cancer prevention and control, such as the efficacy and effectiveness of prostate screening programs or use of self-exams to detect skin cancers. As information on genetic risk becomes available, high-risk groups will be identified and will require information to help individuals decide on behavioral change, whether it be in diet, physical activity, smoking cessation, or seeking out screening programs and making decisions based on the evidence provided to them.

As indicated in Figure 25.1, genetics and genomics might in the future provide the link between risk factors and behavioral choices. Genetics can be used to identify those at increased risk for developing one or more cancers, and to determine prognosis and likelihood of recurrence. In many cases, personal genetic factors may dictate behaviors that are necessary to reduce risk in ways that are different from those recommended for the general population. For example, persons carrying *breast cancer genetic mutation 1* or (*BRCA1*) or *BRCA2* and hereditary nonpolyposis colorectal cancer (*HNPCC*) mutations are at high risk for developing breast and colorectal cancer, respectively. These individuals must begin cancer screening at a much younger age, adhere to more intensive screening regimens, and even contemplate prophylactic surgical removal of affected organs to prevent early death from cancer. Modifying other behaviors, such as diet, physical activity, and smoking, may be critically important for those whose genetic susceptibility to cancer is higher than average. For those diagnosed with cancer, tumor gene expression is increasingly being seen as an important prognostic marker and has been used to modify treatment (e.g., human epidermal growth factor receptor 2 [*HER2/neu*] status in breast cancer). Social and behavioral researchers have only recently begun to grapple with issues on how to help the public, cancer patients, and even clinicians interpret and use genetically based cancer risk information. A great deal of research is needed to understand better the factors influencing individuals' acceptance of genetic tests, and to help clinicians effectively utilize tests based on their analytic validity and clinical utility.

As pharmacological and nonpharmacological chemopreventive agents for cancer are developed, assessment of their outcomes in terms of cost and quality of life are important and difficult considerations. It is important to focus attention on three key types of outcomes experienced by cancer patient survivors: chronic problems with fatigue, pain, and depression. Access to state-of-the-art care is essential for people of all genders, races, ethnic groups, ability or disability levels, and sexual orientations. Considerable challenges exist in reaching vulnerable populations with cancer prevention information, screening, and treatments. A knowledge base and culturally sensitive interventions are required for every group at risk for excess incidence or death from cancer.

No single scientific discipline can effectively address the tremendous array of relevant issues in 21st-century cancer prevention and control. Moreover, the degree of specialization that has become necessary in the basic and clinical sciences often comes at the expense of training about how attitudes, behaviors, and, more broadly, the culture influence cancer prevention and control.

Most prevention and intervention programs in behavior change have focused on the importance of key individual risk factor considerations, psychosocial variables, and individual-level change in both the short and the long term. However, this focus on individual change and maintenance has not been successful in achieving long-term improvements in behavior. Attention is thus shifting to environmental and societal contributions to the maintenance of healthy lifestyles and behaviors. The obesity epidemic is one such case, but there are others, such as maintenance of initial smoking prevention gains. Needed is improved understanding of the mechanisms by which established risk factors for obesity operate. Identifying new and malleable risk factors for obesity will help in the design of interventions for preventing or reducing use of personal health services and public health interventions. This focus on social, built, economic, and cultural environments is relatively new to cancer prevention, and we predict that it will be incorporated on more research into the basic mechanisms of understanding health behavior and interventions designed to improve health outcomes.

Finally, research into dissemination of our success stories lags behind the research to identify efficacious methods of improving health outcomes. The National Cancer Institute has put considerable investment into identifying pathways and mechanisms for dissemination of tested interventions, as indicated on their website (see *www.nci.nih.gov* for complete dissemination discussions). Rogers's theory of diffusion of innovations has been the guide for design, implementation, and evaluation of past health promotion packages (Brink et al., 1995; Brink, Levenson-Gingiss, & Gottlieb, 1991; Parcel et al., 1995). As stated by Rogers (1995), "Diffusion is the process by which an innovation is communicated through certain channels over time among the members of a social system." This process of dissemination has only been applied selectively to cancer prevention and control. Most of the programs that we have reported here have yet to be put into place in clinical or public health practice. Recent references on program dissemination into public health settings begin this process (Bowen et al., 2009), but more needs to be done in this area.

Conclusions

Much work has been done to apply psychological and behavioral findings to the problem of cancer prevention and control. This field is exciting because it provides opportunity to see our basic science actually used in real-life problems in an important health setting. Greater use of social and behavioral findings in cancer prevention and control could result in more lives saved and reduced morbidity. This is an invitation for all of us to increase our efforts in understanding and applying social and behavioral issues to this critically important health problem.

Further Reading

Holland, J. (1998). *Psycho-oncology*. New York: Oxford University Press.

Miller, S. M., Bowen, D. J., Croyle, R. T., & Rowland, J. H. (Eds.). (2008). *Handbook of cancer control and behavioral science: A resource for researchers, practitioners, and policymakers*. Washington, DC: American Psychological Association Press.

Smedley, D. B., & Syme, S. L. (Eds.). (2000). *Pro-

moting health: Intervention strategies from social and behavioral research. Washington, DC: National Academies Press.

References

Ammerman, A. S., Lindquist, C. H., Lohr, K. N., & Hersey, J. (2002). The efficacy of behavioral interventions to modify dietary fat and fruit and vegetable intake: A review of the evidence. *Preventive Medicine, 35,* 25–41.

Backinger, C., Fagan, P., Matthews, E., & Grana, R. (2003). Adolescent and young adult tobacco prevention and cessation: Current status and future directions. *Tobacco Control, 12,* 46–53.

Baker, T. B., Cummings, K. M., Hatsukami, D. K., Johnson, C. A., Lerman, C., Niaura, R., et al. (2009). Transdisciplinary Tobacco Use Research Centers: Research achievements and future implications. *Nicotine and Tobacco Research, 10,* 1231–44.

Baron, R. C., Rimer, B. K., Coates, R. J., Kerner, J., Kalra, G. P., Melillo, S., et al. (2008). Client-directed interventions to increase community access to breast, cervical, and colorectal cancer screening a systematic review. *American Journal of Preventive Medicine, 35*(Suppl. 1), S56–S66.

Bowen, D. J., & Beresford, S. A. A. (2002). Dietary intervention to prevent disease. *Annual Review of Public Health, 23,* 255–286.

Bowen, D. J., Sorensen, G., Weiner, B., Campbell, M., Emmons, K., & Melvin, C. (2009). Dissemination research in cancer control: Where are we and where should we go? *Cancer Causes and Control, 24,* 473–485.

Braveman, P. (2006). Health disparities and health equity: Concepts and measurement. *Annual Review of Public Health, 27*(1), 167–194.

Brink, S. G., Basen-Engquist, K. M., O'Hara-Tompkins, N. M., Parcel, G. S., Gottlieb, N. H., & Lovato, C. Y. (1995). Diffusion of an effective tobacco prevention program: Part I. Evaluation of the dissemination phase. *Health Education Research, 10*(3), 283–295.

Brink, S. G., Levenson-Gingiss, P., & Gottlieb, N. H. (1991). An evaluation of the effectiveness of a planned diffusion process: The Smoke-Free Class of 2000 Project in Texas. *Health Education Research, 6*(3), 353–362.

Buller, D. B. (2008). Interventions to modify skin cancer-related behaviors. In S. M. Miller, D. J. Bowen, R. T. Croyle, & J. H. Rowland (Eds.), *Handbook of cancer control and behavioral science: A resource for researchers, practitioners, and policymakers.* Washington, DC: American Psychological Association Press.

Committee on Health and Behavior: Research and Health. (2002). *Health and behavior: The interplay of biological, behavioral, and soci-etal influences.* Washington, DC: National Academy of Science.

Cozier, Y. C., Palmer, J. R., Horton, N. J., Fredman, L., Wise, L. A., & Rosenberg, L. (2007). Relation between neighborhood median housing value and hypertension risk among black women in the United States. *American Journal of Public Health, 97*(4), 718–724.

Curry, S. J., Wetter, D. W., Grothaus, L. C., McClure, J. B., & Taplin, S. M. (2008). Designing and evaluating individual-level interventions for cancer prevention and control. In S. M. Miller, D. J. Bowen, R. T. Croyle, & J. H. Rowland (Eds.), *Handbook of cancer control and behavioral science: A resource for researchers, practitioners, and policymakers.* Washington, DC: American Psychological Association Press.

Department of Health and Human Services. (1994). *Preventing tobacco use among young people: A report of the Surgeon General.* Atlanta, GA: U.S. Department of Health and Human Services, Public Health Service, Centers for Disease Control and Prevention, National Center for Chronic Disease Prevention and Health Promotion, Office on Smoking and Health.

Dhingra, L. A., & Ostroff, J. A. (2008). Interventions for smoking cessation. In S. M. Miller, D. J. Bowen, R. T. Croyle, & J. H. Rowland (Eds.), *Handbook of cancer control and behavioral science: A resource for researchers, practitioners, and policymakers.* Washington, DC: American Psychological Association Press.

Fiore, M. C., Novotny, T. E., Pierce, J. P., Giovino, G. A., Hatziandreu, E. J., Newcomb, P. A., et al. (1990). Methods used to quit smoking in the United States: Do cessation programs help? *Journal of the American Medical Association, 263*(20), 2760–2765.

Gerberding, J. (2005). Protecting health: The new research imperative. *Journal of the American Medical Association, 294,* 1403–1406.

Glasgow, R. E., & Emmons, K. M. (2007). How can we increase translation of research into practice?: Types of evidence needed. *Annual Reviews in Public Health, 28,* 418–433.

Hiatt, R. A., & Rimer, B. K. (1999). A new strategy for cancer control research. *Cancer Epidemiology, 8,* 957–964.

Kelley, E., Moy, E., Stryer, D., Burstin, H., & Clancy, C. (2005). The National Healthcare Quality and Disparities Reports: An overview. *Medical Care, 43*(Suppl. 3), I3–I8.

Marion, M. S., & Schover, L. R. (2006). Behavioral science and the task of resolving health disparities in cancer. *Journal of Cancer Education, 21*(Suppl. 1), S80–S86.

McQueen, A., Tiro, J. A., & Vernon, S. W. (2008). Construct validity and invariance of four factors associated with colorectal cancer screening across gender, race, and prior screening. *Cancer Epidemiology, Biomarkers and Prevention, 17*(9), 2231–2237.

Mermelstein, R. W., & Wahl, S. K. (2008). Prevention of tobacco use. In S. Miller, D. J. Bowen, R. T. Croyle, & J. H. Rowland (Eds.), *Handbook of cancer control and behavioral science: A resource for researchers, practitioners, and policymakers.* Washington, DC: American Psychological Association Press.

Miles, A., Waller, J., & Wardle, J. (2008). Psychological Consequences of Cancer Screening. In S. M. Miller, D. J. Bowen, R. T. Croyle, & J. H. Rowland (Eds.), *Handbook of cancer control and behavioral science: A resource for researchers, practitioners, and policymakers.* Washington, DC: American Psychological Association Press.

Murray, D. M., Pals, S. L., & Blitstein, J. L. (2008). Design and analysis of group-randomized trials in cancer prevention and control. In S. M. Miller, D. J. Bowen, R. T. Croyle, & J. H. Rowland (Eds.), *Handbook of cancer control and behavioral science: A resource for researchers, practitioners, and policymakers.* Washington, DC: American Psychological Association Press.

Myung, S. K., McDonnell, D. D., Kazinets, G., Seo, H. G., & Moskowitz, J. M. (2009). Effects of Web- and computer-based smoking cessation programs: Meta-analysis of randomized controlled trials. *Archives of Internal Medicine, 169*(10), 929–937. [Erratum in *169*(13), 1194]

Neumark-Sztainer, D., Wall, M., Guo, J., Story, M., Haines, J., & Eisenberg, M. (2006). Obesity, disordered eating, and eating disorders in a longitudinal study of adolescents: How do dieters fare 5 years later? *Journal of the American Dietetic Association, 106*(4), 559–568.

Ockene, J. K., Emmons, K. M., Mermelstein, R. J., Perkins, K. A., Bonollo, D. S., Voorhees, C. C., et al. (2000). Relapse and maintenance issues for smoking cessation. *Health Psychology, 19*(Suppl. 1), 17–31.

Parcel, G. S., O'Hara-Tompkins, N. M., Harrist, R. B., Basen-Engquist, K. M., McCormick, L. K., Gottlieb, N. H., et al. (1995). Diffusion of an effective tobacco prevention program: Part II. Evaluation of the adoption phase. *Health Education Research, 10*(3), 297–307.

Pignone, M. P., Ammerman, A., Fernandez, L., Orleans, C. T., Pender, N., Woolf, S., et al. (2003). Counseling to promote a healthy diet in adults: A summary of the evidence for the U.S. Preventive Services Task Force. *American Journal of Preventive Medicine, 24,* 75–92.

Rogers, E. M. (1995). *Diffusion of innovations* (4th ed.). New York: Free Press.

Sabatino, S. A., Habarta, N., Baron, R. C., Coates, R. J., Rimer, B. K., Kerner, J., et al. (2008). Interventions to increase recommendation and delivery of screening for breast, cervical, and colorectal cancers by healthcare providers systematic reviews of provider assessment and feedback and provider incentives. *American Journal of Preventive Medicine, 35*(Suppl. 1), S67–S74.

Saraiya, M., Glanz, K., Briss, P. A., Nichols, P., White, C., Das, D., et al. (2004). Interventions to prevent skin cancer by reducing exposure to ultraviolet radiation: A systematic review. *American Journal of Preventive Medicine, 27,* 422–466.

Smedley, B., & Syme, L. (2000). *Promoting health: Intervention strategies from social and behavioral research.* Washington, DC: National Academies Press.

Stein, C. J., & Colditz, G. A. (2008). Trends in modifiable risk factors for cancer and the potential for cancer prevention In S. M. Miller, D. J. Bowen, R. T. Croyle, & J. H. Rowland (Eds.), *Handbook of cancer control and behavioral science: A resource for researchers, practitioners, and policymakers.* Washington, DC: American Psychological Association.

Task Force on Community Preventive Services. (Ed.). (2005). *The guide to community preventive services: What works to promote health?* New York: Oxford University Press.

Taylor, S. E., Repetti, R. L., & Seeman, T. (1997). Health psychology: What is an unhealthy environment and how does it get under the skin? *Annual Review of Psychology, 48,* 411–447.

The President's Cancer Panel. (2008). *Promoting healthy lifestyles: Policy, program, and personal recommendations for reducing cancer risk: Annual Report 2006–2007.* Washington, DC: U.S. Department of Health and Human Services.

Turner, L., Mermelstein, R., & Flay, B. (2004). Individual and contextual influences on adolescent smoking. *Annals of the New York Academy of Sciences, 1021,* 1–23.

Warnecke, R. B., Oh, A., Breen, N., Gehlert, S., Paskett, E., Tucker, K. L., et al. (2008). Approaching health disparities from a population perspective: The National Institutes of Health Centers for Population Health and Health Disparities. *American Journal of Public Health, 98*(9), 1608–1615.

Wenzel, L., Reina-Patton, A., & De Alba, I. (2008). Behavioral science applications to gynecologic cancer prevention. In S. M. Miller, D. J. Bowen, R. T. Croyle, & J. H. Rowland (Eds.), *Handbook of cancer control and behavioral science: A resource for researchers, practitioners, and policymakers.* Washington, DC: American Psychological Association.

CHAPTER 26

Community HIV Preventive Interventions

María Luisa Zúñiga
Steffanie A. Strathdee
Estela Blanco
Jose L. Burgos
Thomas L. Patterson

Since the beginning of the human immunodeficiency virus (HIV) epidemic in the early 1980s, psychologists, behavioral scientists, and other health care practitioners and researchers have devoted substantial attention to developing and evaluating HIV prevention interventions, which may be defined as public health projects, programs, or other initiatives whose principal goals are to prevent transmission of HIV, and promote the health and well-being of persons living with HIV (e.g., by preventing comorbidities associated with HIV disease). From 1990 to the time of this publication, over 2,000 peer-reviewed, English-language scientific articles about HIV prevention interventions have been published in the United States alone. Given that nearly 40 million people are living with HIV worldwide (with about one-fourth of infected persons in the United States not knowing they are HIV-positive) and in the absence of effective biologically based measures to prevent HIV (e.g., vaccines or microbicides) (Lagakos & Gable, 2008), the implementation of effective HIV prevention interventions remains a paramount concern.

The breadth and scope of available information about HIV prevention interventions necessitate that psychologists, other practitioners, and researchers be equipped to discern characteristics of effective interventions, so that they can adapt or develop interventions to meet the changing prevention needs of specific communities, both those at risk of acquiring HIV and those at risk of transmitting it.

Guided by established tenets of public health practice, HIV prevention interventions typically work on two levels. Primary prevention aims to keep uninfected persons from becoming infected. Applied to HIV, this can include promoting HIV testing, so that persons know their HIV status and can take measures to reduce risk of future infection; it can also include behavioral counseling for HIV-negative persons who engage in behaviors that place them at risk for HIV infection. In the case of HIV-positive persons, HIV testing is considered a part of secondary prevention, since it detects an existing health problem. Secondary prevention among persons living with HIV may also include appropriate treatment and follow-up care, including access to antiretroviral medications (ARVs) and promotion of medication adherence. Among populations whose members know that they are living with HIV, secondary prevention strategies also include reducing potential transmission risk behaviors and prevention of reinfection ("prevention with positives"). With the advent of powerful ARV regimens that can lower HIV viral load below the level of detection, researchers are also considering "treatment as prevention," in the hope that widespread coverage of ARVs among HIV-infected populations will have a significant impact on HIV incidence at the community level. The "test and treat" approach is gaining momentum among health agencies (e.g., the U.S. Centers for Disease Control and Prevention, or CDC) as a middle course between prevention and treatment.

Through HIV prevention research, we continue to improve our understanding of what works and what does not to reduce transmission of HIV. For public health practitioners, this highly stigmatized disease is a "moving target" that can both reemerge in populations where it was previously controlled and move to new populations. In the United States over the last 15 years, the epidemic has spread from a population of primarily white men who have sex with men (MSM) to MSM from communities of color, to women—primarily African Americans and Latinas—and to injection drug users (IDUs) (CDC, 2003, 2008a). This broadening of the epidemic necessitates meaningful involvement of members of the affected communities in developing and evaluating HIV interventions to ensure that the interventions will be relevant and grounded in the communities' realities (Minkler & Wallerstein, 2003). Bearing in mind this critical principle of community involvement in HIV prevention, we provide examples and tips for community engagement.

The first part of this chapter provides an overview of HIV prevention interventions, with discussions of theoretical underpinnings (behavior change theories and models) and a summary of characteristics shared by effective interventions. The second part addresses how to adapt or develop an intervention, with emphasis on community and environmental considerations that the prac-titioner should take into account in tailoring interventions to the intended community. Many of the areas covered in this chapter are relevant to prevention efforts for other health topics.

Theoretical Bases and Characteristics of Effective HIV Prevention Interventions

HIV prevention interventions can be categorized into three general domains: *biomedical* (e.g., vaccines, topical microbicides, pre- or postexposure prophylaxis); *behavioral*, which can operate at individual, dyad, group, or community levels to change either individual behavior or social norms; and *structural* (e.g., changing environmental factors or intervening in sociopolitical forces that facilitate HIV prevention behavior). The effectiveness of an intervention within one domain may depend on its combination with an intervention from another domain; for example, the effectiveness of a vaccine to prevent HIV (biomedical) requires, among other conditions, that individuals and at-risk communities know about and choose to receive the vaccine (behavioral), that they have access to the vaccine (structural), and that it be sufficiently efficacious to reduce susceptibility to infection. This chapter emphasizes behavioral and structural interventions to prevent HIV infection.

In the United States, the CDC has devoted substantial resources to developing and evaluating interventions that are "evidence-based," that is, interventions conducted with scientific rigor that have demonstrated efficacy in reducing HIV-related behavioral risk within specific at-risk communities (CDC, 2008c; Lyles, Crepaz, Herbst, Kay, & the HIV/AIDS Prevention Research Synthesis Team, 2007). Prevention efforts conducted by health practitioners in large part focus on behavioral and structural interventions whose success is mediated by certain key characteristics that we describe below.

Summary of Behavioral Theories and Models

A common characteristic of successful interventions to change behavior is the application of at least one behavioral health theory or model that provides a rigorous and scientifically valid framework. Many theories about changing health behavior have been successfully adapted to HIV prevention (Michie et al., 2005; Munro, Lewin, Swart, & Volmink, 2007; Washington State Department of Health, 2008). A *health behavior theory* is a set of principles or conditions that helps to predict health behavior change; such a theory helps to explain *why* people do what they do. A *health behavioral model* also has predictive capacity and offers a framework for understanding *how* people do what they do. Table 26.1 summarizes health behavior theories and models that have figured most prominently in the HIV prevention literature.

Many effective interventions have common elements or combine multiple models or theories to achieve a specific behavioral change. Drawing from these theories and models, we can summarize what effective behavior change requires:

1. A clearly defined target behavior (e.g., consistent condom use for vaginal sex with a new sex partner).
2. Knowledge on the individual's part about the behavior (e.g., what a condom can prevent; how a condom is properly used).
3. Sufficient importance to the individual or community to warrant adoption of the behavior (this incorporates elements of perceived risk and motivation to change).
4. Adequate skill and confidence on the individual's part to carry out the behavior on his or her own (e.g., self-efficacy).
5. Individual belief in the value of the anticipated outcome (i.e., outcome expectancy).
6. Adequate access to materials (e.g., condoms, sterile needles for IDUs) or environments (e.g., HIV testing centers) needed to carry out or adopt the behavior.
7. Ability to anticipate barriers beyond the individual's control that could inhibit change in behavior, and to formulate plans to overcome those barriers (e.g., prohibitive cost, laws or regulations, cultural beliefs or taboos, stigma).

Characteristics of Effective HIV Prevention Interventions

Several scholarly articles have identified characteristics of effective HIV prevention interventions among specific target communities (e.g., youths, IDUs, persons with high-risk sexual behavior) (Kirby, Laris, & Rolleri, 2007; Lyles, Crepaz, et al., 2007; Lyles, Kay, et al., 2007; Nation et al., 2003). The challenge in identifying effective interventions lies in their complexity and in variations in the following factors: design; data reporting methods; and evaluation methods (Lyles, Kay, et al., 2007). Importantly, intervention outcomes must be clearly defined and measurable, and must match the intended outcome (Lyles, Kay, et al., 2007). For example, an intervention to improve ARV adherence should consider biological markers such as cluster of differentiation (CD4) cell counts, viral load, or viral resistance, whereas an intervention to reduce needle sharing among IDUs should consider whether the outcome of interest is receptive sharing (i.e., using a borrowed or rented syringe that someone else has already used), distributive needle sharing (i.e., passing on a used syringe to others), or both. Clearly, receptive sharing poses a risk to self, whereas distributive sharing poses a risk to others. Behavioral interventions aimed at reducing the odds of receptive and distributive needle sharing among IDUs at risk of acquiring and transmitting hepatitis C virus (HCV) infection have been reported in the literature (Garfein et al., 2007; Latka et al., 2008), and may have a bearing on HIV transmission as well, since these viruses share certain risk factors. Interestingly, reductions in distributive needle sharing among HCV-infected IDUs that could be attributed to the intervention were mediated through increases in self-efficacy rather than through altruistic behavior, contrary to the authors' hypotheses (Latka et al., 2008).

Using a "review-of-reviews" methodology, Nation and colleagues (2003) identified several principles that are common to successful programs, many of which were similar to those published elsewhere (Dreifuss, 1998). First, programs should be comprehensive. For example, since knowledge alone does not necessarily translate into sustained

TABLE 26.1. Overview of Prominent Health Behavior Theories and Models in HIV Prevention Interventions

Theory or model	Principal characteristics that promote behavior change	Applications in HIV prevention
Health belief model (Becker, 1974; Rosenstock, 1966, 1974)	Based on the premise that behavior change is mediated by knowledge and attitudes about the behavior, individuals must: 1. Perceive that they are at risk. 2. Perceive that the condition is a serious threat. 3. Believe that new behavior is effective. 4. Perceive cues to take action (e.g., by observing friends or family who are affected). 5. Perceive a direct benefit from participating in the behavior. 6. Be able to overcome barriers to taking action.	Promote every-time condom use among HIV-positive MSM.
Social cognitive theory (Bandura, 1986; Lyles, Kay, et al., 2007)	Focuses on knowledge and skills necessary to change behavior: 1. Knowledge of risk. 2. Ability to carry out the skill. 3. Confidence to self-regulate risk. 4. Social support to continue the behavior.	Promote use of clean needles and condoms among female sex workers who are also injection drug users.
Theory of reasoned action (Fishbein & Ajzen, 1975; Fisher & Fisher, 1992)	Based on the assumption that people usually make rational decisions based on consideration of available information. Similar conceptually to the health belief model, but also includes behavioral intention, that is, the intention to adopt or change the behavior.	Promote high level of adherence to ARVs among persons living with HIV.
Diffusion of innovation theory (Beilenson, 2005; Rogers, 2000)	Theory that explains how a new idea is propagated in a community: 1. Must have an advantage to replace existing behavior or "business as usual." 2. Must be compatible with existing social values, infrastructure, and resources of persons who may adopt it. 3. Relatively easy to carry out and is perceived as being so. 4. Must be amenable to evaluation. 5. The results must be observable by others in the community.	Promote HIV testing in pregnant women (*One Test, Two Lives* campaign; CDC, 2007b)
Transtheoretical (TTM) or stages-of-change model (Cabral, Cotton, Semaan, & Gielen, 2004; Prochaska & Velicer, 1997)	Identifies six stages related to a specific behavior that individuals or groups may go through: 1. Precontemplation—change in behavior is not under consideration. 2. Contemplation—change in behavior has been considered. 3. Preparation—decision to change behavior has been made; individual decides what he or she needs to carry out the behavior. 4. Action—individual successfully initiates the behavior. 5. Maintenance—behavior is sustained over time. 6. Relapse—behavior is no longer being sustained, or is sustained inconsistently.	Every-time condom use when engaging in anal sex
Theory of gender and power (Connell, 1987; Lyles, Crepaz, et al., 2007; Lyles, Kay, et al., 2007)	Addresses social and environmental factors that may affect a desired behavior, including power imbalances between genders. This theory recognizes how gender relations, culturally influenced perceptions of gender, and economic power can influence people's ability to protect themselves.	Condom negotiation for women of color

Note. Adapted with permission from the Population Council (2006).

behavioral change, rather than provide only didactic information (e.g., how to use a condom), successful programs should also include skills-building activities (e.g., role playing the negotiation of condom use with a partner) as well as provide pertinent health or social services. Second, programs should incorporate a variety of teaching techniques to maintain participant interest. Effective programs might have a single group facilitator, but this leader should encourage different types of learning (e.g., videos, games, role playing, and practicing risk reduction negotiations using different scenarios). Third, any prevention program needs to provide enough instruction (the so-called "intervention dose") to produce the desired effect. The calculation of this amount should be based on the literature and on relevant experience with the target population. For example, it would be unrealistic to expect children of elementary school age to stay interested in a lecture about HIV/AIDS that lasted an entire day. Fourth, effective programs optimally should match the target population's needs. This includes strategies such as initiating the intervention at the time of highest possible impact (e.g., education about sexual health and HIV risk behaviors prior to sexual debut in youths). Additional characteristics of effective interventions include a theoretical basis or framework; responsiveness to needs of the target community; availability of culturally and linguistically competent staff; a well-developed protocol; implementation monitoring and midprogram evaluation; a process for modifying the protocol as needed; and adequate human, temporal, and financial resources to ensure full and effective implementation (Holtgrave et al., 1995).

Examples of Effective HIV Prevention Interventions

Through the CDC and the National Institutes of Health (NIH), the U.S. federal government has devoted considerable resources to studying what works in HIV prevention interventions and under what conditions. Detailed descriptions of evidence-based HIV prevention interventions have been compiled by the CDC's HIV/AIDS Prevention Research Synthesis (PRS) project,

which conducts ongoing efficacy reviews of promising HIV prevention interventions and, as of November 2007, had identified 49 evidence-based behavioral—both individual- and group-level—interventions (CDC, 2008b). In conjunction with the PRS, Lyles, Crepaz, and colleagues (2007) described specific individual- and group-level HIV interventions. For example, at the group level, the "choices" intervention (Baker et al., 2003), a skills-based program for heterosexual adults to reduce transmission of sexually transmitted infections (STIs) and HIV, is delivered in 16 two-hour sessions by teams of psychotherapists. At the individual level, the "personalized cognitive risk-reduction counseling" intervention (Dilley et al., 2002) for MSMs is designed to reduce unprotected anal intercourse. It is delivered in one session, total time 1 hour, by licensed mental health counselors in HIV testing clinics. It is worth bearing in mind that given the criteria deemed necessary for most scientific reviews, some interventions that fall short on one or more criteria may nevertheless be effective and merit rigorous evaluation (Bollinger, Cooper-Arnold, & Stover, 2004).

Adapting and Developing HIV Interventions

HIV interventions adapted from existing and scientifically efficacious interventions may have a better chance of achieving their goals than interventions developed "from scratch" (Lyles, Kay, et al., 2007). However, the intervention approach should ultimately be driven by the prevention needs and environment of the target population. For example, communities of color that have been hardest hit by the epidemic urgently need interventions that are culturally and linguistically relevant, and prevention programs designed for white MSM, for example, may not be suitable. Another factor that can influence intervention effectiveness is the degree to which members of the target community are meaningfully included in the intervention's development, implementation, evaluation, and dissemination (Minkler & Wallerstein, 2003; Olshefsky, Zive, Scolari, & Zúñiga, 2007). In some cases, affected communities have developed documents to support the meaningful inclusion of HIV-infected and

HIV-affected community members, such as "Nothing about Us without Us," a report that provides guidelines for developing harm reduction interventions for substance-using populations (Jürgens, 2008). Table 26.2 provides a list of recommendations to increase the likelihood that an intervention will be appropriate and effective for a given community.

TABLE 26.2. Steps to Meaningful Engagement of Communities in Interventions

1. Enlist the support of community members, community partners, or both, who are interested in the HIV prevention activity. (Consider potential partnerships with communities as long-term commitments.)
2. Determine behavior or intervention area and relevance to the target population or community.
3. Choose a theory or model that either has been applied successfully in different cultural settings or provides sufficient flexibility to be culturally or linguistically adapted to the target community. (Do not assume that "one size fits all.")
4. Ask community partners for recommendations on intervention implementation. (Pilot-test the intervention for cultural and linguistic relevance with the target community.)
5. Identify at least two representatives of the target community who are willing to participate in the prevention design and to provide feedback on the proposed intervention. (Providing honoraria or stipends to community members is highly recommended and, if at all possible, include this in the budget.)
6. Create a time line for intervention rollout and evaluation.
7. Develop an evaluation plan (see University of Kansas, 2007).
8. If an intervention proves effective, consider ways to sustain or propagate it (e.g., prior to the end of the intervention's funding period, discuss with community partners whether they are willing to take up the intervention or one of its components into routine patient care).
9. Provide evaluative feedback to community partners and other interested parties and collaborators. (e.g., host a feedback forum for community collaborators who may have helped collect data or recruit participants).
10. Include community members and partners in diffusion of intervention results (e.g., as copresenters at meetings and conferences and coauthors on abstracts and papers).

Note. Based on Minkler and Wallerstein (2003) and Zúñiga (2007).

Structural Interventions and Their Role in Effective HIV Prevention

Structural interventions in HIV prevention operate beyond individual- or group-level behavior change and include factors such as physical, social, cultural, community, organizational, economic, and legal or policy elements of the environment that can influence behavior (Rhodes, Singer, Bourgois, Friedman, & Strathdee, 2005; Sumartojo, 2000; Sumartojo, Doll, Holtgrave, Gayle, & Merson, 2000). Structural interventions are designed to address environmental factors and to consider the way the interplay of these factors influences adoption of HIV-related preventive behaviors. For example, an intervention to reduce HIV transmission among IDUs (e.g., availability of syringes in pharmacies without a prescription, syringe exchange programs, syringe vending machines, or safe injection facilities) must consider, among other things, the cost of sterile syringes; availability of bleach to clean syringes when sterile equipment cannot be obtained (e.g., in most jails or prisons); the legality of purchasing sterile syringes at a pharmacy; laws or regulations that may prohibit possession of sterile or used syringes; and the intervention's overall social acceptability. The social, legal, and political environment can vary tremendously between and even within countries, as well as over time, creating major hurdles in the path of implementing an intervention that has repeatedly been shown to be efficacious. An excellent example is ongoing U.S. Congressional opposition to federal funding of needle exchange programs (Vlahov et al., 2001).

Although structural interventions can have individual behavior change as a desired outcome, their macro-level approach helps to promote thinking about the "bigger picture" and provides a useful framework for adapting and developing effective HIV prevention interventions. In light of the stigma and politicization surrounding many HIV prevention initiatives, practitioners would be well served to consider structural and environmental factors of their target community that can hinder or foster behavior change (Sumartojo, 2000).

Structural interventions can also draw the practitioner's attention to community perceptions and norms, such as stigma and discrimination, that can impair the effectiveness of individual- or group-based HIV prevention interventions. Structural interventions can also help cause positive political changes, such as increased funding priority for HIV prevention activities or the institution of routine HIV testing during clinical encounters, which encourages destigmatization and broader acceptance of HIV prevention behavior (CDC, 2006). Indeed, since the aim of structural interventions is to eliminate or interrupt a health condition's root causes (e.g., homelessness, poverty, lack of education), they may significantly reduce the incidence of multiple diseases that share risk factors. For these reasons, they should be an attractive option for resource-constrained settings.

Another type of structural intervention is one that intervenes upon the physical or "built" environment. For example, Cuba's early response to the HIV epidemic was to isolate AIDS patients in a discrete region of the country, where there was little opportunity to infect others (Hoffman, 2004). This extreme approach met with harsh criticism, and the corresponding laws were later relaxed. Another example is the move by certain U.S. cities to close bathhouses in an effort to discourage public sex among MSM (Woods & Binson, 2003). Using a less draconian approach, a randomized trial in Nicaragua demonstrated that an intervention providing free condoms in motel rooms was associated with increased condom use during commercial sex encounters (Egger et al., 2000).

Gender Considerations

Globally, women constitute nearly half of those infected with HIV (United Nations Programme or HIV/AIDS and the World Health Organization [UNAIDS/WHO], 2005), with "feminized" HIV epidemics occurring most prominently in sub-Saharan Africa and parts of Asia. Given the important role of gender in influencing sexual health and behavior, gender considerations play a key role in developing effective HIV interventions. Being socially constructed, gender varies from culture to culture, yet in many, if not most, cultural contexts, men and women differ markedly in behavioral norms and in their symbolic places in society (Rao Gupta, 2000). Throughout most of the world, gender norms are determined by patriarchy (i.e., the idea that men are superior to and should dominate women). This principle can be so pervasive that its influence is often invisible. As a consequence of patriarchal attitudes, women in many cultures can be especially vulnerable to several negative health outcomes, including infection with HIV. According to Rao Gupta, who is President of the International Center for Research on Women, in many parts of the world there is a "culture of silence" built around sexual intercourse, according to which women are expected to be ignorant of sex and passive in their sexual interactions, and are often denied recognition of their own sexual urges and desires.

Women's economic dependency on men—another result of patriarchy—also increases vulnerability to HIV. In many countries, women cannot own property, are limited in their movement (e.g., cannot obtain a driver's license), and do not have access to the same educational opportunities as men. Gender inequalities pervade even supposedly advanced Western societies; in the United States, for example, the average woman makes about 77% of what the average man earns—a wage gap that becomes even more pronounced at lower socioeconomic levels and for women of color (Webster & Alemayehu, 2006). Economic inequality, especially in poorer regions, increases the likelihood that women will engage in behaviors that place them at high risk for HIV infection (e.g., exchanging unprotected sex for housing, food, or money; substance use), while decreasing the likelihood that they will engage in protective behaviors (e.g., successfully negotiating condom use with clients or partners; leaving a relationship that may be violent or in which the partner is not monogamous) (Exner, Dworkin, Hoffmann, & Ehrhardt, 2003; Rao Gupta, 2000).

Physical, emotional, and sexual violence against women is of substantial concern worldwide, not least because it places women at increased risk for unprotected sexual intercourse and HIV infection (Greig, Peacock, Jewkes, & Msimang, 2008; Silverman, Decker, Saggurti, Balaiah, & Raj, 2008). Information on the prevalence of violence against women is limited, but some researchers estimate that anywhere between 10 and 50% of women worldwide have suffered physical assault by an intimate partner (Rao Gupta, 2000). Physical assault has also been connected with increased probability of coerced sexual encounters (Heise, Ellsberg, & Gottemoeller, 1999). The threat of violence can create barriers to safe-sex practices, limiting women's ability to negotiate condom use and to demand monogamous relationships of their steady partners (Rao Gupta, 2000). Such circumstances are an everyday occurrence for some subgroups of women, such as female, drug-dependent sex workers (Shannon et al., 2009).

No discussion of patriarchy and its influences on HIV prevention is complete without considering how it also affects men and their vulnerability to HIV infection. Men, like women, are influenced by cultural gender norms. In some cultures, even young men are expected to possess extensive knowledge and experience of sex (often with many different partners), and they are expected to dominate women in their sexual encounters (Rao Gupta, 2000). Given these expectations, men in some cultures may be reluctant to seek out information on sex that could resolve their doubts as to what behaviors place them and their partners at risk for HIV. Additionally, because dominance over women is fundamental to paternalistic ideology, MSM are stigmatized and are often victims of homophobia and violence (Rao Gupta, 2000). Ongoing stigmatization may be related to recent increases in HIV among MSM in the United States, despite the gradual liberalization of societal attitudes toward homosexuality in this country. The recent upsurge in HIV infection rates among MSM of color in the United States, especially young MSM, calls for the urgent expansion of culturally appropriate preventive HIV interventions in these communities, including interventions among men who do not self-identify as gay or bisexual (CDC, 2008b).

To be effective in specific populations, HIV prevention interventions must obviously respect those populations' prevailing concepts of gender, sexual identities, and power relations; nonetheless, structural interventions should also strive to encourage reconceptualization of gender norms and the creation of gender-equitable relationships (Rao Gupta, 2000). Men should be encouraged to view their female partners as equals whose desires and preferences should be considered. Men and women can also be brought into dialogue about the pressures they feel to engage in HIV risk behavior, and be taught to strategize how to overcome those pressures. In situations where it is not feasible to challenge pervasive gender norms or power imbalances, HIV prevention interventions should consider incorporating elements that limit the propagation or reinforcement of such factors.

Cultural and Linguistic Considerations

In the United States, the cultural and linguistic diversity of populations affected by HIV requires interventions that speak to the realities and norms of different communities. Drawing from the public health movement to provide culturally and linguistically competent care, the practitioner is encouraged to consider such approaches (Zúñiga, 2007). Steps to ensure cultural and linguistic effectiveness in interventions largely parallel the recommendations for community involvement provided in Table 26.2, and may also include focus groups involving members of the target community, practitioners who serve the target community, or agency staff members who are familiar with the community. The growing movement of community-based participatory research also provides a rich source of recommendations to engage members from diverse communities in research processes (Minkler & Wallerstein, 2003).

HIV Stigma and Discrimination

Ongoing stigma surrounding HIV poses special challenges for prevention. "Stigma" is a multidimensional construct used to describe individual or societal negative perceptions, attitudes, or actions toward persons or communities with an undesired condition or attribute. In a health context, certain conditions or illnesses, such as leprosy, tuberculosis, and HIV/AIDS, elicit stigmatizing attitudes (e.g., discrimination) that can severely undermine the health and well-being of individuals living with these diseases. For example, HIV-related stigma creates social barriers that may lead to disparities in health between the stigmatized group and the main population (Morin et al., 2002), for example, by causing HIV-positive people to avoid HIV-related services and to delay seeking treatment (Campo, Alvarez, Santos, & Latorre, 2005; Holtgrave, McGuire, & Milan, 2007; Infante et al., 2006; Zúñiga, Brennan, Scolari, & Strathdee, 2008).

HIV-related stigma can discourage HIV testing, impede health care access and utilization among persons living with HIV, and negatively affect mental health and individuals' relationships with and potential support from family and community. Although HIV-related stigma can affect all HIV-positive persons, the manner in which that stigma plays out in U.S. communities of color has markedly affected our ability to address the disease. For example, stigma has been implicated in the decisions by HIV-positive Latinos either to delay seeking HIV care or to forgo it altogether (Levy et al., 2007; Turner et al., 2000; Zúñiga et al. 2008). Latinos frequently present for care at an advanced stage of HIV disease, and they are the ethnic or racial group most likely to receive an AIDS diagnosis within 1 year of being diagnosed HIV-positive (County of San Diego Health and Human Services Agency, 2008; Wallace & Castañeda, 2008). Qualitative studies of Latinos living with HIV, along with their low participation in HIV clinical trials, have led many Latinos and clinicians specializing in HIV to recognize the far-reaching impact of HIV-related stigma on patients and families alike. For example, to avoid disclosure of HIV status or AIDS-related problems, some HIV-positive Latinos and their family members attribute the sufferer's symptoms to diseases other than HIV (e.g., cancer, tuberculosis, pneumonia) (Zúñiga, Blanco, Martínez, Strathdee, Gifford, 2007; Zúñiga, Blanco, Palinkas, Strathdee, Gifford, 2010).

Efforts to identify, measure, and reduce HIV-related stigma are discussed in detail in a publication by the U.S. Agency for International Development (USAID, 2006). This publication describes three primary types of HIV-related stigma: individual or "felt" stigma (feelings of shame or guilt); provider-level stigma (being turned away from, or receiving reduced access to, health services); and community-level stigma (acts of discrimination,

e.g., loss of employment). In some settings, structural interventions, such as provider sensitivity training, have been implemented to reduce the negative impact of stigma on persons living with HIV. Because stigma has been shown to continue affecting the perceptions and behavior of persons already in care (Zúñiga et al., 2008), consideration of how care is delivered as a structural factor is important. Below we discuss two examples of how HIV-related stigma can be addressed as part of both primary and secondary interventions.

Reducing HIV-Related Stigma in Primary Prevention

Interventions to reduce HIV-related stigma at the community level should include educating the community about HIV transmission, reducing risks of transmission, dispelling stereotypes and fear of persons living with HIV, and promoting compassion. These elements were successfully integrated into a comprehensive adolescent HIV, STI, and pregnancy prevention intervention in Southern California (Zúñiga, Blanco, Sanchez, Carroll, & Olshefsky, 2009). The intervention, aptly named the Peer Empowerment Education Program (PEEP), was found to reduce HIV-stigmatizing attitudes significantly among high-risk youths by including persons living with HIV as cofacilitators of the course with a teen peer educator. The HIV-positive cofacilitator disclosed his or her status on the second day of the 5-day training, allowing students to see the facilitator as someone similar to themselves, and promoting reflection on the reasons behind their own stigmatizing attitudes (Zúñiga, Blanco, Sanchez, et al., 2009). Such innovative approaches hold promise to reduce HIV-related stigma in other populations.

Addressing HIV-Related Stigma in Secondary Prevention

One of the most important structural efforts to reduce barriers to HIV testing has been the CDC (2006) recommendation for routine HIV testing during medical encounters. Although routine testing is intended, among other aims, to improve early detection of HIV and to screen for persons living with HIV who may not know they are infected, as a policy, it could also contribute to decreases in HIV-related stigma in the community as a whole. Routine testing "normalizes" HIV and causes it to be associated with other, less-stigmatized diseases, such as diabetes and hypertension, for which routine screenings are performed. Additional opportunities to offer HIV screening include community health fairs, where several screening activities take place in one setting. Because the CDC does not have authority to mandate the new screening policy, efforts to streamline testing in more health settings are ongoing.

Intervention Cost Considerations

Once published, efficacious interventions are rarely implemented in the real world (Apsler, 1991), in part because policymakers understandably require cost-effectiveness data or cost–benefit analyses as evidence to support rational health policy decisions (Kahn & Marseille, 2000). Considering that budgets for public health prevention programs are shrinking worldwide, an important but often elusive calculation in any prevention program is cost. To maximize investments in HIV prevention, an integral part of any HIV prevention intervention trial should be the collection of detailed cost data, along with efficacy indicators (Pinkerton, Pearson, Eachus, Berg, & Grimes, 2008).

To support rational public health policy decisions, health economists have devised various types of analyses that weigh costs of competing interventions against their health impacts. This leads us to an important characteristic of effective HIV prevention interventions, namely, that the likely benefits (e.g., individual healthy years gained, HIV infections averted) should warrant the resources expended to implement and sustain the intervention (e.g., staff or intervention specialist time, cost of outreach, cost of materials).

The types of economic analysis used most frequently are the following.

1. *Cost analysis* involves systematic collection, processing, and analysis of program costs (CDC, 2008a). Also called "cost-minimization analysis," cost analysis is often used to identify the least expensive strategy to achieve an equivalent health outcome (Eisenberg, 1989).

2. *Cost-effectiveness analysis* refers to the process of comparing two or more health care interventions in terms of the incremental increases in effectiveness (or health outcomes) per unit of added cost (Coffield et al., 2001). Costs are measured in monetary terms, whereas effectiveness or outcome is measured as degrees or rates of change in individual behavior or biomedical status (Yates, 1999). A cost-effectiveness analysis is useful when the goal is to compare competing interventions, and it is often favored by health care professionals (CDC, 2007a).

3. *Cost–benefit analysis* measures both the health outcomes and the costs of an intervention in terms of a common currency. This type of analysis is preferred by some economists, since it provides a more definite end point (Muennig, 2008). Some critics object to placing what can seem to be an arbitrary "dollar" value on human suffering, disease, functional impairment, and mortality (Gold, Siegel, Russel, & Weinstein, 1996).

A further consideration in economic analysis is deciding what costs to include. Several analysts, as well as the Panel on Cost-Effectiveness in Health and Medicine of the U.S. Public Health Service, recommend using a broad perspective that includes not only the costs associated directly with the intervention but also those incurred by everyone affected by the intervention. For example, the analysis of a behavioral intervention to prevent HIV in female IDUs should include not only the direct costs of implementation but also the time that patients and unpaid caregivers spend participating in the intervention. This "societal perspective" encompasses all costs and resources expended in connection with the intervention, regardless of who pays them, although it is usually restricted to costs incurred within a single country (Gold, 1998).

Other perspectives that consider costs relevant to decision makers include a "government perspective," which might include some costs incurred by intervention participants but not by their family members or caregivers (e.g., for transporting the participant to the intervention site); a "private insurance perspective" will probably not include costs outside of the intervention (Grosse, 2006; Muennig, 2008). Examples of various perspectives are presented in Table 26.3.

TABLE 26.3. Costs Included in a Cost-Effectiveness Analysis of a Harm Reduction Behavioral Program for Female IDUs, Conducted from Three Perspectives

	Costs included by perspective		
Cost category	Insurance	Government	Society
Counseling sessions	All	All	All
Laboratory tests	All	All	All
Participant's time	None	Some	All
Transportation	None	Some	All
Family's time for caring for children during counseling sessions	None	None	All

Note. Data from Muennig (2008).

It is important to distinguish between these perspectives on interventions to understand the context of cost-related assessment. Debate continues on whether some HIV prevention measures ultimately save society money (Cohen, Neumann, & Weinstein, 2008; Holtgrave et al., 1995). Economic evaluation is complex, and it is not always possible to state whether an intervention results in a net financial gain to society. Most prevention programs do add to health care costs, as in the case of many screening programs, yet they are seen as worthwhile when the health outcomes are considered (Cofield et al., 2001). Many elements of such programs cannot be assigned a clear dollar or effectiveness value (e.g., family stability, health care equity, reduction in HIV-related stigma) and are therefore difficult to include in cost-effectiveness models (Center for AIDS Prevention Studies, 2002). However, with the introduction of highly active antiretroviral therapy (HAART) in 1996, and the dramatic improvements in survival, have come significant increases in HIV-related medical costs, with current lifetime medical costs of care for one person living with HIV in the United States estimated at over $200,000. More than 50% of health care expenditures related to HIV care are due to outpatient costs (Andresen & Boyd, 2010; Schackman et al., 2006). Given these facts, the cost of preventing new cases of HIV is an area that merits further research. Many HIV behavioral interventions directed at high-risk groups in the United States have been shown to save society money (Center

for AIDS Prevention Studies, 2002; Holtgrave, 2007).

What Is Known about the Cost-Effectiveness of HIV Prevention Interventions?

Work by health economists has focused on what can be called a "unified prevention theory" (Bautista, Gadsden, & Bertozzi, 2007). According to this theory, determining which target population should get priority depends on the prevalence of HIV infection in both special populations and the general population. In areas where overall HIV prevalence is either low or concentrated in specific populations, the bulk of intervention efforts should be directed at high-risk groups. The more HIV prevalence becomes generalized, the more resources and study designs should focus on the general population, and the more justification for directing large expenditures to high-cost items, such as major media campaigns. Attention must also be given to the differential effectiveness of similar interventions among different subpopulations.

Given the importance of evaluating the costs of preventing new cases of HIV, the NIH recently funded the study Prevent AIDS: Network for Cost-Effectiveness Analysis (PANCEA), which examined prevention efforts in five countries: India, Mexico, Russia, South Africa, and Uganda. Collaborators (Marseille et al., 2007) collected information from 228 programs in the five countries to evaluate the relationship between program efficiency (measured as the cost per participant) and scale (measured in number of services delivered). They found that program efficiency increases with the scale of the intervention, with an average cost reduction of 34% per doubling in scale. This implies that as HIV prevention programs across the globe continue to grow, they will likely become less costly per participant.

Conclusions

In this chapter, we have discussed the theoretical underpinnings of the development of HIV prevention interventions, characteristics of effective interventions, the importance of structural interventions, and key considerations for adapting or developing community- and gender-specific interventions for different cultural and environmental settings.

Although "frontline," theory-based behavioral interventions at both individual and community levels will continue to be important, greater emphasis is needed on structural interventions to address societal vulnerabilities to HIV (e.g., reducing HIV-related stigma) and to improve health care service infrastructures (El-Sadr & Hoos, 2008). Effective approaches to HIV prevention include integrated approaches that combine different strategies to strengthen the overall impact on the target behavior (El-Sadr & Hoos, 2008). Integrated approaches to HIV prevention, coupled with meaningful engagement of members of the target community, may allow for development of more effective HIV prevention interventions in the United States and in global settings.

Further Reading

Bowie, C. R., Reichenberg, A., Patterson, T. L., Heaton, R. K., & Harvey, P. D. (2006). Determinants of real-world functioning performance in schizophrenia: Correlations with cognition, functional capacity, and symptoms. *American Journal of Psychiatry, 163*, 418–425.

Harvey, P. D., Helldin, L., Bowie, C. R., Heaton, R. K., Olsson, A. K., et al. (2009). Performance-based measurement of functional disability in schizophrenia: A cross-national study in the United States and Sweden. *American Journal of Psychiatry, 166*, 821–827.

Patterson, T. L., Goldman, S., McKibbin, C. L., Hughs, T., & Jeste, D. V. (2001). UCSD Performance-Based Skills Assessment: Development of a new measure of everyday functioning for severely mentally ill adults. *Schizophrenia Bulletin, 27*, 235–245.

Additional Resources

U.S. Settings

Centers for Disease Control and Prevention. (1999, revised 2001). Compendium of HIV prevention interventions with evidence of effectiveness. Atlanta, GA: Author. Retrieved August 13, 2008, from *www.cdc.gov/hiv/resources/reports/hiv_compendium*.

HIV Prevention Trials Network. (2008). Behavioral science research strategy. Retrieved August 13, 2008, from *www.hptn.org/prevention_science/behavioral.asp*.

Global Settings

Family Health International. (2008). Behavior change communication for HIV/AIDS. Durham, NC: Author. Retrieved August 13, 2008, from *www.fhi.org/en/hivaids/pub/fact/bcchiv.htm*.

Health Communication Partnership. (no date). HIV/AIDS information: A selection of HCP's HIV/AIDS programs. Baltimore: Author. Retrieved August 13, 2008, from *www.hcpartnership.org/Topics/hivaids.php*.

References

Andresen, M. A., & Boyd, N. (2010). A cost–benefit and cost-effectiveness analysis of Vancouver's supervised injection facility. *International Journal of Drug Policy, 21*(1), 70–76.

Apsler, R. (1991). Evaluating the cost-effectiveness of drug abuse treatment services. *NIDA Research Monograph, 113*, 57–66.

Baker, S. A., Beadness, B., Stoner, S., Morrison, D. M., Gordon, J., Collier, C., et al. (2003). Skills training versus health education to prevent STDs/HIV in heterosexual women: A randomized controlled trial utilizing biological outcomes. *AIDS Education and Prevention, 14*, 1–5.

Bandura, A. (1986). *Social foundations of thought and action: A social cognitive theory.* Englewood Cliffs, NJ: Prentice-Hall.

Bautista, S., Gadsden, P., & Bertozzi, S. M. (2007). Optimizing HIV/AIDS prevention programs: Towards multidimensional allocative efficiency. Retrieved August 19, 2008, from *info.worldbank.org/etools/library/lat-estversion.asp?243423.*

Becker, M. (1974). The health belief model and personal health behavior. *Health Education Monographs, 2,* 324–508.

Beilenson, J. (2005). Diffusion of innovation: How National Council on Aging is developing a better way to disseminate evidence-based health programs. Retrieved August 13, 2008, from *www.ncoa.org/downloads/diffusion-ofinnovations.pdf.*

Bollinger, L., Cooper-Arnold, K., & Stover, J. (2004). Where are the gaps?: The effects of HIV-prevention interventions on behavioral change. *Studies in Family Planning, 35,* 27–38.

Cabral, R. J., Cotton, D., Semaan, S., & Gielen, A. C. (2004). Application of the transtheoretical model for HIV prevention in a facility-based and community-level behavioral intervention research study. *Health Promotion Practice, 5,* 199–207.

Campo, R. E., Alvarez, D., Santos, G., & Latorre, J. (2005). Antiretroviral treatment considerations in Latino patients. *AIDS Patient Care and STDs, 19*(6), 366–374.

Center for AIDS Prevention Studies at the University of California, San Francisco (CAPS). (2002). Can cost-effectiveness analysis help in HIV prevention? Retrieved August 15, 2008, from *www.caps.ucsf.edu/pubs/FS/costeffectiverev.php.*

Centers for Disease Control and Prevention (CDC). (2003). Advancing HIV prevention: New strategies for a changing epidemic—United States, 2003. *Morbidity and Mortality Weekly Report, 52,* 239–332.

Centers for Disease Control and Prevention (CDC). (2006). Revised recommendations for HIV testing of adults, adolescents, and pregnant women in health-care settings. *Morbidity and Mortality Weekly Report, 55,* 1–17. Retrieved August 18, 2008, from *www.cdc.gov/mmwr/preview/mmwrhtml/rr5514a1.htm.*

Centers for Disease Control and Prevention (CDC). (2007a). HIV cost-effectiveness. Atlanta, GA: Author. Retrieved August 17, 2008, from *www.cdc.gov/hiv/topics/prev_prog/ce/index.htm.*

Centers for Disease Control and Prevention (CDC). (2007b). One Test, Two Lives. Atlanta, GA: Author. Retrieved August 14, 2008, from *www.cdc.gov/hiv/topics/perinatal/1test2lives/about.htm.*

Centers for Disease Control and Prevention (CDC). (2008a). Economic evaluation of public health preparedness and response efforts. Atlanta, GA: Author. Retrieved on August 17, 2008, from *www.cdc.gov/owcd/eet/seriestoc/seriestoc.html.*

Centers for Disease Control and Prevention (CDC). (2008b). Trends in HIV/AIDS diagnoses among men who have sex with men—33 States, 2001–2006. *Morbidity and Mortality Weekly Report, 57,* 681–686.

Centers for Disease Control and Prevention (CDC). (2008c). Updated compendium of evidence-based interventions. Atlanta, GA: Author. Retrieved August 13, 2008, from *www.cdc.gov/hiv/topics/research/prs/evidence-based-interventions.htm.*

Coffield, A. B., Maciosek, M. V., McGinnis, J. M., Harris, J. R., Caldwell, M. B., Teutsch, S. M., et al. (2001). Priorities among recommended clinical preventive services. *American Journal of Preventive Medicine, 21*(1), 1–9.

Cohen, J. T., Neumann, P. J., & Weinstein, M. C. (2008). Does preventive care save money?: Health economics and the presidential candidates. *New England Journal of Medicine, 358,* 661–663.

Connell, R. W. (1987). *Gender and power.* Stanford, CA: Stanford University Press.

County of San Diego Health and Human Services Agency. (2008). AIDS in Hispanics, County of San Diego, 2008. Retrieved June 1, 2009, from *www.sdcounty.ca.gov/hhsa/programs/phs/documents/aids_in_hispanics2008.pdf.*

Dilley, J. W., Woods, W. J., Sabatino, J., Lihatsh, T., Adler, B., Casey, S., et al. (2002). Changing sexual behavior among gay male repeat testers for HIV: A randomized, controlled trial of single-session intervention. *Journal of Acquired Immune Deficiency Syndromes, 30,* 177–186.

Dreifuss, R. (1998). AIDS prevention: Switzerland. *Integration, 57,* 6–7.

Egger, M., Pauw, J., Lopatatzidis, A., Medrano, D., Paccaud, F., & Smith, G. D. (2000). Promotion of condom use in a high-risk setting in Nicaragua: A randomised controlled trial. *Lancet, 355,* 2101–2105.

Eisenberg, J. M. (1989). Clinical economics: A guide to the economic analysis of clinical practices. *Journal of the American Medical Association, 262*(20), 2879–2886.

El-Sadr, W. M., & Hoos, D. (2008). The President's emergency plan for AIDS relief: Is the emergency over? *New England Journal of Medicine, 359,* 553–555.

Exner, T. M., Dworkin, S. L., Hoffman, S., & Ehrhardt, A. A. (2003). Beyond the male condom: The evolution of gender-specific HIV interventions for women. *Annual Review of Sex Research, 14,* 114–136.

Fishbein, M., & Ajzen, I. (1975). *Belief, attitude, intention, and behavior: An introduction to theory and research.* Reading, MA: Addison-Wesley.

Fisher, J. D., & Fisher, W. A. (1992). Changing

AIDS-risk behaviour. *Psychological Bulletin,* 11, 455–474.

Garfein, R. S., Golub, E. T., Greenberg, A. E., Hagan, H., Hanson, D. L., Hudson, S. M., et al. (2007). A peer-education intervention to reduce injection risk behaviors for HIV and hepatitis C virus infection among young injection drug users. *AIDS,* 21, 1923–1932.

Gold, M. (1998). Standardizing cost-effectiveness analyses: The panel on cost-effectiveness in health and medicine. *Academic Radiology,* 5, S351–S354.

Gold, M., Siegel, J., Russel, L., & Weinstein, M. (1996). *Cost-effectiveness in health and medicine.* New York: Oxford University Press.

Greig, A., Peacock, D., Jewkes, R., & Msimang, S. (2008). Gender and AIDS: Time to act. *AIDS,* 22(Suppl. 2), S35–S43.

Grosse, S. (2006, June). *Towards a consistent payer perspective: A microeconomic approach to economic evaluation.* Paper presented at the annual meeting of the Economics of Population Health: Inaugural Conference of the American Society of Health Economists, Madison, WI. Retrieved August 15, 2008, from *www.allacademic.com/meta/p93449_index.html.*

Heise, L., Ellsberg, M., & Gottemoeller, M. (1999). Ending violence against women (Population Reports, Series L, No. 11). Baltimore: Johns Hopkins University School of Public Health, Population Information Program. Retrieved August 15, 2008, from *www.infoforhealth.org/pr/l11/l11creds.shtml.*

Hoffman, S. Z. (2004). HIV/AIDS in Cuba: A model for care or an ethical dilemma? *African Health Sciences,* 4, 208–209.

Holtgrave, D. (2007). Evidence-based efforts to prevent HIV infection: An overview of current status and future challenges. *Clinical Infectious Diseases,* 45(Suppl. 4), S293–S299.

Holtgrave, D., McGuire, J. F., & Milan, J. (2007). The magnitude of key HIV prevention challenges in the United States: Implications for a new national HIV prevention plan. *American Journal of Public Health,* 92(7), 1163–1167.

Holtgrave, D. R., Qualls, N. L., Curran, J. W., Valdiserri, R. O., Guinan, M. E., & Parra, W. C. (1995). An overview of the effectiveness and efficiency of HIV prevention programs. *Public Health Reports,* 110, 134–146.

Infante, C., Zarco, A., Magali Cuadra, S., Morrison, K., Caballero, M., Bronfman, M., et al. (2006). El estigma asociado al VIH/SIDA: El caso de los prestadores de servicios de salud en México [HIV/AIDS-related stigma and discrimination: The case of a health care providers in Mexico]. *Salud Pública de México,* 48(2), 141–150.

Jürgens, R. (2008). "Nothing about Us without Us: Greater, meaningful involvement of people who use illegal drugs: A public health, ethical, and human rights imperative [International edition]. Toronto: Canadian HIV/AIDS Legal Network, International HIV/AIDS Alliance, Open Society Institute. Retrieved August 17, 2008, from *www.soros.org/initiatives/health/focus/ihrd/articles_publications/publications/nothingaboutus_20080603/int%20nothing%20about%20us%20%28may%20 2008%29.pdf.*

Kahn, J. G., & Marseille, E. (2000). Fighting global AIDS: The value of cost-effectiveness analysis. *AIDS,* 14(16), 2609–2610.

Kirby, D. B., Laris, B. A., & Rolleri, L. A. (2007). Sex and HIV education programs: Their impact on sexual behaviors of young people throughout the world. *Journal of Adolescent Health,* 40, 206–217.

Lagakos, S. W., & Gable, A. R. (2008). Challenges to HIV prevention: Seeking effective measures in the absence of a vaccine. *New England Journal of Medicine,* 358, 1543–1545.

Latka, M. H., Kapadia, F., Golub, E. T., Bonner, S., Campbell, J. V., Coady, M. H., et al. (2008). Effect of randomized intervention trials to reduce lending of used injection equipment among HCV-infected injection drug users. *American Journal of Public Health,* 98, 853–861.

Levy, V., Prentiss, D., Balmas, G., Chen, S., Israelski, D., Katzenstein, D., et al. (2007). Factors in the delayed HIV presentation of immigrants in Northern California: Implications for voluntary counseling and testing programs. *Journal of Immigrant Health,* 9, 49–54.

Lyles, C. M., Crepaz, N., Herbst, J. H., Kay, L. S., & the HIV/AIDS Prevention Research Synthesis Team. (2007). Evidence-based behavioral prevention from the perspective of the CDC's HIV/AIDS Prevention Research Synthesis Team. *AIDS Education and Prevention,* 18(4SSA), 21–31.

Lyles, C. M., Kay, L. S., Crepaz, N., Herbst, J. H., Passin, W. F., Kim, A. S., et al. (2007). Best-evidence interventions: Findings from a systematic review of HIV behavioral interventions for US populations at high risk, 2000–2004. *American Journal of Public Health,* 97, 133–143.

Marseille, E., Dandona, L., Marshall, N., Gaist, P., Bautista-Arredondo, S., Rollins, B., et al. (2007). HIV Prevention Costs and Program Scale: Data from the PANCEA project in five low- and middle-income countries. *BMC Health Services Research,* 7, 108.

Michie, S., Johnston, J., Abraham, C., Lawton, R., Parker, D., Walker, A., et al. (2005). Making psychological theory useful for implementing evidence based practice: A consensus approach. *Quality and Safety in Health Care, 14*, 26–33.

Minkler, M., & Wallerstein, N. (Eds.). (2003). *Community-based participatory research for health.* San Francisco: Jossey-Bass.

Morin, S. F., Sengupta, S., Cozen, M., Richards, T. A., Shriver, M. D., Palacio, H., et al. (2002). Responding to racial and ethnic disparities in use of HIV drugs: Analysis of state policies. *Public Health Reports, 117*, 263–272.

Muennig, P. (2008). *Cost-effectiveness analysis in health* (2nd ed.). San Francisco: Jossey-Bass.

Munro, S., Lewin, S., Swart T., & Volmink, J. (2007). A review of health behaviour theories: How useful are they for developing interventions to promote long-term medication adherence for TB and HIV/AIDS? *BMC Public Health, 7*, 104. Retrieved August 13, 2008, from *www.pubmedcentral.nih.gov/picrender. fcgi?artid=1925084&blobtype=pdf.*

Nation, M., Crusto, C., Wandersman, A., Kumpfer, K. L., Seybolt, D., Morrissey-Kane, E., et al. (2003). What works in prevention: Principles of effective prevention programs. *American Psychologist, 58*, 449–456.

Olshefsky, A. M., Zive, M. M., Scolari, R., & Zúñiga, M. L. (2007). Promoting HIV risk awareness and testing in Latinos living on the U.S.–Mexico border: The *Tú No Me Conoces* social marketing campaign. *AIDS Education and Prevention, 19*, 422–435.

Pinkerton, S. D., Pearson, C. R., Eachus, S. R., Berg, K. M., & Grimes, R. M. (2008). Proposal for the development of a standardized protocol for assessing the economic costs of HIV prevention interventions. *Journal of Acquired Immune Deficiency Syndromes, 47*(Suppl. 1), S10–S14.

Population Council. (2006). AIDSQuest: The HIV/AIDS survey library: Behavioral and social theories commonly used in HIV research. Retrieved August 13, 2008, from *www.popcouncil.org/horizons/AIDSquest/cmnbehvrtheo/index.html.*

Prochaska, J. O., & Velicer, W. F. (1997). The transtheoretical model of health behavior change. *American Journal of Health Promotion, 12*, 38–48.

Rao Gupta, G. (2000, August). *Gender, sexuality and HIV/AIDS: The what, the why and the how.* Plenary address delivered at the 13th International AIDS Conference, Durban, South Africa.

Rhodes, T., Singer, M., Bourgois, P., Friedman, S. R., & Strathdee, S. A. (2005). The social structural production of HIV risk among injecting drug users. *Social Science and Medicine, 61*, 1026–1044.

Rogers, E. (2000). Diffusion theory: A theoretical approach to promote community-level change. In J. L. Peterson & R. J. DiClemente (Eds.), *Handbook of HIV prevention* (pp. 57–65). New York: Kluwer Academic/Plenum Press.

Rosenstock, I. M. (1966). Why people use health services. *Milbank Memorial Fund Quarterly, 44*, 94–124.

Rosenstock, I. M. (1974). Historical origins of the health belief model. *Health Education Monographs, 2*, 328–335.

Schackman, B. R., Gebo, K. A., Walensky, R. P., Losina, E., Muccio, T., Sax, P. E., et al. (2006). The lifetime cost of current human immunodeficiency virus care in the United States. *Medical Care, 44*(11), 990–997.

Shannon, K., Strathdee, S. A., Shoveller, J., Gobson, K., Kerr, T., & Tyndall, M. W. (2009). Structural and environmental barriers to condom use negotiation with clients among women in survival sex work: Implications for HIV prevention and policy. *American Journal of Public Health, 99*(4), 659–665.

Silverman, J. G., Decker, M. R., Saggurti, N., Balaiah, D., & Raj, A. (2008). Intimate partner violence and HIV infection among married Indian women. *Journal of the American Medical Association, 300*(6), 703–710.

Sumartojo, E. (2000). Structural factors in HIV prevention: Concepts, examples, and implications for research. *AIDS, 14*(Suppl. 1), S3–S10.

Sumartojo, E., Doll, L., Holtgrave, D., Gayle, H., & Merson, M. (2000). Enriching the mix: Incorporating structural factors into HIV prevention. *AIDS, 14*(Suppl. 1), S1–S2.

Turner, B. J., Cunningham, W. E., Duan, N., Andersen, R. M., Shapiro, M. F., Bozzette, S. A., et al. (2000). Delayed medical care after diagnosis in a U.S. probability sample of persons infected with the human immunodeficiency virus. *Archives of Internal Medicine, 160*, 2614–2622.

United Nations Programme on HIV/AIDS (UNAIDS) and World Health Organization (WHO). (2005). AIDS epidemic update: December 2005. Geneva: Authors. Retrieved August 14, 2008, from *www.unaids.org/epi/2005/doc/epiupdate2005_pdf_en/epiupdate2005_en.pdf.*

United States Agency for International Development (USAID). (2006). Can we measure HIV/AIDS-related stigma and discrimination? Washington, DC: Author. Retrieved August 14, 2008, from *www.icrw.org/docs/2006_canwemeasurehivstigmareport.pdf.*

University of Kansas. (2007). Community Toolbox. Lawrence, KS: Author. Retrieved August 14, 2008, from *ctb.ku.edu/en.*

Vlahov, D., Des Jarlais, D. C., Goosby, E., Hollinger, P. C., Lurie, P. G., Shriver, M. D., et al. (2001). Case study: Needle exchange programs for the prevention of HIV infection. *American Journal of Epidemiology, 154*, S70–S77.

Wallace, S. P., & Castañeda, X. (2008). Health Policy Fact Sheet: HIV/AIDS and Latinos in the United States. Retrieved June 1, 2009, from *hia.berkeley.edu/documents/hiv_aids.pdf*.

Washington State Department of Health, HIV/AIDS Prevention and Education Services. (2008). *Effective interventions and strategies: Definitions of theories and models*. Retrieved August 10, 2008, from *www.doh.wa.gov/cfh/hiv_aids/prev_edu/effective_interventions/6_def_theor_models.htm*.

Webster, B. H., & Alemayehu, B. (2006). *Income, earnings, and poverty data from the 2005 American Community Survey* (American Community Survey Report No. ACS-02). Washington, DC: U.S. Census Bureau.

Woods, W. J., & Binson, D. (2003). Public health policy and gay bathhouses. *Journal of Homosexuality, 44*(3–4), 1–21.

Yates, B. T. (1999). *Measuring and improving cost, cost-effectiveness, and cost-benefit for substance abuse treatment programs*. Bethesda, MD: National Institute of Drug Abuse.

Zúñiga, M. L. (2007). Tools for culturally effective care gleaned from community-based research. *Virtual Mentor, 9*, 547–551. Retrieved August 18, 2008, from *virtualmentor.ama-assn.org/2007/08/pdf/jdsc1-0708.pdf*.

Zúñiga, M. L., Blanco, E., Martínez, P., Strathdee, S. A., & Gifford, A. L. (2007). Perceptions of barriers and facilitators to clinical trials participation in HIV-positive Latinas. *Journal of Women's Health, 16*(9), 1322–1330.

Zúñiga, M. L., Blanco, E., Palinkas, L. A., Strathdee, S. A., & Gifford, A. L. (in press). Cross-cultural considerations in the recruitment of Latinos of Mexican-origin into HIV/AIDS clinical trials in the US–Mexico border region: Clinician and patient perspectives. *Immigrant and Refugee Studies*.

Zúñiga, M. L., Blanco, E., Sanchez, L., Carroll, S., & Olshefsky, A. (2009). Preventing HIV and other sexually transmitted infections and reducing HIV-stigmatizing attitudes in high-risk youth: Evaluation of a comprehensive community-based and peer facilitated curriculum. *Vulnerable Children and Youth Studies, 4*(4), 333–342.

Zúñiga, M. L., Brennan, J., Scolari, R., & Strathdee, S. A. (2008). Barriers to HIV care in the context of cross-border health care utilization among HIV-positive persons living in the California/Baja California US–Mexico border region. *Journal of Immigrant and Minority Health, 10*, 219–227.

CHAPTER 27

The Contribution of Health Psychology to the Advancement of Global Health

Brian Oldenburg
Maximilian de Courten
Emma Frean

As public health challenges become ever more complex and influenced by the economic, political, social, and ecological circumstances of the world in which we live, it is more and more the case that solutions require global approaches. Clearly, the behavioral and social sciences, and the intersecting fields of behavioral medicine, health psychology, and public health, have a very important role to play in helping us to understand and address these challenges.

This chapter summarizes some of the most important contemporary global health issues and discusses how health psychology and related fields can contribute to the understanding, prevention, and management of these. This chapter stresses the importance of improving our knowledge of (1) those factors and influences in the global and local environment that affect health, (2) the social determinants of health and disease, (3) multilevel explanations for health and disease, and (4) how to improve the translation of research evidence into effective policy and health practice.

The Global Burden of Disease: Trends and Progress in Communicable and Chronic Disease

While the past 50 years have shown significant improvements in health and changes in the pattern of disease burden, both social and economic disparities remain a major cause of poor health and disease. The Global Burden of Disease (GBD) framework, developed in 1992 with the support of the World Bank and World Health Organization (WHO), was an attempt to summarize the wide-ranging and sometimes seemingly contradictory information available on morbidity, mortality, and other health outcomes. Looking at global population data from 1990, as well as data specific to eight global regions, the 1990 GBD study initiated a new way of informing intervention priorities for improved health. Prior to this study, evidence for policymaking was limited primarily to disease-specific mortality statistics. The initial and subsequent GBD studies provide a comprehensive measure that aggregates and standardizes measures of mortality, disability, impairment, and illness that arise from disease, injury and risk factors. Using the disability-adjusted life year (DALY) measure, GBD studies combine the years of life lost due to premature mortality and equivalent healthy years of life lost due to disability (Lopez, Mathers, Ezzati, Jamison, & Murray, 2006). One DALY, therefore, is equal to 1 year of full health lost. This allows for comparison of diseases that cause early death with those that cause prolonged suffering or disability in any country or region of the world.

The majority of countries have experienced an increase in life expectancy over the past 50 years, with an ever-increasing proportion of people expected to live until late adulthood. Between 1950 and 1990, life expectancy at birth increased from 40 years to 63 years in developing countries (World Bank, 1993). More recently still, average life expectancy increased in 2007 to 68 years globally, with a disproportionately large component of that increase occurring in countries in Asia (WHO, 2009b). However, there have been some important exceptions to this average increase in life expectancy around the world, particularly in a number of countries in sub-Saharan Africa, such as Botswana, Congo, Kenya and Lesotho, where HIV/AIDS has until very recently been poorly controlled (WHO, 2009b). A number of these and similar countries have experienced a decline in life expectancy of more than 10 years and a doubling of infant death rates over the past 15 years (Centers for Disease Control and Prevention, 2001).

Despite the inexorable rise in noncommunicable disease in low- and middle-income countries (LMICs),[1] infectious diseases, undernutrition, and perinatal conditions also remain important public health issues in many countries (Figure 27.1). While the number of children who die before 5 years of age decreased from 91 to 67 per 1,000 live births from 1990 to 2007, there still remains great inequality between low- and high-income countries (WHO, 2009b). By way

of comparison with high-income countries, child deaths from perinatal conditions (prematurity, birth trauma, and infection), acute respiratory infections, diarrheal diseases, and malaria account for 16% of all mortality in LMICs, compared to less than 1% in high-income countries (WHO, 2008b). Developing regions account for 99% of all global deaths in children younger than 15 years; the proportion of death between birth and 15 years of age ranges from 1.2% in high-income countries to 23% in LMICs (WHO, 2008b). Importantly, many of these conditions are preventable; for example, more than 1 million children die each year from diseases for which vaccines are available (WHO, 2008b).

Of the eight Millennium Development Goals (MDGs) chartered in 2000 by the United Nations (UN) for achievement by 2015, three are directly related to health: to reduce child mortality; to improve maternal health; and to combat HIV/AIDS, malaria, and tuberculosis (UN, 2008). Despite having already passed the halfway mark on the MDG time line, success in reaching these goals has been only minimal and there remains an ever-present gap in the health status of people in high-income countries and those in LMICs. For example, in developing countries, more than 500,000 women die annually due to pregnancy-related complications or childbirth, indicating little change since 1990; a woman in Africa may face a 1 in 26 lifetime risk of death during pregnancy and childbirth, compared with only 1 in 7,300 in more developed countries (UN, 2008; WHO, 2007).

However, as we have already suggested, significant gains are being achieved in a number of countries in Asia, Latin America, and the Caribbean. There is also recent progress in relation to global deaths from AIDS, which fell from 2.2 million in 2005 to 2.0 million in 2007, while the number of estimated new infections dropped from 3.0 million in 2001 to 2.7 million in 2007 (UN, 2008). Furthermore, 3.0 million of the 9.7 million people in developing countries that need treatment for HIV/AIDS were receiving it in 2007, thanks largely to the development of the Global Fund to Fight AIDS, Tuberculosis and Malaria (UN, 2008). Malaria prevention has expanded, with a threefold increase in insecticide-treated nets among

---

[1] The World Bank (2009) defines national economies according to gross national income (GNI) per capita: GNIs for low-, lower middle-, upper middle-, and high-income countries are $935 or less, $936–$3,705, $3,706–$11,455, and $11,456 or more, respectively.

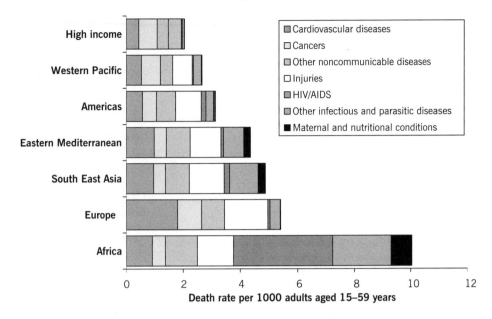

FIGURE 27.1. Adult mortality rates by major cause group and WHO region, 2004. From World Health Organization (2008a). Copyright 2008 by the World Health Organization. Reprinted by permission.

children under age 5 in sub-Saharan Africa since 2000, and 27 countries globally reported a reduction of up to 50% in the number of malaria cases between 1990 and 2006 (UN, 2008; WHO, 2009b). Deaths from measles fell by 74% between 2000 and 2006, with 82% of children in developing countries receiving the measles vaccine in 2007 and, impressively, the incidence of tuberculosis is expected to halt and decline before 2015; the whole-world target for incidence reduction was reached in 2004 (UN, 2008; WHO, 2009b).

The global decline of deaths attributable to communicable diseases has, however, occurred concurrently with a marked increase in noncommunicable diseases (NCDs). In 2000, ischemic heart disease and cerebrovascular disease were identified as the leading causes of mortality, together accounting for 42.4% of all deaths globally (WHO, 2001). The WHO estimates that without action to address the underlying risk factors, chronic diseases will account for an additional 17% of deaths globally by 2015 (WHO, 2005). Additionally, accidents and injuries—both intentional and nonintentional—are a significant and neglected cause of health prob-

lems internationally, accounting for 12% of the GBD (WHO, 2008b). In high-income countries, road traffic accidents are among the 10 leading causes of disease burden, and in LMICs, road traffic accidents are the most significant cause of injuries, with war, violence, and self-inflicted injuries also leading to reductions in quality of life (WHO, 2008b).

NCDs will account for an increasing proportion of GBD; their prevalence is expected to rise from 43% in 1998 to 66% in 2030 (WHO, 2008b). These are expected to include psychosocial disorders, and both cardiovascular and respiratory diseases (Figure 27.2). The primary behavioral risk factors for NCDs are unhealthy diet (including alcohol consumption), physical inactivity, and tobacco use, all three of which can be modified to reduce and prevent disease burden (WHO, 2005). Indeed, it is predicted that tobacco use will cause more premature death and disability than any other single factor, with mortality projected to increase from 5.4 million deaths in 2004 to 8.3 million deaths in 2030 as a result of the increased uptake of tobacco use in very populous countries such as China (WHO, 2008b).

2004 Disease or injury	Rank		Rank	2030 Disease or injury
Lower respiratory infections	1		1	Unipolar depressive disorders
Diarrheal diseases	2		2	Ischemic heart disease
Unipolar depressive disorders	3		3	Road traffic accidents
Ischemic heart disease	4		4	Cerebrovascular disease
HIV/AIDS	5		5	COPD
Cerebrovascular disease	6		6	Lower respiratory infections
Prematurity and low birthweight	7		7	Hearing loss, adult onset
Birth asphyxia and birth trauma	8		8	Refractive errors
Road traffic accidents	9		9	HIV/AIDS
Neonatal infections and other	10		10	Diabetes mellitus
COPD	13		11	Neonatal infections and other
Refractive errors	14		12	Prematurity and low birthweight
Hearing loss, adult onset	15		15	Birth asphyxia and birth trauma
Diabetes mellitus	19		18	Diarrheal disease

FIGURE 27.2. Ten leading causes of burden of disease, world, 2004 and 2030. From World Health Organization (2008a). Copyright 2008 by the World Health Organization. Reprinted by permission.

Behavioral and Social Epidemiology of Health and Disease

Understanding the potentially alterable causes of national and global health trends can help to inform responses to these challenges not only nationally, regionally, and internationally but also within population subgroups. However, a "human rights" view of health that prioritizes emphasis on more upstream determinants of health, as these particularly impact on more vulnerable and disadvantaged populations, is also important to consider alongside the more traditional approach that has emanated from much social and behavioral epidemiological research. Indeed, this human equity and a human rights perspective on health is reflected in the UN Universal Declaration of Human Rights (1948) and the Alma Ata Declaration, which advocated achievement of "health for all" (International Conference on Primary Health Care, 1978). More recently, the WHO (2005) brought together policymakers, researchers, and civil society organizations to establish the Commission on Social Determinants of Health, chaired by Sir Michael Marmot. The Commission conducted a 3-year review of the evidence surrounding global health inequalities and

the "causes of the causes," culminating in the final report, *Closing the Gap in a Generation* (WHO, 2008a). The three main recommendations proposed to reduce ill health and disadvantage are (1) improving daily living conditions; (2) redressing the inequitable distribution of power, money, and resources; and (3) improving measurement and understanding of the problem and assessing the impact of action.

In summary, a multitude of factors explains the changing patterns of morbidity, mortality, and the spread of disease globally, and between regions and countries. Some of these are related to population growth, aging, and changes to family, social structures, education, and reproductive patterns, while others are more related to changes in ecological and living environments. Huynen, Martens, and Hilderink (2005) have developed a comprehensive framework to illustrate the influence of globalization on health, highlighting the range of environmental, cultural, social, and economic factors that have been shown to affect lifestyle and health behaviors (Figure 27.3).

An evidence base for these multilevel determinants of health has been extensively developed over the past decade. In 2004, Mokdad, Marks, Stroup, and Gerberding

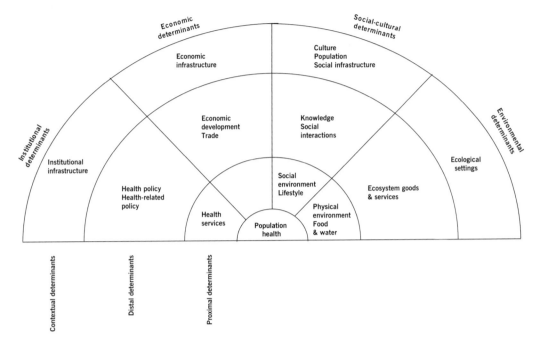

FIGURE 27.3. Framework for determinants of population health. From Huynen, Martens, and Hilderink (2005). Copyright 2005 by BioMed Central. Reprinted by permission.

demonstrated the relative contribution of alterable health behaviors and social factors to mortality and morbidity in the United States, and concluded that the primary causes of death in 2000 were tobacco and alcohol use, poor diet, and physical inactivity (Figure 27.4; WHO, 2005). More recently, the U.S. Centers for Disease Control and Prevention released a key report estimating that 14 of the top 15 causes of death in the United States are attributable to modifiable behaviors, including physical inactivity, diet, smoking, alcohol and other drug use, injury control, sun protective behaviors, appropriate use of medicines, immunization, sexual and reproductive health, oral hygiene, and mental health (Heron et al., 2009). An increased understanding of the social, economic, and environmental influences on behaviors leading to health (and ill-health) from an individual to a neighborhood/community level right up to a global level is consistent with a social ecological model used to explain the rapid increase in chronic NCDs from tobacco, poor diet, and sedentariness (Sallis & Owen, 1997).

Global Approaches to Health Challenges

The rapid increase in knowledge concerning the important links between social and behavioral determinants of health and the related strategies for addressing these has recently been used to establish two relatively new global health programs. The first of these is a global approach to tobacco control, with the establishment and "signing off" of the WHO (2009a) Framework Convention for Tobacco Control (FCTC) by 156 countries. The FCTC has successfully raised the priority of tobacco as a leading cause of preventable illness, and it has been suggested that further frameworks be designed, based on this model, to address other causes of chronic disease (Magnusson, 2007). The second global program related to diet and physical activity is in response to the rapidly rising rate of obesity/overweight and physical inactivity in nearly all countries. In 2004, the WHO adopted the Global Strategy on Diet, Physical Activity and Health (GSDPAH) as an advocacy tool to encourage the development of food- and exercise-related policy at the national level. However,

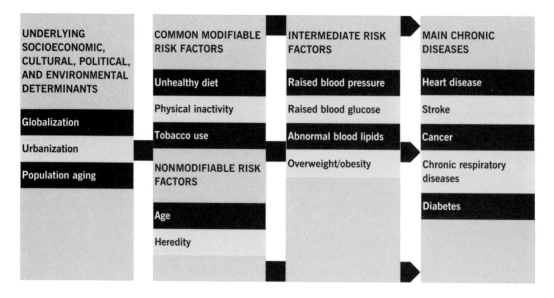

FIGURE 27.4. Causes of chronic disease. From World Health Organization (2005). Copyright 2005 by the World Health Organization. Reprinted by permission.

the absence of a legally binding agreement has meant that progress has been slow, with only 25 of the 192 WHO member states having implemented recommended policies (WHO, 2006a). For the success of the GD-SPAH, strong advocacy is needed to raise the profile of obesity to a level comparable to that of tobacco. Despite worldwide recognition that the adulteration and overconsumption of energy-dense food and beverages are harmful to health, the power and influence of the food industry, in some ways protected by the World Trade Organization, ensures that highly processed, calorie-rich products are widely available and often more affordable than fresh produce. To navigate such determinants of health, there remains a need for capacity-building interventions to address the life skills and competencies of the individual and communities. Such a "bottom-up" approach, through engagement with the population at the community level, allows a comprehensive strategy for disease prevention and health promotion.

The interconnectedness among the health challenges confronting all nations will certainly increase with the continuing globalization of the world's economy, increasing international travel, expanding global migration, the degree of (economic) inequality and consumption, and the widespread use of technology (Beaglehole & Bonita, 2008; McMichael, 2001; McMichael & Beaglehole, 2000). McMichael (2001) further identifies the impact of changes in the natural ecological environment, including climate change, as key determinants of health that pose challenges to disease prevention. Climate change brings with it thermal extremes, increases in the incidence of natural disasters, and a greater propensity toward the spread of vector-, food-, and water-borne disease (McMichael, Woodruff, & Hales, 2006). Furthermore, the spread of vector-borne disease is likely to grow due to the vast number of people traversing international borders; figures show that over 2 billion passengers were carried on the world's airlines in 2006 alone (International Air Transport Association, 2006). With the ability of infectious diseases to be carried across geographically defined borders during the contagious phase, one can see the potential for their wide and rapid dissemination. Severe acute respiratory syndrome (SARS) and the avian and swine influenza viruses are recent examples of the global movement of communicable disease.

The issue of climate change, and additionally, the mortality and morbidity associated with injury and air pollution, is further impacted by our reliance upon motorized transport. Motor vehicle incidents account for nearly 1.2 million global deaths annually, with urban pollution estimated to cause a further 800,000 deaths (Heinrich et al., 2005; WHO & World Bank, 2004). Furthermore, the failures of cities to accommodate pedestrians and cyclists safely contributes to the growing rates of physical inactivity and burden of obesity, diabetes, and cardiovascular disease (Haines et al., 2007; National Heart Forum, 2007).

Despite the ever-growing evidence base concerning the overwhelming impact of chronic NCDs on all countries, the development of a global leadership to address such challenges is still in an embryonic stage. The current policy approach that is supported by strong international agencies, such as the International Monetary Fund and the World Bank, assumes a strong, market-based approach to health interventions, favoring "best buys" over "greatest need" (Beaglehole & Bonita, 2008; Homedes & Ugalde, 2005; Katz, 2008). This approach is then further reflected in the goals set by donors, politicians, and development agencies; that is, they tend to adopt a disease-specific and vertical approach for two major reasons. First, programs focused on targeting a particular disease are comparatively quick and easy to roll out, and they are more likely to provide the measurable returns that are most likely to satisfy the donor (Reid & Pearse, 2003). Second, diseases portrayed as the greatest problem are likely to gain the greatest support of donors, who undoubtedly have to justify funding allocation. Historically, those who set disease priorities have typically advocated for infectious disease control over the prevention and management of chronic NCDs. Summarizing the current and projected global burden of diseases and the precursors to progress made in some regions, the WHO (2006b) stated in the World Health Report:

> The world community has sufficient financial resources and technologies to tackle most of these health challenges; yet today many national health systems are weak, unresponsive, inequitable—even unsafe. What is needed now is political will to implement national plans, together with international cooperation to align resources, harness knowledge and build robust health systems for treating and preventing disease and promoting population health. (p. xv)

Translating What We Already Know into Effective Policy and Health Practice

Until recently, models and frameworks for research and evidence development have identified a number of overlapping stages in the development, research, and evaluation of approaches to address a defined health problem. Typically, these include hypothesis development, methods development, controlled intervention trials, population studies, and both demonstration and implementation studies. A framework such as that developed by Oldenburg, Hardcastle, and Ffrench (1996) can be useful in tracking the accumulating evidence base of an innovation or intervention from its initial development to its institutionalization, in order to assess its utility in the public health area (Figure 27.5). This framework, with four key stages, ranges from identifying interventions that may have been tried on individuals or small groups to their broadest application at a population level, including changes in legislation and the policy environment. While these four general stages are conceptually different, the incremental accumulation of the evidence base from stage to stage may be bidirectional, and stages often overlap. For example, should sustained program use not be achieved, it may be necessary to tailor an existing innovation—such as simplifying a procedure—to the needs of the target adopters.

Oldenburg, Sallis, Ffrench, and Owen (1999) applied this framework to assess the staging and quality of research in behavioral medicine, health promotion, health psychology, and public health. Not surprisingly, results indicated a paucity of research extending beyond the basic research, program development, and innovation development stages, although this has started to change in more recent years. Clearly, there is a need for more research that focuses on dissemination and diffusion of the evidence base, so that the findings are more effectively translated into practice.

The ultimate value of research is determined by the extent to which the knowledge generated is disseminated, adopted, implemented, and maintained by users, and by its impact on systems and policy at a regional, state, and/or national level (i.e., "institutionalization"). With the necessity to improve

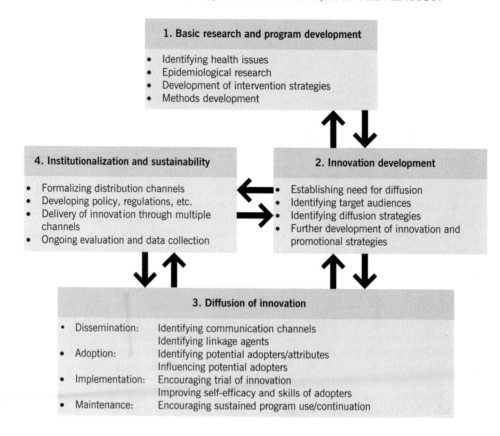

FIGURE 27.5. A staged approach to innovation development and diffusion. From Oldenburg, Hardcastle, and Ffrench (1996). Copyright 1996 by the Australian Health Promotion Association. Adapted by permission.

global health and achieve the health-related MDGs, it is imperative that health systems be able to adapt evidence for use within the local context (Kaul & Faust, 2001). The availability of relevant research findings does not, however, guarantee their use in the practical setting. For example, studies in the United States suggest that only half of patients receive recommended health care treatments, and that preventive measures are given even less attention (Glasgow & Strycker, 2000; McGlynn et al., 2003). Knowledge transfer requires formal development of research policies, organizational structural support, appropriate and targeted funding, monitoring of activity, and ongoing training and education.

"Knowledge brokering" is an important initiative of the Canadian Health Service Research Foundation (2003) and the impact of this novel concept has yet to be properly measured. Knowledge brokering stems from a need to formalize the knowledge transfer process and seeks to bring key individuals together who will compile an evidence-based solution to a particular issue (Canadian Health Services Research Foundation, 2003). This concept is central to the discussion on how best to disseminate, translate, and utilize research findings; the definitions of these actions themselves need clarification. In diffusion theory, "dissemination" may be thought of as the conscious and co-ordinated spread of research, ideas, policy, and practice through mass communication, marketing, literature, and health education channels (Green, Ottoson, Garcia, & Hiatt, 2009). Such information can be "translated" as theory on which effectiveness studies can be based before the knowledge is implemented in real practice (i.e., "utilized"). However, there is a need for continuous monitoring and evaluation processes to ensure that, upon reaching the target audience, the knowledge is correctly translated and avoids deviation from its intended purpose and efficacy (Green et al., 2009).

The spread of knowledge is not an end point itself but a process leading to the further development of policy and practice options for use by public health practitioners and clinicians. Given that they have the ultimate power in determining how health research knowledge is put to use, it is important that they be given due consideration or, better yet, be included in the research design process (Berwick, 2003). Additionally, public health practitioners and clinicians must have support from government and society for the implementation of best practice (Berwick, 2003; Landry, Lamari, & Amara, 2003). For example, health promotion campaigns should serve to create awareness within society and reinforce the message of the health professional, while government policy should reinforce the importance of certain health practices or preventive measures. However, the growing burden of chronic disease requires a multisectoral approach to develop interventions that address causality at the population level (Chopra, Galbraith, & Darnton-Hill, 2002; Reddy, Shah, Varghese, & Ramadoss, 2005; Yach, Hawkes, Gould, & Hofman, 2004). Sorensen, Emmons, Hunt, and Johnston (1998) have identified what they believe to be the key directions for population-level interventions in different settings, such as communities, worksites, and schools. They argue that to be effective such interventions need to (1) target multiple levels of influence, (2) address social inequalities in disease risk, (3) involve communities in program planning and implementation, (4) incorporate approaches for tailoring interventions, and (5) utilize rigorous process tracking.

Physical activity research and population-based interventions directed at reducing levels of sedentary behavior are now also focusing on the impact of local environments in terms of urban planning and neighborhood design, and identifying determinants, such as population density, interconnectedness of streets, and mixed land use (Sallis, Bauman, & Pratt, 1998). For example, in recognition that there is now sufficient evidence that policies to promote more active lifestyles will en-

able children and adolescents to achieve the recommended 60 minutes of daily physical activity, the American Academy of Pediatrics in 2009 released a policy statement "The Built Environment: Designing Communities to Promote Physical Activity in Children." This document gives health professionals, as well as local governments, specific recommendations that by working together with community partners, they can participate in establishing communities designed for activity and health (Committee on Environmental Health, 2009). The recommendations for pediatricians include the following:

1. Ask patients and families about opportunities for recreational and incidental physical activity in nearby parks, playgrounds, or open spaces. Identify barriers that could prevent children from using community locations and offer suggestions when possible.
2. Encourage patients to advocate on behalf of their children and their schools for relevant environmental improvements, such as Safe Routes to School programs or a Walking School Bus. Encourage families to participate and use these programs in their communities. Encourage families who are considering a move of residence to consider the opportunities for physical activity at the new location.
3. Advocate for environmental improvements that promote physical activity in children. Become involved in local community planning processes to encourage cities and local governments to prioritize space for parks. Emphasize the need for built structures, such as playgrounds, that provide more opportunities for physical activity. Advocate for safe routes for incidental activity opportunities, including walking or biking to school.

Population-level interventions to reduce salt intake and tobacco use have also been both successful and cost-effective in addressing people with chronic NCDs. Hypertension accounts for 80% of the chronic disease burden in LMICs; however, this can be reduced by 15% with simple measures, such as limiting the salt content of processed food and introducing long-term mass media campaigns for dietary change (Asaria, Chisholm, Mathers, Ezzati, & Beaglehole, 2007). Likewise, the introduction of the FCTC has successfully reduced the prevalence of tobacco-related illness through effective population-based policies: increasing taxes on tobacco products; introducing mandatory smoke-free public environments; requiring that health risks and outcomes be clearly labeled on tobacco products; and banning tobacco advertising, promotion, and sponsorship (Shibuya et al., 2003).

In reviewing efficacious evidence-to-practice translation, multiple barriers keep the process from being simple, straightforward, and effective (Glasgow & Emmons, 2007). The most sustainable programs for replication are those with minimal intensity, that is, those that do not make heavy demands on coordinators and the target group, that are straightforward to implement, and that consider both cost-effectiveness and availability of resources. Furthermore, interventions are typically hypothesized and tested to work within internally validated guidelines. Their implementation for research purposes is done in a controlled environment and is unlikely to replicate the real-world context, thereby limiting the efficacious utilization of evidence in the external setting (Green et al., 2009). Additionally, comprehensive review of diffusion theory suggests that many interventions do not address what health practitioners want and need because they neither account for the situation in which the intervention is applied nor validate the methods for intervention design (Goodman & Mills, 1999; Green et al., 2009; Oldenburg & Glanz, 2008).

Conclusions

The methods and approaches used to address health challenges that currently confront countries need to focus more on the upstream economic, social, and environmental determinants of health, in addition to the more traditional focus on individual-level determinants. To address these issues, nations require health policies and health care systems that are more prevention-focused and public health-oriented. Additionally, there needs to be increased exchange of knowledge across traditional disciplinary, cultural, and national boundaries. We have already begun to see such international efforts in relation to areas such as tobacco control and obesity prevention.

Finally, it is very important to reiterate the importance of addressing health disparities between and within countries. Many interventions have failed to address the inequalities within populations, and to account for the social and economic causes of ill health. Indeed, the performance of our health care systems, and our teaching and research efforts, should not be judged solely by whether we have contributed to improving the health of the whole population. Rather, our performance should be judged by the extent to which our efforts have also benefited those disadvantaged individuals and population subgroups—nationally and internationally—for whom the disparities are greatest, and who are most in need of focused, coordinated, long-term efforts by health researchers, policymakers, and practitioners around the world.

Further Reading

Beaglehole, R., & Bonita, R. (2009). *Global public health: A new era*. New York: Oxford University Press.

Commission on Social Determinants of Health. (2008). *Closing the gap in a generation: Health equity through action on the social determinants of health: Final Report of the Commission on Social Determinants of Health*. Geneva: World Health Organization.

Huynen, M. M., Martens, P., & Hilderink, H. B. (2005). The health impacts of globalization: A conceptual framework. *Globalization and Health, 1*, 14.

Magnusson, R. (2007). Non-communicable diseases and global health governance: Enhancing global processes to improve health development. *Globalization and Health, 3*, 2.

McMichael, A. J., & Beaglehole, R. (2000). The changing global context of public health. *Lancet, 356*, 495–499.

Oldenburg, B., & Glanz, K. (2008). Diffusions of innovation. In K. Glanz, B. K. Rimer, & K. Viswanath (Eds.), *Health behavior and health education: Theory, research and practice* (4th ed.). San Francisco: Jossey-Bass.

United Nations. (2008). *The Millennium Development Goals Report 2008*. New York: UN Department of Economic and Social Affairs.

World Health Organization. (2008). *The global burden of disease: 2004 update*. Geneva: Author.

References

Asaria, P., Chisholm, D., Mathers, C., Ezzati, M., & Beaglehole, R. (2007). Chronic disease prevention: Health effects and financial costs of strategies to reduce salt intake and control tobacco use. *Lancet, 370,* 2044–2053.

Beaglehole, R., & Bonita, R. (2008). Global public health: A scorecard. *Lancet, 372,* 1988–1996.

Berwick, D. (2003). Disseminating evidence innovations in health care. *Journal of the American Medical Association, 289,* 1969–1975.

Canadian Health Services Research Foundation. (2003). *The theory and practice of knowledge brokering in Canada's health system.* Ottawa: Author.

Centers for Disease Control and Prevention. (2001). The 20th year of AIDS: A time to re-energize prevention. *Morbidity and Mortality Weekly Report, 50*(21), 444–445.

Chopra, M., Galbraith, S., & Darnton-Hill, I. (2002). A global response to a global problem: The epidemic of over-nutrition. *Bulletin of the World Health Organization, 80*(12), 952–958.

Committee on Environmental Health. (2009). The built environment: Designing communities to promote physical activity in children. *Pediatrics, 123*(6), 1591–1598.

Glasgow, R. E., & Emmons, K. M. (2007). How can we increase translation of research into practice?: Types of evidence needed. *Annual Review of Public Health, 28,* 413–33.

Glasgow, R. E., & Strycker, L. A. (2000). Preventive care practices for diabetes management in two primary care samples. *American Journal of Preventive Medicine, 19*(1), 9–14.

Goodman, C. A., & Mills, A. J. (1999). The evidence base on the cost-effectiveness of malaria control measures in Africa. *Health Policy and Planning, 14,* 301–312.

Green, L. W., Ottoson, J. M., Garcia, C., & Hiatt, R. A. (2009). Diffusion theory and knowledge dissemination, utilization, and integration in public health. *Annual Review of Public Health, 30,* 151–174.

Haines, A., Smith, K. R., Anderson, D., Epstein, P. R., McMichael, A. J., Roberts, I., et al. (2007). Policies for accelerating access to clean energy, improving health, advancing development, and mitigating climate change. *Lancet, 370,* 1264–1281.

Heinrich, J., Schwarze, P. E., Stillanakis, N., Momas, I., Medina, S., Totlandsdal, A. I., et al. (2005). Studies on health effects of transport-related air pollution. In M. Krzyzanowski, B. Kuna-Dibbert, & J. Schneider (Eds.), *Health effects of transport-related air pollution.* Geneva: World Health Organization.

Heron, M., Hoyert, D. L., Murphy, S. L., Xu, J., Kochanek, K. D., & Tejada-Vera, B. (2009). Deaths: Final Data for 2006. *National Vital Statistics Reports, 57*(14).

Homedes, N., & Ugalde, A. (2005). Why neoliberal health reforms have failed in Latin America. *Health Policy, 71,* 83–96.

Huynen, M. M., Martens, P., & Hilderink, H. B. (2005). The health impacts of globalization: A conceptual framework. *Globalization and Health, 1,* 14.

International Air Transport Association. (2006). World industry statistics. Montreal: Author. Retrieved June 17, 2009, from *www.iata.org.*

Katz, A. (2008). New global health: A reversal of logic, history and principles (Editorial). *Social Medicine, 3*(1), 1–3.

Kaul, I., & Faust, M. (2001). Global public goods and health: Taking the agenda forward. *Bulletin of the World Health Organization, 79,* 869–874.

Landry, R., Lamari, M., & Amara, N. (2003). The extent and determinants of the utilization of university research in government agencies. *Public Administration Review, 63,* 192–205.

Lopez, A. D., Mathers, C. D., Ezzati, M., Jamison, D. T., & Murray, C. J. L. (Eds.). (2006). *Global burden of disease and risk factors.* Washington, DC: Oxford University Press and the World Bank.

Magnusson, R. (2007). Non-communicable diseases and global health governance: Enhancing global processes to improve health development. *Globalization and Health, 3,* 2.

McGlynn, E. A., Asch, S. M., Adams, J., Keesey, J., Hicks, J., DeCristofaro, A., et al. (2003). The quality of health care delivered to adults in the United States. *New England Journal of Medicine, 348*(26), 2635–2645.

McMichael, A. J. (2001). *Human frontiers, environments and disease: Past patterns, uncertain futures.* New York: Cambridge University Press.

McMichael, A. J., & Beaglehole, R. (2000). The changing global context of public health. *Lancet, 356,* 495–499.

McMichael, A. J., Woodruff, R. E., & Hales, S. (2006). Climate change and human health: Present and future risks. *Lancet, 367,* 859–869.

Mokdad, A. H., Marks, J. S., Stroup, D. F., & Gerberding, J. L. (2004). Actual causes of death in the United States, 2000. *Journal of the American Medical Association, 291*(10), 1238–1245.

National Heart Forum. (2007). *Building health: Creating and enhancing places for active, healthy lives.* London: Author.

Oldenburg, B., & Glanz, K. (2008). Diffusions of innovation. In K. Glanz, B. K. Rimer, & K.

Viswanath (Eds.), *Health behavior and health education: Theory, research and practice* (4th ed.). San Francisco: Jossey-Bass.

Oldenburg, B., Hardcastle, D., & Ffrench, M. (1996). How does research contribute to evidence-based practice in health promotion? *Health Promotion Journal of Australia, 6,* 15–20.

Oldenburg, B., Sallis, J., Ffrench, M., & Owen, N. (1999). Health promotion research and the diffusion and institutionalisation of interventions. *Health Education Research, 14*(1), 121–130.

Reddy, K. S., Shah, B., Varghese, C., & Ramadoss, A. (2005). Responding to the threat of chronic diseases in India. *Lancet, 366,* 1746–1751.

Reid, M., & Pearse, E. J. (2003). Whither the WHO. *Medical Journal of Australia, 178*(1), 9–12.

Sallis, J. F., Bauman, A., & Pratt, M. (1998). Environmental and policy interventions to promote physical activity. *American Journal of Preventive Medicine, 15*(4), 379–397.

Sallis, J. F., & Owen, N. (1997). Ecological models. In K. Glanz, F. M. Lewis, & B. K. Rimer (Eds.), *Health behavior and health education: Theory, research and practice* (pp. 403–424). San Francisco: Jossey-Bass.

Shibuya, K., Ciecierski, C., Guindon, E., Bettcher, D. W., Evans, D. B., Murray, C. J., et al. (2003). WHO Framework Convention on Tobacco Control: Development of an evidence based global public health treaty. *British Medical Journal, 327,* 154–157.

Sorensen, G., Emmons, K., Hunt, M. K., & Johnston, D. (1998). Implications of the results of community intervention trials. *Annual Review of Public Health, 19,* 379–416.

United Nations. (2008). *The Millennium Development Goals Report 2008.* New York: UN Department of Economic and Social Affairs.

World Health Organization (WHO). (2001). *World Health Report—Mental health: New understanding, new hope.* Geneva: Author.

World Health Organization (WHO). (2004). *Global strategy on diet, physical activity and health.* Geneva: Author.

World Health Organization (WHO). (2005). *Preventing chronic diseases: A vital investment.* Geneva: Author.

World Health Organization (WHO). (2006a, May 11). Implementation of resolutions: Report by the secretariat [A59/23]. World Health Assembly. Retrieved October 22, 2008, from *www.who.int/gb/ebwha/pdf_files/wha59/a59_23-en.pdf.*

World Health Organization (WHO). (2006b). *World Health Report: Working together for health.* Geneva: Author.

World Health Organization (WHO). (2007). *Maternal mortality in 2005: WHO, UNICEF, UNFPA, and the World Bank.* Geneva: Author.

World Health Organization (WHO). (2008). *The Global Burden of Disease: 2004 update.* Geneva: Author.

World Health Organization (WHO). (2008). *Closing the gap in a generation: Health equity through action on the social determinants of health: Final report of the Commission on Social Determinants of Health.* Geneva: World Health Organization.

World Health Organization (WHO). (2009a). Parties to the WHO Framework Convention on Tobacco Control. Retrieved June 28, 2009, from *www.who.int/fctc/signatories_parties/en/index.html.*

World Health Organization (WHO). (2009b). *World health statistics 2009.* Geneva: Author.

World Health Organization (WHO), & the World Bank (2004). *World Report on Road Traffic Injury Prevention.* Geneva: World Health Organization.

World Bank. (1993). *World Development Report 1993: Investing in health.* New York: Oxford University Press.

World Bank. (2009). Country classification. Retrieved June 27, 2009, from *www.worldbank.org.*

Yach, D., Hawkes, C., Gould, C. L., & Hofman, K. J. (2004). The global burden of chronic diseases: Overcoming impediments to prevention and control. *Journal of the American Medical Association, 291,* 2616–2622.

PART V

HEALTH PSYCHOLOGY AND THE MEDICAL SPECIALTIES

CHAPTER 28

Cardiology

Manjunath Harlapur
Dennis Abraham
Daichi Shimbo

Coronary heart disease (CHD) is one of the leading causes of mortality and morbidity in industrialized nations (Braunwald, 1997; Fuster & Vedanthan, 2008; Fuster & Voute, 2007). It is estimated that the absolute mortality due to CHD will increase as the average age of the population rises (Braunwald, 1997). Acute coronary syndrome (ACS), defined as myocardial infarction with or without S and T wave (ST)–segment elevation or unstable angina, represents a spectrum of CHD events with similar underlying mechanisms. Despite advances in treatment, the cardiovascular event rate remains relatively high after an ACS event (Anderson et al., 2007; Fraker et al., 2007). Furthermore, quality of life is impaired in many patients with CHD despite optimal treatment (Ruo et al., 2003).

A large proportion of CHD events can be attributed to behavioral or lifestyle factors, including cigarette smoking, poor diet, and physical inactivity, which indicates that CHD is preventable (Mokdad, Marks, Stroup, & Gerberding, 2004; Yusuf et al., 2004). Also, psychosocial factors such as depression, anxiety, and hostility/anger, which are prevalent in patients with CHD,

adversely affect cardiovascular prognosis (Rozanski, Blumenthal, Davidson, Saab, & Kubzansky, 2005; Rozanski, Blumenthal, & Kaplan, 1999). Psychosocial factors influence the course of CHD by either encouraging poor lifestyle behaviors or directly affecting underlying biological CHD pathways. (See Weidner and Kendel, Chapter 24, this volume.)

This chapter reviews the underlying pathophysiological mechanisms that explain the onset of ACS events, current concepts in CHD risk prediction, and selected treatment approaches.

Pathophysiology of Disease

"Atherosclerosis" is a diffuse disease characterized by the deposition of lipid and other blood-borne material within the arterial wall (Corti, Fuster, & Badimon, 2003). Substantial advances over the past decade have demonstrated the important role of inflammation and the underlying cellular and molecular mechanisms in promoting the formation and progression of atherosclerosis (Fuster, Moreno, Fayad, Corti, & Badimon, 2005). Chronic inflammation has been a topic of immense interest in the field of atherosclerosis (Fuster et al., 2005). Early in the disease process, endothelial cells express surface adhesion molecules, such as vascular cell adhesion molecule–1 (VCAM-1) and intercellular adhesion molecule–1 (ICAM-1), which allow for leukocyte binding and entrance into the vessel wall (Blake & Ridker, 2001; Robbie & Libby, 2001). Once inside the vessel wall, these cells stimulate a local inflammatory response, promoting atherosclerotic plaque development (Robbie & Libby, 2001). Inflammation also contributes to plaque vulnerability and subsequent rupture (Robbie & Libby, 2001). Macrophages in the plaque produce proteolytic enzymes that structurally weaken the plaque's fibrous cap, making it prone to rupture (Falk, Shah, & Fuster, 1995). Large, population-based prospective studies have indeed confirmed that inflammation is central to ACS development (Ridker, Buring, & Rifai, 2001; Ridker, Hennekens, Buring, & Rifai, 2000; Ridker, Hennekens, Roitman-Johnson, Stampfer, & Allen, 1998; Ridker, Rifai, Stampfer, & Hennekens, 2000). These studies have found increased ACS risk associated with increased levels of cytokines, such as interleukin-6 (IL-6) and tumor necrosis factor–alpha (TNF-alpha); cell adhesion molecules, such as ICAM-1 and P-selectin; and downstream acute-phase reactants, such as C-reactive protein (CRP).

Evidence indicates that occlusive platelet thrombus formation over a ruptured coronary plaque is fundamental for the development of ischemia and/or infarction characteristic of an ACS event (Badimon, Zaman, Helft, Fayad, & Fuster, 1999; Fuster, Badimon, Badimon, & Chesebro, 1992a, 1992b). ACS events are not typically caused by slow growth of a coronary atherosclerotic plaque, with eventual limitation of blood flow once the stenosis become critical. Instead, ACS events are mostly caused by the acute limitation of blood flow due to occlusive thrombus formation over a ruptured atherosclerotic plaque. A major determinant of thrombus formation is platelet aggregation (Corti et al., 2003), which depends on the interaction of membrane glycoproteins (GPs) that are receptors for adhesive proteins (Coller, 1997). The most abundant receptor is the GPIIb/IIIa integrin. Platelet agonists such as

serotonin, adenosine diphosphate, collagen, and thromboxane A_2 bind to their respective receptors, facilitating the activation of the platelet GPIIb/IIIa receptors necessary to bind a number of ligands, including fibrinogen (Gresele, Page, Fuster, & Vermylen, 2002; Vorchheimer, Badimon, & Fuster, 1999). Fibrinogen binds to GPIIb/IIIa receptors on adjacent platelets, resulting in crosslinking necessary for platelet aggregation and subsequent thrombus formation (Gresele et al., 2002). The importance of platelet reactivity and its inhibition in the onset of the ACS is demonstrated by the clinical benefits associated with the use of antiplatelet agents (Lewis et al., 1983; Mehta et al., 2001; Sabatine et al., 2005; Theroux et al., 1988; Yusuf et al., 2001).

High-Risk or Vulnerable Plaque

The term "high-risk" or "vulnerable" plaque refers to a plaque that is at increased risk of thrombosis and rapid stenosis progression (Fuster et al., 2005; Little, 1990; Muller & Tofler, 1992; Viles-Gonzalez, Fuster, & Badimon, 2006). The identification of these high-risk plaques has been a source of intense investigation, and we have learned a great deal about the nature of these plaques and the processes underlying ACS onset.

Plaques that are prone to rupture are typified by a large lipid core, thin fibrous cap, and high macrophage content (Fuster, Fayad, & Badimon, 1999; Fuster et al., 2005; Kolodgie et al., 2001). Evidence suggests that high cholesterol content in the plaque, associated with active inflammation and macrophage infiltration, is associated with a higher risk of rupture (Felton, Crook, Davies, & Oliver, 1997). Virmani, Kolodgie, Burke, Farb, and Schwartz (2000) noted that ruptured plaques often had the largest cores, suggesting that plaque size is also important. Autopsy studies have shown that the degree of macrophage infiltration in an atherosclerotic plaque is greater in those plaques that rupture (Moreno et al., 1994; Virmani et al., 2000). Finally, the average number of thin-capped atheromas is higher in those dying of an ACS event (Virmani et al., 2000). These observations formed the basis for how we initially defined high-risk plaques.

Coronary angiography is widely considered to be the "gold standard" methodology for the evaluation and diagnosis of obstructive coronary lesions. A lesion that is severely stenotic (i.e., greater than 70%) is often deemed to be at increased risk for future thrombosis. However, numerous studies have brought into question the utility of coronary angiography in identifying atherosclerotic plaques for the prediction of future ACS events (Ambrose et al., 1988; Little et al., 1988; Nobuyoshi et al., 1991). Although severely stenotic lesions are associated with increased risk of an ACS event compared to less obstructive lesions, the majority of ACS events are associated with a nonobstructive lesion (Ambrose et al., 1988; Little et al., 1988; Nobuyoshi et al., 1991). One explanation is that despite lower risk of an ACS event, less obstructive plaques give rise to more ACS events because of their far greater number (Nobuyoshi et al., 1991). Another explanation is that these nonobstructive high-risk lesions as imaged on coronary angiography are actually relatively large atheromas (Nissen & Yock, 2001). Investigators have demonstrated that some atherosclerotic arterial vessels undergo positive remodeling, in which the external elastic membrane adjacent to an atheroma is outwardly displaced compared to an adjacent reference site, thus preserving the lumen from obstruction of blood flow (Glagov, Weisenberg, Zarins, Stankunavicius, & Kolettis, 1987; Schoenhagen, Ziada, Vince, Nissen, & Tuzcu, 2001). In positively remodeled atherosclerotic arteries, the plaque volume is actually greater than that observed in vessels that undergo negative remodeling (i.e., a smaller external elastic membrane at the lesion site compared to an adjacent reference site) (Schoenhagen et al., 2000, 2001). Furthermore, positive remodeling is associated with ruptured plaques (Smits, Pasterkamp, de Jaegere, de Feyter, & Borst, 1999; Yamagishi et al., 2000).

Studies utilizing intravascular ultrasound, a modality that can image the vascular wall, in addition to the lumen, have indicated that the coronary arteries of patients with unstable angina are characterized by positive remodeling and larger plaque size, while the coronary arteries of patients with stable angina are characterized by negative remodeling and smaller plaque size (Schoenhagen et al., 2000). Positive remodeling, which allows for considerable plaque accumulation despite a relatively normal luminal size, may

be associated with an increased risk for an ACS event. In contrast, negative remodeling may be associated with more stable plaques, despite more significant coronary obstruction. The biological mechanisms linking positive remodeling to plaque vulnerability have not been established. A proinflammatory state may play a major role because as histological studies suggest a relationship between inflammation and positive remodeling (Pasterkamp et al., 1998).

The apparent disconnect between lesion severity and subsequent ACS risk highlights the inherent limitations of diagnostic angiography (Topol & Nissen, 1995). Coronary angiography assesses intraluminal stenoses and is not able to determine wall thickness or precise vascular morphology. A number of other imaging modalities, including intravascular ultrasound (see Table 28.1), have been tested in characterizing and identifying plaques prone to rupture. These mostly experimental modalities are supported by a wide range of evidence (Lerakis et al., 2008). A major limitation of these imaging modalities is the dearth of natural history studies linking specific characteristics of a high-risk plaque (e.g., thin-capped, lipid-rich, ruptured) with subsequent plaque rupture, and the onset of an ACS event directly attributable to the ruptured plaque (Ambrose, 2008).

While the identification of such high-risk lesions has been an intense area of research, a number of more recent studies suggest that this paradigm is incomplete (Naghavi et al., 2003a, 2003b). Studies that use imaging to identify high-risk plaques in patients with ACS (e.g., ruptured plaques on intravascular ultrasound or yellow, lipid-rich plaques on angioscopy) have shown that a second or even a third high-risk plaque can be present at another nonculprit coronary site or vessel (Libby, 2005; Rioufol et al., 2002). These findings confirm that atherosclerosis is a diffuse systemic process, and highlight the difficulty in accurately determining whether a specific high-risk plaque is the culprit lesion for a future ACS event.

Furthermore, evidence from pathological studies indicates that an intracoronary thrombus can form over a nonruptured, superficially eroded plaque, which is less lipid-rich, less infiltrated by macrophages, and characterized by a greater predominance of

TABLE 28.1. Imaging Modalities for the Detection of High-Risk Plaques

- Intravascular ultrasound (catheter-based technique that provides a cross-sectional ultrasonographic image of the coronary artery, including the arterial wall and surface components)
- Angioscopy (catheter-based technique that allows for direct visualization of the intravascular surface of the coronary arteries using optical fiber technology)
- Optical coherence tomography (catheter-based technique that allows for high-resolution intravascular imaging by measuring back-reflected infrared light)
- Virtual histology (allows for plaque characterization including size, density, and compressibility using the intravascular ultrasound technique)
- Near infrared spectroscopy (a catheter-based technique that allows for characterization of the plaque components based on light absorbance and scatter properties)
- Thermography (a catheter-based technique that assesses heat emitted from a plaque as a marker of inflammation)
- Electron beam computed tomography (noninvasive technique that assesses coronary artery stenoses and the arterial wall including the degree of calcification)
- Magnetic resonance imaging (a technique that can be performed both noninvasively and invasively, and provide high spatial and temporal resolution of the arterial wall and plaque components; noninvasive method has some limitations in imaging the coronary arteries due to their size and motion)

smooth muscle cells compared to the typical ruptured plaque (Farb et al., 1996; van der Wal, Becker, van der Loos, & Das, 1994; Virmani et al., 2000). One study showed that a large proportion (44%) of sudden deaths due to coronary thrombosis can be explained by an eroded plaque without rupture (Farb et al., 1996). In addition to eroded plaques, a plaque with a calcified nodular component is another (but infrequent) cause of intracoronary thrombosis (Virmani et al., 2000). Studies utilizing imaging modalities have not focused on the detection of either superficially eroded plaques or plaques with a calcified nodular component. Overall, these three types of atherosclerotic plaques (ruptured plaques, eroded plaques, plaques with a calcified nodular component) all can lead to thrombus formation and ACS event onset. The term "high-risk" or "vulnerable"

should and does describe these types of atherosclerotic plaques (Fuster et al., 2005; Naghavi et al., 2003a, 2003b).

As ACS onset can be explained by thrombus formation over a non-ruptured plaque, it is plausible that increased blood thrombogenicity also plays an essential role (Sambola et al., 2003). Although the focus has been on the atherosclerotic coronary plaque, it is intriguing the blood itself may be "vulnerable" or "high-risk." The concept of vulnerable blood, as proposed by others (Naghavi et al., 2003a, 2003b), encompasses a spectrum of prothrombotic or hypercoagulable states that increases the risk of thrombus formation overlying a nonruptured plaque, leading to an ACS event. Alterations in the balance of prothrombotic and antithrombotic processes are probably central to the development of vulnerable blood (Faxon et al., 2004; Rauch et al., 2001; Sambola et al., 2003).

In summary, although a multitude of studies have investigated the underlying mechanisms that explain the onset of ACS events, much remains unknown (Ambrose, 2008). It is unclear how best to identify atherosclerotic plaques that will go on to rupture and induce an ACS event, and how to identify eroded plaques or plaques with a calcified nodular component and predict their risk of thrombosis. Also, it remains unclear whether it is best to treat these high-risk plaques with optimal medical therapy alone or with adjunctive coronary revascularization.

CHD Risk Prediction

Population-based studies have identified multiple, independent risk factors for the development of CHD events, including age, male sex, hypertension, hypercholesterolemia, low high-density lipoprotein (HDL) cholesterol, cigarette smoking, and diabetes (Wilson et al., 1998). The identification of these risk factors has enabled the assessment of 10-year CVD absolute risk through the use of prediction models, the most common of which is the Framingham Risk Score, based on age, total cholesterol (or low-density lipoprotein [LDL] cholesterol), HDL cholesterol, blood pressure levels, diabetes, and cigarette smoking (Wilson, 2005; Wilson et al., 1998).

Because traditional risk factors do not account for all patients who develop CHD events, novel biomarkers have been proposed to identify better individuals at future risk for cardiovascular events (Tsimikas, Willerson, & Ridker, 2006). For instance, given the role of inflammation in atherosclerosis development and progression, elevated inflammatory biomarkers have been proposed as novel risk markers for CHD events. CRP remains the most extensively investigated of these in clinical studies. A multitude of large epidemiological studies have shown that CRP predicts future CHD events, independent of traditional risk factors (Ridker, Buring, Shih, Matias, & Hennekens, 1998; Ridker, Cushman, Stampfer, Tracy, & Hennekens, 1997; Ridker, Hennekens, et al., 2000).

Some controversy exists about what proportion of the risk of a CHD event is explained by traditional risk factors (Khot et al., 2003). Some investigators have suggested that one or more conventional risk factors are present in only 50% of patients with CHD (Braunwald, 1997; Tavazzi, 1999), while others have suggested that the percentage is much higher (i.e., 80–90%) (Khot et al., 2003). However, a large proportion of subjects (i.e., 70%) who do not develop CHD also have one or more major risk factors (Greenland et al., 2003; Khot et al., 2003; Root & Cobb, 2004). Thus, even if the sensitivity of traditional risk factors is high, the specificity is low. These findings indicate that conventional risk factors do not accurately predict the development of CHD events.

Beside novel biomarkers of future CHD events, investigators have recently proposed routine screening for subclinical atherosclerosis. As demonstrated by intravascular ultrasound of the coronary arteries in transplanted hearts (Tuzcu et al., 2001), subclinical atherosclerotic CHD is relatively prevalent even in donor hearts obtained from young adults and adolescents. Examples of proposed screening tools for the detection of subclinical atherosclerosis include carotid intima media thickness (IMT) and plaque assessed by ultrasound or magnetic resonance imaging, coronary calcium quantification by computed tomography, ankle–brachial index, flow-mediated vasodilation assessed by ultrasound, vascular compliance measured by tonometry, and/or left ventricular mass assessed by echocardiography or magnetic resonance imaging (Naghavi et al., 2006). Investigators from the SHAPE (Screening for Heart Attack Prevention and Education) Task Force (Naghavi et al., 2006) have proposed that a subclinical atherosclerosis test be performed in individuals without cardiovascular disease history, and if positive, be used to risk stratify individuals as very high risk, high risk, and moderately high risk. If the atherosclerosis test is negative, then traditional risk factors can be used to stratify individuals as moderate risk and lower risk. Future studies that examine the internal and external validity of this predictive model, risk–benefit ratios, and cost-effectiveness in the general population should be performed to give greater support to these somewhat controversial recommendations. (See Weidner & Kendel, Chapter 24, this volume, for additional discussion of risk factors.)

Mechanistic Pathways Linking Psychosocial Factors to CHD Events

Psychosocial factors, such as depression and anger/hostility, increase the risk of CHD events. Two main pathways linking psychosocial factors to CHD events have been proposed. First, psychosocial factors encourage unhealthy behavioral or lifestyle patterns, such as eating an unhealthy diet, reduced physical activity, smoking, and obesity promotion. Second, given that psychosocial factors appear to confer additional risk, over and above behavioral or lifestyle factors (Rosengren et al., 2004; Yusuf et al., 2004), it is likely that a more direct mechanistic link also exists between psychosocial factors and CHD risk onset. A large body of research has shown associations between psychosocial factors and biological mechanisms underlying ACS event onset, including exaggerated platelet reactivity, inflammation, autonomic imbalance, procoagulant factors, endothelial dysfunction, reduced levels of omega-3 fatty acids, anabolic–catabolic hormonal imbalance, sleep architecture disruption, accelerated cellular aging, and circadian rhythm disruption (Carney, Freedland, Miller, & Jaffe, 2002; Goldston & Baillie, 2008; Parissis et al., 2007; Rozanski et al., 2005; Shimbo, Davidson, Haas, Fuster, & Badimon, 2005). These are only some of the mechanisms that have undergone intensive investigation. The relative contributions of these biological pathways in the relation between psychosocial factors and CHD events, as well as whether a specific biological pathway is unique to a particular psychosocial factor, remains unknown.

Management of Behavioral and Psychosocial Factors in Patients with CHD

In addition to influencing CHD incidents, behavioral and psychological factors influence cardiovascular prognosis in patients with established CHD (Rozanski et al., 2005). Most practicing cardiologists are involved in the secondary prevention of CHD. Thus, cardiologists need to be aware of how these factors influence a patient's cardiovascular prognosis, as well as the potential to modify these risks. This section reviews some of the interventions targeted to improve healthy behaviors, including smoking cessation, diet modification, and exercise in patients with CHD. We also discuss some of the studies that have tested psychosocial interventions in these patients.

Overview of Implementing Behavioral or Lifestyle Interventions

In addition to knowledge, motivation is needed to change behavior. Many interventions incorporate an educational, didactic component and are not tailored to different learning styles, self-regulation, and levels of motivation to change behavior. Research into the "stages of change" (i.e., precontemplation, contemplation, preparation, action, and maintenance) has yielded insights into the processes underlying patient-level behavior change (Prochaska, DiClemente, & Norcross, 1992). Self-regulation is needed not only to initiate but also to maintain behavior change. Unfortunately, intervention studies often demonstrate improvements in the targeted behavior only in the short-term (i.e., few weeks to months), which is not sustained at long-term follow-up (i.e., months to years). The ability to sustain long-term treatment effects is an important priority for obvious reasons.

Ideally, behavioral and lifestyle factors should be addressed collaboratively. CHD is a chronic disease, and its successful man-

---

TABLE 28.2. Techniques for Implementing Behavioral or Lifestyle Interventions

- Identifying treatment goals and reasonable time lines
- Assigning each task to small, manageable steps
- Building "contracts" with the patient to reach self-care goals
- Evaluating patient's readiness for change
- Providing personalized feedback to the patient
- Enlisting the social support of the patient
- Encouraging and teaching self-monitoring behaviors
- Follow-up of patient's commitment to goal-related tasks

---

agement requires collaborations between patients and their clinicians. Patients often lack the knowledge and motivation to make behavioral or lifestyle changes, and the training of cardiologists or other health care providers does not typically include knowledge about successful implementation of evidence-based behavioral interventions. Furthermore, behavioral interventions are rarely reimbursed. Despite these limitations, clinicians should strive to use various techniques to aid in the successful implementation of behavioral or lifestyle interventions (see Table 28.2), given the strong relation between behavioral factors and CHD event risk. Incorporation of a multidisciplinary team to implement behavioral and lifestyle factors is a primary goal.

Smoking Cessation Interventions

Active smoking in patients with established CHD is associated with an increased risk of recurrent cardiovascular events, including sudden cardiac death (Goldenberg et al., 2003; Rea et al., 2002). After a myocardial infarction, smoking cessation is associated with a reduction in coronary events, with the risk approaching that of nonsmokers by 3-year follow-up (Rea et al., 2002). A systematic review of 20 prospective cohort studies indicated a 36% reduction in mortality in patients with CHD who quit smoking compared to those who continued smoking (Critchley & Capewell, 2003).

Given the evidence base, guidelines from the American Heart Association and American College of Cardiology highly recommend smoking cessation in patients with cardiovascular disease (Antman et al., 2008; Smith et al., 2006). Several Class I recommendations (i.e., should be performed/administered in all patients) (Antman et al., 2008; Smith et al., 2006) include asking about smoking use at every clinic visit, advising smokers to quit, assessing the patient's willingness to quit (i.e., stages of change), counseling and developing a plan to quit, and arranging follow-up and referral for therapy. Given the known effects of passive smoking (Glantz & Parmley, 1995; Wells, 1998), another important goal is for the patient to avoid exposure to environmental smoke.

A number of treatment options are available. Pharmacological therapy, including nicotine replacement and/or bupropion hydorchloride, may be effective. Meine, Patel, Washam, Pappas, and Jollis (2005) showed that in a registry of patients admitted after an ACS event, transdermal nicotine patch placement did not increase subsequent short- and long-term mortality. Similarly, bupropion therapy has been shown to be safe in patients with CHD (Rigotti et al., 2006; Tonstad et al., 2003) and may be associated with sustained smoking abstinence (Tonstad et al., 2003). A systematic review and meta-analysis (Barth, Critchley, & Bengel, 2006) indicated that although there was some heterogeneity in the trials, smoking cessation interventions, such as behavioral approaches (group or individual counseling), support by telephone, and self-help approaches (educational material), were associated with increased abstinence from smoking in patients with CHD after a period of 6–12 months. (See Perkins, Chapter 35, and Bricker, Chapter 36, this volume.)

Dietary Interventions

Dietary factors have a substantial impact on the prognosis of CHD (Levine, Keaney, & Vita, 1995). The National Cholesterol Education Program (NCEP) and the American Heart Association (AHA) recommend that dietary counseling should be the foundation of the treatment of patients with CHD ("Executive Summary of the Third Report of the National Cholesterol Education Program," 2001; Krauss et al., 2000). These guidelines recommend restricting the composition of total fat to an upper limit of 30%, and reducing the intake of saturated fat to

an upper limit of 7–10% of the daily caloric intake and cholesterol to less than 200 mg a day. A reduction in trans fatty acids is also recommended (Smith et al., 2006).

Several diets have been examined in patients with CHD, including low-fat diets; very low-fat diets; increased fish oil consumption; a glycemic index diet; increased consumption of fruits and vegetables; increased consumption of whole grains, legumes, and nuts; and combined interventions, including the Mediterranean style diet. A detailed discussion of these diets are beyond the scope of this chapter; we refer the reader to an excellent review in this area (Parikh et al., 2005; see Weidner and Kendel, Chapter 24, this volume, for information on very low-fat diets). We briefly discuss one dietary intervention—increased fish oil consumption.

Increased Fish Oil Consumption

The dietary benefit of consuming fish is hypothesized to be due to the presence of omega-3 fatty acids, including eicosapentanoic acid and decosahexaenoic acid. Several randomized controlled trials have indicated that omega-3 fatty acid supplementation reduces the risk of cardiovascular mortality, including sudden cardiac death and nonfatal events in patients with cardiovascular disease (Kris-Etherton, Harris, & Appel, 2002; Tavazzi et al., 2008). Some recent studies have been negative, particularly in high-risk patients with cardiovascular disease (Brouwer et al., 2009). Regardless, based on the weight of evidence, it is recommended that patients with CHD take omega-3 fatty acid supplementation (1 gram/day) either by eating fish or by taking a capsule (Kris-Etherton, Harris, & Appel, 2003; Smith et al., 2006).

Exercise Intervention (Cardiac Rehabilitation)

It is recommended that clinically stable patients with CHD undergo a moderate level of aerobic activity for a minimum of 30–60 minutes, preferably on a daily basis (Antman et al., 2008; Smith et al., 2006). Exercise training as part of a cardiac rehabilitation program is also recommended. Cardiac rehabilitative programs are typically multifaceted, often including several intervention components, such as education and counseling, the optimization of medical therapy, and implementation of other lifestyle changes in addition to exercise training. Thus, the effects of exercise training on prognosis may be difficult to ascertain from the other interventional components. A number of studies have shown that exercise-based rehabilitation programs are safe (Franklin, Bonzheim, Gordon, & Timmis, 1998; Pavy, Iliou, Meurin, Tabet, & Corone, 2006; Vongvanich, Paul-Labrador, & Merz, 1996). Furthermore, in addition to a reduction in symptoms and improvement in exercise tolerance and physical capacity, exercise-based rehabilitation improves the prognosis of patients with cardiovascular disease (Taylor et al., 2004).

Prior to actually performing aerobic exercise, patients should be risk-stratified by a health care provider, who should inquire carefully about the level of baseline physical activity and/or conduct a symptom-limited exercise test. Depending on the patient's baseline performance, the physician should tailor the level of supervision and monitoring needed, and formulate an individualized exercise program. Exercise training should include aerobic exercise, with or without resistance training (2 days per week) (Antman et al., 2008; Smith et al., 2006). Within these parameters, patients are expected to achieve increased cardiorespiratory fitness, and increased flexibility and physical strength.

Psychosocial Interventions

Evidence indicates that psychosocial factors increase the risk of cardiovascular event recurrence. Of the multitude of psychosocial factors, the one that has been examined most extensively in intervention trials is depression (Berkman et al., 2003; Glassman et al., 2002; Lespérance et al., 2007; van Melle et al., 2007). Randomized controlled trials addressing anxiety and anger/hostility in patients with CHD are much less common (Rozanski et al., 2005). In contrast to depression, no intervention trials have examined the effects of anxiety or anger/hostility treatment on recurrent cardiovascular events. Thus, we focus our discussion on depression treatment trials in patients with CHD.

The effect of cognitive-behavioral therapy on adverse cardiac events in depressed patients with CHD was examined in the Enhancing Recovery in Coronary Heart Disease (ENRICHD) trial (Berkman et al., 2003). Although there were significant improvements in depression and the level of social support associated with treatment, there were no differences in mortality or nonfatal myocardial infarction at a mean follow-up of 41 months. In addition, there were no differences in outcome among the patients who had low perceived social support, depression, or both (see Korin, Kaplan, & Davidson, Chapter 20, this volume).

Because the selective serotonin reuptake inhibitors (SSRIs) are the best studied medications, they are considered the first choice for the pharmacological treatment of depressed patients with CHD (Roose & Spatz, 1999). In SADHART (Sertraline Antidepressant Heart Attack Randomized Trial; Glassman et al., 2002), 369 patients with post–myocardial infarction or unstable angina and depression were randomized to the SSRI sertraline or placebo for 24 weeks. There was no difference in left ventricular ejection fraction, the primary safety end point, between the two arms. Sertraline use was associated with modest reductions in Clinical Global Impression Improvement scores compared with placebo. Also, there were also no differences in the rates of adverse cardiovascular events. However, this trial was not powered to detect differences in the occurrence of adverse cardiac outcomes.

The effect of the antidepressant, mirtazapine, a serotonin and norepinephrine reuptake inhibitor, on cardiovascular events was assessed in MIND-IT (Myocardial INfarction and Depression-Intervention Trial; van Melle et al., 2007). Three hundred thirty-one patients with post–myocardial infarction depression were enrolled and randomized to either usual care or staged pharmacological therapy. In the therapy arm, patients were further randomized to the antidepressant mirtazapine or placebo. In case of refusal or nonresponse, treatment with the SSRI citalopram was offered. Tailored referral was conducted in patients whose symptoms did not respond to citalopram administration. Compared to the usual care condition, depression treatment decreased neither depression nor cardiovascular events (i.e., cardiac death or hospital admission for documented nonfatal myocardial infarction, myocardial ischemia, coronary revascularization, heart failure, or ventricular tachycardia) at 18-month follow-up. Although originally powered for cardiovascular outcomes, the investigators concluded that due to overly optimistic estimates, the study was ultimately underpowered to detect differences in cardiac outcomes. Also, it is entirely possible that the lack of reduction in cardiovascular events was primarily explained by a lack of depression reduction.

Another published trial (Lespérance et al., 2007) assessed the short-term efficacy of pharmacological treatment (the SSRI citalopram) and interpersonal psychotherapy in 284 patients with CHD and major depression. The CREATE (Canadian Cardiac Randomized Evaluation of Antidepressant and Psychotherapy Efficacy; Lespérance et al., 2007) trial was a randomized controlled trial with a 2 × 2 factorial design that assessed 12 weekly sessions of interpersonal psychotherapy plus clinical management, or clinical management alone, and 12 weeks of citalopram or placebo. Citalopram was associated with a significant reduction in depressive symptoms. However, there was no advantage of interpersonal psychotherapy over and above clinical management alone. Cardiovascular events were low in each of the groups, and there were no differences between citalopram and placebo relative to blood pressure and electrocardiographic measures. Whereas a small increase (~2 mmHg) in systolic blood pressure was associated with interpersonal psychotherapy, a small decrease (~2 mmHg) in systolic blood pressure was observed in the clinical management control group. However, like SADHART, CREATE was not designed to examine differential effects on cardiovascular outcomes.

Overall, at the time of this writing, there is little published evidence to support the contention that depression treatment improves cardiovascular prognosis after an ACS event. Calls for the next sufficiently powered trial have been issued, as well as depression intervention trials involving important intermediary cardiovascular biomarkers (Davidson et al., 2006; Rozanski et al., 2005).

Despite the dearth of large, randomly assigned psychosocial interventions showing beneficial effects on cardiovascular outcomes in patients with CHD, there is evidence that improvement in psychosocial functioning can be obtained in therapeutic protocols administered by mental health professionals. Improving quality of life and decreasing the psychological distress of cardiac patients may have additional benefits relative to their behavior. For instance, improving symptoms associated with psychosocial factors may decrease smoking rates, increase engagement in physical activity, and improve dietary habits. For these reasons, it is recommended that screening for psychosocial factors, especially depression, be routine in patients with CHD. Additionally, antidepressant treatment and psychotherapy may improve these patients' quality of life, if not their cardiovascular outcomes. Referring such patients to mental health specialists for further management is a reasonable treatment option.

Many barriers exist in the assessment and treatment of psychosocial factors (Grissom & Phillips, 2005). Lack of training, skepticism that treatment will improve medical outcomes, limitations of current screening tools, reimbursement issues, and lack of time are common impediments to successful management of psychosocial factors in patients with CHD. Nonetheless, detecting and treating psychosocial factors, especially depression, will increasingly become a priority in cardiovascular medicine. Systematic detection and management of psychosocial factors that integrate well with busy cardiology practices are reachable goals that will improve the health and well-being of patients with CHD.

Conclusions

The potential applications of behavioral and psychosocial interventions in cardiovascular medicine are far-reaching. In principle, they help to prevent CHD onset and progression and can be used in conjunction with other cardiovascular interventions. In practice, a number of barriers prevent the successful implementation of behavioral and psychosocial interventions in patients with CHD. Future success depends on better education of physicians, incorporation of a multidisciplinary team approach, recognition of the value of behavioral and psychosocial interventions, and a focus on bidirectional collaboration between patients and physicians.

Further Reading

Davidson, K. W., Kupfer, D. J., Bigger, J. T., Califf, R. M., Carney, R. M., Coyne, J. C., et al. (2006). Assessment and treatment of depression in patients with cardiovascular disease: National Heart, Lung, and Blood Institute Working Group Report. *Psychosomatic Medicine, 68*(5), 645–650.

Fuster, V., Fayad, Z. A., Moreno, P. R., Poon, M., Corti, R., & Badimon, J. J. (2005). Atherothrombosis and high-risk plaque: Part II. Approaches by noninvasive computed tomographic/magnetic resonance imaging. *Journal of the American College of Cardiology, 46*(7), 1209–1218.

Fuster, V., Moreno, P. R., Fayad, Z. A., Corti, R., & Badimon, J. J. (2005). Atherothrombosis and high-risk plaque: Part I. Evolving concepts. *Journal of the American College of Cardiology, 46*(6), 937–954.

Naghavi, M., Falk, E., Hecht, H. S., Jamieson, M. J., Kaul, S., Berman, D., et al. (2006). From vulnerable plaque to vulnerable patient: Part III. Executive summary of the Screening for Heart Attack Prevention and Education (SHAPE) Task Force report. *American Journal of Cardiology, 98*(2A), 2H–15H.

Naghavi, M., Libby, P., Falk, E., Casscells, S. W., Litovsky, S., Rumberger, J., et al. (2003a). From vulnerable plaque to vulnerable patient: A call for new definitions and risk assessment strategies: Part I. *Circulation, 108*(14), 1664–1672.

Naghavi, M., Libby, P., Falk, E., Casscells, S. W., Litovsky, S., Rumberger, J., et al. (2003b). From vulnerable plaque to vulnerable patient: A call for new definitions and risk assessment strategies: Part II. *Circulation, 108*(15), 1772–1778.

Schaar, J. A., Muller, J. E., Falk, E., Virmani, R., Fuster, V., Serruys, P. W., et al. (2004). Terminology for high-risk and vulnerable coronary artery plaques: Report of a meeting on the vulnerable plaque, June 17 and 18, 2003, Santorini, Greece. *European Heart Journal, 12*, 1077–1082.

References

Ambrose, J. A. (2008). In search of the "vulnerable plaque": Can it be localized and will focal regional therapy ever be an option for cardiac prevention? *Journal of the American College of Cardiology, 51*(16), 1539–1542.

Ambrose, J. A., Tannenbaum, M. A., Alexopoulos, D., Hjemdahl-Monsen, C. E., Leavy, J., Weiss, M., et al. (1988). Angiographic progression of coronary artery disease and the development of myocardial infarction. *Journal of the American College of Cardiology, 12*(1), 56–62.

Anderson, J. L., Adams, C. D., Antman, E. M., Bridges, C. R., Califf, R. M., Casey, D. E., Jr., et al. (2007). ACC/AHA 2007 guidelines for the management of patients with unstable angina/non-ST-elevation myocardial infarction: A report of the American College of Cardiology/American Heart Association Task Force on Practice Guidelines (writing committee to revise the 2002 guidelines for the management of patients with unstable angina/non-ST-elevation myocardial infarction) developed in collaboration with the American College of Emergency Physicians, the Society for Cardiovascular Angiography and Interventions, and the Society of Thoracic Surgeons endorsed by the American Association of Cardiovascular and Pulmonary Rehabilitation and the Society for Academic Emergency Medicine. *Journal of the American College of Cardiology, 50*(7), 652–726.

Antman, E. M., Hand, M., Armstrong, P. W., Bates, E. R., Green, L. A., Halasyamani, L. K., et al. (2008). 2007 Focused update of the ACC/AHA 2004 guidelines for the management of patients with ST-elevation myocardial infarction. *Circulation, 117*(2), 296–329.

Badimon, J. J., Zaman, A., Helft, G., Fayad, Z., & Fuster, V. (1999). Acute coronary syndromes: Pathophysiology and preventive priorities. *Joural of Thrombosis and Haemostasis, 82*(2), 997–1004.

Barth, J., Critchley, J., & Bengel, J. (2006). Efficacy of psychosocial interventions for smoking cessation in patients with coronary heart disease: A systematic review and meta-analysis. *Annals of Behavioral Medicine, 32*(1), 10–20.

Berkman, L. F., Blumenthal, J., Burg, M., Carney, R. M., Catellier, D., Cowan, M. J., et al. (2003). Effects of treating depression and low perceived social support on clinical events after myocardial infarction: The Enhancing Recovery in Coronary Heart Disease Patients (ENRICHD) randomized trial. *Journal of the American Medical Association, 289*(23), 3106–3116.

Blake, G. J., & Ridker, P. M. (2001). Novel clinical markers of vascular wall inflammation. *Circulation Research, 89*(9), 763–771.

Braunwald, E. (1997). Shattuck lecture—Cardiovascular medicine at the turn of the millennium: Triumphs, concerns, and opportunities. *New England Journal of Medicine, 337*(19), 1360–1369.

Brouwer, I. A., Raitt, M. H., Dullemeijer, C., Kraemer, D. F., Zock, P. L., Morris, C., et al. (2009). Effect of fish oil on ventricular tachyarrhythmia in three studies in patients with implantable cardioverter defibrillators. *European Heart Journal, 30*(7), 820–826.

Carney, R. M., Blumenthal, J. A., Freedland, K. E., Youngblood, M., Veith, R. C., Burg, M. M., et al. (2004). Depression and late mortality after myocardial infarction in the Enhancing Recovery in Coronary Heart Disease (ENRICHD) study. *Psychosomatic Medicine, 66*(4), 466–474.

Carney, R. M., Freedland, K. E., Miller, G. E., & Jaffe, A. S. (2002). Depression as a risk factor for cardiac mortality and morbidity: A review of potential mechanisms. *Journal of Psychosomatic Research, 53*(4), 897–902.

Coller, B. S. (1997). Platelet GPIIb/IIIa antagonists: The first anti-integrin receptor therapeutics. *Journal of Clinical Investigation, 99*(7), 1467–1471.

Corti, R., Fuster, V., & Badimon, J. J. (2003). Pathogenetic concepts of acute coronary syndromes. *Journal of the American College of Cardiology, 41*(4, Suppl. S), 7S–14S.

Critchley, J. A., & Capewell, S. (2003). Mortality risk reduction associated with smoking cessation in patients with coronary heart disease: A systematic review. *Journal of the American Medical Association, 290*(1), 86–97.

Davidson, K. W., Kupfer, D. J., Bigger, J. T., Califf, R. M., Carney, R. M., Coyne, J. C., et al. (2006). Assessment and treatment of depression in patients with cardiovascular disease: National Heart, Lung, and Blood Institute Working Group Report. *Psychosomatic Medicine, 68*(5), 645–650.

Executive Summary of the Third Report of the National Cholesterol Education Program (NCEP) Expert Panel on Detection, Evaluation, and Treatment of High Blood Cholesterol in Adults (Adult Treatment Panel III). (2001). *Journal of the American Medical Association, 285*(19), 2486–2497.

Falk, E., Shah, P. K., & Fuster, V. (1995). Coronary plaque disruption. *Circulation, 92*(3), 657–671.

Farb, A., Burke, A. P., Tang, A. L., Liang, T. Y., Mannan, P., Smialek, J., et al. (1996). Coronary plaque erosion without rupture into a lipid core: A frequent cause of coronary thrombosis in sudden coronary death. *Circulation, 93*(7), 1354–1363.

Faxon, D. P., Fuster, V., Libby, P., Beckman, J. A., Hiatt, W. R., Thompson, R. W., et al. (2004). Atherosclerotic Vascular Disease Conference: Writing Group III. Pathophysiology. *Circulation, 109*(21), 2617–2625.

Felton, C. V., Crook, D., Davies, M. J., & Oliver, M. F. (1997). Relation of plaque lipid composition and morphology to the stability of human aortic plaques. *Arteriosclerosis, Thrombosis, and Vascular Biology, 17*(7), 1337–1345.

Fraker, T. D., Jr., Fihn, S. D., Gibbons, R. J., Abrams, J., Chatterjee, K., Daley, J., et al. (2007). 2007 Chronic Angina Focused Update of the ACC/AHA 2002 Guidelines for the Management of Patients with Chronic Stable Angina: A report of the American College of Cardiology/American Heart Association Task Force on Practice Guidelines Writing Group to develop the focused update of the 2002 Guidelines for the Management of Patients with Chronic Stable Angina. *Journal of the American College of Cardiology, 50*(23), 2264–2274.

Franklin, B. A., Bonzheim, K., Gordon, S., & Timmis, G. C. (1998). Safety of medically supervised outpatient cardiac rehabilitation exercise therapy: A 16-year follow-up. *Chest, 114*(3), 902–906.

Fuster, V., Badimon, L., Badimon, J. J., & Chesebro, J. H. (1992a). The pathogenesis of coronary artery disease and the acute coronary syndromes (1). *New England Journal of Medicine, 326*(4), 242–250.

Fuster, V., Badimon, L., Badimon, J. J., & Chesebro, J. H. (1992b). The pathogenesis of coronary artery disease and the acute coronary syndromes (2). *New England Journal of Medicine, 326*(5), 310–318.

Fuster, V., Fayad, Z. A., & Badimon, J. J. (1999). Acute coronary syndromes: Biology. *Lancet, 353*(Suppl. 2), S115–S119.

Fuster, V., Moreno, P. R., Fayad, Z. A., Corti, R., & Badimon, J. J. (2005). Atherothrombosis and high-risk plaque: Part I. Evolving concepts. *Journal of the American College of Cardiology, 46*(6), 937–954.

Fuster, V., & Vedanthan, R. (2008). Cardiovascular disease and the UN Millennium Development Goals: Time to move forward. *Nature Clinical Practice Cardiovascular Medicine, 5*(10), 593.

Fuster, V., & Voute, J. (2007). Expanding the cardiovascular mandate: From treatment to the protection of health. *Nature Clinical Practice Cardiovascular Medicine, 4*(3), 117.

Glagov, S., Weisenberg, E., Zarins, C. K., Stankunavicius, R., & Kolettis, G. J. (1987). Compensatory enlargement of human atherosclerotic coronary arteries. *New England Journal of Medicine, 316*(22), 1371–1375.

Glantz, S. A., & Parmley, W. W. (1995). Passive smoking and heart disease: Mechanisms and risk. *Journal of the American Medical Association, 273*(13), 1047–1053.

Glassman, A. H., O'Connor, C. M., Califf, R. M., Swedberg, K., Schwartz, P., Bigger, J. T., Jr., et al. (2002). Sertraline treatment of major depression in patients with acute MI or unstable angina. *Journal of the American Medical Association, 288*(6), 701–709.

Goldenberg, I., Jonas, M., Tenenbaum, A., Boyko, V., Matetzky, S., Shotan, A., et al. (2003). Current smoking, smoking cessation, and the risk of sudden cardiac death in patients with coronary artery disease. *Archives of Internal Medicine, 163*(19), 2301–2305.

Goldston, K., & Baillie, A. J. (2008). Depression and coronary heart disease: A review of the epidemiological evidence, explanatory mechanisms and management approaches. *Clinical Psychology Review, 28,* 288–306.

Greenland, P., Knoll, M. D., Stamler, J., Neaton, J. D., Dyer, A. R., Garside, D. B., et al. (2003). Major risk factors as antecedents of fatal and nonfatal coronary heart disease events. *Journal of the American Medical Association, 290*(7), 891–897.

Gresele, P., Page, C. P., Fuster, V., & Vermylen, J. (2002). *Platelets in thrombotic and non-thrombotic disorders: Pathophysiology, pharmacology and therapeutics.* Cambridge, UK: Cambridge University Press.

Grissom, G. R., & Phillips, R. A. (2005). Screening for depression: This is the heart of the matter. *Archives of Internal Medicine, 165*(11), 1214–1216.

Khot, U. N., Khot, M. B., Bajzer, C. T., Sapp, S. K., Ohman, E. M., Brener, S. J., et al. (2003). Prevalence of conventional risk factors in patients with coronary heart disease. *Journal of the American Medical Association, 290*(7), 898–904.

Kolodgie, F. D., Burke, A. P., Farb, A., Gold, H. K., Yuan, J., Narula, J., et al. (2001). The thin-cap fibroatheroma: A type of vulnerable plaque: the major precursor lesion to acute coronary syndromes. *Current Opinion in Cardiology, 16*(5), 285–292.

Krauss, R. M., Eckel, R. H., Howard, B., Appel, L. J., Daniels, S. R., Deckelbaum, R. J., et al. (2000). AHA Dietary Guidelines: Revision 2000. A statement for healthcare professionals from the Nutrition Committee of the American Heart Association. *Circulation, 102*(18), 2284–2299.

Kris-Etherton, P. M., Harris, W. S., & Appel, L. J. (2002). Fish consumption, fish oil, omega-3 fatty acids, and cardiovascular disease. *Circulation, 106*(21), 2747–2757.

Kris-Etherton, P. M., Harris, W. S., & Appel, L. J. (2003). Omega-3 fatty acids and cardiovascular disease: New recommendations from the American Heart Association. *Arteriosclerosis, Thrombosis, and Vascular Biology, 23*(2), 151–152.

Lauzon, C., Beck, C. A., Huynh, T., Dion, D., Racine, N., Carignan, S., et al. (2003). Depression and prognosis following hospital admission because of acute myocardial infarc-tion. *Canadian Medical Association Journal, 168*(5), 547–552.

Lerakis, S., Synetos, A., Toutouzas, K., Vavuranakis, M., Tsiamis, E., & Stefanadis, C. (2008). Imaging of the vulnerable plaque: Noninvasive and invasive techniques. *American Journal of the Medical Sciences, 336*(4), 342–348.

Lespérance, F., Frasure-Smith, N., Koszycki, D., Laliberte, M. A., van Zyl, L. T., Baker, B., et al. (2007). Effects of citalopram and interpersonal psychotherapy on depression in patients with coronary artery disease: The Canadian Cardiac Randomized Evaluation of Antidepressant and Psychotherapy Efficacy (CREATE) trial. *Journal of the American Medical Association, 297*(4), 367–379.

Levine, G. N., Keaney, J. F., Jr., & Vita, J. A. (1995). Cholesterol reduction in cardiovascular disease: Clinical benefits and possible mechanisms. *New England Journal of Medicine, 332*(8), 512–521.

Lewis, H. D., Jr., Davis, J. W., Archibald, D. G., Steinke, W. E., Smitherman, T. C., Doherty, J. E., III, et al. (1983). Protective effects of aspirin against acute myocardial infarction and death in men with unstable angina: Results of a Veterans Administration Cooperative Study. *New England Journal of Medicine, 309*(7), 396–403.

Libby, P. (2005). Act local, act global: Inflammation and the multiplicity of "vulnerable" coronary plaques. *Journal of the American College of Cardiology, 45*(10), 1600–1602.

Little, W. C. (1990). Angiographic assessment of the culprit coronary artery lesion before acute myocardial infarction. *American Journal of Cardiology, 66*(16), 44G–47G.

Little, W. C., Constantinescu, M., Applegate, R. J., Kutcher, M. A., Burrows, M. T., Kahl, F. R., et al. (1988). Can coronary angiography predict the site of a subsequent myocardial infarction in patients with mild-to-moderate coronary artery disease? *Circulation, 78*(5, Pt. 1), 1157–1166.

Mehta, S. R., Yusuf, S., Peters, R. J., Bertrand, M. E., Lewis, B. S., Natarajan, M. K., et al. (2001). Effects of pretreatment with clopidogrel and aspirin followed by long-term therapy in patients undergoing percutaneous coronary intervention: The PCI-CURE study. *Lancet, 358,* 527–533.

Meine, T. J., Patel, M. R., Washam, J. B., Pappas, P. A., & Jollis, J. G. (2005). Safety and effectiveness of transdermal nicotine patch in smokers admitted with acute coronary syndromes. *American Journal of Cardiology, 95*(8), 976–978.

Mokdad, A. H., Marks, J. S., Stroup, D. F., & Gerberding, J. L. (2004). Actual causes of death in the United States, 2000. *Journal of the American Medical Association, 291*(10), 1238–1245.

Moreno, P. R., Falk, E., Palacios, I. F., Newell, J. B., Fuster, V., & Fallon, J. T. (1994). Macrophage infiltration in acute coronary syndromes: Implications for plaque rupture. *Circulation, 90*(2), 775–778.

Muller, J. E., & Tofler, G. H. (1992). Triggering and hourly variation of onset of arterial thrombosis. *Annals of Epidemiology, 2*(4), 393–405.

Naghavi, M., Falk, E., Hecht, H. S., Jamieson, M. J., Kaul, S., Berman, D., et al. (2006). From vulnerable plaque to vulnerable patient: Part III. Executive summary of the Screening for Heart Attack Prevention and Education (SHAPE) Task Force report. *American Journal of Cardiology, 98*(2A), 2H–15H.

Naghavi, M., Libby, P., Falk, E., Casscells, S. W., Litovsky, S., Rumberger, J., et al. (2003a). From vulnerable plaque to vulnerable patient: A call for new definitions and risk assessment strategies: Part I. *Circulation, 108*(14), 1664–1672.

Naghavi, M., Libby, P., Falk, E., Casscells, S. W., Litovsky, S., Rumberger, J., et al. (2003b). From vulnerable plaque to vulnerable patient: A call for new definitions and risk assessment strategies: Part II. *Circulation, 108*(15), 1772–1778.

Nissen, S. E., & Yock, P. (2001). Intravascular ultrasound: Novel pathophysiological insights and current clinical applications. *Circulation, 103*(4), 604–616.

Nobuyoshi, M., Tanaka, M., Nosaka, H., Kimura, T., Yokoi, H., Hamasaki, N., et al. (1991). Progression of coronary atherosclerosis: Is coronary spasm related to progression? *Journal of the American College of Cardiology, 18*(4), 904–910.

Parikh, P., McDaniel, M. C., Ashen, M. D., Miller, J. I., Sorrentino, M., Chan, V., et al. (2005). Diets and cardiovascular disease: An evidence-based assessment. *Journal of the American College of Cardiology, 45*(9), 1379–1387.

Parissis, J. T., Fountoulaki, K., Filippatos, G., Adamopoulos, S., Paraskevaidis, I., & Kremastinos, D. (2007). Depression in coronary artery disease: Novel pathophysiologic mechanisms and therapeutic implications. *International Journal of Cardiology, 116*(2), 153–160.

Pasterkamp, G., Schoneveld, A. H., van der Wal, A. C., Haudenschild, C. C., Clarijs, R. J., Becker, A. E., et al. (1998). Relation of arterial geometry to luminal narrowing and histologic markers for plaque vulnerability: The remodeling paradox. *Journal of the American College of Cardiology, 32*(3), 655–662.

Pavy, B., Iliou, M. C., Meurin, P., Tabet, J. Y., & Corone, S. (2006). Safety of exercise training for cardiac patients: Results of the French registry of complications during cardiac rehabilitation. *Archives of Internal Medicine, 166*(21), 2329–2334.

Prochaska, J. O., DiClemente, C. C., & Norcross, J. C. (1992). In search of how people change: Applications to addictive behaviors. *American Psychologist, 47*(9), 1102–1114.

Rauch, U., Osende, J. I., Fuster, V., Badimon, J. J., Fayad, Z., & Chesebro, J. H. (2001). Thrombus formation on atherosclerotic plaques: Pathogenesis and clinical consequences. *Annals of Internal Medicine, 134*(3), 224–238.

Rea, T. D., Heckbert, S. R., Kaplan, R. C., Smith, N. L., Lemaitre, R. N., & Psaty, B. M. (2002). Smoking status and risk for recurrent coronary events after myocardial infarction. *Annals of Internal Medicine, 137*(6), 494–500.

Ridker, P. M., Buring, J. E., & Rifai, N. (2001). Soluble P-selectin and the risk of future cardiovascular events. *Circulation, 103*(4), 491–495.

Ridker, P. M., Buring, J. E., Shih, J., Matias, M., & Hennekens, C. H. (1998). Prospective study of C-reactive protein and the risk of future cardiovascular events among apparently healthy women. *Circulation, 98*(8), 731–733.

Ridker, P. M., Cushman, M., Stampfer, M. J., Tracy, R. P., & Hennekens, C. H. (1997). Inflammation, aspirin, and the risk of cardiovascular disease in apparently healthy men. *New England Journal of Medicine, 336*(14), 973–979.

Ridker, P. M., Hennekens, C. H., Buring, J. E., & Rifai, N. (2000). C-reactive protein and other markers of inflammation in the prediction of cardiovascular disease in women. *New England Journal of Medicine, 342*(12), 836–843.

Ridker, P. M., Hennekens, C. H., Roitman-Johnson, B., Stampfer, M. J., & Allen, J. (1998). Plasma concentration of soluble intercellular adhesion molecule 1 and risks of future myocardial infarction in apparently healthy men. *Lancet, 351,* 88–92.

Ridker, P. M., Rifai, N., Stampfer, M. J., & Hennekens, C. H. (2000). Plasma concentration of interleukin-6 and the risk of future myocardial infarction among apparently healthy men. *Circulation, 101*(15), 1767–1772.

Rigotti, N. A., Thorndike, A. N., Regan, S., McKool, K., Pasternak, R. C., Chang, Y., et al. (2006). Bupropion for smokers hospitalized with acute cardiovascular disease. *American Journal of Medicine, 119*(12), 1080–1087.

Rioufol, G., Finet, G., Ginon, I., Andre-Fouet, X., Rossi, R., Vialle, E., et al. (2002). Multiple atherosclerotic plaque rupture in acute coronary syndrome: A three-vessel intravas-cular ultrasound study. *Circulation, 106*(7), 804–808.

Robbie, L., & Libby, P. (2001). Inflammation and atherothrombosis. *Annals of the New York Academy of Sciences, 947,* 167–180.

Roose, S. P., & Spatz, E. (1999). Treatment of de-pression in patients with heart disease. *Journal of Clinical Psychiatry, 60*(Suppl. 20), 34–37.

Root, M., & Cobb, F. (2004). Traditional risk factors for coronary heart disease. *Journal of the American Medical Association, 291–300.*

Rosengren, A., Hawken, S., Ounpuu, S., Sliwa, K., Zubaid, M., Almahmeed, W. A., et al. (2004). Association of psychosocial risk fac-tors with risk of acute myocardial infarction in 11,119 cases and 13,648 controls from 52 countries (the INTERHEART Study): Case–control study. *Lancet, 364,* 953–962.

Rozanski, A., Blumenthal, J. A., Davidson, K. W., Saab, P. G., & Kubzansky, L. (2005). The epidemiology, pathophysiology, and manage-ment of psychosocial risk factors in cardiac practice: The emerging field of behavioral car-diology. *Journal of the American College of Cardiology, 45*(5), 637–651.

Rozanski, A., Blumenthal, J. A., & Kaplan, J. (1999). Impact of psychological factors on the pathogenesis of cardiovascular disease and implications for therapy. *Circulation, 99*(16), 2192–2217.

Ruo, B., Rumsfeld, J. S., Hlatky, M. A., Liu, H., Browner, W. S., & Whooley, M. A. (2003). Depressive symptoms and health-related qual-ity of life: The Heart and Soul Study. *Journal of the American Medical Association, 290*(2), 215–221.

Sabatine, M. S., Cannon, C. P., Gibson, C. M., Lopez-Sendon, J. L., Montalescot, G., Ther-oux, P., et al. (2005). Addition of clopidogrel to aspirin and fibrinolytic therapy for myo-cardial infarction with ST-segment elevation. *New England Journal of Medicine, 352*(12), 1179–1189.

Sambola, A., Osende, J., Hathcock, J., Degen, M., Nemerson, Y., Fuster, V., et al. (2003). Role of risk factors in the modulation of tis-sue factor activity and blood thrombogenicity. *Circulation, 107*(7), 973–977.

Schoenhagen, P., Ziada, K. M., Kapadia, S. R., Crowe, T. D., Nissen, S. E., & Tuzcu, E. M. (2000). Extent and direction of arterial re-modeling in stable versus unstable coronary syndromes: An intravascular ultrasound study. *Circulation, 101*(6), 598–603.

Schoenhagen, P., Ziada, K. M., Vince, D. G., Nissen, S. E., & Tuzcu, E. M. (2001). Arte-rial remodeling and coronary artery disease: The concept of "dilated" versus "obstructive"

coronary atherosclerosis. *Journal of the Amer-ican College of Cardiology, 38*(2), 297–306.

Shimbo, D., Davidson, K. W., Haas, D. C., Fus-ter, V., & Badimon, J. J. (2005). Negative impact of depression on outcomes in patients with coronary artery disease: Mechanisms, treatment considerations, and future direc-tions. *Journal of Thrombosis and Haemosta-sis, 3*(5), 897–908.

Smith, S. C., Jr., Allen, J., Blair, S. N., Bonow, R. O., Brass, L. M., Fonarow, G. C., et al. (2006). AHA/ACC guidelines for secondary preven-tion for patients with coronary and other ath-erosclerotic vascular disease: 2006 update: Endorsed by the National Heart, Lung, and Blood Institute. *Circulation, 113*(19), 2363–2372.

Smits, P. C., Pasterkamp, G., de Jaegere, P. P., de Feyter, P. J., & Borst, C. (1999). Angioscopic complex lesions are predominantly compen-satory enlarged: An angioscopy and intrac-oronary ultrasound study. *Cardiovascular Re-search, 41*(2), 458–464.

Tavazzi, L. (1999). Clinical epidemiology of acute myocardial infarction. *American Heart Journal, 138*(2, Pt. 2), S48–S54.

Tavazzi, L., Maggioni, A. P., Marchioli, R., Barlera, S., Franzosi, M. G., Latini, R., et al. (2008). Effect of n-3 polyunsaturated fatty acids in patients with chronic heart failure (the GISSI-HF trial): A randomised, double-blind, placebo-controlled trial. *Lancet, 372,* 1223–1230.

Taylor, R. S., Brown, A., Ebrahim, S., Jolliffe, J., Noorani, H., Rees, K., et al. (2004). Ex-ercise-based rehabilitation for patients with coronary heart disease: Systematic review and meta-analysis of randomized controlled tri-als. *American Journal of Medicine, 116*(10), 682–692.

Theroux, P., Ouimet, H., McCans, J., Latour, J. G., Joly, P., Levy, G., et al. (1988). Aspi-rin, heparin, or both to treat acute unstable angina. *New England Journal of Medicine, 319*(17), 1105–1111.

Tonstad, S., Farsang, C., Klaene, G., Lewis, K., Manolis, A., Perruchoud, A. P., et al. (2003). Bupropion SR for smoking cessation in smok-ers with cardiovascular disease: A multicentre, randomised study. *European Heart Journal, 24*(10), 946–955.

Topol, E. J., & Nissen, S. E. (1995). Our preoc-cupation with coronary luminology: The dis-sociation between clinical and angiographic findings in ischemic heart disease. *Circulation, 92*(8), 2333–2342.

Tsimikas, S., Willerson, J. T., & Ridker, P. M. (2006). C-reactive protein and other emerg-ing blood biomarkers to optimize risk stratification of vulnerable patients. *Journal of the American College of Cardiology, 47*(Suppl. 8), C19–C31.

Tuzcu, E. M., Kapadia, S. R., Tutar, E., Ziada, K. M., Hobbs, R. E., McCarthy, P. M., et al. (2001). High prevalence of coronary atherosclerosis in asymptomatic teenagers and young adults: Evidence from intravascular ultrasound. *Circulation, 103*(22), 2705–2710.

van der Wal, A. C., Becker, A. E., van der Loos, C. M., & Das, P. K. (1994). Site of intimal rupture or erosion of thrombosed coronary atherosclerotic plaques is characterized by an inflammatory process irrespective of the dominant plaque morphology. *Circulation, 89*(1), 36–44.

van Melle, J. P., de Jonge, P., Honig, A., Schene, A. H., Kuyper, A. M., Crijns, H. J., et al. (2007). Effects of antidepressant treatment following myocardial infarction. *British Journal of Psychiatry, 190*, 460–466.

Viles-Gonzalez, J. F., Fuster, V., & Badimon, J. J. (2006). Links between inflammation and thrombogenicity in atherosclerosis. *Current Molecular Medicine, 6*(5), 489–499.

Virmani, R., Kolodgie, F. D., Burke, A. P., Farb, A., & Schwartz, S. M. (2000). Lessons from sudden coronary death: A comprehensive morphological classification scheme for atherosclerotic lesions. *Arteriosclerosis, Thrombosis, and Vascular Biology, 20*(5), 1262–1275.

Vongvanich, P., Paul-Labrador, M. J., & Merz, C. N. (1996). Safety of medically supervised exercise in a cardiac rehabilitation center. *American Journal of Cardiology, 77*(15), 1383–1385.

Vorchheimer, D. A., Badimon, J. J., & Fuster, V. (1999). Platelet glycoprotein IIb/IIIa receptor antagonists in cardiovascular disease. *Journal of the American Medical Association, 281*(15), 1407–1414.

Wells, A. J. (1998). Heart disease from passive smoking in the workplace. *Journal of the American College of Cardiology, 31*(1), 1–9.

Wilson, P. W. (2005). Estimating the risk for atherothrombosis: Are current approaches sufficient? *European Journal of Cardiovascular Prevention and Rehabilitation, 12*(5), 427–432.

Wilson, P. W., D'Agostino, R. B., Levy, D., Belanger, A. M., Silbershatz, H., & Kannel, W. B. (1998). Prediction of coronary heart disease using risk factor categories. *Circulation, 97*(18), 1837–1847.

Yamagishi, M., Terashima, M., Awano, K., Kijima, M., Nakatani, S., Daikoku, S., et al. (2000). Morphology of vulnerable coronary plaque: Insights from follow-up of patients examined by intravascular ultrasound before an acute coronary syndrome. *Journal of the American College of Cardiology, 35*(1), 106–111.

Yusuf, S., Hawken, S., Ounpuu, S., Dans, T., Avezum, A., Lanas, F., et al. (2004). Effect of potentially modifiable risk factors associated with myocardial infarction in 52 countries (the INTERHEART Study): Case–control study. *Lancet, 364*, 937–952.

Yusuf, S., Zhao, F., Mehta, S. R., Chrolavicius, S., Tognoni, G., & Fox, K. K. (2001). Effects of clopidogrel in addition to aspirin in patients with acute coronary syndromes without ST-segment elevation. *New England Journal of Medicine, 345*(7), 494–502.

CHAPTER 29

The Management of Diabetes

Ian M. Kronish
Devin Mann

History and Evolution of Behavioral Treatment of Diabetes

Since the discovery of insulin in 1921, the management of diabetes has been marked by incredible scientific advancements, ranging from the development of novel oral diabetic medications to the manufacture of devices that allow for continuous glucose monitoring. This growth in the understanding of the biology, genetics, and pharmacology of diabetes has enhanced the importance of behavioral science in diabetes management. Diabetes is now clearly understood as a chronic illness whose outcomes are dependent on the behavior of individual patients within the context of their surrounding health environment.

A pivotal step that led to the current relationship between behavioral medicine and diabetes care was based on the findings from the National Institute of Health Diabetes Control and Complications Trial (DCCT), first published in 1993 (Lasker, 1993). The DCCT was a clinical trial in which more than 1,400 adults and adolescents with Type 1 diabetes were randomized either to an in-

tensive insulin regimen aimed at achieving tighter glucose control or to a less intensive insulin regimen with looser glucose control. The study found that the subjects in the more intensive arm had up to 70% reductions in many of the complications of diabetes.

From the point of view of behavioral scientists, the success of the intervention in the DCCT was not merely the prescription for a more intensive insulin regimen. A key component was the increased behavioral support given to patients in the intervention group. To help participants in the intervention group sustain the demanding health behaviors required in the more intensive insulin strategy, the intervention group received increased follow-up contacts and personalized problem-solving strategies. By the end of the study, the intensive group reported receiving one and a half times the level of support from staff compared to participants in the conventional treatment group (Davis & Fisher, 1997).

After the publication of the DCCT results, providers caring for individuals with diabetes were suddenly expected to devise their own techniques for helping their patients achieve the targets set in the DCCT (Rubin & Peyrot, 1994). Few providers had access to the behavioral resources provided in the DCCT. Providers soon discovered that most patients found it difficult to adhere to more intensive insulin regimens and these regimens were putting their patients at increased risk for hypoglycemic episodes. As a result, health care providers and policymakers looked to behavioral scientists to help them understand how to help individuals with diabetes modify their behavior to achieve the targets set in the DCCT.

Behavioral scientists quickly responded with a number of useful resources (Anderson & Rubin, 2002; Bradley, 1994). The field subsequently continued to expand, taking into account not only the role of behavioral science in modifying diabetes behavior but also the psychological impact of living with diabetes. Moreover, behavioral scientists began considering diabetes from a public health perspective, in addition to the individual patient level.

The goal of this chapter is, first, to provide a concise review of the pathophysiology, epidemiology, and treatment of diabetes. Second, we review important theoretical models that behavioral scientists have designed to help understand diabetes self-management behavior. Third, we discuss several significant interventions designed to improve diabetics' behavior. We conclude by considering the challenges and opportunities for continued growth of behavioral science in the field of diabetes.

Pathophysiology of Disease

"Diabetes mellitus" refers to chronic endocrine disorders that result in abnormally high levels of sugar (glucose) in the blood. There are several types of diabetes. Type 1 diabetes is characterized by insufficient insulin production, and Type 2 diabetes, by an inappropriate response to insulin by target cells (particularly muscle cells) in the body (also known as "insulin resistance"). A third type of diabetes, known as gestational diabetes, is caused by insulin resistance that only develops during pregnancy and usually resolves after the delivery of the child. "Insulin," a hormone released by the pancreas,

is responsible for the uptake of glucose into the cells of the body for use as energy. The presence of abnormally high levels of glucose in the blood causes glucose to overflow into the urine, which in turn produces the sweet-smelling urine from which diabetes mellitus gets its name. If untreated, high levels of glucose cause frequent urination, dehydration, increased thirst, blurry vision, and fatigue.

Type 1 diabetes was previously called insulin-dependent diabetes or juvenile-onset diabetes. It is caused by autoimmune destruction of the pancreatic insulin-producing cells and usually develops in childhood or adolescence, making it the most common chronic disease of childhood. The reasons for this autoimmune destruction are still unclear and appear to be related to a combination of genetic and environmental factors, such as viruses. As a result of the lack of insulin, individuals with Type 1 diabetes are unable to utilize glucose as a nutrient for cells and must instead rely on the breakdown of fat as a nutrient. This reliance on fat metabolism can lead to a buildup of ketone acids in the blood (known as "diabetic ketoacidosis"), and this can lead to a diabetic coma and death. The treatment for Type 1 diabetes requires the delivery of insulin through injections into the body. Before the discovery of insulin, Type 1 diabetes was universally fatal.

Previously referred to as non-insulin-dependent diabetes or adult-onset diabetes, Type 2 diabetes is by far the most common type of diabetes, accounting for more than 90% of all cases (National Institute of Diabetes and Digestive and Kidney Diseases [NIDDK], 2008). Type 2 diabetes is initially caused by resistance to insulin by the body's cells. This leads the pancreas to try to compensate by increasing its production of insulin. While the exact causes of this insulin resistance are currently being investigated, both genetic and environmental factors have been implicated. Risk factors associated with Type 2 diabetes include older age, physical inactivity, obesity, prior history of gestational diabetes, certain ethnicities, family history of diabetes, and since the sequencing of the human genome, a growing number of genetic markers (Florez et al., 2006; Saxena et al., 2007). Prolonged periods of elevated glucose in the blood from insulin resistance eventually lead to damage of the blood vessels and nerves in the body, and can impair the body's ability to fight off infections. Treatments for Type 2 diabetes are geared toward helping the pancreas produce more insulin or the body to utilize insulin more effectively by decreasing insulin resistance. Other strategies include trying to minimize the production of glucose by the liver or preventing the absorption of large loads of carbohydrates (precursors of glucose) by the digestive system. These treatments can involve medications or nonpharmacological approaches, such as modifying diet or trying to lose weight through exercise. Over time, the pancreatic cells may not be able to keep up with the needed insulin production, and individuals with Type 2 diabetes may need insulin injections as well.

Epidemiology

Overall, diabetes represents one of the largest health care problems in the United States. It was estimated in 2007, that over 23 million Americans, nearly 8% of the population, had diabetes, of which nearly one-fourth were undiagnosed (NIDDK, 2008). The predicted total cost of diabetes in 2006 was $174 billion, and in 2007, diabetes was the seventh leading cause of death. People with diabetes have twice the risk for death and increased rates of comorbid illnesses and disability. For example, diabetes is the leading cause of blindness, kidney failure (44% of new cases in 2005), and nontraumatic lower limb amputations (60% of all cases).

While the incidence of Type 1 diabetes has remained relatively stable, the incidence of Type 2 diabetes has been rising in epidemic fashion. Between 1980 and 2005, the number of cases of newly diagnosed diabetes in adults nearly tripled, from about 500,000 cases per year to 1.4 million cases per year (Centers for Disease Control and Prevention [CDC], 2007). Current estimates from the CDC suggest that 1 person in 3 born in the United States in the year 2000 will go on to develop diabetes in his or her lifetime. The reasons behind this increase have to do with rising rates of obesity and inactivity in the U.S. population, as well as faster growth of minority populations, such as Latinos, who are affected by diabetes at about twice the rate of European Americans. Diabetes is not just an issue in developed countries such as the United States. The World Health Organization (WHO; 2008) estimates that 180 million people are living with diabetes worldwide, and this number is expected to double by the year 2030. Almost 80% of diabetes deaths occur in low- and middle-income nations (WHO, 2008).

Treatment

With the development of insulin, physicians began to be able to prevent the acute, life-threatening impact of severe uncontrolled hyperglycemia, allowing patients with diabetes to live longer. This led to an appreciation of the more delayed-onset yet still serious complications of diabetes. "Delayed-onset complications" are often divided into two categories: macrovascular (large blood vessel) disease, including heart disease and stroke; and microvascular (small blood vessel) disease, including kidney failure, blindness from retinopathy, and limb amputations from peripheral vascular disease. Avoiding these diabetic complications involves careful control of not only glucose but also the associated cardiovascular risk factors. Traditional cardiovascular disease risk factors include smoking, high blood pressure, and high cholesterol. Hence, in addition to taking glucose-lowering medications, patients with diabetes often require several medications, including aspirin, to achieve good control of their cardiovascular risk factors.

While the DCCT gave a rationale for tighter glucose control, subsequent research has verified a role for tighter control of the other cardiovascular risk factors as well, such that patients with diabetes are expected to achieve lower blood pressure and cholesterol targets than average patients (American Diabetes Association [ADA], 2008). It should be noted that while tight glucose control has been proven to reduce microvascular complications and improve wound healing (U.K. Prospective Diabetes Study [UKPDS] Group, 1998), it has not been proven to reduce macrovascular complications, such as strokes or heart attacks. Recently, the debate over the utility of tight glucose control for preventing macrovascular complications has intensified as a result of the findings from two large randomized controlled trials (called Action to Control Cardiovascular Risk in Diabetes [ACCORD] and Action in Diabetes and Vascular Disease [ADVANCE]); Gerstein et al., 2008; Patel et al., 2008). The more aggressive glucose control strategies employed by both studies did not lead to reductions in macrovascular complications, and in the ACCORD study, tight glucose control was actually associated with *increased* overall mortality. As such, the limits of how far to push glucose control in Type 2 diabetes with drug therapy is still uncertain, and behavioral interventions to encourage tight glucose control need to acknowledge this uncertainty.

Lifestyle (diet, exercise, and other health habits) changes are also essential tools for controlling diabetes risk factors and for reducing subsequent diabetic complications. To achieve control, the provider or nutritionist puts many patients on specialized risk factor diets. For example, Dietary Approaches to Stop Hypertension (DASH) targets high blood pressure (Sacks et al., 2001) and the low sugar "diabetic diet" helps to control blood glucose. Patients with diabetes are also expected to incorporate regular physical activity into their weekly routine. If they are smokers, they are expected to quit. In addition, they need to monitor their risk factors with blood testing and, specifically, their blood glucose with a hemoglobin A1c (HbA1c; which measures the average blood glucose over the prior 3 months) and home-based blood glucose monitoring (fingersticks). Other key diabetes management responsibilities include annual eye and foot exams. Careful management of these risk factors requires substantial effort by the patient and provider, but it is the key to preventing serious diabetic complications.

Behavioral Issues in the Management of Diabetes Mellitus

As described earlier, after diagnosis with diabetes, patients are expected to perform a complicated set of health behaviors. While health care providers can make evidence-based recommendations on medications, diet, and exercise, the patients are the ones who actually have to implement and sustain these behaviors. Accordingly, diabetes represents a chronic illness whose successful management is dependent on the self-management behavior of patients.

Behavioral scientists have made significant contributions to understanding the determinants of diabetes self-management. These determinants can be organized into models starting at the personal level (e.g., health beliefs) and extending more broadly to incorporate interpersonal factors (e.g., social support), health care system factors (e.g., physician behavior, insurance costs), and finally, environmental factors (e.g., workplace environment) (see Table 29.1). The goal of these models is to understand the determinants of diabetes health behavior better and to use this knowledge to derive targets for interventions that may alter behavior in a way that enables patients to control their diabetes better. We first provide an overview of how these models have been utilized in the diabetes field, and we then review some of the major interventions based on the lessons learned from these behavioral models.

TABLE 20.1. Determinants of Diabetes Self-Care Management Behavior

Personal level
- Health beliefs
- Self-efficacy
- Locus of control
- Past illness experience
- Motivation for change
- Negative affect

Interpersonal level
- Social support
- Family environment
- Peer relationships

Health care system level
- Physician communication
- Cost of treatment
- Access to medical care
- Chronic disease management programs

Environmental level
- Worksite policies
- Neighborhood
- Media messages

Personal Factors

Health Belief Model

One of the most prominent models used to explain self-management in diabetes at the personal level is known as the health belief model (HBM; Rosenstock, 1966). Like other social learning theory models, the theoretical basis for the HBM is that behavior is determined by an interaction between an individual's incentives and expectancies. More specifically, according to the HBM model, a person will take a health-related action (e.g., monitor blood sugar) if he or she (1) has an incentive to make the change (e.g., perceives that he or she is at increased risk for a serious complication like kidney failure if the diabetes goes uncontrolled), and (2) has an expectation that by taking a recommended action, he or she can avoid a negative outcome without paying too high a price (e.g., expects that careful glucose monitoring by simple finger testing will allow better control of blood sugar intake, which in turn helps to prevent serious diabetes-related kidney damage). Hence, incentives are based on beliefs about perceived risk and severity of the illness, and expectancies pertain to beliefs about perceived costs and benefits of behavior change.

Self-Efficacy

The HBM was later expanded to incorporate the concept of self-efficacy that was simultaneously being developed by cognitive psychologists (Bandura, 1977; Rosenstock, Strecher, & Becker, 1988). The theory underlying self-efficacy is that, to make a successful behavior change, patients must not only expect a behavior to help prevent a serious complication of a disease to which they are susceptible, but also believe they have the skills to perform the behavior. For example, some patients believe that uncontrolled blood sugars can cause complications, and that a diabetic diet can help lower their blood sugars, but according to self-efficacy theory, these same patients will not change their eating habits if they do not feel confident they can change the way they obtain and prepare their meals.

The HBM has had mixed success in terms of its ability to explain diabetic health behavior. For example, Polley, Jakicic, Venditti, Barr, and Wing (1997) did not find that perceived risk of developing diabetes was associated with adherence to a behavioral weight loss program aimed at preventing Type 2 diabetes. In contrast, Nelson, McFarland, and Reiber (2007) and McCaul, Glasgow, and Schafer (1987) found that higher self-efficacy scores were associated with greater adherence to a range of diabetic health behaviors.

Locus of Control

Other theories that have been developed are complementary to the HBM. The locus of control theory posits that some people attribute events in life (e.g., diabetes outcomes) to be in their control (internal locus of control), while others are more likely to believe that events are out of their personal control and due to fate or health professionals (external locus of control) (Rotter, 1966). The theory is that patients with greater internal locus of control are more likely to perform recommended self-management behaviors. While self-efficacy theory applies to confidence in performing specific behaviors, locus of control refers to a more generalized concept of the self. Several studies in the diabetes literature have confirmed a modest association between locus of control and self-management (Peyrot & Rubin, 1994; Tillotson & Smith, 1996).

Self-Regulation

Another model that has been tested to predict diabetes-related health behavior is the self-regulation model (Leventhal, Nerenz, & Steele, 1984). While this model overlaps with the HBM, in that personal perceptions of the consequences of the disease and the efficacy of treatment are relevant to behavior change, the self-regulation model also integrates the patient's past illness experience into current interpretation of disease. Furthermore, this model incorporates the patient's emotional response to disease and treatment. This model appears to complement the predictive ability of the HBM (Hampson, Glasgow, & Foster, 1995; Senecal, Nouwen, & White, 2000).

Other Personal Models of Health Behavior

Several other personal models of health behavior have been applied to diabetes, including the theory of planned behavior (Azjen, 1991), the theory of reasoned action (Azjen & Fishbein, 1980) and the transtheoretical model (Prochaska & DiClemente, 1983). These models emphasize that before making a behavior change, individuals first have to develop intentions to perform the health behavior, and the strength of these intentions are based on a consideration of the perceived costs and benefits of the behavior change. Some of these models also incorporate the concept of how external factors, such as social pressures for behavior change or lack of control over environment, can influence behavior. Some have shown that these models predict not only initiation but also maintenance of diabetic behaviors (Shankar, Conner, & Bodansky, 2007).

Psychopathology

While the self-regulation model emphasizes the emotional impact of an illness, health psychologists have separately considered the impact of common mental disorders on diabetes health behavior. The best studied disorder has been depression. The relevance of understanding the relationship of depression to adherence in diabetes derives from the fact that people with diabetes have two to three times the rate of depression compared to people in the general population (Anderson, Freedland, Clouse, & Lustman, 2001; Lloyd, Dyer, & Barnett, 2000; Thomas, Jones, Scarinci, & Brantley, 2003). Moreover, depression is a risk factor for poor glycemic control (Lustman, Anderson, et al., 2000) and increased mortality among patients with diabetes (Katon et al., 2005). The primary mechanism to explain how depression may be associated with worse outcomes is that depressed patients have poorer self-care. The literature has shown that even mild depressive symptoms are associated with decreased diabetes self-care (Ciechanowski, Katon, Russo, & Hirsch, 2003; Gonzalez et al., 2007; Lin et al., 2006; Park, Hong, Lee, Ha, & Sung, 2004). Accordingly, a number of researchers have sought to determine whether enhanced screening and treatment of depression can improve diabetic outcomes.

Less is known about the association between other emotional states and diabetes self-care behaviors (Rubin & Peyrot, 2001). There is a growing understanding that just being given a diagnosis of diabetes can cause significant subsyndromal distress to patients, and the added burden of expectations for health behavior changes can intensify this distress. In some studies, diabetes-specific distress was more closely linked to diabetes behaviors than to a formal diagnosis of major depression (Fisher et al., 2007). Diabetes distress is more prevalent than depression and may require a different set of interventions than traditional depression treatments. Similar to depression, the presence of diabetes can be associated with an increased level of anxiety (Peyrot & Rubin, 1997), and an anxious coping style may be associated with decreased adherence (Peyrot, McMurry, & Kruger, 1999). However, anxiety disorders have a less clear association with adherence to self-care behaviors.

Interpersonal Factors

While the patient is ultimately responsible for the behaviors required to manage diabetes, behavioral scientists have explored the impact of interpersonal relationships on patient behavior. *Social support* is a concept researchers have used to understand the impact of interpersonal relationships. Social support can be subdivided into different components: (1) emotional support (e.g., expressing empathy and encouragement for the need repeatedly to self-test blood sugar), and (2) practical support (e.g., assistance with picking up diabetic medications from the pharmacy or bringing the patient to appointments) (Berkman, Leo-Summers, & Horwitz, 1992; Seeman & Berkman, 1988). In addition, particularly in pediatric and adolescent populations, behavioral scientists have considered social support in terms of the influence of the *family environment* (Hanson, De Guire, Schinkel, & Kolterman, 1995; Jacobson et al., 1994) and *peer relationships*. The impact of social support may vary depending on the self-care behavior (Wang & Fenske, 1996). While social support is commonly shown to be an independent predictor of some aspects of self-care management (Lewandowski & Drotar, 2007; Skinner, John, & Hampson, 2000; Tang, Brown, Funnell, & Anderson, 2008), overall, it has a modest relationship with diabetes-related health behavior (Burroughs, Harris, Pontious, & Santiago, 1997; Gallant, 2003; Tillotson & Smith, 1996).

Health System Factors

Physician Communication

Abundant research has gone into understanding how health system factors in general and physician behavior in particular can influence diabetic self-management. While the majority of diabetes treatment must be carried out by patients, health care providers play an important role in educating and motivating patients. Over the last 20 years, there has been a paradigm shift away from a model of disease in which patients are perceived to comply with their physicians' advice, a paternalistic model based on the precepts of acute medical care. Instead, patients with chronic illnesses such as diabetes are now viewed as collaborating with their providers, who share information to develop personalized strategies to control their chronic illness (Funnell et al., 1991; Glasgow et al., 1999). Indeed, several authors have been able to show that physician communication that incorporates more shared decision making is associated with improved diabetes self-management (Stewart, 1995; Williams, Freedman, & Deci, 1998). Other measures of enhanced provider–patient communication have also been shown to be associated with better patient self-management (Golin, DiMatteo, & Gelberg, 1996; Heisler, Bouknight, Hayward, Smith, & Kerr, 2002).

Risk Communication

Another lens through which behavioral scientists have begun to understand the influence of physician communication is the concept of risk communication. Decades of research have produced a growing understanding of how personal risk is perceived by individuals, and how differences in communicating risk to patients can influence behavior change (Fagerlin, Ubel, Smith, & Zikmund-Fisher, 2007). Patient understanding of risk

entails several steps: knowing relevant risk factors, establishing the likelihood of getting the disease (or complication) based on these risk factors (a probability function), understanding the consequences and severity of the disease, comprehending the positive or negative aspects of the potential preventive behaviors, and the affective reactions to the risk information (Weinstein, 1999). Patients also form mental models based on personal or learned experience of diseases and comprehend risk information based on these experiences. While the relationship between risk perception and risk-reducing behavior is complex and not always consistent, the association is considered integral to behavioral counseling, and was supported by a recent meta-analysis (Brewer et al., 2007; Gerrard, Gibbons, & Reis-Bergan, 1999; Weinstein, 2003).

Health Care System Organizational and Financial Factors

While the provider plays an important role, there is a growing appreciation of the importance of other health system factors. A well-described example of how health system factors can influence behavior is through cost. The rising price of medications adversely affects adherence to pharmacological treatment, as well as other aspects of diabetes management (Piette, Heisler, & Wagner, 2004). Beyond cost, health care system policies, regulations, and structures serve to facilitate or impair behavioral diabetes management. For example, institutional policies such as automatic telephone appointment reminders have been found to be associated with improved treatment adherence (Macharia, Leon, Rowe, Stephenson, & Haynes, 1992).

Environmental Factors

Diabetes behavior is also affected by more distal influences than the health system, such as the worksite, the neighborhood, and the media. The worksite has the potential to present special challenges for workers living with diabetes (e.g., finding time and privacy for monitoring blood glucose or injecting insulin, eating within certain time periods or when symptoms suggest a snack, experiencing social pressure to eat similarly to coworkers or appear "different") (Trief, Aquilino, Paradies, & Weinstock, 1999; Wood & Jacobson, 2008). The environment can affect behavior by raising the barriers to sustaining healthy behaviors. For example, living in neighborhoods that have less access to affordable, healthy food choices (Horowitz, Colson, Hebert, & Lancaster, 2004) may make it more difficult for patients with diabetes to adhere to recommended diets.

Diabetes Behavioral Interventions

Behavioral scientists have devised a number of plausible models to help explain how patients perform diabetes-related self-management behaviors. Accordingly, the next step has been to test a series of interventions based on these models. Behavioral interventions aimed at the personal level focus on enhancing patient self-management knowledge, affect, and skills; interpersonal interventions seek to fill in gaps in social support; health care system interventions try to improve provider–patient communication and, in accordance with the chronic disease model, aim to foster coordinated care across domains. We now review key interventions and approaches at each level.

Personal-Level Interventions

Behavioral diabetes interventions frequently work to enhance self-efficacy by teaching diabetics skills and boosting their confidence to perform the numerous disease management activities. Studies focused on self-management training have demonstrated positive effects on knowledge, frequency, and accuracy of self-monitoring of blood glucose, self-reported dietary habits, and glycemic control (Norris, Engelgau, & Venkat Narayan, 2001). The impact of self-efficacy interventions on clinical outcomes and behaviors, such as blood lipids, physical activity, weight, and blood pressure, has been positive but less consistent. In general, collaborative patient education interventions that emphasize shared decision making have shown superior results in comparison to more didactically based educational interventions (Norris et al., 2001). In addition, group-based self-management interventions have demonstrated efficacy in many tri-

als (Deakin, McShane, Cade, & Williams, 2005).

Stanford Chronic Disease Self-Management Program

One of the best studied self-management training programs is the Stanford Chronic Disease Self-Management Program. Drawing heavily on Bandura's self-efficacy theory, the diabetes version helps people with diabetes develop skills for dealing with the symptoms of diabetes, appropriate exercise regimens, healthy eating habits, appropriate medication usage, and better communication with their health care providers. The model relies on participants' generation of weekly action plans, then use of a group format to share their experiences and develop solutions to overcome personal behavior change obstacles. The success of this self-management program has been demonstrated in many studies of adults with diabetes and other chronic illnesses (Lorig, Hurwicz, Sobel, Hobbs, & Ritter, 2005; Lorig, Ritter, & Gonzalez, 2003; Lorig, Ritter, Laurent, & Plant, 2006; Lorig, Ritter, Villa, & Piette, 2008). The program, which is now used on an international scale, has led to improvements in weekly exercise, physician communication, self-reported health, health distress, fatigue, and disability (Lorig et al., 2001, 2006).

Diabetes Prevention Program

In the seminal Diabetes Prevention Program (DPP), another key program that demonstrated the effectiveness of enhancing behavioral self-management, weight loss is the single therapy proven to prevent or delay diabetes, and 5–10% weight loss is enough to produce significant reductions in cardiovascular risk (ADA & NIDDK, 2003; Nathan et al., 2007). Accordingly, the DPP was designed as a randomized controlled trial to test the effectiveness of a lifestyle intervention (to lose 7% of body weight via diet and exercise) on incident diabetes. The lifestyle intervention, a structured program involving weekly behavioral self-management training classes and intensive exercise promotion activities, was led by a case manager trained in nutrition, exercise, and behavior modification. Borrowing from the self-regulation, HBM, and social cognitive-behavioral theories, counseling sessions included instruction and modeling of self-monitoring, goal setting, stimulus control, problem solving, and relapse prevention techniques. In addition, a flexible "toolbox" approach helped to personalize the training to meet the needs of each participant (Diabetes Prevention Program, 1999). Over a 2-year period, 50% of the lifestyle intervention participants lost 7% or more of total body weight, and 74% engaged in at least 150 minutes of physical activity. More importantly, these behavior changes led to a 58% reduction in the incidence of diabetes (Diabetes Prevention Program Research Group, 2002; Hamman et al., 2006). The DPP showed that a behavioral management program can be an effective method for preventing diabetes.

Pathways Study

Since depression has been clearly linked with elevated risk of uncontrolled diabetes, researchers hoped that enhancing treatment for depression could lead to improved self-management and diabetic outcomes. While the majority of studies have shown that enhanced depression strategies improve depressive symptoms, improvements in depression have not always been associated with better adherence to diabetes self-management behaviors or to diabetic control (Lustman et al., 1997; Lustman, Freedland, Griffith, & Clouse, 2000; Lustman, Griffith, Freedland, Kissel, & Clouse, 1998). For example, the Pathways Study showed that a proven depression intervention relying on a collaborative, stepped-care case management approach was effective at improving depressive symptoms and quality-of-life scores (Katon et al., 2004). However, the intervention did not lead to improvements in HbA1c tests or self-care activities based on the Summary of Diabetes Self-Care Activities (SDSCA) scale compared to usual care (Lin et al., 2006). The authors concluded that an integrated biopsychosocial approach that simultaneously seeks to improve depression care and to address self-management behaviors directly would be necessary.

Interpersonal Interventions

Interpersonal interventions specifically target the relationship between the patient and other critical players in diabetes management, such as family and friends. For example, Ingram and colleagues (2007) designed a study in which they trained culturally concordant *promotoras* to perform a community-based intervention, including increased support groups, telephone visits, and advocacy for patients with diabetes in a farming community on the U.S.–Mexico border, with the overall goal of supplementing preexisting social support. Participants in the intervention reported increased social support from friends and family, and high-risk patients lowered their HbA1c by 1%. Overall, there is evidence that some forms of social support, particularly those based in new technologies such as the Internet or text-messaging, can improve diabetes self-care (Franklin, Greene, Waller, Greene, & Pagliari, 2008; van Dam et al., 2005).

Health Care Provider and Organizational Interventions

Traditional didactic, paternalistic education from provider to patient is often not sufficient to change behavior (Clement, 1995; Padgett, Mumford, Hynes, & Carter, 1988). Accordingly, provider communication interventions seek to promote shared decision making, to enhance understanding of risks and benefits, to be tailored to patient beliefs and preferences, and to incorporate teaching on problem-solving and coping strategies. In addition, institutional interventions have been designed to alter the manner in which diabetes care is delivered and to promote successful behavioral management.

Provider Communication

Behavioral interventions often rely on a patient's understanding of the risks of diabetes and interpreting this risk as a threat that will lead to behavior change. While risk perception is a complicated cognitive and emotional process, many behavioral interventions seek to improve the communication of risk to enhance patient uptake of risk-reducing behaviors. Most of these efforts have relied on traditional patient education models, in which risk information is presented in an unstructured oral or written format. This methodology has led to small improvements in disease knowledge, risk perception, and behavior change (Montori, Gafni, & Charles, 2006). More recently, in accordance with the tenets of shared decision making, provider communication interventions are being designed to facilitate a bidirectional discussion of diabetes risks and treatment benefits, and to present the information in formats that use proven methods to improve comprehension, such as graphic presentations and careful framing of numerical data (Montori et al., 2006).

A recent example of this type of intervention was a provider communication tool that graphically displayed the risks and benefits of taking cholesterol medication among diabetics. The intervention guided the provider through a series of steps designed to promote discussion and comprehension of the rationale for taking the medication, its benefits and side effects, as well as the need for daily adherence. The tool improved understanding of the risks and benefits of diabetes, reduced anxiety about taking the medication, and enhanced participants' adherence to the medications (Weymiller et al., 2007). Furthermore, videotapes of the sessions demonstrated increased use of shared decision making and more extensive discussion of behavior modification (Montori, Breslin, Maleska, & Weymiller, 2007).

Health Care Organizations

Beyond individuals with diabetes and their health care providers, organizations play a critical role in diabetes management. Within the U.S. health care system, this is often conducted in a poorly coordinated fashion that can lead to oversights and gaps in care. However, the past decade has seen major efforts to improve the quality and efficiency of diabetes care at provider and organizational levels. These health care systems level interventions have led to increased monitoring of processes of care (i.e., checking of HbA1c or referral for eye exams), along with attempts to change systems of care to promote provider and patient adherence to established guidelines and performance measures. In a review of 41 studies, comprehensive interventions targeting health care providers and organizations were found to improve significantly the aforementioned processes of care, but the final impact on patient behaviors and outcomes was not clear (Renders et

al., 2001). While these organizational-Type 1nterventions are important, combining them with concurrent patient-oriented behavioral programs led by counselors, nurses, and psychologists substantially increases their impact. The data clearly support this synergistic relationship, and have demonstrated that organizational- and provider-level interventions, when combined with patient education interventions and collaborative nurse-monitoring programs, can deliver significant improvement in diabetes outcomes (Renders et al., 2001).

Environmental Interventions

Environmental interventions aimed at the community, the workplace, and society at large have the potential for enormous impact on health behavior and diabetes management. While there are numerous examples of environmental interventions, a case in point is the recent mandatory labeling of calories at all chain restaurants throughout New York City. This type of public-health-level intervention has enormous promise for reducing weight and thereby improving diabetes prevention and control. Another avenue of environmental approaches is workplace interventions. In a workplace-based diabetes prevention and control program, a comprehensive behavioral intervention modeled on the DPP demonstrated sustained improvements in both glucose and cardiovascular risk factors 2 years after its initiation (Aldana et al., 2006).

The Chronic Care Model

The chronic care model is a unified framework that integrates individual, interpersonal, health care system, and environmental approaches. It has six components: community resources and policies, health care organization, self-management support, delivery system design, decision support, and clinical information systems (Bodenheimer, Wagner, & Grumbach, 2002a; Wagner et al., 2001). This organizational system has translated into programs that simultaneously utilize diverse methods, such as disease registries, self-management education, group-based counseling, enhanced electronic medical records, automated telephone follow-up, case management, and other methods for improving care at each level of the model (Boden-heimer, Wagner, & Grumbach, 2002b). Using various combinations of these methodologies within the chronic care framework, interventions have been implemented in large and small health care settings. Significant improvements in diabetes outcomes include better glycemic control, as well as fewer hospitalizations and doctors visits (Bodenheimer et al., 2002b; Bodenheimer, Lorig, Holman, & Grumbach, 2002).

Conclusions

Health psychologists have made important contributions to understanding health behavior in diabetes and have led the way in designing effective behavioral interventions that can improve diabetes outcomes. In research settings, behavioral interventions that seek to enhance diabetes self-management have improved diabetes outcomes as effectively as the addition of any medication. The current challenge and opportunity in the field is to integrate more broadly the lessons learned from clinical trials into the world of clinical practice (Fisher & Glasgow, 2007). In the current U.S. health care environment, a minority of patients with diabetes ever attend or complete a diabetes behavioral program (Graziani, Rosenthal, & Diamond, 1999). Furthermore, few health care providers employ the lessons learned from health behavior theory in their clinical practice.

Incorporating the lessons of behavioral medicine into clinical care requires its own set of interventions. At the provider level, there is the need to advocate for curriculum in medical training and continuing education that teaches the precepts of health behavior theory, emphasizing the shift away from the acute care model of illness to a collaborative, shared decision-making approach that is conducive to operating within a health system with a chronic care model (Glasgow et al., 1999). Health psychologists could facilitate the uptake of health behavior theory into clinical practice by distilling health behavior models into practical, time-efficient approaches that can be taught to busy clinicians (Peyrot & Rubin, 2007). Similarly, behavioral scientists could work toward incorporating behavioral factors into diabetes guidelines. In addition, as elec-

tronic information systems and genetic data become widespread, behavioral scientists will be able to help providers find effective ways of utilizing and communicating this information to support continued behavior modification.

At the health organization level, there is a need to move forward from research testing the efficacy of individual interventions and disseminating proven interventions into actual clinical practice (Glasgow et al., 2001). Moreover, behavioral scientists should advocate for changes in reimbursement to allow the lessons of behavioral science to be incorporated more broadly into clinical care. For example, developing a mechanism to support chronic care managers financially as part of proven chronic care model–based interventions may facilitate broader adoption into clinical practice. In this vein, research on the cost-effectiveness of behavior change interventions will be important to convince health insurers of the merits of these programs. Already, a number of health insurance companies are beginning to support these programs.

At a public health level, incentives to implement the lessons of behavioral medicine will be critical. Policies aimed at increasing food choices, labeling food, providing access to physical activity, and creating diabetes media campaigns all will have roles in changing behavior on a societal scale. The next generation of behavioral scientists and practitioners have the opportunity to utilize the theoretical frameworks developed over the past 50 years and build on previous diabetes interventions, in addition to continuing to play a prominent role in managing, and we hope, reversing the epidemic of diabetes and its complications.

Further Reading

Diabetes Control and Complications Trial Research Group. (1993). The effect of intensive treatment of diabetes on the development and progression of long-term complications of insulin-dependent diabetes mellitus. *New England Journal of Medicine, 329*, 997–986.

Diabetes Prevention Program Research Group. (2002). Reduction in the incidence of Type 2 diabetes with lifestyle intervention or metformin. *New England Journal of Medicine, 346*(6), 393–403.

Fisher, L., & Glasgow, R. E. (2007). A call for more effectively integrating behavioral and social science principles into comprehensive diabetes care. *Diabetes Care, 30*(10), 2746–2749.

Glasgow, R. E., Fisher, E. B., Anderson, B. J., LaGreca, A., Marrero, D., Johnson, S. B., et al. (1999). Behavioral science in diabetes: Contributions and opportunities. *Diabetes Care, 22*(5), 832–843.

Gonder-Frederick, L. A., Cox, D. J., & Ritterband, L. M. (2002). Diabetes and behavioral medicine: The second decade. *Journal of Consulting and Clinical Psychology, 70*(3), 611–625.

Lustman, P. J., Anderson, R. J., Freedland, K. E., de Groot, M., Carney, R. M., & Clouse, R. E. (2000). Depression and poor glycemic control: A meta-analytic review of the literature. *Diabetes Care, 23*(7), 934–942.

Norris, S. L., Engelgau, M. M., & Venkat Narayan, K. M. (2001). Effectiveness of self-management training in Type 2 diabetes: A systematic review of randomized controlled trials. *Diabetes Care, 24*(3), 561–587.

Peyrot, M., & Rubin, R. R. (2007). Behavioral and psychosocial interventions in diabetes: A conceptual review. *Diabetes Care, 30*(10), 2433–2440.

Snoek, F. J., & Skinner, T. C. (Eds.). (2005). *Psychology in diabetes care* (2nd ed.). Chichester, UK: Wiley.

References

Aldana S., Barlow M., Smith R., Yanowitz F., Adams T., Loveday L., et al. (2006). A worksite diabetes prevention program: Two-year impact on employee health. *AAOHN Journal, 54*(9), 389–395.

American Diabetes Association (ADA). (2008). Executive summary: Standards of medical care in diabetes. *Diabetes Care, 31*(Suppl. 1), S5–S11.

American Diabetes Association (ADA), & National Institute of Diabetes and Digestive Kidney Diseases (NIDDK). (2003). The prevention or delay of Type 2 diabetes. *Diabetes Care, 26,* S62–S69.

Anderson, B. J., & Rubin, R. R. (Eds.). (2002). *Practical psychology for diabetes clinicians* (2nd ed.). Alexandria: American Diabetes Association.

Anderson, R. J., Freedland, K. E., Clouse, R. E., & Lustman, P. J. (2001). The prevalence of comorbid depression in adults with diabetes: A meta-analysis. *Diabetes Care, 24*(6), 1069–1078.

Azjen, I. (1991). The theory of planned behavior. *Organizational Behavior and Human Decision Processes, 50,* 179–211.

Azjen, I., & Fishbein, M. (1980). *Understanding attitudes and predicting social behavior.* Englewood Cliffs, NJ: Prentice-Hall.

Bandura, A. (1977). Self-efficacy: Toward a unifying theory of behavioral change. *Psychological Review, 84*(2), 191–215.

Berkman, L. F., Leo-Summers, L., & Horwitz, R. I. (1992). Emotional support and survival after myocardial infarction: A prospective, population-based study of the elderly. *Annals of Internal Medicine, 117*(12), 1003–1009.

Bodenheimer, T., Lorig, K., Holman, H., & Grumbach, K. (2002). Patient self-management of chronic disease in primary care. *Journal of the American Medical Association, 288*(19), 2469–2475.

Bodenheimer, T., Wagner, E. H., & Grumbach, K. (2002a). Improving primary care for patients with chronic illness. *Journal of the American Medical Association, 288*(14), 1775–1779.

Bodenheimer, T., Wagner, E. H., & Grumbach, K. (2002b). Improving primary care for patients with chronic illness: The chronic care model, Part 2. *Journal of the American Medical Association, 288*(15), 1909–1914.

Bradley, C. (1994). *Handbook of psychology and diabetes: A guide to psychological measurement in diabetes research and management.* New York: Psychology Press.

Brewer, N. T., Chapman, G. B., Gibbons, F. X., Gerrard, M., McCaul, K. D., & Weinstein, N. D. (2007). Meta-analysis of the relationship between risk perception and health behavior: The example of vaccination. *Health Psychology, 26*(2), 136–145.

Burroughs, T. E., Harris, M. A., Pontious, S. L., & Santiago, J. V. (1997). Research on social support in adolescents with IDDM: A critical review. *Diabetes Education, 23*(4), 438–448.

Centers for Disease Control and Prevention [CDC]. (2007). *Diabetes data and trends.* Atlanta, GA: Author. Retrieved from *www.cdc.gov/diabetes/statistics/incidence/fig1.htm.*

Ciechanowski, P. S., Katon, W. J., Russo, J. E., & Hirsch, I. B. (2003). The relationship of depressive symptoms to symptom reporting, self-care and glucose control in diabetes. *General Hospital Psychiatry, 25*(4), 246–252.

Clement, S. (1995). Diabetes self-management education. *Diabetes Care, 18*(8), 1204–1214.

Davis, K. H. J., & Fisher, E. B., Jr. (1997). *Types of social support deemed important by participants in the DCCT.* Boston: American Diabetes Association.

Deakin, T., McShane, C. E., Cade, J. E., & Williams, R. (2005). Group based training for self-management strategies in people with Type 2 diabetes mellitus. *Cochrane Database Systems*

Review, Issue 2 (Article No. CD003417), DOI: 10.1002/14651858.CD003417.pub2.

Diabetes Prevention Program. (1999). Design and methods for a clinical trial in the prevention of Type 2 diabetes. *Diabetes Care, 22*(4), 623–634.

Diabetes Prevention Program Research Group. (2002). Reduction in the incidence of Type 2 diabetes with lifestyle intervention or metformin. *New England Journal of Medicine, 346*(6), 393–403.

Fagerlin, A., Ubel, P. A., Smith, D. M., & Zikmund-Fisher, B. J. (2007). Making numbers matter: Present and future research in risk communication. *American Journal of Health Behavior, 31*(Suppl. 1), S47–S56.

Fisher, L., & Glasgow, R. E. (2007). A call for more effectively integrating behavioral and social science principles into comprehensive diabetes care. *Diabetes Care, 30*(10), 2746–2749.

Fisher, L., Skaff, M. M., Mullan, J. T., Arean, P., Mohr, D., Masharani, U., et al. (2007). Clinical depression versus distress among patients with Type 2 diabetes: Not just a question of semantics. *Diabetes Care, 30*(3), 542–548.

Florez, J. C., Jablonski, K. A., Bayley, N., Pollin, T. I., de Bakker, P. I. W., Shuldiner, A. R., et al. (2006). TCF7L2 polymorphisms and progression to diabetes in the Diabetes Prevention Program. *New England Journal of Medicine, 355*(3), 241–250.

Franklin, V. L., Greene, A., Waller, A., Greene, S. A., & Pagliari, C. (2008). Patients' engagement with "Sweet Talk"—a text messaging support system for young people with diabetes. *Journal of Medical Internet Research, 10*(2), e20.

Funnell, M. M., Anderson, R. M., Arnold, M. S., Barr, P. A., Donnelly, M., Johnson, P. D., et al. (1991). Empowerment: An idea whose time has come in diabetes education. *Diabetes Education, 17*(1), 37–41.

Gallant, M. P. (2003). The influence of social support on chronic illness self-management: A review and directions for research. *Health Education and Behavior, 30*(2), 170–195.

Gerrard, M., Gibbons, F. X., & Reis-Bergan, M. (1999). The effect of risk communication on risk perceptions: The significance of individual differences. *Journal of the National Cancer Institute Monographs, 25*, 94–100.

Gerstein, H. C., Miller, M. E., Byington, R. P., Goff, D. C., Jr., Bigger, J. T., Buse, J. B., et al. (2008). Effects of intensive glucose lowering in Type 2 diabetes. *New England Journal of Medicine, 358*(24), 2545–2559.

Glasgow, R. E., Fisher, E. B., Anderson, B. J., LaGreca, A., Marrero, D., Johnson, S. B., et al. (1999). Behavioral science in diabetes: Contributions and opportunities. *Diabetes Care, 22*(5), 832–43.

Glasgow, R. E., Hiss, R. G., Anderson, R. M., Friedman, N. M., Hayward, R. A., Marrero, D. G., et al. (2001). Report of the Health Care Delivery Work Group: Behavioral research related to the establishment of a chronic disease model for diabetes care. *Diabetes Care, 24*(1), 124–130.

Golin, C., DiMatteo, M., & Gelberg, L. (1996). The role of patient participation in the doctor visit: Implications for adherence to diabetes care. *Diabetes Care, 19*(10), 1153–1164.

Gonzalez, J. S., Safren, S. A., Cagliero, E., Wexler, D. J., Delahanty, L., Wittenberg, E., et al. (2007). Depression, self-care, and medication adherence in type 2 diabetes: Relationships across the full range of symptom severity. *Diabetes Care, 30*(9), 2222–2227.

Graziani, C., Rosenthal, M. P., & Diamond, J. J. (1999). Diabetes education program use and patient-perceived barriers to attendance. *Family Medicine, 31*(5), 358–363.

Hamman, R. F., Wing, R. R., Edelstein, S. L., Lachin, J. M., Bray, G. A., Delahanty, L., et al. (2006). Effect of weight loss with lifestyle intervention on risk of diabetes. *Diabetes Care, 29*(9), 2102–2107.

Hampson, S. E., Glasgow, R. E., & Foster, L. S. (1995). Personal models of diabetes among older adults: Relationship to self-management and other variables. *Diabetes Education, 21*(4), 300–307.

Hanson, C. L., De Guire, M. J., Schinkel, A. M., & Kolterman, O. G. (1995). Empirical validation for a family-centered model of care. *Diabetes Care, 18*(10), 1347–1356.

Heisler, M., Bouknight, R. R., Hayward, R. A., Smith, D. M., & Kerr E. A. (2002). The relative importance of physician communication, participatory decision making, and patient understanding in diabetes self-management. *Journal of General Internal Medicine, 17*(4), 243–252.

Horowitz, C. R., Colson, K. A., Hebert, P. L., & Lancaster, K. (2004). Barriers to buying healthy foods for people with diabetes: Evidence of environmental disparities. *American Journal of Public Health, 94*(9), 1549–1554.

Ingram, M., Torres, E., Redondo, F., Bradford, G., Wang, C., & O'Toole, M. L. (2007). The impact of *promotoras* on social support and glycemic control among members of a farmworker community on the US–Mexico border. *Diabetes Education, 33*(Suppl. 6), 172S–178S.

Jacobson, A. M., Hauser, S. T., Lavori, P., Willett, J. B., Cole, C. F., Wolfsdorf, J. I., et al. (1994). Family environment and glycemic control: A four-year prospective study of children and adolescents with insulin-dependent diabetes mellitus. *Psychosomatic Medicine, 56*(5), 401–409.

Katon, W. J., Rutter, C., Simon, G., Lin, E. H., Ludman, E., Ciechanowski, P., et al. (2005). The association of comorbid depression with mortality in patients with Type 2 diabetes. *Diabetes Care, 8*(11), 2668–2672.

Katon, W. J., Von Korff, M., Lin, E. H., Simon, G., Ludman, E., Russo, J., et al. (2004). The Pathways Study: A randomized trial of collaborative care in patients with diabetes and depression. *Archives of General Psychiatry, 61*(10), 1042–1049.

Lasker, R. D. (1993). The diabetes control and complications trial: Implications for policy and practice. *New England Journal of Medicine, 329,* 1035–1036.

Leventhal, H., Nerenz, D. R., & Steele, D. J. (1984). Illness representation and coping with health threats. In A. Baum & J. E. Singer (Eds.), *Handbook of psychology and health* (pp. 219–252). Hillsdale, NJ: Erlbaum.

Lewandowski, A., & Drotar, D. (2007). The relationship between parent-reported social support and adherence to medical treatment in families of adolescents with Type 1 diabetes. *Journal of Pediatric Psychology, 32*(4), 427–436.

Lin, E. H., Katon, W., Rutter, C., Simon, G. E., Ludman, E. J., Von Korff, M., et al. (2006). Effects of enhanced depression treatment on diabetes self-care. *Annals of Family Medicine, 4*(1), 46–53.

Lloyd, C. E., Dyer, P. H., & Barnett, A. H. (2000). Prevalence of symptoms of depression and anxiety in a diabetes clinic population. *Diabetic Medicine, 17*(3), 198–202.

Lorig, K. R., Hurwicz, M. L., Sobel, D., Hobbs, M., & Ritter, P. L. (2005). A national dissemination of an evidence-based self-management program: A process evaluation study. *Patient Education Counseling, 59*(1), 69–79.

Lorig, K. R., Ritter, P. L., & Gonzalez, V. M. (2003). Hispanic chronic disease self-management: A randomized community-based outcome trial. *Nursing Research, 52*(6), 361–369.

Lorig, K. R., Ritter, P. L., Laurent, D. D., & Plant, K. (2006). Internet-based chronic disease self-management: A randomized trial. *Medical Care, 44*(11), 964–971.

Lorig, K. R., Ritter, P. L., Stewart, A. L., Sobel, D. S., Brown, B. W., Jr., Bandura, A., et al. (2001). Chronic disease self-management program: 2-year health status and health care utilization outcomes. *Medical Care, 39*(11), 1217–1223.

Lorig, K. R., Ritter, P. L., Villa, F., & Piette, J. D. (2008). Spanish diabetes self-management with and without automated telephone reinforcement: Two randomized trials. *Diabetes Care, 31*(3), 408–414.

Lustman, P. J., Anderson, R. J., Freedland, K. E., de Groot, M., Carney, R. M., & Clouse, R. E. (2000). Depression and poor glycemic control: A meta-analytic review of the literature. *Diabetes Care, 23*(7), 934–942.

Lustman, P. J., Freedland, K. E., Griffith, L. S., & Clouse, R. E. (2000). Fluoxetine for depression in diabetes: A randomized double-blind placebo-controlled trial. *Diabetes Care, 23*(5), 618–623.

Lustman, P. J., Griffith, L. S., Clouse, R. E., Freedland, K. E., Eisen, S. A., Rubin, E. H., et al. (1997). Effects of nortriptyline on depression and glycemic control in diabetes: Results of a double-blind, placebo-controlled trial. *Psychosomatic Medicine, 9*(3), 241–250.

Lustman, P. J., Griffith, L. S., Freedland, K. E., Kissel, S. S., & Clouse, R. E. (1998). Cognitive behavior therapy for depression in Type 2 diabetes mellitus: A randomized, controlled trial. *Annals of Internal Medicine, 129*(8), 613–621.

Macharia, W. M., Leon, G., Rowe, B. H., Stephenson, B. J., & Haynes, R. B. (1992). An overview of interventions to improve compliance with appointment keeping for medical services. *Journal of the American Medical Association, 267*(13), 1813–1817.

McCaul, K. D., Glasgow, R. E., & Schafer, L. C. (1987). Diabetes regimen behaviors: Predicting adherence. *Medical Care, 25*(9), 868–881.

Montori, V., Breslin, M., Maleska, M., & Weymiller, A. (2007). Creating a conversation: Insights from the development of a decision aid. *PLoS Medicine, 4*(8), e233.

Montori, V. M., Gafni, A., & Charles, C. (2006). A shared treatment decision-making approach between patients with chronic conditions and their clinicians: The case of diabetes. *Health Expectations, 9*(1), 25–36.

Nathan, D. M., Davidson, M. B., DeFronzo, R. A., Heine, R. J., Henry, R. R., Pratley, R., et al. (2007). Impaired fasting glucose and impaired glucose tolerance: Implications for care. *Diabetes Care, 30*(3), 753–759.

National Institute of Diabetes and Digestive and Kidney Diseases [NIDDK]. (2008). *National diabetes statistics, 2007 fact sheet.* Bethesda, MD: Author.

Nelson, K. M., McFarland, L., & Reiber, G. (2007). Factors influencing disease self-management among veterans with diabetes and poor glycemic control. *Journal of General Internal Medicine, 22*(4), 442–447.

Norris, S. L., Engelgau, M. M., & Venkat Narayan, K. M. (2001). Effectiveness of self-management training in Type 2 diabetes: A systematic review of randomized controlled trials. *Diabetes Care, 24*(3), 561–587.

Padgett, D., Mumford, E., Hynes, M., & Carter, R. (1988). Meta-analysis of the effects of educational and psychosocial interventions on management of diabetes mellitus. *Journal of Clinical Epidemiology, 41*(10), 1007–1030.

Park, H., Hong, Y., Lee, H., Ha, E., & Sung, Y. (2004). Individuals with Type 2 diabetes and depressive symptoms exhibited lower adherence with self-care. *Journal of Clinical Epidemiology, 57*(9), 978–984.

Patel, A., MacMahon, S., Chalmers, J., Neal, B., Billot, L., Woodward, M., et al. (2008). Intensive blood glucose control and vascular outcomes in patients with Type 2 diabetes. *New England Journal of Medicine, 358*(24), 2560–2572.

Peyrot, M., McMurry, J. F., Jr., & Kruger, D. F. (1999). A biopsychosocial model of glycemic control in diabetes: Stress, coping and regimen adherence. *Journal of Health and Social Behavior, 40*(2), 141–158.

Peyrot, M., & Rubin, R. R. (1994). Structure and correlates of diabetes-specific locus of control. *Diabetes Care, 17*(9), 994–1001.

Peyrot, M., & Rubin, R. R. (1997). Levels and risks of depression and anxiety symptomatology among diabetic adults. *Diabetes Care, 20*(4), 585–590.

Peyrot, M., & Rubin, R. R. (2007). Behavioral and psychosocial interventions in diabetes: A conceptual review. *Diabetes Care, 30*(10), 2433–2440.

Piette, J. D., Heisler, M., & Wagner, T. H. (2004). Problems paying out-of-pocket medication costs among older adults with diabetes. *Diabetes Care, 27*(2), 384–391.

Polley, B. A., Jakicic, J. M., Venditti, E. M., Barr, S., & Wing, R. R. (1997). The effects of health beliefs on weight loss in individuals at high risk for NIDDM. *Diabetes Care, 20*(10), 1533–1538.

Prochaska, J. O., & DiClemente, C. C. (1983). Stages and processes of self-change of smoking: Toward an integrative model of change. *Journal of Consulting and Clinical Psychology, 51*(3), 390–395.

Renders, C. M., Valk, G. D., Griffin, S. J., Wagner, E. H., Eijk van, J. T., & Assendelft, W. J. J. (2001). Interventions to improve the management of diabetes in primary care, outpatient, and community settings: A systematic review. *Diabetes Care, 24*(10), 1821–1833.

Rosenstock, I. M. (1966). Why people use health services. *Milbank Memorial Fund Quarterly, 44*(Suppl. 3), 94–127.

Rosenstock, I. M., Strecher, V. J., & Becker, M. H. (1988). Social learning theory and the health belief model. *Health Education Quarterly, 15*(2), 175–183.

Rotter, J. B. (1966). Generalized expectancies for internal versus external control of reinforcement. *Psychological Monographs, 80*(1), 1–28.

Rubin, R. R., & Peyrot, M. (1994). Implications of the DCCT: Looking beyond tight control. *Diabetes Care, 17*(3), 235–236.

Rubin, R. R., & Peyrot, M. (2001). Psychological issues and treatments for people with diabetes. *Journal of Clinical Psychology, 57*(4), 457–478.

Sacks, F. M., Svetkey, L. P., Vollmer, W. M., Appel, L. J., Bray, G. A., Harsha, D., et al. (2001). Effects on blood pressure of reduced dietary sodium and the Dietary Approaches to Stop Hypertension (DASH) diet. *New England Journal of Medicine, 344*(1), 3–10.

Saxena, R., Voight, B. F., Lyssenko, V., Burtt, N. P., de Bakker, P. I., Chen, H., et al. (2007). Genome-wide association analysis identifies loci for Type 2 diabetes and triglyceride levels. *Science, 316*, 1331–1336.

Seeman, T. E., & Berkman, L. F. (1988). Structural characteristics of social networks and their relationship with social support in the elderly: Who provides support? *Social Science and Medicine, 26*(7), 737–749.

Senecal, C., Nouwen, A., & White, D. (2000). Motivation and dietary self-care in adults with diabetes: Are self-efficacy and autonomous self-regulation complementary or competing constructs? *Health Psychology, 19*(5), 452–457.

Shankar, A., Conner, M., & Bodansky, H. J. (2007). Can the theory of planned behaviour predict maintenance of a frequently repeated behaviour? *Psychology, Health and Medicine, 12*(2), 213–224.

Skinner, T. C., John, M., & Hampson, S. E. (2000). Social support and personal models of diabetes as predictors of self-care and well-being: A longitudinal study of adolescents with diabetes. *Journal of Pediatric Psychology, 25*(4), 257–267.

Stewart, M. A. (1995). Effective physician-patient communication and health outcomes: A review. *Canadian Medical Association Journal, 152*(9), 1423–1433.

Tang, T. S., Brown, M. B., Funnell, M. M., & Anderson, R. M. (2008). Social support, quality of life, and self-care behaviors among African Americans with Type 2 diabetes. *Diabetes Education, 34*(2), 266–276.

Thomas, J., Jones, G., Scarinci, I., & Brantley, P. (2003). A descriptive and comparative study of the prevalence of depressive and anxiety disorders in low-income adults with Type 2 diabetes and other chronic illnesses. *Diabetes Care, 26*(8), 2311–2317.

Tillotson, L. M., & Smith, M. S. (1996). Locus of control, social support, and adherence to the diabetes regimen. *Diabetes Education, 22*(2), 133–139.

Trief, P. M., Aquilino, C., Paradies, K., & Weinstock, R. S. (1999). Impact of the work environment on glycemic control and adaptation to diabetes. *Diabetes Care, 22*(4), 569–574.

U.K. Prospective Diabetes Study [UKPDS] Group. (1998). Intensive blood-glucose control with sulphonylureas or insulin compared with conventional treatment and risk of complications in patients with Type 2 diabetes. *Lancet, 352*, 837–853.

van Dam, H. A., van der Horst, F. G., Knoops, L., Ryckman, R. M., Crebolder, H. F., van den Borne, B. H. (2005). Social support in diabetes: A systematic review of controlled intervention studies. *Patient Education Counseling, 59*(1), 1–12.

Wagner, E. H., Austin, B. T., Davis, C., Hindmarsh, M., Schaefer, J., & Bonomi, A. (2001). Improving chronic illness care: Translating evidence into action. *Health Affairs (Millwood), 20*(6), 64–78.

Wang, C. Y., & Fenske, M. M. (1996). Self-care of adults with non-insulin-dependent diabetes mellitus: Influence of family and friends. *Diabetes Education, 22*(5), 465–470.

Weinstein, N. D. (1999). What does it mean to understand a risk?: Evaluating risk comprehension. *Journal of the National Cancer Institute Monographs, 25*, 15–20.

Weinstein, N. D. (2003). Exploring the link between risk perceptions and preventive health behaviors. In J. M. Suls & K. Wallston (Eds.), *Psychological foundations of health and illness* (pp. 22–53). Malden, MA: Blackwell.

Weymiller, A. J., Montori, V. M., Jones, L. A., Gafni, A., Guyatt, G. H., Bryant, S. C., et al. (2007). Helping patients with Type 2 diabetes mellitus make treatment decisions: Statin Choice Randomized Trial. *Archives of Internal Medicine, 167*(10), 1076–1082.

Williams, G. C., Freedman, Z. R., & Deci, E. L. (1998). Supporting autonomy to motivate patients with diabetes for glucose control. *Diabetes Care, 21*(10), 1644–1651.

Wood, F. G., & Jacobson, S. (2008). Educating supervisors of employees with diabetes. *AAOHN Journal, 56*(6), 262–267.

World Health Organization [WHO]. (2008). *Diabetes*. Geneva: Author. Retrieved from *www.who.int/diabetes/en/index.html*.

CHAPTER 30

Sleep Medicine

Amy M. Sawyer
Terri E. Weaver

From his text *The Philosophy of Sleep*, published in 1834, Robert MacNish (as cited in Dement, 2000, p. 1) defined sleep as "the intermediate state between wakefulness and death; wakefulness being regarded as the active state of all the animal and intellectual functions, and death as that of their total suspension." Although our understanding of sleep has substantially changed since this early definition, sleep is defined similarly today as "a reversible behavioral state of perceptual disengagement from and unresponsiveness to the environment" (Carskadon & Dement, 2000, p. 15). Throughout the past century, scientists have discovered many of the physiological and behavioral mechanisms that control and contribute to sleep–wake states. Much of what we understand about the function of sleep is derived from animal and human studies of sleep deprivation and sleep restriction.

Human studies of total and partial sleep deprivation, or sleep restriction, provide evidence of the critical nature of sleep in cognitive and motor function, physiological homeostasis, and mood (Banks & Dinges, 2007; Pilcher & Huffcutt, 1996; Van Don-gen, Maislin, Mullington, & Dinges, 2003). In a meta-analysis of 19 studies published between 1984 and 1992, Pilcher and Huffcutt (1996) identified significant differences in performance between a sleep-deprived group and a non-sleep-deprived group on measures of motor function, cognitive function, and mood under the conditions of short-term sleep deprivation (≤ 45 hours), long-term sleep deprivation (> 45 hours), and partial sleep deprivation (sleep period < 5 hours/24-hour period). Partial sleep deprivation was shown to have the greatest negative effect on both cognitive function and mood (Pilcher & Huffcutt, 1996). Yet all conditions of sleep deprivation caused large negative effects on cognitive and motor function tests and mood evaluations (Pilcher & Huffcutt, 1996). Recognizing societal tendencies to chronically restrict sleep (i.e., partial sleep deprivation), Van Dongen and colleagues (2003) examined the dose–response effects of chronic sleep deprivation on neurobehavioral functions and sleep physiology. Among a sample of 48 healthy adults, sleep restriction of even 6 hours per night resulted in cognitive performance deficits compared to

8 hours per night, suggesting that even modest reductions in sleep time affect daytime function. Furthermore, subjects' self-ratings of sleepiness were not reflective of objectively measured impairment (Van Dongen et al., 2003).

In a comprehensive review of recent research examining the effects of chronic sleep restriction on neurobehavioral and physiological functions, Banks and Dinges (2007) discuss the impact of varying doses of sleep restriction (3 hours, 4 hours, 5 hours, etc.) on behavioral alertness, cognitive performance, subjective sleepiness, driving, and physiological functions. Their review verified that chronic sleep restriction contributes to significant and cumulative neurobehavioral impairments and physiological dysfunction. Physiological effects of sleep restriction include increased risk of all-cause mortality, obesity, and cardiovascular disease (Banks & Dinges, 2007). Thus, the cumulative effects of sleep restriction possibly explain not only impaired function but also poor health outcomes among those who have chronically reduced sleep time.

Normal Sleep and Circadian Rhythms

Normal sleep is characterized by a repetitive cycle of sleep stages. Sleep architecture, or the organization of sleep into sleep stages that are distributed across time, is composed of non–rapid eye movement [NREM] sleep (Stages 1, 2, 3, and 4) and rapid eye movement [REM] sleep (Harris, 2005). Sleep stages are identified by characteristic patterns on simultaneously recorded electroencephalogram [EEG] measuring brain activity, electro-oculogram [EOG] measuring eye movements, and electromyelogram [EMG] measuring muscle tone. The recording of these physiological measures is the "gold standard" technique, called polysomnogram, used to identify sleep stages and abnormalities during sleep (Markov & Goldman, 2006). Normal sleep consists of progression from Stages 1 and 2 to Stages 3 and 4 (referred to as "delta sleep" or "slow-wave sleep"), then a brief transition to Stage 3 followed by Stage 2 just prior to the onset of REM sleep. This cyclic progression of sleep recurs throughout the sleep period with some variation in the order/occurrence of sleep stages. Each sleep cycle lasts approximately 60–120 minutes (Harris, 2005). Sleep disruption can occur throughout the sleep cycle, primarily through the mechanism of arousals. The frequency and duration of arousals contribute to impaired sleep quality and duration, and are caused by a variety of factors, including age, sleep environment, substances such as nicotine and alcohol, medications, and comorbid conditions (i.e., mood disorders, pain, cardiopulmonary conditions). In addition to these influential factors that affect sleep duration and quality, many sleep disorders cause arousals and sleep fragmentation, or the impedance of what is normally a time-based cumulative process, leading to abnormal sleep architecture, and impaired health and functional outcomes.

Circadian rhythms are cyclic processes that, in humans, have an intrinsic period of just over 24 hours (Markov & Goldman, 2006). The human circadian clock has an important role in sleep–wake regulation, consolidating sleep–wake cycles into "discrete and contiguous blocks of time" (Zee & Manthena, 2006, p. 60). The sleep–wake cycle in humans is a circadian rhythm regulated by the suprachiasmatic nuclei (SCN). Located in the hypothalamus, the SCN are essentially bilaterally paired nuclei located just above the optic chiasm in the anterior hypothalamus (Markov & Goldman, 2006). Environmental cues influence the synchronization of circadian rhythms. Possibly the most influential environmental cue on circadian clock setting is light–dark cycles (Markov & Goldman, 2006). Exposure to light and dark maintains the circadian clock relatively consistent with day–night and wake–sleep cycles. Other environmental influences on the circadian clock include melatonin and physical activity (Zee & Manthena, 2006). The SCN, though, without environmental influence, maintains its circadian clock because total darkness studies have provided evidence that circadian rhythmicity persists, albeit shifted from what is socially deemed wake and sleep time (Markov & Goldman, 2006). Furthermore, a homeostatic process within mammals defines the need for sleep, which is influenced by previous periods of sleep and wake (Turek, 2000). Essentially, if sleep has recently occurred, the homeostatic drive to sleep is relatively low; if sleep occurred less recently, the homeostatic drive to sleep is greater, and increases over time until sleep recurs. This homeostatic process is called Process S, mediating sleep propensity during waking hours and its dissipation during sleep (Borbely & Achermann, 1999). Process S is balanced with the circadian clock, or Process C (Borbely & Achermann, 1999; Turek, 2000), which is a clocklike mechanism that determines the altering phases of high and low sleep propensity, independent of prior sleep and wake cycles (Borbely & Achermann, 1999).

Sleep Disorders

Disorders of sleep vary by type, cause, and underlying physiology. However, all sleep disorders directly contribute to fragmented sleep (poor sleep quality), shortened sleep duration (total sleep time), and/or impaired wakefulness (Thorpy, 2000). Sleep disorders have traditionally been categorized as dyssomnias, parasomnias, and secondary sleep phenomena. "Parasomnias" include disorders characterized by undesirable physical phenomena that occur primarily during sleep. Secondary sleep phenomena are attributed to a primary non-sleep-disorder/disease, which contributes to impaired sleep quality, quantity, or impaired wakefulness. "Dyssomnias" include insomnias and disorders of excessive sleepiness, and extrinsic and intrinsic sleep disorders, including sleep-disordered breathing, and circadian rhythm sleep disorders (Table 30.1). In large part, the successful treatment and management of this group of sleep disorders is complemented by behavioral medicine, which is therefore the focus of the remainder of this chapter.

TABLE 30.1. Dyssomnias: International Classification of Sleep Disorders (ICSD-2) Diagnostic Categories and International Classification of Diseases (ICD-9) Classification Codes

Extrinsic	Intrinsic	Circadian rhythm disorders
Inadequate sleep hygiene (307.41-1)	Psychophysiological insomnia (307.42-0)	Time zone change (jet lag) syndrome (307.45-0)
Environmental sleep disorder (780.52-6)	Sleep state misperception (307.49-1)	Shift work sleep disorder (307.45-1)
Altitude insomnia (289.0)	Idiopathic insomnia (780.52-7)	Irregular sleep–wake pattern (307.45-3)
Adjustment sleep disorder (307.41-0)	Narcolepsy (347)	Delayed sleep phase syndrome (780.55-0)
Insufficient sleep syndrome (307.49-4)	Idiopathic hypersomnia (780.54-7)	Advanced sleep phase syndrome (780.55-1)
Limit-setting sleep disorder (307.42-4)	Recurrent hypersomnia (780.54-2)	Non-24-hour sleep–wake disorder (780.55-2)
Sleep-onset association disorder (307.42-5)	Posttraumatic hypersomnia (780.54-8)	
Food allergy insomnia (780.52-8)	Obstructive sleep apnea (780.53-0)	
Nocturnal eating (drinking) syndrome (780.52-8)	Central sleep apnea syndrome (780.51-1)	
Hypnotic-dependent sleep disorder (780.52-8)	Central alveolar hypoventilation (780.51-1)	
Stimulant-dependent sleep disorder (780.52-1)	Periodic limb movement disorder (780.52-4)	
Alcohol-dependent sleep disorder (780.52-3)	Restless legs syndrome (780.52-5)	
Toxin-induced sleep disorder (780.55-1)		

From the American Academy of Sleep Medicine. (2006). *Crosswalk from ICSD-2 to ICD-9.* Available at *www.aasmnet.org/PDF/CrosswalkCard.pdf.*

Insomnia

Insomnia is increasingly prevalent among adults, with approximately 33% of adults reporting insomnia symptoms and nearly 6% of the adult population meeting criteria for the diagnosis of insomnia (Morin et al., 2006). Insomnia is characterized by subjective complaints of difficulty falling asleep or staying asleep that contributes to daytime impairment and/or marked distress (Morin et al., 2006). The onset of insomnia is often insidious and affected by physiological, psychological, and behavioral factors. Although some individuals may be predisposed to the development of insomnia, the sleep disorder typically occurs with exposure to precipitating factors (e.g., familial stress, job-related stress, childbirth) and persists with the influence of perpetuating factors (e.g., sleep practices, beliefs about sleep) (Hauri, 2000; Yang, Spielman, & Glovinsky, 2006). A conceptual model of insomnia proposed by Yang and colleagues (2006) provides an overview of psychological and behavioral factors that contribute to the onset and persistence of insomnia. These factors include sleep cognition, maladaptive sleep practices, and emotional arousal.

Sleep cognition includes not only worries and traumatic events that contribute to excessive cognitive arousal during sleep (Yang et al., 2006) but also one's beliefs about sleep, often described by those with insomnia as the belief that their quality and duration of sleep are inevitably poor. These beliefs contribute to both cognitive and emotional burdens, which often become pervasive with efforts to initiate or return to sleep. Abnormal sleep cognition also contributes to accommodating behaviors that perpetuate the cycle of difficulties in initiating or maintaining sleep (Yang et al., 2006). For example, in anticipation of difficulties with sleep at night, a daily planned nap may be thought to be helpful in the total accrual of sleep time; however, daytime napping is widely recognized as a poor sleep practice that contributes to difficulty initiating sleep at night.

Maladaptive sleep practices are a second factor contributing to insomnia in Yang and colleagues' model of insomnia (2006). Behaviors around bedtime are essential to healthy sleep. Persons with insomnia recognize their own difficulties in initiating or maintaining sleep and often implement daily compensatory behaviors that are believed to improve sleep. Many such behaviors, including spending more time in bed, napping, and "make up" sleep, are actually detrimental to sleep and promote the ongoing cycle of insomnia.

Emotional arousal is the third factor that contributes to poor sleep in insomnia (Yang et al., 2006). Anticipating poor sleep, individuals with insomnia worry about getting to sleep or attaining a certain desired amount of sleep. Emotional arousal precludes the individual's ability to get to sleep. Not only do worries and stress about sleep complicate sleep initiation, but also learned responses to the environmental and emotional cues about sleep, commonly associated with sleeplessness, perpetuate the cycle of insomnia (Yang et al., 2006).

Diagnosis and Treatment

The diagnosis of insomnia is established with the clinical interview and diagnostic polysomnogram. Persons diagnosed with insomnia must have a complaint of disturbed sleep that interferes with daytime functioning. The diagnostic polysomnogram reveals increased sleep latency (amount of time to fall asleep), reduced sleep efficiency (percentage of time in bed that is spent sleeping), and arousals and awakenings (Hauri, 2000). The clinical interview is possibly most helpful in establishing the diagnosis of insomnia, providing information about daily routines, sleep practices, functional abilities, history of the current complaint, medical and psychological history, familial medical and psychological history, prior treatments, and medications (Yang et al., 2006). To complement the clinical interview, sleep diaries maintained for 1 to 2 weeks provide insight into the person's sleep complaint and daily routines/practices that may contribute to the sleep complaint. A sleep diary typically includes self-reported bedtime, length of time to fall asleep, number and reason for awakenings from sleep, time of awakening for the day, caffeine and alcohol intake record, medications, and time/duration of any naps (refer to *www.sleepeducation.com* for a free, publicly available sleep diary).

Treating insomnia is challenging because physiological, psychological, and behavioral contributors need to be recognized and considered in the treatment plan. A multidisciplinary approach to the treatment of insomnia is generally most effective and acknowledges the multifactorial causes of insomnia. Empirical studies of the management of insomnia are increasingly prevalent in the literature and have led to new practice parameters for the treatment of insomnia (Morgenthaler et al., 2006). An extensive review of evidence-based practices in the treatment of insomnia has identified the importance of both psychological and behavioral interventions in the treatment of chronic insomnia (Morin et al., 2006). Accordingly, stimulus control therapy, relaxation, and cognitive-behavioral therapy are evidence-based treatment standards for the effective management of insomnia.

Stimulus Control Therapy

Stimulus control therapy is a behavioral intervention that is intended to eliminate the maladaptive association between bedtime cues and conditioned arousal that occurs with persistent sleeplessness at bedtime (Yang et al., 2006), and to reestablish a consistent sleep–wake schedule (Morgenthaler et al., 2006). First described by Bootzin in 1972, stimulus control therapy includes the following instructions:

> (1) go to bed only when sleepy and not before the scheduled bedtime; (2) use the bed only for sleeping; sexual activity is the only exception. Do not watch television, listen to the radio, eat, or read in bed; (3) if you do not fall asleep within 15–20 minutes, get up and go to another room; stay up as long as you wish and return to bed when sleepy. Repeat this step as often as is necessary during the night; (4) set your alarm and get up at the same time every morning; (5) do not nap during the day. (Lichstein, Wilson, & Johnson, 2000, pp. 234–235)

Stimulus control therapy has been a mainstay of insomnia treatment since the mid-1970s and continues to be incorporated in combination treatment regimens and used in isolation to manage effectively negative cues commonly associated with sleeping.

Sleep Restriction Therapy

Sleep restriction therapy limits the total time in bed and potentially makes the individual excessively sleepy, increasing the likelihood of falling and staying asleep. Thus, it changes the perception of the time in bed to a more positive experience, reducing the associated anxiety and promoting sleep. Sleep restriction therapy results in an overall increase in the amount of time sleeping in bed (Harvey, Tang, & Browning, 2005). Estimation of the amount of time "permitted" in bed is based on the individual's average total sleep time. Typically, this management strategy requires frequent follow-up for positive reinforcement and a practitioner-provided review of small increments of positive response to the treatment.

Relaxation Training

Relaxation training incorporates methods to reduce overall somatic tension and intrusive thoughts at bedtime, and has been shown to be effective in the treatment of insomnia (Morin et al., 2006). Though relaxation training may include numerous strategies, those that have been empirically tested and found to be effective in the treatment of insomnia include (1) progressive muscle relaxation (Edinger, Wohlgemuth, Radtke, Marsh, & Quillian, 2001; Means, Lichstein, Epperson, & Johnson, 2000; Pallesen et al., 2003; Rybarczyk, Stepanski, Fogg, Lopez, Barry, & Davis, 2005; Viens, De Koninck, Mercier, St. Onge, & Lorrain, 2003; Waters et al., 2003); (2) hybrid or combination relaxation programs, including relaxing one's attitude, deep breathing, passive relaxation, and/or autogenic phrasing (Lichstein et al., 2000; Lichstein, Reidel, Wilson, Lester, & Aguillard, 2001); and (3) audiotaped relaxation guides, including progressive relaxation, passive focal attention, active expiration, deep breathing, and/or imagery (Pallesen et al., 2003; Rybarczyk et al., 2005). Many empirical studies include relaxation therapy within other interventions and have been shown to be highly effective. Yet even when relaxation therapy was examined, independent of other insomnia interventions, subjects' sleep onset latency, sleep quality, sleep efficiency, and total sleep time improved compared with controls or placebo (Edinger et al., 2001; Lichstein et al., 2001; Means et al., 2000; Rybarczyk et al., 2005).

Cognitive-Behavioral Therapy

Cognitive-behavioral therapy (CBT) includes both cognitive and behavioral interventions. The cognitive interventions focus on changing beliefs and attitudes about sleep and insomnia, while the behavioral interventions focus on sleep practices and sleep-associated cues that interfere with initiating or maintaining sleep (Morganthaler et al., 2006). Studies that examined the effectiveness of CBT in the treatment of insomnia have demonstrated that multiple treatment components are more effective than single-component treatment regimens (Wang, Wang, & Tsai, 2005). To date, though, no study has examined individual components of CBT in the treatment of insomnia (Morin et al., 2006). Furthermore, there is no "standard" set of components deemed to be effective in studies that have tested the effectiveness of CBT. Ideally, the components included in any CBT program will be individualized and address specifically the precipitating and perpetuating factors of insomnia. The clinician's assessment of these factors guide the tailored program of CBT.

Cognitions about sleep that disrupt initiation or maintenance of sleep are widely varied and include a broad range of cognitive processes, including beliefs, attributions, expectations, perception, and attention (Harvey et al., 2005). Yang and colleagues (2006) suggest that broad categories of dysfunctional cognitions interfere with normal sleep, classified as (1) misconceptions concerning the causes of insomnia; (2) misattributions or amplifications of its consequences; (3) unrealistic sleep expectations; (4) diminished perceptions of control; and (5) mistaken beliefs about the predictability of sleep (p. 909). Cognitive therapies target these maladaptive beliefs and perceptions to increase control over sleep and subjective improvement of symptoms (Wang et al., 2005).

Behavioral therapy components of CBT address activities that are maladaptive to sleep. These activities are often perpetuating factors in insomnia, yet they are not recognized as problematic by the individual with insomnia. Specific behavioral interventions include sleep restriction therapy, stimulus control therapy, and sleep hygiene education. Sleep restriction therapy and stimulus control therapy have been primary treatments with empirically established effectiveness in the management of insomnia (Morin et al., 2006). Sleep hygiene education is frequently combined with other behavioral therapies to bring to awareness daily behaviors that are detrimental or beneficial for sleep (Figure 30.1). Although frequently included in CBT, sleep hygiene education, in isolation, has not been identified as effective in the treatment of insomnia (Morganthaler et al., 2006). Yet sleep hygiene education is important, providing insomnia patients those daily behaviors that help create a positive environment for sleep. The majority of studies that have used CBT as a treatment for insomnia commonly "combine educational (sleep hygiene), behavioral (stimulus control, sleep restriction, relaxation), and cognitive components" to address the multiplicity of contributing factors in the management of insomnia (Morin et al., 2006, p. 1408). A combination approach to treating insomnia in various insomnia groups is presently the most effective intervention strategy for managing insomnia (Table 30.2).

1. Maintain a regular bedtime and wake time schedule, including weekends.
2. Establish a regular, relaxing bedtime routine.
3. Create a sleep-conducive environment (dark, quiet, cool, and comfortable).
4. Sleep on a comfortable mattress and pillow(s).
5. Use your bedroom only for sleep and sex.
6. Finish eating at least 2–3 hours before your regular bedtime.
7. Exercise regularly, but be sure your exercise is not within 2–3 hours of your regular bedtime.
8. Avoid caffeine (coffee, tea, soft drinks, chocolate) too close to bedtime.
9. Avoid nicotine.
10. Avoid alcohol too close to bedtime.

FIGURE 30.1. Sleep hygiene educational components. From National Sleep Foundation (2009). Used with permission of the National Sleep Foundation. For further information, please visit *www.sleepfoundation.org*.

TABLE 30.2. Adult and Older Adult Insomnia Studies Examining the Effectiveness of Cognitive-Behavioral Therapy (CBT) in the Treatment of Insomnia and Specific Components of Treatment Included in Study Protocol

Study	Sample	Design	Cognitive-behavioral component(s)	Results
Perlis et al. (2004)	Adults with primary insomnia (*N* = 30)	Randomized controlled trial (RCT) comparing placebo with CBT delivered individually across eight weekly sessions, modafanil (Provigil) + CBT, or modafanil (Provigil) + weekly contact control	*Cognitive therapy*—cognitive restructuring *Behavioral therapy*—sleep restriction and stimulus control therapy + *Sleep hygiene education*	CBT > contact controls
Morgan et al. (2003)	Adults with primary, chronic insomnia using hypnotic drugs for at least 1 month (*N* = 290)	RCT comparing CBT of six 50-minute sessions or control	*Cognitive therapy*—focus on control of presleep mentation and strategies to deal with intrusive and ruminative thoughts *Behavioral therapy*—stimulus control therapy + *Sleep hygiene education* + *Relaxation therapy* (progressive muscle relaxation or autogenic training)	CBT > control
Edinger et al. (2001)	Adults with sleep maintenance insomnia (*N* = 75)	RCT comparing CBT of 6 weekly individual sessions of 30–60 minutes, progressive muscle relaxation, or placebo	*Cognitive therapy*—standardized audiocassette module to correct misconceptions about sleep requirements, aging, circadian rhythms, and sleep loss on wake function *Behavioral therapy*—sleep restriction therapy and stimulus control therapy	CBT > relaxation > placebo
Rybarczyk et al. (2002)	Older adults with comorbid insomnia and medical illness (*N* = 38)	RCT comparing classroom CBT of eight 1.5-hour weekly group sessions, home-based audio relaxation treatment, or delayed-treatment control	*Cognitive therapy*—discussion emphasizing changing unrealistic beliefs and irrational fears regarding sleep and sleep loss *Behavioral therapy*—sleep restriction therapy and stimulus control therapy + *Relaxation therapy* (deep breathing, progressive muscle relaxation, autogenic training, and imagery) + *Sleep hygiene education*	CBT > delayed-treatment control
Morin et al. (2004)	Older adults with chronic insomnia and chronic benzodiazepine use (*N* = 76)	RCT comparing 10-week intervention of supervised benzodiazepine withdrawal, CBT of weekly 90-minute group sessions, or supervised withdrawal + CBT	*Cognitive therapy*—education about sleep and aging to highlight normal physiological changes during sleep with aging; discussion about "faulty" beliefs and attitudes that impact on sleep *Behavioral therapy*—sleep restriction and stimulus control therapy + *Sleep hygiene education*	CBT > medication taper

Circadian Rhythm Disorders

Circadian rhythm disorder types include delayed sleep phase, advanced sleep phase, irregular sleep–wake phase, free-running, jet lag, and shift work. This group of disorders is characterized by a "persistent or recurrent pattern of sleep disturbance due primarily to alterations in the circadian timekeeping system or a misalignment between the endogenous circadian rhythm and exogenous factors that affect the timing or duration of sleep" (Sack et al., 2007a, p. 1461). The disturbance in the sleep pattern must be accompanied by impairment relative to the individual's ability to participate in "normal activities and responsibilities," and the disturbance cannot be explained by another primary sleep disorder (Sack et al., 2007a). Scientific study of circadian rhythm biology has led to a greater understanding of this group of disorders. Yet the clinical applicability of these findings is presently not clear. Furthermore, the relatively infrequent occurrence of the majority of these disorders, with the exception of shift work and jet lag types, presents obvious barriers to identifying evidence-based guidelines and standards in the clinical treatment of circadian rhythm disorders.

Delayed sleep phase disorder is a circadian rhythm disorder characterized by a stable delay in the major sleep period (i.e., sleep onset and wakeup times hours later than socially desirable). Adolescents tend to have a delayed sleep schedule; however, it is not known whether this tendency is due to intrinsic physiology or socially reinforced sleep–wake schedules (Sack et al., 2007b). Common complaints of delayed sleep phase disorder include difficulty falling asleep and sleepiness in the morning: "...Attempts to fall asleep earlier than desired are usually unsuccessful and can result in prolonged sleep latency and promote the development of behaviors associated with psychophysiologic insomnia" (Reid & Burgess, 2005, p. 454). In advanced sleep phase disorder, a stable advance in the major sleep period occurs (i.e., early sleep onset and early morning wake-up times inconsistent with conventional waking hours). Although data are inconclusive about age as a risk for advanced sleep phase disorder, such complaints are more common among older individuals (Sack et al., 2007b). Common complaints include early sleep onset, early morning awakenings, sleep maintenance insomnia, and sleepiness in the late afternoon and evening (Reid & Burgess, 2005).

Diagnosis and Treatment

Both delayed and advanced type phase disorders are diagnosed only after other primary sleep disorders are excluded. Clinical history, sleep diaries maintained over at least 7 days, and/or activity monitoring with actigraphy are useful in the diagnosis of either phase type disorder. Polysomnography is useful to exclude other primary sleep disorders in the setting of circadian rhythm disorders.

Treatment options for either phase type disorder include prescribed sleep scheduling (i.e., chronotherapy), timed light exposure, and timed melatonin administration. According to an extensive review of the scientific literature on the treatment of circadian rhythm disorders (Sack et al., 2007b) and practice parameters supported by the American Academy of Sleep Medicine (Morgenthaler et al., 2007), there are no established standards for the treatment of both advanced and delayed sleep phase disorders; rather, evidence-based guidelines suggest that timed light exposure and timed melatonin administration be used, but the effectiveness of these treatments are not well documented. Furthermore, although phase type disorders are commonly treated with planned sleep schedules or chronotherapy (i.e., treatment incorporating environmental cues that influence circadian rhythmicity), no consistent evidence suggests that chronotherapy is effective (Morgenthaler et al., 2007).

Application of Behavioral Strategies in the Management of Phase Type Disorders

Treatment of phase type circadian rhythm disorders is difficult and requires consistent effort from the individual and positive reinforcement from the provider for seemingly small improvements. As with insomnia, individuals with circadian rhythm disorders develop a conditioned response to efforts to sleep, perpetuating accompanying sleep-onset insomnia. In many cases, the conditioned responses contribute to worsened phase delay. Behavioral strategies of treatment for sleep-onset insomnia include stimulus control therapy and sleep hygiene education (Lack & Wright, 2007). Because individuals with circadian rhythm disorders usually present long after the onset of symptoms, many have developed poor sleep hygiene practices that further complicate their difficulties with sleep.

Adherence to behavioral treatment strategies for circadian rhythm disorders is often low. Consistency and commitment to sleep–wake schedule changes are necessary for treatment to be effective. Identifying realistic treatment goals and recognizing the individual's motivation to change the sleep–wake schedule are imperative first steps in treating phase shift type disorders. It is important to discuss daytime schedule commitments, such as work hours, family activities, use of leisure time, and social routines, so that chronotherapy and/or sleep–wake schedules can be realistically implemented and adherence to the regimen maximized. If the treatment demands conflict with usual daily activities and commitments, then treatment adherence is likely to be low. Even when the prescribed sleep–wake time is consistent with activities of daily living and social engagement routines, individuals need anticipatory guidance with regard to expected treatment responses. For example, if the individual studies in the evening and feels this is his or her best cognitive performance time of the day, then evening sleepiness may occur with advancement of the phase. Mornings now, rather than evenings, are the time to schedule these types of activities. By collaboratively setting treatment goals and providing anticipatory guidance, patients are more likely to adhere to and find treatment regimens effective (Lack & Wright, 2007).

Relapse prevention is critical to maintaining positive treatment responses in phase shift type disorders. Strict adherence to good sleep hygiene practices should be emphasized. Depending on the phase type, sleeping in, retiring early to bed, or late night engagements may cause a shift response (Lack & Wright, 2007). Recognizing shift responses and returning to a strict sleep–wake schedule is imperative, particularly maintaining the target wake-up time. Stimulus control therapy should remain a consistent part of the daily routine, so that sleep-onset insomnia does not recur (Lack & Wright, 2007).

The emphasis of relapse prevention should be on maintaining consistency in the sleep–wake schedule and remaining vigilant in performing positive sleep habits.

Adherence in the Management of Sleep Disorders

Adherence to treatment in the management of sleep disorders has been identified as a research priority by a panel of experts convened in 2003 for a National Institutes of Health (NIH) workshop, *Effects of Sleep Disorders and Sleep Restriction on Adherence to Cardiovascular and Other Disease Treatment Regimens: Research Needs.* The panel identified 30 research issues deemed critical to better understanding, "factors essential for effective adherence to treatments for sleep disorders and the role of sleep factors in adherence to treatments for non-sleep disorders" (p. 1). Over the past 10 years, a substantial body of literature reporting the systematic examination of adherence to treatment in sleep disorders has emerged. The complex nature of adherence as a health behavior has yet to be explained, but empirical studies examining adherence to the treatment of sleep-disordered breathing with continuous positive airway pressure (CPAP) therapy have provided a significant foundation on which future studies can build.

Sleep-Disordered Breathing

"Obstructive sleep apnea" (OSA), characterized by repetitive closures of the upper pharyngeal wall during sleep, resulting in intermittent nocturnal oxyhemoglobin desaturation and recurrent sleep fragmentation (Chesson et al., 1997), results in excessive daytime sleepiness, impaired cognition and mentation, decreased daytime functional status, and alterations in mood (Dinges et al., 1997; Weaver et al., 1999). OSA is also an independent risk factor for hypertension and is associated with increased risk of cardiovascular accidents, myocardial infarction, congestive heart failure, and insulin resistance (Harsch et al., 2004; Nieto et al., 2000; Peppard, Young, Palta, & Skatrud, 2000). Treatment of OSA with CPAP is highly effective in eradicating the upper airway closures, thereby reducing the daytime sequelae of OSA (Sullivan & Grunstein, 1989).

Treatment Effectiveness and Adherence to CPAP

First described in 1981 by Sullivan, Issa, Berthon-Jones, and Eves, CPAP was identified as a "safe, simple treatment for the obstructive sleep apnoea syndrome" (p. 862). After this first description of treating OSA with CPAP, many studies followed that described the efficacy of the treatment. Yet, as early as 1986, adherence to CPAP was recognized as a potentially significant limitation to the effective treatment of OSA (Sanders, Gruendl, & Rogers, 1986). Following this first study to identify the potential problem of adherence to treatment, three seminal studies were published, each identifying poor adherence as a significant limitation in the effective treatment of OSA with CPAP (Engleman, Martin, & Douglas, 1994; Kribbs et al., 1993; Reeves-Hoche, Meck, & Zwillich, 1994).

In a prospective cohort study, Kribbs and colleagues (1993) identified 46% of their sample ($N = 35$) that met criteria for "regular use" of CPAP (defined as 4 hours' use on 70% of days). Similarly, Reeves-Hoche, Meck, and Zwillich (1994) conducted a prospective descriptive study in which they identified, at 6 months, 4.7 mean hours of nightly use for the sample ($N = 38$) represented an adherence rate of 68%. Engleman and colleagues (1994) also identified newly diagnosed patients with OSA ($N = 54$) who used CPAP 4.7 ± 0.4 hours/night on average over the first 3 months of treatment. These early CPAP adherence studies identified the problem of "underuse" of CPAP (i.e., 4.7 hours/night) among patients with OSA, who were expected to use it all night, every night, both in the United States and the United Kingdom. From these seminal works suggesting that adherence was an obstacle to the effective treatment of OSA, investigations have further substantiated and described the problem of nonadherence to CPAP.

DESCRIBING THE PROBLEM

Only about half of patients with OSA prescribed CPAP use the treatment all night, every night as prescribed (Kribbs et al., 1993; Weaver et al., 1997). Although the average daily use of persons who are adherent to CPAP is approximately 6 hours, those who routinely skip nights of use average only about 3 hours (Weaver et al., 1997). In other words, patients who are not adherent to CPAP not only fail to use it on many nights but also even when they apply it, nightly duration of use is shorter than that of patients who are adherent. Although most CPAP users apply CPAP for the same duration on the first night of treatment, nonadherent users begin skipping nights of treatment in the first week (Aloia, Arnedt, Stanchina, & Millman, 2007; Rosenthal et al., 2000; Weaver et al., 1997). More alarming is the fact that patients who become nonadherent in the first few days of CPAP treatment generally remain nonadherent (Krieger, 1992; McArdle et al., 1999; Weaver et al., 1997). The return of symptoms and other manifestations of OSA with nonuse of CPAP, even for one night (Grunstein et al., 1996; Kribbs et al., 1993), underscores the need for adherence to treatment to realize positive physiological and behavioral outcomes.

CORRELATES OF USE

With an empirically derived description of the problem of adherence to CPAP, scientists sought to identify correlates of adherence to CPAP. Although often a presenting complaint from CPAP users, self-reported side effects of CPAP do not distinguish between adherers and nonadherers (Engleman et al., 1994, 1996; Hui et al., 2001; Massie, Hart, Peralez, & Richards, 1999; Meurice et al., 1994; Sanders et al., 1986). The more consistent, yet weak, correlates of adherence to CPAP include (1) subjective sleepiness (Engleman et al., 1996; Kribbs et al., 1993; McArdle et al., 1999; Sin, Mayers, Man, & Pawluk, 2002); (2) severity of OSA, as determined by the Apnea–Hypopnea Index (AHI; Fletcher & Luckett, 1991; McArdle et al., 1999; Rauscher, Formanek, Popp, & Zwick, 1993; Reeves-Hoche et al., 1994; Rolfe, Olson, & Saunders, 1991; Rosenthal et al., 2000; Schweitzer, Chambers, Birkenmeier, & Walsh, 1987), and (3) severity of nocturnal hypoxia (Kribbs et al., 1993; Krieger, 1992; Reeves-Hoche et al., 1994; Rosenthal et al., 2000; Schweitzer et al., 1987).

In a comprehensive review of studies that have examined predictors of adherence to

CPAP and preliminary intervention studies to enhance CPAP adherence, Engleman and Wild (2003) found that empirical studies to date that have sought to identify predictors of CPAP adherence explain only 4–25% of the variance in CPAP use. These authors suggest that the biomedical model traditionally applied to studies seeking to identify the determinants of CPAP adherence may actually be limited in both scope and application. For example, although severe OSA (AHI > 30 events/hour) typically contributes to significant morbidity and impairment among the OSA population, disease severity does not serve *consistently* to predict adherence to CPAP treatment. Many such studies have been developed on what Engleman and Wild term, the "use and need" model. Specifically, the authors suggest that the biomedical model of inquiry has contributed to identifying OSA patients likely to use and benefit from CPAP, but it has not similarly contributed to identifying patients with OSA who are at risk of stopping the treatment or being less than optimally adherent.

MOVING TOWARD A MULTIFACTORIAL, THEORY-BASED PERSPECTIVE

Recognizing that adherence to CPAP is a health behavior to which many factors likely contribute a theory-based approach has more recently been systematically examined to explain and predict adherence to CPAP. The incorporation of theoretical frameworks (i.e., transtheoretical model [TTM; Prochaska & DiClemente, 1983], active ways of coping [Lazarus & Folkman, 1984], social cognitive theory [SCT; Bandura, 1977]) has been suggested to guide future research on adherence to CPAP treatment. Stemming from conceptually driven inquiries about adherence to CPAP, cognitive perceptions are emerging as a more robust predictor of adherence and contributing to a new body of scientific work in adherence to CPAP (Aloia, Arnedt, Stepnowsky, Hecht, & Borrelli, 2005; Stepnowsky, Bardwell, Moore, Ancoli-Israel, & Dimsdale, 2002; Weaver et al., 2003; Weaver & Grunstein, 2008).

Weaver and colleagues (2003) have identified concepts derived from Bandura's SCT that may contribute to early adherence determination and be predictive of CPAP adherence outcomes, including "perceived risk,"

"outcome expectancies," and "self-efficacy," or perceptions of one's volition to use CPAP. The stimulus for this proposition stems from the development of an instrument, the Self-Efficacy Measure in Sleep Apnea (SEMSA; Weaver et al., 2003). Although yet untested as a predictor of CPAP adherence outcomes, Weaver and colleagues' perspective is consistent with published studies examining theoretical constructs as predictive of adherence, including the cognitive domains from SCT.

Stepnowsky, Bardwell, and associates (2002) built on SCT and the TTM to identify the following cognitive perception variables: outcome expectancies for CPAP, perceived self-efficacy, social support, knowledge, decisional balance, and individual utilization of change processes. Cognitive perception measures were timed at pretreatment exposure intervals and early treatment intervals (i.e., first week of treatment) in 23 CPAP-naive patients with OSA. Pretreatment cognitive perceptions were not associated with early CPAP use. At 1 week, self-efficacy, outcomes expectations, social support, and knowledge variables (SCT), and the decisional balance variable (TTM) were examined in a model including CPAP pressure and subjective sleepiness and found to be significantly associated with CPAP adherence, accounting for 38 and 31% of the variability in adherence, respectively. At 1 month, both SCT and TTM variables still played a statistically significant role in adherence (Stepnowsky, Bardwell, et al., 2002).

Aloia and colleagues (2005) conducted a prospective longitudinal study to determine the relative predictive utility of measures of behavior change principles on CPAP adherence among 98 subjects with moderate to severe OSA. Behavioral change principles, including readiness to change, perceived self-efficacy, and decisional balance, measured at 1 week, and CPAP treatment at 3 months predicted CPAP adherence at 6 months. Pretreatment measures of the same behavioral change principles were not predictive of CPAP adherence at 6 months (Aloia et al., 2005).

Collectively, these theory-derived correlates of adherence are behavioral change factors that are potentially modifiable risk factors for low CPAP adherence. Furthermore, this empirical line of inquiry has provided insight about the factors that influence the health behavior of adherence to CPAP. It is from this perspective that recent studies of adherence-promoting interventions have shown promise as influencing treatment adherence among patients with OSA.

INTERVENTION TO IMPROVE ADHERENCE

Relatively few published intervention studies have promoted adherence to CPAP. The majority of these studies have employed support, education, or, most recently, cognitive-behavioral strategies to influence CPAP adherence (Table 30.3). With a better understanding of salient factors that predict adherence to CPAP, recent studies have increasingly focused on adherence as a health behavior influenced by psychological, social, and cognitive factors. With this focus, several studies have incorporated theoretically derived interventions and identified improved adherence outcomes.

One of the earliest published intervention studies aimed at improving CPAP adherence was highly effective yet not cost-effective or practically applicable. Hoy, Vennelle, Kingshott, Engleman, and Douglas (1999) compared standard support with intensive support. Standard support was based on their usual care for newly diagnosed patients

TABLE 30.3. Intervention Study Strategies to Improve CPAP Adherence

Intervention strategy	Study	Design	Result: Change in CPAP adherence outcome
Support	Fletcher & Luckett (1991)	Crossover RCT	No
	Chervin et al. (1997)	RCT	No
	Hoy et al. (1999)	RCT	Yes (5.4 ± 0.3 vs. 3.8 ± 0.4 hours/night, intervention group vs. control group ($p = .003$)
	Hui et al. (2000)	RCT	No
	Palmer et al. (2004)	RCT	No
	DeMolles et al. (2004)	RCT	No
	Smith et al. (2006)	RCT	No
	Stepnowsky et al. (2007)	RCT	No
Education	Wiese et al. (2005)	RCT	No
	Golay et al. (2006)	RCT	No
	Meurice et al. (2007)	RCT	No
Cognitive-behavioral	Aloia et al. (2001)	RCT	Yes (experimental group with greater number of compliant CPAP users [$\chi^2 = 5.3$; $p < .03$])
	Richards et al. (2007)	RCT	Yes (average nightly use of CPAP CBT group higher than treatment-as-usual group at both 7 days and 28 days [$p < .0001$ and $p < .0001$, respectively])
	Aloia, Arnedt, Millman, et al. (2007)	RCT	Yes (standard of care group more likely to discontinue treatment [< 1-hour use for 2 weeks] [41%] than education group [30%] and motivational enhancement therapy group [26%]; $\chi^2 = 6.61$; $p = .04$. No other differences were identified for levels of CPAP use defined as > 4 hours/night for 2 weeks and > 6 hours/night for 2 weeks)

with OSA and included verbal explanation for CPAP treatment, a 20-minute educational video, a 20-minute acclimatization to CPAP during waking hours, one-night CPAP titration in the laboratory, and telephone follow-up on Day 2 and Day 21 of treatment, followed by clinical visits at 1, 3, and 6 months. Intensive support included the standard support, with CPAP education provided in subjects' homes with partners, two additional nights of CPAP titration in the sleep center for CPAP troubleshooting during initial CPAP exposure, and home visits by sleep nurses at Days 7, 14, and 28, and at 4 months. The intervention strategy combined support, education, and the concept of self-efficacy promotion through the initial CPAP exposure under supervised conditions. Although Hoy's group identified significant improvement in CPAP adherence at 6 months (5.4 ± 0.3 hours/night vs. 3.8 ± 0.4 hours/night, intensive vs. standard support, respectively; $p = .003$), the applicability of the intervention to clinical practice is limited because the intervention is labor- and time-intensive. Furthermore, in the current climate of limited health care resources, particularly for sleep diagnostics, this intervention strategy is not cost-effective nor does it promote access to sleep services. The study does reflect the importance of addressing adherence from a multidimensional perspective and highlights the importance of education, experiences during initial exposure to CPAP, and social support (i.e., partner or spouse) in patients' decisions to use CPAP and persist with the treatment.

Other early intervention studies incorporated the concept of support as an intervention strategy to influence adherence. Early studies reporting supportive interventions to promote CPAP adherence compared positive reinforcement with usual care (Chervin, Theut, Bassetti, & Aldrich, 1997; Fletcher & Luckett, 1991; Hui et al., 2000). Although these studies varied the timing of intervention delivery and the mechanism of support (i.e., phone call, printed documents, clinical follow-up), there were no differences in CPAP adherence between experimental and control groups. With the advancement of technology, more recent supportive intervention studies have used telecommunications mechanisms of delivery (DeMolles,

Sparrow, Gottlieb, & Friedman, 2004; Smith et al., 2006; Stepnowsky, Palau, Marler, & Gifford, 2007). Both DeMolles and colleagues (2004) and Stepnowsky and colleagues (2007) used telecommunications interventions with CPAP-naive subjects, monitoring CPAP use and providing feedback (reinforcement) and supportive information in response to the telemonitored pattern of CPAP use. Although both studies reported no differences in CPAP adherence at 2 months, there was improvement in adherence in the treatment group, though it was not statistically significant (4.4 hours/night vs. 2.9 hours/night, $p = .076$; 4.1 hours/night vs. 2.8 hours/night, $p = .07$, respectively). It is possible that both pilot studies were underpowered to detect differences between the groups and with a larger sample size, this intervention would positively influence CPAP adherence.

Smith and colleagues (2006) found that CPAP users who were exposed to a telecommunications intervention after their first 3 months demonstrated significantly greater CPAP use at 12 weeks than the control group ($\chi^2 = 4.55$, $p = .033$). Adherence to CPAP was analyzed as a dichotomous variable: greater than 4 hours/night on 9 of 14 nights (80% use rate) or less than 4 hours/night or less than 9/14 nights of CPAP use (< 80% use rate). All subjects were experienced CPAP users who had demonstrated poor adherence to the treatment in the first 3 months. Although statistically significant differences were identified, the sampling technique of self-selection may have biased the findings. Furthermore, these subjects were not CPAP-naive; this study is one of the first published adherence intervention studies to focus on experienced, nonadherent CPAP users, and it is not known whether adherence interventions affect experienced CPAP users, or whether this group may be affected differently by such interventions compared to CPAP-naive patients.

These intervention studies suggest that supportive, simplistic, unidirectional (provider to patient; investigator to participant) reinforcement of CPAP use is not adequate to improve overall adherence rates to CPAP. However, when combined with real-time assessment of CPAP use (CPAP adherence records) and support for problem-solving or troubleshooting difficulties with CPAP, supportive interventions may be useful in promoting adherence to CPAP.

Although education is clinically recognized as an essential part of treating OSA with CPAP, education-alone interventions have not been extensively examined in the literature. Three clinical trials (Golay et al., 2007; Meurice et al., 2007; Wiese, Boethel, Phillips, Wilson, Peters, & Viggiano, 2005), using three different educational strategies, have been published to date, each of which identified no significant difference in adherence outcomes among CPAP users. The largest study, conducted in France (Meurice et al., 2007), compared three different educational interventions with standard education in 112 severe OSA, CPAP-naive participants. The educational interventions were (1) reinforced education by both prescriber and home care provider; (2) reinforced education by prescriber and standard care by the home care provider; (3) standard education by prescriber and reinforced education by the home care provider; and (4) the control group, which received standard education by both the prescriber and the home care provider. The content of the reinforced educational interventions differed from the standard educational interventions by an increased frequency of delivery (reinforced education) and by the expansiveness of explanation and demonstration (reinforced education). CPAP adherence was measured at 3, 6, and 12 months, without statistically significant differences between intervention groups compared with the control group (Meurice et al., 2007). The overall, average adherence for all groups at 3 months and 6 months was 5.6 hours/night and 5.8 hours/night at 12 months (nonsignificant). As evidenced by the high adherence rates across all groups, both groups included relatively few nonadherers, which may have contributed to the absence of an intervention effect. It is also not known whether the educational intervention enhanced participants' knowledge of their diagnosis and treatment because no direct measure of knowledge was reported. Participants may not have gained any direct benefit from the intended educational intervention.

In a smaller study of 35 patients with severe OSA, Golay and colleagues (2006) sought to evaluate a newly developed, interdisciplinary educational intervention for CPAP users. Applying a variety of educational strategies (i.e., video, demonstration, discussion), some of which were based on the health belief model (Rosenstock, 1966), participants and their spouses participated in a 1-day program, followed by a single night of in-hospital CPAP exposure. Participants in the study had used CPAP on average for 1 year. Following participation in the educational program, CPAP adherence, measured 3 months after intervention, did not differ from baseline (Golay et al., 2006). In this pilot study, likely underpowered to detect differences in adherence to CPAP, there was a trend toward higher CPAP adherence after the intervention. The cost-effectiveness of the intervention, however, must be addressed because the utility of this intervention may be limited by personnel, time, and patient burden costs.

Wiese and colleagues (2005) examined a more simplistic educational intervention, a 15-minute videotaped program delivered to patients with mild OSA. The content of the videotaped intervention defined OSA, described symptoms of OSA, CPAP, and the sensation of wearing CPAP, and the benefits of using CPAP. After randomization to treatment group, the experimental group (N = 51) was exposed to the videotaped educational intervention after an initial clinical visit with a sleep provider, and the control group (N = 49) completed the initial clinical visit and a set of questionnaires. CPAP use for participants who returned for a 4-week follow-up visit was not associated with treatment group (Wiese et al., 2005). Rate of follow-up, however, was associated with the videotaped educational program, with 72.9% of the experimental group versus 48.9% of the control group returning for follow-up (χ^2 = 5.65; p = .017) (Wiese et al., 2005). A simple videotaped educational program may reduce attrition at clinical follow-up, yet it is not clear that CPAP adherence improves with this educational strategy.

Collectively, educational interventions alone do not influence future use of CPAP among patients with OSA. It is not clear from this small group of studies that the intervention influenced the mediating variable of interest, knowledge, because none of the studies measured this variable. Instead, the studies examined the outcome of CPAP adherence, or return to clinic, as a surrogate outcome, with the underlying assumption that CPAP adherence is amenable to influence through the process of knowledge acquisition. As Bandura (2004) describes it, knowledge is a precondition for health behavior or change in health behavior. Knowledge alone, however, is unlikely to produce exacting healthful behaviors (Bandura, 2004).

A strategy of intervention that has shown significant promise in improving adherence to CPAP is cognitive-behavioral intervention. Prediction studies examining cognitive-behavioral variables as correlates of CPAP use have provided a critically important understanding of measurable constructs from which interventions have been developed (Aloia et al., 2005; Stepnowsky, Bardwell, et al., 2002; Stepnowsky, Marler, & Ancoli-Israel, 2002; Wild, Engleman, Douglas, & Espie, 2004). Although limited in number, these intervention studies provide some consistency with regard to influencing actual acceptance of and persistence with CPAP treatment.

The earliest study to examine cognitive-behavioral intervention strategies, published in 2001, was a pilot randomized clinical trial in older adults, naive to CPAP, with OSA (Aloia et al., 2001). The intervention group received two 45 minute sessions, one-on-one, wherein subject-specific information about OSA, symptoms, performance on cognitive tests, treatment relevance, goal development, symptom change with CPAP, troubleshooting advice, treatment expectations, and treatment goal refinement were provided. Theoretically, the investigators suggested that by providing individual specific education and information that influences self-efficacy and decisional balance, adherence to CPAP would be enhanced (Aloia et al., 2001). The control group received a placebo intervention consisting of two 45-minute sessions, in which general information about sleep, sleep architecture, and patient opinions regarding sleep clinic experience were discussed. At 1 week and at 4 weeks, there was no difference in CPAP use between the groups ($p = .48$ and $p = .22$, respectively). At 12 weeks, the experimental group used CPAP for 3.2 hours more than the control

group ($p < .04$) with a large effect size ($d = 1.27$). This small pilot study suggests that an intervention based on cognitive-behavioral constructs potentially influences CPAP adherence behaviors over time.

In a larger, randomized controlled trial, Aloia, Arnedt, Millman, and colleagues (2007) applied the same intervention strategy, focusing on education to promote self-efficacy and decisional balance compared with motivational enhancement therapy and usual standard of care. Interventions were delivered after 1 week of CPAP use. Both motivational enhancement therapy and education groups had lower discontinuation rates over the 13-week protocol than did the standard of care group ($\chi^2 = 6.62$; $p < .05$) (Aloia, Arnedt, Millman, et al., 2007). There were no differences in higher levels of CPAP use (i.e., > 4 hours/night, > 6 hours/night) among the groups. Together with Aloia and colleagues' earlier work (2001), these cognitive-behavioral interventions may influence the overall risk of very poor adherence (i.e., ≤ 1 hour/night) and abandonment of the treatment altogether.

Richards, Bartlett, Wong, Malouff, and Grunstein (2007) similarly identified that "uptake" or acceptance of CPAP treatment was greater among their experimental group, which received two 1-hour CBT sessions at baseline (i.e., prior to CPAP titration in the sleep center), compared with usual care ($p < .02$). In this randomized controlled trial of 100 moderately severe subjects with OSA, the intervention group did exhibit higher CPAP adherence both at 1 week and at 1 month than the control group (5.90 hours/night vs. 2.97 hours/night, $p < .0001$; 5.38 hours/night vs. 2.51 hours/night, $p < .0001$, respectively). These investigators also demonstrated that the specific cognitive-behavioral variables of interest, self-efficacy ($p < .0001$) and social support ($p < .008$) but not outcome expectations ($p = .60$), differed between the groups as well, suggesting that the outcome of interest, adherence to CPAP, increased as a result of the cognitive-behavioral intervention.

Empirical studies of interventions to promote adherence to CPAP have provided some insight into both theoretical underpinnings and interventions that may likely affect CPAP-treated patients' patterns and overall use of the treatment. The complexity in addressing adherence is notably significant. Some of the most promising, recent research suggests that psychological correlates (i.e., risk perception, decision making, self-efficacy) are not only predictive of CPAP adherence but also are amenable to intervention, as is suggested by the cognitive-behavioral intervention studies. Furthermore, although intervention studies do not identify educational interventions as independently effective in promoting adherence, knowledge is widely recognized as imperative to health behaviors (Bandura, 2004). With more empirical studies emerging that address the phenomenon of adherence to treatment of OSA, a more dynamic understanding of this complex health behavior is permitted. Although much of the scientific work to date has been in the area of adherence to CPAP, it may be possible to broadly apply the underlying theoretical constructs to adherence behaviors across the disorders of sleep that are treated by an increasingly interdisciplinary practice of sleep medicine.

Conclusions

Over the past half-century, scientists and practitioners have made significant contributions to our current understanding of normal sleep, the functions of sleep and sleep loss, and sleep disorders. The complex nature of achieving a healthy "dose" of sleep, coupled with the demands of a 24-hour society, has necessitated an increasingly interdisciplinary approach to the study of sleep and treatment of sleep disorders. Behavioral specialists are critically important to the successful management of many sleep disorders, including promoting and maintaining adherence to treatments that are often challenging. Through multidisciplinary sleep centers that include behavioral specialists, patients receive medical care and management strategies for dyssomnias. As a result of this interdisciplinary approach, health, functional, and quality of life outcomes in sleep disorder patients are further enhanced and cross-discipline empirical study of sleep and sleep disorders will contribute to our ongoing pursuit of understanding and promoting normal sleep.

Further Reading

Normal Sleep and Sleep Regulation

Banks, S., & Dinges, D. F. (2007). Behavioral and physiological consequences of sleep restriction. *Journal of Clinical Sleep Medicine*, 3(5), 519–528.

Borbely, A. A., & Achermann, P. (1999). Sleep homeostasis and models of sleep regulation. *Journal of Biological Rhythms*, 14(6), 559–570.

Zee, P. C., & Manthena, P. (2007). The brain's master circadian clock: Implication and opportunities for therapy of sleep disorders. *Sleep Medicine Reviews*, 11, 59–70.

Circadian Rhythm Disorders

Sack, R. L., Auckley, D., Auger, R. R., Carskadon, M. A., Wright, K. P., Vitiello, M. V., et al. (2007). Circadian rhythm sleep disorders: Part I. Basic principles, shift work, and jet lag disorders. *Sleep*, 30, 1460–1483.

Sack, R. L., Auckley, D., Auger, R. R., Carskadon, M. A., Wright, K. P., Vitiello, M. V., et al. (2007). Circadian rhythm sleep disorders: Part II. Advanced sleep phase disorder, delayed sleep phase disorder, free-running disorder, and irregular sleep–wake rhythm. *Sleep*, 30, 1484–1501.

Insomnia

Harvey, A. G., Tang, N. K. Y., & Browning, L. (2005). Cognitive approaches to insomnia. *Clinical Psychology Review*, 25, 593–611.

Morin, C. M., Bootzin, R. R., Buysse, D. J., Edinger, J. D., Espie, C. A., & Lichstein, K. L. (2006). Psychological and behavioral treatment of insomnia: Update of the recent evidence (1998–2004). *Sleep*, 29, 1398–1414.

Wang, M.-Y., Wang, S.-Y., & Tsai, P.-S. (2005). Cognitive behavioural therapy for primary insomnia: A systematic review. *Journal of Advanced Nursing*, 50, 553–564.

Sleep-Disordered Breathing: Adherence to CPAP

Gay, P., Weaver, T. E., Loube, D., & Iber, C. (2006). Evaluation of positive airway pressure treatment for sleep related breathing disorders in adults. *Sleep*, 29, 381–401.

Haniffa, M., Lasserson, T. J., & Smith, I. (2005). Interventions to improve compliance with continuous positive airway pressure for obstructive sleep apnoea. *Cochrane Database System Reviews*, Issue 3 (Article No. CD003531), DOI: 10.1002/14651858.CD003531.pub3.

Weaver, T. E., & Sawyer, A. (2009). Management of obstructive sleep apnea by continuous positive airway pressure. *Oral Maxillofacial Surgery Clinics of North America, 21*(4), 403–412.

Weaver, T. E., & Sawyer, A. (2010). Adherence to continuous positive airway pressure treatment for obstructive sleep apnea: Current state of the science and implications for future intervention research. *Indian Journal of Medical Research, 131,* 245–258.

References

Aloia, M. S., Arnedt, J. T., Millman, R. P., Stanchina, M., Carlisle, C., Hecht, J., et al. (2007). Brief behavioral therapies reduce early positive airway pressure discontinuation rates in sleep apnea syndrome: Preliminary findings. *Behavioral Sleep Medicine, 5,* 89–104.

Aloia, M. S., Arnedt, J. T., Stanchina, M., & Millman, R. P. (2007). How early in treatment is PAP adherence established?: Revisiting night-to-night variability. *Behavioral Sleep Medicine, 5,* 229–240.

Aloia, M. S., Arnedt, J., Stepnowsky, C., Hecht, J., & Borrelli, B. (2005). Predicting treatment adherence in obstructive sleep apnea using principles of behavior change. *Journal of Clinical Sleep Medicine, 1*(4), 346–353.

Aloia, M. S., Di Dio, L., Ilniczky, N., Perlis, M. L., Greenblatt, D. W., & Giles, D. E. (2001). Improving compliance with nasal CPAP and vigilance in older adults with OAHS. *Sleep and Breathing, 5*(1), 13–21.

Bandura, A. (1977). Self-efficacy: Toward a unifying theory of behavioral change. *Psychology Reviews, 84,* 191–215.

Bandura, A. (2004). Health promotion by social cognitive means. *Health Education and Behavior, 31,* 143–164.

Banks, S., & Dinges, D. F. (2007). Behavioral and physiological consequences of sleep restriction. *Journal of Clinical Sleep Medicine, 3*(5), 519–528.

Bootzin, R. R. (1972). A stimulus control treatment for insomnia. *Proceedings of the American Psychological Association, 7,* 395–396.

Borbely, A. A., & Achermann, P. (1999). Sleep homeostasis and models of sleep regulation. *Journal of Biological Rhythms, 14*(6), 559–570.

Carskadon, M. A., & Dement, W. C. (2000). Normal human sleep: An overview. In M. H. Kryger, T. Roth, & W. C. Dement (Eds.), *Principles and practice of sleep medicine* (3rd ed., pp. 15–25). Philadelphia: Saunders.

Chervin, R. D., Theut, S., Bassetti, C., & Aldrich, M. S. (1997). Compliance with nasal CPAP can be improved by simple interventions. *Sleep, 20,* 284–289.

Chesson, A., Ferber, R., Fry, J., Grigg-Damberger, M., Hartse, K., Hurwitz, T., et al. (1997). Practice parameters for the indications for polysomnography and related procedures. *Sleep, 20,* 406–422.

Dement, W. C. (2000). History of sleep physiology and medicine. In M. H. Kryger, T. Roth, & W. C. Dement (Eds.), *Principles and practice of sleep medicine* (3rd ed., pp. 1–25). Philadelphia: Saunders.

DeMolles, D. A., Sparrow, D., Gottlieb, D. J., & Friedman, R. (2004). A pilot trial of a telecommunications system in sleep apnea management. *Medical Care, 42,* 764–769.

Dinges, D., Pack, F., Williams, K., Gillen, K., Powell, J., Ott, G., et al. (1997). Cumulative sleepiness, mood disturbance, and psychomotoer vigilance performance decrements during a week of sleep restricted to 4–5 hours per night. *Sleep, 20,* 267–277.

Edinger, J. D., Wohlgemuth, W. K., Radtke, R. A., Marsh, G. R., & Quillian, R. E. (2001). Cognitive behavioral therapy for treatment of chronic primary insomnia: A randomized controlled trial. *Journal of American Medical Association, 285,* 1856–1864.

Engleman, H. M., Asgari-Jirandeh, N., McLeod, A. L., Ramsay, C. F., Deary, I. J., & Douglas, N. J. (1996). Self-reported use of CPAP and benefits of CPAP therapy. *Chest, 109,* 1470–1476.

Engleman, H. M., Martin, S. E., & Douglas, N. J. (1994). Compliance with CPAP therapy in patients with the sleep apnoea/hypopnoea syndrome. *Thorax, 49,* 263–266.

Engleman, H. M., & Wild, M. (2003). Improving CPAP use by patients with the sleep apnoea/hypopnoea syndrome (SAHS). *Sleep Medicine Reviews, 7*(1), 81–99.

Fletcher, E. C., & Luckett, R. A. (1991). The effect of positive reinforcement on hourly compliance in nasal continuous positive airway pressure users with obstructive sleep apnea. *American Reviews in Respiratory Disease, 143,* 936–941.

Golay, A., Girard, A., Grandin, S., Metrailler, J.-C., Victorion, M., Lebas, P., et al. (2006). A new educational program for patients suffering from sleep apnea syndrome. *Patient Education and Counseling, 60,* 220–227.

Grunstein, R. R., Stewart, D. A., Lloyd, H., Akinci, M., Cheng, N., & Sullivan, C. E. (1996). Acute withdrawal of nasal CPAP in obstructive sleep apnea does not cause a rise in stress hormones. *Sleep, 19*(10), 774–782.

Harris, C. D. (2005). Neurophysiology of sleep and wakefulness. *Respiratory Care Clinics of North America, 11,* 567–586.

Harsch, I. A., Schahin, S. P., Radespiel-Troger, M., Weintz, O., Jahreib, H., Fuchs, F. S., et al. (2004). CPAP treatment rapidly improves insulin sensitivity in patients with obstructive sleep apnea syndrome. *American Journal of Respiratory and Critical Care Medicine, 169,* 156–162.

Harvey, A. G., Tang, N. K. Y., & Browning, L. (2005). Cognitive approaches to insomnia. *Clinical Psychology Review, 25,* 593–611.

Hauri, P. J. (2000). Primary insomnia. In M. H. Kryger, T. Roth, & W. C. Dement (Eds.), *Principles and practice of sleep medicine* (3rd ed., pp. 633–639). Philadelphia: Saunders.

Hoy, C. J., Vennelle, M., Kingshott, R. N., Engleman, H. M., & Douglas, N. J. (1999). Can intensive support improve continuous positive airway pressure use in patients with the sleep apnea/hypopnea syndrome? *American Journal of Respiratory and Critical Care Medicine, 159,* 1096–1100.

Hui, D., Chan, J., Choy, D., Ko, F., Li, T., Leung, R., et al. (2000). Effects of augmented continuous positive airway pressure education and support on compliance and outcome in a Chinese population. *Chest, 117,* 1410–1416.

Hui, D., Choy, D., Li, T., Ko, F., Wong, K., Chan, J., et al. (2001). Determinants of continuous positive airway pressure compliance in a group of Chinese patients with obstructive sleep apnea. *Chest, 120,* 170–176.

Kribbs, N. B., Pack, A. I., Kline, L. R., Smith, P. L., Schwartz, A. R., Schubert, N. M., et al. (1993). Objective measurement of patterns of nasal CPAP use by patients with obstructive sleep apnea. *American Reviews in Respiratory Diseases, 147,* 887–895.

Krieger, J. (1992). Long-term compliance with nasal continuous positive airway pressure (CPAP) in obstructive sleep apnea patients and nonapneic snorers. *Sleep, 15*(Suppl. 6), S42–S46.

Lack, L. C., & Wright, H. R. (2007). Clinical management of delayed sleep phase disorder. *Behavioral Sleep Medicine, 5,* 57–76.

Lazarus, R., & Folkman, S. (1984). Coping and adaptation. In W. Gentry (Ed.), *The handbook of behavioral medicine* (pp. 282–325). New York: Guilford Press.

Lichstein, K. L., Riedel, B. W., Wilson, N. M., Lester, K. W., & Aguillard, R. N. (2001). Relaxation and sleep compression for late-life insomnia: A placebo controlled trial. *Journal of Consulting and Clinical Psychology, 69,* 227–239.

Lichstein, K. L., Wilson, N. M., & Johnson, C. T. (2000). Psychological treatment of secondary insomnia. *Psychology and Aging, 15*(2), 232–240.

Markov, D., & Goldman, M. (2006). Normal sleep and circadian rhythms: Neurobiologic mechanisms underlying sleep and wakefulness. *Psychiatric Clinics of North America, 29,* 841–853.

Massie, C., Hart, R., Peralez, K., & Richards, G. (1999). Effects of humidification on nasal symptoms and compliance in sleep apnea patients using continuous positive airway pressure. *Chest, 116,* 403–408.

McArdle, N., Devereux, G., Heidarnejad, H., Engleman, H., Mackay, T., & Douglas, N. (1999). Long-term use of CPAP therapy for sleep apnea/hypopnea syndrome. *American Journal of Respiratory and Critical Care Medicine, 159,* 1108–1114.

Means, M. K., Lichstein, K. L., Epperson, M. T., & Johnson, C. T. (2000). Relaxation therapy for insomnia: Nighttime and daytime effects. *Behaviour Research and Therapy, 38,* 665–678.

Meurice, J. C., Dore, P., Paquereau, J., Neau, J. P., Ingrand, P., Chavagnat, J. J., et al. (1994). Predictive factors of long-term compliance with nasal continuous positive airway pressure treatment in sleep apnea syndrome. *Chest, 105*(2), 429–434.

Meurice, J.-C., Ingrand, P., Portier, F., Arnulf, I., Rakotonanahari, D., Fournier, E., et al. (2007). A multicentre trial of education strategies at CPAP induction in the treatment of severe sleep apnoea–hypopnoea syndrome. *Sleep Medicine, 8,* 37–42.

Morgan, K., Dixon, S., Mathers, N., Thompson, J., & Tomeny, M. (2003). Psychological treatment for insomnia in the management of long-term hypnotic drug use: A pragmatic randomized controlled trial. *British Journal of General Practice, 53,* 923–928.

Morgenthaler, T., Kramer, M., Alessi, C., Friedman, L., Boehlecke, B., Brown, T., et al. (2006). Practice parameters for the psychological and behavioral treatment of insomnia: An update. *Sleep, 29,* 1415–1419.

Morgenthaler, T., Lee-Chiong, T., Alessi, C., Friedman, L., Aurora, R. N., Boehlecke, B., et al. (2007). Practice parameters for the clinical evaluation and treatment of circadian rhythm sleep disorders. *Sleep, 30,* 1445–1459.

Morin, C. M., Bastien, C., Guay, B., Radouco-Thomas, M., Leblanc, J., & Vallieres, A. (2004). Randomized clinical trial of supervised tapering and cognitive behavior therapy to facilitate benzodiazepine discontinuation in older adults with chronic insomnia. *American Journal of Psychiatry, 161,* 332–342.

Morin, C. M., Bootzin, R. R., Buysse, D. J., Edinger, J. D., Espie, C. A., & Lichstein, K. L. (2006). Psychological and behavioral treatment of insomnia: Update of the recent evidence (1998–2004). *Sleep, 29*(11), 1398–1414.

National Institutes of Health. (2003, March). *Effects of sleep disorders and sleep restriction on adherence to cardiovascular and other disease treatment regimens: Research needs* (NTIS No. PB2007106839). Bethesda, MD: Author.

National Sleep Foundation. (2009). Healthy sleep tips. Retrieved January 11, 2010, from *www.sleepfoundation.org/article/sleep-topics/healthy-sleep-tips*.

Nieto, F. J., Young, T. B., Lind, B. K., Shahar, E., Samet, J. M., Redline, S., et al. (2000). Association of sleep-disordered breathing, sleep apnea, and hypertension in a large community-based study. *Journal of the American Medical Association, 283,* 1829–1836.

Pallesen, S., Nordhus, I. H., Kvale, G., Nielson, G. H., Havik, O. E., Johnsen, B. H., et al. (2003). Behavioral treatment of insomnia in older adults: An open clinical trial comparing two interventions. *Behaviour Research and Therapy, 41,* 31–48.

Palmer, S., Selvaraj, S., Dunn, C., Osman, L. M., Cairns, J., Franklin, D., et al. (2004). Annual review of patients with sleep apnea/hypopnea syndrome: A pragmatic randomized trial of nurse home visit versus consultant clinic review. *Sleep Medicine, 5*(1), 61–65.

Peppard, P. E., Young, T., Palta, M., & Skatrud, J. (2000). Prospective study of the association between sleep-disordered breathing and hypertension. *New England Journal of Medicine, 342,* 1378–1384.

Perlis, M., Smith, M. T., Orff, H., Enright, T., Nowakowski, S. Jungquist, C., et al. (2004). The effects of modafanil and cognitive behavior therapy on sleep continuity in patients with chronic insomnia. *Sleep, 27,* 715–725.

Pilcher, J. J., & Huffcutt, A. I. (1996). Effects of sleep deprivation on performance: A meta-analysis. *Sleep, 19*(4), 318–326.

Prochaska, J. O., & DiClemente, C. C. (1983). Stages and processes of self-change of smoking: Toward an integrative model of change. *Journal of Consultative Clinical Psychology, 51,* 390–395.

Rauscher, H., Formanek, D., Popp, W., & Zwick, H. (1993). Self-reported vs. measured compliance with nasal CPAP for obstructive sleep apnea. *Chest, 103*(6), 1675–1671.

Reeves-Hoche, M. K., Meck, R., & Zwillich, C. W. (1994). Nasal CPAP: An objective evaluation of patient compliance. *American Journal of Respiratory and Critical Care Medicine, 149,* 149–154.

Reid, K. J., & Burgess, H. J. (2005). Circadian rhythm sleep disorders. *Primary Care Clinics in Office Practice, 32,* 449–473.

Richards, D., Bartlett, D. J., Wong, K., Malouff, J., & Grunstein, R. R. (2007). Increased adherence to CPAP with a group cognitive behavioral treatment intervention: A randomized trial. *Sleep, 30,* 635–640.

Rolfe, I., Olson, L. G., & Saunders, N. A. (1991). Long-term acceptance of continuous positive airway pressure in obstructive sleep apnea. *American Reviews in Respiratory Diseases, 144,* 1130–1133.

Rosenstock, I. M. (1966). Why people use health services. *Millbank Memorial Fund Quarterly, 44*(3, Pt. 2), 94–127.

Rosenthal, L., Gerhardstein, R., Lumley, A., Guido, P., Day, R., Syron, M. L., et al. (2000). CPAP therapy in patients with mild OSA: Implementation and treatment outcome. *Sleep Medicine, 1,* 215–220.

Rybarczyk, B., Lopez, M., Benson, R., Alsten, C., & Stepanski, E. (2002). Efficacy of two behavioral treatment programs for comorbid geriatric insomnia. *Psychology and Aging, 17,* 288–298.

Rybarczyk, B., Stepanski, E., Fogg, L., Lopez, M., Barry, P., & Davis, A. (2005). A placebo-controlled test of cognitive-behavioral therapy for comorbid insomnia in older adults. *Journal of Consulting and Clinical Psychology, 73,* 1164–1174.

Sack, R. L., Auckley, D., Auger, R., Carskadon, M. A., Wright, K. P., Vitiello, M. V., et al. (2007a). Circadian rhythm sleep disorders: Part I. Basic principles, shift work, and jet lag disorders. *Sleep, 30,* 1460–1483.

Sack, R. L., Auckley, D., Auger, R., Carskadon, M. A., Wright, K. P., Vitiello, M. V., et al. (2007b). Circadian rhythm sleep disorders: Part II. Advanced sleep phase disorder, delayed sleep phase disorder, free-running disorder, and irregular sleep–wake rhythm. *Sleep, 30,* 1484–1501.

Sanders, M. H., Gruendl, C. A., & Rogers, R. M. (1986). Patient compliance with nasal CPAP therapy for sleep apnea. *Chest, 90*(3), 330–333.

Schweitzer, P., Chambers, G., Birkenmeier, N., & Walsh, J. (1987). Nasal continuous positive airway pressure (CPAP) compliance at six, twelve, and eighteen months. *Sleep Research, 16,* 186.

Sin, D., Mayers, I., Man, G., & Pawluk, L. (2002). Long-term compliance rates to continuous positive airway pressure in obstructive sleep apnea: A population-based study. *Chest, 121,* 430–435.

Smith, C. E., Dauz, E. R., Clements, F., Puno, F. N., Cook, D., Doolittle, G., et al. (2006). Telehealth services to improve nonadherence: A placebo-controlled study. *Telemedicine and e-Health, 12,* 289–296.

Stepnowsky, C., Bardwell, W. A., Moore, P. J., Ancoli-Israel, S., & Dimsdale, J. E. (2002). Psychologic correlates of compliance with continuous positive airway pressure. *Sleep, 25*(7), 758–762.

Stepnowsky, C. J., Marler, M. R., & Ancoli-Israel, S. (2002). Determinants of nasal CPAP compliance. *Sleep Medicine, 3*, 239–247.

Stepnowsky, C. J., Palau, J. J., Marler, M. R., & Gifford, A. L. (2007). Pilot randomized trial of the effect of wireless telemonitoring on compliance and treatment efficacy of obstructive sleep apnea. *Journal of Medical Internet Research, 9*(2), e14.

Sullivan, C. E., & Grunstein, R. R. (1989). Continuous positive airway pressure in sleep-disordered breathing. In M. H. Kryger, T. Roth, & W. E. Dement (Eds.), *Principles and practice of sleep medicine* (pp. 559–570). Philadelphia: Saunders.

Sullivan, C. E., Issa, F. G., Berthon-Jones, M., & Eves, L. (1981). Reversal of obstructive sleep apnoea by continuous positive airway pressure applied through the nares. *Lancet, 1*, 862–865.

Thorpy, M. J. (2000). Classification of sleep disorders. In M. H. Kryger, T. Roth, & W. C. Dement (Eds.), *Principles and practice of sleep medicine* (3rd ed., pp. 547–557). Philadelphia: Saunders.

Turek, F. W. (2000). Introduction to chronobiology: Sleep and the circadian clock. In M. H. Kryger, T. Roth, & W. C. Dement (Eds.), *Principles and practice of sleep medicine* (3rd ed., pp. 319–320). Philadelphia: Saunders.

Van Dongen, H. P. A., Maislin, G., Mullington, J. M., & Dinges, D. F. (2003). The cumulative cost of additional wakefulness: Dose-response effects on neurobehavioral functions and sleep physiology from chronic sleep restriction and total sleep deprivation. *Sleep, 26*(2), 117–126.

Viens, M., De Koninck, J., Mercier, P., St. Onge, M., & Lorrain, D. (2003). Trait anxiety and sleep-onset insomnia: Evaluation of treatment using anxiety management training. *Journal of Psychosomatic Research, 54*, 31–37.

Wang, M.-Y., Wang, S.-Y., & Tsai, P.-S. (2005). Cognitive behavioural therapy for primary insomnia: A systematic review. *Journal of Advanced Nursing, 50*, 553–564.

Waters, W. F., Hurry, M. J., Binks, P. G., Carney, C. E., Lajos, L. E., Fuller, K. H., et al. (2003). Behavioral and hypnotic treatments for insomnia subtypes. *Behavioral Sleep Medicine, 1*, 81–101.

Weaver, T., Honbo, B., Maislin, G., Chugh, D., Mahowald, M., Kader, G., et al. (1999). Improvement in affect after 3-month CPAP: Multicenter study. *American Journal of Respiratory and Critical Care Medicine, 159*, A770.

Weaver, T. E., & Grunstein, R. R. (2008). Adherence to continuous positive airway pressure therapy: The challenge to effective treatment. *Proceedings of the American Thoracic Society, 5*(2), 173–178.

Weaver, T. E., Kribbs, N. B., Pack, A. I., Kline, L. R., Chugh, D. K., Maislin, G., et al. (1997). Night-to-night variability in CPAP use over first three months of treatment. *Sleep, 20*, 278–283.

Weaver, T. E., Maislin, G., Dinges, D. F., Younger, J., Cantor, C., McCloskey, S., et al. (2003). Self-efficacy in sleep apnea: Instrument development and patient perceptions of obstructive sleep apnea risk, treatment benefit, and volition to use continuous positive airway pressure. *Sleep, 26*, 727–732.

Wiese, H. J., Boethel, C., Phillips, B., Wilson, J. F., Peters, J., & Viggiano, T. (2005). CPAP compliance: Video education may help! *Sleep Medicine, 6*, 171–174.

Wild, M. R., Engleman, H. M., Douglas, N. J., & Espie, C. A. (2004). Can psychological factors help us to determine adherence to CPAP?: A prospective study. *European Respiratory Journal, 24*, 461–465.

Yang, C.-M., Spielman, A. J., & Glovinsky, P. (2006). Nonpharmacologic strategies in the management of insomnia. *Psychiatric Clinics of North America, 29*, 895–919.

Zee, P. C., & Manthena, P. (2007). The brain's master circadian clock: Implications and opportunities for therapy of sleep disorders. *Sleep Medicine Reviews, 11*, 59–70.

CHAPTER 31

Psychosocial Interventions for Patients with Cancer

Michael A. Diefenbach
Nihal E. Mohamed
Gina Turner
Catherine S. Diefenbach

Cancer is a serious health threat, with an expected 1,479,350 new cancer cases in the United States in 2009 (and about 562,340 expected deaths—more than 1,500 people a day), and worldwide deaths of 7.6 million people in 2007. With the growth and aging of the population, worldwide deaths are expected to rise to 17.5 million by 2050 (American Cancer Society, 2009). Despite increasing efforts by researchers worldwide to eradicate the disease, cancer rates have not been reduced as much as was hoped when President Nixon declared the "War on Cancer" on December 23, 1971, when he signed the National Cancer Act.

Cancer not only affects the physical self but also impacts the psychological self and reduces the well-being of patients and their family members. To address these issues, behavioral scientists have developed numerous interventions to assist patients in their effort to cope with the clinical and psychological sequelae of the disease and its treatment. A majority of interventions aims to lessen the emotional impact of cancer, particularly anxiety and depression. A recent summary of this literature by Jacobsen and Jim (2008) comprehensively focuses on the systematic reviews and meta-analyses that have evaluated evidence-based interventions designed to decrease anxiety and depression among cancer patients.

Building on Jacobson and Jim's (2008) excellent review, this chapter provides an overview of the most important psychosocial issues covering the cancer continuum from diagnosis and treatment to survivorship. Overall findings indicate a great heterogeneity in intervention approaches, with successes in psychoeducation, problem solving, stress management training, and cognitive-behavioral approaches delivered either to groups or to single patients. However, Jacobson and Jim also noted areas of weakness in the current literature; they found that conclusions are restricted because most studies are based on samples of patients with several different types of cancer. Very few studies are limited to a single form of cancer (except for breast cancer). Another methodological limitation is that over 70% of studies reviewed did not include or focus on specific disease stages of cancer, thus restricting overall conclusions that can be drawn from the existing literature. To address this shortcoming we focus the current review on studies examining the most prevalent cancers (American Cancer Society, 2009) among men and women (i.e., prostate, breast, and lung cancer).

To review the literature exhaustively for the three types of cancer would require separate chapters for each; instead, we focus on publications that provide Level I and Level II evidence for each cancer and phases of the disease. This evidence rating system is based on the recommendations for interventions studies by the Standing Committee on Quality of Care and Health Outcomes (QCHOC) of the National Health and Medical Research Council (1999), which adapted a rating system developed by the U.S. Preventive Services Task Force. These levels are defined as follows: Level I evidence is obtained from a systematic review of all relevant randomized controlled trials (RCTs); Level II evidence is obtained from at least one properly designed RCT. According to these guidelines, we present Level I evidence, and resort to Level II evidence only if that for Level I is not available. However, as previously noted, Level I evidence is quite rare because most of the reviews do not distinguish among cancer types or stages.

An Overview of Psychosocial Interventions

"Cancer patient" is a generic term that subsumes a great variability among individuals' demographic, social, emotional, and cognitive characteristics, including clinical variables such as cancer site, cancer treatment, and location in the cancer trajectory (Andrykowski & Manne, 2006). Consequently, psychological care needs vary among individuals, depending on factors such as the person's location in the cancer trajectory (i.e., from prevention to cancer diagnosis and survivorship); cancer site; treatment received; and treatment side effects. Although psychological interventions in cancer patients are a recent development, research in this area is growing (Petrie & Revenson, 2005). Interventions for patients with cancer are generally designed to (1) enhance cancer screening; (2) enhance cancer treatment decision making when patients are faced with several treatment options, and no definite and uniform treatment recommendations exist (e.g., prostate and breast cancer); (3)

improve patients' adjustment to cancer and facilitate coping with symptoms and treatment side effects; and (4) help patients cope with challenges in health self-care and cancer treatments and therapies (Petrie & Revenson, 2005). Interventions that address these areas vary widely in content and application. For example, some interventions focus on changing behavior or cognition to become more adaptive and work toward psychological adjustment. Other interventions focus on interpersonal relationships, such as working with family members, or becoming part of a support group. Still others might target stress with relaxation therapies, using music, guided imagery, breathing exercises, or other techniques. While many approaches have been used, it is important to have empirical evidence for their efficacy (Jacobsen & Jim, 2009).

Breast Cancer

Breast cancer is the most frequently diagnosed cancer and the second highest cause of cancer death in women. According to the American Cancer Society statistics, there will be an estimated 192,370 new breast cancer cases, and 40,170 deaths in U.S. women in 2009 (American Cancer Society, 2009).

Medical Approach

Treatment for breast cancer is based on disease factors such as tumor size, clinical stage at diagnosis, and tumor histopathology, as well as patient comorbidity, age (pre- vs. postmenopausal), and patient preferences. Choices for treatment may involve one or more of the following: "mastectomy" (surgical removal of the breast and underlying tissue) or "lumpectomy" (surgical removal of the tumor), with sentinel lymph node biopsy, with or without removal of axillary (underarm) lymph node; radiation therapy (most commonly combined with lumpectomy); and chemotherapy; hormone therapy, or targeted biological therapy, either in the adjuvant setting in early stages (I, II) of the disease, or to treat micrometastatic or metastatic disease for patients who present in advanced stages (III, IV).

Potential side effects of surgery include postoperative pain and fatigue, swelling of the arm on the affected side due to disruption of lymphatic drainage channels ("lymphedema"), decreased arm mobility, and cosmetic changes. General side effects of chemotherapy include fatigue, malaise, and increased susceptibility to infection. Hormonal therapies can cause muscle and bone aches, as well as menopausal symptoms in premenopausal woman. Short-term side effects of radiation therapy include fatigue and skin damage. Various physiological effects of cancer and its treatment may affect cognitive function, including attentional problems (Cimprich & Ronis, 2001) commonly reported by patients during and following cancer treatment (e.g., "chemo brain"; see Hede, 2008).

Interventions to Enhance Screening

Evaluation of the efficacy of cancer screening is usually based on the reduction of cancer mortality, but it should also take into consideration morbidity and quality of life. There is sufficient evidence from several RCTs to demonstrate mortality reduction as a result of breast and colon cancer screening (e.g., Hakama, Coleman, Alexe, & Auvinen, 2008). However, in the United States, where a universal health care program does not exist, studies have shown that lack of insurance is a significant barrier to breast cancer screening (e.g., Rodríguez, Ward, & Pérez-Stable, 2005).

Despite increased public interest in breast cancer genetic risk and genetic testing, there are a few RCTs to enhance patients' decision making on breast cancer genetic testing (e.g., Green, McInerney, Biesecker, & Fost, 2001; Green et al., 2004; Lerman et al., 1997; Miller et al., 2005; Schwartz et al., 2001). For example, in an RCT among women, Lerman and colleagues (1997) examined the impact of an educational intervention, a decisional aid brochure, including oral and visual aids, and nondirective decisional counseling versus usual care on decision, knowledge, risk perception, perceived benefits, and perceived limitations of genetic testing. Study findings indicated that although there were no significant differences between the control and intervention groups in the decision to undergo genetic testing, the intervention effectively increased women's knowledge about screening, risk perception, and reports of perceived benefits of testing, and decreased perceived limitations of genetic testing. In another RCT, conducted with female callers to the National Cancer Institute's Atlantic Region Cancer Information Service, Miller and colleagues (2005) developed and evaluated a theory-based educational intervention designed to increase callers' understanding of genetic testing for breast cancer, risks and benefits of genetic testing, and to determine what information women used to determine the risks. Callers requesting information were randomized to one of two groups: (1) standard care or (2) an educational intervention. The educational intervention changed the women's intention to obtain genetic testing, based on their objective level of risk; intention decreased among average-risk women but increased among high-risk women.

Interventions to Address Issues during Diagnosis and Treatment

The diagnosis of breast cancer is threatening for many reasons (e.g., Derogatis, 1986; Sinsheimer & Holland, 1987; Taylor, 1983), among which are the risk of losing one's life and worries about treatment-related disfigurement. Social and emotional concerns are equally prevalent, often represented by fear of stigmatization and/or rejection; worries about responsiveness to treatment and cancer spread; as well as worries about future fertility and body image. Also emotionally taxing are decisions to undergo breast-conserving surgery (BCS) or mastectomy (MT); whether to continue with adjuvant treatment or to have reconstructive surgery; and, finally, financial cost to one's family.

Although treatment decision aids have been developed to assist women's treatment decision making, very few RCTs evaluate the efficacy of decision aids to enhance early-stage breast cancer treatment decision (e.g., BCS vs. MT). These studies have used various methods to enhance patients' treatment decision making, including audiotaped workbooks (Goel, Sawka, Thiel, Gort, & O'Connor, 2001) and interactive computer programs (Jibaja-Weiss et al., 2006). Goel and colleagues (2001) examined the impact of an audiotape and workbook that included explicit presentation of probabilities, photographs and graphics, and a values clarification exercise on patients' treatment decisions. Their results, however, showed no significant impact of the intervention on study outcomes (i.e., anxiety, knowledge, and decisional regret). Jibaja-Weiss and colleagues (2006) examined the impact of two computer-based components comprising didactic soap opera episodes and interactive learning modules versus a usual-care group on early-stage breast cancer treatment decision making among low-literate, multiethnic women making initial surgical treatment decisions. Patients in the intervention group found the computer components easy to use and to understand, informative, and enjoyable. In addition, intervention patients reported increased knowledge of breast cancer treatment and reduced uncertainty about their treatment preferences and values regarding positive and negative aspects of their treatment options.

Severe emotional reactions, such as depression, anxiety, and anger, have often been reported (Meyerowitz, 1980; Miller, 1980), although other studies suggest that women with no prior psychiatric disorder are unlikely to develop chronic and severe psychological symptoms (Bloom et al., 1987; Penman et al., 1987). Addressing the emotional impact of breast cancer therapy, Schnur and colleagues (2009) combined cognitive-behavioral therapy and hypnosis (CBTH) to reduce negative affect and increase positive affect in 40 women undergoing breast cancer radiotherapy. Participants who were randomized to receive CBTH versus standard care had reduced levels of negative affect and increased levels of positive affect during radiotherapy treatment. The CBTH group also reported more days during which they experienced higher levels of positive versus negative affect.

Interventions to Enhance Survivorship

Long-term survivorship has increased for patients with breast cancer; the 5-year relative survival rate for female breast cancer patients has greatly improved over time, increasing from a rate of 63% in the early 1960s to a rate of 89% today (American Cancer Society, 2009). The current survival rate for women diagnosed with localized breast cancer (which has not spread to lymph nodes or other locations) is 98%. However, cancer survivors are also at increased risk for other diseases, such as cardiovascular disease, diabetes, osteoporosis, and second primary tumors. Demark-Wahnefried and colleagues (2007) attempted to improve overall health and well-being of survivors by developing a tailored intervention in which healthful lifestyle practices were taught to survivors. The intervention succeeded in improving health behaviors in a newly diagnosed population of breast (and prostate) cancer survivors versus those randomly assigned to receive nontailored mailed materials about diet and exercise, who did not improve their health behaviors.

Prostate Cancer

Cancer of the prostate is the most common cancer affecting men in the United States. The National Institute of Cancer estimated that 192,280 men would be diagnosed with prostate cancer and 27,360 men would die from the disease in 2009 (American Cancer Society, 2009). Despite its prevalence, public perception about prostate cancer screening and treatment is complicated by many factors, including the controversy regarding the guidelines for screening; the debate about efficacy of treatment versus active surveillance/watchful waiting; and the lack of standard of care, which is often reflected in contradictory treatment recommendations from physicians (Germino, 2001).

Medical Approach

Similar to breast cancer, treatment of prostate cancer depends on multiple factors, including disease stage, the patient's age, comorbidities, and patient preferences (National Comprehensive Cancer Network [NCCN], 2009). Management options for localized disease (i.e., confined to the prostate, without nodal involvement or metastases) include radical prostatectomy, external beam radiation, brachytherapy, and active surveillance (AS; also referred to as observation, watchful waiting, expectant management). Although either of these management options is quite effective, with an average 5-year survival rate of 95%, treatment-related side effects are common. Sexual and urinary dysfunction, for example, are known potential complications of radical prostate-ctomy, whereas problems with bowel function are typical complaints reported by patients undergoing external beam radiation and brachytherapy (Eton & Lepore, 2002; NCCN, 2009; van Andel et al., 2004). Any of these side effects might have a significant impact on patients' functioning and overall quality of life (Eton & Lepore, 2002). AS, the close monitoring of prostate-specific antigen (PSA) levels without active treatment, may be associated with psychological implications of not treating cancer; cancer progression; chances of missed opportunity for cure; and later treatment of a larger tumor (NCCN, 2009).

Treatment of advanced-stage prostate cancer includes androgen deprivation therapy (ADT) and chemotherapy to slow tumor growth. Potential complications of ADT can include mood changes, fatigue, hot flashes (i.e., vasomotor symptoms), loss of muscle strength, redistribution of body fat, thinning of the bones, and breast tenderness or enlargement (NCCN, 2009). Side effects associated with chemotherapy can include fatigue, loss of appetite, loss of hair, reduced resistance to infection, and nausea and vomiting (NCCN, 2009).

Psychological Interventions

Although the majority of the interventions in cancer patients have focused on relieving psychological distress, anxiety, and depression (Jacobsen & Jim, 2008), previous reviews indicate that some of the interventions among men with prostate cancer focused on psychoeducational and/or psychosocial aspects of the prostate cancer trajectory. These include interventions designed to enhance prostate cancer screening (e.g., Gattellari & Ward, 2003, 2005; Partin et al., 2004); treatment decision making (e.g., Auvinen et al., 2001, 2004; Davison & Degner, 1997); and coping with treatment, symptoms, and side effects (e.g., Lepore, Helgeson, Eton, & Schulz, Mishel et al., 2002; Zhang, Strauss, & Siminoff, 2006).

Prostate Cancer Screening

During the past two decades, the widespread use and application of PSA screening has led to a dramatic increase in the diagnosis of low-volume, low-risk, nonpalpable, early-stage prostate cancer (Albertsen et al., 2005). However, several autopsy studies of men dying of causes other than prostate cancer have documented the high prevalence of histological evidence of prostate cancer, with a significant portion of the tumors being small and possibly clinically insignificant (Dall'Era et al., 2008). These findings created many challenges and debates regarding (1) whether to treat low-grade prostate cancer, (2) the definition of PSA reference range outside of which the test can be reliably classified as abnormal, and (3) the merits of using other clinical PSA-related parameters in prostate cancer diagnosis, such as PSA velocity and density and PSA free-to-total ratio (Sriprasad et al., 2001).

In spite of this controversy, PSA screening is becoming more frequent, and men diagnosed with low-grade prostate cancer are facing decisions regarding whether to undergo frequent PSA testing without undergoing active treatment, whether to undergo active treatment, and what type of management options to choose (i.e., surgery, radiation therapy). Studies on the psychosocial impact of prostate cancer screening on men's emotional adjustment (i.e., anxiety and depression levels) showed that the psychological health of the men being screened was the same as, or better than, population norms (e.g., Brindle et al., 2006; Essink-Bot et al., 1998). However, other research findings showed higher levels of intrusive thoughts about cancer among men who received a positive screening test result, although no differences between the groups in quality of life were found (Taylor, Shelby, Gelmann, & McGuire, 2004). Given the prevalence of distress, anxiety, and depression related to cancer screening among other cancer populations (e.g., breast cancer: Gilbert et al., 1998), these results might suggest that the measures of psychological health used in prostate cancer research were not sensitive enough to men's psychological reactions. Thus, valid assessments for measuring men's cognitive and emotional reactions to prostate cancer screening are needed.

Interventions to Enhance Prostate Cancer Screening

Interventions related to prostate cancer screening have focused on helping men make informed decisions about the PSA test (Mc-Cormack, Bann, Williams-Piehota, Driscoll, & Kuo, 2005) and/or establishing the habit of regular screening for prostate cancer (i.e., health behavior change; Germino, 2001). The literature reviews on prostate cancer decision aids/interventions in both screening and treatment-related contexts showed some consistency in intervention outcomes. These include O'Connor and colleagues (2001), Evans and colleagues (2005), and Volk and colleagues (2006) reviews on decision aids among different cancer populations, including prostate cancer patients. These reviews, however, have either examined decision aids in other broader medical contexts (i.e., non-cancer diseases; O'Connor et al., 2003) or included randomized and nonrandomized studies in prostate cancer patients (Evans et al., 2005; Volk et al., 2006).

In this chapter we focus on O'Brien and colleagues' (2009) systematic review and meta-analysis of RTCs of prostate cancer-related decisional aids for screening. Their review showed significant effects of the decision aids/interventions on patients' cognitive, behavioral, and emotional outcomes. The included RCTs represented decision aids with different formats and used various methodologies, such as brochures (Gattellari & Ward, 2003, 2005; Partin et al., 2004), counseling (Davison et al., 1997), and videotapes (Gattellari & Ward, 2005; Partin et al., 2004; Taylor et al., 2004; Volk et al., 2006). These approaches were compared to usual appointment or waiting-list controls. All decision aids presented information about risks and benefits of prostate cancer screening, and chances of false-positive screening results, and used diagrams and illustrations to convey probabilities and medical information. Results of this systematic review indicated that prostate cancer screening decision aids were effective in increasing patients' knowledge of prostate cancer screening and their participation in the decision making, and in decreasing decisional conflict. No significant effect of the reviewed decision aids on reducing emotional distress and anxiety were found (O'Brien et al., 2009). These findings were consistent with previous reviews of decision aids among other cancer patients and patients with noncancer diseases (Evans et al., 2005; O'Connor et al., 2003; Volk et al., 2007).

In spite of the growing diversity of clinical populations including prostate cancer patients in the United States, many prostate cancer screening studies are conducted in homogenous study populations, thus limiting the generalizability and usefulness of the study findings (Germino, 2001). A study that examined factors associated with intention to be tested for prostate cancer risk among African American men showed that older age, having had a prostate cancer screening examination in the past year, perceived susceptibility of one's prostate cancer, and fatalistic beliefs about prostate cancer prevention were negatively associated with intention to be tested for risk (Myers et al., 2000). These findings highlight the need for more culturally sensitive interventions that address the needs of minorities such as African American and Latino patients. Furthermore, challenges regarding the controversial nature of prostate cancer screening need to be addressed. Patients need to be informed about this issue, and their screening decisions should be congruent with their values and goals.

Interventions on Prostate Cancer Treatment Decisions: AS or Active Treatment?

AS, as mentioned earlier, offers the opportunity to delay active treatment and its associated morbidity (e.g., incontinence, erectile dysfunction), and allows the patient entry into a management protocol with frequent monitoring and the option of curative therapy should the cancer progress. Research, however, showed that within 3 years, approximately 33% of men develop more aggressive cancers and have to discontinue AS protocols to receive active treatment. Because there are no medical standards that allow physicians to predict who will develop aggressive cancer and who will continue to have a low-grade tumor, patients may decide not to consider AS, or they may terminate AS programs and opt for active treatment to avoid the uncertainty, worries, and anxiety caused by having untreated cancer (Dall'Era et al., 2008). Developing better prognostic tools to determine which patient will develop aggressive disease and to address the psychosocial management of prostate cancer patients is an ongoing area of need and active research.

ACTIVE TREATMENT: RADICAL PROSTATECTOMY, EXTERNAL BEAM RADIATION, OR BRACHYTHERAPY?

For most patients diagnosed with localized prostate cancer, or for those who terminate an AS protocol, radical prostatectomy, external beam radiation, or brachytherapy remain the most common treatment options (Eton & Lepore, 2002). Decisions among prostate cancer treatment options for these patients, however, are complicated because patients are likely to receive different treatment recommendations depending on the specialty physician they are consulting. Disagreements among physicians are common and can be traced to lack of consensus about a standard of care and a poor evidence base that lacks the necessary RCTs to compare the various treatment options (Dall'Era et al., 2008; Eton & Lepore, 2002; O'Brien et al., 2009). Treatment decisions are further complicated by the frequent side effects (e.g., urinary incontinence, sexual and bowel dysfunction) that to a certain degree accompany all treatment options.

Interventions to Enhance Prostate Cancer Treatment Decisions

Only a very few RCTs have examined the influence of decision aids/interventions on enhancing prostate cancer treatment decisions (O'Brien et al., 2009). Davison and Degner (1997) examined the efficacy of providing patients with written prostate cancer treatment information, a list of questions to ask their physicians during consultation, and an audiotape of their discussions. The study findings indicated that men in the intervention group assumed a significantly more active role in treatment decision making and had lower state anxiety levels at 6 weeks following the intervention compared to patients in the control group (i.e., written information package alone). However, no significant differences between the two groups in levels of reported depression were found at 6 weeks.

Although printed educational materials and videotape/audiotape-based decision-making interventions have the advantage of being affordable, widely available, and easy to use in medical setting, their feasibility is limited by their one-size-fits-all approach, lack of interactivity in the selection of in-

formation relevant to personal values and goals in treatment of side effects, and lack of information regarding the psychoeducational needs of men for whom AS is the recommended management option. These limitations, however, were addressed in studies that used advanced software and media tools, such as CD-ROM and Internet-based programs (e.g., DePalma, 2000; Diefenbach & Butz, 2004; Kim et al., 2001). Interactive CD-ROM and Internet-based intervention programs can tailor prostate cancer information to patients' needs and to clinical and demographic characteristics (e.g., age, early-stage prostate cancer), elicit patient treatment preferences by providing value clarification exercise, and offer social support through patients testimonials. Study of non-RCT results in prostate cancer patients and patients with benign prostatic hyperplasia (BPH) showed that use of the CD-ROM and Internet-based intervention increased patient satisfaction, and patient and physician communication about the benefits and risks of various treatment options, and decreased the rate of transurethral prostatectomy (TURP). In spite of their feasibility and positive results, CD-ROM and Internet-based intervention programs have some limitations that could reduce the generalizability of their use, including the lack of an RCT study design to examine the efficacy of the multimedia programs used, the need for computer literacy, and face-to face sessions to introduce and implement the multimedia programs (Kim et al., 2001).

Interventions to Enhance Psychosocial Adaptation with Treatment and Side Effects

Previous studies in prostate cancer patients indicated that the psychological adjustment of men with prostate cancer is influenced by different demographic, psychosocial, and clinical factors, including the patient's age, availability of social support, coping, cancer stage, time since diagnosis, and treatment effects on sexual and urinary function (Bloch et al., 2007). However, a recent study by Sharpley, Bitsika, and Christie (2008) that "reviewed the reviews" of psychological distress among patients with prostate cancer showed contradictory conclusions in three major reviews regarding whether patients with prostate cancer do experience elevated levels of psychological distress compared to other cancer patients or age-matched healthy men (Bennett & Badger, 2005; Bloch et al., 2007; Katz, 2007; Sharpley et al., 2008). Whereas two of the reviews indicated increased depression and anxiety, and decreased quality of life among patients with prostate cancer compared to their nonpatient peers, one review showed no significant differences in reported psychological distress between a prostate cancer sample and an age-matched healthy sample (Bennett & Badger, 2005; Bloch et al., 2007; Katz, 2007; Sharpley et al., 2008). This contradiction in findings on psychological distress among patients with prostate cancer might be associated with the methods used to select studies included in the reviews. The three reviews differ in that their outcomes/dependent variables (mood, quality of life, depression, anxiety), focused on mood rather than clinical measures of depression or anxiety (Bennett & Badger, 2005), used quality-of-life measures as the principal component rather than psychological distress–related measures (Katz, 2007), included all relevant studies regardless of their methodological weakness (Katz, 2007), and depended on a very few studies to examine the difference between patients and an age-matched sample in the study outcomes (Bloch et al., 2007).

Despite these contradictory research findings, the majority of psychosocial interventions operates under the assumption that patients diagnosed with prostate cancer are in need of psychosocial support, and hence has focused on alleviating psychological distress and anxiety, and improving coping and adjustment to treatment and side effects (Jacobsen & Jim, 2008). Our review of RCTs that address these issues showed significant effects on psychosocial interventions designed to improve patients' adjustment and quality of life. Lepore and colleagues (2003) examined the influence of an educational intervention in RCTs of men treated for early-stage prostate cancer to improve adjustment and quality of life that included biological and epidemiological information; discussed physical side effects, as well as issues surrounding nutrition and cancer, stress and coping, relationships and sexuality; and follow-up care and future health concerns. Their results indicated that patients in the study group reported increased knowledge

about prostate cancer, adoption of healthy behaviors, improvements in general physical functioning, greater employment stability, and less distress about sexual dysfunction than those in the control condition. Penedo and colleagues (2002) examined the impact of a cognitive-behavioral stress management (CBSM; Antoni, 2003) intervention to improve quality of life. The researchers' approach was to help patients identify and effectively manage stressful experiences related to treatment and side effects by identifying distorted thoughts related to cancer and treatment side effects, rational thought replacement, effective coping, anger management, assertive training, and utilization of social support. The intervention, tested in an RCT, showed that significant improvement in quality of life was mediated by greater perceived stress management skills in the study group compared to a comparison group.

Interventions to Enhance Sexual and Urinary Function Following Prostate Cancer Treatment

Sexual Function Following Prostate Cancer Treatment

Reports of erectile dysfunction (ED) and incontinence following prostate cancer treatment vary considerably. One of the determining factors of sexual functioning after treatment is the status of functioning before treatment. In general, ED and incontinence rates among patients treated with surgery are slightly higher than rates of those treated with radiation treatment (60–93% with ED after surgery vs. 67–85% with ED after external beam; 20–70% with incontinence after surgery vs. 58–64% with incontinence after external beam) (Grise & Thurman, 2001; Leng & Chancellor, 2001). Some reports of functional erections without medication are as low as 18% of men who underwent bilateral nerve-sparing surgery (Schover, 2007). This variation in ED and reported incontinence might be associated with difficulty in assessing these complications; lack of precise definitions of incontinence or impotence in the literature; data obtained by widely divergent methods, including questionnaires, telephone interviews, or surgeon assessment; bias in selecting study participants (i.e., continence and potency rates are improved when the patient are younger and have fewer comorbidities (Michaelson et al., 2008).

Efforts to increase sexual functioning among patients and their spouses showed some progress. In an RCT for men with prostate cancer that was directed at managing uncertainty and improving symptom control, Mishel and colleagues (2002) evaluated a psychoeducational phone intervention. Compared to the control group (i.e., usual care), the intervention group reported lower certainty, improved urinary and sexual function, satisfaction with sexual function, and a decrease in the number of treatment side effects reported. Canada, Neese, Sui, and Schover (2005) examined in an RCT the effects of information provision about prostate cancer and sexual functioning, and options to treat ED, as well as sexual communication and stimulation skills, among couples dealing with prostate cancer. Their results showed improvements in patients' overall distress levels and global sexual function, and spouses' global sexual function, and an increase in the utilization of ED treatments.

In summary, because ED involves both biological and psychosocial processes, interventions designed to reduce ED use medical treatments and sexual aids (e.g., oral drugs, local injections, vacuum devices) and/or psychoeducation, psychotherapy, and counseling (Melnik, Soares, & Nasello, 2007; Schover, 2007; Schover et al., 2002). However, there is a gap in the literature concerning long-term efficacy of ED interventions following prostate cancer treatment because patients are more likely to discontinue use of sexual aids, and research on the impact of psychoeducation- and counseling-based interventions is scant (Chambers et al., 2008; Melnik et al., 2007; Schover, 2007; Schover et al., 2002).

Urinary Function Following Prostate Cancer Treatment

A significant decline in urinary function following prostate cancer treatment is not uncommon. This decline is more pronounced among patients treated with surgery than among those treated with external beam radiation and brachytherapy (Eton & Lepore, 2002). Urinary dysfunction or incontinence can reduce the patient's quality of life and may lead to embarrassment, loss of a sense of control, depression, and decreased social

interactions (Eton & Lepore, 2002; Ko & Sawatzky, 2008). Medications and physiotherapy-based interventions (e.g., pelvic muscle exercise) are the most common first-line treatments of urinary incontinence and are often used together (Grise & Thurman, 2001). Several interventions were designed to enhance urinary function through pelvic muscles exercise and biofeedback. Zhang and colleagues (2006) examined the effect of combined pelvic floor muscle exercises (PFME) and support group on quality of life of patients following prostate cancer treatment in an RCT. Patients learned PFME through biofeedback and were randomized to control and support groups. Study results indicated that the PFME and support group experienced significantly enhanced functioning and reduced perception of illness intrusiveness compared to the control group (PFME only). Improved urinary continence was significantly associated with reduced depression and symptom distress over time. These results were consistent with previous study findings (e.g., Moore, Griffiths, & Hughton, 1999; Opsomer et al., 1994; Von Kampen et al., 2001).

Lung Cancer

For both men and women, lung cancer accounts for the most cancer-related deaths. According to American Cancer Society (2009) statistics, an estimated 219,440 new lung cancer cases, and 159,390 deaths will occur in the United States in 2009.

Treatment options vary based on the type (small-cell or non-small-cell) and stage of cancer. Options include surgery, radiation therapy, chemotherapy, and targeted biological therapies.

Medical Approach

Treatment planning for a patient with newly diagnosed lung cancer is determined by three main issues: cancer cell type (small-cell lung cancer [SCLC] vs. non-small-cell lung cancer [NSCLC]), the stage of disease, and the functional status of the patient. For patients with NSCLC with resectable lesions and acceptable cardiac and pulmonary function, curative surgery is the mainstay of treatment. Postoperative adjuvant chemotherapy has been shown to improve survival in patients with pathological Stage II disease and may have a role for patients with localized disease. Patients with Stage I or Stage II disease who are not candidates for surgical resection, or who refuse surgery, may be candidates for radiation therapy. For patients with Stage III disease, a combined modality approach of chemotherapy and radiation therapy is preferred; surgery following chemoradiotherapy is currently under active investigation. Patients with Stage IV disease are generally treated with systemic chemotherapy or with palliative approaches. Patients with limited-stage SCLC (disease limited to one hemithorax) are primarily treated with chemoradiotherapy. Surgery for patients with all-stage SCLC is rare. For patients with both limited and extensive disease, prophylactic cranial irradiation (PCI) is used in patients who respond to their initial treatment. Side effects of treatment include decreased pulmonary capacity in patients who undergo removal of significant lung parenchyma, fatigue and increased susceptibility to infection with chemotherapy, and short-term pulmonary toxicity in patients who undergo pulmonary radiation therapy. Patients who undergo PCI may experience fatigue and cognitive deficits.

Interventions to Enhance Screening

RCTs of lung cancer screening based on chest X-ray and sputum cytology have demonstrated a lack of effect. These tests have not shown mortality reduction, which may be due to low sensitivity in detecting early-stage tumors (Hakama et al., 2008).

Interventions to Address Issues during Diagnosis and Treatment

Level I or Level II psychosocial interventions for patients with lung cancer are scarce. Indeed, the levels and types of supportive care needs of patients with lung cancer are relatively unknown, with little published literature compared to other cancer populations (Houts, Yasko, Kahn, Schelzel, & Marconi, 1986). Not until recently have researchers focused on remedying this lack of information. Li and Girgis (2006) examined and

compared the psychosocial need of lung cancer patients to those of other cancer patients recruited from nine major public cancer treatment centers in New South Wales, Australia. Their study findings showed that patients with lung cancer reported a higher average number of unmet psychological needs, particularly psychological, physical, and daily living needs, than did patients coping with other types of cancers, suggesting that this subgroup of cancer survivors could use some focused attention (Li & Girgis, 2006).

A second study (Kenny et al., 2008) examined quality of life before surgery, at discharge, and at 1 month, 4 months, and 2 years thereafter among patients with early-stage NSCLC (Stage I or II). The study results showed that surgery significantly and negatively impacted patients' quality of life.

Interventions to Address Side Effects and Enhance Survivorship

Given the relatively poor prognosis associated with a lung cancer diagnosis, with 5-year overall survival rates of less than 15%, perhaps the findings of Li and Girgis (2006) and high levels of reported need in this population are not surprising. The 1-year relative survival rate for lung cancer increased from 35% in 1975–1979 to 41% in 2001–2004, largely due to improvements in treatment, and the 5-year survival rate improves to 50% for cases in which the disease is still localized; unfortunately, only 16% of lung cancers are diagnosed this early. Although guidelines for treating Stage IV NSCLC suggest that the patient's values should be considered in decision making, there are no practical tools available to assist with their decision making (Fiset et al., 2000).

Conclusions

The number of studies that apply psycho-educational and psychosocial approaches to diverse cancer populations is growing. These include interventions designed to enhance screening and treatment decision making, coping and adjustment to cancer and related side effects, symptom management, and interventions that address issues pertinent to cancer survivors. The multitude of intervention applications suggests that a "one size fits all" approach is not appropriate. Yet the specialization of interventions to address a circumscribed set of problems is not conducive to addressing issues that extend beyond the particular issue investigated. For example, interventions designed to facilitate treatment decision making are not likely to address potential problems that might occur during survivorship. However, a patient's decision might be better informed if issues that might emerge during a later stage of the cancer trajectory were addressed at an earlier stage, thus preparing the patient to anticipate and to deal with the potential problem. Thus, researchers might consider developing interventions that include components that address potential future issues of survivorship.

Another shortcoming of this body of work is that too few interventions are guided by theory. Too often, if a theoretical approach is chosen at all, researchers resort to established theories, without assessing the appropriateness of their chosen approach. A better approach to comprehensive theory development and evaluation is needed, and the inclusion of psychologists of various disciplines might be useful during intervention development.

Finally, given the growing diversity of the cancer population, there is a need for culturally sensitive and targeted research that addresses the needs of an increasingly diverse cancer population. Cancer remains a universally feared and highly stigmatizing disease with culturally diverse beliefs about its origin, causes, and possibilities for treatment. Interventions that do not take these individualized beliefs into account and incorporate them into a wider cultural system are more likely to fail.

In summary, increasingly the psychosocial needs of cancer patients are being recognized by researchers and clinicians, and addressed with the development of specialized interventions. Beyond these promising developments, more attention is needed to evaluate such efforts using stringent methodological approaches in the form of RCTs. Attention should also be focused on the enhancement of health behavior theory, taking into account approaches from neighboring disciplines.

Further Reading

Eton, D. T., & Lepore, S. J. (2002). Prostate cancer and quality of life: A review of the literature. *Psycho-Oncology, 11,* 307–326.

Jacobsen, P. B., & Jim, H. S. (2008). Psychosocial interventions for anxiety and depression in adult cancer patients: Achievements and challenges. *CA: A Cancer Journal for Clinicians, 58,* 214–230.

O'Brien, M. A., Whelan, T. J., Villasis-Keever, M., Gafni, A., Charles, C., Roberts, R., et al. (2009). Are cancer-related decision aids effective?: A systematic review and meta-analysis. *Journal of Clinical Oncology, 27*(6), 974–985.

O'Connor, A. M., Bennett, C. L., Stacey, D., Barry, M., Col, N. F., Eden, K. B., et al. (2001). Decision aids to help people who are facing health treatment or screening decisions. *Cochrane Database of Systematic Reviews,* Issue 3 (Article No. CD001431), DOI: 10.1002/14651858.CD001431.pub2.

Sharpley, C. F., Bitsika, V., & Christie, D. H. R. (2008). Psychological distress among prostate cancer patients: Fact or fiction? *Clinical Medicine: Oncology, 2,* 563–572.

References

Albertsen, P. C., Hanley, J. A., Barrows, G. H., Penson, D. F., Kowalczyk, P. D. H., Sanders, M. M., et al. (2005). Prostate cancer and the Will Rogers phenomenon. *Journal National Cancer Institute, 97,* 1248–1253.

American Cancer Society. (2009). *Cancer facts and figures.* Retrieved March 15, 2010, from *www.cancer.org/downloads/STT/500809web.pdf.*

Andrykowski, M., & Manne, S. (2006). Are psychological interventions effective and accepted by cancer patients?: I. Standards and levels of evidence. *Annals of Behavioral Medicine, 32*(2), 93–97.

Antoni, M. H. (2003). *Stress management intervention for women with breast cancer.* Washington, DC: American Psychological Association.

Auvinen, A., Hakama, M., Ala-Opas, M., Vornanen, T., Leppilahti, M., Salminen, P., et al. (2004). A randomized trial of choice of treatment in prostate cancer: The effect of intervention on the treatment chosen. *British Journal of Urology International, 93*(1), 52–56.

Auvinen, A., Vornanen, T., Tammela, T. L. J., Ala-Opas, M., Leppilahti, M., Salminen, P., et al. (2001). A randomized trial of the choice of treatment in prostate cancer: Design and baseline characteristics. *British Journal of Urology International, 88*(7), 708–715.

Bennett, G., & Badger, T. A. (2005). Depression in men with prostate cancer. *Oncology Nursing, 32,* 545–556.

Bloch, S., Love, A., Macvean, M., Duchesne, G., Couper, J., & Kissane, D. (2007). Psychological adjustment of men with prostate cancer: A review of the literature. Retrieved April 3, 2009, from *www.bpsmedicine.com/content/1/1/2.*

Bloom, J. R., Cook, M., Fotopoulos, S., Flamer, D., Gates, C., Holland, J. C., et al. (1987). Psychological response to mastectomy: A prospective comparison study. *Cancer, 59,* 189–196.

Brindle, L. A., Oliver, S. E., Dedman, D., Donovan, J. L., Neal, D. N., Hamdy, F. C., et al. (2006). Measuring the psychosocial impact of population-based prostate-specific antigen testing for prostate cancer in the UK. *British Journal of Urology International, 98*(4), 777–782.

Canada, A. L., Neese, L. E., Sui, D., & Schover, L. R. (2005). Pilot intervention to enhance sexual rehabilitation for couples after treatment for localized prostate carcinoma. *Cancer, 104*(12), 2689–2700.

Chambers, S. K., Schover, L., Halford, K., Clutton, S., Ferguson, M., Gordon, L., et al. (2008). ProsCan for Couples: Randomised controlled trial of a couples-based sexuality intervention for men with localised prostate cancer who receive radical prostatectomy. *BMC Cancer, 8,* 226–234.

Cimprich, B., & Ronis, D. L. (2001). Attention and symptom distress in women with and without breast cancer. *Nursing Research, 50*(2), 86–94.

Dall'Era, M. A., Cooperberg, M. R., Chan, J. M., Davis, B. J., Albertsen, B., Klotz, L. H., et al. (2008). Active surveillance for early-stage prostate cancer: Review of the current literature. *Cancer, 112*(8), 1650–1659.

Davison, B. J., & Degner, L. F. (1997). Empowerment of men newly diagnosed with prostate cancer. *Cancer Nursing, 20,* 187–196.

Demark-Wahnefried, W., Clipp, E. C., Lipkus, I. M., Lobach, D., Clutter Snyder, D., Sloane, R., et al. (2007). Main outcomes of the FRESH START trial: A sequentially tailored, diet and exercise mailed print intervention among breast and prostate cancer survivors. *Journal of Clinical Oncology, 25*(19), 2709–2718.

DePalma, A. (2000). Prostate cancer shared decision: A CD-ROM educational and decision-assisting tool for men with prostate cancer. *Seminars in Urologic Oncology, 18*(3), 178–181.

Derogatis, L. R. (1986). The unique impact of breast and gynecologic cancers on body image and sexual identity in women: A reassessment. In J. M. Vaeth (Ed.), *Body image, self-esteem, and sexuality in cancer patients* (2nd ed., pp. 1–14). Basel: Karger.

Diefenbach, M. A., & Butz, B. P. (2004). The development of an interactive multimedia software program for prostate cancer patients. *Journal of Medical Internet Research, 6*(1), e3. Retrieved from *www.jmir.org/2004/1/e3.*

Essink-Bot, M. L., de Koning, H. J., Nijs, H. G., Kirkels, W. J., van der Maas, P. J., & Schroder, F. H. (1998). Short-term effects of population-based screening for prostate cancer on health-related quality of life. *Journal of the National Cancer Institute, 90,* 925–931.

Eton, D. T., & Lepore, S. J. (2002). Prostate cancer and quality of life: A review of the literature. *Psycho-Oncology, 11,* 307–326.

Evans, R., Edwards, A., Brett, J., Bradburn, M., Watson, E., Austoker, J., et al. (2005). Reduction in uptake of PSA tests following decision aids: Systematic review of current aids and their evaluations. *Patient Education and Counseling, 58,* 13–26.

Fiset, V., O'Connor, A. M., Evans, W., Graham, I., Degrasse, C., & Logan, J. (2000). Development and evaluation of a decision aid for patients with stage IV non-small cell lung cancer. *Health Expectations, 3*(2), 125–136.

Gattellari, M., & Ward, J. E. (2005). A community-based randomised controlled trial of three different educational resources for men about prostate cancer screening. *Patient Education and Counseling, 57*(2), 168–182.

Germino, B. (2001). Educational and psychosocial intervention trials in prostate cancer. *Seminars in Oncology Nursing, 17*(2), 129–137.

Gilbert, F. G., Cordiner, C. M., Affleck, I. R., Hood, I., Mathieson, D., & Walker, L. G. (1998). Breast screening: The psychological sequelae of false-positive recall in women with and without a family history of breast cancer. *European Journal of Cancer, 34*(13), 2010–2014.

Goel, V., Sawka, A., Thiel, E. C., Gort, E. H., & O'Connor, A. M. (2001). Randomized trial of a patient decision aid for choice of surgical treatment for breast cancer. *Medical Decision Making, 21,* 1–6.

Green, M. J., McInerney, A. M., Biesecker, B. B., & Fost, N. (2001). Education about genetic testing for breast cancer susceptibility: Patient preferences for a computer program or genetic counselor. *American Journal of Medical Genetics, 103*(1), 24–31.

Green, M. J., Peterson, S. K., Baker, M. W., Harper, G. R., Friedman, L. C., Rubinstein, W. S., et al. (2004). Effect of a computer-based decision aid on knowledge, perceptions, and intentions about genetic testing for breast cancer susceptibility: A randomized controlled trial. *Journal of the American Medical Association, 292*(4), 442–452.

Grise, P., & Thurman, S. (2001). Urinary incontinence following treatment of localized prostate cancer. *Cancer Control, 28*(6), 532–539.

Hakama, M., Coleman, M. P., Alexe, D., & Auvinen, A. (2008). Cancer screening: Evidence and practice in Europe. *European Journal of Cancer, 44*, 1404–1413.

Hede, K. (2008). Chemobrain is real but may need new name. *Journal of the National Cancer Institute, 100*(3), 162–163, 169.

Houts, P. S., Yasko, J. M., Kahn, S. B., Schelzel, G. W., & Marconi, K. M. (1986). Unmet psychological, social, and economic needs of persons with cancer in Pennsylvania. *Cancer, 58*(10), 2355–2361.

Jacobsen, P. B., & Jim, H. S. (2008). Psychosocial interventions for anxiety and depression in adult cancer patients: Achievements and challenges. *CA: A Cancer Journal for Clinicians, 58*, 214–230.

Jibaja-Weiss, M., Volk, R. J., Granch, T. S., Nefe, N. E., Spann, S. J., Aoki, N., et al. (2006). Entertainment education for informed breast cancer treatment decisions in low-literate women: Development and initial evaluation of a patient decision aid. *Journal of Cancer Education, 21*(3), 133–139.

Katz, A. (2007). Quality of life for men with prostate cancer. *Cancer Nursing, 30*, 302–308.

Kenny, P. M., King, M. T., Viney, R. C., Boyer, M. J., Pollicino, C. A., McLean, J. M., et al. (2008). Quality of life and survival in the 2 years after surgery for non-small-cell lung cancer. *Journal of Clinical Oncology, 26*(2), 233–241.

Kim, S. P., Knight, S. J., Tomori, C., Colella, K. M., Schoor, R. A., Shih, L., et al. (2001). Health literacy and shared decision making for prostate cancer patients with low socioeconomic status. *Cancer Investigation, 19*(7), 684–691.

Ko, W., & Sawatzky, J. (2008). Understanding urinary incontinence after radical prostatectomy: A nursing framework. *Clinical Journal of Oncology Nursing, 4*, 647–654.

Leng, W. W., & Chancellor, M. B. (2001). Comparison of incontinence risk after radical prostatectomy versus hysterectomy. *Reviews in Urology, 3*(3), 156–159.

Lepore, S. J., Helgeson, V. S., Eton, D. T., & Schulz, R. (2003). Improving quality of life in men with prostate cancer: A randomized controlled trial of group education interventions. *Health Psychology, 22*(5), 443–452.

Lerman, C., Biesecker, B., Benkendorf, J. L., Kerner, J., GomezCaminero, A., Hughes, C.,

et al. (1997). Controlled trial of pretest education approaches to enhance informed decision-making for BRCA1 gene testing. *Journal of the National Cancer Institute, 89*(2), 148–157.

Li, J., & Girgis, A. (2006). Supportive care needs: Are patients with lung cancer a neglected population?, *Psycho-Oncology, 15*, 509–516.

McCormack, L., Bann, C., Williams-Piehota, P., Driscoll, D., & Kuo, M. (2005). *Knowledge about prostate cancer screening and treatment results of a community-based evaluation.* Paper presented at the Third RTI Fellow Symposium. Retrieved from *www.rti.org/pubs/Fellows_Sym_06_Abst_Bios.pdf*

Melnik, T., Soares, B., & Nasello, A. G. (2007). Psychosocial interventions for erectile dysfunction. *Cochrane Database of Systematic Reviews*, Issue 3 (Article no. CD004825), DOI: 10.1002/14651858.CD004825.pub2.

Meyerowitz, B. E. (1980). Psychosocial correlates of breast cancer and its treatments. *Psychological Bulletin, 87*, 108–131.

Michaelson, M. D., Cotter, S. E., Gargollo, P. C., Zietman, A. L., Dahl, D. M., & Smith, M. R. (2008). Management of complications of prostate cancer treatment. *CA: A Cancer Journal for Clinicians, 58*(4), 196–213.

Miller, P. J. (1980). Mastectomy: A review of psychosocial research. *Health and Social Work, 4*, 60–65.

Miller, S. M., Fleisher, L., Roussi, P., Buzaglo, J. S., Schnoll, R., Slater, E., et al. (2005). Facilitating informed decision making about breast cancer risk and genetic counseling among women calling the NCI's cancer information service. *Journal of Health Communication, 10*(Suppl. 1), 119–136.

Mishel, M. H., Belyea, M., Germino, B. B., Stewart, J. L., Bailey, D. E., Robertson, C., et al. (2002). Helping patients with localized prostate cancer manage uncertainty and treatment side effects: Nurse delivered psycho-education intervention over the telephone. *Cancer, 94*, 1854–1866.

Moore, K. N., Griffiths, D., & Hughton, A. (1999). Urinary incontinence after radical prostatectomy: A randomized controlled trial comparing pelvic muscle exercises with or without electrical stimulation. *British Journal of Urology, 83*, 57–65.

Myers, R. E., Hyslop, T., Wolf, T. A., Burgh, D., Kunkel, E. J., Oyesanmi, O. A., et al. (2000). African-American men and intention to adhere to recommended follow-up for an abnormal prostate cancer early detection examination result. *Urology, 55*(5), 716–720.

National Comprehensive Cancer Network Clinical Practice Guidelines in Oncology. (2009). *Prostate cancer.* Retrieved April 3, 2009, from *www.nccn.org/professionals/physician_gls/pdf/prostate.pdf.*

National Health and Medical Research Council. (1999). *A guide to the development, implementation and evaluation of clinical practice guidelines.* Canberra: Australian Government Publishing Service.

O'Brien, M. A., Whelan, T. J., Villasis-Keever, M., Gafni, A., Charles, C., Roberts, R., et al. (2009). Are cancer-related decision aids effective?: A systematic review and meta-analysis. *Journal of Clinical Oncology, 27*(6), 974–985.

O'Connor, A. M., Bennett, C. L., Stacey, D., Barry, M., Col, N. F., Eden, K. B., et al. (2001). Decision aids to help people who are facing health treatment or screening decisions. *Cochrane Database of Systematic Reviews*, Issue 3 (Article No. CD001431), DOI: 10.1002/14651858.CD00143.pub2.

Opsomer, R. J., Castille, Y., Abi-Aad, A. S., Long, F., Wese, F., & Van Langh, P. J. (1994). Urinary incontinence after radical prostatectomy: Is professional pelvic floor training necessary? *Neurourology and Urodynamics, 13*(4), 382–384.

Partin, M. R., Nelson, D., Radosevich, D., Nugent, S., Flood, A. B., Dillon, N., et al. (2004). Randomized trial examining the effect of two prostate cancer screening educational interventions on patient knowledge, preferences, and behaviors. *Journal of General Internal Medicine, 19*(8), 835–842.

Penedo, F. J., Dahn, J. R., Molton, I., Gonzalez, J. S., Kinsinger, D., Roos, B. A., et al. (2002). Cognitive-behavioral stress management improves stress-management skills and quality of life in men recovering from treatment of prostate carcinoma. *Cancer, 94*, 1854–1866.

Penman, D. T., Bloom, J. R., Fotopoulos, S., Cook, M. R., Holland, J. C., Gates, C., et al. (1987). The impact of mastectomy on self-concept and social function: A combined cross-sectional and longitudinal study with comparison groups. *Women and Health, 11*, 101–130.

Petrie, K. J., & Revenson, T. A. (2005). Editorial: New psychological interventions in chronic illness: Towards examining mechanisms of action and improved targeting. *Journal of Health Psychology, 10*(2), 179–184.

Rodríguez, M. A., Ward, L. M., & Pérez-Stable, E. J. (2005). Breast and cervical cancer screening: Impact of health insurance status, ethnicity, and nativity of Latinas. *Annals of Family Medicine, 3*(3), 235–241.

Schnur, J. B., David, D., Kangas, M., Green, S., Bovbjerg, D. H., & Montgomery, G. H. (2009). A randomized trial of a cognitive-behavioral therapy and hypnosis intervention on positive and negative affect during breast cancer radiotherapy. *Journal of Clinical Psychology, 65*(4), 443–455.

Schover, L. R. (2007). Reproductive complications and sexual dysfunction in cancer survivors. In P. A. Ganz (Ed.), *Cancer survivorship: Today and tomorrow* (pp. 251–271). New York: Springer.

Schover, L. R., Fouladi, R. T., Warneke, C. L., Neese, L., Klein, E. A., Zippe, C., et al. (2002). Defining sexual outcomes after treatment for localized prostate cancer. *Cancer, 95*, 1773–1785.

Schwartz, M. D., Benkendorf, J., Lerman, C., Isaacs, C., Ryan-Robertson, A., & Johnson, L. (2001). Impact of educational print materials on knowledge, attitudes, and interest in BRCA1/BRCA2: Testing among Ashkenazi Jewish women. *Cancer, 92*(4), 932–940.

Sharpley, C. F., Bitsika, V., & Christie, D. H. R. (2008). Psychological distress among prostate cancer patients: Fact or fiction? *Clinical Medicine: Oncology, 2*, 563–572.

Sinsheimer, L. M., & Holland, J. C. (1987). Psychological issues in breast cancer. *Seminars in Oncology, 14*, 75–82.

Sriprasad, S., Dew, T. K., Muir, G. H., Thompson, P. M., Mulvin, D., Choi, W. H., et al. (2001). Validity of PSA, free/total PSA ratio and complexed/total PSA ratio measurements in men with acute urinary retention. *Prostate Cancer and Prostatic Diseases, 4*(3), 167–172.

Taylor, K. L., Shelby, R., Gelmann, E., & McGuire, C. (2004). Quality of life and trial adherence among participants in the prostate, lung, colorectal, and ovarian cancer screening trial. *Journal of National Cancer Institute, 96*, 1083–1094.

Taylor, S. E. (1983). Adjustment to threatening events: A theory of cognitive adaptation. *American Psychologist, 38*, 1161–1173.

van Andel, G., Visser, A. P., Zwinderman, A. H., Hulshof, M. C., Horenblas, S., & Kurth, K. H. (2004). A prospective longitudinal study comparing the impact of external radiation therapy with radical prostatectomy on health related quality of life in prostate cancer patients. *Prostate, 58*(4), 354–365.

Volk, R. J., Hawley, S. T., Kneuper, S., Holden, E. W., Stroud, L. A., Cooper, C. P., et al. (2006). Trials of decision aids for prostate cancer screening: A systematic review. *American Journal of Preventive Medicine, 33*, 428–434.

Von Kampen, M., De Weerdt, W., Van Poppel, H., et al. (2001). Effect of pelvic-floor re-education on duration and degree of incontinence after radical prostatectomy: A randomised controlled trial. *Lancet, 355*, 98–102.

Zhang, A. Y., Strauss, G. J., & Siminoff, L. A. (2006). Intervention of urinary incontinence and quality of life outcome in prostate cancer patients. *Journal of Psychosocial Oncology, 24*(2), 17–30.

CHAPTER 32

Pain and Painful Syndromes (Including Rheumatoid Arthritis and Fibromyalgia)

David A. Williams

There is no single organ responsible for pain; rather, it is best thought of as a conscious experience—an integration of nociceptive sensory awareness with genetic, affective, and cognitive (including memories) factors. Each of these factors is needed for pain perception; however, the relative contribution of each factor differs between individuals and across time within individuals.

Pain is a universal experience affecting all ages, from infants (American Academy of Pediatrics, 2001) to older adults (Horgas, 2003), both males and females (Greenspan et al., 2007), and extends beyond humans into much of the animal kingdom (Rollin, 2008). A random Harris Poll (2007) of U.S. adults ($N = 1,486$) revealed that 72% of respondents reported experiencing some form of pain within the last 12 months, and 42% were experiencing some form of pain at the time of the random call. A second study using advanced environmental momentary assessment methods to assess pain found greater average pain intensity to be associated with increasing age, lower income, and less education (Krueger & Stone, 2008).

While nearly everyone experiences episodes of acute pain throughout their lives, not everyone will experience chronic pain. The prevalence of chronic pain is estimated at between 15 and 20% in adults (Breivik, Collett, Ventafridda, Cohen, & Gallacher, 2006; Verhaak, Kerssens, Dekker, Sorbi, & Bensing, 1998) and accounts for 17% of primary care physician office visits (Gureje, Von, Simon, & Gater, 1998). Estimates place economic costs associated with chronic pain treatment, loss in productivity, and compensation to be between $50 and $70 billion per annum in the United States (Brennan, Carr, & Cousins, 2007).

Throughout history, human societies have differed in the meanings they ascribe to the experience of pain. As such, treatments for pain often reflect a given society's conceptualization of pain. This chapter begins with a brief history of pain and its treatment, along with an overview of current thinking about pain, emphasizing the integration of the biomedical and biopsychosocial models. Consistent with the biopsychosocial model of pain, this chapter reviews neurobiological mechanisms associated with acute and chronic pain, multidimensional approaches to pain assessment, and psychosocial interventions for chronic pain. The chapter concludes with some ideas about future opportunities for health psychologists in the management of pain conditions.

Historical Perspectives on Pain and Its Treatment

Human beings have long pondered the origin of pain, its purpose, its value, and its role in life and survival. Some of the earliest writings about pain trace back to 2,600 B.C. (Bonica, 1990). Early recorded accounts on stone tablets indicate that pain was as much a part of early humanity as it is today. Early conceptualizations of pain, however, reflected a strong societal belief in the supernatural. Pain was thought to be the product of evil, magic, and demons that entered the body though orifices such as nostrils, the mouth, or wounds. For example, evil spirits were thought to enter the body when an arrow pierced the skin. The experience of pain resulting from the arrow was not dissociable from the activity of the evil spirits stirring within the body. Given a supernatural understanding of pain, interventionists of the time were often sorcerers, shamans, priests and priestesses. To relieve pain, the evil spirits needed to leave the body; thus, interventionists encouraged the spirits to leave the body in bodily fluids (e.g., vomiting, sneezing, urinating, sweating), by gashing new wounds in the skin or drilling holes in the skull to set the spirits free. Other early approaches to pain management included the use of pressure, heat, water, exposure to the sun, electric fish (e.g., an intervention that predates today's use of electrical stimulation), and use of the poppy berry (Clipper, 2008; Rey, 1993).

Greek and Roman societies placed a value on empiricism and, as such, were able to advance theories of sensation involving nerves for both movement and sensation. While there was not consensus as to whether pain was perceived in the brain (i.e., Hippocrates) or in the heart (i.e., Plato), there was consensus that pain was produced within the body and not attributable to evil spirits (Clipper, 2008; Rey, 1993). As the Roman Empire fell, so did a focus on the physiological basis of pain perception.

During the Middle Ages, much of the Western World was under the control of the Christian church, which imbued pain with religious meaning (Meldrum, 2003; Morris, 1994). Pain was thought to be God's punishment of humanity for Adam's original sin in the Garden of Eden. Thus, bodily defects, painful illnesses, and death were attributed to the will of God. As might be presumed, interventions for pain were less common during this period given a reluctance to interfere with or question the will of a greater power. Comfort from pain could be had if great suffering on earth was interpreted as a sign of future reward in heaven.

The Renaissance and Classical periods saw resurgence in rational scientific endeavors and a resurfacing of Greek and Roman ideas from some 1,000 years earlier. During this period, work resumed that supported the brain and spinal cord working together to produce sensations of pain. Applications of scientific methods to the study of pain transformed pain into a medical condition, and physicians began using opium and sherry to control pain. Initially, the intent of medical treatment for pain was not to eradicate it. On the contrary, while scientists were defining pain as a physiological process (i.e., not supernatural or religious), pain was believed to play an important role in healing, and pain was therefore encouraged in a controlled manner (Meldrum, 2003).

Not until the 18th and 19th centuries would relief from pain become a desirable outcome of medical practice. Surgeons capable of performing procedures quickly, with as little pain as possible, became valued and were considered to be the most skilled. The introduction of surgical anesthesia, however, enabled physicians to control pain while turning their primary focus toward curing the many diseases and deformities for which physiological causes were emerging. In part due to the ease of administering anesthesia, the study of pain per se declined in importance compared to curative interventions that could now be performed under anesthesia. As the study of pain declined in importance, knowledge about pain become fragmented across many medical specialties and medical conditions—a philosophical legacy that still exists today to some degree.

It was not until 1953 when John Bonica, an anesthesiologist, published his book *The Management of Pain* that pain reemerged as something other than a side effect of otherwise effective medical treatment. This was followed by the introduction of the gate control theory of pain (Melzack & Wall, 1965), a neurobiological model that helped to reconcile how the experience of pain could be inconsistent with observable physical damage. This was the first model that required and integrated important roles for learning, behavior, cognition, and affect in the perception and modulation of pain.

In 1972, the International Association for the Study of Pain (IASP) held its first scientific meeting. The organization comprised not only physicians but also multidisciplinary professionals capable of addressing the many factors now thought to contribute to pain and its management.

The current definition espoused by the IASP defines pain as "an unpleasant sensory and emotional experience associated with actual or potential tissue damage, or described in terms of such damage" (Merskey & Bogduk, 1994, p. 211). This definition emphasizes the current understanding of pain as an integrated subjective experience. Currently, there is a strong sense in the United States and the world at large that pain needs to be treated aggressively when possible (Brennan et al., 2007). No longer a side effect of successful medical treatment, pain is now considered a symptom worthy of treatment in its own right (Liebeskind, 1991).

The current practice of pain medicine is a mix of evidence-based approaches and many nonempirical, legacy-based approaches from the past. The challenge facing individuals in pain today is the need to ensure that practitioners are educated in the latest models of pain, and that the economic incentives for delivering pain treatments are consistent with evidence-based approaches. The health psychologist, trained as a clinician, a researcher, or both, is nicely positioned to impact pain management meaningfully from multiple perspectives (e.g., assessment, treatment, mechanisms, and policy). To do so, however, requires that the health psychologist possess knowledge that goes beyond traditional psychological concepts to include all aspects of the biopsychosocial model of pain. The remainder of this chapter attempts to provide the most essential information.

Acute and Chronic Pain

In acute form, pain acts as a warning signal of actual or imminent damage to the body; as such, pain is thought to function adaptively by helping individuals learn about and avoid dangers that could harm the body (Wiertelak et al., 1994). Thus, although unpleasant, pain, like sneezing, coughing, and fever, serves a useful and protective function in survival. Its complete eradication would not be adaptive.

Acute pain often results from injury, disease, or medical procedure. By definition it resolves within about 3 months of onset (IASP, 1986). Currently medical science possesses many pharmacological approaches that effectively control most forms of acute pain. The challenges facing the treatment of acute pain are not to find medications that work, but to get the effective interventions into the hands of patients. Both lack of availability and fear of misuse dampen broader distribution and application of many medications capable of controlling acute pain (Brennan et al., 2007). The need for education is great on the parts of both patients and clinicians about how and when it is best to use these effective interventions for acute pain (Gordon et al., 2005).

Many patients and many clinicians are unaware that chronic and recurrent pain conditions are not simply temporal extensions of acute pain. These persistent forms of pain appear to have no inherent value for survival, are functionally distinct from acute pain, and are best thought of as diseases (the position taken by the European Federation of IASP chapters [www.epic.org/eap.htm]). As such, extending the application of effective acute pain interventions to the context of chronic pain should not be expected to work, but it is often attempted.

Most interventions for chronic pain are still based on the biomedical model, which aims philosophically to eradicate, cure, or correct malfunctioning nerves or tissues thought to be causing the pain. Often based on successful use with acute pain, these methods can include pharmacological agents (e.g., nonsteroidal anti-inflammatory drugs [NSAIDs], opiates, anticonvulsants, antidepressants, N-methyl-D-aspartate [NMDA] antagonists, and topical agents such as capsaicin); physical modalities (e.g., ultrasound, transcutaneous electrical nerve stimulation [TNS], therapeutic nerve blocks, and neurostimulation [e.g., spinal cord stimulation, deep brain stimulation]; implantable drug delivery [IDD] devices; and operative procedures [e.g., corrective surgery, neuroablation]).

Despite the vast number of interventions available, patients are often left with unsatisfactory relief from chronic pain. For example, pain medications are the second most commonly prescribed class of drug, but they do not eliminate chronic pain (e.g., long-term opiates tend to produce only a 32% reduction in pain on average). Corrective surgery, such as spinal fusion or repairs of herniated discs, leaves 70–75% of recipients still in pain. Pain relief from spinal cord stimulators across studies is only 19% on average, with the majority of patients still reporting "horrible" pain after 4 years; and epidural injections, despite being commonly applied, have been shown to produce little long-term relief (Armon, Argoff, Samuels, & Backonja, 2007; Turk, 2002).

Our increasingly sophisticated understanding of the pathophysiology of pain continues to draw into question the gap between our understanding of chronic pain and the widespread use of non-evidence-based interventions in clinical practice (Brennan et al., 2007). The next section provides an overview of the pathophysiology of pain.

Mechanisms of Pain

To distinguish between "acute pain" (i.e., a properly functioning bodily experience) and "chronic pain" (i.e., a disorder), one must remember that pain is an integrated experience originating from and impacting not one but many systems within the body. When the body detects a noxious stimulus, the nervous system responds with a host of autonomic changes (e.g., rise in blood pressure, activation of the hypothalamus–pituitary–adrenal axis, pupil dilation, and excitatory neural impulses discriminating and localizing the stimulus). This sensory response, called "nociception" may or may not lead to the experience of pain. Biomedical interventions for acute pain tend to target the nociceptive system by masking or quieting these responses.

Nociception

Noxious events occur in many forms (e.g., heat, cold; mechanical pressure; chemical and metabolic stimuli, such as low pH). These events impinge upon nerve endings that transduce the noxious event into sensory neural signals that then travel along a variety of A-delta nerve fibers (i.e., thinly myelinated and fast moving) or c-fibers (i.e., unmylenated and slower moving) (Torebjork, 1994). These afferent A-delta and C-fibers enter the spinal cord via the dorsal root and terminate in laminae I, II, and V of the superficial dorsal horn, where excitatory neurotransmitters at the terminals of these nerve fibers activate secondary projection neurons that ascend the spinal cord.

Pain Processing

The secondary neurons originating in the dorsal horn ascend to the brain via several tracts. The spinothalamic tract is the one most studied regarding pain processing. This tract provides nociceptive information to thalamic nuclei (Jones, 1999) as well as to the primary (SI) and secondary (SII) somatosensory cortices. SI and SII are cortical regions thought to play a role in the sensory–discriminative aspects of pain, as well as in the anticipation of painful stimuli (Sawamoto et al., 2000). Projections from this tract are also thought to provide nociceptive input to the insular cortex (IC), a region thought to integrate homeostatic input with emotional responses (Craig, 2003, 2009), which in turn links to the amygdala, a region thought to be involved in emotional processing and learning (especially fear and anxiety); the prefrontal cortex (PFC); regions involved in the cognitive-evaluative aspects of pain; and the anterior cingulate cortex (ACC), a region key to executive functioning.

Other tracts include the spinomesencephalic, spinoreticular, spinolimbic, spinocervical, and postsynaptic dorsal column tracts (Bourgeais, Gauriau, & Bernard, 2001; Desbois & Villanueva, 2001; Koyama, Kato, & Mikami, 2000; Koyama, McHaffie, Laurienti, & Coghill, 2005; Rainville, 2002; Watanabe, Kakigi, Kayama, Hoshiyama, & Kaneoke, 1998; Willis & Westlund, 1997). Like aspects of the spinothalamic tract, these other pathways also help to mediate the interactions between nociceptive signals and memory, affective responses, and the meaning of past and potentially threatening stimuli (Coghill, Sang, Maisog, & Iadarola, 1999; Peck, 1986; Treede, Kenshalo, Gracely, & Jones, 1999).

Given that no single organ or structure is responsible for pain processing, researchers have referred to the complex network of cortical structures involved in pain processing as the "pain matrix," or the "cerebral signature for pain" (Tracey & Mantyh, 2007). It should be noted, however, that all regions are not uniformly active during pain perception/processing; rather, the great variability as to which regions are involved in processing pain depend on the type of pain and variance within and between individuals. The most consistent regions involved in normal pain processing include the spinal cord, thalamus, SI and SII, insula, ACC, and the PFC. Other secondary regions that appear to be involved in at least some aspects of pain processing include the amygdala, the hippocampus, the posterior parietal cortex (PPC), basal ganglia, and elements of the brainstem (Tracey, 2008). Chronic pain states, on the other hand, have been more difficult to study. Relative to acute pain processing, chronic pain cortical processing often reflects *decreased* sensory processing (e.g., SI, SII) in favor of enhanced activation of regions associated with cognitive, emotional, and introspective processing of events (Apkarian, Bushnell, Treede, & Zubieta, 2005).

The Relevance of Psychological Factors in Pain

Due in part to historical biases, pain associated with unobservable damage or pain of medically unexplainable origin is often attributed to psychiatric illness. This dualistic view of pain as being either somatically explained or psychogenic in nature has not been helpful. It has unnecessarily stigmatized many individuals with pain as being psychiatrically ill, hampered more rapid advancement of evidence-based interdisciplinary approaches to pain management, and perpetuated an overly simplistic model of pain upon which medical and legal decision making has been based.

Psychological factors affecting pain can be divided into two types: (1) psychiatric disorders and (2) psychosocial influences. Psychiatric disorders, such as major depression, anxiety disorders, and personality disorders, are diagnosable concerns that can coexist with and negatively impact pain. For example, depression occurs in the general population at a rate of 5–10% (Narrow, Rae, Robins, & Regier, 2002) but has been shown to co-occur with pain 52% of the time in pain clinics, 27% of the time in primary care clinics, and 18% of the time in population-based studies (Bair, Robinson, Katon, & Kroenke, 2003). Anxiety disorders occur in the general population at a rate of 12–19% (Narrow et al., 2002) but occur with pain and depression 23% of the time (Bair, Wu, Damush, Sutherland, & Kroenke, 2008). Personality disorders have been associated with poorer treatment outcomes and poorer adherence to pain treatment (Gatchel, 1997; Gatchel, Polatin, & Kinney, 1995; Gatchel, Polatin, & Mayer, 1995). Occurring 14.8% of the time in the general population (Grant et al., 2004), personality disorders are seen in pain clinics at rates of 51–58% (Fishbain, Goldberg, Meagher, Steele, & Rosomoff, 1986; Polatin, Kinney, Gatchel, Lillo, & Mayer, 1993).

While chronic pain and psychiatric conditions frequently co-occur, they should not be confused with one another or be viewed as the same condition. Treatment of coexisting psychiatric disorders in a patient with chronic pain is highly appropriate; but is not likely to address fully the chronic pain problem. Both conditions need to be addressed, often with different interventions. Neuroimaging studies suggest that augmented pain perception (e.g., as seen in fibromyalgia, irritable bowel syndrome, and low back pain) occurs whether comorbid depression is present or not (Giesecke et al., 2005), refuting claims that "unexplainable pain" is simply a manifestation of depression (Alfici, Sigal, & Landau, 1989).

A person need not be psychiatrically disturbed to perceive pain in a manner that exceeds that of other individuals given comparable levels of tissue damage or deformity. It is quite possible that some individuals are genetically predisposed toward greater pain sensitivity. Some of the best work supporting this notion is with individuals with "temporomandibular disorder," a chronic pain condition affecting the face and head. While there does not appear to be a single gene responsible for chronic pain, there are a number of genes that, together, predispose certain individuals to developing chronic pain conditions. These genetic influences appear to cluster into two camps: polymorphisms associated with heightened pain sensitivity, and polymorphisms associated with affective vulnerability (Diatchenko et al., 2005; Diatchenko, Nackley, Slade, Fillingim, & Maixner, 2006). In genetically predisposed individuals, psychosocial factors influence pain modulation and maintenance. Such factors include, but are not limited to, ethnic and cultural influences, patient appraisals/beliefs about pain, and emotional stress/distress.

Ethnic/Cultural Factors

Cultural affiliation has been shown to influence perception and response to pain (Bates, Edwards, & Anderson, 1993; Greenwald, 1991; Lipton & Marbach, 1984; Zborowski, 1952). Important factors include a culture's normative tolerance for affective expression and stoicism, beliefs about the meaning of pain, and normative responses to pain. Cultural norms influencing the expression of pain appear to be learned at an early age (Zborowski, 1952) and may influence the experience of pain to an extent similar to that of physiological factors. A study of healthy females compared responses to a standardized experimental pain stimulus in a sample representing four different ethnic/cultural backgrounds: Anglo-Saxon, Irish, Italian, and Jewish (Sternbach & Tursky, 1965). "Pain thresholds" (i.e., the point at which a stimulus becomes painful) did not differ between groups, but "tolerances" (i.e., the maximum amount of the stimulus allowed by the subject) did differ. Italian women had the lowest tolerance for pain, whereas stoic or neutral responses were characteristic of the Irish and Anglo groups. Diminished reactivity was found in the members of the Jewish sample, who tended to minimize the significance (i.e., personal relevance) of the experimental pain stimulus. Several studies have found that African American samples report greater pain than do European American samples undergoing similar acute medical procedures (Edwards & Fillingim, 1999; Faucett, Gordon, & Levine, 1994; Rahim-Williams et al., 2007).

Appraisals, Beliefs, and Coping

The appraisal process is highly relevant to understanding individual differences in pain perception. Once a nociceptive event occurs, individuals make an appraisal of that event. This first or primary appraisal is used to determine whether the nociceptive event is harmful, threatening, or of some benefit. If judged to be harmful or threatening, a secondary appraisal process helps to determine whether the necessary resources for controlling the nociceptive event can be accessed. If resources are adequate and available, then appropriate coping with pain commences. If resources are inadequate, affective responses, such as anxiety or fear, can further heighten the perception of pain until appropriate resources for quieting the pain are brought to bear on the problem (e.g., help from others, medications, etc.) (Lazarus & Folkman, 1984). When adaptive resources for comfort are not forthcoming, then responses such as helplessness, isolation, avoidance of work and social activities, and prolonged inactivity may be adopted. In the short term, these behavioral responses may actually be successful in reducing pain. Unfortunately, early success in reducing pain with these responses can operantly condition individuals with pain to expect relief from such responses in the long term. Unfortunately, the same behaviors that were temporarily successful in reducing acute pain may prove maladaptive for long-term adaptation to chronic pain. For example, prolonged rest reduces pain acutely, but with time, leads to physical deconditioning. Deconditioning makes functioning more painful in the long term. The early adoption of maladaptive behavioral responses to pain is thought to account (in part) for how acute pain states transition into chronic pain conditions (Gatchel, 1996).

Awareness of individuals' cognitions about pain (i.e., beliefs) can importantly influence adherence to treatment, treatment responsivity, and long-term outcomes to both physical and psychologically oriented treatments (Jensen, Turner, & Romano, 2007; Stroud, Thorn, Jensen, & Boothby, 2000; Williams & Keefe, 1991; Williams, Robinson, & Geisser, 1994). Underscoring the importance of considering individual beliefs about pain, 40% of the variance in physical functional status and around 30% of the variance in affective symptoms may be attributed to how individuals think about their pain (Turner, Jensen, & Romano, 2000).

Two cognitive factors that have received a great deal of research attention are locus of pain control and catastrophizing. The general concept of "personal control" is central to many prominent theories that attempt to explain human motivation, learning, behavior, and emotion (Bandura, 1977; Rotter, 1954; Thompson, 1981). These theories share the notion that perceived personal control over life events positively impacts psychological and behavioral functioning. Beliefs in personal control are thought to evolve from multiple learning experiences supporting the general belief that personal effort is associated with positive outcomes and avoidance of negative effects.

"Locus of control for pain" refers to patients' perceptions about whether pain is something that can fall under personal control. In studies of patients with chronic pain conditions, a stronger belief in internal locus of control for pain has repeatedly been associated with lower levels of physical and psychological symptoms, and better response to therapy (Crisson & Keefe, 1988; Flor & Turk, 1988; Gibson & Helme, 2000; Hagglund, Haley, Reveille, & Alarcon, 1989; Jensen, Turner, Romano, & Karoly, 1991; Lipchik, Milles, & Covington, 1993; Parker et al., 1988; Rudy, Kerns, & Turk, 1988; Strong, Ashton, Cramond, & Chant, 1990).

"Pain catastrophizing," or the tendency to think about pain as being awful, horrible, and unbearable, is recognized as being an extremely important contributor to the experience of pain. Early research suggested that catastrophizing might be a thinking style associated with depression (Rosenstiel & Keefe, 1983; Sullivan & D'Eon, 1990), but later studies found catastrophizing to be associated with pain and pain-related disability in a manner that is independent of depressive influences (Geisser, Robinson, Keefe, & Weiner, 1994; Geisser, Robinson, Miller, & Bade, 2003; Geisser & Roth, 1998; Jensen et al., 2007; Keefe, Brown, Wallston, & Caldwell, 1989; Keefe et al., 1990b; Sullivan, Stanish, Waite, Sullivan, & Tripp, 1998). Catastrophizing appears to play an important role in the transition of acute pain to chronic pain, with 47% of the variance in

transition being attributed to catastrophizing (Burton, Tillotson, Main, & Hollis, 1995).

Emotional Stress/Distress

Emotional stress/distress can also facilitate the transition from acute to chronic pain and help to maintain the chronic condition. Environmental stressors associated with chronic pain are broad and varied, and include topics such as family discord, work demands, fear of reinjury, litigation issues, comorbid illnesses, and loss of independence. Although these stressors are varied, common to each are the psychological factors of environmental lack of control, lack of support, and lack of predictability. For chronic pain conditions, personally relevant stressors appear to play a more salient role in symptom exacerbation than do more global stressors. For example, at the time of the September 11, 2001, terrorist attacks, two pain studies using daily symptom monitoring were being conducted in New York City and in Washington, DC (Raphael, Natelson, Janal, & Nayak, 2002; Williams, Brown, Clauw, & Gendreau, 2003). In each study, symptoms on the days immediately before, during, and following the terrorists' attacks were compared. Both studies failed to find any relationship between global stressors (i.e., the terrorist attacks) and symptom worsening; rather, symptom fluctuations were much more strongly associated with personal activities and personally relevant stressors.

Assessing Pain

There is no machine or sensor capable of measuring directly the conscious perception of pain. To assess pain, clinicians must rely on the patient's verbal report, a potentially biased behavioral observation that is at best an indirect corollary of the patient's full experience of pain. Currently, the most common method of assessing pain is to have patients report their pain on a quantitative pain scale, where one end of the scale represents *No pain* and the other represents *Extreme pain* (Agency for Healthcare Policy and Research [AHCPR], 1992). Despite its apparent simplicity, there are many variations of this strategy that can lead to differing clinical impressions in a given patient (Litcher-Kelly,

Martino, Broderick, & Stone, 2007). The following is a description of several common approaches to clinical pain assessment.

Pain Intensity Ratings

The most common methods of assessing pain use the numeric rating scale (NRS), the verbal rating scale (VRS), or the visual analogue scale (VAS). When using an NRS, patients are asked to rate the intensity of their pain along a single numeric dimension (e.g., 0–10 or 0–100). The end points typically have verbal descriptors, such as *No pain* and *Worst pain*, and can be administered verbally, in written form, or over the phone. The NRS can be completed in less than 10 seconds and is easily administered repeatedly over time, with little patient burden. One disadvantage of the NRS stems from the inability of some patients (e.g., older adults and some cultural groups) to conceptualize a perception (e.g., pain) as a number.

VRSs comprise a list of adjectives arranged along a linear dimension. The number of adjectives along the dimension has varied across different instruments, with some having as few as four adjectives (Seymour, 1982) and others as many as 15 (Gracely, McGrath, & Dubner, 1978). Each adjective is arranged semantically to represent increasing intensity along a line and is assigned a numeric value as a function of its rank order. An advantage of the VRS is that linguistic descriptors of pain represent the experience better than do numbers. A disadvantage, however, is that this method is limited to written administration, since committing multiple adjectives to memory, as would be needed in a verbal or phone administration, would be difficult.

The VAS is a straight line, usually 10 cm in length, with verbal descriptors only at the ends. Patients are asked simply to place a mark on the line to indicate the intensity of pain. Scoring of the VAS requires measuring where the mark occurred on the paper and translating the value into a quantitative rating of pain. The VAS is especially useful when working with children, who may not be able to conceptualize pain as a number, or with cognitively impaired populations, who are unable to make the fine verbal discriminations of pain intensity required by the verbal scales (Varni, Jay, Masek, & Thompson, 1986). Like the NRS, some individuals may not be able to translate the experience of pain into a mark on a line. In a study of 218 physicians, it was found that 56% preferred NRSs, 19.5% preferred VRSs, and only 7% preferred VASs (Price, Bush, Long, & Harkins, 1994).

Qualitative Pain Measurement

Some measures of pain focus more heavily on the nature of the pain experience than on its intensity. One such measure is the McGill Pain Questionnaire (MPQ; Melzack, 1975) or its validated short form (Melzack, 1987). The full version of the MPQ consists of 78 pain descriptors (adjectives) grouped into 20 categories, each representing a different quality of the pain experience (e.g., pressure sensations, burning sensations, tearing sensations). The 20 categories may be consolidated into sensory descriptors, affective descriptors, and evaluative descriptors. The MPQ has a demonstrated ability to discriminate between different pain conditions based on how patients reported experiencing the pain (e.g., Grushka & Sessle, 1984; Masson, Hunt, Gem, & Boulton, 1989; Melzack, Terrence, Fromm, & Amsel, 1986).

Pictorial Pain Assessment

Picture or face scales use series of photographs or drawings that illustrate increasing amounts of pain. With these scales, patients are asked to choose the face that best depicts the expression representing the amount of pain that they are experiencing (Keck, Gerkensmeyer, Joyce, & Schade, 1996). This method can be particularly useful when assessing pain in pediatric populations or populations with questionable literacy. However, patients must be able to comprehend that they are being asked to translate their personal pain experience into the facial expression of another individual, a task that may be differentially challenging to individuals.

Environmental Momentary Assessment of Pain

Much of pain research has relied on asking individuals with pain to report their average pain over a specified time period (e.g., the past week). While some studies suggest that this approach is reasonably accurate and acceptable for clinical use (e.g., Hunter,

Philips, & Rachman, 1979; Smith, Salovey, Turk, Jobe, & Willis, 1993), others have questioned whether individuals are capable of creating an accurate mental average of their pain experience over time (Hufford & Shiffman, 2002). This debate has led to the introduction of a new method of pain assessment into pain research and practice.

Ecological momentary assessment (EMA) is an alternative approach to the assessment of clinical pain (Shiffman, Stone, & Hufford, 2008; Stone & Shiffman, 1994). EMA allows researchers to study patients in the environments they typically inhabit and under conditions representative of their daily lives. It focuses on repeated and dense data collection of real-time reports of patients' "current" pain over time. Aggregating these data is thought to minimize recall biases (Bradburn, Rips, & Shevell, 1987), and to maximize real-world generalization. Electronic diaries that patients carry into real-world settings are often used to apply EMA in clinical pain research.

Other Relevant Assessment Domains

While it is important to assess the symptom of pain in chronic pain conditions, often many other health-related domains contribute to the well-being of individuals with pain. The Initiative on Methods, Measurement, and Pain Assessment in Clinical Trials (IMMPACT) is a working group that focuses on identifying the domains that should be assessed in research involving chronic pain. This group identified four core areas for assessment: (1) pain intensity, (2) physical functioning, (3) emotional functioning, and (4) overall improvement/well-being (Dworkin et al., 2005). In addition, this group has produced scholarly recommendations regarding the choice of assessment instruments for pain and determinations of clinical improvement (Dworkin et al., 2008), approaches to analyzing multiple end points (Turk et al., 2008), and approaches to pain measurement in pediatric populations (McGrath et al., 2008).

Psychosocial Interventions for Chronic Pain

Early attempts to apply psychosocial interventions in chronic pain were based on adaptations of traditional mental health interventions with foundations in psychoanalytic, psychodynamic, and behavioral theory. In these initial applications, it was not clear whether the psychological intervention directly targeted the pain, the affective and cognitive processes modulating pain, the functional limitations of pain, or the comorbid psychiatric illnesses accompanying pain. As such, these interventions were quite broad in scope and required a number of sessions to accomplish all the possible objectives. Over time, evidence from treatment studies has helped to clarify the contributions of psychological interventions for specific forms of chronic pain. Interventions based on behavioral and cognitive-behavioral theory currently have the broadest base of empirical support for the management of pain (Chambless et al., 1998; Compas, Haaga, Keefe, Leitenberg, & Williams, 1998; Hoffman, Papas, Chatkoff, & Kerns, 2007; Morley, Eccleston, & Williams, 1999; Morley, Williams, & Hussain, 2008). This is not to say that more traditional psychodynamic (or insight-oriented) approaches do not benefit patients with pain; rather, the majority of methodologically rigorous studies on pain have used behavioral and cognitive-behavioral approaches. It is likely that insight can be of great benefit for individuals who fail to respond adequately to behaviorally oriented interventions, or who suffer from pain conditions evolving from traumatic or highly affectively charged events (Grzesiak, Ury, & Dworkin, 1996).

As stated earlier, there is strong empirical support for the efficacy of behavioral therapy (BT) and cognitive-behavioral therapy (CBT) in the management of chronic pain (Hoffman et al., 2007; Morley et al., 1999, 2008). Versions of BT/CBT appear to share a common theoretical underpinning and a common process for engaging patients in making lifestyle adaptations consistent with improved management of pain and functional status with pain. Such interventions have been developed for many forms of pain, including osteoarthritis (Keefe et al., 1990a, 1990b) and rheumatoid arthritis (Keefe et al., 1991), low back pain (Reid, Otis, Barry, & Kerns, 2003), sickle-cell disease pain (Gil, Williams, Thompson, & Kinney, 1991), fibromyalgia (Williams, 2003), and irritable bowel syndrome (Lackner et al., 2008).

Common Components of Evidence-Supported Psychosocial Interventions

While each of these pain syndromes benefits from skills specific to the given condition, many of the skills sets utilized in the treatment of these conditions hold relevance for any type of chronic pain. A brief description of shared processes and some of the most common skill sets utilized in BT and CBT follows.

BT and CBT interventions typically include three phases: (1) an educational phase, in which patients are introduced to a model for understanding their pain and the role they can play in the management of the condition (e.g., the biopsychosocial model); (2) a skills training phase, in which training is provided in a variety of cognitive and behavioral skills useful for managing pain and improving function (e.g., relaxation training, activity pacing etc.); and (3) an application phase, in which patients learn to apply their skills in progressively more challenging real-life situations (Keefe, 1996). Each application of BT/CBT for chronic pain needs to be tailored to the needs of the individual patient, and a clear treatment target needs to be agreed upon by both therapist and patient (a focus on pain, function, sleep, etc.). The most common behavioral changes attempted through BT/CBT for chronic pain include the following: (1) adoption of the relaxation response into daily practice for pain and stress reduction, (2) adoption of graded activation and pleasant activity scheduling as a means of improving functional status, (3) behavioral methods to improve sleep and cognition, (4) problem-solving and cognitive restructuring techniques to increase productivity and reduce stress, and (5) communication skills to facilitate more beneficial relationships between patients and their physicians, family members, and friends.

The Relaxation Response

The human body naturally relaxes in the absence of perceived threat. Pain, however, is a persistent stressor that precludes opportunities for natural relaxation to occur. Patients with chronic pain must therefore learn to trigger relaxation under their own conscious control. The relaxation response is considered a highly beneficial nonpharmacological method of reducing pain through diminished autonomic arousal (National Institutes of Health, 1996).

The relaxation response is a physiologically based learned response that involves quieting physiological activity (e.g., muscle tension, heart rate, and breathing) through active and focused mental effort. Learning the response requires the individual to practice the techniques repeatedly until his or her body acquires the desired response. While there is no consensus as to the best method of teaching the relaxation response (e.g., progressive muscle relaxation, visual imagery, hypnosis, biofeedback, mindfulness meditation), all appear to be useful modalities for learning this response.

Graded Activation and Pleasant Activity Scheduling

For many individuals, chronic pain impairs multiple aspects of life, including work productivity, social engagement, and personal hobbies/pleasant activities. Most individuals with pain will attempt to pace their activities by placing essential tasks before personal pleasures. While this strategy results in getting the essentials accomplished, daily denial of personal pleasures can have devastating effects on mood and motivation. Denial of pleasurable activities augments pain and further reduces function.

Taking time to engage in pleasant activities should not be viewed as a selfish indulgence. Instead, enjoyment of pleasant activities is a natural way to elevate mood (Lewinsohn, 1975) and invites confidence in one's body to function at a higher level. This behavioral change encourages one to schedule pleasant activities into one's day, placing the same priority on a meeting, a doctor's appointment, or a deadline. Scheduling is preferable to spontaneity given that, with spontaneity, the activity may never occur or it may occur at a time when the individual is vulnerable to overdoing and at risk for increased pain.

To avoid overdoing, pleasant activity scheduling is often paired with skills in graded activation. Many patients unwittingly worsen pain on "good days" by doing more than personal limitations allow. This overactivity is followed by several "bad days" of symptom flares. An intermittent burst of activity followed by increased pain can be a source of frustration for patients and limits the ability to plan and commit to accomplishing future activities. Graded activation is a method of pacing that can improve physical functioning while minimizing the likelihood of pain flare-ups. This approach has been successfully applied in low back pain populations (Lindstrom et al., 1992), rheumatological populations (Gil, Ross, & Keefe, 1988), individuals with fibromyalgia (Williams et al., 2002), and patients with chronic fatigue syndrome (Deale, Chalder, Marks, & Wessely, 1997). The key to this strategy is to limit activities based on time rather than on patients' subjective experience of pain or task completion. Active time can be as short as several minutes or as long as several hours, depending on what the patient can initially tolerate without exacerbation. Once patient and therapist agree on a time-based activity program, subsequent goals for steadily increasing the time spent on specified targeted behaviors can proceed. Time-based pacing can be used as a complementary skill to help ensure the long-term adoption of exercise regimens; work-related activities; and pleasant activities, such as social outings and sporting activities.

Behavioral Methods for Improving Sleep and Cognition

Individuals with chronic pain have a number of problems related to getting a good night's sleep, including difficulty falling asleep, being awakened by pain or discomfort, or awakening from sleep feeling unrefreshed and unrestored. There exists a number of behavioral strategies that, if used regularly, can help individuals get needed restorative sleep, with additional benefits in improved mood, better management of pain, less fatigue, and improved mental clarity (Morin, Culbert, & Schwartz, 1994). Some of these skills focus on timing strategies (e.g., having regular sleep routines), sleep behaviors (e.g., attempting to sleep only when in need of sleep), and behavioral avoidance of stimulating activities before bed, such as emotionally charged conversations, watching action movies, or consuming nicotine or caffeine. CBT targeting sleep appears to have a direct impact on pain symptoms and on functional interference resulting from nonrestorative sleep (Affleck et al., 1996, 1998; Edinger,

Wohlgemuth, Krystal, & Rice, 2005). Like the relaxation response, behavioral strategies for improving sleep are physiological self-regulation skills that require repeated practice and consistency to train the body to respond in the desired manner under conscious control.

Some pain conditions are associated with memory and concentration difficulties (Dick & Rashiq, 2007). The cause of dyscognition in chronic pain is not well understood but is likely to be associated with the lack of restorative sleep architecture and the distracting effect of persistent pain on information processing (Eccleston & Crombez, 1999, 2005). Behavioral approaches (e.g., the relaxation response for pain and behavioral methods to improve sleep) are likely to benefit dyscognition, but more study is needed in this area.

Problem-Solving Strategies and Cognitive Restructuring

Individuals with chronic pain face interpersonal and functional challenges that rarely affect healthy individuals. The daily barrage of seemingly novel and unsolvable challenges adds to the fatigue and burden of chronic pain. Programmatic problem-solving strategies that can be taught to patients help to break large problems down into solvable pieces (D'Zurilla & Goldfried, 1971; Nezu, Nezu, & Perri, 1989). What is taught in therapy is a strategy for solving problems rather than specific solutions; thus, patients learn a strategy that can be carried into the future as new problems arise. When applied successfully, patients learn to overcome barriers and attain a greater sense of control over the process of adapting to a chronic illness.

Solutions to problems often reflect beliefs about the nature of the problem and about one's personal ability to execute solutions effectively. Strong belief in one's helplessness, the futility of trying to control illness, and the inability to contribute meaningfully to others are examples of learned automatic thinking patterns that impede successful adaptation. Cognitive restructuring (Beck, Rush, Shaw, & Emery, 1979) is a cognitive skill that challenges the rationality of negative automatic thoughts and seeks to instill alternative thinking that promotes greater functioning and well-being. Cognitive restructuring is often confused with "positive thinking," which can be perceived as ingenuous and unrealistic if the suggested thinking patterns fall too far outside the perceived reality of the patient with pain. Cognitive restructuring invites individuals to explore the origin of learned automatic thinking patterns that promote maladaptive behavior in response to pain. Fortunately, with practice, the new thinking patterns that replace old ones are more consistent with well-being and functioning, even with the discomforts associated with pain.

Communication Skills

Individuals with chronic pain frequently report unsatisfying visits with their physicians. The basis for this perception is multifaceted, including factors such as too little time, becoming disorganized and forgetting to mention all that was important, the physician's own agenda and questions, and interpersonal factors (e.g., a desire to please the physician or fear of the physician).

Regardless of the cause, patients need to feel adequately understood by the clinicians providing care, in order to partner with the physician in carrying out a pain management plan. While it is unlikely that the patient will be able to change the behavior of the clinician, many behavioral strategies can be used by the patient to improve doctor–patient communication.

Family members also need to understand what they can do to be most helpful to the patient. A common mistake of family members is to remove all responsibility from the patient to facilitate rest and reduce stress. This is often the wrong approach because individuals with chronic pain need to be able to engage in activities that empower them to feel efficacious and productive. Communicating with family and friends about how best to support such efforts can require tact and a good bit of assertiveness. Assertive communication skills training (Goldfried & Davidson, 1976; Gombeski et al., 2002) represents a skills set that is easily communicated to individuals but best implemented with consistent practice or role playing with a therapist. Typically, a bit of trial and error helps to refine one's personal strengths in being appropriately assertive.

Conclusions

Health psychologists walk a line between the models, philosophies, and biases of mental health and those of traditional medicine. As such, the health psychologist is in a perfect position to draw from both to understand better and predict pain, and to provide better comprehensive care to patients. By virtue of a health psychologist's training, he or she can contribute in a variety of ways to the exploration and treatment of chronic pain conditions. As previously described, there is a great need for improved measurement of pain and its associated symptoms. Health psychologists trained in psychometric and scaling methods are ideally positioned to contribute to advances in this area. Knowledge of the interfaces among the practices of mental health, medicine, and biological psychology/neuroscience facilitates health psychologists' crucial roles as collaborators with physicians in treating pain conditions. The health psychologist can also help to improve the lives of patients either through direct clinical intervention or by facilitating other professionals in the development of comprehensive therapeutic programs to serve the needs of individuals in pain. Pain is one of the medical conditions in which health psychologists have played important roles both in shaping the contemporary conceptualization of the condition and developing evidence-based comprehensive treatments.

Acknowledgments

Preparation of this chapter was supported in part by Grant Nos. R01-AR050044 (National Institute of Arthritis and Musculoskeletal and Skin Diseases, National Institutes of Health), AR053207 (National Institute of Arthritis and Musculoskeletal and Skin Diseases, National Institutes of Health), U01AR55069 (National Institute of Arthritis and Musculoskeletal and Skin Diseases, National Institutes of Health), and DAMD 17-00-2-0018 (U.S. Department of Defense).

Further Reading

Fransen, J., & Russell, I. J. (1996). *The fibromyalgia help book: Practical guide to living better with fibromyalgia.* St. Paul, MN: Smith House Press.

Mease, P., Arnold, L. M., Choy, E. H., Clauw, D. J., Crofford, L. J., Glass, J. M., et al. (2009). Fibromyalgia syndrome module at OMER-ACT 9: Domain construct. *Journal of Rheumatology, 36*(10), 2318–2329.

Thieme, K., Turk, D. C., & Flor, H. (2007). Responder criteria for operant and cognitive-behavioral treatment of fibromyalgia syndrome. *Arthritis and Rheumatism, 57*(5), 830–836.

Wallace, D. J., & Clauw, D. J. (2005). *Fibromyalgia and other central pain syndromes.* Philadelphia: Lippincott, Williams & Wilkins.

Williams, D. A., & Clauw, D. J. (2009). Understanding fibromyalgia: Lessons from the broader pain research community. *Journal of Pain, 10*(8), 777–791.

Williams, D. A., & Schilling, S. (2009). Advances in the assessment of fibromyalgia. *Rheumatic Disease Clinics of North America, 35*(2), 339–357.

References

Affleck, G., Tennen, H., Urrows, S., Higgins, P., Abeles, M., Hall, C., et al. (1998). Fibromyalgia and women's pursuit of personal goals: A daily process analysis. *Health Psychology, 17,* 40–47.

Affleck, G., Urrows, S., Tennen, H., Higgins, P., & Abeles, M. (1996). Sequential daily relations of sleep, pain intensity, and attention to pain among women with fibromyalgia. *Pain, 68,* 363–368.

Agency for Health Care Policy and Research (AHCPR). (1992). *Acute pain management: Operative or medical procedures and trauma* (Clinical Practice Guideline No. 1, Rep. No. 92-0032). Rockville, MD: U.S. Department of Health and Human Services.

Alfici, S., Sigal, M., & Landau, M. (1989). Primary fibromyalgia syndrome—a variant of depressive disorder? *Psychotherapy and Psychosomatics, 51,* 156–161.

American Academy of Pediatrics. (2001). The assessment and management of acute pain in infants, children, and adolescents. *Pediatrics, 108,* 793–797.

Apkarian, A. V., Bushnell, M. C., Treede, R. D., & Zubieta, J. K. (2005). Human brain mechanisms of pain perception and regulation in health and disease. *European Journal of Pain, 9,* 463–484.

Armon, C., Argoff, C. E., Samuels, J., & Backonja, M. M. (2007). Assessment: Use of epidural steroid injections to treat radicular lumbosacral pain: Report of the Therapeutics and Technology Assessment Subcommittee of the American Academy of Neurology. *Neurology, 68,* 723–729.

Bair, M. J., Robinson, R. L., Katon, W., & Kroenke, K. (2003). Depression and pain co-morbidity: A literature review. *Archives of Internal Medicine, 163,* 2433–2445.

Bair, M. J., Wu, J., Damush, T. M., Sutherland, J. M., & Kroenke, K. (2008). Association of depression and anxiety alone and in combination with chronic musculoskeletal pain in primary care patients. *Psychosomatic Medicine, 70,* 890–897.

Bandura, A. (1977). Self-efficacy: Towards a unifying theory of behavioral change. *Psychological Review, 2,* 191–215.

Bates, M. S., Edwards, W. T., & Anderson, K. O. (1993). Ethnocultural influences on variation in chronic pain perception. *Pain, 52,* 101–112.

Beck, A. T., Rush, A. J., Shaw, B. F., & Emery, G. (1979). *Cognitive therapy of depression.* New York: Guilford Press.

Bonica, J. J. (1953). *The management of pain: With special emphasis on the use of analgesic block in diagnosis, prognosis, and therapy.* Philadelphia: Lea & Febiger.

Bonica, J. J. (1990). History of pain concepts and theories. In J. J. Bonica, J. D. Loeser, C. R. Chapman, & W. E. Fordyce (Eds.), *The management of pain* (pp. 2–17). Philadelphia: Lea & Febiger.

Bourgeais, L., Gauriau, C., & Bernard, J. F. (2001). Projections from the nociceptive area of the central nucleus of the amygdala to the forebrain: A PHA-L study in the rat. *European Journal of Neuroscience, 14,* 229–255.

Bradburn, N. M., Rips, L. J., & Shevell, S. K. (1987). Answering autobiographical questions: The impact of memory and inference on surveys. *Science, 236,* 157–161.

Breivik, H., Collett, B., Ventafridda, V., Cohen, R., & Gallacher, D. (2006). Survey of chronic pain in Europe: Prevalence, impact on daily life, and treatment. *European Journal of Pain, 10,* 287–333.

Brennan, F., Carr, D. B., & Cousins, M. (2007). Pain management: A fundamental human right. *Anesthesia and Analgesia, 105,* 205–221.

Burton, A. K., Tillotson, K. M., Main, C. J., & Hollis, S. (1995). Psychosocial predictors of outcome in acute and subchronic low back trouble. *Spine, 20,* 722–728.

Chambless, D. L., Baker, M. J., Baucom, D. H., Beutler, L. E., Calhoun, K. S., Crist-Christoph, P., et al. (1998). Update on empirically validated therapies, II. *Clinical Psychologist, 51,* 3–16.

Clipper, S. E. (2008). *A brief history of pain* [Office of Communications and Public Relations, NINDS/NIH]. Retrieved October 1, 2008, from *www.nihds.nih.gov*.

Coghill, R. C., Sang, C. N., Maisog, J. M., & Iadarola, M. J. (1999). Pain intensity processing within the human brain: A bilateral, distributed mechanism. *Journal of Neurophysiology, 82*, 1934–1943.

Compas, B. E., Haaga, D. A., Keefe, F. J., Leitenberg, H., & Williams, D. A. (1998). Sampling of empirically supported psychological treatments from health psychology: Smoking, chronic pain, cancer, and bulimia nervosa. *Journal of Consulting and Clinical Psychology, 66*, 89–112.

Craig, A. D. (2003). A new view of pain as a homeostatic emotion. *Trends in Neuroscience, 26*, 303–307.

Craig, A. D. (2009). How do you feel—now?: The anterior insula and human awareness. *Nature Reviews Neuroscience, 10*, 59–70.

Crisson, J. E., & Keefe, F. J. (1988). The relationship of locus of control to pain coping strategies and psychological distress in chronic pain patients. *Pain, 35*, 147–154.

Deale, A., Chalder, T., Marks, I., & Wessely, S. (1997). Cognitive behavior therapy for chronic fatigue syndrome: A randomized controlled trial. *American Journal of Psychiatry, 154*, 408–414.

Desbois, C., & Villanueva, L. (2001). The organization of lateral ventromedial thalamic connections in the rat: A link for the distribution of nociceptive signals to widespread cortical regions. *Neuroscience, 102*, 885–898.

Diatchenko, L., Nackley, A. G., Slade, G. D., Fillingim, R. B., & Maixner, W. (2006). Idiopathic pain disorders—pathways of vulnerability. *Pain, 123*, 226–230.

Diatchenko, L., Slade, G. D., Nackley, A. G., Bhalang, K., Sigurdsson, A., Belfer, I., et al. (2005). Genetic basis for individual variations in pain perception and the development of a chronic pain condition. *Human Molecular Genetics, 14*, 135–143.

Dick, B. D., & Rashiq, S. (2007). Disruption of attention and working memory traces in individuals with chronic pain. *Anesthia and Analgesia, 104*, 1223–1229.

Dworkin, R. H., Turk, D. C., Farrar, J. T., Haythornthwaite, J. A., Jensen, M. P., Katz, N. P., et al. (2005). Core outcome measures for chronic pain clinical trials: IMMPACT recommendations. *Pain, 113*, 9–19.

Dworkin, R. H., Turk, D. C., Wyrwich, K. W., Beaton, D., Cleeland, C. S., Farrar, J. T., et al. (2008). Interpreting the clinical importance of treatment outcomes in chronic pain clinical trials: IMMPACT recommendations. *Journal of Pain, 9*, 105–121.

D'Zurilla, T. J., & Goldfried, M. R. (1971). Problem solving and behavior modification. *Journal of Abnormal Psychology, 78*, 107–126.

Eccleston, C., & Crombez, G. (1999). Pain demands attention: A cognitive–affective model of the interruptive function of pain. *Psychological Bulletin, 125*, 356–366.

Eccleston, C., & Crombez, G. (2005). Attention and pain: Merging behavioural and neuroscience investigations. *Pain, 113*, 7–8.

Edinger, J. D., Wohlgemuth, W. K., Krystal, A. D., & Rice, J. R. (2005). Behavioral insomnia therapy for fibromyalgia patients: A randomized clinical trial. *Archives of Internal Medicine, 165*, 2527–2535.

Edwards, R. R., & Fillingim, R. B. (1999). Ethnic differences in thermal pain responses. *Psychosomatic Medicine, 61*, 346–354.

Faucett, J., Gordon, N., & Levine, J. (1994). Differences in postoperative pain severity among four ethnic groups. *Journal of Pain and Symptom Management, 9*, 383–389.

Fishbain, D. A., Goldberg, M., Meagher, B. R., Steele, R., & Rosomoff, H. (1986). Male and female chronic pain patients categorized by DSM-III psychiatric diagnostic criteria. *Pain, 26*, 181–197.

Flor, H., & Turk, D. C. (1988). Chronic back pain and rheumatoid arthritis: Predicting pain and disability from cognitive variables. *Journal of Behavioral Medicine, 11*, 251–265.

Gatchel, R. J. (1996). Psychological disorders and chronic pain: Cause-and-effect relationships. In R. J. Gatchel & D. C. Turk (Eds.), *Psychological approaches to pain management: A practitioner's handbook* (pp. 33–52). New York: Guilford Press.

Gatchel, R. J. (1997). The significance of personality disorders in the chronic pain population. *Pain Forum, 6*, 12–15.

Gatchel, R. J., Polatin, P. B., & Kinney, R. K. (1995). Predicting outcome of chronic back pain using clinical predictors of psychopathology: A prospective analysis. *Health and Psychology, 14*, 415–420.

Gatchel, R. J., Polatin, P. B., & Mayer, T. (1995). The dominant role of psychosocial risk factors in the development of chronic low back pain disability. *Spine, 20*, 2702–2709.

Geisser, M. E., Robinson, M. E., Keefe, E. J., & Weiner, M. L. (1994). Catastrophizing, depression and the sensory, affective and evaluative aspects of chronic pain. *Pain, 59*, 79–83.

Geisser, M. E., Robinson, M. E., Miller, Q. L., & Bade, S. M. (2003). Psychosocial factors and functional capacity evaluation among persons with chronic pain. *Journal of Occupational Rehabilitation, 13*, 259–276.

Geisser, M. E., & Roth, R. S. (1998). Knowledge of and agreement with chronic pain diagnosis:

Relation of affective distress, pain beliefs and coping, pain intensity, and disability. *Journal of Occupational Rehabilitation, 8,* 73–88.

Gibson, S. J., & Helme, R. D. (2000). Cognitive factors and the experience of pain and suffering in older persons. *Pain, 85,* 375–383.

Giesecke, T., Gracely, R. H., Williams, D. A., Geisser, M., Petzke, F., & Clauw, D. J. (2005). The relationship between depression, clinical pain, and experimental pain in a chronic pain cohort. *Arthritis and Rheumatism, 52,* 1577–1584.

Gil, K. M., Ross, S. L., & Keefe, F. J. (1988). Behavioral treatment of chronic pain: Four pain management protocols. In R. D. France & K. R. Krishnan (Eds.), *Chronic pain* (pp. 376–413). New York: American Psychiatric Press.

Gil, K. M., Williams, D. A., Thompson, R. J. J., & Kinney, T. R. (1991). Sickle cell disease in children and adolescents: The relation of child and parent pain coping strategies to adjustment. *Journal of Pediatric Psychology, 16,* 643–663.

Goldfried, M. R., & Davidson, G. (1976). *Clinical behavioural therapy.* New York: Holt, Rinehart & Winston.

Gombeski, W. R., Jr., Kramer, K., Wilson, T., Krauss, K., Taylor, J., Colihan, L., et al. (2002). Women's Heart Advantage program: Motivating rapid and assertive behavior. *Journal of Cardiovascular Management, 13,* 21–28.

Gordon, D. B., Dahl, J. L., Miaskowski, C., McCarberg, B., Todd, K. H., Paice, J. A., et al. (2005). American Pain Society recommendations for improving the quality of acute and cancer pain management: American Pain Society Quality of Care Task Force. *Archives of Internal Medicine, 165,* 1574–1580.

Gracely, R. H., McGrath, P., & Dubner, R. (1978). Validity and sensitivity of ratio scales of sensory and affective verbal pain descriptors: Manipulation of affect by diazepam. *Pain, 5,* 19–29.

Grant, B. F., Hasin, D. S., Stinson, F. S., Dawson, D. A., Chou, S. P., Ruan, W. J., et al. (2004). Prevalence, correlates, and disability of personality disorders in the United States: Results from the National Epidemiologic Survey on Alcohol and Related Conditions. *Journal of Clinical Psychiatry, 65,* 948–958.

Greenspan, J. D., Craft, R. M., LeResche, L., Rendt-Nielsen, L., Berkley, K. J., Fillingim, R. B., et al. (2007). Studying sex and gender differences in pain and analgesia: A consensus report. *Pain, 132*(Suppl. 1), S26–S45.

Greenwald, H. P. (1991). Interethnic differences in pain perception. *Pain, 44,* 157–163.

Grushka, M., & Sessle, B. J. (1984). Applicability of the McGill Pain Questionnaire to the differentiation of "toothache" pain. *Pain, 19,* 49–57.

Grzesiak, R. C., Ury, G. M., & Dworkin, R. H. (1996). Psychodynamic psychotherapy with chronic pain patients. In R. J. Gatchel & D. C. Turk (Eds.), *Psychological approaches to pain management: A practitioner's handbook* (pp. 148–178). New York: Guilford Press.

Gureje, O., Von, K. M., Simon, G. E., & Gater, R. (1998). Persistent pain and well-being: A World Health Organization study in primary care. *Journal of the American Medical Association, 280,* 147–151.

Hagglund, K. J., Haley, W. E., Reveille, J. D., & Alarcon, G. S. (1989). Predicting individual differences in pain and functional impairment among patients with rheumatoid arthritis. *Arthritis and Rheumatism, 32,* 851–858.

Harris Poll. (2007). A survey of 1,484 U.S. adults sponsored by the National Pain Foundation with the assistance of a grant provided by Alpharma Pharmaceuticals LLC. *National Pain Foundation,* pp. 1–3.

Hoffman, B. M., Papas, R. K., Chatkoff, D. K., & Kerns, R. D. (2007). Meta-analysis of psychological interventions for chronic low back pain. *Health Psychology, 26,* 1–9.

Horgas, A. L. (2003). Pain management in elderly adults. *Journal of Infusion Nursing, 26,* 161–165.

Hufford, M. R., & Shiffman, S. S. (2002). Methodological issues affecting the value of patient-reported outcomes data. *Expert Review of Pharmacoeconomics and Health Outcomes, 2,* 119–128.

Hunter, M., Philips, C., & Rachman, S. (1979). Memory for pain. *Pain, 6,* 35–46.

International Association for the Study of Pain [IASP], Subcommittee on Taxonomy. (1986). Classification of chronic pain: Descriptions of chronic pain syndromes and definitions of pain terms. *Pain Supplement, 3,* S1–S226.

Jensen, M. P., Turner, J. A., & Romano, J. M. (2007). Changes after multidisciplinary pain treatment in patient pain beliefs and coping are associated with concurrent changes in patient functioning. *Pain, 131,* 38–47.

Jensen, M. P., Turner, J. A., Romano, J. M., & Karoly, P. (1991). Coping with chronic pain: A critical review of the literature. *Pain, 47,* 249–283.

Jones, A. K. (1999). The contribution of functional imaging techniques to our understanding of rheumatic pain. *Rheumatic Disease Clinics of North America, 25,* 123–152.

Keck, J. F., Gerkensmeyer, J. E., Joyce, B. A., & Schade, J. G. (1996). Reliability and validity of the faces and word descriptor scales to measure procedural pain. *Pediatric Nursing, 11,* 368–374.

Keefe, F. J. (1996). Cognitive behavioral therapy for managing pain. *Clinical Psychologist, 49,* 4–5.

Keefe, F. J., Brown, G. K., Wallston, K. A., & Caldwell, D. S. (1989). Coping with rheumatoid arthritis pain: Catastrophizing as a maladaptive strategy. *Pain, 37,* 51–56.

Keefe, F. J., Caldwell, D. S., Martinez, S., Nunley, J., Beckham, J., & Williams, D. A. (1991). Analyzing pain in rheumatoid arthritis patients: Pain coping strategies in patients who have had knee replacement surgery. *Pain, 46,* 153–160.

Keefe, F. J., Caldwell, D. S., Williams, D. A., Gil, K. M., Mitchell, D., Robertson, C., et al. (1990a). Pain coping skills training in the management of osteoarthric knee pain: I. A comparative study. *Behavior Therapy, 21,* 49–62.

Keefe, F. J., Caldwell, D. S., Williams, D. A., Gil, K. M., Mitchell, D., Robertson, C., et al. (1990b). Pain coping skills training in the management of osteoarthric knee pain: II. Follow-up results. *Behavior Therapy, 21,* 435–447.

Koyama, T., Kato, K., & Mikami, A. (2000). During pain-avoidance neurons activated in the macaque anterior cingulate and caudate. *Neuroscience Letters, 283,* 17–20.

Koyama, T., McHaffie, J. G., Laurienti, P. J., & Coghill, R. C. (2005). The subjective experience of pain: Where expectations become reality. *Proceedings of the National Academy of Sciences USA, 102,* 12950–12955.

Krueger, A. B., & Stone, A. A. (2008). Assessment of pain: A community-based diary survey in the USA. *Lancet, 371,* 1519–1525.

Lackner, J. M., Jaccard, J., Krasner, S. S., Katz, L. A., Gudleski, G. D., & Holroyd, K. (2008). Self-administered cognitive behavior therapy for moderate to severe irritable bowel syndrome: Clinical efficacy, tolerability, feasibility. *Clinical Gastroenterology and Hepatology, 6,* 899–906.

Lazarus, R. S., & Folkman, S. (1984). *Stress, appraisal, and coping.* New York: Springer.

Lewinsohn, P. M. (1975). The behavioral study and treatment of depression. In M. Hersen, R. M. Eisler, & P. M. Miller (Eds.), *Progress in behavior modification* (pp. 19–64). New York: Academic Press.

Liebeskind, J. C. (1991). Pain can kill. *Pain, 44,* 3–4.

Lindstrom, I., Ohlund, C., Eek, C., Wallin, L., Peterson, L. E., Fordyce, W. E., et al. (1992). The effect of graded activity on patients with subacute low back pain: A randomized prospective clinical study with an operant-conditioning behavioral approach. *Physical Therapy, 72,* 279–290.

Lipchik, G. L., Milles, K., & Covington, E. C. (1993). The effects of multidisciplinary pain management treatment on locus of control and pain beliefs in chronic non-terminal pain. *Clinical Journal of Pain, 9,* 49–57.

Lipton, J. A., & Marbach, J. J. (1984). Ethnicity and the pain experience. *Social Science and Medicine, 19,* 1279–1298.

Litcher-Kelly, L., Martino, S. A., Broderick, J. E., & Stone, A. A. (2007). A systematic review of measures used to assess chronic musculoskeletal pain in clinical and randomized controlled clinical trials. *Journal of Pain, 8,* 906–913.

Masson, E. A., Hunt, L., Gem, J. M., & Boulton, A. J. M. (1989). A novel approach to the diagnosis and assessment of symptomatic diabetic neuropathy. *Pain, 38,* 25–28.

McGrath, P. J., Walco, G. A., Turk, D. C., Dworkin, R. H., Brown, M. T., Davidson, K., et al. (2008). Core outcome domains and measures for pediatric acute and chronic/recurrent pain clinical trials: Ped IMMPACT recommendations. *Journal of Pain, 9,* 771–783.

Meldrum, M. L. (2003). A capsule history of pain management. *Journal of the American Medical Association, 290,* 2470–2475.

Melzack, R. (1975). The McGill Pain Questionnaire: Major properties and scoring methods. *Pain, 1,* 277–299.

Melzack, R. (1987). The short-form McGill Pain Questionnaire. *Pain, 30,* 191–197.

Melzack, R., Terrence, C., Fromm, G., & Amsel, R. (1986). Trigeminal neuralgia and atypical facial pain: Use of the McGill Pain Questionnaire for discrimination and diagnosis. *Pain, 27,* 297–302.

Melzack, R., & Wall, P. D. (1965). Pain mechanisms: A new theory. *Science, 150,* 971–979.

Merskey, H., & Bogduk, N. (1994). *Classification of chronic pain: Description of chronic pain syndromes and definitions of pain terms* (2nd ed.). Seattle, WA: IASP Press.

Morin, C. M., Culbert, J. P., & Schwartz, S. M. (1994). Nonpharmacological interventions for insomnia: A meta-analysis of treatment efficacy. *American Journal of Psychiatry, 151,* 1172–1180.

Morley, S., Eccleston, C., & Williams, A. (1999). Systematic review and meta-analysis of randomized controlled trials of cognitive behaviour therapy and behaviour therapy for chronic pain in adults, excluding headache. *Pain, 80,* 1–13.

Morley, S., Williams, A., & Hussain, S. (2008). Estimating the clinical effectiveness of cognitive behavioural therapy in the clinic: Evaluation of a CBT informed pain management programme. *Pain, 137,* 670–680.

Morris, D. B. (1994). *The culture of pain.* Berkley: University of California Press.

Narrow, W. E., Rae, D. S., Robins, L. N., &

Regier, D. A. (2002). Revised prevalence estimates of mental disorders in the United States: Using a clinical significance criterion to reconcile two surveys' estimates. *Archives of General Psychiatry, 59*, 115–123.

National Institutes of Health. (1996). Integration of behavioral and relaxation approaches into the treatment of chronic pain and insomnia: NIH Technology Assessment Panel on Integration of Behavioral and Relaxation Approaches into the Treatment of Chronic Pain and Insomnia. *Journal of the American Medical Association, 276*, 313–318.

Nezu, A. M., Nezu, C. M., & Perri, M. G. (1989). *Problem-solving therapy for depression: Theory, research and clinical guidelines.* New York: Wiley.

Parker, J. C., Frank, R. G., Beck, N. C., Smarr, K. L., Buescher, K. L., Phillips, L. R., et al. (1988). Pain management in rheumatoid arthritis patients: A cognitive-behavioral approach. *Arthritis and Rheumatism, 31*, 593–601.

Peck, C. L. (1986). Psychological factors in acute pain management. In M. J. Cousins & G. D. Phillips (Eds.), *Acute pain management* (pp. 251–274). New York: Churchill Livingstone.

Polatin, P. B., Kinney, R. K., Gatchel, R. J., Lillo, E., & Mayer, T. (1993). Psychiatric illness and chronic low-back pain: The mind and the spine—which goes first? *Spine, 18*, 66–71.

Price, D. D., Bush, F. M., Long, S., & Harkins, S. W. (1994). A comparison of pain measurement characteristics of mechanical visual analogue and simple numerical rating scales. *Pain, 56*, 217–226.

Rahim-Williams, F. B., Riley, J. L., III, Herrera, D., Campbell, C. M., Hastie, B. A., & Fillingim, R. B. (2007). Ethnic identity predicts experimental pain sensitivity in African Americans and Hispanics. *Pain, 129*, 177–184.

Rainville, P. (2002). Brain mechanisms of pain affect and pain modulation. *Current Opinion in Neurobiology, 12*, 195–204.

Raphael, K. G., Natelson, B. H., Janal, M. N., & Nayak, S. (2002). A community-based survey of fibromyalgia-like pain complaints following the World Trade Center terrorist attacks. *Pain, 100*, 131–139.

Reid, M. C., Otis, J., Barry, L. C., & Kerns, R. D. (2003). Cognitive-behavioral therapy for chronic low back pain in older persons: A preliminary study. *Pain Medicine, 4*, 223–230.

Rey, R. (1993). *History of pain.* Paris: Editions la Découverte.

Rollin, B. E. (2008). *The unheeded cry: Animal consciousness, animal pain and science.* Ames: Iowa State University Press.

Rosenstiel, A. K., & Keefe, F. J. (1983). The use of coping strategies in chronic low back pain patients: Relationship to patient characteristics and current adjustment. *Pain, 17*, 33–44.

Rotter, J. B. (1954). *Social learning and clinical psychology.* Englewood Cliffs, NJ: Prentice-Hall.

Rudy, T. E., Kerns, R. D., & Turk, D. C. (1988). Chronic pain and depression: Toward a cognitive-behavioral mediation model. *Pain, 35*, 129–140.

Sawamoto, N., Honda, M., Okada, T., Hanakawa, T., Kanda, M., Fukuyama, H., et al. (2000). Expectation of pain enhances responses to nonpainful somatosensory stimulation in the anterior cingulate cortex and parietal operculum/posterior insula: An event-related functional magnetic resonance imaging study. *Journal of Neuroscience, 20*, 7438–7445.

Seymour, R. A. (1982). The use of pain scales in assessing the efficacy of analgesics in postoperative dental pain. *European Journal of Clinical Pharmacology, 23*, 441–444.

Shiffman, S., Stone, A. A., & Hufford, M. R. (2008). Ecological momentary assessment. *Annual Review of Clinical Psychology, 4*, 1–32.

Smith, A. F., Salovey, P., Turk, D. C., Jobe, J. B., & Willis, G. B. (1993). Theoretical and methodological issues in assessing memory for pain: A reply. *American Pain Society Journal, 2*, 203–206.

Sternbach, R. A., & Tursky, B. (1965). Ethnic differences among housewives in psychosocial and skin potential responses to electric shock. *Psychophysiology, 1*, 241–246.

Stone, A., & Shiffman, S. (1994). Ecological momentary assessment: Measuring real world processes in behavioral medicine. *Annals of Behavioral Medicine, 16*, 199–202.

Strong, J., Ashton, R., Cramond, T., & Chant, D. (1990). Pain intensity, attitude and function in back pain patients. *Australian Occupational Therapy Journal, 37*, 179–183.

Stroud, M. W., Thorn, B. E., Jensen, M. P., & Boothby, J. L. (2000). The relation between pain beliefs, negative thoughts, and psychosocial functioning in chronic pain patients. *Pain, 84*, 347–352.

Sullivan, M. J., & D'Eon, J. L. (1990). Relation between catastrophizing and depression in chronic pain patients. *Journal of Abnormal Psychology, 99*, 260–263.

Sullivan, M. J., Stanish, W., Waite, H., Sullivan, M., & Tripp, D. A. (1998). Catastrophizing, pain, and disability in patients with soft-tissue injuries. *Pain, 77*, 253–260.

Thompson, S. C. (1981). Will it hurt less if I can control it?: A complex answer to a simple question. *Psychological Bulletin, 90*, 89–101.

Torebjork, E. (1994). Nociceptor dynamics in humans. In G. F. Gebhart, D. L. Hammond, & T. S. Jensen (Eds.), *Proceedings of the 7th World Congress on Pain* (pp. 277–284). Seattle: IASP Press.

Tracey, I. (2008). Imaging pain. *British Journal of Anaesthesia, 101*, 32–39.

Tracey, I., & Mantyh, P. W. (2007). The cerebral signature for pain perception and its modulation. *Neuron, 55*, 377–391.

Treede, R. D., Kenshalo, D. R., Gracely, R. H., & Jones, A. K. (1999). The cortical representation of pain. *Pain, 79*, 105–111.

Turk, D. C. (2002). Clinical effectiveness and cost-effectiveness of treatments for patients with chronic pain. *Clinical Journal of Pain, 18*, 355–365.

Turk, D. C., Dworkin, R. H., McDermott, M. P., Bellamy, N., Burke, L. B., Chandler, J. M., et al. (2008). Analyzing multiple endpoints in clinical trials of pain treatments: IMMPACT recommendations. *Pain, 139*, 481–482.

Turner, J. A., Jensen, M. P., & Romano, J. M. (2000). Do beliefs, coping, and catastrophizing independently predict functioning in patients with chronic pain? *Pain, 85*, 115–125.

Varni, J. W., Jay, S. M., Masek, B. J., & Thompson, K. L. (1986). Cognitive-behavioral assessment and management of pediatric pain. In A. D. Holzman & D. C. Turk (Eds.), *Pain management: A handbook of psychological treatment approaches* (pp. 168–192). New York: Pergamon.

Verhaak, P. F., Kerssens, J. J., Dekker, J., Sorbi, M. J., & Bensing, J. M. (1998). Prevalence of chronic benign pain disorder among adults: A review of the literature. *Pain, 77*, 231–239.

Watanabe, S., Kakigi, R., Koyama, S., Hoshiyama, M., & Kaneoke, Y. (1998). Pain processing traced by magnetoencephalography in the human brain. *Brain Topography, 10*, 255–264.

Wiertelak, E. P., Smith, K. P., Furness, L., Mooney-Heiberger, K., Mayr, T., Maier, S. F., et al. (1994). Acute and conditioned hyperalgesic responses to illness. *Pain, 56*, 227–234.

Williams, D. A. (2003). Psychological and behavioral therapies in fibromyagia and related syndromes. *Bailliere's Best Practice and Research (Clinical Rheumatology), 17*, 649–665.

Williams, D. A., Brown, S. C., Clauw, D. J., & Gendreau, R. M. (2003). Self-reported symptoms before and after September 11 in patients with fibromyalgia. *Journal of the American Medical Association, 289*, 1637–1638.

Williams, D. A., Cary, M. A., Groner, K. H., Chaplin, W., Glazer, L. J., Rodriguez, A. M., et al. (2002). Improving physical functional status in patients with fibromyalgia: A brief cognitive behavioral intervention. *Journal of Rheumatology, 29*, 1280–1286.

Williams, D. A., & Keefe, F. J. (1991). Pain beliefs and the use of cognitive-behavioral coping strategies. *Pain, 46*, 185–190.

Williams, D. A., Robinson, M. E., & Geisser, M. E. (1994). Pain beliefs: Assessment and utility. *Pain, 59*, 71–78.

Willis, W. D., & Westlund, K. N. (1997). Neuroanatomy of the pain system and of the pathways that modulate pain. *Journal of Clinical Neurophysiology, 14*, 2–31.

Zborowski, M. (1952). Cultural components in responses to pain. *Journal of Social Issues, 8*, 16–30.

CHAPTER 33

Coping with Chronic Illness

Austin S. Baldwin
Quinn D. Kellerman
Alan J. Christensen

The past century has seen a dramatic shift in patterns of morbidity and mortality in the United States and other technologically advanced parts of the world. Although deaths from acute illness have dropped dramatically, this decline has been juxtaposed against a steadily increasing prevalence of chronic physical illness (Heron, 2007). People are living longer, but at the cost of increasing morbidity and greater burden of disease and disease management. Given this shifting epidemiology of health and illness, it is increasingly critical to understand the process of coping with chronic illness and how coping influences care delivery and patient outcomes. The central objective of this chapter is to bring psychological theory and research to bear on the issue of coping with chronic illness. We attempt to delineate ways in which theory and empirical research can help researchers and clinicians alike better understand patient coping and its place in a broader context of chronic illness management. In the first part of the chapter, we briefly describe and review the most prevalent theoretical models that have guided research on factors thought to be critical in coping with chronic illness. In the second

part of the chapter, we provide a specific overview of research on two issues that are central to coping with many types of chronic illness: depression and treatment adherence.

Theoretical Models

An understanding of the most prevalent theoretical models in the domain of coping with chronic illness is important because the models guide how researchers think (and have thought) about the issue. Moreover, good theoretical models provide a coherent framework in which to understand the coping process, and they specify the factors on which coping interventions might best be designed. Some of the models we review here are based on broader theories of human behavior that have been applied to coping with chronic illness, whereas others were developed specifically in the context of coping. Notwithstanding these and other important differences, the models share a number of conceptual similarities in the factors and processes they describe. Specifically, all the models suggest that there are critical behavioral, cognitive, and affective responses that influence successful coping, and it is with those similarities in mind that we review the models.

Stress Appraisal and Coping Model

The stress appraisal and coping model (Lazarus & Folkman, 1984) is not specific to the stress and coping associated with chronic illness, but because the concepts of stress and coping articulated in this model have influenced subsequent thinking about coping with chronic illness, we briefly review it here. According to the model, people assess potential stress-inducing situations (e.g., learning one has a chronic illness) through a two-part appraisal process. People engage in a primary appraisal of the situation, in which they assess the threat, harm, or challenge that the situation poses to them. People then engage in a secondary appraisal, in which they assess the resources available to cope with the situation. The subjective experience of stress occurs when people perceive that the threat, harm, or challenge of the situation is greater than the resources they have available to cope with it.

Coping is conceptualized as a dynamic process of interactions between the individual and the environment, in which the effectiveness of a strategy is determined by its outcome in a specific situation (i.e., context) over time. Through this process, people attempt to manage two aspects of the stress: the associated emotions (e.g., anxiety, guilt, depression) and the threat, harm, or challenge itself. Coping with the associated emotions, or emotion-focused coping, often occurs through cognitive efforts to reappraise the situation (e.g., "Having diabetes is not so bad and it's not a death sentence") to minimize the perception of the threat. People can also avoid the threat by attempting not to think about it, or by engaging in distracting activities (e.g., exercise, meditation, drinking). Although people often engage in both emotion- and problem-focused coping, emotion-focused forms of coping are more likely to predominate when people perceive that not much can be done to change or minimize the stress-inducing threat (Lazarus & Folkman, 1984). However, when something tangible can be done about the stressful situation and resources are available, a problem-focused form of coping (e.g., dia-

betics actively managing their blood glucose levels) is likely to predominate (Lazarus & Folkman, 1984). Moreover, people are more likely to be successful in coping with chronic forms of stress, such as those associated with chronic illness, when they focus on actively managing the stress rather than avoiding it (Suls & Fletcher, 1985). Yet when the stress-inducing threat is not modifiable, or when sufficient resources are not available, engaging in problem-focused coping may be detrimental to people's health and well-being (James, Keenan, Strogatz, Browning, & Garrett, 1992).

Cognitive Adaptation Model

The cognitive adaptation model focuses broadly on the processes of adjusting to or coping with threatening situations or events, such as living with a chronic illness (Taylor, 1983; Taylor, Kemeny, Reed, Bower, & Gruenewald, 2000). According to the model, successful coping with the threatening situation revolves around three issues that include behavioral, cognitive, and affective components: finding meaning in the situation, mastery over the situation, and self-enhancement in response to the threatening situation.

For a person living with a chronic illness, finding meaning in the threatening situation includes both trying to understand why it occurred (e.g., "Why did I get sick? What caused my illness?"), and rethinking one's priorities to realign one's life along more satisfying lines (e.g., "Now that I'm sick, I'm not going to spend so much time at work"). Empirical evidence has shown that when people find meaning in their lives following diagnosis of a chronic illness, it can delay progression of heart disease (Affleck, Tennen, Croog, & Levine, 1987) and HIV (Bower, Kemeny, Taylor, & Fahey, 1998). Moreover, evidence suggests that it is finding meaning in the illness that is critical because thinking about one's illness *without* finding meaning (i.e., ruminating) can have harmful effects (Bower et al., 1998). Mastery is realized by asserting control over the illness or over related aspects of the illness, such as treatment. Evidence from patients with HIV suggests that those who had a greater sense of control over the progression of the illness were more likely to engage in healthier behaviors (Taylor et al., 1992). The third issue thought to be critical to successfully coping with a chronic illness is self-enhancement. Because having a chronic illness can result in heightened negative affect and depression (an issue we address later in this chapter), being able to engage in some form of self-enhancement and, as a result, feel good about oneself, has been shown to be an important part of successful coping (de Ridder, Geenen, Kuijer, & van Middendorp, 2008). Much of the research in chronic illness populations has focused on social comparison as a vehicle through which self-enhancement occurs (Taylor & Brown, 1988; Wood & Van der Zee, 1997).

What is remarkable about the evidence based on the cognitive adaptation model is that these three forms of coping are often illusory; that is, people may find meaning in their illness that has no rational basis, they may perceive control over aspects of the illness that in reality are uncontrollable, and they may engage in favorable social comparisons with hypothetical others rather than actual people they know. Yet the evidence suggests that these illusory beliefs are predictive of better physical and mental health (see Taylor et al., 2000).

Self-Regulation Model

The self-regulation model is a broader model of goal-directed behavior that has been applied to understanding people's ability to cope with chronic illness (Carver & Scheier, 1990, 2002). According to the model, human behavior is guided by goals through which people seek to create or maintain desired conditions in their lives, and self-regulation is the process through which people strive to realize their goals. According to this perspective, people experience stress when they encounter impediments to their goals, and coping with stress is conceptualized as efforts at self-regulation under that adversity. Therefore, living with a chronic illness is stressful to the extent that it is perceived to impede a person's goals (e.g., to be a healthy person), and a person's ability to cope successfully with the illness is determined by his or her ability to reassess the goals that have been impeded.

People's goals can differ on two important dimensions: focus and abstraction. In terms

of focus, goals can be construed as either approaching a desired end state (i.e., approach goals) or avoiding an undesired end state (i.e., avoidance goals). For example, some people may have a goal to be a healthy person (an approach goal), whereas others may have a goal to avoid getting sick (an avoidance goal). In terms of abstraction, goals are organized hierarchically, and the most abstract goals (e.g., to be a healthy person) at the top of the hierarchy and related subgoals (e.g., exercising three times per week, avoiding food high in saturated fats) lower in the hierarchy. These different goal dimensions have important implications for behavioral self-regulation. The implications of goal focus are beyond the scope of this chapter, but see Carver and Scheier (2002) for a more detailed discussion. The implications of goal abstraction, however, are central to conceptualization of coping with chronic illness as a form of self-regulation. If the onset of a chronic illness impedes a person's goal to engage in regular exercise, successful coping can be achieved by setting new, lower-order goals that allow continued movement toward the higher-order goal of being healthy (e.g., eat more fruits and vegetables), partially disengaging from the goal by setting a more modest goal (e.g., a daily walk instead of more vigorous exercise), disengaging from the goal if it is unattainable, or setting new goals entirely (e.g., to be a better parent or grandparent). When people's goals are impeded and they fail to establish new goals or remain engaged with goals that are unattainable, they experience distress.

What might help people engage in successful coping when dealing with the stress of impeded goals? Research across various chronic illnesses has shown that differences in dispositional optimism are predictive of successful coping after coronary artery bypass surgery (e.g., Scheier et al., 1999) and among cancer patients (Carver et al., 1993). Moreover, optimism is associated with slower disease progression and lower mortality rates in cancer patients (Watson, Haviland, Greer, Davidson, & Bliss, 1999) and HIV patients (Reed, Kemeny, Taylor, & Visscher, 1999). Although the processes through which these effects occur are not entirely clear, evidence does suggest that optimism is associated with people engaging in more effective behavioral (e.g., setting new goals that allow continued movement toward higher-order goals), as well as effective cognitive and affective (e.g., accepting the situation and reframing one's goals) responses to their impeded goals (Carver et al., 1993; Taylor et al., 2000).

Self-Determination Model

This model of coping with chronic illness is derived from a broader theory of human motivation and behavior called self-determination theory (Ryan & Deci, 2000), which, in short, posits that humans have three innate psychological needs: autonomy, competence, and relatedness to others. It is thought that when these needs are facilitated and met, people experience enhanced self-motivation, development, and well-being. In recognizing that the behavioral and affective aspects of coping with many chronic illnesses are facilitated by self-management (e.g., diabetes, hypertension), the model draws on the tenets of the broader theory to suggest that successful coping is influenced by people's motivations for autonomy and competence (Williams, 2002). In coping with and managing a chronic illness, autonomous motivation occurs when people experience volition and choice in their illness-related behaviors (e.g., how to manage their diabetes), and competence occurs when people feel they are capable of controlling important illness-related outcomes (e.g., glucose levels). The evidence from tests of this model suggests that as people's autonomous motivation and competence increase, they experience better health outcomes across different chronic illnesses, including diabetes (Williams, McGregor, Zeldman, Freedman, & Deci, 2004) and coronary artery disease (Williams, Gagné, Mushlin, & Deci, 2005).

The self-determination model also explicitly accounts for the influence of a patient's relationship with his or her health care provider on successful coping, an aspect about which most theoretical models are silent. Specifically, the model posits that when health care providers elicit and acknowledge patients' perspectives, offer choices, and provide information, while minimizing pressure and control, the providers engage in autonomy support. Evidence across different behavioral domains suggests that when patients view their health care providers as autonomy supportive, patients tend to become more autonomous in their motivations and subsequently feel more competent in coping with their illness. The changes in patients' autonomy and competence translate into better coping and management of their chronic illness (Williams et al., 2006; Williams, Lynch, & Glasgow, 2007).

Patient × Treatment Context Interactive Framework

This model draws on the observation that much variation in human behavior is found in the interaction between the person and the situational context (Bem & Funder, 1978; Dance & Neufeld, 1988). In recognizing that a critical aspect of coping with chronic illness is in the delivery of and adherence to treatment recommendations, the model suggests that successful coping occurs when the effects of individual differences in cognition, behavior, and personality are considered along with characteristics of the chronic illness and medical treatment context (the "person × context interactive perspective"). The central assumption of the model is that relevant contextual or situational features of the treatment context (e.g., How much of the treatment can a patient control and manage?) should interact with patient variables (e.g., Does the patient prefer an active coping style?) to influence coping with and managing the illness (Christensen, 2000).

Several studies conducted with patients who have chronic kidney disease have suggested that regimen adherence and patient satisfaction is highest when patients' preferred styles of coping are consistent with the contextual features or demands of the particular type of dialysis the patient is undergoing (Christensen, 2000). For example, patients who had been classified as high in "information vigilance" (i.e., reflecting a strong preference to seek information and participate actively in treatment) exhibited more favorable adherence when undergoing self-managed, home-based dialysis treatments than did patients with more passive coping preferences (Christensen, Smith, Turner, & Cundick, 1994). The opposite pattern was observed for patients undergoing largely provider-managed, hospital-based dialysis treatment. In fact, in the provider-managed, hospital-based group, more active coping preferences were actually associated with poorer adherence. In more recent work, Cvengros, Christensen, Hillis, and Rosenthal (2007) observed that primary care patients (many of whom were hypertensive and/or diabetic) who believed they had control over their health outcomes reported better treatment regimen adherence and higher satisfaction with care when treated by a physician who also believed patients have control over their health. Moreover, those patients who believed they had little control over their health reported better adherence and higher satisfaction when treated by a physician who also believed that patients have little control over their health. Thus, the degree to which a particular treatment approach or practice style is congruent with patients' preferred coping style or health beliefs can be an important determinant of regimen adherence and satisfaction with care.

Summary

Although the theoretical models we have reviewed here differ in the specific factors that are thought to be most critical in coping with chronic illness, they also share some important conceptual similarities. Many of the models suggest that a sense of control over the situation is important (e.g., mastery, autonomy, proper patient and treatment fit). A greater sense of control should allow for a favorable cognitive framing of the situation (e.g., realignment of one's priorities, setting new goals, feeling competent, satisfied with the treatment course) and result in people experiencing more positive (and fewer negative) emotions in the process of coping with the chronic illness. Moreover, the favorable cognitive and affective response should increase the likelihood that people with chronic illness engage in healthier behaviors (e.g., proper treatment management and adherence). The value of these cognitive, affective, and behavioral responses to successful coping has been borne out in a recent empirical review (de Ridder et al., 2008).

Given the importance of people's cognitive, affective, and behavioral responses to the demands associated with chronic illness, the remainder of the chapter focuses on two prevalent issues that are often asso-

ciated with unfavorable responses to those demands: depression and treatment nonadherence. In both cases, we describe the problem, its implications for coping with chronic illness, and how the problem is assessed, then we briefly review evidence of related interventions.

Depression and Chronic Illness

One common result of a person's failure to cope effectively with the new circumstances of a chronic disease is depression (Carver & Scheier, 2002; de Ridder et al., 2008; Taylor et al., 2000). Approximately 30% of patients with a chronic illness experience comorbid depression at some point during the course of their illness, with variability in reported rates based on the type of illness and the method of assessment used (e.g., self-report, standardized diagnostic interviews) (Evans et al., 2005). Across different illnesses, however, patients with chronic illness are two to three times more likely to experience depression compared to individuals in the general population (American Psychiatric Association, 2000). Taking variability in assessment methods into account, the prevalence of depression has been found to range from 20 to 30% in patients with diabetes (Anderson, Clouse, Freedland, & Lustman, 2001), from 19 to 34% in patients with heart failure (Rutledge, Reis, Linke, Greenberg, & Mills, 2006), and to be about 50% in patients with HIV/AIDS (P. Williams et al., 2005). Rates of depression in patients with cancer vary considerably based on the researchers' definition of depression (e.g., subthreshold symptoms vs. clinical diagnosis), methodology employed, type and stage of cancer, and whether the patient is assessed during a first diagnosis or recurrence, with the highest prevalence rate around 60% (Massie, 2004). In this section, we conceptualize depression in terms of its symptoms, which may or may not meet the severity or frequency criteria required for a clinical diagnosis. Identification and treatment of depressive symptoms (at either subthreshold or clinical levels) in patients with chronic illness are important because of their significant effects on functioning, quality of life, and disease management.

Consequences of Depression in Chronic Illness

Comorbid depression in physical illness is associated with increases in morbidity and mortality across patient populations. A review of the diabetes literature by de Groot, Anderson, Freedland, Clouse, and Lustman (2001) concluded that symptoms of depression were significantly related to long-term diabetes complications (e.g., retinopathy, nephropathy, neuropathy, cardiovascular disease), both in number and severity. Depression may decrease habituation to aversive symptoms such as chronic pain, leading to more severe functional impairment and poorer quality of life (Katon, 2003). For example, results of a study examining patients with comorbid depression and chronic pain found a higher rate of panic disorder and increased symptom severity among these individuals (Arnow et al., 2006). In addition, several studies provide evidence for an association between depression and mortality risk in chronic conditions such as heart failure (Dejonge et al., 2007), HIV/AIDS (Lesserman et al., 2007) and end-stage renal disease (Kimmel, 2002). For patients with a chronic illness, depression may affect morbidity and mortality indirectly through changes in behaviors such as eating habits, smoking, exercise, adherence, and health care utilization. There is also evidence to suggest that depression may influence these outcomes directly through changes in physiology (de Ridder et al., 2008; Katon, 2003).

Coping, Control, and Depression

As we described previously in this chapter, perceptions of control appear to be critical in successful coping and are thought to be generally adaptive (Taylor & Brown, 1988; Walker, Jackson, & Littlejohn, 2004). Problem-focused forms of coping (e.g., information seeking, direct action in problem solving) may be linked to greater perceived control and lower levels of distress. Moreover, when perceptions of illness controllability are low, patients may engage in emotion-focused forms of coping (e.g., escape, avoidance, distancing) that can lead to heightened distress (Walker et al., 2004). Given that perceptions of control appear to act as a buffer against psychological distress (e.g., anxiety, depression), they may moderate the effects of depression on successful coping. For example, a recent study by Kiviruusu, Huurre, and Aro (2007) found that an external locus of control and emotion-focused coping were associated with greater severity of depression in a sample of chronically ill men. However, patients who utilized active coping strategies (e.g., problem solving, seeking social support) were found to have lower levels of depression. Taylor, Helgeson, Reed, and Skokan (1991) found that patients with coronary artery disease who perceived they had less personal control over their illness reported higher levels of distress over time and therefore poorer adjustment to their condition. In addition, for patients with rheumatoid arthritis who perceived they had less control over the daily management of their symptoms, internal and global attributions for negative events led to increases in symptoms of depression (Chaney et al., 1996).

Other research, however, provides evidence to suggest that the positive effects of high perceived control and problem-focused coping may not be present in every illness context. As mentioned previously in this chapter, Lazarus and Folkman (1984) described the effectiveness of a coping response as being determined by its outcome in a specific situation (i.e., context) over time. Similarly, the patient × treatment interactive framework suggests that contextual factors play an important role in understanding how control preferences and coping style may be differentially related to adjustment and adherence (Christensen, 2000). Thus, preference for control and use of problem-focused coping may be adaptive only in treatment contexts conducive to patient control, and may be detrimental when actual opportunities for control are low (Wiebe & Christensen, 1996). This is illustrated in the findings of Affleck, Tennen, Pfeifer, and Fifield (1987), in which patients with severe rheumatoid arthritis who held beliefs about control over their illness course experienced greater mood disturbance in this uncontrollable context. Future research using the patient × treatment interactive framework may elucidate our understanding of how incompatible perceptions of control and coping styles can influence patients' depression.

Assessment of Depression in Chronic Illness

Depression is often difficult to assess in the context of comorbid physical illness because several of the somatic/vegetative symptoms of depression (e.g., fatigue, changes in appetite, sleep disturbance, psychomotor retardation or agitation) may be similar to those associated with the physical illness. DSM-IV criteria for diagnosing depression require clinicians to exclude symptoms that "are due to the direct physiological effects of a general medical condition" (American Psychiatric Association, 2000, p. 356), yet the nonspecific nature of symptoms such as fatigue often preclude clinicians' ability to determine the etiology of somatic indicators in patients with chronic illness. One resolution for this issue has been to exclude the aforementioned somatic symptoms and use only elevated cognitive/nonsomatic item scores on measures to reflect depression. Alternatively, researchers have proposed an emphasis on more subjective indicators of depression, such as social withdrawal or tearfulness (Simon & Von Korff, 2006). There is some evidence to suggest that somatic symptoms show similar relationships to underlying depression severity and improve equally well with treatment in patients with and without comorbid medical conditions (Simon & Von Korff, 2006), yet caution should still be taken when including these symptoms in depression assessments for patients with chronic illness.

Interventions to Improve Depression in Chronic Illness

Given the prevalence and clinical implications of depression in chronic illness, researchers have tested the efficacy of psychosocial interventions to improve mental and physical health outcomes in various patient populations. There has been extensive research on interventions to reduce cancer-related distress, which typically involve some combination of psychoeducation, behavioral training, and group or individual psychotherapy. Cognitive-behavioral stress management (CBSM) interventions appear to be the most common and effective for lowering distress and improving quality of life and well-being. These interventions have potential to moderate the effects of perceptions of control and coping styles on depression. For example, Antoni and colleagues (2001) conducted a CBSM intervention in patients with breast cancer and found significant effects for lower depression, increased optimism, and finding meaning in life. These findings are consistent with Taylor's cognitive adaptation model (1983) regarding how effective coping with a threatening situation (e.g., finding meaning) leads to successful coping.

A recently emerging, coping-based approach to facilitating adjustment in chronic illness involves the systematic, written disclosure of illness-related cognitions and emotions. These interventions were based on the findings that emotional regulation in the form of avoidance, distancing, or inhibition was typically associated with unfavorable psychological or disease-related outcomes (de Ridder et al., 2008). In contrast, acknowledgment or expression of emotions in written disclosure interventions has been found to decrease distress in patients with chronic illness. For example, Broderick, Junghaenel, and Schwartz (2005) found that among patients with fibromyalgia, those in the emotional disclosure intervention arm reported fewer symptoms of depression at posttreatment compared to patients in the neutral writing and usual care conditions (whose reports of depression were unchanged following the intervention). Results of other disclosure interventions also provide strong support for the expression of emotions in decreasing distress and improving mood in cancer and HIV (de Ridder et al., 2008). In addition to alleviating depression, these interventions also have notable effects on objective markers of disease activity, such as reducing chronic pain in rheumatoid arthritis and improving pulmonary function in patients with asthma (Smyth, Stone, Hurewitz, & Kaell, 1999).

Summary

Given the prevalence of depression in patients with chronic illness and its negative impact on quality of life and disease-related outcomes, assessment of depressive symptoms and use of effective interventions to reduce distress should be of high priority to researchers and clinicians. Emphasis on identifying the cognitive/nonsomatic markers of depression through both patient self-report and interview assessments will be important, so that treatments can guide patients in expression of distressing emotions and development of useful coping strategies given the illness context.

Treatment Adherence

Inadequate behavioral coping with the new circumstances of a chronic illness is often manifest in patient nonadherence to treatment regimens (Wiebe & Christensen, 1996). Adherence has been defined in various ways in the literature, but for the purpose of this chapter we define it as the extent to which patients' behavior corresponds with the recommended treatment course. Most chronic conditions require patients to participate actively in the treatment (i.e., self-manage their illness), with some demanding more complex patient involvement (e.g., diabetes) than others (e.g., hypertension). Thus, when patients are diagnosed with a chronic illness, often significant behavioral and lifestyle changes need to occur to achieve favorable outcomes. For some individuals, these tasks are very difficult to accomplish. Although it is important to understand how failure to engage in recommended self-management behaviors may reflect poor coping, we first discuss the extent and consequences of nonadherence in a broader sense.

Nature and Implications of Nonadherence

Rates of nonadherence to chronic illness regimens vary across conditions, but are generally in the range of 30–60% (Christensen, 2004), with medication nonadherence typically around 50% (Haynes, McDonald, & Garg, 2002). A quantitative review by Di-Matteo (2004) revealed that the average nonadherence rate across multiple chronic illness conditions was around 25%. According to this meta-analysis, nonadherence was higher in pulmonary disease, diabetes, and sleep disorders, yet the calculated percentages may underestimate the nature of the problem because of different methods of assessment (i.e., self-report vs. objective measures). Furthermore, assessment of adherence as a single construct, particularly

for conditions that require a complex regimen, is problematic due to the variability in adherence among different components of the regimen. For example, a recent study examining self-care behaviors in patients with end-stage renal disease found that although 70% of patients did not adhere to the fluid-intake restrictions associated with the hemodialysis regimen and 55% were nonadherent to their medications, only 16% of patients did not adequately adhere to their dietary restrictions (O'Connor, Jardine, & Millar, 2008). Complexity of the regimen in general has also been associated with poor adherence in various patient populations (e.g., ulcerative colitis; Kane, 2006).

Consequences of nonadherence at the individual-patient level include deleterious effects on morbidity and mortality. Nonadherence can also affect disease severity in the short term by exacerbating symptoms and increasing the likelihood of treatment failures, and the need for hospitalization (Christensen & Johnson, 2002). Long-term complications associated with nonadherence are also often cited for conditions such as diabetes and end-stage renal disease. For example, chronic elevations in blood glucose levels that, in large part, reflect poor diabetes management (e.g., insufficient monitoring of blood glucose, inaccurate insulin administration, neglecting to take prescribed medications) may lead to cardiovascular disease, neuropathy, retinopathy, and nephropathy (Diabetes Control and Complications Trial Research Group, 1993). For patients with end-stage renal disease receiving hemodialysis as their treatment, nonadherence to fluid intake and dietary restrictions may lead to long-term complications such as pulmonary edema, congestive heart failure, cardiac arrhythmias, and decreased life expectancy (Wolcott, Maida, Diamond, & Nissenson, 1986).

Determinants of Adherence

Many investigators have sought to understand from varying perspectives the determinants of adherence behavior. Perhaps the area that has received the most empirical attention has been attempting to predict nonadherence from the level of individual-patient characteristics. Some individual-difference factors have explained a modest part of the observed variance in nonadherence, yet none of these factors has been a consistently strong predictor across studies and patient populations. For example, a few researchers have reported that personality traits such as high conscientiousness and low neuroticism predict adherence, yet the evidence in this area is mixed (Wiebe & Christensen, 1996). There exists little to no evidence that demographic variables such as age, gender, and race are directly or consistently related to adherence behavior; this conclusion is similar for patients' knowledge about their chronic illness and its treatment (Wiebe, 2004). With regard to health beliefs, preference for control appears to be related to better adherence, but only when the delivery context allows patients to perceive that they have control over their treatment. For example, patients with end-stage renal disease who have a high desire for control displayed better adherence when treated in a context that necessitates extensive patient involvement at home, and poorer adherence when treatment was directed primarily by health care professionals in a center (Christensen, 2000). Given these results and the importance of the treatment context (e.g., type of relationship with provider), the patient × treatment interactive approach and the self-determination approach to coping described earlier are particularly promising avenues for future research in adherence to chronic illness regimens.

Psychological disorders and symptoms (e.g., depression, substance use) have also been studied in terms of their relation to treatment nonadherence. In a review, Lustman and Clouse (2005) concluded that comorbid depression in patients with diabetes was associated with inadequate glycemic control and poor adherence to taking medication and dietary restrictions. A study by Cukor, Newville, and Jindal (2008) reported that depression was a significant predictor of nonadherence to the immunosuppressant therapy regimen in renal transplant patients. In HIV research, results of a systematic review suggested that current substance use in these patients negatively impacted adherence to antiretroviral therapy, as did other psychological problems such as depression and anxiety (Malta, Strathdee, Magnanini, & Bastos, 2008).

Assessment of Adherence

As mentioned previously, reported rates of nonadherence often vary based on the method of assessment used. Given that each method has its limitations, and that the field lacks a "gold standard" for adherence measurement, it is important for researchers and clinicians to obtain assessments from multiple sources when attempting to understand adherence behavior in patients.

Interestingly, physicians appear to be relatively inaccurate in their estimations of the extent to which patients adhere to their treatment regimens (Patel & Davis, 2006). Thus, patient self-report measures of adherence are commonly used in a number of different formats, including single questions, structured questionnaires, and monitoring forms to record daily behavior (e.g., medication use, diet, exercise, blood glucose testing, and fluid intake). Although self-report measures are convenient and inexpensive to administer, they have several limitations regarding the extent to which they provide a complete and accurate depiction of the behaviors under study. For example, patient endorsements on these measures are subject to reporting biases, such as inaccurate recall of past behavior (even over short periods of time), social desirability, and impression management (Wiebe, 2004).

To address these limitations, some researchers have also used more objective methods to measure adherence both directly and indirectly. Examples of indirect adherence measures include pill counting and examination of pharmacy refill records, whereas more direct assessments include use of electronic monitoring devices and checking records of attendance at office visits and/ or laboratory appointments. In addition, biological markers or clinical outcomes are known to reflect behavioral adherence to the prescribed treatment regimen and may be considered the most objective of these measures. In the case of diabetes, hemoglobin A1c is a physiological marker of metabolic control that represents the average blood glucose level over the previous 90-day period (Diabetes Control and Complications Trial Research Group, 1993). Other examples include use of interdialysis weight gains as an adherence marker in end-stage renal disease (which reflects the amount of fluid ingested by patients between treatment sessions), and testing the level of medication or metabolite in the patient's bloodstream to determine whether this corresponds to the recommended dosage. Although objective assessments are not subject to the reporting biases that limit self-report measures, they are also not imperfect measures of adherence. The limitations of these methods are related to unreliability in the case of pill counting and pharmacy refills (e.g., patients may not actually ingest the medication even if they fill the prescription), logistical obstacles (e.g., electronic devices may be expensive or impractical depending on the regimen), and influence of other factors (e.g., metabolic control outcomes may not be fully explained by behavioral adherence).

Adherence Interventions

Considering that nonadherence to treatment regimens is a widespread problem associated with negative outcomes, interventions to promote adherence in chronic illness have been the focus of much empirical attention. The most commonly used interventions have been educational or behavioral in nature. Patient education programs typically involve provision of information about the illness and treatment regimen. Based on a meta-analysis by Weingarten and colleagues (2002), interventions focused only on education have had small effects on management of chronic conditions (e.g., depression, asthma, hypertension). Given the findings that patient knowledge is generally not predictive of more favorable adherence, it seems plausible that education alone would not be sufficient to produce marked changes in adherence behavior. Thus, several researchers have integrated educational components into behavioral interventions, which have had slightly better success. For instance, Christensen, Moran, Wiebe, Ehlers, and Lawton (2002) conducted a pilot study to test the efficacy of a behavioral intervention (including self-monitoring, goal setting, and self-reinforcement techniques) in improving fluid-intake adherence among patients with end-stage renal disease receiving center hemodialysis. Their findings pointed toward a trend in improved adherence at follow-up among the patients in the intervention group compared to those in the control group.

Roter and colleagues (1998) conducted a meta-analysis of 153 studies to investigate the success of educational, behavioral, and affective interventions in improving multiple adherence behaviors across various patient populations. Results differed based on the measure of adherence employed, such that effect sizes were largest for objective indirect (e.g., pill counts and prescription refills) and direct (e.g., blood tracers, weight changes) markers of adherence, particularly in patients with diabetes. Although the effects were smaller, interventions also improved patient health outcomes and care utilization. Patients with cancer typically received educational and affective interventions (emphasizing emotional expression through counseling and utilization of social support), and demonstrated marked improvements in survival, relapse, and many indicators of adherence. Overall, no single type of intervention was more effective than another; rather, the combination of educational, behavioral, and affective components produced the strongest effects on patient outcomes. A more recent meta-analysis, however, concluded that although combined interventions have been successful in improving medication adherence and clinical outcomes, it appears that the current methods are often complex, labor-intensive, and do not have strong, consistent results in terms of effectiveness (McDonald, Garg, & Haynes, 2002).

Although affective coping-related interventions are not as commonly implemented, there has been some research on the efficacy of psychotherapy interventions for improving adherence behavior (as well as psychological distress). For example, Winkley, Landau, Eisler, and Ismail (2006) conducted a systematic review and meta-analysis of randomized controlled trials (mostly cognitive-behavioral therapy interventions) designed to improve metabolic control in diabetes. The authors concluded that there was no significant effect of these interventions in reducing adults' blood glucose levels. However, an emerging body of research has found support for the use of acceptance and commitment therapy (ACT) in improving psychological, behavioral, and clinical outcomes in patients with chronic illness. The acceptance and mindfulness-based techniques used in ACT serve to help individuals develop broad patterns of behavior that are consistent with movement toward important life values (Gregg, Callaghan, Hayes, & Glenn-Lawson, 2007). Results of a recent randomized controlled trial in diabetes found that patients who received both an educational and an ACT intervention (to facilitate effective coping with distressing diabetes-related feelings and thoughts) showed improved self-management behaviors and glycemic control at follow-up compared to patients who received only the educational component of the intervention (Gregg et al., 2007).

Summary

Nonadherence to chronic illness treatment regimens is a pervasive problem associated with deleterious consequences for both the individual patient and the health care system in general. To develop targeted interventions to improve adherence behavior, thorough assessment of the problem through both patient self-report and objective markers is an important first step for researchers and clinicians. Although challenges have arisen with regard to cost-effectiveness and implementation in clinical practice, comprehensive intervention programs that include educational, behavioral, and affective components have demonstrated significant effects on adherence and, when feasible, should be incorporated into patient treatment plans.

Conclusions

An individual's ability to cope successfully with chronic illness includes cognitive (e.g., perceptions of control), affective (e.g., positive emotions), and behavioral (e.g., treatment adherence) responses to the demands associated with the illness. These different types of responses are interrelated, and each influences successful coping (de Ridder et al., 2008). Future theoretical and empirical work should be aimed at elucidating the interrelations among these different types of responses to identify ways in which coping with chronic illness might be facilitated. To the extent that these interrelations are better understood, interventions aimed at improving patients' ability to cope with chronic illness will become more precise and more efficient.

Further Reading

Carver, C. S., & Scheier, M. F. (2002). Coping processes and adjustment to chronic illness. In A. J. Christensen & M. H. Antoni (Eds.), Chronic physical disorders: Behavioral medicine's perspective (pp. 47–68). Oxford, UK: Blackwell.

Christensen, A. J. (2004). Patient adherence with treatment regimens: Bridging the gap between behavioral science and biomedicine. New Haven, CT: Yale University Press.

de Ridder, D., Geenen, R., Kuijer, R., & van Middendorp, H. (2008). Psychological adjustment to chronic disease. Lancet, 372, 246–255.

Detweiler-Bedell, J. B., Friedman, M. A., Leventhal, H., Miller, I. W., & Leventhal, E. A. (2008). Integrating co-morbid depression and chronic physical disease management: Identifying and resolving failures in self-regulation. Clinical Psychology Review, 28, 1426–1446.

Taylor, S. E., Kemeny, M. E., Reed, G. M., Bower, J. E., & Gruenewald, T. L. (2000). Psychological resources, positive illusions, and health. American Psychologist, 55, 99–109.

Williams, G. C. (2002). Improving patients' health through supporting the autonomy of patients and providers. In E. L. Deci & R. M. Ryan (Eds.), Handbook of self-determination research (pp. 233–254). Rochester, NY: University of Rochester Press.

References

Affleck, G., Tennen, H., Croog, S., & Levine, S. (1987). Causal attribution, perceived benefits, and morbidity after a heart attack: An eight-year study. Journal of Consulting and Clinical Psychology, 55, 29–35.

Affleck, G., Tennen, H., Pfeifer, C., & Fifield, J. (1987). Appraisals of control and predictability in adapting to a chronic disease. Journal of Personality and Social Psychology, 53, 273–279.

American Psychiatric Association. (2000). Diagnostic and statistical manual of mental disorders (4th ed., text rev.). Washington, DC: Author.

Anderson, R. J., Clouse, R. E., Freedland, K. E., & Lustman, P. J. (2001). The prevalence of comorbid depression in adults with diabetes. Diabetes Care, 24, 1069–1078.

Antoni, M. H., Lehman, J. M., Kilbourn, K. M., Boyers, A. E., Culver, J. L., Alferi, S. M., et al. (2001). Cognitive-behavioral stress management intervention decreases the prevalence of depression and enhances benefit finding among women under treatment for early-stage breast cancer. Health Psychology, 20, 20–32.

Arnow, B. A., Hunkeler, E. M., Blasey, C. M., Lee, J., Constantino, M. J., Fireman, B., et al. (2006). Comorbid depression, chronic pain, and disability in primary care. *Psychosomatic Medicine, 68,* 262–268.

Bem, D. J., & Funder, D. C. (1978). Predicting more of the people more of the time: Assessing the personality of situations. *Psychological Review, 85,* 485–501.

Bower, J. E., Kemeny, M. E., Taylor, S. E., & Fahey, J. L. (1998). Cognitive processing, discovery of meaning, CD4 decline, and AIDS-related mortality among bereaved HIV-seropositive men. *Journal of Consulting and Clinical Psychology, 66,* 979–986.

Broderick, J. E., Junghaenel, D. U., & Schwartz, J. E. (2005). Written emotional expression produces health benefits in fibromyalgia. *Psychosomatic Medicine, 67,* 326–334.

Carver, C. S., Pozo, C., Harris, S. D., Noriega, V., Scheier, M. F., Robinson, D. S., et al. (1993). How coping mediates the effect of optimism on distress: A study of women with early stage breast cancer. *Journal of Personality and Social Psychology, 65,* 375–390.

Carver, C. S., & Scheier, M. F. (1990). Origins and functions of positive and negative affect: A control–process view. *Psychological Review, 97,* 19–35.

Carver, C. S., & Scheier, M. F. (2002). Coping processes and adjustment to chronic illness. In A. J. Christensen & M. H. Antoni (Eds.), *Chronic physical disorders: Behavioral medicine's perspective* (pp. 47–68). Oxford, UK: Blackwell.

Chaney, J., Mullins, L., Uretsky, D., Doppler, M., Palmer, W., Wees, S., et al. (1996). Attributional style and depression in rheumatoid arthritis: The moderating role of perceived illness control. *Rehabilitation Psychology, 41,* 205–223.

Christensen, A. J. (2000). Patient × treatment context interaction in chronic disease: A conceptual framework for the study of patient adherence. *Psychosomatic Medicine, 62,* 435–443.

Christensen, A. J. (2004). *Patient adherence with treatment regimens: Bridging the gap between behavioral science and biomedicine.* New Haven, CT: Yale University Press.

Christensen, A. J., & Johnson, J. A. (2002). Patient adherence with medical treatment regimens: An interactive approach. *Current Directions in Psychological Science, 11,* 94–97.

Christensen, A. J., Moran, P. J., Wiebe, J. S., Ehlers, S. L., & Lawton, W. (2002). Effect of a behavioral self-regulation intervention on patient adherence in hemodialysis. *Health Psychology, 21,* 393–397.

Christensen, A. J., Smith, T. W., Turner, C. W., & Cundick, K. E. (1994). Patient adherence and adjustment in renal dialysis: A person × treatment interactive approach. *Journal of Behavioral Medicine, 17,* 549–566.

Cukor, D., Newville, H., & Jindal, R. (2008). Depression and immunosuppressive medication adherence in kidney transplant patients. *General Hospital Psychiatry, 30,* 386–389.

Cvengros, J. A., Christensen, A. J., Hillis, S., & Rosenthal, G. (2007). Patient and physician attitudes in the health care context: Attitudinal symmetry predicts patient satisfaction and adherence. *Annals of Behavioral Medicine, 33,* 262–268.

Dance, K. A., & Neufeld, R. W. J. (1988). Aptitude–treatment interaction research in the clinical setting: A review of attempts to dispel the "patient uniformity myth." *Psychological Bulletin, 104,* 192–213.

de Groot, M., Anderson, R., Freedland, K. E., Clouse, R. E., & Lustman, P. J. (2001). Association of depression and diabetes complications: A meta-analysis. *Psychosomatic Medicine, 63,* 619–630.

Dejonge, P., Honig, A., van Melle, J. P., Schene, A. H., Kuyper, A. M. G., Tulner, D., et al. (2007). Nonresponse to treatment for depression following myocardial infarction: Association with subsequent cardiac events. *American Journal of Psychiatry, 164,* 1371–1378.

de Ridder, D., Geenen, R., Kuijer, R., & van Middendorp, H. (2008). Psychological adjustment to chronic disease. *Lancet, 372,* 246–255.

Diabetes Control and Complications Trial Research Group. (1993). The effect of intensive treatment of diabetes on the development and progression of long-term complications in insulin-dependent diabetes mellitus. *New England Journal of Medicine, 329,* 977–986.

DiMatteo, M. R. (2004). Variations in patients' adherence to medical recommendations: A quantitative review of 50 years of research. *Medical Care, 42,* 200–209.

Evans, D. L., Charney, D. S., Lewis, L., Golden, R. N., Gorman, J. M., Krishnan, K. R. R., et al. (2005). Mood disorders in the medically ill: Scientific review and recommendations. *Biological Psychiatry, 58,* 175–189.

Gregg, J. A., Callaghan, G. M., Hayes, S. C., & Glenn-Lawson, J. L. (2007). Improving diabetes self-management through acceptance, mindfulness, and values: A randomized controlled trial. *Journal of Consulting and Clinical Psychology, 75,* 336–343.

Haynes, R. B., McDonald, H. P., & Garg, A. X. (2002). Helping patients follow prescribed treatment: Clinical applications. *Journal of the American Medical Association, 288,* 2880–2883.

Heron, M. (2007). Death: Leading causes for

2004. *National Vital Statistics Report, 56*(5), 1–95.

James, S. A., Keenan, N. L., Strogatz, D. S., Browning, S. R., & Garrett, J. M. (1992). Socioeconomic status, John Henryism, and blood pressure in black adults: The Pitt County Study. *American Journal of Epidemiology, 135,* 59–67.

Kane, S. V. (2006). Systematic review: Adherence issues in the treatment of ulcerative colitis. *Alimentary Pharmacology and Therapeutics, 23,* 577–585.

Katon, W. J. (2003). Clinical and health services relationships between major depression, depressive symptoms, and general medical illness. *Biological Psychiatry, 54,* 216–226.

Kimmel, P. L. (2002). Depression in patients with chronic renal disease: What we know and what we need to know. *Journal of Psychosomatic Research, 53,* 951–956.

Kiviruusu, O., Huurre, T., & Aro, H. (2007). Psychosocial resources and depression among chronically ill young adults: Are males more vulnerable? *Social Science and Medicine, 65,* 173–186.

Lazarus, R., & Folkman, S. (1984). *Stress, coping, and appraisal.* New York: Springer.

Lesserman, J., Pence, B. W., Whetten, K., Mugavero, M. J., Thielman, N. M., Swartz, M. S., et al. (2007). Relation of lifetime trauma and depressive symptoms to mortality in HIV. *American Journal of Psychiatry, 164,* 1707–1713.

Lustman, P. J., & Clouse, R. E. (2005). Depression in diabetic patients: The relationship between mood and glycemic control. *Journal of Diabetes and Its Complications, 19,* 113–122.

Malta, M., Strathdee, S. A., Magnanini, M. M. F., & Bastos, F. I. (2008). Adherence to antiretroviral therapy for human immunodeficiency virus/acquired immune deficiency syndrome among drug users: A systematic review. *Addiction, 103,* 1242–1257.

Massie, M. J. (2004). Prevalence of depression in patients with cancer. *Journal of the National Cancer Institute Monographs, 32,* 57–71.

McDonald, H. P., Garg, A. X., & Haynes, R. B. (2002). Interventions to enhance patient adherence to medication prescriptions: Scientific review. *Journal of the American Medical Association, 88,* 2868–2879.

O'Connor, S. M., Jardine, A. G., & Millar, K. (2008). The prediction of self-care behaviors in end-stage renal disease patients using Leventhal's self-regulatory model. *Journal of Psychosomatic Research, 65,* 191–200.

Patel, U. D., & Davis, M. M. (2006). Physicians' attitudes and practices regarding adherence to medical regimens by patients with chronic illness. *Clinical Pediatrics, 45,* 439–445.

Reed, G. M., Kemeny, M. E., Taylor, S. E., & Visscher, B. R. (1999). Negative HIV-specific expectancies and AIDS-related bereavement as predictors of symptom onset in asymptomatic HIV-positive gay men. *Health Psychology, 18,* 354–363.

Roter, D. L., Hall, J. A., Merisca, R., Nordstrom, B., Cretin, D., & Svarstad, B. (1998). Effectiveness of interventions to improve patient compliance: A meta-analysis. *Medical Care, 36,* 1138–1161.

Rutledge, T., Reis, V. A., Linke, S. E., Greenberg, B. H., & Mills, P. J. (2006). Depression in heart failure: A meta-analytic review of prevalence, intervention effects, and associations with clinical outcomes. *Journal of the American College of Cardiology, 48,* 1527–1537.

Ryan, R. M., & Deci, E. L. (2000). Self-determination theory and the facilitation of intrinsic motivation, social development, and well-being. *American Psychologist, 55,* 68–78.

Scheier, M. F., Matthews, K. A., Owens, J. F., Schulz, R., Bridges, M. W., Magovern, G. J., et al. (1999). Optimism and rehospitalization following coronary artery bypass graft surgery. *Archives of Internal Medicine, 159,* 829–835.

Simon, G. E., & Von Korff, M. (2006). Medical co-morbidity and validity of DSM-IV depression criteria. *Psychological Medicine, 36,* 27–36.

Smyth, J. M., Stone, A. A., Hurewitz, A., & Kaell, A. (1999). Effects of writing about stressful experiences on symptom reduction in patients with asthma or rheumatoid arthritis: A randomized trial. *Journal of the American Medical Association, 281,* 1304–1309.

Suls, J., & Fletcher, B. (1985). The relative efficacy of avoidant and nonavoidant coping strategies: A meta-analysis. *Health Psychology, 4,* 249–288.

Taylor, S., Helgeson, V., Reed, G., & Skokan, L. (1991). Self-generated feelings of control and adjustment to physical illness. *Journal of Social Issues, 47,* 91–109.

Taylor, S. E. (1983). Adjustment to threatening events: A theory of cognitive adaptation. *American Psychologist, 38,* 1161–1173.

Taylor, S. E., & Brown, J. D. (1988). Illusion and well-being: A social psychological perspective on mental health. *Psychological Bulletin, 110,* 193–210.

Taylor, S. E., Kemeny, M. E., Aspinwall, L. G., Scheider, S. C., Rodriguez, R., & Herbert, M. (1992). Optimism, coping, psychological distress, and high-risk sexual behavior among men at risk for AIDS. *Journal of Personality and Social Psychology, 63,* 460–473.

Taylor, S. E., Kemeny, M. E., Reed, G. M., Bower, J. E., & Gruenewald, T. L. (2000). Psychological resources, positive illusions, and health. *American Psychologist, 55,* 99–109.

Walker, J. G., Jackson, H. J., & Littlejohn, G. O. (2004). Models of adjustment to chronic illness: Using the example of rheumatoid arthritis. *Clinical Psychology Review, 24,* 461–488.

Watson, M., Haviland, J. S., Greer, S., Davidson, J., & Bliss, J. M. (1999). Influence of psychological response on survival in breast cancer: A population-based cohort study. *Lancet, 354,* 1331–1336.

Weingarten, S. R., Henning, J. M., Badamgarav, E., Knight, K., Hasselblad, V., Gano, A., et al. (2002). Interventions used in disease management programmes for patients with chronic illness—which ones work?: Meta-analysis of published reports. *British Medical Journal, 325,* 925–932.

Wiebe, J. S. (2004). Patient adherence. In A. J. Christensen, R. Martin, & J. M. Smyth (Eds.), *Encyclopedia of health psychology* (pp. 200–204). New York: Kluwer Academic/Plenum Press.

Wiebe, J. S., & Christensen, A. J. (1996). Patient adherence in chronic illness: Personality and coping in context. *Journal of Personality, 64,* 815–835.

Williams, G. C. (2002). Improving patients' health through supporting the autonomy of patients and providers. In E. L. Deci & R. M. Ryan (Eds.), *Handbook of self-determination research* (pp. 233–254). Rochester, NY: University of Rochester Press.

Williams, G. C., Gagné, M., Mushlin, A. I., & Deci, E. L. (2005). Motivation for behavior change in patients with chest pain. *Health Education, 105,* 304–321.

Williams, G. C., Lynch, M., & Glasgow, R. E. (2007). Computer-assisted intervention improves patient-centered diabetes care by increasing autonomy support. *Health Psychology, 26,* 728–734.

Williams, G. C., McGregor, H. A., Sharp, D., Levesque, C., Kouides, R. W., Ryan, R. M., et al. (2006). Testing a self-determination theory intervention for motivating tobacco cessation: Supporting autonomy and competence in a clinical trial. *Health Psychology, 25,* 91–101.

Williams, G. C., McGregor, H. A., Zeldman, A., Freedman, Z. R., & Deci, E. L. (2004). Testing self-determination theory process model for promoting glycemic control through diabetes self-management. *Health Psychology, 23,* 58–66.

Williams, P., Narciso, L., Browne, G., Roberts, J., Weir, R., & Gafni, A. (2005). The prevalence, correlates, and costs of depression in people living with HIV/AIDS in Ontario: Implications for service directions. *Aids Education and Prevention, 17,* 119–130.

Winkley, K., Landau, S., Eisler, I., & Ismail, K. (2006). Psychological interventions to improve glycaemic control in patients with Type 1 diabetes: Systematic review and meta-analysis of randomised controlled trials. *British Medical Journal, 333,* 65–69.

Wolcott, D. W., Maida, C. A., Diamond, R., & Nissenson, A. R. (1986). Treatment compliance in end-stage renal disease patients on dialysis. *American Journal of Nephrology, 6,* 329–338.

Wood, J. V., & Van der Zee, K. (1997). Social comparisons among cancer patients: Under what conditions are comparisons upward and downward? In B. Buunk & F. X. Gibbons (Eds.), *Health, coping, and well-being: Perspectives from social comparison theory* (pp. 299–328). Mahwah, NJ: Erlbaum.

CHAPTER 34

Managing the Obesity Epidemic

Lucy F. Faulconbridge
Thomas A. Wadden

The prevalence of obesity has been rising sharply over the last 30 years, making it one of our nation's most pressing health concerns. In this chapter, we define obesity and review its epidemiology and complications. Causes of this disorder are discussed, as are methods of treating and preventing the condition.

Obesity and Its Complications

"Obesity" is defined by an excess accumulation of body fat that presents a risk to health. In normal-weight women, 25% of body weight consists of fat. When a woman's percentage of fat rises to 35% of her weight, she is considered obese. In a normal-weight man, 15–18% of body weight is fat, and when 25% or more of weight is fat, he is obese. There are numerous methods to measure body fat, but it is typically estimated by calculating the body mass index (BMI), derived by dividing weight in kilograms by height in meters squared (i.e., kg/m^2). The World Health Organization (WHO), the National Institutes of Health (NIH), and the National Heart, Lung and Blood Institute (NHLBI) all define obesity as a BMI $\geq$ 30 kg/m^2.

Recent data suggest that more than one-third of adults in the United States are obese: 33% of men and 35% of women met criteria for obesity in 2005–2006 (Ogden, Carroll, McDowell, & Flegal, 2007). This survey found that 40- to 59-year-olds had the highest rates of obesity compared to other age groups, with 40% of men and 41% of women in this age range being obese. Fifty-three percent of African American and 51% of Mexican American women in this age group were obese, compared to 39% of European American women, highlighting the significant disparities between ethnic groups. These statistics have been described as "alarming" by the Centers for Disease Control and Prevention. Obesity rates have increased similarly in other developed nations.

Adverse Effects

Obesity is associated with a large burden of physical illness. The criterion for defining "obesity" (i.e., a BMI $\geq$ 30 kg/m^2) was selected principally on the basis of the strong relationship between BMI and mortality. The life expectancy of severely obese people is reduced by an estimated 5–20 years due to cardiovascular disease, Type 2 diabetes, and several cancers (Flegal, Graubard, Williamson, & Gail, 2007). Obesity is also associated with an increased risk of depression and anxiety disorders. Part of this risk appears to result from the prejudice and discrimination to which obese individuals are routinely subjected. Children as young as 4 years of age hold negative attitudes toward their overweight peers, and discrimination against obese individuals has been observed in school, work, and social settings. Remarkably, such discrimination does not violate federal law because obesity is not a protected characteristic (unlike gender, ethnicity, or religious belief).

Positive Effects

Despite the current negative opinion of obesity, fat has many important functions. Stored fat is an efficient reserve of energy, helping the body to maintain a constant temperature and an uninterrupted supply of nutrients to tissues, which is essential when food availability is limited. Fat also plays a critical role in digestion and energy metabolism, cushions and protects vital organs, and is involved in the production and regulation of various hormones. It provides structure to the walls of cells, maintains proper nerve transmission, plays a role in memory storage, and is required for reproduction. Thus, fat is critical to survival, and all humans, including newborn babies, need body fat.

The ability to store fat conferred a particular survival advantage for our prehistoric ancestors. Those who had fat stores were able to survive famines and to reproduce, while those without fat perished, often before having offspring and passing on their genes to the next generation. As such, humans have evolved with biological mechanisms that easily store excess energy as fat, the "thrifty genotype" (Neel, 1962). These mechanisms were extremely useful when food sources were scarce and large amounts of physical activity were required to hunt for food. Now, however, we live in a different environment, one in which the "thrifty genotype" is exposed to a "toxic environment" (Brownell, 1994), characterized by the increased availability of cheap, energy-dense foods and a decreased need for physical activity. As Egger and Swinburn (1997) suggest, obesity is "a normal response to an abnormal environment" (p. 477).

Energy Balance and the Regulation of Body Weight

A constant body weight is maintained by balancing energy intake with energy expenditure. Energy is measured in units called "calories." "Energy intake" refers to the fuel needed by our tissues and organs, and is acquired through consuming food and beverages that contain calories. "Energy expenditure" refers to the energy that our bodies use, and is made up of three components: our basal metabolic rate, the thermic effect of food, and activity thermogenesis. "Basal metabolic rate," which accounts for about 60% of energy expenditure, is the energy required for core bodily functions (e.g., maintaining a constant temperature and heart rate) and is measured at rest in a fasting state (i.e., resting energy expenditure). The "thermic effect of food," which accounts for approximately 10% of all energy expended, is the energy expended in response to eating. Calories are burned in digesting food, absorbing nutrients, and storing excess energy. "Activity thermogenesis" includes the energy used by our bodies when we move around throughout the day and when we undertake deliberate exercise. Activity thermogenesis varies widely depending on an individual's lifestyle and exercise habits, and can account for 5–30% of total energy expended (Levine & Kotz, 2005). When energy intake exceeds energy expenditure, people gain weight as extra fuel is stored as fat. To reduce fat mass, people must ensure that their energy intake is less than their energy expenditure.

Biological Factors in the Regulation of Body Weight

Current evidence suggests that body weight is controlled, in part, by a group of hormones that provide information to the brain about the body's short- and long-term energy needs. This section reviews some of the major hormones that control food intake and body weight.

Leptin

Leptin is a hormone that is synthesized in white adipose (fat) tissue in proportion to the amount of body fat. Released directly into the bloodstream, leptin travels to the hypothalamus, one of the "feeding centers" in the brain,[1] where it serves to increase satiety and prevent further food intake. The discovery of leptin in 1994 by Friedman and colleagues (Zhang et al., 1994) excited researchers, who hoped that increasing leptin levels in overweight humans would reduce food intake and, in turn, body weight. Evidence consistent with this notion came from research with mice that could not produce leptin and were hyperphagic (i.e., excessive eaters), sedentary, and very obese. However, when the animals were given replacement leptin, their obesity was reversed in a matter of weeks (Pellymounter et al., 1995; Zhang et al., 1994). The animals' eating, activity, and body weight all returned to normal.

Researchers quickly began to look for similar mutations in the leptin-producing genes in obese humans, hypothesizing that these individuals, like the leptin-deficient mice, would have low levels of leptin in their blood. However, only a handful of individuals in the world have been found to have such a leptin mutation (Montague et al., 1997), with accompanying low levels of leptin. Paradoxically, obese individuals actually have higher than average leptin levels due to their increased amount of fat tissue. (While this should cause them to reduce their food intake, it is believed that many obese people have become insensitive to circulating leptin.) In other cases of severe childhood obesity, single-gene defects have been identified for different genes involved in the control of energy homeostasis, such as mutations in the melanocortin system (Farooqi et al., 2003). However, these are rare cases, and scientists now believe that the biological factors contributing to obesity are likely to be more complex than can be explained by a mutation in a single gene. Most types of obesity are thought to be due to small mutations in potentially dozens of genes, or parts of

genes, that occur simultaneously and interact with each other.

Ghrelin

The hormone ghrelin, discovered in 1999, was first studied in the context of growth hormone release (Kojima et al., 1999). However, scientists quickly realized that ghrelin had potent effects on energy homeostasis, causing increases in hunger, food intake, and body weight (Tschop, Smiley, & Heiman, 2000). Ghrelin is released in the stomach and small intestine when there is very little food in the gut, with levels rising sharply before each meal, and falling rapidly as soon as food is consumed (Cummings et al., 2002). Administration of ghrelin to rodents dramatically increases food intake by increasing the number of meals the animal eats (Faulconbridge, Cummings, Kaplan, & Grill, 2003), indicating that ghrelin is likely to be a "hunger" (orexigenic) signal. Researchers are working to develop compounds that either block the ghrelin receptor or interfere with the hunger signal downstream to help reduce obesity.

Central Regulation of Feeding

Although ghrelin and leptin are produced in the periphery (i.e., outside the central nervous system), both act in the brain to control energy homeostasis. Each hormone binds to its respective receptor, which sits on two different types of neurons in the hypothalamus (see Figure 34.1). The first type of neuron releases two neuropeptides, neuropeptide Y (NPY) and agouti-related protein (AgRP), which are orexigenic signals that instruct the organism to eat more food and to conserve energy through reduced energy expenditure. Ghrelin stimulates these neurons (increasing their action), while leptin inhibits them (decreasing activity). The second type of neuron contains two different neuropeptides, pro-opiomelanocortin (POMC) and cocaine–amphetamine regulated transcript (CART). These two peptides produce an opposite, anorexigenic (i.e., decreasing appetite) signal, which is associated with a reduction in energy intake and an increase in energy expenditure. Leptin stimulates these neurons and ghrelin inhibits them (Barsh & Schwartz, 2002). The reciprocal action of

---

[1] Another feeding center is a group of nuclei in the hindbrain known as the dorsal vagal complex, which receives information from the mouth and gut, and relays it to the hypothalamus; see Grill and Kaplan (2002) for a review.

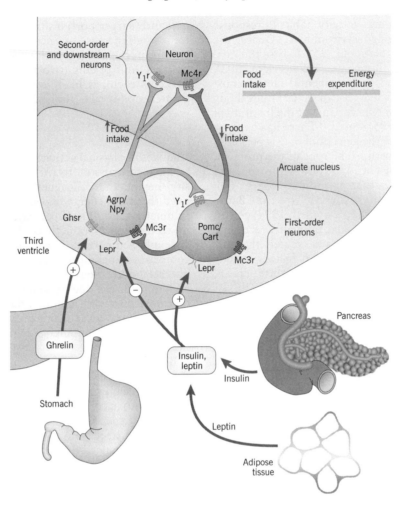

FIGURE 34.1. Two different types of neurons in the arcuate nucleus of the hypothalamus contribute to the control of energy homeostasis. One type of neuron produces NPY/AgRP, which stimulates food intake, while the other produces POMC/CART, which inhibits food intake. From Barsh and Schwartz (2002). Reprinted with permission from Macmillan Publishers Ltd.

these two hormones on these neurons has led some to describe ghrelin as the "yin" to leptin's "yang."

Other circulating factors that play a crucial role in energy homeostasis include insulin, peptide YY (PYY), the incretin hormones—gastric inhibitory peptide (GIP) and glucagon-like peptide (GLP-1)—and cholesystokinin (CCK), which all serve as satiation signals to inhibit food intake. These peptides are but a handful of the large number of biological mediators involved in the regulation of body weight homeostasis. That such redundancy in the system should have evolved is not surprising given that food intake is crucial for survival, and it explains why animals are highly motivated to eat to defend their body weight. The disadvantage of such a defended system, however, is the difficulty of developing effective drug treatments because deletion of one system is followed by up-regulation (i.e., an increase in activity) of a sister system, waiting to compensate for its inaction.

Environmental Factors in the Regulation of Body Weight

Many researchers believe that the high prevalence of obesity can be explained by changes in our eating and activity habits in response to a changing environment. Genes are thought to explain only 25–40% of the variance in BMI (Bouchard, 1994; Price, 2002), indicating that environmental factors must play a significant role in determining body weight. As an expert panel of the Institute of Medicine (1995) stated, "There has been no real change in the gene pool in this period of increasing obesity. The root of the problem, therefore, must lie in the powerful social and cultural forces that promote an energy-rich diet and a sedentary lifestyle" (p. 152). Battle and Brownell (1996; Brownell, 1994) coined the term the "toxic environment," recognizing the factors that have created the current obesogenic mileu. Such factors include constant exposure to energy-dense, cheap, highly accessible foods, combined with significantly decreased needs for physical activity via the development of energy-saving devices such as automobiles, televisions, and computers (Prentice & Jebb, 2003). Together with the explosion of fast-food restaurants, dramatic increases in portion sizes, and strategic marketing campaigns, these forces significantly challenge our capacity to maintain a normal body weight.

Food Intake

The sheer amount of food available for consumption in the United States increased by 523 calories per day from 1970 to 2003 (U.S. Department of Agriculture, 2005). The percentage of calories derived from fat, the most calorically dense macronutrient, increased from 32 to 43% between 1910 and 1985, while the percentage from carbohydrate declined from 57 to 46%. High-calorie foods are available more than ever before in fast-food restaurants, convenience food stores, malls, airports, and school cafeterias. Americans, in record numbers, now eat out instead of cooking at home; in 1970, approximately 26% of total food expenditure dollars were spent on food away from home; this amount increased to 41% in 2005 (U.S. Bureau of Labor Statistics). Several studies have shown that more people eat in fast-food restaurants today than three decades ago (Guthrie, Lin, & Frazao, 2002), and that serving portions in these establishments have grown significantly (Nielsen & Popkin, 2003). Value meals, which offer significantly larger portions of food and sodas for a small increase in price, have continued to gain in popularity. Such supersizing, like multiple-unit pricing (two for $1 instead of 55 cents each), is likely only to encourage greater food intake (Rolls, 2003).

Physical Activity

Changes in physical activity are also thought to have contributed to the increase in obesity. Levine and colleagues (2005) have argued that total energy expenditure varies by as much as 2,000 kcal per day, due primarily to differences in activity thermogenesis. As explained earlier, activity thermogenesis comprises expenditure due to exercise (deliberate bodily exertion to maintain fitness) and expenditure due to nonexercise activity thermogenesis (NEAT; all other activities, e.g., going to work, turning on an appliance, doing grocery shopping, playing a musical instrument).

Because the vast majority of people in the Western World do not engage in intense daily physical exercise, alterations in NEAT are likely to account for the wide variability in energy expenditure. Several environmental factors affect NEAT. In most developed countries, the need for locomotion has been reduced by the introduction of convenience services, such as drive-through banks and restaurants, computers, and escalators. In addition, an increase in the use of automobiles for transportation, instead of walking, has become the cultural norm, even when driving is not necessary. In children, computer games and television have replaced running and playing games outside. Several studies have shown that higher levels of television viewing are associated with increased BMI in both children and adults (e.g., Foster, Gore, & West, 2006). In a recent longitudinal study, Parsons, Manor, and Power (2008) showed that frequent television viewing in adolescence and early adulthood was associated with increased adiposity in later life. Although energy burned by NEAT may seem to be small (e.g., walking to the local store may not seem to burn many calories), a difference of 20 calories per day over the course of a year would result in a significant change in weight. Evidence suggests that lean people stand and walk 152 more minutes per day than do obese people, who tend to be seated for large portions of their day (Levine et al., 2005). Thus, decreased physical activity in our daily lives is likely to be a strong contributor to the rise of obesity.

Benefits of Modest Weight Losses

Many obese individuals seek to lose weight to improve their appearance and to reduce weight-related health complications such as Type 2 diabetes and high blood pressure. Historically, the goal of obesity treatment has been to help people achieve an "ideal" or "normal" weight (Foster, Wadden, Phelan, Sarwer, & Sanderson, 2001). However, a greater appreciation of the biological factors that regulate body weight, described previously, and of the difficulty of achieving and maintaining an "ideal" weight led to new weight loss goals in the late 1990s. Expert panels convened by both the WHO (1998) and the NIH recommended that obese individuals attempt to lose 10% of their initial weight, regardless of their starting point (NIH/NHLBI, 1998). This recommendation was based on the finding that weight loss of 5–10% of initial weight was frequently sufficient to improve previously mentioned health complications of obesity, as well as high triglyceride levels and sleep apnea (Goldstein, 1992). Weight losses of this size also improve mood, body image, and quality of life. Thus, the quest for achieving "ideal" weight was replaced by the more attainable goal of attaining a "healthier" weight.

The strongest evidence to date of the benefits of modest weight loss was provided by the Diabetes Prevention Program Research Group (2002). This study enrolled overweight and obese individuals (mean BMI of 34 kg/m^2) who already had high blood sugar levels and were at risk of developing Type 2 diabetes, which is associated with cardiovascular morbidity and mortality. More than 3,200 participants were randomly assigned to one of three groups: (1) placebo; (2) metformin (an oral medication for diabetes); or (3) a lifestyle intervention designed to induce a 7% reduction in initial weight and to increase physical activity to 150 minutes or more a week. Participants in the lifestyle intervention met these goals during the first year of treatment. After an average of 2.8 years, the study investigators found that participants in the lifestyle intervention had a 58% reduction in their risk of developing Type 2 diabetes compared with people in the placebo group (who lost no weight). The lifestyle participants also were more successful than the participants who received metformin in preventing the occurrence of Type 2 diabetes. Even though most participants in the lifestyle intervention remained overweight or obese after losing their 7% of initial weight (about 15 pounds) and, even though many regained some of their lost weight during the 2.8-year follow-up, they still enjoyed significant improvements in their cardiovascular health and reduced risk of developing Type 2 diabetes. Large, long-term studies from Finland (Tuomilehto, Lindstrom, & Eriksson, 2001) and Sweden (Sjöström et al., 2007) also have provided definitive evidence of the health benefits of intentional weight loss.

Weight Loss Interventions for Obesity

The NIH has provided an algorithm based on an individual's BMI to guide the treatment of obesity (see Table 34.1; NHLBI & the North American Association for the Study of Obesity [NAASO], 2000). Overweight individuals (i.e., BMI of 25.0–29.9 kg/m^2) who have two or more risk factors for cardiovascular disease (e.g., high blood pressure or high cholesterol) are encouraged to follow a program of lifestyle modification (Wadden, Butryn, & Wilson, 2007). It consists of decreasing calorie intake by approximately 500 kcal/day, increasing physical activity (to ≥ 30 minutes a day most days of the week), and modifying inappropriate health habits by using behavioral techniques. As BMI increases, so generally do the health complications of obesity and the need for more intensive interventions. Pharmacotherapy is an option for persons with a BMI of 30 kg/m^2 or greater (or a BMI $\geq$ 27 kg/m^2 in the presence of comorbid conditions) who are unable to lose 10% or more of initial weight with lifestyle modification alone (Yanovski & Yanovski, 2002). Weight loss surgery is an option for individuals with a BMI $\geq$ 40 kg/m^2 (or 35 kg/m^2 with comorbidities) who are unsuccessful with lifestyle modification and pharmacotherapy (Sjöström et al., 2007). Regardless of which

TABLE 34.1. A Guide to Selecting Treatment

	BMI category (kg/m^2)				
Treatment	25–26.9	27–29.9	30–34.9	35–39.9	≥ 40
Diet, physical activity, and behavior therapy	With comorbidities	With comorbidities	+	+	+
Pharmacotherapy		With comorbidities	+	+	+
Surgery				With comorbidities	+

Note. The "+" represents the use of indicated treatment regardless of comorbidities. From National Heart, Lung and Blood Institute and the North American Association for the Study of Obesity (2006).

intervention is selected, all are designed to help patients reduce their calorie intake and increase physical activity to achieve optimal weight loss and cardiovascular health.

Behavioral Treatment

A primary goal of behavioral treatment, also referred to as "lifestyle modification," is to help obese patients identify their problem eating and activity habits (Wadden & Foster, 2000). Behavioral treatment teaches overweight individuals to conduct a functional analysis of the antecedent events and consequences of problem behaviors (Brownell, 2000). Problem behaviors are often triggered by a series of events that are linked together in a chain, as illustrated in Figure 34.2. Mapping the links in a behavioral chain can identify the source of the problem and suggest options for intervention.

Behavioral treatment is typically delivered as a package that includes multiple components, such as self-monitoring, stimulus control, diet, exercise, cognitive restructuring, social support, problem solving, slowing the

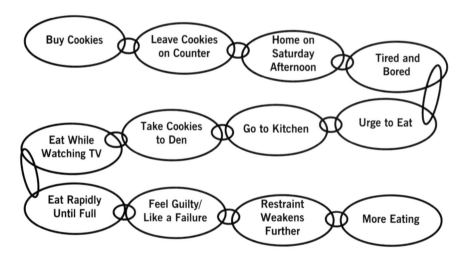

FIGURE 34.2. A behavior chain illustrating how one behavior linked to another can contribute to an overeating episode. What appears to be an unexpected dietary lapse can be traced to a whole series of small decisions and behaviors. The behavior chain also reveals where the individual can intervene in the future to prevent unwanted eating. Thus, the individual might avoid bringing cookies into the house or at least store them out of sight to reduce impulse eating. From Brownell (2000). Reprinted with permission from Kelly D. Brownell.

rate of eating, and relapse prevention. Detailed descriptions of these components are available elsewhere (Brownell, 2000; Wing, 2002). We highlight here self-monitoring and discuss interventions for diet and exercise given that they are the primary targets of behavioral treatment.

Self-Monitoring

Self-monitoring (i.e., recording one's behaviors) is probably the most important component of behavioral treatment for obesity (Wadden & Foster, 2000). Patients keep detailed records of their food intake, physical activity, and weight throughout treatment. They initially record the types, amounts, and caloric value of foods eaten. This information is used to help patients reduce their calorie intake by 500–1,000 kcal/day. As treatment progresses, patients expand their self-monitoring to include additional information about times, places, and feelings associated with eating (Brownell, 2000). This information typically reveals patterns of which patients may not be aware. An individual, for example, may notice that he snacks excessively in the evenings. Another may realize that she often makes poor food choices when upset. Once problem areas have been identified, the individual—alone or with a health professional—can develop a plan to tackle the problem behavior. Individuals who regularly keep food records lose significantly more weight than those who record inconsistently (Berkowitz, Wadden, Tershakovec, & Cronquist, 2003; Wadden, et al., 2005).

Dietary Options

Patients in behavioral programs are usually encouraged to consume a high-carbohydrate, low-fat diet (i.e., fewer than 30% of calories from fat, with no more than 7% from saturated fat) that emphasizes consumption of fruits, vegetables, and whole grains (Brownell, 2000). This diet is consistent with recommendations of the U.S. Department of Agriculture (2005). Patients who weigh ≤ 250 pounds are usually instructed to consume 1,200–1,500 kcal/day, while those who weigh > 250 pounds are prescribed 1,500–1,800 kcal/day (Diabetes Prevention Program, 2002; Look AHEAD

Research Group, 2006). These calorie targets are sufficient to induce a weight loss of approximately 1.0–1.5 pounds/week for 16–26 weeks (Wadden & Foster, 2000). Patients are permitted to consume any foods they wish, including sweet and salty items, provided that they incorporate them into their calorie goal. Most patients reduce their calorie intake by decreasing their portion sizes and eliminating excess sugar (e.g., soft drinks) and fat (e.g., butter or salad dressing) from their diet (Brownell, 2000). They are also encouraged to cook foods by broiling or baking (rather than frying) and to substitute lower-fat for high-fat items (i.e., 2% milk for whole milk). The goal is for patients to make small dietary changes that they can live with long term (Brownell, 2000). Lifestyle modification, however, can be combined with a variety of other dietary approaches, several of which have been designed to produce greater initial weight losses, which are so desired by patients.

MEAL REPLACEMENTS

Meal replacements, such as SlimFast (i.e., liquid shakes) or Lean Cuisine (i.e., frozen-food entrees), provide patients a fixed amount of food with a known calorie content (Tsai & Wadden, 2006). They also simplify food choices, require little preparation, and allow dieters to avoid contact with problem foods. These factors appear to improve patients' adherence to their targeted calorie goals. Obese individuals typically underestimate their calorie intake by 40–50% when consuming a diet of conventional foods (Lichtman et al., 1992). Meal replacements appear to help patients meet their calorie targets. Ditschuneit, Flechtner-Mors, Johnson, and Adler (1999), for example, found that patients who replaced two meals and two snacks a day with a liquid supplement (i.e., SlimFast) lost 8% of their initial weight during 3 months of treatment, compared with a loss of only 1.5% for participants who were prescribed the same number of calories (i.e., 1,200–1,500 kcal/day) but consumed a self-selected diet of conventional foods. A meta-analysis by Heymsfield, van Mierlo, van der Knaap, Heo, and Frier (2003) confirmed the superiority of meal replacements over isocaloric diets composed of conventional foods.

LOW-CARBOHYDRATE DIETS

Low-carbohydrate diets, as developed by Atkins (1998), also appear to facilitate dietary adherence and weight loss. Such diets simplify food choices by virtually eliminating an entire class of macronutrients—carbohydrates. In addition, the high-protein intake may increase satiation (i.e., fullness) (Makris & Foster, 2005). A recent study of severely obese patients, many of whom had Type 2 diabetes, found that participants randomly assigned to a low-carbohydrate versus low-fat diet lost significantly more weight (5.8 kg vs. 1.9 kg, respectively) at 6 months and had significantly greater improvements in triglyceride levels and blood glucose control (Samaha et al., 2003). A second study similarly found significantly greater weight losses on a low-carbohydrate than on a low-fat diet at 6 months (6.9 kg vs. 3.2 kg, respectively) but not at 1 year (4.3 kg vs. 2.5 kg, respectively) because of greater weight regain in the former group (Foster et al., 2003). This pattern of findings was confirmed by the results of a meta-analysis that examined six randomized controlled trials of low-carbohydrate versus low-fat diets (Nordmann et al., 2006). These and other findings (Sachs et al., 2009) suggest that low-carbohydrate diets are safe and relatively effective when used for periods up to 2 years.

There are numerous other dietary options for inducing weight loss, as shown in Figure 34.3 (Wadden et al., 2007). Although these diets may vary dramatically in the amounts of carbohydrate and fat they contain, weight loss results from the reduction in total calories consumed rather than consumption (or avoidance) of specific macronutrients. With this understanding, the choice of a diet may be left in part to patients' preferences. One of the keys to successful weight control is finding a reduced-calorie eating plan that the individual likes and can adhere to long term (Dansinger, Gleason, Griffith, Selker, & Schaefer, 2005).

Physical Activity

Participants in behavioral programs are encouraged to engage in moderate physical activity (e.g., brisk walking) for at least 180 minutes (3 hours) a week (Blair & Leermakers, 2002). Individuals who expect to lose weight from exercising are usually disappointed to learn that they need to walk approximately 35 miles a week (about 10 hours of walking) to lose just 1 pound a week. The principal

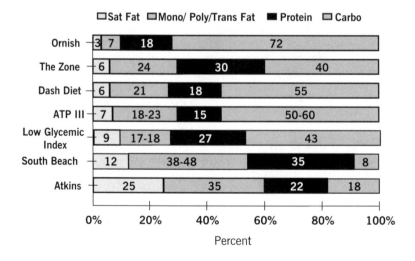

FIGURE 34.3. Macronutrient composition of several popular reducing diets. Data from Atkins (1998); Ornish (2001); Sears (1995); Appel et al. (2006); Adult Treatment Panel III (2001); Pereira, Swain, Goldfine, Rifai, and Ludwig (2004); and Agatston (2003). We thank Dr. Peter Wilson for providing a prototype of the figure.

value of regular exercise is for maintaining rather than inducing weight loss, and for improving cardiovascular health regardless of weight change (Blair & Leermakers, 2002). Regular bouts of aerobic activity may reduce cholesterol, blood pressure, blood sugar (in patients with Type 2 diabetes), and the risk of osteoporosis. Moreover, several studies have suggested that obese individuals who are physically fit have a lower risk of cardiovascular morbidity and mortality than do obese persons who are unfit (Hu et al., 2004; Lee, Blair, & Jackson, 1999; Stevens, Cai, Evenson, & Thomas, 2002). Thus, it is possible to be fat and fit.

PROGRAMMED VERSUS LIFESTYLE ACTIVITY

Obese individuals can increase their energy expenditure in two ways—with programmed or lifestyle activity (Epstein, Wing, Koeske, & Valoski, 1985). "Programmed activity," traditionally referred to as exercise, is usually planned and completed in a discrete period of time (i.e., 30–60 minutes) at a relatively high-intensity level (i.e., 60–80% of maximum heart rate). Examples of programmed activity include jogging, biking, swimming, or exercising to a video. "Lifestyle activity," by contrast, involves increasing energy expenditure throughout the course of the day, without concern for the intensity or duration of the activity (Brownell, 2000). Patients can increase their lifestyle activity by parking farther away from store entrances, taking stairs rather than escalators, or getting off the bus three stops early and walking the remainder of the way. The energy expenditure associated with such events may sum to 300 kcal/day, the equivalent of walking 3 miles.

Epstein and colleagues (1985) found that lifestyle activity was superior to programmed exercise in facilitating the maintenance of weight loss in obese children. Andersen and colleagues (1999), in a study of obese women, found that both types of activity, when combined with a 1,200 kcal/day diet, induced a loss of ~8 kg in 16 weeks. There was a trend ($p = .06$) for lifestyle activity rather than programmed exercise to be associated with less weight regain 1 year after treatment. These findings suggest that lifestyle activity is an ideal option for patients reporting that they hate to exercise.

Weight Loss with Behavioral Treatment

Patients treated by a comprehensive group behavioral program lose approximately 10 kg (about 10% of initial weight) in 26 weeks of treatment (Wadden, Butryn, & Byrne, 2004). In addition, about 80% of patients who begin treatment complete it. Thus, behavioral treatment yields very favorable results, as judged by the current criteria for success (i.e., a 5–10% reduction in initial weight) proposed by expert panels (NIH/NHLBI, 1998; WHO, 1998).

Weight regain, however, is a challenge following virtually all interventions for obesity, but particularly for lifestyle modification. Patients treated by this approach typically regain about 30–35% of weight lost in the year following treatment (Wadden et al., 2004; Wadden & Foster, 2000). Weight regain slows after the first year, but by 5 years, 50% or more of patients are likely to have returned to their baseline weight (Kramer, Jeffery, Forster, & Snell, 1989). Remarkably little is known about factors responsible for weight regain, despite the frequency with which this problem is observed. There are, however, several steps that overweight individuals can take to prevent weight regain: participating in an organized weight loss maintenance program, as well as practicing four key behaviors used by successful maintainers (see below).

Long-Term Treatment

The best way for patients to achieve long-term weight control is by participating in weight maintenance sessions, after losing weight. Perri and colleagues (1988), for example, found that individuals who attended every-other-week group maintenance sessions for the year following weight reduction maintained 13.0 kg of their 13.2 kg end-of-treatment weight loss, whereas those who did not receive such therapy maintained only 5.7 kg of a 10.8 kg loss. Weight maintenance programs encourage people to practice a minimum of four key behaviors: exercise regularly, consume a low-calorie diet, monitor weight regularly, and record (at least periodically) food intake and physical activity. The significance of these behaviors is highlighted by findings from the National

Weight Control Registry (NWCR), founded by Wing and Hill (2001). The NWCR identifies individuals nationwide who have lost a minimum of 13.6 kg (30 pounds) and have kept the weight off for at least 1 year. When first described in 1997, the NWCR had over 2,900 members who had lost an average of 32.4 kg and maintained the loss for 5.5 years (Klem, Wing, McGuire, Seagle, & Hill, 1997). Losses of this size are not representative of those achieved by obese individuals in the general population; NWCR members clearly comprise a highly selective subset of dieters. The NCWR, however, provides valuable descriptive information about the behaviors practiced by successful weight loss maintainers. As shown in Table 34.2, NWCR members report consuming a low-calorie, low-fat diet. Women report eating only 1,302 kcal/day and men, 1,732 kcal/day. They also engage in high levels of physical activity, expending approximately 2,838 calories a week, the equivalent of walking 28 miles. NWCR members also weigh themselves regularly; 44% do so at least once a day, and an additional 33% weigh-in at least once a week. A study by Wing, Tate, Gorin, Raynor, and Fava (2006) demonstrated that weighing daily greatly reduced the risk of regaining weight (5 pounds or more) in the 18 months after losing weight. Patients are encouraged to respond to small increases in weight, by reducing calorie intake and increasing physical activity, before they become large increases.

Pharmacotherapy

Currently only two medications—sibutramine (Meridia) and orlistat (Xenical)—are approved by the U.S. Food and Drug Administration (FDA) for the induction and maintenance of weight loss. Sibutramine, a combined serotonin–norepinephrine reuptake inhibitor, acts on receptors in the hypothalamus that control satiation (i.e., the feeling of fullness that terminates eating). In randomized trials, sibutramine plus diet produced a 7% reduction in initial weight at 1 year, compared with a 2% loss for patients treated by placebo plus diet (Lean, 1997). Losses of 10–15% were achieved when sibutramine was combined with a more intensive program of diet and exercise modification (Wadden et al., 2005), suggesting that behavioral treatment improves the effects of weight loss medication.

Orlistat, a gastric lipase inhibitor, blocks the absorption of about one-third of the fat contained in a meal (Sjöström et al., 1998). The undigested fat (oil) is passed in stool, leading to the loss of about 150–180 kcal/day. In addition, orlistat requires the consumption of a low-fat diet. If patients con-

TABLE 34.2. Eating Habits of National Weight Control Registry Members

Characteristics	Women ($N = 629$)	Men ($N = 155$)
Maximum weight, kg	94.6	121.0
Maximum BMI, kg/m²	34.6	37.2
Current weight, kg	66.0	85.6
Current BMI, kg/m²	24.1	26.4
Energy intake, kcal/day	1,296	1,724
Energy from fat, %	24	23
Energy from protein, %	19	18
Energy from carbohydrates, %	55	56
No. of meals or snacks/day	5.0	4.5
No. of meals at fast-food restaurants/week	0.7	0.8
No. of meals at non-fast-food restaurants/week	2.4	2.9

Note. Data from Klem et al. (1997).

sume more than 20 grams of fat per meal, or a total of 65 grams/day, they increase their risk of adverse gastrointestinal (GI) events that include oily stools, flatus with discharge, and fecal urgency. Thus, patients are negatively reinforced to eat a low-fat diet (to avoid GI affects), which further reduces their caloric intake. In randomized trials, orlistat plus diet produced a 10% reduction in initial weight at 1 year, compared with a 6% loss for placebo plus diet (Davidson et al., 1999; Sjöström et al., 1998). Patients who remained on the drug for an additional year maintained a loss of 8% of weight at the end of this time.

Patients typically regain weight when medications are stopped, leading to the perception that drug treatments for obesity are ineffective. However, obesity is a chronic disease with many causes, and aims to palliate, rather than cure, the condition are likely to be more successful. The long-term use of medications for the control of hypertension, hypercholesterolemia, and diabetes is accepted because when treatment is discontinued, the diseases recur. Likewise, obesity must be considered a chronic and incurable disease that requires continuous treatment, and health care providers should expect effective results only when treatments are used over the long term.

The rising numbers of people with obesity has resulted in an intense search for medications that decrease energy intake and/or increase energy expenditure. Compounds that are currently being targeted include leptin, ghrelin, GLP-1 (see below), and many others (see Table 34.3). The results of initial leptin trials have been disappointing; the highest doses of the protein induced losses of only about 8% of initial weight (Heymsfield et al., 1999). As a result, leptin is now being investigated as a drug that could help weight loss maintenance rather than initial weight loss. In addition, researchers are investigating medications initially established for other disorders, such as topiramate (Topamax) and bupropion (Wellbutrin), or combinations of these agents with those approved for weight loss, such as phentermine, for the treatment of obesity.

Further research on the genetics of body weight regulation is likely to identify additional candidates for intervention. More research is needed on methods of combining pharmacological and behavioral interventions, which may be more effective than using either one alone.

Surgical Treatment of Obesity

The significant health hazards of extreme obesity (BMI $\geq$ 40 kg/m^2) and the modest weight losses produced by traditional treatments led to the development of surgical interventions. In 1969, Mason and Ito developed a gastric bypass (GB) procedure that remains the basis for Roux-en-Y gastric bypass (RYGB), the "gold standard" to which all surgeries are now compared. The RYGB creates a small (15–30 ml) gastric pouch at the base of the esophagus to limit intake. In addition, the stomach and part of the intestine (duodenum) are bypassed by attaching the small pouch to the jejunum, as shown in Figure 34.4. Such procedures have produced average weight losses of approximately 32–38% of initial weight during the first year, with maintenance of 25% up to 10 years later (Sjöström et al., 2004) and 27% at 15 years postsurgery (Sjöström et al., 2007).

Laparoscopic adjustable gastric banding (LAGB), another procedure that is widely used in the United States and Europe, also involves the creation of a small pouch to limit intake, but no alterations are made in the gastrointestinal tract. A band placed around the top portion of the stomach can be adjusted to increase or decrease the aperture through which food passes into the remainder of the stomach.

Surgical intervention is the most effective long-term treatment for obesity. Both procedures described here restrict the amount of food that can be consumed. Weight loss appears to be greater for RYGB than for LAGB (38 vs. 21% at 1-year postsurgery; Sjöström et al., 2004) probably because of malabsorption of food (due to bypassing significant proportions of intestine) and hormonal alterations associated with the former procedure. Well-documented changes in ghrelin, leptin, PYY, and GLP-1 following RYGB are likely responsible for the lack of hunger reported by patients who have had the procedure. In addition, RYGB induces an unpleasant "dumping syndrome" following the ingestion of foods high in fat or refined sugar. Patients experience nausea and other

TABLE 34.3. Potential Targets for New Obesity Treatments.

Target	Action of drug
Appetite suppressants	
Serotonin ($5\text{-}HT_{2C}$ receptor)	Agonists, reuptake inhibitors
Norepinephrine (α_1 and β_2) receptors	Agonists, reuptake inhibitors
Dopamine (D1)	Agonists, reuptake inhibitors
Leptin receptor	Leptin agonists
NPY Y1 and Y5 receptors	Antagonists
$PYY_{3\text{-}36}$	Agonist
Ghrelin	Antagonist
MC3 receptor	Agonist
MC4 receptor	Agonists
α-MSH	Agonist
MCH receptor	Antagonist
CRH receptor/binding proteins	Antagonist
Urocortin	Antagonists
Galanin receptor	Antagonists
Histamine (H3) receptor	Antagonists
CART receptor	Agonist
Amylin	Agonist
Apo (A^{IV}) receptor	Agonists
Orexin receptor	Antagonists
CCK-A receptor	Agonists
GLP-1 receptor	Agonists
Bombesin	Agonists
Enhancers of energy expenditure	
Uncoupling proteins	Stimulator
Protein kinase A	Stimulator
B_3 adrenergic receptor	Agonists
Stimulators of fat mobilization	
Leptin receptor	Leptin agonists
B_3 adrenergic receptor	Agonists
Growth hormone receptor	Agonists
Fatty acid synthease	Inhibitor
Protein kinase A	Stimulator

Note. Apo, apolipoprotein; CART, cocaine- and amphetamine-regulated transcript; CCK, cholecystokinin; CRH, corticotropin-releasing hormone; MC, melanocortin; MCH, melanin-concentrating hormone; MSH, melanocyte-stimulating hormone; $PYY_{3\text{-}36}$, peptide $YY_{3\text{-}36}$. From Thearle and Aronne (2003). Copyright 2003 by Elsevier. Reprinted by permission.

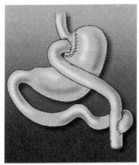

**Roux-en-Y Gastric Bypass
(RYGB)**

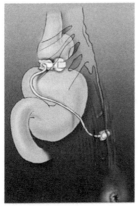

**Adjustable Gastric Band
(Band)**

FIGURE 34.4. Two different surgical procedures, Roux-en-Y gastric bypass (top) and adjustable gastric banding (bottom). From Maggard et al. (2005). Copyright 2005 by the American College of Physicians. Reprinted by permission.

adverse gastrointestinal events that discourage future consumption of sweets.

Prevention and Policy

The various treatments described are likely to benefit individuals who receive them but are inadequate to solve our nation's epidemic obesity. This is because weight reduction therapy is currently available only to a minority of overweight and obese individuals, typically those who can pay for them out of pocket. Even with these persons, earnest efforts to modify eating and activity habits usually are no match in the long term for a toxic environment that explicitly encourag-

es the consumption of high-fat, high-sugar foods and implicitly discourages physical activity as a result of fundamental changes in our nation's work and leisure habits. Clearly, more efforts are needed to improve the treatment of obesity, as well as to obtain reimbursement for treatment of this disorder (Tsai, Asch, & Wadden, 2006). But far greater attention must now be devoted to the prevention of obesity, as proposed by Brownell and Horgen (2004) and Schmitz and Jeffery (2002). Such efforts must attack the environment that lies at the heart of the obesity epidemic.

One approach to prevention is to examine public policy as a means for changing diet and physical activity (Brownell & Horgen, 2004; Jacobson & Brownell, 2000; Nestle & Jacobson, 2000). The prevalence of cigarette smoking has fallen dramatically in the past 50 years in response to federal and state restrictions on the advertisement and sale of tobacco products, and as a result of high taxes on cigarettes and the creation of smoke-free public environments (Mercer et al., 2003). Similar policy approaches could be developed to encourage healthier eating and activity habits. Proposals in this area are in their infancy and largely untested, but they are worthy of further discussion and testing (Wadden, Brownell, & Foster, 2002). The three proposals that follow are drawn from Brownell and Horgen (2004).

1. *Regulate food advertising aimed at children.* The average American child sees 10,000 food advertisements on television each year; 90–95% of these are for sugared cereals, fast food, soft drinks, and candy (Horgen, Choate, & Brownell, 2001). There is clear evidence that exposure relates to food preferences and that content of food ads aimed at children overwhelmingly favors foods of poor nutritional quality (Horgen et al., 2001). Direct regulation might be possible, but perhaps more feasible would be offering equal time for pronutrition messages. This issue is of particular concern in schools, where commercial television now couples food advertisements with education and news programming.

2. *Prohibit fast foods and soft drinks from schools.* School systems in several large U.S. cities, including Los Angeles and Philadelphia, have now banned the sale of soft

drinks in schools, replacing these items with water, low-fat milk, and some juices. This is an encouraging development. However, far too many other schools have imported fast-food franchises into cafeterias and signed contracts with soft drink companies that increase exposure to foods low in nutrition. Research is needed on the effects on weight of banning unhealthy foods, but this approach would appear to have promise.

3. *Provide resources for physical activity.* Given the strong contribution of physical inactivity to obesity, easy access to opportunities to be physically active, additional activity requirements and opportunities in the schools, and other initiatives must be considered (Sallis, Bauman, & Pratt, 1998). Whether additional facilities and opportunities to be active increase activity in sedentary individuals must be studied. Simple, low-cost interventions, such as posting signs that encourage the use of the stairs, should be explored on a broad level (Andersen, Franckowiak, Snyder, Bartlett, & Fontaine, 1998).

It is not known whether any of these or other policy initiatives would be effective, acceptable to the public, or even if effective, would have unanticipated negative consequences. Policy-based approaches can be dismissed as unrealistic and politically naive. Similar reactions, however, initially greeted calls to equip cars with seat belts, to regulate cigarette advertising, and to get tough on drunk driving. Great strides were made in all three areas by virtue of bold public policies.

Conclusions

The dramatic rise in the prevalence of obesity in the last 40 years is the result of a complex interaction between genes and the environment. Studies focusing on biological/genetic and environmental factors converges to yield a picture in which the human body, evolved to conserve body fat, is challenged to its physical limits by the availability of cheap, high-calorie foods and a decrease in physical activity. A number of effective interventions are available for weight loss in the form of behavior therapy, pharmacotherapy, and surgery, but the real challenge lies in effective weight loss maintenance. Despite the

herculean efforts by health care providers to curtail the obesity problem, prevalence rates continue to soar in rich Western countries, a trend that is also apparent in developing countries (James, 2008; Popkin & Doak, 1998), contributing to a now-global epidemic. In the absence of bold policy initiatives, the numbers are likely to rise even further, resulting in an enormous cost to health care systems already stretched thin by the significant increases in mortality and morbidity associated with obesity. Advances in genetics and biology may contribute to the development of effective treatments, although we remain years away from successful manipulation of our own biology. Our best hope may be in preventing the problem at its start. Efforts to educate the population about appropriate nutrition and development of policy initiatives that target the toxic environment are all under way.

Further Reading

Barsh, G. S., & Schwartz, M. W. (2002). Genetic approaches to studying energy balance: Perception and integration. *Nature Reviews Genetics, 3*, 589–600.

Brownell, K. D., & Horgen, K. B. (2004). *Food fight: The inside story of the food industry, America's obesity crisis, and what we can do about it.* Chicago: Contemporary Books.

Cummings, D. E., Overduin, J., Shannon, M. H., & Foster-Schubert, K. E. (2005). Hormonal mechanisms of weight loss and diabetes resolution after bariatric surgery. *Surgery for Obesity and Related Disorders, 1*, 358–368.

Foster, G. D., Sherman, S., Borradaile, K. E., Grundy, K. M., Vander Veur, S. S., Nachmani, J., et al. (2008). A policy-based school intervention to prevent overweight and obesity. *Pediatrics, 121*, 794–802.

Look AHEAD Research Group, Pi-Sunyer, X., Blackburn, G., Brancati, F. L., Bray, G. A., Bright, R., et al. (2007). Reduction in weight and cardiovascular disease risk factors in individuals with Type 2 diabetes: One-year results of the Look AHEAD trial. *Diabetes Care, 30*, 1374–83.

Prospective Studies Collaboration. (2009). Body-mass index and cause-specific mortality in 900 000 adults: Collaborative analyses of 57 prospective studies. *Lancet, 373*, 1083–1096.

Sachs, F. M., Bray, G. A., Carey, V. J., Smith, S. R., Ryan, D. H., Anton, S. D., et al. (2009). Comparison of weight-loss diets with different compositions of fat, protein and carbohydrates. *New England Journal of Medicine, 360,* 859–873.

Sjöström, L., Narbro, K., Sjostrom, C. D., Karason, K., Larsson, B., Wedel, H., et al. (2007). Effects of bariatric surgery on mortality in Swedish obese subjects. *New England Journal of Medicine, 357,* 741–752.

Wadden, T. A., Butryn, M. L., & Wilson, C. (2007). Lifestyle modification for the management of obesity. *Gastroenterology, 132,* 2226–38.

References

Adult Treatment Panel III. (2001). Executive summary of the third report of the National Cholesterol Education Program (NCEP) Expert Panel on Detection, Evaluation, and Treatment of High Blood Cholesterol in Adults. *Journal of the American Medical Association, 285,* 2486–2497.

Agatston, A. (2003). *South Beach diet.* Emmaus, PA: Rodale Press.

Andersen, R. E., Franckowiak, S. C., Snyder, J., Bartlett, S. J., & Fontaine, K. R. (1998). Can inexpensive signs encourage the use of stairs?: Results from a community intervention. *Annals of Internal Medicine, 129,* 363–369.

Andersen, R. E., Wadden, T. A., Bartlett, S. J., Zemel, B., Verde, T. J., & Franckowiak, S. C. (1999). Effects of lifestyle activity vs. structured aerobic exercise in obese women: A randomized trial. *Journal of the American Medical Association, 281,* 335–340.

Appel, L. J., Brands, M. W., Daniels, S. R., Karanja, N., Elmer, P. J., Sacks, F. M., et al. (2006). Dietary approaches to prevent and treat hypertension: A scientific statement from the American Heart Association. *Hypertension, 47,* 296–308.

Atkins, R. C. (1998). *Dr. Atkins' new diet revolution.* New York: Avon Books.

Barsh, G. S., & Schwartz, M. W. (2002). Genetic approaches to studying energy balance: Perception and integration. *Nature Reviews Genetics, 3,* 589–600.

Battle, E. K., & Brownell, K. D. (1996). Confronting a rising tide of eating disorders and obesity: Treatment vs. prevention and policy. *Addictive Behaviors, 21,* 755–765.

Berkowitz, R. I., Wadden, T. A., Tershakovec, A. M., & Cronquist, J. L. (2003). Behavior therapy and sibutramine for the treatment of adolescent obesity: A randomized controlled trial. *Journal of the American Medical Association, 289,* 1805–1812.

Blair, S. N., & Leermakers, E. A. (2002). Exercise and weight management. In T. A. Wadden & A. J. Stunkard (Eds.), *Handbook of obesity treatment* (pp. 283–300). New York: Guilford Press.

Bouchard, C. B. (1994). Genetics of obesity: Overview and research direction. In *The genetics of obesity* (pp. 223–233). Boca Raton, FL: CRC Press.

Brownell, K. D. (1994, December 15). Get slim with higher taxes. *New York Times,* p. A 29.

Brownell, K. D. (2000). *The LEARN program for weight management 2000.* Dallas, TX: American Health Publishing.

Brownell, K. D., & Horgen, K. B. (2004). *Food fight: The inside story of the food industry, America's obesity crisis, and what we can do about it.* Chicago: Contemporary Books.

Cummings, D. E., Weigle, D. S., Frayo, R. S., Breen, P. A., Ma, M. K., Dellinger, E. P., et al. (2002). Plasma ghrelin levels after diet-induced weight loss or gastric bypass surgery. *New England Journal of Medicine, 346,* 1623–1630.

Dansinger, M. L., Gleason, J. A., Griffith, J. L., Selker, H. P., & Schaefer, E. J. (2005). Comparison of the Atkins, Ornish, Weight Watchers, and Zone diets for weight loss and heart disease risk reduction: A randomized trial. *Journal of the American Medical Association, 293,* 43–53.

Davidson, M. H., Hauptman, J., DiGirolamo, M., Foreyt, J. P., Halsted, C. H., Heber, D., et al. (1999). Weight control and risk factor reduction in obese subjects treated for 2 years with orlistat: A randomized controlled trial. *Journal of the American Medical Association, 281,* 235–242.

Diabetes Prevention Program Research Group. (2002). The Diabetes Prevention Program: Description of lifestyle intervention. *Diabetes Care, 25,* 2165–2171.

Ditschuneit, H. H., Flechtner-Mors, M., Johnson, T. D., & Adler, G. (1999). Metabolic and weight loss effects of long-term dietary intervention in obese subjects. *American Journal of Clinical Nutrition, 69,* 198–204.

Egger, G., & Swinburn, B. (1997). An "ecological" approach to the obesity pandemic. *British Medical Journal, 315,* 477–480.

Epstein, L. H., Wing, R. R., Koeske, R., & Valoski, A. (1985). A comparison of lifestyle exercise, aerobic exercise, and calisthenics on weight loss in obese children. *Behavior Therapy, 16,* 345–356.

Farooqi, I. S., Keogh, J. M., Yeo, G. S., Lank, E. J., Cheetham, T., & O'Rahilly, S. (2003). Clinical spectrum of obesity and mutations in the melanocortin 4 receptor gene. *New England Journal of Medicine, 348,* 1085–1095.

Faulconbridge, L. F., Cummings, D. E., Kaplan, J. M., & Grill, H. J. (2003). Hyperphagic effects of brainstem ghrelin administration. *Diabetes, 52,* 2260–2265.

Flegal, K. M., Graubard, B. I., Williamson, D. F., & Gail, M. H. (2007). Cause-specific excess deaths associated with underweight, overweight, and obesity. *Journal of the American Medical Association, 298*, 2028–2037.

Foster, G. D., Wadden, T. A., Phelan, S., Sarwer, D. B., & Sanderson, R. S. (2001). Obese patients' perceptions of treatment outcomes and the factors that influence them. *Archives of Internal Medicine, 161*, 2133–2139.

Foster, G. D., Wyatt, H. R., Hill, J. O., McGuckin, B. G., Brill, C., Mohammed, B. S., et al. (2003). A randomized trial of a low-carbohydrate diet for obesity. *New England Journal of Medicine, 348*, 2082–2090.

Foster, J. A., Gore, S. A., & West, D. S. (2006). Altering TV viewing habits: An unexplored strategy for adult obesity intervention? *American Journal of Health Behavior, 30*, 3–14.

Goldstein, D. J. (1992). Beneficial health effects of modest weight loss. *International Journal of Obesity Related Metabolic Disorders, 16*, 397–415.

Grill, H. J., & Kaplan, J. M. (2002). The neuroanatomical axis for control of energy balance. *Frontiers in Neuroendocrinology, 23*, 2–40.

Guthrie, J. F., Lin, B. H., & Frazao, E. (2002). Role of food prepared away from home in the American diet, 1977-78 versus 1994-96: Changes and consequences. *Journal of Nutrition Education and Behavior, 34*, 140–150.

Heymsfield, S. B., Greenberg, A. S., Fujioka, K., Dixon, R. M., Kushner, R., Hunt, T., et al. (1999). Recombinant leptin for weight loss in obese and lean adults: A randomized, controlled, dose-escalation trial. *Journal of the American Medical Association, 282*, 1568–1575.

Heymsfield, S. B., van Mierlo, C. A., van der Knaap, H. C., Heo, M., & Frier, H. I. (2003). Weight management using a meal replacement strategy: Meta and pooling analysis from six studies. *International Journal of Obesity, 27*, 537–549.

Horgen, K. B., Choate, M., & Brownell, K. D. (2001). Television and children's nutrition. In D. G. Singer & J. L. Singer (Eds.), *Handbook of children and the media* (pp. 447–461). San Francisco: Sage.

Hu, F. B., Willett, W. C., Li, T., Stampfer, M. J., Colditz, G. A., & Manson, J. E. (2004). Adiposity as compared with physical activity in predicting mortality among women. *New England Journal of Medicine, 351*, 2694–2703.

Institute of Medicine. (1995). *Weighing the options: Criteria for evaluating weight management programs.* Washington, DC: National Academy Press.

Jacobson, M. F., & Brownell, K. D. (2000). Small taxes on soft drinks and snack foods to promote health. *American Journal of Public Health, 90*, 854–857.

James, W. P. (2008). The epidemiology of obesity: The size of the problem. *Journal of Internal Medicine, 263*, 336–352.

Klem, M. L., Wing, R. R., McGuire, M. T., Seagle, H. M., & Hill, J. O. (1997). A descriptive study of individuals successful at long-term maintenance of substantial weight loss. *American Journal of Clinical Nutrition, 66*, 239–246.

Kojima, M., Hosoda, H., Date, Y., Nakazato, M., Matsuo, H., & Kangawa, K. (1999). Ghrelin is a growth-hormone-releasing acylated peptide from stomach. *Nature, 402*, 656–660.

Kramer, F. M., Jeffery, R. W., Forster, J. L., & Snell, M. K. (1989). Long-term follow-up of behavioral treatment for obesity: Patterns of weight regain among men and women. *International Journal of Obesity, 13*, 123–136.

Lean, M. E. (1997). Sibutramine—a review of clinical efficacy. *International Journal of Obesity and Related Metabolic Disorders, 21*, 30–36.

Lee, C. D., Blair, S. N., & Jackson, A. S. (1999). Cardiorespiratory fitness, body composition, and cardiovascular disease mortality in men. *American Journal of Clinical Nutrition, 69*, 373–380.

Levine, J. A., & Kotz, C. M. (2005). NEAT—non-exercise activity thermogenesis—egocentric and geocentric environmental factors vs. biological regulation. *Acta Physiologica Scandanavia, 184*, 309–318.

Levine, J. A., Lanningham-Foster, L. M., McCrady, S. K., Krizan, A. C., Olson, L. R., Kane, P. H., et al. (2005). Interindividual variation in posture allocation: Possible role in human obesity. *Science, 307*, 584–586.

Lichtman, S. W., Pisarska, K., Berman, E. R., Pestone, M., Dowling, H., Offenbacher, E., et al. (1992). Discrepancy between self-reported and actual caloric intake and exercise in obese subjects. *New England Journal of Medicine, 327*, 1893–1898.

Look AHEAD Research Group. (2006). The Look AHEAD Study: A description of the lifestyle intervention and the evidence supporting it. *Obesity, 14*, 737–752.

Maggard, M. A., Shugarman, L. R., Suttorp, M., Maglione, M., Sugerman, H. J., Livingston, E. H., et al. (2005). Meta-analysis: Surgical treatment of obesity. *Annals of Internal Medicine, 142*, 547–559.

Makris, A. P., & Foster, G. D. (2005). Dietary approaches to the treatment of obesity. *Psychiatric Clinics of North America, 28*, 117–139.

Mason, E. E., & Ito, C. (1969). Gastric bypass. *Annals of Surgery, 170*, 329–339.

Mercer, S. L., Green, L. W., Rosenthal, A. C.,

Husten, C. G., Khan, L. K., & Dietz, W. H. (2003). Possible lessons from the tobacco experience for obesity control. *American Journal of Clinical Nutrition, 77,* 1073S–1082S.

Montague, C. T., Farooqi, I. S., Whitehead, J. P., Soos, M. A., Rau, H., Wareham, N. J., et al. (1997). Congenital leptin deficiency is associated with severe early-onset obesity in humans. *Nature, 387,* 903–908.

National Heart, Lung and Blood Institute (NHLBI) & the North American Association for the Study of Obesity (NAASO). (2000). *The practical guide: Identification, evaluation, and treatment of overweight and obesity in adults.* Bethesda, MD: National Institutes of Health.

National Institutes of Health (NIH)/National Heart, Lung, and Blood Institute (NHLBI). (1998). Clinical guidelines on the identification, evaluation, and treatment of overweight and obesity in adults. *Obesity Research, 6,* 51S–209S.

Neel, J. V. (1962). Diabetes mellitus: A "thrifty" genotype rendered detrimental by "progress"? *American Journal of Human Genetics, 14,* 353–362.

Nestle, M., & Jacobson, M. F. (2000). Halting the obesity epidemic: A public health policy approach. *Public Health Reports, 115,* 12–24.

Nielsen, S. J., & Popkin, B. M. (2003). Patterns and trends in food portion sizes, 1977–1998. *Journal of the American Medical Association, 289,* 450–453.

Nordmann, A. J., Nordmann, A., Briel, M., Keller, U., Yancy, W. S., Jr., Brehm, B. J., et al. (2006). Effects of low-carbohydrate vs low-fat diets on weight loss and cardiovascular risk factors: A meta-analysis of randomized controlled trials. *Archives of Internal Medicine, 166,* 285–293.

Ogden, C. L., Carroll, M. D., McDowell, M. A., & Flegal, K. M. (2007). *Obesity among adults in the United States—no change since 2003–2004* (NCHS Data Brief No. 1). Hyattsville, MD: National Center for Health Statistics.

Ornish, D. (2001). *Eat more, weigh less: Dr. Dean Ornish's life choice program for losing weight safely while eating abundantly.* New York: Quill.

Parsons, T. J., Manor, O., & Power, C. (2008). Television viewing and obesity: A prospective study in the 1958 British birth cohort. *European Journal of Clinical Nutrition, 62,* 1355–1363.

Pellymounter, M. A., Cullen, M. J., Baker, M. B., Hecht, R., Winters, D., Boone, T., et al. (1995). Effects of the obese gene product on body weight regulation in ob/ob mice. *Science, 269,* 540–543.

Pereira, M. A., Swain, J., Goldfine, A. B., Rifai, N., & Ludwig, D. S. (2004). Effects of a low-glycemic load diet on resting energy expenditure and heart disease risk factors during weight loss. *Journal of the American Medical Association, 292,* 2482–2490.

Perri, M. G., McAllister, D. A., Gange, J. J., Jordan, R. C., McAdoo, G., & Nezu, A. M. (1988). Effects of four maintenance programs on the long-term management of obesity. *Journal of Consulting and Clinical Psychology, 56,* 529–534.

Popkin, B. M., & Doak, C. M. (1998). The obesity epidemic is a worldwide phenomenon. *Nutrition Reviews, 56,* 106–114.

Prentice, A. M., & Jebb, S. A. (2003). Fast foods, energy density and obesity: A possible mechanistic link. *Obesity Reviews, 4,* 187–194.

Price, R. A. (2002). Genetics and common obesities: Background, current status, strategies and future prospects. In T. A. Wadden & A. J. Stunkard (Eds.), *Handbook of obesity treatment* (pp. 73–94). New York: Guilford Press.

Rolls, B. J. (2003). The supersizing of America: Portion size and the obesity epidemic. *Nutrition Today, 38,* 42–53.

Sachs, F. M., Bray, G. A., Carey, V. J., Smith, S. R., Ryan, D. H., Anton, S. D., et al. (2009). Comparison of weight-loss diets with different compositions of fat, protein and carbohydrates. *New England Journal of Medicine, 360,* 859–873.

Sallis, J. F., Bauman, A., & Pratt, M. (1998). Environmental and policy interventions to promote physical activity. *American Journal of Preventative Medicine, 15,* 379–397.

Samaha, F. F., Iqbal, N., Seshadri, P., Chicano, K. L., Daily, D. A., McGrory, J., et al. (2003). A low-carbohydrate as compared with a low-fat diet in severe obesity. *New England Journal of Medicine, 348,* 2074–2081.

Schmitz, K. H., & Jeffery, R. W. (2002). Prevention of obesity. In T. A. Wadden & A. J. Stunkard (Eds.), *Handbook of obesity treatment* (pp. 556–593). New York: Guilford Press.

Sears, B. (1995). *The Zone: A dietary map to lose weight permanently: Reset your genetic code: Prevent disease: Achieve maximum physical performance.* New York: HarperCollins.

Sjöström, L., Lindroos, A. K., Peltonen, M., Torgerson, J., Bouchard, C., Carlsson, B., et al. (2004). Lifestyle, diabetes, and cardiovascular risk factors 10 years after bariatric surgery. *New England Journal of Medicine, 351,* 2683–2693.

Sjöström, L., Narbro, K., Sjöström, C. D., Karason, K., Larsson, B., Wedel, H., et al. (2007). Effects of bariatric surgery on mortality in Swedish obese subjects. *New England Journal of Medicine, 357,* 741–752.

Sjöström, L., Rissanen, A., Andersen, T., Boldrin, M., Golay, A., Koppeschaar, H. P., et al. (1998). Randomised placebo-controlled trial of orlistat for weight loss and prevention of weight regain in obese patients: European Multicentre Orlistat Study Group. *Lancet, 352*, 167–172.

Stevens, J., Cai, J., Evenson, K. R., & Thomas, R. (2002). Fitness and fatness as predictors of mortality from all causes and from cardiovascular disease in men and women in the lipid research clinics study. *American Journal of Epidemiology, 156*, 832–841.

Thearle, M., & Aronne, L. J. (2003). Obesity and pharmacologic therapy. *Endocrinology and Metabolism Clinics of North America, 32*, 1005–1024.

Tsai, A. G., Asch, D. A., & Wadden, T. A. (2006). Insurance coverage on obesity treatment. *Journal of the American Dietetic Association, 106*, 1651–1655.

Tsai, A. G., & Wadden, T. A. (2006). The evolution of very-low-calorie diets: An update and meta-analysis. *Obesity, 14*, 1283–1293.

Tschop, M., Smiley, D. L., & Heiman, M. L. (2000). Ghrelin induces adiposity in rodents. *Nature, 407*, 908–913.

Tuomilehto, J., Lindstrom, J., & Eriksson, J. G. (2001). Prevention of Type 2 diabetes mellitus by changes in lifestyle among subjects with impaired glucose tolerance. *New England Journal of Medicine, 344*, 1343–1350.

U.S. Department of Agriculture, U.S. Department of Health and Human Services. (2005). *Dietary guidelines for Americans.* Washington, DC: Author.

Wadden, T. A., Berkowitz, R. I., Womble, L. G., Sarwer, D. B., Phelan, S., Cato, R. K., et al. (2005). Randomized trial of lifestyle modification and pharmacotherapy for obesity. *New England Journal of Medicine, 353*, 2111–2120.

Wadden, T. A., Brownell, K. D., & Foster, G. D. (2002). Obesity: Responding to the global epidemic. *Journal of Consulting and Clinical Psychology, 70*, 510–525.

Wadden, T. A., Butryn, M. L., & Byrne, K. J. (2004). Efficacy of lifestyle modification for long-term weight control. *Obesity Research, 12*, 151S–162S.

Wadden, T. A., Butryn, M. L., & Wilson, C. (2007). Lifestyle modification for the management of obesity. *Gastroenterology, 132*, 2226–38.

Wadden, T. A., & Foster, G. D. (2000). Behavioral treatment of obesity. *Medical Clinics of North America, 84*, 441–461.

Wing, R. R. (2002). Behavioral weight control. In T. A. Wadden & A. J. Stunkard (Eds.), *Handbook of obesity treatment* (pp. 301–316). New York: Guilford Press.

Wing, R. R., & Hill, J. O. (2001). Successful weight loss maintenance. *Annual Review of Nutrition, 21*, 323–341.

Wing, R. R., Tate, D. F., Gorin, A. A., Raynor, H. A., & Fava, J. L. (2006). A self-regulation program for maintenance of weight loss. *New England Journal of Medicine, 355*, 1563–1571.

World Health Organization. (1998). Obesity: Preventing and managing the global epidemic. *World Health Organization Technical Support Series, 894*, 1–253.

Yanovski, S. Z., & Yanovski, J. A. (2002). Obesity. *New England Journal of Medicine, 346*, 591–602.

Zhang, Y., Proenca, R., Maffei, M., Barone, M., Leopold, L., & Friedman, J. M. (1994). Positional cloning of the mouse obese gene and its human homologue. *Nature, 372*, 425–432.

CHAPTER 35

Pharmacology and Behavior
The Case of Tobacco Dependence

Kenneth A. Perkins

Reducing tobacco use may be the most important public health accomplishment by psychologists working to promote positive behavior change. No other behavior problem has as great an impact on morbidity and mortality. Smoking-related deaths number over 430,000 per year in the United States alone (Mokdad, Marks, Stroup, & Gerberding, 2004) and 5 million people worldwide (Ezzati & Lopez, 2003), or about one person every 6 seconds. The rise of smoking in developing countries indicates that tobacco use will remain a major global public health problem throughout the 21st century.

Overview of Tobacco Dependence

"Tobacco dependence" is defined primarily by persistence of tobacco use despite awareness of tobacco's harm, inability to quit despite a desire to do so, use of greater amounts than intended, and the presence of withdrawal symptoms soon after an attempt to quit (American Psychiatric Association, 1994). Tobacco dependence is a problem not easily or quickly overcome, and repeated cycles of success (quit attempt) followed by fail-ure (i.e., relapse to regular smoking) are the norm. Thus, dependence should be viewed much like chronic disorders, such as diabetes or hypertension, which are generally "managed" rather than permanently "cured." Psychology, the science of human behavior, is critically important to understanding drug dependence, which is similar to other behavioral problems, since it is essentially characterized by a discrete behavior, drug taking, and always occurs in an environmental context that can shape that behavior. However, because of other features of drug dependence, particularly the pharmacological influences, a thorough understanding of dependence requires knowledge from disciplines outside psychology. The multidisciplinary nature of tobacco dependence and the need for health psychologists in this area to collaborate with those in other fields are major emphases of this chapter.

As with any drug dependence, the onset and maintenance of tobacco dependence occurs through the actions of both pharmacological and nonpharmacological factors. Consequently, treating tobacco dependence involves addressing both types of factors. The key pharmacological factor is *nicotine*, the main psychoactive ingredient of tobacco. We know that nicotine intake is necessary but not sufficient to induce tobacco dependence. Nicotine intake is necessary because smoked products not containing nicotine (e.g., clove or herbal cigarettes) do not produce dependence. However, nicotine intake alone is not sufficient because use of non-tobacco nicotine products such as nicotine gum rarely produces dependence-like behavior. The nonpharmacological factors are numerous and include the stimuli that usually accompany nicotine intake when smoking, such as the sight and smell of a lit cigarette (i.e., "cues"); favorite smoking locations, such as a comfortable couch; or complementary activities, such as drinking alcohol with friends (Conklin, 2006). Health psychology researchers need to be familiar with these pharmacological and nonpharmacological factors maintaining tobacco dependence because these are important topics of research themselves, and researchers should understand how to control for these factors in research designs aimed at identifying other influences.

Phases of Dependence

The natural course of dependence generally follows three phases: onset (usually in one's teens), maintenance, and, for many, cessation. Health psychology research focuses on understanding and controlling the factors that influence dependence at each phase. For example, most teens in the United States try cigarette smoking at least once, but only about one-third of these teens ever become dependent (Anthony, Warner, & Kessler, 1994). Thus, many health psychologists interested in the onset of dependence try to understand what factors lead some teens to continue and escalate tobacco use, while others quickly or gradually discontinue use before ever becoming dependent. Results of this research can help in the development of smoking prevention programs.

Maintenance of dependence describes the phase of the vast majority of adult smokers, about 90%. (The remaining 10% or so are able to smoke occasionally or at a low level that does not meet dependence criteria [American Psychiatric Association, 1994].) So, not surprisingly, much health psychology

research focuses on the factors that maintain this dependence, such as the relative contributions of nicotine versus non-nicotine aspects of smoking (e.g., cues, environmental context, social factors). Manipulation of these factors may lead to methods to reduce smoking behavior or otherwise prepare smokers for quitting.

Finally, clinical health psychology research focuses on the last phase, cessation. Because reduction in smoking amount has not been shown to reduce the health risks of smoking substantially, complete cessation of smoking is the treatment goal in health care. Yet, even though perhaps 70% of smokers say they want to quit, only about one-third make a quit attempt in any given year. Of those who try to quit on their own, without counseling or medication, fewer than 5% will stay quit permanently; 95% will resume smoking (termed "relapse"), half of them within a few weeks. Because very few smokers quit abruptly and never relapse, cessation is really a long-term process with intermittent progress and setbacks. This process involves preparing to quit, making the attempt, coping with the difficulty in staying quit, usually failing, then eventually trying again. Although most are eventually successful in staying quit, "success" can take years and many quit attempts, and many others die of smoking-related illnesses before they can successfully quit. Formal treatments involving professional counseling and medication can substantially increase the quit rate during a given attempt, but even these aids fail to help a majority of smokers who use them. Clinical health psychology research is aimed at understanding the intractability of smoking and developing improved interventions to enable smokers to quit permanently.

These phases really represent continua across the natural course of dependence, and dependence is often not neatly divided into distinct phases. For example, when does dependence "onset" end and "maintenance" begin? Research suggests that onset may give way to maintenance far earlier than previously assumed (Colby, Tiffany, Shiffman, & Niaura, 2000). Similarly, because most adult smokers claim to want to quit and often do try to quit, when does "maintenance" clearly give way to "abstinence," and vice versa (upon relapse)? Moreover, most health psychology research at all three phases of dependence is essentially concerned with one thing—the factors that promote persistence of smoking behavior—regardless of smokers' past experience with tobacco or stated interest in quitting. Nevertheless, consideration of the phases of dependence being studied is relevant because each involves many of its own independent and dependent variables of interest, requiring expertise with different methods and subdisciplines. Also, much of the research on each phase is examined at a different "level of analysis," as noted next.

Levels of Analysis

In addition to its focus on one or more of these three phases of dependence, health psychology research on tobacco dependence is generally approached from three "levels of analysis": (1) basic research on the mechanisms of dependence, often conducted in the laboratory and almost always with small groups of nonquitting adult dependent smokers (i.e., in the maintenance phase); (2) clinical research in larger groups of smokers usually trying to quit (i.e., cessation phase); and (3) epidemiological and communitywide research on the onset, maintenance, or control of tobacco use (all three phases). Basic research with nonhuman animal models addresses all three levels but mostly focuses on maintenance. Basic research in humans also focuses on maintenance and rarely examines the onset or cessation phases for several reasons. Identifying processes in both phases often requires longitudinal assessment (i.e., escalation of smoking in onset, quitting and remaining abstinent in cessation), and basic research usually does not track changes in subjects over long periods of time. Also, onset typically occurs in teens, and ethical and practical concerns inhibit studies of the acute effects of teens smoking, with a few exceptions (e.g., Kassel et al., 2007). Basic research on dependence onset does exist but is likely to involve cross-sectional comparisons between self-identified smoking and nonsmoking teens on characteristics believed to increase risk of dependence, such as measures of impulsivity (Reynolds et al., 2007), without having subjects actually smoke. In research on the cessation phase, of key interest is the ex-smoker's long-term adjustment to difficulties that result from

stopping smoking, and the time course of this adjustment is difficult to simulate with basic research procedures in the laboratory. However, basic research has begun to assess certain measures in smokers at one point in time before quitting, then determine whether responses on those measures predict success during a subsequent quit attempt (e.g., Perkins et al., 2002; Waters et al., 2003). These responses could be markers of dependence that improve our understanding of dependence and aid identification of those requiring greater assistance in quitting.

Yet in many respects these distinctions among levels of analysis are artificial, as the separations among them are somewhat arbitrary. The National Institutes of Health (NIH) and other research funders have recognized that a very narrow focus on a topic specific to one level of analysis can provide only a limited knowledge of dependence (Turkkan, Kaufman, & Rimer, 2000). They realize that a comprehensive understanding of nicotine dependence requires integrated collaborations among researchers with expertise across a wide range of scientific disciplines. Thus, much of the health psychology research on tobacco dependence is *multidisciplinary* or *transdisciplinary* in nature. Multidisciplinary research incorporates findings from individual disciplines to present a more complete picture of the phenomenon of interest (e.g., rapid escalation of smoking in teens). Thus, developmental and clinical psychologists might team up with geneticists, pharmacologists, and sociologists to study basic biological, behavioral, and social influences on smoking escalation. Each investigator, largely working independently, would generate data from research within his or her own discipline, and evaluation of these separate results would form a picture of smoking escalation. In transdisciplinary research, a newer concept, such researchers would work jointly within a shared conceptual model that combines concepts and study approaches from the various disciplines to examine the issue of smoking escalation (Turkkan et al., 2000).

Regardless of the approach, the complexity of nicotine dependence highlights the need to incorporate knowledge from many different disciplines to develop effective tobacco control policies informed by science. What this means for health psychology research is that psychologists who study tobacco dependence are increasingly likely to collaborate with scientists from other disciplines, which requires some familiarity with concepts and methods from those disciplines and an ability to convey concepts and methods from health psychology to others outside the field. Moreover, tobacco control is a very active policy area within public health, as public institutions continue to develop stronger policies to reduce tobacco use and other exposure (i.e., secondhand smoke). Thus, health psychology tobacco researchers need to be able to communicate with nonresearchers such as health practitioners, policy leaders (local government officials, business leaders, etc.), and public health advocates to ensure that tobacco control efforts in the community are guided effectively by the research findings (National Cancer Institute, 2007).

This chapter describes health psychology research on tobacco dependence, primarily the factors that influence smoking behavior and its psychological effects. This research focuses on the first two of the three levels of analysis noted earlier, basic and clinical levels because epidemiological or community-based smoking research is adequately described elsewhere (Bricker, Chapter 36, this volume). This chapter does not attempt to review all health psychology research on nicotine dependence, but it does provide a few illustrative examples of these approaches. It also does not cover the extensive research in health psychology that focuses on the disease risks of smoking (e.g., psychological factors in cancer [Diefenbach, Mohamed, Turner, & Diefenbach, Chapter 31] or heart disease in smokers [Harlapur, Abraham, & Shimbo, Chapter 28]), which is addressed in other chapters. Finally, because of its overwhelming risks, cigarette smoking is the form of tobacco use examined in these examples, and other forms, such as smokeless tobacco use, are not discussed.

Health Psychology Basic Research on Mechanisms of Dependence

Research with nonhuman animal models, mostly rats, has clearly demonstrated the importance of pharmacological and non-pharmacological factors in drug-taking behavior (Caggiula et al., 2002). Findings from animal models on nicotine self-administration, or reinforcement, can guide laboratory research on tobacco dependence in humans. For example, rats repeatedly press a bar to receive intravenous infusions of nicotine (i.e., they self-administer nicotine), and environmental cues, such as lights or tones that predict the availability of nicotine, can have at least as great an influence on that bar pressing as the presence of nicotine itself (Caggiula et al., 2002). Congruent with these findings, humans engage in simple lever pulling to receive intravenous infusions of nicotine (Harvey et al., 2004), and the presence of smoking cues, such as a lit cigarette, can increase responding to receive puffs on a cigarette (Perkins, Epstein, Grobe, & Fonte, 1994). Cross-species consistency in these influences on nicotine self-administration illustrates the fundamental nature of this behavior and supports the idea that health psychology researchers, particularly those involved in basic research, should be familiar with findings from animal studies. Animal research can also invasively examine brain mechanisms that influence nicotine self-administration in a way not yet possible ethically or practically in humans, and such research can inform early testing of medications or other treatments for smoking cessation before they are known to be safe for humans.

Laboratory-based basic research on tobacco dependence in humans can involve manipulation of many "independent" variables, or factors that are hypothesized to influence smoking. These can include short-term manipulations, such as the duration of tobacco deprivation, the nicotine content of cigarettes, presence of a psychological stressor (e.g., challenging computer task), or concurrent intake of alcohol, as well as long-term or fixed individual differences, such as the amount of lifetime smoking exposure, family history of tobacco dependence, history of a psychiatric disorder, or a smoker's sex. However, laboratory research generally focuses on just a few key "dependent" variables or measures, primarily, smoking behavior, self-report or other measures of urge to smoke (i.e., craving), and responses to smoking or nicotine intake, such as mood or cognitive processing. Several studies are described in detail to illustrate laboratory studies on factors that contribute to tobacco dependence.

Smoking and Mood

Virtually all smokers, and most nonsmokers, believe that smoking is strongly influenced by mood. Smokers observe that being in a negative mood increases smoking behavior and perhaps, as a consequence of that observation, readily claim that smoking relieves negative affect (i.e., self-reported mood) during stressful situations. Many studies support the first observation, that negative mood increases smoking behavior, but not the second, that smoking relieves negative affect. A key exception to the latter is that smoking does relieve negative affect that arises due to withdrawal symptoms during smoking abstinence. Thus, broad relief of negative affect due to stress is a very common explanation for why smokers say they like to smoke, but it has not been established as a reliable effect of smoking.

In a study that specifically tested the relationship between mood and smoking behavior (Conklin & Perkins, 2005), 48 smokers were randomly divided into two groups, one that was allowed during each session to smoke and another that was only allowed to drink water (as a control procedure). All participants completed three laboratory sessions on different days during which one of three moods (positive, neutral, or negative) was induced by use of emotional pictures and mood-congruent music (i.e., pleasant classical music for positive scenes, dramatic classical music for negative scenes, innocuous music for neutral scenes). As shown in Figure 35.1, negative affect for both groups was sharply increased by the negative mood induction. However, no differences in affect were seen between participants allowed to drink water and those allowed to smoke briefly (after Time 1 [T1]) during the mood induction on any of the days, although smoking sharply decreased self-reported craving. Participants were told later in each session, after T3, to smoke (or drink, depending on their group) as much as they wanted as the mood induction continued, so that the influence of mood on smoking behavior could be determined. Smokers did light up more quickly and smoked more puffs during negative versus positive mood, with smoking behavior during neutral mood midway between the other two (see Figure 35.1). Participants in the water-drinking group showed no change in water consumption across moods, demonstrating that negative mood induction affected smoking but did not broadly influence other consummatory behaviors, such as drinking water.

This study showed that although negative mood acutely increases smoking behavior, this increase cannot be due to any short-term effect of smoking on relieving negative affect. Prior research observing an increase in smoking behavior due to being in a negative mood often inferred that this must have occurred because smoking relieves negative affect. Such a view assumes a symmetrical relationship between negative mood and smoking: Negative mood increases smoking, and smoking relieves negative affect. However, this study suggests that the relationship between smoking and negative mood is more complicated and, perhaps, asymmetrical. In other words, being in a negative mood often increases smoking behavior, but smoking does not appear to relieve negative affect from most causes, other than withdrawal. A more recent study confirmed these findings, as smoking fully relieved negative affect due to withdrawal but had little influence on negative affect due to several laboratory challenges (Perkins, Karelitz, Conklin, Sayette, & Giedgowd, 2010). Thus, other explanations for why smokers smoke more when in a negative mood need to be explored.

Sex and Genetic Effects on Smoking

A major direction of tobacco research is identification of individual differences associated with dependence onset and persistence, including sex or genetic factors. Recent research suggests that the smoking behavior of women, relative to that of men, may be influenced less by nicotine intake and more by nonpharmacological factors, such as smoking cues (Perkins, 2009c). Genetic influences on different phases of dependence have been examined, but to date few genes show reliable associations. However, one recent study found effects of both subject sex and a genetic factor on a measure of the reinforcing

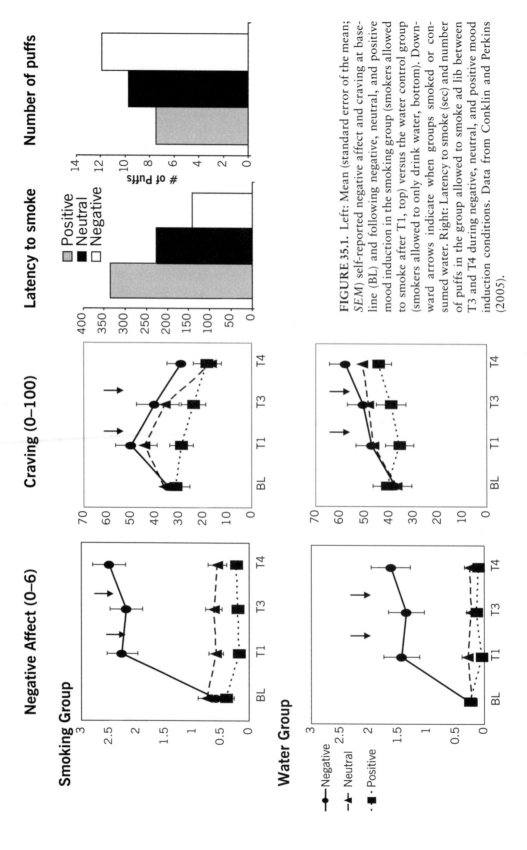

FIGURE 35.1. Left: Mean (standard error of the mean; *SEM*) self-reported negative affect and craving at baseline (BL) and following negative, neutral, and positive mood induction in the smoking group (smokers allowed to smoke after T1, top) versus the water control group (smokers allowed to only drink water, bottom). Downward arrows indicate when groups smoked or consumed water. Right: Latency to smoke (sec) and number of puffs in the group allowed to smoke ad lib between T3 and T4 during negative, neutral, and positive mood induction conditions. Data from Conklin and Perkins (2005).

value of nicotine via smoking, suggesting that failure to consider interactions among factors may obscure individual differences in smoking behavior.

Ray and colleagues (2006), who tested the degree to which nicotine itself is reinforcing, used a choice procedure in which smokers intermittently chose puffs between a regular nicotine cigarette and a cigarette that looked and tasted the same but had no nicotine (denicotinized). The number of times the nicotine cigarette was chosen over the denicotinized cigarette was a measure of preference for nicotine, or the relative reinforcing effects of nicotine. The gene of interest was OPRM1, which is associated with the function of the mu opioid receptor, important for determining responses to opiate drugs such as morphine or heroin and perhaps other drugs of abuse (e.g., nicotine and alcohol). Differences in this gene have been related to ability to quit smoking using the nicotine patch (Lerman et al., 2004). Male and female smokers of either OPRM1 genotype (absence vs. presence of the G allele, which is associated with weaker activity of the mu opioid receptor gene) participated in two study sessions, one following administration of naltrexone, a medication that blocks opiate receptors, and the other following placebo. One study hypothesis was that naltrexone would have a stronger effect in lowering nicotine choice depending on genotype. Results showed no effect of naltrexone on nicotine cigarette choice, contrary to hypotheses, as well as no overall difference in choice between men and women. However, choice was influenced marginally by OPRM1 genotype and significantly by the interaction of sex by OPRM1 genotype. Genotype had no influence on choice in men, as they chose the nicotine cigarette about 75% of the time regardless of OPRM1 genotype, but women with the G allele chose nicotine significantly less often than did women without the G allele (approximately 57 and 82%, respectively).

This finding suggests that at least one genetic influence on nicotine reinforcement may vary by sex, and other gene × sex interactions also likely exist (Perkins, 2009a). If replicated (i.e., repeated) by other researchers, these results could suggest that looking for simple relationships between dependence markers and one individual difference may overlook the complexity of the etiology of dependence, and interactions among individual differences may reveal stronger associations than each taken individually.

Expectancy to Smoke and Neural Responses to Smoking Cues

Craving for cigarettes can be viewed as the result of two broad influences: (1) abstinence from tobacco, which causes a longer-term rise in craving over hours and days, and (2) the presence of cues, which cause craving to fluctuate over minutes. Although both influences can occur simultaneously (i.e., when recently quit smokers encounter smoking cues), these types are probably due to different mechanisms and affected differently by cessation medications; for example, a nicotine patch can relieve abstinence-induced but not cue-induced craving (Waters et al., 2004).

Some of the strongest evidence that tobacco dependence involves nonpharmacological factors, and not just nicotine intake, is the observation that smokers routinely respond to smoking cues with robust increases in craving (Conklin, 2006). Smoking cues can include seeing and smelling a lit cigarette, seeing pictures of smoking paraphernalia, and being in situations previously associated with smoking, such as drinking alcohol in a bar. This craving usually decreases rapidly when the cues are removed. Because these quick changes in craving occur without any change in blood nicotine, they must be due to nonpharmacological factors. Moreover, because nonsmokers do not respond to such cues, the responses of smokers to these cues are likely the result of learned associations between the cues and smoking over the course of years of smoking in the presence of these cues (i.e., conditioning). These cues are believed to elicit responses, such as pleasure or distress, at least in part because they signal the availability of cigarettes. Consistent with this notion, craving responses to cues are larger when smokers believe they will be allowed to smoke soon (i.e., that smoking is available), compared to when they believe they will not be allowed to smoke (Wertz & Sayette, 2001).

"Cue reactivity" research is the name usually applied to studies examining the influence of cues on desire to use a drug, measured by not only self-reported craving measures but also behavior (i.e., actual drug use), psychophysiology (e.g., electrodermal or startle responses), cognition (e.g., information processing tasks), and, recently, changes in neural activity detected by neuroimaging. An excellent example of the latter is from McBride, Barrett, Kelly, Aw, and Dagher (2006), who examined neural changes in response to smoking cues as functions of brief smoking abstinence versus no abstinence, and of the presence versus absence of expectations of being able to smoke. Twenty smokers participated in two separate sessions, the first after abstaining from smoking for 12 hours and the second after smoking normally beforehand. At the start of both sessions, half the subjects were told they would be able to smoke right after the neuroimaging scan (functional magnetic resonance imaging, or fMRI), and half were told they would have to wait 4 hours before smoking, leading these subgroups to differ in whether they expected to smoke soon. During scanning on each session, subjects watched a series of 2-minute videos of either smoking cues (e.g., people lighting and smoking a cigarette) or control cues (e.g., people getting a haircut).

Results of the study showed that self-reported craving increased in response to smoking cues (vs. control cues) in all conditions, regardless of abstinence or expectancy to smoke. However, virtually all the neural changes in response to smoking cues—increases in activation of the anterior cingulate, parietal, prefrontal cortex, and so forth—were observed only in the subjects expecting to smoke after the scan, not in those not expecting to smoke. The authors interpreted the pattern of increases in neural activation as reflecting greater arousal and attention. These findings show that mere exposure to cues is not sufficient to elicit craving, that for cues to elicit the conditioned responses of interest, smokers must expect to be able to smoke. Moreover, this study demonstrates that cue effects are not uniform across all response domains of craving because results differed between self-report versus neural activation measures. Thus, reliance on only one type of measure may not provide a complete picture of the influence of

smoking cues on responses that could maintain tobacco dependence (Perkins, 2009b; see also Perkins et al., 2010).

Summary of Laboratory-Based Research on Tobacco Dependence

Although these three studies are far from an exhaustive demonstration of the kinds of laboratory-based research on smoking by health psychologists, they are exemplary of this research in many ways. What should be particularly notable is the multidisciplinary nature of this research, combining genetics, neuroscience, psychophysiology, and other disciplines with psychology to provide a comprehensive examination of a phenomenon relevant to understanding tobacco dependence. Yet these studies also are limited in a number of ways, such as providing only a snapshot of responses over a short interval and being conducted in an "artificial" setting away from the smoker's natural environment. Future studies need to find ways to improve the generalizability of findings from laboratory studies of influences on smoking to the natural environment, and to determine the reliability of those findings across time.

At the same time, laboratory-based studies offer much better control over sources of error in measurement, so that the effects of the manipulations of interest can be determined more clearly. (Imagine the complexity of measuring neural activation as smokers view smoking stimuli in their natural environments!) Because of this advantage, laboratory-based approaches need to be applied more commonly to the study of the other two phases of dependence, onset and abstinence, which are typically avoided in laboratory-based research for reasons noted earlier. For example, a study examining predictors of cessation in smokers before quitting (Perkins et al., 2002) assessed choice of nicotine versus placebo via nasal spray using the same choice procedure as that described earlier with cigarettes (Ray et al., 2006). Those choosing nicotine more often during laboratory testing later had more severe withdrawal during the first week of quitting and relapsed more quickly (i.e., failed to stay quit). Other laboratory-based research is also searching for behavioral markers of dependence that predict difficulty quitting, such as differences in attentional processes (e.g., Waters et al., 2003). Such markers could identify those smokers needing more intense treatment and could help us better understand the intractability of tobacco dependence (see Lerman, Perkins, & Gould, 2009).

Clinical Health Psychology Research on Tobacco Dependence

Because tobacco dependence involves both pharmacological and nonpharmacological factors, treatment to help smokers quit requires us to address both types of factors. Clinical health psychology is perhaps uniquely suited to conduct research on the intersection of these factors given its multidisciplinary nature. Until the 1980s, the only treatment demonstrated to be effective in aiding cessation was behavioral counseling, much of it by pioneers in health psychology. Such counseling, which has changed remarkably (and perhaps distressingly) little over the decades, generally involves teaching smokers how to cope with urges to smoke by avoiding or escaping situations that elicit craving, or by otherwise engaging in behaviors that aid coping (e.g., relaxation exercises) or are incompatible with smoking (e.g., keeping one's hands busy). Other common techniques are self-monitoring of smoking behavior to understand how often and in what situations one smokes and getting rid of as many smoking cues as possible prior to quitting, such as removing ashtrays from the home. Cognitive techniques have been added, such that most counseling of this type is referred to as cognitive-behavioral treatment (see Perkins, Conklin, & Levine, 2007). These techniques include steps in "relapse prevention" (Marlatt & Gordon, 1985), such as preparing smokers for the possibility of lapses (brief instances of smoking) by instilling the attitude that such lapses constitute danger signs and require greater coping efforts but should not be viewed as evidence of failure. Cognitive strategies are also used to increase motivation to quit and to cope with craving (e.g., redirecting thoughts toward nonsmoking concepts often cause craving to recede).

Since the 1980s, however, by far the main thrust of research into new cessation treatments has been in the area of medication development, led by large pharmaceutical companies. Although dozens of medications have been tested for efficacy in smoking cessation, only three have been sufficiently effective and safe to be approved by the U.S. Food and Drug Administration (FDA): the varieties of nicotine replacement therapy (NRT; gum, patch, lozenge, etc.), the antidepressant bupropion (Zyban), and the newer drug varenicline (Chantix). In general, cessation medications are believed to effectively relieve withdrawal symptoms during abstinence, blunt the pleasurable effects of smoking during a lapse, or both (see Perkins, Stitzer, & Lerman, 2006).

The development of cessation treatments over the past several decades has appeared to swing from reliance on one approach, counseling, to another, medications. Yet a more appropriate way to view this history is to see the advent of medications as offering new components of a comprehensive counseling intervention. It can be argued that professional counseling is a more important component of treatment than medication because medications are rather limited in how they aid cessation. Medications can reduce the severity of withdrawal and craving in the week or two after quitting, but relapse beyond that point typically has little to do with these symptoms that normally abate (i.e., return to prequit levels). Relapse later on is often triggered by failure to cope with smoking cues or expectations of feeling better by smoking, and medications cannot help much with these issues. They cannot reduce craving in response to cues or enhance motivation to quit, for example (Waters et al., 2004). Furthermore, smokers often do not know what reasonably to expect from medications and how to use them, and counseling can help to fill these gaps in knowledge (Perkins et al., 2007).

For health psychologists involved in smoking cessation research, the most important measure is biochemical validation of smoking status, such as expired air carbon monoxide or saliva cotinine (a metabolite of nicotine). Self-report of smoking status is not a sufficient measure in clinical trials because smokers are often reluctant to admit they have relapsed (i.e., "failed") and often misrepresent their current smoking status.

Validation of success or failure in quitting is critical to interpreting the results of a clinical trial.

For example, among smokers in the Multiple Risk Factor Intervention Trial (MRFIT), whose aim was to reduce several risk factors for cardiovascular disease, 42% of those given the special cessation intervention reported being abstinent from all tobacco at the final 6-year follow-up, compared to only 26% in the control group (Ockene, Hymowitz, Lagus, & Shaten, 1991). However, biochemical validation indicated that about 1 in 7 persons in the intervention group claiming to be quitters were still smoking, compared to few in the control group. Thus, the true difference in abstinence between the intervention and control groups was 36 versus 24%, a smaller, if still significant, difference. This observation is important to interpreting the medical outcomes in this study because the difference between groups in morbidity was far less than expected, based on the self-reported quit rates of 42 versus 26%. If biochemical validation had not been done, the investigators might have had to conclude that quitting smoking does little to prevent adverse health effects. Recognizing that the quit rates between groups were actually much narrower enabled them to determine not only that quitting does in fact reduce risk of health effects but also that getting at-risk smokers to quit is much more difficult than anticipated. This difference between self-reported and validated abstinence illustrates the point that smokers are reluctant to admit relapse to health care or research personnel, especially those who have worked with them to encourage abstinence, making biochemical validation essential. Yet even 20% or more of self-quitters, or those receiving no help from study personnel, claimed to be continuously abstinent at 6 months despite biochemical evidence of recent smoking (Hughes et al., 1992).

Because the vast majority of smokers fail to maintain abstinence after trying to quit, research continues to explore new or improved approaches to aid cessation. Health psychologists are well-qualified to examine virtually all facets of the quitting process and to develop methods to control smoking. This section presents a few examples of clinical health psychology research aimed at improving interventions to help smokers quit.

Scheduled Reduction in Cigarettes per Day Prior to Quitting

Part of what makes quitting difficult is inability to cope with the influence of cues, or environmental stimuli associated with smoking, on increasing smoking reinforcement. Before quitting, smokers have no need to cope with cues; they simply smoke when they want to, depending on indoor smoking restrictions. One way to try to reduce the influence of cues on smoking in the weeks prior to quitting is essentially to take control over the timing of smoking away from the smoker via "scheduled reduction" (Cinciripini et al., 1995). Procedurally, scheduled reduction involves systematically reducing the amount of smoking over time by gradually lengthening the time between each cigarette. However, the efficacy of this approach relies not on smokers getting used to smoking less—the "reduction" part of the approach—but rather on their being forced to cope with urges without smoking, as a result of "scheduling." Instead of smoking whenever they desire throughout the day, as cues occur and the urge arises, smoking is done only on a predetermined time schedule. Theoretically, this approach weakens the association between cues and smoking, which presumably enhances the ex-smoker's ability to cope with those cues after quitting.

In a test of this idea, Cinciripini and colleagues (1995) randomized smokers wanting to quit to one of four groups that varied in the pattern of smoking during the 3 weeks leading up to their quit day. The groups involved each combination of scheduling versus no scheduling of the timing of smoking, and reduction versus no reduction in the number of cigarettes per day (i.e., 2 × 2). Thus, subjects in the "scheduled reduction" group could smoke only according to a time schedule that gradually lengthened the time between each cigarette (one per hour for a few days, then one every 90 minutes for a few days, etc.), so that fewer and fewer cigarettes could be smoked in a day. Subjects in the "scheduled nonreduction" group also smoked only according to a time schedule, but the time interval between cigarettes remained the same across weeks (e.g., remained fixed at one per hour). Members of the "nonscheduled reduction" group were instructed to smoke fewer and fewer cigarettes per day but could do so as they wanted, in response to cues and urges, as long as they did not exceed their daily allotment. The "nonscheduled non-reduction" (control) group members essentially smoked as they normally did. Subjects in the reduction groups had their cigarettes prepackaged into daily allotments to increase compliance with the instructed amount of smoking per day.

At the end of the 3-week manipulation of smoking patterns, all subjects received the same cognitive-behavioral treatment to quit smoking (and no medication), and the outcome of primary interest was success in staying quit over the next year. The 1-year quit rates were 44 and 32% in scheduled reduction and scheduled nonreduction, respectively, versus 18 and 22% for nonscheduled reduction and nonscheduled nonreduction, respectively. Thus, reducing the number of cigarettes per day by itself had no effect; "scheduling" was the key component. Interestingly, both scheduled groups also experienced milder withdrawal and craving after quitting, suggesting improved ability to cope with cues. The scheduled reduction group also reported higher self-efficacy to stay quit throughout follow-up, while the nonscheduled reduction group (i.e., those simply told to smoke less, but however they wanted) reported lower self-efficacy.

This novel behavioral intervention serves to prepare smokers to deal effectively with cues and urges, and shows the power of a fairly simple behavioral procedure; the quit rates compare very favorably to quit rates commonly found in medication trials. Additional research is needed to understand precisely why this approach to smoking before quitting has such a robust effect in fostering sustained abstinence after quitting, and to explore how this approach could be applied in a widespread and efficient way.

Monetary Reinforcement of Abstinence in Smokers Not Interested in Quitting

Tobacco dependence has rightly been considered a highly intractable problem, a view supported by the observation that very few smokers succeed in staying quit for long after a given quit attempt. Consequently, researchers interested in the causes of dependence often focus on the chronic brain changes due to persistent exposure to nicotine and attribute smokers' inability to quit to these changes. However, many health psychologists recognize that smoking behavior is not really atypical compared to other persistent behaviors and can be influenced by the same contingencies that alter most other behaviors. A clear demonstration of this idea comes from studies showing that monetary contingencies for staying quit can result in very high rates of abstinence, at least while the contingencies are in effect.

An increasingly common component of behavioral treatment of drug dependence involves providing positive reinforcement, in the form of vouchers for goods and services, to those patients who are able to maintain abstinence from drugs. Vouchers, rather than actual money, are used to reinforce abstinence to guard against patients' use of the monetary reinforcement to buy drugs or alcohol. Biochemical measures are used to detect drugs in the body (e.g., urine drug screen) or to verify the patient's claim of abstinence, just as biochemical validation is done to confirm smoking cessation. This treatment approach, usually called "contingency management," was first developed by Maxine Stitzer at Johns Hopkins University, and refined and applied to the treatment of several drug-using populations, including cocaine and opiate abusers, by Stephen Higgins at the University of Vermont, among others. Contingency management, an approach derived directly from behavioral psychology, has proven to be one of the few effective drug abuse treatments of any kind, including treatment with medications (Higgins, Heil, & Lussier, 2004).

Contingency management has been applied to smoking cessation, primarily over relatively brief periods of days or weeks rather than months, as in drug abuse treatment. The purpose of most studies has been to demonstrate that smoking is a behavior that can be effectively controlled, even among those not trying to quit permanently, if the proper reinforcing contingencies can be identified. Studies have shown that over half of smokers not interested in quitting will nevertheless abstain continuously for 2 weeks if abstinence results in monetary payment. Typically, payments escalate with continuous abstinence and average about $30 per day (Alessi, Badger, & Higgins,

2004). This approach has also been used to initiate abstinence in those with strong reason to quit, such as pregnant women, in the hope that long-term maintenance of abstinence will be more likely in those induced to quit right away compared to those given standard counseling alone, with its variable degree of success. (Use of medications can be problematic with pregnant women, so that cognitive-behavioral approaches are the most desirable interventions [Perkins et al., 2007].)

One example of contingency management with pregnant women who smoke was published by Higgins, Heil, Solomon, and colleagues (2004). Women about 12–15 weeks pregnant were randomly assigned to a contingent voucher condition, in which continuous abstinence was reinforced by an escalating value of vouchers exchangeable for commercial products, or a noncontingent voucher condition, in which vouchers comparable in value to those earned by the contingent group were given to patients independent of whether they abstained from smoking. (This control condition ensures that sustained quitting in the contingent group is due explicitly to the reinforcement of abstinence, and not simply because patients are getting vouchers for participating in the study.) For those in the contingent group, the voucher value started at $6.25 and escalated by $1.25 for each consecutive visit at which the patient was verified to be abstinent, as determined by biochemical validation, up to a maximum of $45. If a patient was found to have smoked, the voucher value was reset to the initial level, a common procedure that strongly encourages maintaining abstinence as time goes on. All women were followed up over the end of the prepartum period and for 24 weeks postpartum. Abstinence rates for the contingent versus noncontingent voucher groups were 37 versus 9%, respectively, at the end of pregnancy, and 27 versus 0%, respectively, at 24 weeks postpartum. Although the absolute quit rates seem disappointing given that pregnant women smokers should have a natural incentive to quit, the effect of contingent vouchers, a purely behavioral intervention, rivaled that of medications or comprehensive counseling to quit smoking.

A variation on contingency management is to shape abstinence gradually by reinforcing successively lower levels of biochemical indices of smoking, such as expired air carbon monoxide, across time. This approach has been used to induce most smokers who are unable and unwilling to quit on their own to become completely abstinent within a few weeks and to sustain this abstinence for several more weeks (Lamb, Morral, Galbicka, Kirby, & Iguchi, 2005). Contingency management has also been used to increase compliance with the use of nicotine gum during quit attempts (Mooney, Babb, Jensen, & Hatsukami, 2005), demonstrating the versatility of this one approach to changing behaviors relevant to fostering smoking cessation.

Addressing Quitting Smokers' Concerns about Weight Gain

Many smokers, about 50% of women and 25% of men, are reluctant to quit out of concern about gaining weight after they quit. Smokers gain on average about 8–10 pounds in the year after quitting, although smokers with more concern about weight gain before quitting typically gain more than this amount of weight after quitting (Perkins, 1993). The typical approach in counseling to address this issue has been to recommend dieting and exercise concurrent with the quit attempt, in an effort to prevent the weight gain. The assumption here is that preventing any weight gain will reduce the concern, thereby increasing chances of staying quit. However, other evidence suggests this is not a prudent method to enhance abstinence in weight-concerned smokers. First, several studies show that this approach does not help ex-smokers to stay quit, and it may even be counterproductive and hasten relapse (see Perkins, Levine, Marcus, & Shiffman, 1997). Among possible explanations for the failure of a concurrent weight control and smoking cessation program are increased feelings of deprivation (i.e., being both food-deprived and giving up smoking), the behavioral complexity of following simultaneous programs to change two important health behaviors (smoking and eating), and loss of food as a coping strategy to deal with urges to smoke (Perkins et al., 1997). Second, it is the amount of *concern* about weight gain rather than the amount of the weight gain itself that seems to be related to difficulty staying quit. Thus, altering the amount of weight gain without affecting the concern may have little impact on quit success. Moreover, the amount of weight gain is fairly benign from the standpoint of worsening health, compared to the dramatically increased health risks of smoking. So to quit smoking despite gaining weight results is a substantial improvement in health, compared to continuing to smoke and not gaining weight.

For these reasons, we decided to try a different approach, that of developing a cognitive-behavioral treatment that focused directly on reducing weight gain concerns rather than trying to alter the weight gain (Perkins et al., 2001). Weight-concerned women smokers wanting to quit ($N = 219$) received a 10-session, group-based counseling intervention without medication. Only women were included because of their much higher prevalence of weight concern compared to men. The intervention involved standard cessation counseling supplemented by one of three additional counseling components: (1) cognitive-behavioral therapy for weight concerns (CBT); (2) behavioral weight control (DIET); or (3) non-weight-related informal discussion (i.e., STANDARD only).

Thus, all the groups received comprehensive counseling but differed in the additional component designed to address weight gain. In the CBT component, we addressed women's concerns about weight gain due to quitting by using cognitive-behavioral techniques that changed their attitudes and challenged their assumptions about the consequences of the weight gain. This approach was adapted from more intensive counseling used in treating women with eating disorders. Note that although dieting was discouraged, moderation in snacking was encouraged. In the DIET component, women were told that preventing weight gain by dieting was a way to manage their concerns. These women were given behavioral weight control information and instructed to decrease overall calorie intake. In the STANDARD component, women were advised to focus their efforts solely on the problem of quitting smoking and to set aside for much later the issue of weight gain. So that all three treatment conditions received equal amounts of attention from the counselors, women in the STANDARD component spent additional time

discussing the importance of social support in preparing to quit and staying quit. The rationales for these treatments are presented in more detail in Perkins and colleagues (1997). We followed up each group for 1 year after the quit date, assessing weight gain and verifying abstinence with expired air carbon monoxide.

As shown in Figure 35.2 (left), the CBT group had significantly better quit rates at most follow-up points relative to the STANDARD group, but the DIET group was no better than the STANDARD group (i.e., dieting did not improve quit rates). Although quit rates dropped over the year, as is always found with any drug abuse treatment, these quit rates due to counseling alone were similar to quit rates with medication alone and were several times the quit rates of those who try to quit on their own, without formal assistance (under 5%). Results for weight gain were also interesting, as also shown in Figure 35.2 (right). Women in the DIET condition did not gain any weight during the first month after quitting, while counseling was still going on, as intended by the dieting intervention. However, this effort to prevent weight gain was very short-lived because abstinent women in the DIET (and STANDARD) condition subsequently gained more weight than those in the CBT condition.

In summary, a CBT approach to reducing weight concerns was more effective than standard counseling alone, while behavioral weight control to prevent weight gain (DIET) was not, and CBT, unexpectedly, was superior to the other two conditions in attenuating long-term weight gain. This latter effect may have been due to the emphasis on moderation of between-meal snacking, typically the main source of weight gain after quitting (Perkins, 1993). However, the attenuation in weight gain is not likely the reason the CBT group was more likely to stay quit; they were already more likely than the DIET group to quit in the first month, even though they had gained more weight than the DIET group at that point (see Figure 35.2). This study illustrates how the simple approach to addressing a concern about quitting smoking, such as dieting to prevent weight gain after quitting in, weight-concerned smokers, may not be the best approach. It also shows how varied and rich are the treatments enlisted in health psychology to help smokers quit;

Continuous abstinence rates (%) by group   **Weight gain (kg) in abstinent subjects by group**

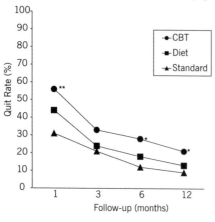 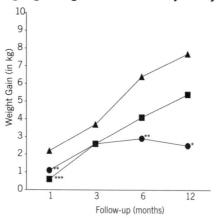

FIGURE 35.2. Left: Continuous smoking abstinence across the 1-year follow-up period in weight-concerned women smokers given cessation counseling plus one of three adjunct components—cognitive-behavioral therapy to reduce weight concerns (CBT), behavioral weight control (DIET), or nonspecific discussion unrelated to weight concerns (STANDARD). Right: Weight gain across the 1-year follow-up period in abstinent smokers of each treatment group. *$p < .05$; **$p < .01$; ***$p < .001$ for the difference from the STANDARD (reference) group. Data from Perkins et al. (2001).

there are many different ways to help smokers quit, and if one way does not work, then others are available that might work. Health psychology research needs to continue refining and testing these methods to determine for whom they work best.

Summary of Clinical Health Psychology Research on Tobacco Dependence

These studies represent just a few of the directions taken in clinical health psychology research to improve interventions for smoking cessation. Although absolute quit rates remain stubbornly low, cessation counseling—with or without medications—represents one of the most cost-effective treatments in medicine, on the order of a few thousand dollars per year of life saved compared to $10,000 to $50,000 per year of life saved for commonly accepted procedures such as giving aspirin after a heart attack and implanting defibrillators in those with arrhythmias (Parrott & Godfrey, 2004). Other relevant research is aimed at maximizing the efficacy of existing medications for cessation. One example here is improving compliance with cessation medications, so that patients obtain the full benefit of their actions. Another

is pharmacogenetics, or examining whether certain medications may be more effective in smokers with a particular genetic makeup compared to those with a different genetic makeup (Munafo, Shields, Berrettini, Patterson, & Lerman, 2005).

Conclusions

Although cigarette smoking is a deceptively simple and discrete behavior, its persistence in the face of life-threatening risks (i.e., dependence) results from a complex multitude of factors. Influences on tobacco-dependence onset, maintenance, and cessation include genetic, early environmental, personality, and other long-term "trait-like" factors, as well as acute and chronic effects of pharmacological and nonpharmacological components of cigarette smoke inhalation. No single discipline can provide a comprehensive explanation of dependence, but health psychologists are well-positioned to oversee and integrate research on dependence, if they understand the importance of the multifactorial nature of tobacco dependence. Psychology as the science of human behavior recognizes the diverse biological and environmental influences on behavior, and health psychology applies this focus to understanding and controlling important health behaviors such as smoking. Increased emphasis is on understanding how findings from this varied field of research fit together to explain basic phenomenon in dependence, somewhat contrary to the long-term trend of greater specialization in science (Turkkan et al., 2000).

Standout contributions from health psychology to date include (1) characterization of the onset and persistence of smoking and consequences of abstinence (i.e., withdrawal and craving), and (2) virtually all elements of standard counseling used widely to help smokers quit, as well as evaluation of the mechanisms of action of new medications for cessation. Despite this progress, the vast majority of smokers make many unsuccessful quit attempts before finally succeeding, and the death toll from smoking is still rising worldwide. Thus, considerably more research effort is needed from health psychologists and others before tobacco dependence can be sufficiently understood and controlled.

Acknowledgments

Preparation of this chapter was supported by National Institute on Drug Abuse Grant Nos. DA019478, DA027449, and P50 CA143187.

Further Reading

Baker, T. B., Piper, M. E., McCarthy, D. E., Majeskie, M. R., & Fiore, M. C. (2004). Addiction motivation reformulated: An affective processing model of negative reinforcement. *Psychological Review, 111*(1), 33–51.

Everitt, B. J., & Robbins, T. W. (2005). Neural systems of reinforcement for drug addiction: From actions to habits to compulsion. *Nature Neuroscience, 8*(11), 1481–1489.

Higgins, S. T., Heil, S. H., & Lussier, J. P. (2004). Clinical implications of reinforcement as a determinant of substance use disorders. *Annual Review of Psychology, 55*, 431–461.

Kassel, J. D., Stroud, L. R., & Paronis, C. A. (2003). Smoking, stress, and negative affect: Correlation, causation, and context across stages of smoking. *Psychological Bulletin, 129*(2), 270–304.

Lerman, C., Perkins, K. A., & Gould, T. (2009) Nicotine dependence endophenotypes in chronic smokers. *National Cancer Institute Tobacco Control Monographs, 20*, 403–484.

McBride, D., Barrett, S. P., Kelly, J. T., Aw, A., & Dagher, A. (2006). Effects of expectancy and abstinence on the neural response to smoking cues in cigarette smokers: An fMRI study. *Neuropsychopharmacology, 31*(12), 2728–2738.

Munafo, M. R., Shields, A. E., Berrettini, W. H., Patterson, F., & Lerman, C. (2005). Pharmacogenetics and nicotine addiction treatment. *Pharmacogenomics, 6*(3), 211–223.

Perkins, K. A. (2009) Does smoking cue-induced craving tell us anything important about nicotine dependence? *Addiction, 104*, 1610–1616.

References

Alessi, S. M., Badger, G. J., & Higgins, S. T. (2004). An experimental examination of the initial weeks of abstinence in cigarette smokers. *Experimental and Clinical Psychopharmacology, 12*, 276–287.

American Psychiatric Association. (1994). *Diagnostic and statistical manual of mental disorders* (4th ed.). Washington, DC: Author.

Anthony, J. C., Warner, L. A., & Kessler, R. C. (1994). Comparative epidemiology of dependence on tobacco, alcohol, controlled substances, and inhalants: Basic findings from the National Comorbidity Survey. *Experimental and Clinical Psychopharmacology, 2*, 244–268.

Caggiula, A. R., Donny, E. C., Chaudhri, N., Perkins, K. A., Evans-Martin, F. F., & Sved, A. F. (2002). Importance of nonpharmacological factors in nicotine self-administration. *Physiology and Behavior, 77*, 683–687.

Cinciripini, P. M., Lapitsky, L., Seay, S., Wallfisch, A., Kitchens, K., & Van Vunakis, H. (1995). The effects of smoking schedules on cessation outcome: Can we improve on common methods of gradual and abrupt nicotine withdrawal? *Journal of Consulting and Clinical Psychology, 63*, 388–399.

Colby, S. M., Tiffany, S. T., Shiffman, S., & Niaura, R. S. (2000). Are adolescent smokers dependent on nicotine?: A review of the evidence. *Drug and Alcohol Dependence, 59*(Suppl. 1), S83–S95.

Conklin, C. A. (2006). Environments as cues to smoke: Implication for human extinction-based research and treatment. *Experimental and Clinical Psychopharmacology, 14*, 12–19.

Conklin, C. A., & Perkins, K. A. (2005). Subjective and reinforcing effects of smoking during negative mood induction. *Journal of Abnormal Psychology, 114*, 153–164.

Ezzati, M., & Lopez, A. D. (2003). Estimates of global mortality attributable to smoking in 2000. *Lancet, 362*, 847–852.

Harvey, D. M., Yasar, S., Heishman, S. J., Panlilio, L. V., Henningfield, J. E., & Goldberg, S. R. (2004). Nicotine serves as an effective reinforcer of intravenous drug-taking behavior in human cigarette smokers. *Psychopharmacology, 175*(2), 134–142.

Higgins, S. T., Heil, S. H., & Lussier, J. P. (2004). Clinical implications of reinforcement as a determinant of substance use disorders. *Annual Review of Psychology, 55*, 431–461.

Higgins, S. T., Heil, S. H., Solomon, S. J., Bernstein, I. M., Lussier, J. P., Abel, R. L., et al. (2004). A pilot study on voucher-based incentives to promote abstinence from cigarette smoking during pregnancy and postpartum. *Nicotine and Tobacco Research, 6*, 1015–1020.

Hughes, J. R., Gulliver, S. B., Fenwick, J. W., Valliere, W. A., Cruser, K., Pepper, S., et al. (1992). Smoking cessation among self-quitters. *Health Psychology, 11*, 331–334.

Kassel, J. D., Greenstein, J. E., Evatt, D. P., Wardle, M. C., Yates, M. C., Veilleux, J. C., et al. (2007). Smoking topography in response to denicotinized and high-yield nicotine cigarettes in adolescent smokers. *Journal of Adolescent Health, 40*, 54–60.

Lamb, R. J., Morral, A. R., Galbicka, G., Kirby, K. C., & Iguchi, M. Y. (2005). Shaping reduced smoking in smokers without cessation plans. *Experimental and Clinical Psychopharmacology, 13*, 83–92.

Lerman, C., Perkins, K. A., & Gould, T. (2009). Nicotine dependence endophenotypes in chronic smokers. *National Cancer Institute Tobacco Control Monographs, 20*, 403–484.

Lerman, C., Wileyto, E. P., Patterson, F., Rukstalis, M., Audrain-McGovern, J., Restine, S., et al. (2004). The functional mu opioid receptor (OPRM1) Asn40Asp variant predicts short-term response to nicotine replacement therapy in a clinical trial. *Pharmacogenomics Journal, 4*(3), 184–192.

Marlatt, G. A., & Gordon, J. R. (Eds.). (1985). *Relapse prevention: Maintenance strategies in the treatment of addictive behaviors.* New York: Guilford Press

McBride, D., Barrett, S. P., Kelly, J. T., Aw, A., & Dagher, A. (2006). Effects of expectancy and abstinence on the neural response to smoking cues in cigarette smokers: An fMRI study. *Neuropsychopharmacology, 31*(12), 2728–2738.

Mokdad, A. H., Marks, J. S., Stroup, D. F., & Gerberding, J. L. (2004). Actual causes of death in the United States, 2000. *Journal of the American Medical Association, 291*, 1238–1245.

Mooney, M., Babb, D., Jensen, J., & Hatsukami, D. (2005). Interventions to increase use of nicotine gum: A randomized, controlled, single-blind trial. *Nicotine and Tobacco Research, 7*, 565–579.

Munafo, M. R., Shields, A. E., Berrettini, W., Patterson, F., & Lerman, C. (2005). Pharmacogenetics and nicotine addiction treatment. *Pharmacogenomics, 6*, 211–223.

National Cancer Institute. (2007). *Tobacco Control Monograph 18: Greater than the sum: Systems thinking in tobacco control.* Washington, DC: U.S. Public Health Service.

Ockene, J. K., Hymowitz, N., Lagus, J., & Shaten, B. J. (1991). Comparison of smoking behavior change for SI and UC study groups. *Preventive Medicine, 20*, 564–573.

Parrott, S., & Godfrey, C. (2004). ABC of smoking cessation: Economics of smoking cessation. *British Medical Journal, 328*, 947–949.

Perkins, K. A. (1993). Weight gain following smoking cessation. *Journal of Consulting and Clinical Psychology, 61*, 768–777.

Perkins, K. A. (2009a). Acute responses to nicotine and smoking: Implications for prevention and treatment of smoking in lower SES women. *Drug and Alcohol Dependence, 104S*, S79–S86.

Perkins, K. A. (2009b). Does smoking cue-induced craving tell us anything important about nicotine dependence? *Addiction, 104*, 1610–1616.

Perkins, K. A. (2009c). Sex differences in nicotine reinforcement and reward: Influences on the persistence of tobacco smoking. In R. Bevins & A. R. Caggiula (Eds.), *The motivational impact of nicotine and its role in tobacco use* (pp. 143–169). New York: Springer-Verlag.

Perkins, K. A., Broge, M., Gerlach, D., Sanders, M., Grobe, J. E., Cherry, C., et al. (2002). Acute nicotine reinforcement, but not chronic tolerance, predicts withdrawal and relapse after quitting smoking. *Health Psychology, 21*(4), 332–339.

Perkins, K. A., Conklin, C. A., & Levine, M. D. (2007). *Cognitive-behavioral treatment of smoking cessation.* New York: Routledge.

Perkins, K. A., Epstein, L. H., Grobe, J., & Fonte, C. (1994). Tobacco abstinence, smoking cues, and the reinforcing value of smoking. *Pharmacology Biochemistry and Behavior, 47*(1), 107–112.

Perkins, K. A., Karelitz, J. L., Conklin, C. A., Sayette, M. A., & Giedgowd, G. E. (2010). Acute negative affect relief from smoking depends on the affect measure and situation, but not on nicotine. *Biological Psychiatry, 67*, 707–714.

Perkins, K. A., Levine, M. D., Marcus, M. D., & Shiffman, S. (1997). Addressing women's concerns about weight gain due to smoking cessation. *Journal of Substance Abuse Treatment, 14*, 173–182.

Perkins, K. A., Marcus, M. D., Levine, M. D., D'Amico, D., Miller, A., Broge, M., et al. (2001). Cognitive-behavioral therapy to reduce weight concerns improves smoking cessation outcome in weight concerned women. *Journal of Consulting and Clinical Psychology, 69*, 604–613.

Perkins, K. A., Stitzer, M., & Lerman, C. (2006). Medication screening for smoking cessation: A proposal for new methodologies. *Psychopharmacology, 184*, 628–636.

Ray, R., Jepson, C., Patterson, F., Strasser, A. A., Rukstalis, M., Perkins, K., et al. (2006). Association of OPRM1 Asn40Asp variant with the relative reinforcing value of nicotine in female smokers. *Psychopharmacology, 188*, 355–363.

Reynolds, B., Patak, M., Shroff, P., Penfold, R. B., Melanko, S., & Duhig, A. M. (2007). Laboratory and self-report assessments of impulsive behavior in adolescent daily smokers and nonsmokers. *Experimental and Clinical Psychopharmacology, 15*, 264–271.

Turkkan, J. S., Kaufman, N. J., & Rimer, B. K. (2000). Transdisciplinary tobacco use research centers: A model collaboration between public and private sectors. *Nicotine and Tobacco Research, 2*, 9–14.

Waters, A. J., Shiffman, S., Sayette, M. A., Paty, J. A., Gwaltney, C. J., & Balabanis, M. H. (2003). Attentional bias predicts outcome in smoking cessation. *Health Psychology, 22*(4), 378–387.

Waters, A. J., Shiffman, S., Sayette, M. A., Paty, J. A., Gwaltney, C. J., & Balabanis, M. H. (2004). Cue-provoked craving and nicotine replacement therapy in smoking cessation. *Journal of Consulting and Clinical Psychology, 72*(6), 1136–1143.

Wertz, J. M., & Sayette, M. A. (2001). A review of the effects of perceived drug use opportunity of self-reported urge. *Experimental and Clinical Psychopharmacology, 9*(1), 3–13.

CHAPTER 36

Theory-Based Behavioral Interventions for Smoking Cessation
Efficacy, Processes, and Future Directions

Jonathan B. Bricker

Despite great progress in the reduction of U.S. smoking prevalence (American Cancer Society, 2000), this decline has recently stalled (Centers for Disease Control and Prevention, 2006). Currently, 21% of American adults smoke, far above the Healthy People 2010 national goal of 12% (Centers for Disease Control and Prevention, 2006). Cigarette smoking remains the leading cause of preventable death in the United States, accounting for over 400,000 deaths annually (Centers for Disease Control and Prevention, 2006). Worldwide, there are now about 1.2 billion smokers (Mackay, Ericksen, & Shafey, 2006). Smoking causes 5 million deaths per year, and if the present trends continue, 10 million smokers per year are projected to die by 2025. The prevalence of smoking tends to be highest in Eastern Europe and in Asia, with men smoking more than women (Hatsukami, Stead, & Gupta, 2008).

Smoking causes a large number of cancers. The first cancer known to be caused by smoking was lung cancer. Since then, the types of cancers found to be caused by smoking have increased dramatically and now include cancer of the oral cavity, oropharynx and hypopharynx; esophagus, stomach, liver, pancreas, larynx, and nasopharynx; nasal cavity and nasal sinuses; urinary bladder, kidney, and uterine cervix; and myeloid leukemia. More than 1.3 million new lung cancer cases and 644,000 cancers of the oral cavity, nasopharynx, other pharynx, or larynx are diagnosed annually (Parkin, Bray, Ferlay, & Pisani, 2005). Most of these cancers are attributable to smoking. Nearly 1.2 million lung cancer patients and 352,000 patients with cancer of the oral cavity, nasopharynx, other pharynx, or larynx die each year. Most of these deaths are caused by cancer (Parkin et al., 2005). The International Agency for Research on Cancer (2004), the U.S. Surgeon General, the National Academy of Sciences, the U.S. Environmental Protection Agency, and many other authorities have determined that exposure to secondhand smoke (SHS) causes lung cancer in humans (National Research Council, 1986; U.S. Department of Health and Human Services, 2006).

Current Smoking Cessation Intervention Approaches

A key ingredient in reducing U.S. and worldwide morbidity and mortality attributed to smoking is directly helping individuals to quit (Fiore et al., 2008; Hatsukami et al., 2008), in addition to effective government policy and media interventions to control tobacco use and exposure (Bala, Strzeszynski, & Cahill, 2008; National Cancer Institute, 2008; World Health Organization, 2005). The current standard in smoking cessation interventions is the combination of some form of behavioral intervention and pharmacotherapy, reviews of which are covered in detail in recent publications (see, e.g., Fiore et al., 2008; Ranney, Melvin, Lux, McClain, & Lohr, 2006). Regarding pharmacotherapies, there are a number of effective drugs for smoking cessation (Fiore et al., 2008), including the innovative nicotine partial agonists (e.g., varenicline), which partially block the binding of nicotine to neurotransmitter receptors in the brain that stimulate smoking-induced feelings of pleasure (for a recent review, see Cahill, Stead, & Lancaster, 2008). Through this mechanism, these innovative pharmacotherapies are designed to undermine the positively reinforcing (i.e., rewarding) functions of smoking. Of the various types of behavioral intervention available, most focus on a variety of topics: (1) enhancing motivation and social support for quitting; (2) providing basic information about the health risks of smoking and health benefits of quitting; (3) helping smokers set a quit date; and (4) teaching basic skills on how to cope with situations, cravings, and emotions that trigger smoking and withdrawal symptoms (Fiore et al., 2008).

What is the efficacy of the standard behavioral interventions? Based on calculations derived from four recent Cochrane Library Reviews of behavioral interventions for smoking cessation, the weighted average of the 30-day point prevalence (i.e., not smoking at all in the past 30 days) quit rates at the 1-year postintervention follow-up are 14 and 20% for counseling and counseling combined with pharmacotherapy, respectively, *across all modes of intervention delivery* (Lancaster & Stead, 2005; Silagy, Lancaster, Stead, Mant, & Fowler, 2004; Stead & Lancaster, 2005; Stead, Perera, & Lancast-

er, 2006). While it is clear that the standard behavioral interventions do help smokers to quit, the fact that these interventions were not able to help 80–86% of smokers to quit permanently means that there is a lot room for improvement. These low cessation rates partly reflect the serious lack of progress made in behavioral interventions for smoking cessation (Brandon, 2001; Hajek, 1996; Niaura & Abrams, 2002; Shiffman, 1993). These efficacy rates raise the question: What role can health psychology researchers have in *improving* these quit rates, thereby helping to reduce the U.S. and worldwide burden of tobacco-attributed morbidity and mortality?

The Value of Psychological Theory in Smoking Cessation Interventions

A core mission of health psychology is the testing and refinement of mainstream and emerging psychological theories applied to clinical/public health interventions for health behavior change (Leventhal, Musumeci, & Contrada, 2007). Psychological theories are critical for planning and evaluating behavioral interventions (Bartholomew, Parcel, Kok, & Gottlieb, 2006). Theories state which mediating variables require intervention to effect a behavior change (e.g., smoking cessation intervention) (Lippke, Ziegelmann, & Schwarzer, 2005). Theory development and refinement provide valuable guides to the development of smoking cessation interventions (Rothman, 2004). Overall, theories applied to smoking cessation interventions help to (1) determine why an intervention works, (2) why an intervention does not work, and (3) by revealing what processes need to be targeted more effectively, provide guidance on specifically how to improve future smoking cessation interventions. In the words of Kurt Lewin (1951, p. 169), one of the founders of social psychology, "There is nothing so practical as a good theory."

Health psychology researchers can address the great U.S. and worldwide need for improving the quit rates of behavioral interventions for smoking cessation (delivered alone or in combination with pharmacotherapy) by conducting programmatic research that tests and refines mainstream and emerging psychological theories applied to smoking cessation. The purpose of this chapter is to (1) briefly review major and newly emerging psychological theories that have been applied to smoking cessation interventions, (2) report on the overall efficacy of behavioral interventions that have applied each of these theories to smoking cessation, (3) report evidence that these interventions influence their underlying theory-based processes, and (4) offer directions for how to use theory-based interventions to advance the science of behavioral interventions for smoking cessation. The approaches reviewed here (1) provide common examples of major and emerging theory-based approaches that have been applied to smoking cessation, and (2) highlight critical issues in the field that are common to all intervention research on behavioral approaches (e.g., methodological quality and testing of underlying processes).

Social Cognitive Approaches

One of the most influential health behavior change theories is Albert Bandura's social cognitive theory (SCT; Bandura, 1986). At the broadest level, SCT posits that human behavior reciprocally interacts with personal factors (e.g., cognitions) and the environment. When applied to the individual attempting to quit smoking, SCT suggests that the critical psychological processes to change are (1) outcome expectancies of quitting (i.e., the value, or *importance*, that a person places on quitting smoking); (2) quitting self-efficacy (i.e., belief in one's ability to quit smoking); (3) smoking outcome *expectations* (i.e., beliefs about the most likely positive and negative consequences of smoking and quitting smoking); (4) behavioral capability (i.e., knowledge and skills to quit and prevent relapse); and (5) perceptions of social norms for smoking (i.e., beliefs about the prevalence of smoking in a given social environment, such as a same-age peer group) (Bandura, 1997; Glanz, Rimer, & Lewis, 2002; Mackay, Donovan, & Marlatt, 1991).

Cognitive-Behavioral Therapy

Within the context of smoking cessation, SCT has historically been the main theoretical model linked to cognitive-behavioral

therapy (CBT). CBT is a generic term for a variety of behavior change techniques that share in common a focus on teaching specific skills for (1) modifying the thoughts that trigger a dysfunctional behavior and (2) using classical and operant conditioning principles to reduce dysfunctional behaviors (e.g., smoking). Techniques for modifying thoughts that trigger smoking come from a variety of sources, including basic strategies from Beck's cognitive therapy (Beck, 1993) and Ellis's rational emotive behavior therapy (Ellis & Dryden, 2007). For example, if one has the thought, "I will fail at quitting smoking," ways to dispute this thought would be to ask one's self the following questions: (1) What is the evidence for this thought?; (2) What is the evidence against this thought?; (3) If this thought were true, what would I then do about it?; (4) What would I tell a friend who is having this thought? (Abrams et al., 2003). Other cognitive techniques include examining the downsides of continuing to smoke and the benefits of quitting (i.e., decisional balance) (Janis & Mann, 1977). Major behavioral techniques for smoking cessation include (1) self-monitoring the situational, physical, emotional, and cognitive triggers for smoking behavior; (2) gradual exposure to nicotine withdrawal symptoms (e.g., nicotine fading); (3) setting a definite quit date; (4) signing a behavioral contract to quit smoking; and (5) avoiding situations that commonly trigger smoking behavior (Perkins, Conklin, & Levine, 2008). Both cognitive and behavioral techniques are believed to target five core SCT theoretical processes: (1) outcome expectancies, (2) quitting self-efficacy, (3) smoking outcome expectations, (4) behavioral capability, and (5) perceptions of social norms for smoking. However, in practice, CBT interventions for smoking cessation usually encompass a very broad array of theoretical constructs, with only vague links to a wide number of specific intervention techniques.

Efficacy of CBT for Smoking Cessation

A number of meta-analyses have examined the efficacy of CBT for smoking cessation. Four major meta-analyses are reviewed here. First, in the 2008 Clinical Practice Guideline, Fiore and colleagues (2008) rereported their meta-analysis, originally published in the 2000 Guideline (Fiore et al., 2000), of 64 controlled trials of CBT-type interventions for smoking cessation. The results of the meta-analysis showed that compared to no behavioral intervention, problem solving, skills training, and stress management were modestly effective for smoking cessation (104 study arms: estimated odds ratio [OR] = 1.5, 95% confidence interval [CI] = 1.3, 1.8; estimated abstinence rate = 16.2%, 95% CI = 14.0, 18.5). Nicotine fading, compared to no behavioral intervention, was not shown to be beneficial for smoking cessation (25 study arms: estimated OR = 1.1, 95% CI = 0.8–1.5; estimated abstinence rate = 11.8% [8.4, 15.8]). Second, in a meta-analysis of randomized trials published up to December 2004 (the majority of which were CBT interventions with at least 6-month follow-up since the start of therapy), Lancaster and Stead (2005) reported a similar pattern of results for *individually* delivered behavioral interventions. The 15 randomized trials they reviewed that compared behavioral intervention with minimal contact controls showed a mildly beneficial effect of the behavioral intervention on long-term abstinence (OR = 1.56; 95% CI = 1.30, 1.88). Third, a meta-analysis of randomized trials published up to January 2005 also reported a similar pattern of results for *group*-delivered CBT interventions with at least 6 months of follow-up since the start of therapy (Stead & Lancaster, 2005). Specifically, they reviewed eight studies that compared programs with added CBT components to control programs of the same duration. These comparisons overall show a moderate benefit of adding the CBT components (OR = 1.36; 95% CI = 1.03, 1.79). However, when they deleted the Stevens and Hollis (1989) study, which, with almost 400 participants added most of the weight to the analysis, the effect of adding CBT components became nonsignificant (OR = 1.36; 95% CI = 0.94, 1.98). Only one trial (Goldstein, Niaura, Follick, & Abrams, 1989) showed a statistically significant benefit at long-term follow-up. Fourth, in an update on an earlier meta-analysis (Sussman, Sun, & Dent, 2006), Sussman and Sun (2009) conducted a meta-analysis of 23 controlled smoking cessation trials of CBT for adolescents (i.e., ages 12–19) published up to December 2007. The results showed that CBT interventions for adolescents had

overall a statistically significant and modest 4.51% absolute risk reduction effect, pooled across a broad range of postintervention follow-up lengths (ranging from 0 to over 12 months).

Fiore and colleagues (2008) observed and other meta-analyses concurred (e.g., (Stead & Lancaster, 2005) that interpreting the results of meta-analyses of CBT for smoking cessation presents a number of challenges. First, rarely did the reviewed studies examine the effect of one type of CBT technique in isolation because nearly all of the CBT intervention studies tested a whole multicomponent treatment package. Second, these CBT interventions were heterogeneous, making it difficult to compare results across studies that used different numbers and types of CBT intervention components. Third, all of these types of counseling and behavioral therapies were compared with no-contact/control conditions. Therefore, the control conditions in these meta-analyses did not account for nonspecific or placebo effects of treatment. This feature of the studies made it difficult to attribute effectiveness to particular types of CBT interventions. Finally, nearly all of the reviewed interventions, as well as nearly all those published since then, had a longer total intervention contact time compared to the control groups, making it difficult to determine whether the higher abstinence rates were due to the interventions themselves or to the nonspecific factor of having more treatment contact.

Summary and Recommendations for Future Directions

Overall, the meta-analyses of controlled trials of CBT for smoking cessation have modest effects when examined across multiple modes of delivery and multiple study populations. One key way these analyses could have shown the effect of CBT interventions more definitely is if they had included a separate analysis of only randomized controlled trials. Moreover, Fiore and colleagues (2008) observed serious design limitations that made it very difficult to isolate the effects of CBT treatments and their specific components from nonspecific factors, such as longer treatment contact time. Also lacking in this research literature is a full reporting of intervention fidelity, that is, the degree to which the counselors delivered the intervention as intended. Finally, a paucity of research reports on the extent to which the effects of these CBT intervention trials on smoking cessation are mediated by core processes of SCT (e.g., self-efficacy). Future research is therefore needed that focuses on the following areas: (1) using randomized controlled trial designs, (2) demonstrating that the intervention was delivered with fidelity, (3) testing specific CBT intervention components, (4) controlling for nonspecific factors, and (5) testing the degree to which the intervention effects were mediated by theory-based processes, and (6) and specifying the type of CBT being tested, since CBT is only a generic term for a variety of broadly related intervention techniques.

Relapse Prevention

CBT for smoking cessation often includes a component that focuses on the prevention of relapse. It is common for individuals trying to quit smoking to slip up by having a cigarette (i.e., a lapse); therefore, it is important to keep a slip from leading to a complete return to regular smoking (i.e., a relapse). CBT for relapse prevention (RP) was designed specifically to address this issue through the use of cognitive and behavioral strategies to help individuals avoid returning to regular smoking (or any other addictive behavior) following successful treatment (Marlatt & Gordon, 1985). The basic premise of RP is that smoking (or any other addictive behavior) is a learned behavior driven by dysfunctional ways of thinking, feeling, and behaving. To change this learned behavior, RP teaches an individual skills in anticipating, coping, and cognitive restructuring. Specifically, RP adopts a reattributional approach to help individuals see that a slip does not necessarily lead to relapse. For example, if an individual attributes a slip to internal, stable, and global factors within him- or herself ("I am always weak"), the chances of preventing relapse will be lower. This concept is described as the "abstinence violation effect" (AVE; Marlatt & George, 1984). While the empirical evidence for the existence of the AVE for smoking relapse is both supportive (e.g., Curry, Marlatt, & Gordon, 1987) and nonsupportive (Shiffman et al., 1996), RP nonetheless uses techniques to help smokers cope with the AVE. Specifically, RP helps individuals reattribute a slip to

external, unstable, and specific factors (i.e., "I smoked today because I was drinking at a bar"), thereby raising the chances of preventing relapse.

The most common type of RP program, which was developed by Alan Marlatt and Judith Gordon, has been conceptualized within the theoretical framework of SCT (Marlatt & Gordon, 1985). RP posits that high-risk situations (e.g., being with a friend who is smoking) can lead to either effective or ineffective coping responses. An ineffective coping response can lead to decreased self-efficacy to quit smoking and increased positive outcome expectancies for smoking, which in turn can lead to a slip, the AVE, then an increased probability of relapsing. In contrast, an effective coping response can lead to increased self-efficacy to quit smoking and decreased positive outcome expectancies to smoke, which can in turn prevent (1) a slip, (2) a subsequent AVE, and (3) a relapse. More recently, RP has been conceptualized within the framework of a systems theory focusing on reciprocal relationships between relapse risk factors and smoking (Witkiewitz & Marlatt, 2004). This new theory includes both distal and proximal relapse risks. In this theory, "distal risks" are defined as stable predispositions that increase an individual's vulnerability to relapse (e.g., family history of smoking), whereas "proximal risks" are defined as immediate precipitants that increase the statistical probability of relapse. The reciprocal relationships between these risk factors and smoking (e.g., coping skills influence smoking, and smoking in turn influences coping) create continuous feedback loops that either increase or decrease the probability of a lapse. These feedback loops highlight the interaction among coping skills, cognitions, craving, affect, and smoking behavior. In the theory, contextual factors (e.g., drinking coffee) moderate the relationship between the risk factors and smoking behavior. To date, no published studies have applied this recent systems theory conceptualization of RP (Witkiewitz & Marlatt, 2004) to a smoking cessation intervention.

Efficacy of RP for Smoking Cessation

A 2005 Cochrane Review conducted a meta-analysis of 40 controlled trials of RP interventions published up to September 2004, with a minimum follow-up of 6 months (Hajek, Stead, West, Jarvis, & Lancaster, 2005). Among trials that included individuals who had already stopped smoking, the review reported that the six trials of postpartum relapse prevention showed no evidence for the benefit of RP ($N = 1,183$, OR = 1.17, 95% CI = 0.90, 1.53), the two trials of hospitalized inpatient showed no RP intervention benefit ($N = 558$, OR = 0.86, 95% CI = 0.60, 1.22), and the two trials of military personnel showed no RP intervention benefit. There was also no benefit of RP for interventions of (1) unaided abstainers, (2) aided abstainers, and (3) smokers randomized prior to their quit date. In a subsequent meta-analysis by the same research team, Lancaster, Hajek, Stead, West, and Jarvis (2006), reviewing studies published up to August 2005, showed the same pattern of results. They commented that the challenge of interpreting these null results is that the reviewed studies tended to be underpowered, used brief interventions, and did not randomize after a person made a successful quit attempt (which would have provided a true test of the RP concept).

While some of the studies of RP for smoking cessation published since August 2005 are more powered, they still have serious methodological limitations (Japuntich et al., 2006; Schröter, Collins, Frittrang, Buchkremer, & Batra, 2006; van Osch, Lechner, Reubsaet, Wigger, & de Vries, 2008). For example, van Osch and colleagues (2008) used a randomized controlled trial design to examine the efficacy of brief coping planning to prevent smoking relapse among 1,566 individuals participating in a Quit and Win smoking cessation incentive intervention. Participants were randomly assigned to either a control group or a planning group. The control group participated in the Quit and Win incentive intervention, and the planning group completed a planning intervention that included the formation of three coping plans for how to refrain from smoking in personal-risk situations. Among the 571 individuals remaining (36.5% retention) in the 7-month follow-up, intent-to-treat continuous abstinence rates were 10.5% for the control group and 13.4% for the coping planning group (OR = 1.41, 95% CI = 1.00, 1.98), suggesting a modest effect of coping planning to prevent relapse. Like the studies reviewed in Hajek and colleagues (2005),

this study was a brief intervention and did not randomize after a sustained period of quitting (e.g., 4 weeks). Moreover, this study also had a very low level of participant retention (i.e., 36.5%).

Summary and Recommendations for Future Research

The RP intervention research literature is relatively small in comparison to the broader CBT intervention research literature. As the RP intervention research literature grows, there are a number of potentially fruitful opportunities to conduct research on improving the efficacy of RP interventions. RP interventions have usually been added as components of broader CBT intervention packages. The downside is that this approach does not give sufficient regard to the potential impact of the added RP components. Indeed, few RP trials randomized participants after they made a successful quit attempt. In addition to designing a study with adequate power, adding this feature to the experimental design would be a critical step toward learning whether RP intervention components do in fact prevent relapse. A further step toward improving RP interventions would be to test specific components of these interventions in isolation (e.g., using only an AVE intervention) to understand both their underlying processes of change and efficacy in preventing relapse.

Integrating findings from basic research on smoking relapse would be valuable. For example, a study using ecological momentary analysis found that SCT-based constructs of (1) decreases in daily abstinence self-efficacy and (2) increases in daily positive smoking outcome expectancies predicted the occurrence of a first lapse in a sample of 305 smokers who achieved initial abstinence from smoking (Gwaltney, Shiffman, Balabanis, & Paty, 2005). The study demonstrates the important role of dynamic factors in smoking relapse, thereby highlighting the need to develop and test RP interventions within the framework of a dynamic systems theory (Witkiewitz & Marlatt, 2004).

Motivational Approaches

A major focus of smoking cessation intervention research has been on *motivating* individuals to quit smoking (Fiore et al.,

2008). The most commonly applied motivational approach, motivational interviewing (MI; Miller & Rollnick, 1991, 2002), is a client-centered directive method for helping people work through ambivalence and develop motivation to change (Miller & Rollnick, 1991). An adaptation of Carl Rogers's (1959) client-centered therapy approach, MI combines a supportive and empathetic counseling style with a method of intentionally directing the client toward changing dysfunctional behavior. Emphasis is placed upon creating a collaborative relationship and affirming the client's autonomy to change. Therapists elicit motivation for change by drawing on the client's goals and values. Major principles of the MI therapeutic stance include expressing empathy, developing an awareness of discrepancy between current behavior and important goals or values, avoiding the struggle or "rolling with" resistance, and supporting self-efficacy for change. The therapeutic techniques that illustrate these principles include asking open-ended questions, affirming, listening reflectively, and summarizing. The counselor uses techniques such as making selectively reflective statements to reinforce expressions of the client's desire, ability, reasons, and need for change—what is known as "change talk." Furthermore, the counselor offers periodic summaries of what the client has said—a kind of bouquet comprising the client's own self-motivational statements (Miller & Rollnick, 2002).

While not originally derived from a psychological theory, MI's core hypothesized processes are consistent with specific psychological theories. The first core hypothesis is that the MI therapeutic stance is predictive of behavior change (Miller & Rollnick, 2002). The foundation of MI is the context of a working alliance between client and counselor, known as "MI spirit" (Miller & Rollnick, 2002). This spirit (1) is collaborative rather than authoritarian, (2) evokes the client's own motivation rather than trying to install it, and (3) honors the client's autonomy. The second and third core hypotheses focus on the client's verbalizations to change. A strong working therapeutic alliance facilitates conditions for clients to verbalize arguments for change (i.e., change talk) (Miller & Rollnick, 2002). Miller and Rollnick hypothesize that an increase in

change talk predicts a higher likelihood of behavior change. Their converse hypothesis is that evoking counterchange arguments (i.e., resistance) predicts a lower likelihood of behavior change. These hypotheses are both consistent with two major social psychological theories: (1) cognitive dissonance theory (Festinger, 1957) and (2) self-perception theory (Bem, 1972). Both theories hypothesize that leading a client to verbalize arguments for change predicts a higher likelihood of future behavior change, whereas leading the client to verbalize reasons not to change predicts a lower likelihood of behavior change.

Efficacy of MI for Smoking Cessation

Three major MI meta-analyses including smoking cessation and published since 2003 are reviewed here. First, Burke, Arkowitz, and Menchola (2003) reviewed randomized controlled trials (RCTs) of MI delivered in a face-to-face, individual context. The two trials of MI for smoking cessation that met their selection criteria both reported no significant differences between MI and the control arm at long-term follow-up (Butler et al., 1999; Colby et al., 1998). For example, the Butler and colleagues (1999) study, an RCT for 536 adult, primary care patients who smoked daily, compared a 2-minute standard advice-to-quit-smoking intervention to a 10-minute motivational consulting intervention (i.e., brief MI without reflective listening) delivered by primary care physicians. In the intent-to-treat analysis at the 6-month follow-up (78% retention), the 24-hour point prevalence was 8.1% in the experimental arm versus 3.0% in the control arm (OR = 2.86, 95% CI = 1.21, 6.76). However, results were nonsignificant (3.0% in the experimental arm vs. 1.5% in the control arm; OR = 2.00, 95% CI = 0.63, 6.29) for 30-day point prevalence.

A second meta-analysis by Rubak, Sandbaek, Lauritzen, and Christensen (2005), selected RCTs of MI delivered in any treatment context (e.g., telephone, face-to-face) published up until January 2004. The meta-analysis of the 12 studies of MI for smoking cessation that met this study's selection criteria showed a nonsignificant trend toward a reduction in the number of cigarettes smoked per day ($N = 190$; effect estimate = 1.32, 95% CI = −0.25–2.88). The third meta-analysis selected all MI studies, published up until 2004, with any kind of comparison group design (e.g., randomized, quasi-experimental design) and a posttreatment measure (Hettema, Steele, & Miller, 2005). The two trials of MI for smoking cessation that met their selection criteria and included a follow-up of at least 3 months showed a nonsignificant mean Cohen's *d* effect size of 0.04 (95% CI = −0.08, 0.16).

The RCTs published since the period covered by these three meta-analyses have shown a largely similar pattern of outcome results (Ahluwalia et al., 2006; Baker et al., 2006; Borrelli et al., 2005; Colby et al., 2005; Horn, Dino, Hamilton, & Noerachmanto, 2007; McCambridge & Strang, 2004; Okuyemi et al., 2007; Prochaska et al., 2008; Prokhorov et al., 2008; Rigotti et al., 2006; Soria, Legido, Escolano, Lopez Yeste, & Montoya, 2006; Tappin et al., 2005; Wakefield, Olver, Whitford, & Rosenfeld, 2004). Some have reported that MI is significantly more effective than the comparison arms for smoking cessation (Colby et al., 2005; McCambridge & Strang, 2004; Soria et al., 2006). Regarding MI for *adolescent* smoking cessation, in an update on Sussman and colleagues (2006), Sussman and Sun (2009) conducted a meta-analysis of 21 controlled trials of MI smoking cessation for adolescents (i.e., ages 12–19), published up to December 2007. The results showed that MI interventions for adolescents had overall a statistically significant and modest 4.60% absolute risk reduction effect, pooled across a broad range of postintervention follow-up lengths (ranging from 0 to over 12 months).

The challenge of interpreting the trials of MI for smoking cessation is that they tend to have serious methodological weaknesses, including small sample sizes, lack of long-term (i.e., at least 6 months) follow-up, use of nonrandomized designs, and a lack of reporting on MI treatment fidelity. One study, while reporting encouraging results, reflects many of these primary methodological weaknesses. Specifically, Soria and colleagues (2006) randomized 200 smokers (114 in experimental arm; 86 in control arm) to either a three-session (20 minutes per session) primary care, physician-delivered MI intervention (114 participants) or a one-session (3 minutes) physician-delivered generic antismoking advice intervention. Participants

who scored 7 or higher on the Fagerstrom Test of Nicotine Dependence were offered a prescription of bupropion. The intent-to-treat results showed that at the 12-month postintervention follow-up (87% retention), the objectively verified abstinence point prevalence was 18.4% in the MI experimental arm and 3.5% in the antismoking advice control arm (OR = 6.25, 95% CI = 1.8, 21.7). Major methodological limitations of this study were the following. First, there was no reporting of MI intervention fidelity, so the extent to which the intervention actually was a test of MI is unclear. Second, a higher percentage of control participants were in the precontemplation stage at baseline, thereby potentially biasing the results in favor of the MI experimental arm. Third, since all five patients who were prescribed bupropion participated in the MI intervention, this pharmacotherapy addition may have contributed to a higher percentage of abstainers in the MI arm. Fourth, the antismoking control arm intervention was shorter (up to 3 minutes) than the MI intervention arm (up to 60 minutes). Therefore, the results may simply be due to a longer contact time in the MI intervention arm.

Finally, it is worth recalling the intended purpose of MI: *to develop motivation to change* (Miller & Rollnick, 1991). Keeping this in mind, it may be unreasonable to expect that MI *alone* would be efficacious for smoking cessation. Instead, it may be more reasonable to examine the efficacy of MI for its intended purpose. Indeed, the 2008 Clinical Practice Guideline (Fiore et al., 2008) reviewed three trials that reported the efficacy of MI for various broad indicators of motivation to change. These trials showed that MI significantly increased (1) quit attempts of cancer patients (Wakefield et al., 2004), (2) the proportion of patients with schizophrenia who contacted a tobacco-dependence treatment provider and attended an initial treatment session (Steinberg, Ziedonis, Krejci, & Brandon, 2004), and (3) levels of intention to quit smoking among adolescents (Brown et al., 2003). While, these results suggest the promise of MI for advancing individuals' *motivation to change* their smoking behavior, other interventions combined with MI may be needed to help individuals achieve the important outcome of long-term smoking cessation.

Evidence of Underlying Processes

Miller and Rollnick (2002) hypothesized that the therapist's spirit of empathetic understanding, genuineness, and unconditional positive regard predict positive behavior change. This hypothesis is consistent with client-centered therapy (Rogers, 1959, 1980), which posits that these same factors create an atmosphere of safety and acceptance in which clients can change. Regarding evidence for this hypothesis, Gaume, Gmel, Faouzi, and Daeppen (2008) reported a positive correlation between therapist empathy and 12-month drinking outcomes. Investigations with adult smokers found that overall MI spirit (a composite of acceptance, egalitarianism, warmth, genuineness, empathy, and overall adherence to the MI "spirit") was a strong predictor of a greater working alliance, client engagement in treatment (Boardman, Catley, Grobe, Little, & Ahluwalia, 2006), and positive within-session client behaviors (i.e., expression of affect, cooperation, disclosure, and engagement; Catley et al., 2006). Additionally, Catley and colleagues (2006) found that listening reflectively and reframing statements were significantly and positively associated with clients' verbalization of change (e.g., "I think am ready to quit smoking").

Partial evidence for the hypothesis that an increase in change talk predicts a higher likelihood of behavior change has come from research in the context of interventions for substances other than smoking. For example, a psycholinguistic analysis of specific components of change talk found that the strength of client *commitment* to change language predicted drug abstinence. A positive slope of increasing commitment strength across the MI session was associated with a higher percentage of abstinent days during the subsequent year, with the strongest prediction derived from utterances during the closing segment of the session (Amrhein, Miller, Yahne, Palmer, & Fulcher, 2003).

Summary and Recommendations for Future Research

Overall, there is a lack of evidence that MI has long-term efficacy for smoking cessation. Two primary factors may account for this pattern of results. The first is that the majority of empirical studies have serious methodological limitations that make it difficult to interpret the overall body of results. The second factor is that MI is intended to motivate change and this, therefore, may be the more appropriate measure of its intended purpose. One potentially valuable direction for future outcome research, in addition to methodological rigor, would be to examine the efficacy of MI for increasing various indicators of motivation to change. A second valuable direction would be develop and test a coherent theoretical model that combines MI's focus on developing the *willingness* to change with the focus of a CBT-type intervention on teaching individuals *how* to change once they are willing. Such a model would focus on the pathway toward quitting smoking (e.g., making a quit attempt) and the overall impact of the intervention on the smoking cessation outcome. One way to test this model would be to randomize unmotivated individuals to receive (vs. not receive) MI and, among those who show a defined increase in motivation to change, to rerandomize them to receive (vs. not receive) CBT for smoking cessation.

There is a current lack of research on the role of underlying MI processes predictive of smoking cessation. Therapeutic relationship processes that appear promising are the overall MI spirit, as well as specific processes that make up this spirit, including the therapist's accurate empathy. Client-focused processes that appear promising include the role of an increase in commitment-to-change language and a decrease in resistance-to-change language as potential predictors of positive behavior change. Examining both the therapeutic relationship and client-focused processes together in one meditational analysis may lead to a theoretically coherent model of the underlying processes of MI, enhancements of MI treatment techniques, and future advancements in MI's efficacy for smoking cessation.

Transtheoretical/Stages-of-Change Approaches

The transtheoretical model/stages of change (TTM/SOC), a health behavior change theory, posits that individuals progress through five stages of change on the pathway toward changing an unhealthy behavior (e.g., smoking). These stages are (1) precontemplation (not intending to change), (2) contemplation (intending to change in the foreseeable future), (3) preparation (planning to change very soon and currently taking measurable steps to change), (4) action (changed in the past 6 months), and (5) maintenance (changed and sustained the behavior change for 6 months or more). The major psychological factors hypothesized to move individuals through the stages of change are similar to core constructs of SCT (Bandura, 1986): (1) increase the perception of positive outcomes and decrease the perception of negative outcomes for engaging in the behavior change (outcome expectations; Prochaska et al., 1994) and (2) increase individuals' confidence that they have the skills to make the change (self-efficacy) (Prochaska, Redding, & Evers, 2002). The TTM/SOC suggests that because individuals' outcome expectations and self-efficacy levels vary depending on stage of change they are in, interventions should be uniquely tailored to that stage to move individuals forward effectively through the stages of change (Prochaska, DiClemente, Velicer, & Rossi, 1993).

Efficacy of TTM/SOC for Smoking Cessation

A recent meta-analysis that included 14 TTM/SOC-based, print-tailored interventions for smoking cessation tested in randomized or quasi-experimental designs showed that this approach had a weighted mean smoking cessation effect size of $r = .086$ (Noar, Benac, & Harris, 2007), which according to Cohen's (1988) criteria would be considered a small effect size. A second meta-analysis included a focus on the efficacy of TTM/SOC interventions for facilitating *forward stage progression* in smoking cessation, but not the important outcome of long-term smoking cessation (Bridle et al., 2005). The analysis reported that 12 trials (only four of which reported an RCT design) compared a stage-based intervention with a non-stage-based intervention or usual care control. The 12 trials reported data on 14 comparisons. Overall, four comparisons favored the stage-based intervention, three of which were compared with usual care. Two comparisons (both compared with a non-stage-based intervention) were inconclusive, and eight comparisons (three of which were

compared with usual care) showed no significant differences between groups.

Since the publication of these meta-analyses, two notable randomized trials of TTM/SOC for smoking cessation have been reported. The first is a three-group RCT that included results on the efficacy of TTM/SOC for smoking cessation (Prochaska et al., 2008). The first group, called the Health Risk Assessment and Intervention (HRI) group, provided feedback on participants' stages of change for smoking and the single most important step they could take to begin progressing toward smoking cessation. The second group received HRI plus TTM/SOC assessments and tailored feedback on core TTM/SOC processes (e.g., pros and cons of changing, self-efficacy) relevant to participants' stage of smoking cessation. In the first session, an algorithm generated normative feedback comparing participants' efforts to those of peers who made the most progress for their current stage. Remaining sessions provided feedback on variables in which participants were improving and those in which they needed to make better efforts. The third group received HRI plus an MI-based intervention. Results showed no significant differences in smoking cessation rates between the three groups (Prochaska et al., 2008). The authors interpreted this nonsignificant result as an indication of a lack of statistical power.

The second randomized trial (Aveyard, Massey, Parsons, Manaseki, & Griffin, 2009) tested the TTM/SOC hypothesis that stage-matched interventions cause a greater increase in forward movement through the stages of change relative to interventions that are not stage matched (Hypothesis 1). The study also tested the hypothesis that the relative effectiveness of stage matched interventions is greater for people in precontemplation or contemplation (stage matched for TTM/SOC but not for control) than for those in preparation (where both intervention and control were stage matched; Hypothesis 2). The study tested both hypotheses, in a sample of 2,471 adult smokers in a four-group randomized trial. The first was the control group, which provided (1) a manual on how to stop smoking, (2) a written review of different smoking aids, and (3) two small cards covering the benefits of smoking cessation and tips for staying quit.

In the second group, participants were sent the TTM/SOC-based pro-change self-help booklet, which explained how participants could stage themselves. It has chapters for each stage, with exercises that engage the appropriate processes of change. These participants received a feedback letter on TTM/SOC constructs, which was generated from their responses to a baseline questionnaire, providing stage-appropriate advice and feedback. In the third group, participants received the self-help booklet plus scripted telephone calls at baseline and at 3 and 6 months postrandomization that was designed to remind and motivate them to use the self-help materials, but did not provide additional behavioral support. In the fourth group, participants were sent the self-help booklet and were asked to see their nurse at baseline and at 3 and 6 months postrandomization. The nurse group participants withdrew from the study at high rates. Therefore, the researchers dropped this arm part way through, so that later waves of recruitment were randomized only to control, TTM/SOC-based manual, or TTM/SOC-based manual plus phone.

Regarding Hypothesis 1, results showed participants in the TTM/SOC arms were not significantly more likely to make positive stage changes in smoking cessation compared to the control arm. Regarding Hypothesis 2, there was no significant evidence that the relative benefit of the TTM/SOC-based materials was greater for participants in precontemplation or contemplation than for participants in preparation: The stage change score difference between control and the TTM/SOC groups was not significantly larger in precontemplation or contemplation than in preparation. Moreover, the likelihood of participants to stop smoking in the TTM/SOC arms relative to the control arm was not significantly greater for participants in precontemplation or contemplation than for participants in preparation.

Summary and Recommendations for Future Research

Overall, the weak, mixed, and null findings from the meta-analyses and randomized trials reviewed here are consistent with serious concerns of some in the field about the overall utility of TTM/SOC as a theory and model to guide intervention (see, e.g., West, 2005). However, health psychology researchers who see promise in testing TTM/SOC interventions can make a major contribution to improving their methodological design, thereby helping to provide more definitive evidence about the utility of TTM/SOC for smoking cessation. Major methodological problems in the current empirical TTM/SOC literature include (1) nonrandomized trials, (2) underpowered sample sizes, (3) low participant recruitment and retention, and (4) lack of data on fidelity of intervention delivery. Future research should directly address these methodological weaknesses. Other areas of improvement would be to (1) examine the mediating role of processes other than pros and cons of change (outcome expectations) and confidence of change (self-efficacy), and (2) revise the stage-matching algorithms.

Emerging Theory: Acceptance-Focused Approaches

Over the past 15 years, there has been a rising interest in the field of behavioral clinical psychology toward what can be described as "acceptance-focused" interventions, or those that focus on helping individuals to be willing to experience their unpleasant physical sensations, emotions, and cognitions rather than trying to change or otherwise control these internal states (Hayes, 2004). In the context of smoking cessation, promising evidence suggests that teaching individuals to be willing to experience urges, emotions, and thoughts—without responding to these internal states by smoking—helps them quit smoking (Gifford et al., 2004, 2009; Hernandez-Lopez, Luciano, Bricker, Roales-Nieto, & Montesinos, 2009). Moreover, increased willingness to experience these internal states is associated with lower levels of stress, negative affect, and depression (Brown & Ryan, 2003; Carlson, Speca, Patel, & Goodey, 2004; Speca, Carlson, Goodey, & Angen, 2000), which are major cues for smoking behavior and relapse (Baker, Piper, McCarthy, Majeskie, & Fiore, 2004; Niaura, Shadel, Britt, & Abrams, 2002; Piasecki, Jorenby, Smith, Fiore, & Baker, 2003; Siahpush & Carlin, 2006). People who smoke are very interested in trying such approaches (Sood, Ebbert, Sood, & Stevens, 2006), some of which are increasingly being applied in the context of smoking cessation (see, e.g., Brown et al., 2008). Acceptance-focused approaches that have recently been applied to smoking cessation include acceptance and commitment therapy (Gifford et al., 2009; Hernandez-Lopez et al., 2009), mindfulness meditation (Davis, Fleming, Bonus, & Baker, 2007), and yoga (McIver, O'Halloran, & McGartland, 2004). This section reviews (1) a theory that is consistent with the acceptance-focused approaches and (2) the application of acceptance-focused approaches to smoking cessation.

Relational Frame Theory

The acceptance-focused approaches are consistent with relational frame theory (RFT), a contemporary operant conditioning theory of human language (Hayes, Barnes-Holmes, & Roche, 2001). Over 70 studies provide strong empirical support for RFT's basic tenets (Hayes et al., 2001; Hayes, Luoma, Bond, Masuda, & Lillis, 2006). RFT focuses on a key feature of human language, the learned ability to relate events arbitrarily, mutually, and in combination. For example, very young children learn that a nickel is larger than a dime in terms of physical size, but not until they get a little older do they develop the ability to apply the relation of comparative *value* to these coins arbitrarily, such as when a child will label a dime as "bigger" than a nickel. Because of this relational response, a dime develops a more reinforcing function than does a nickel. This and other forms of relational responding are incredibly useful for many domains of everyday functioning, including communication, problem solving, and creativity.

Given the great utility of such relational skills, once learned they become a more common way for people to regulate their behavior. The problem is that this process means people can begin, in a sense, to "live in their heads" rather than in their present awareness of the world around them. RFT theorists have labeled the tendency for people to live in their heads as "cognitive fusion." Cognitive fusion can help individuals avoid experiencing their physical sensations, emotions, thoughts, and overall awareness of the world around them. Individuals

begin behaving more automatically, without awareness of what they are doing. Their behavior becomes more habitual, with a narrow range of responses.

However, efforts to avoid physical sensations, emotions, and thoughts that cue smoking can paradoxically result in an increase of these internal states. For example, smokers scoring high on measures of the avoidance of internal states that cue smoking had 1.5 times higher odds of subsequently relapsing (Gifford et al., 2004). Moreover, there is evidence that mean scores on suppression of thoughts were significantly higher ($p < .05$) for smokers than for ex-smokers (Toll, Sobell, Wagner, & Sobell, 2001). This result suggests that coping with thoughts by suppressing them may interfere with smoking cessation. Similarly, people who tend to engage in avoidant forms of coping with life stress (e.g., trying not to think about the problem) also tend to smoke more and to have higher levels of other substance use (Pirkle & Richter, 2006). A lower tolerance for stress in general, higher levels of depressive symptoms, and greater self-reported tendency to react to stress with negative affect were associated with not being able to remain quit beyond 24 hours (Brown, Lejuez, Kahler, & Strong, 2002).

Overall, RFT suggests that *attempts to avoid, control, or change* sensations, emotions, and thoughts have, through operant conditioning processes, the following *consequences*: (1) increase in the frequency of these sensations, emotions, and thoughts; (2) increase in the strength of the link between these internal states and maladaptive behavior; and (3) decrease in an ability to commit to behaviors consistent with long-term values due to the short-term focus on trying to avoid, control, or change internal states. Patterns of action that are detached from long-term desired qualities of living emerge and gradually dominate in the person's repertoire. In contrast, RFT suggests that *accepting* sensations, emotions, and thoughts has, through operant conditioning processes, the following beneficial *consequences*: (1) decrease in the frequency of unpleasant sensations, emotions, and thoughts, (2) weakened link between these internal states and maladaptive behavior, and (3) increased freedom to *commit* to doing the things the person most wants in life.

Acceptance and Commitment Therapy

Acceptance and commitment therapy (ACT) is explicitly based on RFT (Hayes, Strosahl, & Wilson, 1999). ACT is fully described in a number of books (Harris, 2008; Hayes et al., 1999; Luoma, Hayes, & Walser, 2007), so only a brief summary is provided here. The core interdependent therapeutic processes of ACT are acceptance and commitment. In accordance with its Latin root *capere*, meaning "take," *acceptance* in ACT is the act of receiving or "taking what is offered." (This is not the same as tolerance or resignation, which are passive and fatalistic.) Acceptance in ACT refers to taking completely, in the moment, without defense. The process of commitment in ACT helps individuals articulate what they want to do with their lives, make a plan to do it, then use that plan to guide specific actions. ACT is designed to help individuals stop controlling or avoiding unpleasant sensations or emotions, and instead allow the things that are deeply important to guide their behavior. Indeed, the goal of ACT is not to *decrease* the occurrence of unpleasant sensations, emotions, and thoughts, but to increase willingness and openness to experience them. Willingness to experience these sensations, emotions, and thoughts (e.g., as simply "sensations" or "thoughts")—and to respond with *acceptance* rather than avoidance—is hypothesized to facilitate individuals' *commitment* to behaviors guided by their values (Wilson & Murrell, 2004).

Efficacy of ACT for Smoking Cessation

The effect of ACT on accepting internal smoking cues and on smoking cessation has been tested in three promising trials of ACT for smoking cessation. First, Gifford and colleagues (2004) conducted a pilot study comparing individual plus group therapy ACT (with no nicotine patch) intervention to a nicotine patch (with no behavioral treatment) intervention in an RCT of 76 adult nicotine-dependent smokers. Compared to nicotine patch participants, ACT participants at the end of treatment had higher levels of acceptance of internal smoking cues overall ($p < .05$). In intent-to-treat analyses of the 12-month posttreatment follow-up data, ACT participants showed a 24-hour biochemically supported abstinence rate of 21 versus 9% for the nicotine patch control arm (OR = 2.62, 95% CI = 0.70, 9.88). In a second randomized trial of 302 smokers, Gifford and colleagues (2009) compared face-to-face ACT plus bupropion (a pharmacotherapy) to bupropion alone in a nicotine dependent sample of adults. Compared to participants receiving bupropion alone, ACT participants at end of treatment had higher levels of acceptance of internal smoking cues ($p < .001$). In intent-to-treat analyses, the ACT intervention group had a 7-day biochemically supported point prevalence quit rate of 32% at 12 months postintervention versus 18% in the comparison group ($p < .05$). While results were encouraging, the control group in both trials did not include counseling. The cessation effects of both ACT interventions were significantly mediated by overall increases in acceptance of internal smoking cues (Gifford et al., 2004, 2009). Importantly, recent analyses of both trials show that the ACT intervention groups, compared to the control groups, had significantly higher ($p < .01$ for Trial 1, and $p < .001$ for Trial 2) levels of acceptance of physical cravings and withdrawal symptoms at end of treatment. A third trial compared a seven-session, face-to-face group therapy for ACT to CBT counseling for smoking cessation in a sample of 81 nicotine-dependent adult smokers (Hernandez-Lopez et al., 2009). At posttreatment, participants in the ACT intervention had significantly higher levels of acceptance of internal cues to smoke ($p < .05$) than those in the CBT intervention. In intent-to-treat analyses, results showed that participants in the ACT condition had a biochemically supported 30-day point prevalence quit rate of 30% at the 12-month posttreatment endpoint versus 13% in the CBT group (OR adjusted for baseline group differences = 5.13, 95% CI = 1.28, 24.47; OR unadjusted = 2.86, 95% CI = 0.96, 9.79).

One fundamental reason why some smokers lapse early (Abrantes et al., 2008) is that they have difficulty tolerating internal cues to smoke (Brown et al., 2008). Fortunately, face-to-face ACT showed promise for improving tolerance of these internal cues in a one-arm study of early lapse nicotine-dependent smokers (Brown et al., 2008). The majority ($N = 13$, 81%) were able to remain quit for longer than 72 hours, and 7 individuals (43%) for longer than 1 month. Given that participants had not been abstinent for longer than 72 hours in the preceding 10 years, these results are encouraging. Overall, these studies demonstrate the promise of ACT for smoking cessation, and their methodological limitations emphasize the need to test this promise in rigorous, well-powered randomized trials of both ACT's efficacy and RFT-based mediating processes.

Meditation

RFT is also consistent with the over 5,000-year-old tradition of meditation. The word "meditation" comes from the Latin *meditari*, which means "to engage in contemplation or reflection" (Perez-de-Albeniz & Holmes, 2000). While there are many types of meditation, all share a focus on (1) observing one's thoughts, emotions, and physical sensations; (2) training one's level of awareness; and (3) developing an attitude of observing processes rather than content (e.g., noticing that one is having thoughts as opposed to focusing on the content of one's thoughts) (Ospina et al., 2007). One type of meditation that is now being tested for smoking cessation is mindfulness meditation (MM). "Mindfulness" means focusing one's attention on a particular aspect of one's internal experiences (e.g., physical sensations, emotions, and thoughts) without trying to alter, judge, or otherwise control these experiences. The purpose of practicing MM is to help individuals develop the mental clarity and flexibility that facilitate effective handling of life challenges (Segal, Williams, & Teasdale, 2002). MM may be useful for helping smokers to accept the physical sensations (e.g., urges), emotions, and thoughts that usually cue smoking. In a recent pilot study with 18 adult daily smokers given a commonly researched form of MM intervention called mindfulness-based stress reduction (MBSR; Segal et al., 2002), the results showed that a promising 56% of participants reported abstinence at the 6-week follow-up (Davis et al., 2007). MM is also now being testing in a National Institutes of Health (NIH)-funded RCT of MM in comparison with RP. While MM is a promising approach to smoking cessation, there is no evidence to date of its efficacy for smoking

cessation or effect on processes that mediate smoking cessation.

Yoga

RFT is also consistent with the over 5,000-year-old tradition of yoga (Perez-de-Albeniz & Holmes, 2000). All of the many types of yoga share a common focus on physical postures, breathing techniques, and meditation. The term "postures" refers both to types used specifically for gaining greater strength and flexibility and those used specifically to achieve proper concentration for meditation. During each posture, attention is directed to the breathing, as well as the part of the body that is being stretched. The practitioner simply observes, while suspending judgment, the physical or psychical sensations and emotions that arise (Ospina et al., 2007). The focus on the breathing and meditation in yoga may be useful in helping smokers cope with the physical sensations (e.g., urges), emotions, and thoughts that usually cue smoking. Rather than respond to these cues by smoking, the breathing and meditation may instead help smokers to accept these cues without acting upon them. In the only published research to date on yoga for smoking cessation, McIver and colleagues (2004) had 20 smokers (18 male, 2 female) participate in a five-session (60 minutes per session) yoga intervention to increase the motivation to quit smoking. While not providing results on the important outcome of long-term smoking cessation, the study did show that intervention participants' TTM/SOC-based stages of change increased from baseline to end of treatment ($p < .014$). In addition to this study, currently there is an NIH-funded study to examine the feasibility, acceptability, and initial effectiveness of adding yoga to a traditional, group-based treatment for smoking cessation in women smokers. While yoga is also a promising approach to smoking cessation, there is to date no evidence of its efficacy for smoking cessation or its effect on processes that mediate smoking cessation.

Summary and Recommendations for Future Research

Acceptance-focused interventions comprise an emerging approach to smoking cessation and share a focus on helping individuals develop a willingness to experience the physical sensations, emotions, and thoughts that cue their smoking. RFT, a theoretical model, is explicitly linked to ACT and is also consistent with the acceptance-focused approaches of meditation and yoga. RFT may therefore serve as a useful theoretical model for conceptualizing and testing the core processes that underlie the acceptance-focused interventions. While ACT has had three promising RCTs to date for smoking cessation and has shown evidence that its efficacy is at least partially mediated by acceptance of internal smoking cues, all of the acceptance approaches are at very early stages of empirical study. Overall, the acceptance-focused approaches present new opportunities for health psychology researchers to (1) determine the shared and distinct core processes that underlie the various acceptance-focused approaches for smoking cessation, (2) form clear linkages between theories (e.g., RFT) and specific acceptance-focused interventions, and (3) determine the efficacy of these approaches for long-term smoking cessation.

General Discussion and Recommendations

Need for Rigorous Intervention Research

This chapter has reviewed three commonly applied theoretical approaches to smoking cessation intervention (i.e., SCT, TTM/SOC, and MI), an emerging approach to smoking cessation intervention (i.e., acceptance), and their corresponding intervention techniques. One of the main themes in the meta-analyses and reviews of specific studies is that there are serious methodological limitations in this wide body of research. These limitations make it difficult to evaluate the efficacy of theory-based approaches to smoking cessation and the degree to which they influence their underlying theory-based processes. Future research can greatly advance the science of theory-based behavioral interventions for smoking cessation by including the following intervention design features: (1) Clearly develop and articulate the theory guiding the intervention and its link to specific intervention components; (2) provide a "clean test" of the specific theory-based intervention

by testing only that intervention approach; and (3) control for nonspecific factors. Trial design features include (1) use of an RCT design, (2) high recruitment and retention rates, (3) adequate statistical power to test the hypotheses of the study, and (4) demonstration that the intervention was delivered with fidelity. Using these intervention and trial design features for both the commonly used and emerging theory-based interventions would be highly valuable.

Research Underlying Processes

A second broad theme of this chapter is the lack of research on the degree to which theory-based interventions influence their underlying processes. Determining *whether* an intervention works is just as important as *how* an intervention works. For interventions that did not impact smoking cessation outcomes, it is very instructive to learn whether the intervention successfully impacted underlying processes. Reasons why an intervention did not work may be that (1) it did not successfully impact its underlying processes or (2) it did impact these processes, but the processes were not predictive of smoking cessation, which suggests that the theory underlying the intervention needs to be revised. As this review has shown, there is a lack of research on theory-based mediators of smoking cessation interventions. Indeed, in a meta-analysis, Sussman and colleagues (2006) stated that, in the context of *adolescent* smoking cessation intervention research, there is only one published paper on mediation (McCuller, Sussman, Wapner, Dent, & Weiss, 2006). My own literature search confirms that this is the only published study to date that has examined the degree to which an adolescent smoking cessation intervention was mediated by theory-based mechanisms. For the broader research area of interventions for all smokers, the Clinical Practice Guidelines published in 2000 (Fiore et al., 2000) recommended research on processes underlying behavioral interventions for smoking cessation. There has been little progress in this area in the 8 years since that publication. Indeed the 2008 practice guidelines (Fiore et al., 2008) continue to make this same recommendation. Research that focuses on theory-based mediators of behavioral interventions for smoking cessation is a relatively unexplored area, with the potential to reveal key mechanisms for *improving* smoking cessations interventions.

An Important Role for Theory Component and Intervention Technique Testing

The major theories reviewed here, and the interventions based on them, comprise a diverse set of theoretical constructs and intervention techniques. A major problem in smoking cessation intervention research is that specific behavioral intervention techniques are not closely linked to specific theoretical constructs. For example, CBT interventions for smoking cessation encompass a very broad array of theoretical constructs, with usually vague links to a wide number of specific intervention techniques. While researchers may intend that an intervention technique be based on a given theory, this link needs to be proven in order to compare results from an intervention with other interventions said to be linked to the same theory. Moreover, it may be that certain intervention techniques, even if actually linked to a theoretical construct, have no influence, little influence, or (worse) counteract the influence of other intervention techniques that have important influences on the mediators of smoking cessation.

Recent health psychology research on theory mapping and coding (see, e.g., Abraham & Michie, 2008; Michie, Johnston, Francis, Hardeman, & Eccles, 2008) is taking an important step toward addressing these critical issues. This work is attempting to (1) link health behavior theories to specific therapeutic interventions (e.g., SCT is linked to the technique of setting graded tasks) and (2) define specific intervention techniques. To enrich this important new direction of research, needed now is basic, small-scale experimental research to link specific theoretical constructs to specific intervention techniques, then to test the efficacy of each technique on changing specific theory-based mediators of smoking cessation. Such a program of experimental research would also contribute significantly to the new theories of health behavior as they make the critically important link from theoretical construct to intervention technique. This research could

prove especially valuable in (1) tightening the links between specific theoretical constructs and intervention techniques, (2) revising existing intervention techniques so that they are more consistent with specific theoretical constructs, (3) developing new intervention techniques consistent with specific theoretical constructs, (4) deleting unhelpful intervention techniques, and (5) creating more theoretically coherent and efficacious behavioral interventions for smoking cessation. This small-scale experimental research can run parallel with large-scale RCTs because each can inform the other and make unique contributions to science.

Role of Emerging Theories to Guide in the Development of New Interventions

RFT is one theory that is consistent with the newly emerging acceptance-focused interventions for smoking cessation. While RFT is already being linked to the acceptance-based approach, health psychologists looking to the future might also find it valuable to continue searching for other theories that prove useful for the development of new interventions for smoking cessation. One example is the PRIME theory of motivation (West, 2006) which articulates the synthesis of plans (P), reflex responses (R), impulses (I), and motives (M), evaluations (E) in directing individuals toward addictive behaviors (e.g., smoking). In addition to making predictions about what leads individuals to develop addictive behaviors, the PRIME theory includes some potentially original hypotheses about what helps individuals to stop their addictive behaviors. For example, it posits that major changes (e.g., long-term smoking cessation) can be chaotic, unstable, and triggered by very small changes. Observational and small-scale experimental data collected now to test the PRIME theory's major hypotheses may serve as a useful basis for building new behavioral interventions for smoking cessation.

Role of Combining Behavioral and Pharmacological Interventions

The combination of behavioral intervention and pharmacotherapy is now regarded as the standard of care, and empirical research supports this standard (Fiore et al., 2008). For example, the 2008 Clinical Practice Guideline conducted a meta-analysis of nine studies that evaluated the impact of adding medication to behavioral interventions. The results of this meta-analysis showed that behavioral intervention alone had an estimated abstinence rate of 14.6%, while the combination of medication and behavioral intervention had an estimated abstinence rate of 22.1%. These estimates are similar to the one, mentioned earlier, derived from four recent Cochrane Library Reviews of behavioral interventions for smoking cessation (Lancaster & Stead, 2005; Silagy et al., 2004; Stead & Lancaster, 2005; Stead et al., 2006). From the point of view of standards of care, this combination is practical and sensible.

From the point of view of theory testing, this combination may or may not make sense. Researchers should be careful to consider why they are combining a behavioral intervention with pharmacotherapy. Besides the obvious reasons an individual would not be given pharmacotherapy in an intervention (e.g., strong side effects, failure to respond in previous attempts), questions to consider include the following:

1. Is this combination theoretically consistent and coherent?
2. Does the addition of pharmacotherapy unintentionally undermine the behavioral intervention or vice versa?
3. To what extent does adding a pharmacotherapy intervention to a behavioral intervention make it difficult to determine the extent to which the intervention's efficacy was mediated by the behavioral intervention?

Pharmacotherapy clearly has an important role in research testing behavioral interventions for smoking cessation, but care needs to be taken in deciding on this combination, so that results of such trials are interpretable and can thus significantly advance the science. Moreover, behavioral interventions can play a key role in increasing adherence to smoking cessation pharmacotherapy (Fiore et al., 2008). Health psychology researchers in close collaboration with experts in pharmacotherapy might provide a fruitful way address these important scientific issues.

High-Risk Population Research

Theory-based behavioral interventions should be adapted and tested in the populations that need them most: currently, those with the highest rates of smoking. As articulated in the 2008 *Clinical Practice Guidelines* (Fiore et al., 2008), critically needed now is intervention research dedicated to helping the following populations of individuals who smoke at high rates to quit smoking: (1) HIV positive; (2) hospitalized; (3) lesbian, gay, bisexual, or transexual (LGBT); (4) low-income/low education; (5) medically comorbid (e.g., cancer patients); (6) older individuals; (7) psychiatrically disordered (e.g., schizophrenia); (8) substance abusers; (9) racial/ethnic minorities; and (10) women. The Guidelines recommend research on the efficacy of behavioral interventions for all of these high-risk populations. While there is need for intervention research in all of these populations, the populations for which *no* long-term RCTs have examined efficacy include (1) HIV positive, (2) LGBT, and (3) Asian and Pacific Islanders (Fiore et al., 2008). Understanding the unique characteristics and needs of these populations will help in determining which theoretical approach is the best fit and how to tailor the intervention to these specific characteristics and needs. Overall, theory-based research on high-risk populations will serve the dual role of testing theory and addressing a critically important U.S. public health need.

Culturally Relevant Adaptations of Theory-Based Interventions

Nearly all of the research on theory-based behavioral interventions for smoking cessation has been conducted on the continents of North America, Europe (except Eastern Europe), and Australia (Fiore et al., 2008; Sussman & Sun, 2009; World Health Organization, 2005). This research has helped to address the great need for smoking cessation intervention development and testing in these parts of the world. But as I mentioned earlier, smoking is a global health problem. The prevalence of smoking is now the highest in Eastern Europe and the continent of Asia (Hatsukami et al., 2008). The tobacco industry is now interested in expanding its presence in these parts of the world, in addition to the continent of Africa (Yach & Bettcher, 2000). In response to this serious global health problem, the World Health Organization (2005) adopted a Framework Convention on Tobacco Control (FCTC), an agreement that commits member countries to adopt tobacco control policies that include taxation, no-smoking policies, tobacco education, and cessation programs.

Theory-based behavioral interventions for smoking cessation can play an important role in the overall tobacco control polices of the countries in Eastern Europe, Asia, and Africa. However, the application of these interventions worldwide is unlikely to be so straightforward as simply translating prepackaged interventions and exporting them to a new country. Behavioral theories and techniques of a smoking cessation intervention implicitly reflect universal processes of human behavior change, but this assumption needs to be tested in cross-cultural research. Interventions that make a lot of sense to an American may run contrary to other cultural beliefs and prove ultimately ineffective. Therefore, tailoring and modifying theory-based interventions to fit the cultural values, beliefs, and social structure of these countries would be highly important. Ways to do that may include close collaboration with anthropologists who have expertise in the given culture, collaboration with other behavioral scientists who are natives of the given culture, focus groups with individuals who match your study population, and pilot studies of intervention feasibility. Overall, there are many potential opportunities for health psychology researchers to develop and test cultural adaptations of theory-based smoking cessation interventions, especially in countries where the smoking prevalence is now the highest.

Conclusions

Theory-based research on behavioral interventions for smoking cessation provides numerous opportunities for programmatic research in health psychology. These opportunities range broadly from linking specific theoretical constructs and specific interventions to testing innovative interventions. The focus on the application and testing of *theory* capitalizes on a key strength of

health psychologists, thereby making important unique contributions to the overall body of research on smoking cessation intervention. When conducted rigorously, this research can lead to new discoveries in how to improve the efficacy of behavioral interventions for smoking cessation both in the United States and worldwide.

Acknowledgments

I thank Robert West and Susan Michie for their helpful comments on a draft of this chapter. I also acknowledge my colleague Art Peterson for teaching me the value and practice of rigorous research methodology.

Further Reading

Fiore, M. C., Jaén, C. R., Baker, T. B., Bailey, W. C., Benowitz, N. L., Curry, S. J., et al. (2008). *Treating tobacco use and dependence: 2008 update. Clinical Practice Guidelines*. Rockville, MD: U.S. Department of Health and Human Services, Public Health Service.

Gifford, E. V., Kohlenberg, B. S., Hayes, S. C., Antonuccio, D. O., Piasecki, M. M., Rasmussen-Hall, M. L., et al. (2004). Acceptance-based treatment for smoking cessation. *Behavior Therapy, 35*, 689–705.

Lancaster, T., Hajeck, P., Stead, L. F., West, R., & Jarvis, M. J. (2006). Prevention of relapse after quitting smoking: A systematic review of trials. *Archives of Internal Medicine, 166*, 828–835.

Michie, S., Johnston, M., Francis, J., Hardeman, W., & Eccles, M. (2008). From theory to intervention: Mapping theoretically derived behavioural determinants to behaviour change techniques. *Applied Psychology: An International Review, 57*, 660–680.

Noar, S. M., Benac, C. N., & Harris, N. S. (2007). Does tailoring matter?: Meta-analytic review of tailored print health behavior change interventions. *Psychological Bulletin, 133*, 673–693.

Perkins, K. A., Conklin, C. A., & Levine, M. D. (2008). *Cognitive-behavioral therapy for smoking cessation: A practical guide to the most effective treatments*. New York: Routledge.

Rubak, S., Sandbæk, A., Lauritzen, T., & Christensen, B. (2005). Motivational interviewing: A systematic review and meta-analysis. *British Journal of General Practice, 55*(513), 305–312.

Sussman, S., Sun, P., & Dent, C. W. (2005). A

meta-analysis of teen cigarette smoking cessation. *Health Psychology, 25*(5), 549–557.

West, R. (2006). *Theory of addiction.* Oxford, UK: Blackwell.

World Health Organization. (2005). *WHO framework convention on tobacco control.* Geneva: Author. Retrieved August 25, 2008, from *www.fctc.org.*

References

Abraham, C., & Michie, S. (2008). A taxonomy of behavior change techniques used in interventions. *Health Psychology, 27,* 379–387.

Abrams, D. B., Niaura, R., Brown, R. A., Emmons, K. M., Goldstein, M. G., & Monti, P. M. (2003). *The tobacco dependence treatment handbook: A guide to best practices.* New York: Guilford Press.

Abrantes, A. M., Strong, D. R., Lejuez, C. W., Kahler, C. W., Carpenter, L. L., Price, L. H., et al. (2008). The role of negative affect in risk for early lapse among low distress tolerance smokers. *Addictive Behaviors, 33,* 1394–1401.

Ahluwalia, J. S., Okuyemi, K., Nollen, N., Choi, W. S., Kaur, H., Pulvers, K., et al. (2006). The effects of nicotine gum and counseling among African American light smokers: A 2 × 2 factorial design. *Addiction, 101,* 883–891.

American Cancer Society. (2000). *Cancer facts and figures—2000.* Atlanta, GA: Author.

Amrhein, P. C., Miller, W. R., Yahne, C. E., Palmer, M., & Fulcher, L. (2003). Client commitment language during motivational interviewing predicts drug use outcomes. *Journal of Consulting and Clinical Psychology, 71,* 862–878.

Aveyard, P., Massey, L., Parsons, A., Manaseki, S., & Griffin, C. (2009). The effect of transtheoretical model based interventions on smoking cessation. *Social Science and Medicine, 68,* 397–403.

Baker, A., Richmond, R., Haile, M., Lewin, T. J., Carr, V. J., Taylor, R. L., et al. (2006). A randomized controlled trial of a smoking cessation intervention among people with a psychotic disorder. *American Journal of Psychiatry, 163,* 1934–1942.

Baker, T. B., Piper, M. E., McCarthy, D. E., Majeskie, M. R., & Fiore, M. C. (2004). Addiction motivation reformulated: An affective processing model of negative reinforcement. *Psychology Review, 111,* 33–51.

Bala, M., Strzeszynski, L., & Cahill, K. (2008). Mass media interventions for smoking cessation in adults (Review). *Cochrane Database Systematic Reviews,* Issue 1 (Article No. CD004704), DOI: 10.1002/14652858. CD004704.pub2.

Bandura, A. (1986). *Social foundations of thought and action: A social cognitive theory.* Englewood Cliffs, NJ: Prentice-Hall.

Bandura, A. (1997). *Self-efficacy: The exercise of control.* New York: Freeman.

Bartholomew, L. K., Parcel, G. S., Kok, G., & Gottlieb, N. H. (2006). *Planning health promotion programs: An intervention mapping approach* (2nd ed.). San Francisco: Jossey-Bass.

Beck, A. (1993). *Cognitive therapy and the emotional disorders.* New York: Penguin.

Bem, D. J. (1972). Self-perception theory. In L. Berkowitz (Ed.), *Advances in experimental social psychology* (Vol. 6, pp. 1–62). New York: Academic Press.

Boardman, T., Catley, D., Grobe, J. E., Little, T. D., & Ahluwalia, J. S. (2006). Using motivational interviewing with smokers: Do therapist behaviors relate to engagement and therapeutic alliance? *Journal of Substance Abuse Treatment, 31,* 329–339.

Borrelli, B., Novak, S., Hecht, J., Emmons, K., Papandonatos, G., & Abrams, D. (2005). Home health care nurses as a new channel for smoking cessation treatment: Outcomes from project cares (community-nurse assisted research and education on smoking). *Preventive Medicine, 41,* 815–821.

Brandon, T. H. (2001). Behavioral tobacco cessation treatments: Yesterday's news or tomorrow's headlines? *Journal of Clinical Oncology, 19*(Suppl. 18), 64S–68S.

Bridle, C., Riemsma, C., Pattenden, J., Sowden, A. J., Mather, L., Watt, I. S., et al. (2005). Systematic review of the effectiveness of health behavior interventions based on the transtheoretical model. *Psychology and Health, 20,* 283–301.

Brown, K. W., & Ryan, R. M. (2003). The benefits of being present: Mindfulness and its role in psychological well-being. *Journal of Personality and Social Psychology, 84,* 822–848.

Brown, R. A., Lejuez, C. W., Kahler, C. W., & Strong, D. R. (2002). Distress tolerance and duration of past smoking cessation attempts. *Journal of Abnormal Psychology, 111,* 180–185.

Brown, R. A., Palm, K. M., Strong, D. R., Lejuez, C. W., Kahler, C. W., Zvolensky, M. J., et al. (2008). Distress tolerance treatment for early-lapse smokers: Rationale, program description, and preliminary findings. *Behavior Modification, 32,* 302–332.

Brown, R. A., Ramsey, S. E., Strong, D. R., Myers, M. G., Kahler, C. W., Lejuez, C. W., et al. (2003). Effects of motivational interviewing on smoking cessation in adolescents with psychiatric disorders. *Tobacco Control, 12*(Suppl. 4), IV3–IV10.

Burke, B. L., Arkowitz, H., & Menchola, M. (2003). The efficacy of motivational interviewing: A meta-analysis of controlled clinical trials. *Journal of Consulting and Clinical Psychology, 71,* 843–861.

Butler, C. C., Rollnick, S., Cohen, D., Bachmann, M., Russell, I., & Stott, N. (1999). Motivational consulting versus brief advice for smokers in general practice: A randomized trial. *British Journal of General Practice, 49,* 611–616.

Cahill, K., Stead, L. F., & Lancaster, T. (2008). Nicotine receptor partial agonists for smoking cessation: *Cochrane Database of Systematic Reviews,* Issue 3 (Article No. CD006103), DOI: 10.1002/14651858.CD0047054.pub2.

Carlson, L. E., Speca, M., Patel, K. D., & Goodey, E. (2004). Mindfulness-based stress reduction in relation to quality of life, mood, symptoms of stress and levels of cortisol, dehydroepiandrosterone sulfate (DHEAS) and melatonin in breast and prostate cancer outpatients. *Psychoneuroendocrinology, 29,* 448–474.

Catley, D., Harris, K. J., Mayo, M. S., Hall, S., Okuyemi, K. S., Boardman, T., et al. (2006). Adherence to principles of motivational interviewing and client within-session behavior. *Behavioural and Cognitive Psychotherapy, 34,* 43–56.

Centers for Disease Control and Prevention. (2006). Tobacco use among adults—United States, 2005. *MMWR Morbidity and Mortality Weekly Report, 55*(42), 1145–1148.

Cohen, J. (1988). *Statistical power analysis for the behavioral sciences* (2nd ed.). Hillsdale, NJ: Erlbaum.

Colby, S. M., Monti, P. M., Barnett, N. P., Rohsenow, D. J., Weissman, K., Spirito, A., et al. (1998). Brief motivational interviewing in a hospital setting for adolescent smoking: A preliminary study. *Journal of Consulting and Clinical Psychology, 66,* 574–578.

Colby, S. M., Monti, P. M., O'Leary Tevyaw, T., Barnett, N. P., Spirito, A., Rohsenow, D. J., et al. (2005). Brief motivational intervention for adolescent smokers in medical settings. *Addictive Behaviors, 30,* 865–874.

Curry, S., Marlatt, G. A., & Gordon, J. R. (1987). Abstinence violation effect: Validation of an attributional construct with smoking cessation. *Journal of Consulting and Clinical Psychology, 55,* 145–149.

Davis, J. M., Fleming, M. F., Bonus, K. A., & Baker, T. B. (2007). A pilot study on mindfulness based stress reduction for smokers. *BMC Complementary and Alternative Medicine, 7,* 2.

Ellis, A., & Dryden, W. (2007). *The practice of rational emotive behavior therapy* (2nd ed.). New York: Springer.

Festinger, L. (1957). *A theory of cognitive dissonance.* Evanston, IL: Row, Peterson.

Fiore, M. C., Bailey, W. C., Cohen, S. J., Dorfman, S. F., Goldstein, M. G., Gritz, E. R., et al. (2000). *Treating tobacco use and dependence. Clinical Practice Guidelines.* Rockville, MD: U.S. Department of Health and Human Services. Public Health Service.

Fiore, M. C., Jaén, C. R., Baker, T. B., Bailey, W. C., Benowitz, N. L., Curry, S. J., et al. (2008). Treating tobacco use and dependence: 2008 update. In *Clinical practice guidelines.* Rockville, MD: U.S. Department of Health and Human Services, Public Health Service.

Gaume, J., Gmel, G., Faouzi, M., & Daeppen, J. B. (2008). Counsellor behaviours and patient language during brief motivational interventions: A sequential analysis of speech. *Addiction, 103,* 1793–1800.

Gifford, E. V., Kohlenberg, B. S., Hayes, S. C., Antonuccio, D. O., Piasecki, M. M., Rasmussen-Hall, M. L., et al. (2004). Acceptance-based treatment for smoking cessation. *Behavior Therapy, 35,* 689–705.

Gifford, E. V., Kohlenberg, B. S., Hayes, S. C., Pierson, H. M., Piasecki, M. M., Antonuccio, D. O., et al. (2009). *Applying the acceptance and relationship context model to smoking cessation: A randomized controlled trial integrating acceptance and commitment therapy and buproprion for adult nicotine dependent smokers.* Manuscript in review.

Glanz, K., Rimer, B. K., & Lewis, F. M. (2002). *Health behavior and health education: Theory, research and practice* (3rd ed.). San Francisco: Jossey-Bass.

Goldstein, M. G., Niaura, R., Follick, M. J., & Abrams, D. B. (1989). Effects of behavioral skills training and schedule of nicotine gum administration on smoking cessation. *American Journal of Psychiatry, 146,* 56–60.

Gwaltney, C. J., Shiffman, S., Balabanis, M. H., & Paty, J. A. (2005). Dynamic self-efficacy and outcome expectancies: Prediction of smoking lapse and relapse. *Journal of Abnormal Psychology, 114,* 661–675.

Hajek, P. (1996). Current issues in behavioral and pharmacological approaches to smoking cessation. *Addictive Behaviors, 21,* 699–707.

Hajek, P., Stead, L. F., West, R., Jarvis, M., & Lancaster, T. (2005). Relapse prevention interventions for smoking cessation. *Cochrane Database of Systematic Reviews,* Issue 1 (Article No. CD003999), DOI: 10.1002/14651858/CD003999.pub3.

Harris, R. (2008). *The happiness trap.* Boston: Trumpeter.

Hatsukami, D. K., Stead, L. F., & Gupta, P. C. (2008). Tobacco addiction. *Lancet, 371,* 2027–2038.

Hayes, S. C. (2004). Acceptance and commitment therapy, relational frame theory, and the third wave of behavioral and cognitive therapies. *Behavior Therapy, 35,* 639–665.

Hayes, S. C., Barnes-Holmes, D., & Roche, B. (2001). *Relational frame theory: A post-Skinnerian account of human language and cognition.* New York: Plenum Press.

Hayes, S. C., Luoma, J. B., Bond, F. W., Masuda, A., & Lillis, J. (2006). Acceptance and commitment therapy: Model, processes and outcomes. *Behaviour Research and Therapy, 44,* 1–25.

Hayes, S. C., Strosahl, K. D., & Wilson, K. G. (1999). *Acceptance and commitment therapy: An experimental approach to behavior change.* New York: Guilford Press.

Hernandez-Lopez, M. C., Luciano, C., Bricker, J. B., Roales-Nieto, J. G., & Montesinos, F. (2009). Acceptance and commitment therapy for smoking cessation: Preliminary study of its effectiveness in comparison with cognitive behavioral treatment. *Psychology of Addictive Behaviors, 23,* 723–730.

Hettema, J., Steele, J., & Miller, W. R. (2005). Motivational interviewing. *Annual Review of Clinical Psychology, 1,* 91–111.

Horn, K., Dino, G., Hamilton, C., & Noerachmanto, N. (2007). Efficacy of an emergency department-based motivational teenage smoking intervention. *Prevention of Chronic Disease, 4*(1), A08.

International Agency for Research on Cancer. (2004). *Monographs on the evaluation of carcinogenic risks to humans: Vol. 83. Tobacco smoke and involuntary smoking.* Lyon: IARC Press.

Janis, I. L., & Mann, L. (1977). *Decision making: A psychological analysis of conflict, choice, and commitment.* New York: Free Press.

Japuntich, S. J., Zehner, M. E., Smith, S. S., Jorenby, D. E., Valdez, J. A., Fiore, M. C., et al. (2006). Smoking cessation via the Internet: A randomized clinical trial of an Internet intervention as adjuvant treatment in a smoking cessation intervention. *Nicotine and Tobacco Research, 8*(Suppl. 1), S59–S67.

Lancaster, T., Hajek, P., Stead, L. F., West, R., & Jarvis, M. J. (2006). Prevention of relapse after quitting smoking: A systematic review of trials. *Archives of Internal Medicine, 166,* 828–835.

Lancaster, T., & Stead, L. F. (2005). Individual behavioural counselling for smoking cessation. *Cochrane Database of Systematic Reviews,* Issue 2 (Article No. CD001292), DOI: 10/1002/14651858.CD001292.pub2.

Leventhal, H., Musumeci, T. J., & Contrada, R. J. (2007). Current issues and new directions in psychology and health: Theory, translation, and evidence-based practice. *Psychology and Health, 22,* 381–386.

Lewin, K. (1951). *Field theory in social science: Selected theoretical papers.* New York: Harper & Row.

Lippke, S., Ziegelmann, J. P., & Schwarzer, R. (2005). Initiation and maintenance of physical exercise: Stage-specific effects of a planning intervention. *Research in Sports Medicine, 12,* 221–240.

Luoma, J. B., Hayes, S. C., & Walser, R. D. (2007). *Learning act: An acceptance and commitment therapy skills training manual for therapists.* Oakland, CA: New Harbinger.

Mackay, J., Ericksen, M., & Shafey, O. (2006). *The tobacco atlas* (2nd ed.). Atlanta, GA: American Cancer Society.

Mackay, P. W., Donovan, D. M., & Marlatt, G. A. (1991). Cognitive behavioral approaches to alcohol abuse. In R. J. Frances & S. I. Miller (Eds.), *Clinical textbook of addictive disorders* (pp. 452–481). New York: Guilford Press.

Marlatt, G. A., & George, W. H. (1984). Relapse prevention: Introduction and overview of the model. *British Journal of Addiction, 79,* 261–273.

Marlatt, G. A., & Gordon, J. R. (Eds.). (1985). *Relapse prevention: Maintenance strategies in the treatment of addictive behaviors.* New York: Guilford Press.

McCambridge, J., & Strang, J. (2004). The efficacy of single-session motivational interviewing in reducing drug consumption and perceptions of drug-related risk and harm among young people: Results from a multi-site cluster randomized trial. *Addiction, 99,* 39–52.

McCuller, W. J., Sussman, S., Wapner, M., Dent, C., & Weiss, D. J. (2006). Motivation to quit as a mediator of tobacco cessation among at-risk youth. *Addictive Behaviors, 31,* 880–888.

McIver, S., O'Halloran, P., & McGartland, M. (2004). The impact of hatha yoga on smoking behavior. *Alternative Therapies in Health and Medicine, 10,* 22–23.

Michie, S., Johnston, M., Francis, J., Hardeman, W., & Eccles, M. (2008). From theory to intervention: Mapping theoretically derived behavioural determinants to behaviour change techniques. *Applied Psychology: An International Review, 57,* 660–680.

Miller, W. R., & Rollnick, S. (1991). *Motivational interviewing: Preparing people to change addictive behavior.* New York: Guilford Press.

Miller, W. R., & Rollnick, S. (2002). *Motivational interviewing: Preparing people for change* (2nd ed.). New York: Guilford Press.

National Cancer Institute. (2008). *The role of the media in promoting and reducing tobacco use. Tobacco Control Monograph No. 19* [NIH

Publication No. 07-6242]. Bethesda, MD: U.S. Department of Health and Human Services, National Institutes of Health, National Cancer Institute.

National Research Council. (1986). *Environmental tobacco smoke. Measuring exposures and assessing health effects.* Washington, DC: National Academy Press.

Niaura, R., & Abrams, D. B. (2002). Smoking cessation: Progress, priorities, and prospectus. *Journal of Consulting and Clinical Psychology, 70,* 494–509.

Niaura, R., Shadel, W. G., Britt, D. M., & Abrams, D. B. (2002). Response to social stress, urge to smoke, and smoking cessation. *Addictive Behaviors, 27,* 241–250.

Noar, S. M., Benac, C. N., & Harris, M. S. (2007). Does tailoring matter?: Meta-analytic review of tailored print health behavior change interventions. *Psychological Bulletin, 133,* 673–693.

Okuyemi, K. S., James, A. S., Mayo, M. S., Nollen, N., Catley, D., Choi, W. S., et al. (2007). Pathways to health: A cluster randomized trial of nicotine gum and motivational interviewing for smoking cessation in low-income housing. *Health Education and Behavior, 34,* 43–54.

Ospina, M. B., Bond, T. K., Karkhaneh, M., Tjosvold, L., Vandermeer, B., Liang, Y., et al. (2007). *Meditation practices for health: State of the research* [Evidence Report/Technology Assessment No. 155, AHRQ Publication No. 07-E010]. Rockville, MD: Agency for Healthcare Research and Quality.

Parkin, D. M., Bray, F., Ferlay, J., & Pisani, P. (2005). Global cancer statistics, 2002. *CA: A Cancer Journal for Clinicians, 55,* 74–108.

Perez-de-Albeniz, A., & Holmes, J. (2000). Meditation: Concepts, effects and uses in therapy. *Internal Journal of Psychotherapy, 5,* 49–58.

Perkins, K. A., Conklin, C. A., & Levine, M. D. (2008). *Cognitive-behavioral therapy for smoking cessation: A practical guide to the most effective treatments.* New York: Routledge.

Piasecki, T. M., Jorenby, D. E., Smith, S. S., Fiore, M. C., & Baker, T. B. (2003). Smoking withdrawal dynamics: I. Abstinence distress in lapsers and abstainers. *Journal of Abnormal Psychology, 112,* 3–13.

Pirkle, E. C., & Richter, L. (2006). Personality, attitudinal and behavioral risk profiles of young female binge drinkers and smokers. *Journal of Adolescent Health, 38,* 44–54.

Prochaska, J. O., Butterworth, S., Redding, C. A., Burden, V., Perrin, N., Leo, M., et al. (2008). Initial efficacy of MI, TTM tailoring and HRI's with multiple behaviors for employee health promotion. *Preventive Medicine, 46,* 226–231.

Prochaska, J. O., DiClemente, C. C., Velicer, W. F., & Rossi, J. S. (1993). Standardized, individualized, interactive, and personalized self-help programs for smoking cessation. *Health Psychology, 12,* 399–405.

Prochaska, J. O., Redding, C. A., & Evers, K. (2002). The transtheoretical model and stages of change. In K. Glantz, B. K. Rimer, & F. M. Lewis (Eds.), *Health behavior and health education: Theory, research, and practice* (pp. 99–120). San Francisco: Jossey-Bass.

Prochaska, J. O., Velicer, W. F., Rossi, J. S., Goldstein, M. G., Marcus, B. H., Rakowski, W., et al. (1994). Stages of change and decisional balance for 12 problem behaviors. *Health Psychology, 13,* 39–46.

Prokhorov, A. V., Yost, T., Mullin-Jones, M., de Moor, C., Ford, K. H., Marani, S., et al. (2008). "Look at your health": Outcomes associated with a computer-assisted smoking cessation counseling intervention for community college students. *Addictive Behaviors, 33,* 757–771.

Ranney, L., Melvin, C., Lux, L., McClain, E., & Lohr, K. N. (2006). Systematic review: Smoking cessation intervention strategies for adults and adults in special populations. *Annals of Internal Medicine, 145,* 845–856.

Rigotti, N. A., Park, E. R., Regan, S., Chang, Y., Perry, K., Loudin, B., et al. (2006). Efficacy of telephone counseling for pregnant smokers: A randomized controlled trial. *Obstetrics and Gynecology, 108,* 83–92.

Rogers, C. (1959). A theory of therapy, personality and interpersonal relationships as developed in the client-centered framework. In S. Koch (Ed.), *Psychology: A study of a science: Vol. 3. Formulations of the person and the social context.* New York: McGraw-Hill.

Rogers, C. (1980). *A way of being.* Boston: Houghton Mifflin.

Rothman, A. J. (2004). "Is there nothing more practical than a good theory?": Why innovations and advances in health behavior change will arise if interventions are used to test and refine theory. *International Journal of Behavior Nutrition and Physical Activity, 1,* 11.

Rubak, S., Sandbaek, A., Lauritzen, T., & Christensen, B. (2005). Motivational interviewing: A systematic review and meta-analysis. *British Journal of General Practice, 55*(513), 305–312.

Schröter, M., Collins, S. E., Frittrang, T., Buchkremer, G., & Batra, A. (2006). Randomized controlled trial of relapse prevention and a standard behavioral intervention with adult smokers. *Addictive Behaviors, 31,* 1259–1264.

Segal, Z. V., Williams, J. M. G., & Teasdale, J. D. (2002). *Mindfulness-based cognitive therapy for depression: A new approach to preventing relapse*. New York: Guilford Press.

Shiffman, S. (1993). Smoking cessation treatment: Any progress? *Journal of Consulting and Clinical Psychology, 61*, 718–722.

Shiffman, S., Hickcox, M., Paty, J. A., Gnys, M., Kassel, J. D., & Richards, T. J. (1996). Progression from a smoking lapse to relapse: Prediction from abstinence violation effects, nicotine dependence, and lapse characteristics. *Journal of Consulting and Clinical Psychology, 64*, 993–1002.

Siahpush, M., & Carlin, J. B. (2006). Financial stress, smoking cessation and relapse: Results from a prospective study of an Australian national sample. *Addiction, 101*, 121–127.

Silagy, C., Lancaster, T., Stead, L., Mant, D., & Fowler, G. (2004). Nicotine replacement therapy for smoking cessation. *Cochrane Database of Systematic Reviews*, Issue 3 (Article No. CD000146), DOI: 10.1002/14651858. CD000146.pub2.

Sood, A., Ebbert, J. O., Sood, R., & Stevens, S. R. (2006). Complementary treatments for tobacco cessation: A survey. *Nicotine and Tobacco Research, 8*, 767–771.

Soria, R., Legido, A., Escolano, C., Lopez Yeste, A., & Montoya, J. (2006). A randomised controlled trial of motivational interviewing for smoking cessation. *British Journal of General Practice, 56*, 768–774.

Speca, M., Carlson, L. E., Goodey, E., & Angen, M. (2000). A randomized, wait-list controlled clinical trial: The effect of a mindfulness meditation-based stress reduction program on mood and symptoms of stress in cancer outpatients. *Psychosomatic Medicine, 62*, 613–622.

Stead, L. F., & Lancaster, T. (2005). Group behaviour therapy programmes for smoking cessation. *Cochrane Database of Systematic Reviews*, Issue 2 (Article No. CD001007), DOI: 10.1002/14651858.CD0001002.pub2.

Stead, L. F., Perera, R., & Lancaster, T. (2006). Telephone counseling for smoking cessation. *Cochrane Database of Systematic Reviews*, Issue 3 (Article No. CD002850), DOI: 10.1002/14651858.CD002850.pub2.

Steinberg, M. L., Ziedonis, D. M., Krejci, J. A., & Brandon, T. H. (2004). Motivational interviewing with personalized feedback: A brief intervention for motivating smokers with schizophrenia to seek treatment for tobacco dependence. *Journal of Consulting and Clinical Psychology, 72*, 723–728.

Stevens, V. J., & Hollis, J. F. (1989). Preventing smoking relapse, using an individually tailored skills-training technique. *Journal of Consulting and Clinical Psychology, 57*, 420–424.

Sussman, S., & Sun, P. (2009). Youth tobacco use cessation: 2008 update. *Tobacco Induced Diseases, 5*, 3.

Sussman, S., Sun, P., & Dent, C. W. (2006). A meta-analysis of teen cigarette smoking cessation. *Health Psychology, 25*(5), 549–557.

Tappin, D. M., Lumsden, M. A., Gilmour, W. H., Crawford, F., McIntyre, D., Stone, D. H., et al. (2005). Randomized controlled trial of home based motivational interviewing by midwives to help pregnant smokers quit or cut down. *British Medical Journal, 331*, 373–377.

Toll, B. A., Sobell, M. B., Wagner, E. F., & Sobell, L. C. (2001). The relationship between thought suppression and smoking cessation. *Addictive Behaviors, 26*, 509–515.

U.S. Department of Health and Human Services. (2006). *The health consequences of involuntary exposure to tobacco smoke: A report of the Surgeon General*. Atlanta, GA: Author.

van Osch, L., Lechner, L., Reubsaet, A., Wigger, S., & de Vries, H. (2008). Relapse prevention in a national smoking cessation contest: Effects of coping planning. *British Journal of Health Psychology, 13*(Pt. 3), 525–535.

Wakefield, M., Olver, I., Whitford, H., & Rosenfeld, E. (2004). Motivational interviewing as a smoking cessation intervention for patients with cancer: Randomized controlled trial. *Nursing Research, 53*, 396–405.

West, R. (2005). Time for a change: Putting the transtheoretical (stages of change) model to rest. *Addiction, 100*, 1036–1039.

West, R. (2006). *Theory of addiction*. Oxford, UK: Blackwell.

Wilson, K. G., & Murrell, A. R. (2004). Values work in acceptance and commitment therapy: Setting a course for behavioral treatment. In S. C. Hayes, V. M. Follette, & M. M. Lindan (Eds.), *Mindfulness and acceptance: Expanding the cognitive-behavioral tradition* (pp. 120–151). New York: Guilford Press.

Witkiewitz, K., & Marlatt, G. A. (2004). Relapse prevention for alcohol and drug problems: That was zen, this is tao. *American Psychologist, 59*, 224–235.

World Health Organization. (2005). *WHO Framework Convention on Tobacco Control*. Retrieved August 25, 2008, from *www.fctc. org*.

Yach, D., & Bettcher, D. (2000). Globalisation of tobacco industry influence and new global responses. *Tobacco Control, 9*, 206–216.

Author Index

Subject Index

Page numbers followed by *f* indicate figure, *t* indicate table